PAIN
ASSESSMENT
and Pharmacologic
Management

Chris Pasero, MS, RN-BC, FAAN

Pain Management Educator and Clinical Consultant

Margo McCaffery, MS, RN-BC, FAAN

Consultant in the Nursing Care of Patients with Pain

ELSEVIER
MOSBY

3251 Riverport Lane
St. Louis, Missouri 63043

PAIN ASSESSMENT AND PHARMACOLOGIC
MANAGEMENT

ISBN: 978-0-323-05696-0

Library of Congress Cataloging-in-Publication Data

Pasero, Chris.
  Pain assessment and pharmacologic management / Chris Pasero, Margo McCaffery.
    p. ; cm.
  Includes bibliographical references and index.
  ISBN 978-0-323-05696-0 (pbk. : alk. paper) 1. Pain–Chemotherapy.   2. Pain–Measurement.
3. Analgesics. I. McCaffery, Margo.   II. Title.
  [DNLM: 1. Pain–drug therapy. 2. Analgesics–administration & dosage. 3. Pain–nursing.
4. Pain Measurement–methods. WL 704 P281p 2011]
  RB127.P368 2011
  616'.0472–dc22

                                                                              2010014538

Acquisitions Editor: Tamara Myers
Publishing Services Manager: Jeff Patterson
Senior Project Manager: Clay S. Broeker
Design Direction: Amy Buxton

Printed in the United States

Last digit is the print number: 9 8 7 6 5 4 3 2 1

In memory of
Melissa Mielke
1970-2001
Margo's daughter

In memory of
Rick Brewer
1947-2003
Margo's husband

Contributors

Jan Frandsen, MSN, CNP
Nurse Practitioner
Palliative Care Program
Hillcrest Hospital
Mayfield Heights, Ohio

Keela A. Herr, PhD, RN, FAAN, AGSF
Professor and Chair
Adult and Gerontological Nursing
College of Nursing
University of Iowa
Iowa City, Iowa

Karen Snow Kaiser, PhD, RN-BC, AOCN, CHPN
Clinical Practice Coordinator
Division of Clinical Quality Systems
University of Maryland Medical Center
Baltimore, Maryland

Kenneth L. Kirsh, PhD
Assistant Professor
Department of Pharmacy Practice and Science
College of Pharmacy
University of Kentucky
Lexington, Kentucky

Allison T. Nisbet, MSN, RN-BC, CPN
Clinical Specialist
Pediatric Hematology and Oncology
Adolescent Unit
Inova Fairfax Hospital for Children
Falls Church, Virginia

Steven D. Passik, PhD
Psychiatry and Behavioral Sciences
Memorial Sloan-Kettering Cancer Center
New York, New York

Rosemary C. Polomano, PhD, RN, FAAN
Associate Professor of Pain Practice
School of Nursing
University of Pennsylvania
Philadelphia, Pennsylvania

Russell K. Portenoy, MD
Chairman
Department of Pain Medicine and Palliative Care
Beth Israel Medical Center
New York, New York

Thomas E. Quinn, APRN, MSN, AOCN, CHPN
Advanced Practice Nurse and Lecturer
Supportive Oncology
Yale Cancer Center
Yale School of Nursing
Yale University
New Haven, Connecticut

Albert Rizos, PharmD
System Senior Clinical Pharmacy Specialist
Sharp Healthcare
San Diego, California

Foreword

Reading the pages of this book is a profound reflection for me on the progress in our field. I began my work in pain management in 1977 on a 40-bed oncology unit. Most of the patients had extreme pain from our early attempts at treatment and late-stage disease. As a new graduate on the evening shift, my options for responding to the call bell voices of "I'm in pain" (long before a pain scale was used) were limited. We had three analgesics available: oral codeine, intramuscular meperidine, and morphine. We watched the clock closely so not to medicate early; we believed that adding promethazine to the meperidine was sophisticated practice, and we gave placebos on a far more common basis than I would ever like to admit. There was no such thing as pain certification or a pain service, and I can promise you that there was not a textbook on pain management at the nurses' station.

Two years later, I attended a lecture given by Ada Rogers, RN, from the Memorial Sloan Kettering Pain Service. She described their pioneering work to aggressively treat pain and the scientific basis of their evolving practice, but most of all she spoke with a passionate commitment and belief that pain could be relieved. She spoke for an hour, and my professional life was changed forever.

Some years later, I read an article from a nurse, Margo McCaffery, and her profound message that "pain is what the person says it is, existing when he or she says it does." Again, my understanding of pain changed completely. Pain was no longer just a physiologic response awaiting a pharmacologic treatment. Pain became a human response; pain was a suffering person in need of both competent treatment and compassionate attention. There are times when I, and I think many of my colleagues, are outraged at the slow progress in pain management. It is now 2010, and this book will be released 33 years from my entre to the world of those in pain. There are other days when I marvel at the progress that has been made in the relief of pain: the understanding of the physiology of pain, the abundance of treatment options, the development of the specialty, and the progress toward addressing the truly enormous cultural, social, and regulatory hurdles that must be faced to do the work of relieving pain

and suffering. Holding this book reminds even the cynics and the weary among us that much has been achieved.

There are many books now written about pain, but the book before you is in a class of its own. As I reviewed this work, I was reminded of an experience I had some years ago (outside my professional life) as an avid fan of theater, music, and art. I was attending a performance of a popular play in a Los Angeles theater that included two very seasoned and successful actors. The two actors were beyond wonderful; as the play progressed, they moved beyond their superb performance, clearly having perfected their roles, and as the audience responded to their art, the two rose to the moment, providing a performance beyond description. As observers of the performance, the audience felt as if we were witnessing an intimate moment in these performers' lives, a career achievement. After the performance, my theater companion commented that these performers had "mastered their craft."

This book by Chris Pasero and Margo McCaffery is a master work. It is far above the quality of what we expect in a book. These authors wisely recognized that the field of pain has become so diverse and the literature to be reviewed so vast that they could not possibly cover all aspects of pain. This book focuses on the essentials of pain physiology, assessment, and management, but in a scientifically rigorous way that creates a solid foundation for the field. The book is a masterful combination of an exquisitely written critique of the evidence combined with clinical application to the real world of patients in pain and the clinicians who care for them.

As a fellow author and editor of texts, I recall the words of one of my most cherished mentors when a book I edited was published. She told me that publication of a major book for a field is a synthesis of the science and a statement of the integrity of that area of science. In the era of sound bites, instant messages, e-mails, and brief reports, a book means something.

Professionals who are within the field of pain management as researchers, clinicians, and educators owe a great thanks to Pasero and McCaffery. Master works such as this can take over a good bit of your life for many months or years. I personally believe that most excellent books simply can't be written in daylight hours; precise writing such as this happens late at night, over agonizing weekends, and only after drafts far too numerous to count. This is a masterful performance, one that should inspire readers to a new level of what it means to be a professional who has been given the great opportunity to serve people in pain.

Betty Ferrell, PhD, MA, FAAN, FPCN
Research Scientist
City of Hope Medical Center
Duarte, California

Acknowledgements

Without the support of our families, friends, and colleagues, we would not have been able to write this book. Our families and friends encouraged us every step of the way. Writing a book can be a lonely experience for both the authors and their families, but our families as well as our friends tolerated the social isolation we imposed, and they were there when the writing was over.

Chris wishes to thank David, her husband, best friend, and partner in all aspirations. Without his unending and immeasurable support, this book would not have been possible. Chris would also like to acknowledge the person who introduced her to the specialty of pain management and inspired and continues to inspire her passion for it, her mentor and friend Dr. Lex Hubbard. She also expresses appreciation to Dr. Russell Portenoy for his many hours of counsel in writing this book.

You cannot write a book without a computer these days, but Margo acknowledges that she is computer impaired. She wishes to thank her two friends and computer consultants, Mel Vincent and Craig Colbert, who were willing to consult at all hours of the day and night when her anxiety rose to a panic level. She is also especially grateful for the patience of her brother, Don Smith, over the years of writing books.

We wish to express our deep gratitude to our colleagues, Russell Portenoy, Keela Herr, Thomas Quinn, Albert Rizos, Rosemary Polomano, Allison Nisbet, Jan Frandsen, Stephen Passik, Kenneth Kirsh, and Karen Kaiser who coauthored and otherwise contributed to this book. Their insights, knowledge, and hard work were invaluable.

We also appreciate the many hours our library researcher, Chan Thai, spent obtaining and tracking down articles for us. It took a load off our shoulders. Thank you, Chan, for your thoroughness and promptness.

Many people at Elsevier contributed to the publication of this book. In particular we wish to thank our superb editors, Tamara Myers and Clay Broeker, for their expertise, attention to detail, and willingness and ability to find solutions to every problem we encountered.

The comments and patient stories shared with us by our colleagues across the country have always been a great source of inspiration and have helped us keep abreast of the challenges and misconceptions related to pain management. They helped us identify what the health care team needs to know to improve the care of people with pain. Let us continue to hear from you.

Chris Pasero, MS, RN-BC, FAAN
Pain Management Educator and Clinical Consultant
1252 Clearview Drive
El Dorado Hills, CA 95762
Phone: 916-933-2023
E-mail: cpasero@aol.com

Margo McCaffery, MS, RN-BC, FAAN
Consultant in the Nursing Care of Patients with Pain
8347 Kenyon Avenue
Los Angeles, CA 90045
Phone: 310-649-2219
E-mail: margopain@aol.com

Contents

Neurophysiology of Pain and Analgesia and the Pathophysiology of Neuropathic Pain

Chris Pasero and Russell K. Portenoy

Terminology

Afferent Neuron that carries information to the central nervous system.

Allodynia Pain with a nonnoxious stimulus (e.g., touch); a common characteristic of some neuropathic pain.

Central disinhibition A central mechanism of neuropathic pain that occurs when control mechanisms along inhibitory (modulatory) pathways are lost or suppressed, leading to abnormal excitability of central neurons.

Central sensitization A key central mechanism of neuropathic pain; the abnormal hyperexcitability of central neurons in the spinal cord, which results from complex changes induced by the incoming afferent barrages of nociceptors.

Cross excitation See ephaptic conduction.

Cross talk See ephaptic conduction.

Efferent A neuron that carries information away from the central nervous system.

Ephaptic conduction Also called cross-excitation or cross-talk; a peripheral mechanism that may sustain neuropathic pain through the creation of chemically mediated connections between nerve fibers, causing the abnormal activation of nociceptive neurons, ultimately producing pain.

GABAergic Increased function of the gamma aminobutyric acid (GABA) inhibitory pathways; increased GABA (GABAergic) function may help to relieve neuropathic pain.

Hyperalgesia Increased sensation of pain in response to a normally painful stimulus.

Neuroplasticity The ability of the peripheral and central nervous systems to change both structure and function as a result of noxious stimuli.

Nociceptor Primary afferent neurons that exist throughout the body and have the intrinsic ability to respond selectively to specific noxious stimuli.

Peripheral sensitization A key peripheral mechanism of neuropathic pain that occurs when there are changes in the number and location of ion channels, in particular sodium channels, which abnormally accumulate in injured nociceptors, producing a lower nerve depolarization threshold, ectopic discharges, and an increase in the response to stimuli.

Sympathetically maintained pain Pain that is identified through a very positive response to sympathetic nerve blocks; likely to be part of the syndrome known as complex regional pain syndrome (CRPS); underlying mechanism is unclear but thought to be related to ephaptic conduction.

Wind-up The progressive increase in response of central neurons that may be induced by high-intensity activity in the peripheral nociceptors that synapse on these neurons.

There are many ways to classify pain, and clear distinctions are not always possible. Simple classifications invariably result in some omissions and overlap. General discussions of pain refer simply to three types: (1) acute pain (e.g., postoperative or trauma pain), (2) cancer pain, and (3) noncancer pain (e.g., osteoarthritis pain, postherpetic neuralgia, painful diabetic neuropathy). Pain can also be classified by its inferred pathophysiology: (1) nociceptive (physiologic) pain (normal neural processing of noxious stimuli), or (2) neuropathic pain (stimuli abnormally processed by the nervous system (Figure I-1). The types of neuropathic pain are often divided into categories on the basis of the mechanism thought to be primarily responsible for causing the

pain (i.e., peripheral nervous system [PNS] or central nervous system [CNS] activity). Note that in some cases the original injury occurs in the peripheral nerves (e.g., amputation), but the mechanisms that underlie the pain (e.g., phantom pain) seem to be generated primarily in the CNS. Some patients have both nociceptive and neuropathic pain, for example, nociceptive pain resulting from tumor growth and metastasis and neuropathic pain resulting from tumor compression of neural structures (see Section II for more on classifications and assessment of types of pain).

Appropriate pharmacologic management of nociceptive and neuropathic pain requires an understanding of their complex underlying mechanisms. This section

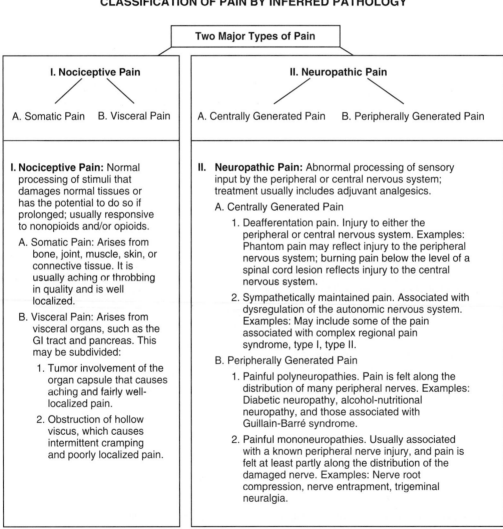

Figure I-1 | A method of classifying pain is by inferred pathophysiology: **I,** Nociceptive pain, stimuli from somatic and visceral structures; **II,** Neuropathic pain, stimuli abnormally processed by the nervous system.

From Pasero, C., & McCaffery, M. *Pain assessment and pharmacologic management*, p. 2, St. Louis, Mosby. Data from Max, M. B., & Portenoy, R. K. (2003). Methodological challenges for clinical trials of cancer pain treatments. In C. R. Chapman, & K. M. Foley (Eds), *Current and emerging issues in cancer pain: Research and practice*, New York, Raven Press; Portenoy, R. K. (1996). Neuropathic pain. In R. K. Portenoy, & R. M. Kanner (Eds), *Pain management: Theory and practice,* Philadelphia, FA Davis. © 2011, Pasero C, McCaffery M. May be duplicated for use in clinical practice.

presents an overview of nociception, which is followed by a discussion of the pathophysiology of neuropathic pain. The action sites of various analgesics are presented throughout the section.

Nociception

Nociception refers to the normal functioning of physiologic systems that leads to the perception of noxious stimuli as being painful. In short, it means "normal" pain transmission and includes four specific processes: transduction, transmission, perception, and modulation (Figure I-2).

Transduction

Transduction refers to the processes by which noxious events activate nociceptors, the primary afferent neurons that exist throughout the body (skin, subcutaneous tissue, and visceral or somatic structures) and have the intrinsic ability to respond selectively to specific noxious stimuli. Nociceptors have free nerve endings with specific channels that can respond to different kinds of stimuli. Different subtypes are activated when tissue damage or potential damage results from mechanical stimuli (e.g., incision, tumor growth); thermal stimuli (e.g., burn, frostbite); or chemical stimuli (e.g., toxins, chemotherapy) (Argoff, Albrecht, Irving, et al., 2009; Marchand, 2008). These stimuli activate nociceptors directly and also cause the release of a number of excitatory compounds (e.g., serotonin, bradykinin, histamine, substance P, and prostaglandins) that facilitate the further activation of nociceptors. These compounds, which may originate from local tissues, immune cells, or nerve endings themselves, may be collectively labeled an inflammatory soup (Marchand, 2008; see Figure I-2, A).

The prostaglandins are a particularly important group of compounds in the inflammatory soup that accompanies tissue injury. Prostaglandins are formed when the enzyme phospholipase breaks down phospholipids into arachidonic acid. The arachidonic acid, in turn, is acted upon by the enzyme cyclooxygenase (COX) to produce a set of compounds known as the prostaglandins (Figure I-3).

Cyclooxygenase is actually a small family of enzymes, each one of which is known as an isoenzyme. The two best characterized COX isoenzymes are COX-1 and COX-2. These isoenzymes are widely distributed in tissues and are known to play important roles in the effects produced by the nonopioid analgesics. The existence of other COX isoenzymes is likely, including a COX-3 isoenzyme that appears to predominate in the CNS.

The nonopioid analgesics act peripherally and centrally to inhibit the COX isoenzymes; various drugs have varying selectivities (see Chapter 6 and Figure 6-1 on p. 198). Peripheral actions reduce nociception in part by

diminishing the facilitory effect of inflammation-related compounds on transduction. Central actions may be involved in pain transmission and other effects such as reduction of fever.

The importance of the central effects of nonopioid analgesics is most clearly demonstrated by the efficacy of acetaminophen, which is a COX inhibitor that has minimal peripheral effect, is not antiinflammatory, and can both relieve pain and reduce fever by preventing the formation of prostaglandins in the CNS (Muth-Selbach, Tegeder, Brune, et al., 1999). The antipyretic effect of this drug and nonsteroidal antiinflammatory drugs (NSAIDs) may involve COX-3 inhibition (Botting, 2003). Research is ongoing to elucidate all of the underlying mechanisms of NSAIDs, but spinal COX-2 inhibition has been found to reduce not only prostaglandin production but also endocannabinoid breakdown (Telleria-Diaz, Schmidt, Kreusch, et al., 2010). Endocannabinoids have analgesic properties; however, they are subject to rapid breakdown, which limits their analgesic action. Recent research suggests that endocannabinoid analgesia may be enhanced by the action of COX-2 selective NSAIDs and that this may be a primary underlying mechanism of these NSAIDs (Telleria-Diaz, Schmidt, Kreusch, et al., 2010).

The ability to reduce nociception by partially blocking transduction is the mode of action of other types of analgesics as well. For example, sodium (NA$^+$) channels are closed and inactive at rest but undergo structural changes in response to membrane depolarization. Transient channel opening leads to an influx of sodium ions and subsequent nerve conduction (Dib-Hajj, Black, Waxman, 2009). Nociceptor activation may be reduced by local anesthetics, which block sodium (Na$^+$) channels and reduce the likelihood that the nerve will generate an action potential (see Chapter 23, Sodium Channel Blockers and Local Anesthetics). Similarly, compounds that change the flux of other ions, such as calcium (CA^{++}) or potassium (K$^+$), may have the potential to reduce transduction (see Chapter 23, Anticonvulsants). A variety of topical therapies, including topical NSAIDs and local anesthetics, have been developed with the goal of relieving pain through the lessening of transduction (see Chapter 7, Topical NSAIDs and Chapter 24, Topical Local Anesthetics).

Transmission

Transmission is the second process involved in nociception (see Figure I-2, B). Nociceptors are neurons that, compared with other sensory neurons, have small-diameter axons— either A-delta (δ) or C fibers (Argoff, Albrecht, Irving, et al., 2009). Effective transduction generates an action potential that is transmitted in these fibers toward the CNS. A-δ fibers are lightly myelinated, larger, and faster conducting than unmyelinated C fibers. The endings of A-δ fibers detect thermal and mechanical injury. These neurons typically

Figure I-2: Nociception
• The neural processing of noxious stimuli
• Described in four processes:
  - Transduction (A)
  - Transmission (B)
  - Perception (C)
  - Modulation (D)

Figure I-2A: Transduction
• Conversion of one energy form to another.
• Starts at the periphery when noxious stimulus causes tissue damage.
• Primary nociceptive fibers (afferents) are activated.
• Numerous excitatory substances are released and facilitate the further activation of nociceptors. These substances are collectively labeled an "inflammatory soup" and include:
  - Prostaglandins
  - Bradykinin
  - Substance P
  - Serotonin
  - Histamine
• Ion transfers (e.g., CA^{++}, NA^+, K^+) generate an action potential

Figure I-2B: Transmission
• Primary afferents continue the impulse via A-delta (δ) and C fibers (nerve axons) from the periphery to the spinal cord
  - Aδ fibers: Larger, myelinated, fast conduction: "first pain" (withdrawal)
  - C fibers: Smaller, unmyelinated, slow conduction: "second pain"
  - A-beta (β) fibers respond to touch, vibration, and movement; largest of the fibers, myelinated, fast conduction; A-β fibers do not normally transmit pain
• Afferent information passes through dorsal root ganglia to the spinal cord where it synapses in the dorsal horn and connects to the "second order" neuron (see INSET below)
• The stimulus is continued from the spinal cord via multiple ascending pathways to the brainstem and higher cortical levels

Figure I-2B Inset
In the dorsal horn, incoming information is extensively modulated through complex neurophysiologic and neurochemical mechanisms. The primary Aδ and C afferents release a variety of transmitters, among the most important of which are excitatory amino acids, such as glutamate, neurokinins, and substance P. Glutamate binds to the N-methyl-D-aspartate (NMDA) receptor and promotes pain transmission. Note that dorsal horn modulation involves both local, segmental systems and descending systems.

Figure I-2C: Perception
• End result of the neural activity of pain transmission
• Conscious awareness of pain
• Requires activation of higher brain structures, e.g., thalamus, limbic system
• Generates a network of cortical and subcortical gray matter
• Includes processes that influence movement, emotions, and drives related to pain

Figure I-2D: Modulation
• Inhibitory mechanisms
• Local and descending processes occur in multiple sites from the periphery to the cortex, most importantly in the spinal cord
• Involves the release of numerous neurochemicals which include:
  - Endogenous opioids
  - Serotonin
  - Norepinephrine

Continued

Figure I-2 | Nociception: "normal" pain transmission.

From Pasero, C., & McCaffery, M. *Pain assessment and pharmacologic management*, pp. 4-5, St. Louis, Mosby. © 2011, Pasero C, McCaffery M. May be duplicated for use in clinical practice.

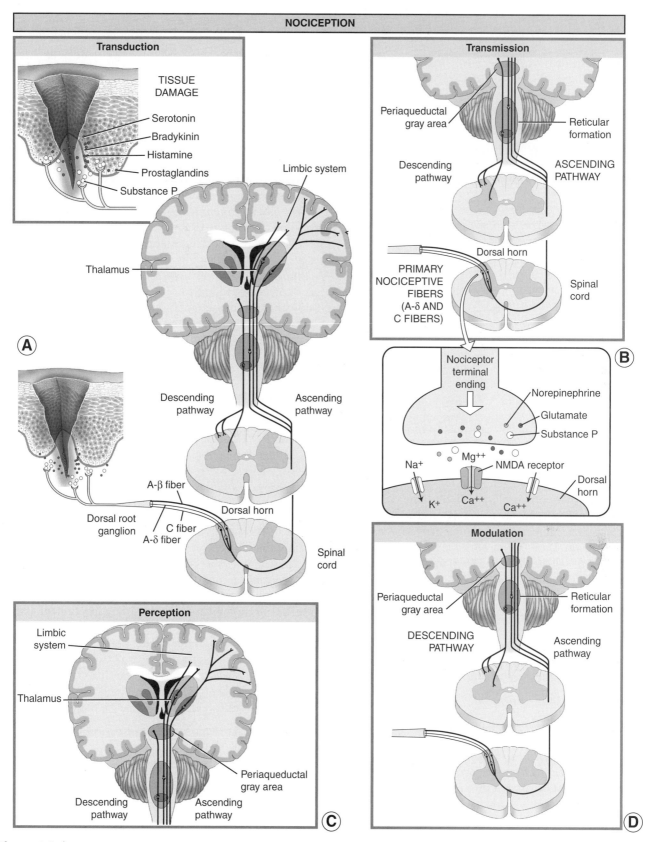

Figure I-2. Cont'd.

ENZYME PATHWAY: COX-1 AND COX-2

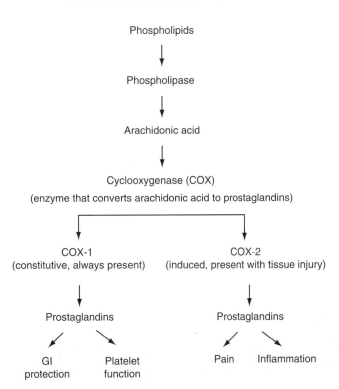

Figure I-3 | Enzyme pathway: COX-1 and COX-2.

From Pasero, C., & McCaffery, M. *Pain assessment and pharmacologic management*, p. 6, St. Louis, Mosby. © 2011, Pasero C, McCaffery M. May be duplicated for use in clinical practice.

transmit information that allows relatively quick localization of pain and an appropriately rapid protective response. The sensation accompanying A-δ fiber activation has been termed first pain (Dahl, Moiniche, 2004; Marchand, 2008). It is sharp and well-localized and leads to reflex withdrawal from the painful stimuli.

Unmyelinated C fibers are slow conductors and may respond to mechanical, thermal, or chemical stimuli. Activation after acute injury yields a poorly localized, typically aching or burning pain, which often is referred to as second pain (Dahl, Moiniche, 2004; Marchand, 2008). A-beta (β) fibers, the largest of the fibers, do not normally transmit pain but respond to touch, movement, and vibration.

The cell bodies of the nociceptive neurons that subserve the processes of transduction and transmission of information about noxious events are in dorsal root ganglia, which lie outside the spinal cord (see Figure I-2, *A*). Afferent information passes through the cell body to a central process, which synapses in the dorsal horn of the spinal cord. This synapse connects the nociceptor with the so-called second-order neuron in the dorsal horn. The second-order neuron, in turn, generates an action potential that ascends up the spinal cord and transmits information to the brain, where pain is perceived (see Figure I-2, *B*).

In the dorsal horn, incoming information is extensively modulated through complex neurophysiologic and neurochemical mechanisms. The primary A-δ and C afferents release a variety of transmitters, among the most important of which are excitatory amino acids, such as glutamate, neurokinins, and substance P. Glutamate binds to the *N*-methyl-D-aspartate (NMDA) receptor and promotes pain transmission (see inset of Figure I-2, *B*) (Carlton, 2009). NMDA receptors may contribute to the sensory disturbances experienced by patients with the neuropathic pain state known as *complex regional pain syndrome* (CRPS) (Finch, Knudsen, Drummond, 2009). Ketamine, an NMDA receptor antagonist, is an example of a drug that produces pain relief by preventing glutamate from binding to the NMDA receptor sites and thereby blocking the transmission of pain (see Chapter 23 for more on ketamine).

Dorsal horn modulation involves both local, segmental systems and descending systems. The neurochemistry is complex and not yet fully understood. Endogenous opioid compounds bind to opioid receptor sites and help to slow the transmission of pain. Opioid analgesics also bind to opioid receptor sites throughout the nervous system to produce analgesia and other effects, such as constipation, sedation, and respiratory depression (see Section IV).

Perception

The third broad process involved in nociception is termed perception. Perception, which may be viewed as the end result of the neural activity associated with transmission of information about noxious events, involves conscious awareness of pain (see Figure I-2, *C*). It requires the activation of higher brain structures, presumably including the cortex. It involves both awareness and related cognitions and the occurrence of emotions and drives associated with pain. These complex processes generate a network of cortical and subcortical gray matter when transmission of information about noxious events reaches the threshold for perception.

The physiology subserving the perception of pain is very poorly understood, but presumably can be targeted by therapies that activate higher cortical functions in the service of pain control or coping. Cognitive-behavioral therapy and specific approaches such as distraction and imagery have been developed based on evidence that brain processes can strongly influence pain perception.

Modulation

As noted, modulation of afferent input generated in response to noxious stimuli happens at every level, from the periphery to the cortex (see Figure I-2). Given the importance of this physiology, modulation usually is considered the last of the key processes of nociception (Marchand, 2008).

Peripheral and central systems and dozens of neurochemicals are involved in these modulatory processes. The endogenous opioids, for example, are found throughout the PNS and CNS and, like the exogenous opioids administered therapeutically, they inhibit neuronal activity through actions initiated by binding to opioid receptors. Other central inhibitory neurotransmitters important in the modulation of pain include serotonin and norepinephrine, which are released in the spinal cord and brainstem by the descending fibers of the modulatory system (see Figure I-2, *D*). Antidepressants relieve pain by blocking the body's reuptake (resorption) of serotonin and norepinephrine, making them more available to fight pain (see Chapter 22 for more information about antidepressants).

Pathophysiology of Pain: Neuropathic Pain

Neuropathic pain, like nociceptive pain, is a descriptive term used to refer to pain that is believed to be sustained by a set of mechanisms that is driven by damage to, or dysfunction of, the PNS or CNS. In contrast to nociceptive pain, which reflects the clinical judgment that pain is sustained by ongoing activation of essentially normal neural systems that exist to subserve the perception of noxious events, neuropathic pain is sustained by the abnormal processing of stimuli from the PNS or CNS or both (Adler, Nico, VandeVord, et al., 2009; Argoff, Albrecht, Irving, et al., 2009; Beydoun, Backonja, 2003; Dworkin, Backonja, Rowbotham, et al., 2003). Injury to the PNS can irreversibly alter central signaling mechanisms, and disturbances of these central signaling mechanisms can alter peripheral signaling mechanisms (Argoff, Albrecht, Irving, et al., 2009). Whereas nociceptive pain involves tissue damage or inflammation (Pasero, 2004), neuropathic pain may occur in the absence of either. Acute nociceptive pain, such as that which follows trauma,

serves to warn and protect individuals from further injury; neuropathic pain, even when acute, reflects a pathophysiology that is believed to serve no useful purpose (Beydoun, Backonja, 2003; Pasero, 2004). The peripheral and central mechanisms that initiate and maintain neuropathic pain are discussed subsequently and in Table I-1.

Peripheral Mechanisms

As described earlier, primary afferent neurons, called nociceptors, are distributed throughout the PNS. Nociceptors have free nerve endings that have the capacity to distinguish noxious and innocuous stimuli. They are activated when tissue damage or potential damage results from stimuli that are mechanical (e.g., surgical or nonsurgical trauma, tumor growth); thermal (e.g., burn, frostbite); or chemical (e.g., toxins, chemotherapy) (Marchand, 2008). Infection, viruses, metabolic disease, nutritional deficiencies, ischemia, and stroke are among the many other sources of tissue injury (Pasero, 2004). When noxious stimuli exceed the threshold required to activate the nociceptor (transduction), an electric signal (action potential) is set up in the nerve and is then transmitted to the CNS (see Figures I-2, *A* and I-2, *B*). In the periphery, transduction involves numerous substances (e.g., serotonin, bradykinin, histamine, substance P, prostaglandins) that may lead to activation of nociceptors. The inflammatory process that occurs with tissue damage produces these and other substances and also causes the transfer of ions (e.g., sodium, potassium, calcium) that support the creation of an action potential in the nerve.

Once an electric signal is established in the neuron, ion channels are responsible for conduction of

Table I-1	**Mechanisms of Neuropathic Pain**
Peripheral Mechanisms	**Central Mechanisms**
Peripheral sensitization initiated by release of substances from damaged cells (e.g., prostaglandins, bradykinin, serotonin, norepinephrine, substance P)	Central sensitization (hyperexcitability of central neurons) initiated by prolonged binding of neurotransmitters (e.g., glutamate, substance P)
Alteration in ion channel expression	NMDA receptor activation and influx of intracellular calcium
Collateral sprouting	Lowered threshold for nerve conduction
Recruitment of "silent" nociceptors	Increased response to stimuli
Ephaptic conduction	Enlarged receptor field
Lowered threshold for nerve depolarization → spontaneous ectopic neuronal discharges	Collateral sprouting
Coupling between sensory and central nervous systems	Coupling between sensory and central nervous systems
Clinical signs: primary hyperalgesia, burning pain, dysesthesias, paresthesias, allodynia	Central disinhibition
	Clinical signs: secondary hyperalgesia, allodynia, sympathetically maintained pain

From Pasero C, McCaffery M. (2011). *Pain assessment and pharmacologic management*, p. 7, St. Louis, Mosby. Data from Adler, J. E., Nico, L., VandeVord, P., et al. (2009). Modulation of neuropathic pain by glial-driven factor. *Pain Med, 10*(7), 1229-1236; Argoff, C. E., Albrecht, P., Irving, G., et al. (2009). Multimodal analgesia for chronic pain: Rationale and future directions. *Pain Med, 10*(Suppl 2), S53-S66; Beydoun, A., & Backonja, M. M. (2003). Mechanistic stratification of antineuralgic agents. *J Pain Symptom Manage, 25*(Suppl 5), S18-S30; Bridges, D., Thompson, S. W. N.,

& Rice, A. S. C. (2001). Mechanisms of neuropathic pain. *Br J Anaesth, 87*(1), 12-26; Carlton, S. M. (2009). NMDA receptors revisted—Hope floats. *Pain, 146*(1-2), 1-2; Dickenson, A. H., Matthews, E. A., & Suzuki, R. (2002). Neurobiology of neuropathic pain: Mode of action of anticonvulsants. *Eur J Pain, 6*(Suppl A), 51-60; Mao, J., & Chen, L. L. (2000). Gabapentin in pain management. *Anesth Analg, 91*(3), 680-687; Pasero, C. (2004). Pathophysiology of neuropathic pain. *Pain Manage Nurs, 5*(4), 3-8. © 2004, Pasero C. May be duplicated for use in clinical practice.

that electric signal along the nerve axon (Beydoun, Backonja, 2003). Transmission of information about noxious events occurs along both large-diameter A-δ nerve fibers and along the slow-conducting C fibers. The largest and most rapidly conducting A-β peripheral nerve fibers do not carry information about noxious events (see Figure I-2, *B*).

In this normal process of transduction and transmission of information about noxious stimuli, several processes could occur that lead to the development of neuropathic pain. For example, hyperexcitable epidermal nerve endings in the periphery, which have been damaged by noxious stimuli, and nearby keratinocytes are thought to be factors in abnormal reorganization of the CNS, an underlying mechanism of some persistent neuropathic pain states (Argoff, Albrecht, Irving, et al., 2009; Fishman, 2009). Changes can occur in the number and location of ion channels. Sodium channels, in particular, abnormally accumulate in injured nociceptors (Beydoun, Backonja, 2003; Jensen, 2002). The nerve depolarization threshold is lowered, leading to ectopic discharges, and the response to stimuli is increased (Bridges, Thompson, Rice, 2001). These processes, which may lead to peripheral sensitization, may be important contributors to the maintenance of neuropathic pain (Beydoun, Backonja, 2003; Fishman, 2009). Drugs, such as anticonvulsants, antidepressants, and sodium channel blockers (including those applied locally as local anesthetics), may act in the periphery to relieve pain by modulating ion channels and suppressing ectopic discharges (see Section V).

Another peripheral mechanism that may sustain neuropathic pain is the creation of chemically mediated connections between nerve fibers. These connections, or ephapses, are the substrates of an abnormal excitatory process, which is known as ephaptic conduction (cross-excitation or cross-talk) (Bridges, Thompson, Rice, 2001). This process may cause the abnormal activation of nociceptive neurons, ultimately producing pain (Pasero, 2004). Ephaptic conduction between afferent sensory nerves that transmit information about pain and efferent sympathetic nerves that exist in the same nerve bundle has been speculated to be involved in the pathophysiology of so-called sympathetically maintained pain (Bridges, Thompson, Rice, 2001). Because sympathetically maintained pain, identified through a very positive response to sympathetic (local anesthetic) nerve blocks, is likely to be part of CRPS, the recommended early treatment of the syndrome usually includes a trial of sympathetic nerve blocks.

Hyperalgesia, which is the increased sensation of pain in response to a normally painful stimulus, is seen clinically in patients with neuropathic pain. The mechanisms underlying hyperalgesia continue to be the focus of research but are thought to be multifaceted and mediated in part by sensitization of C-fiber primary afferent neurons (Byers, Bonica, 2001).

Central Mechanisms

Central mechanisms also play a critical role in the development and maintenance of neuropathic pain. A key mechanism is called *central sensitization*, which is defined as abnormal hyperexcitability of central neurons, and that results from complex changes induced by the incoming afferent barrages of nociceptors (Bridges, Thompson, Rice, 2001). This can occur at any level of the CNS (Argoff, Albrecht, Irving, et al., 2009). The best-characterized mechanism linked to central sensitization involves the prolonged release and binding of excitatory neurotransmitters, such as substance P and glutamate, which activate the NMDA receptor (see inset in Figure I-2, *B*). Activation of this receptor causes an increase in intracellular calcium levels by moving calcium into the cell through the so-called N-type calcium channel (Jensen, 2002). The N-type calcium channel is thought to play a key role in the processing of painful stimuli; when blocked, abnormal pain sensation is inhibited (Dickenson, Matthews, Suzuki, 2002). An increase in intracellular calcium lowers the cells threshold for firing, the substrate for central sensitization.

Research also has demonstrated expression of sodium channels on dorsal horn neurons near spinal cord lesions, which were linked to central pain behaviors (Finnerup, Biering-Sorensen, Johannesen, et al., 2005; Hains, Klein, Saab, et al., 2003). An increase in the influx of sodium also could lead to a lowered threshold for activation, an increased response to stimuli, and enlargement of the receptive field served by the affected neuron (Beydoun, Backonja, 2003; see inset in Figure I-2, *B*). Research is ongoing, but all of these outcomes could contribute to sensitization.

Central sensitization often is considered to be closely allied, or even synonymous, with a phenomenon known as *wind-up* (Dickenson, Matthews, Suzuki, 2002). *Wind-up* refers to the progressive increase in the response of central neurons, and it may be induced by high-intensity activity in the peripheral nociceptors that synapse on these neurons (see Figure I-2) (Argoff, Albrecht, Irving, et al., 2009). The relationship between the relatively short-lived wind-up phenomenon observed in cellular modules and the persistent state of central sensitization that can occur in animals, presumably including humans, is not completely understood (Adler, Nico, VandeVord, et al., 2009; Bridges, Thompson, Rice, 2001).

Injured or intensely activated peripheral neurons may undergo synaptic reorganization or change anatomically, sprouting new processes. These processes also occur in the CNS and are thought to be sustained by an increased or inappropriate responsiveness of central neurons to relatively mild peripheral stimuli (Adler, Nico, VandeVord, et al., 2009). Loss of C-fiber afferents into the CNS, such as may follow an injury to a nerve root, leads to reorganization in the dorsal horn of the spinal cord. Large myelinated fibers sprout and invade other areas where nociceptive-specific neurons were located, and this change may correlate with the development of abnormal sensation in the area of the body served by the injured nerve (Jensen, 2002). Allodynia, or pain with a nonnoxious stimulus (e.g., touch), is one such type of abnormal sensation and is common in some patients with neuropathic pain (Pasero, 2004).

The ability of the PNS and CNS to change both structure and function as a result of noxious stimuli is called neuroplasticity (Byers, Bonica, 2001; Dickenson, Matthews, Suzuki, 2002; Jensen, 2002). Neuroplasticity is exceedingly complex but appears to be a key feature in many diseases of the nervous system, including persistent pain.

Another central mechanism, called central disinhibition, occurs when control mechanisms along inhibitory (modulatory) pathways are lost or suppressed, leading to abnormal excitability of central neurons (Pasero, 2004). Among the possible causes of disinhibition is dysfunction in gamma aminobutyric acid (GABA) pathways. GABA is the most abundant neurotransmitter in the CNS (Dickenson, Matthews, Suzuki, 2002) and composes a major inhibitory neurotransmitter system (Bridges, Thompson, Rice, 2001). When GABA receptor inhibition is suppressed, abnormal pain processing occurs (Bridges, Thompson, Rice, 2001). Conversely, increased GABA function (GABAergic) may help to relieve neuropathic pain.

Other supraspinal processes that modulate and inhibit the transmission of nociceptive impulses also may be involved in central disinhibition (Beydoun, Backonja, 2003). Abnormal functioning in the descending fibers containing the inhibitory neurotransmitters serotonin and norepinephrine may be one such process.

As mentioned, hyperalgesia, or increased pain sensation, is common in patients with neuropathic pain. Two types of hyperalgesia are described. Primary hyperalgesia is thought to be the result of peripheral changes and is seen clinically as increased pain and sensitivity at the site of the injury. Secondary hyperalgesia is the result of central neural events and is seen clinically as allodynia and increased pain and sensitivity in areas extending outside of the site of injury (Pasero, 2004).

Most of the drugs used to treat neuropathic pain produce effects through their actions on the CNS. Anticonvulsants, sodium channel blockers, and other drugs, including some antidepressants and ziconotide, produce analgesia by blocking central neuron ion channels. Local anesthetics are sodium channel blockers that can work locally when applied directly to nerves; when taken systemically, their effects appear to be related primarily to CNS actions. Antidepressants inhibit synaptic reuptake of the biogenic amines serotonin and norepinephrine, thereby increasing activity in monoaminergic pain modulating pathways that originate in the brainstem and descend to every level of the spinal cord. Ketamine produces pain relief by antagonizing activity at the NMDA receptor site. Midazolam enhances GABAergic function to produce analgesia for conditions like muscle spasm (see Section V).

Multimodal Analgesia

Multimodal therapy is a relatively new concept. It was first proposed in the early 1990s and was applied primarily to the treatment of acute pain and the prevention of persistent post-surgical pain (Gartner, Kroman, Callesen, et al., 2008; Kehlet, Jensen, Woolf, 2006; Pasero, 2003; Polomano, Rathmell, Krenzischek, et al., 2008). Multimodal pain treatment involves the use of two or more classes of analgesics to target different pain mechanisms in the PNS or CNS. It relies on the thoughtful and rational combination of analgesics to maximize pain relief and prevent analgesic gaps that may lead to worsening pain or unnecessary bouts of uncontrolled pain (Argoff, Albrecht, Irving, et al., 2009; Carr, Reines, Schaffer, et al., 2005; Tang, Evans, Chaput, et al., 2009).

A multimodal approach may allow lower doses of each of the drugs in the treatment plan, and lower doses have the potential to produce fewer adverse effects (Ashburn, Caplan, Carr, et al., 2004; Brodner, Van Aken, Hertle, et al., 2001; Tang, Evans, Chaput, et al., 2009). Further, multimodal analgesia can result in comparable or greater pain relief than can be achieved with any single analgesic (Busch, Shore, Bhandari, et al., 2006; Butterfield, Schwarz, Ries, et al., 2001; Cassinelli, Dean, Garcia, et al., 2008; Huang, Wang, Wang, et al., 2008; White, 2005). In the setting of postoperative pain, the use of combination therapy to prevent both inflammatory and neuropathic pain is likely to yield the best immediate results and also offers the promise of reducing the incidence of prolonged or persistent postsurgical pain (Kehlet, Jensen, Woolf, 2006) (see Sections III, IV, and V).

The multimodal strategy also has a role in the management of persistent pain. This is true in all of the various practice settings, including the emergency department (Baker, 2005), outpatient treatment sites (Gatchel, Okifuji, 2006), and settings providing specialist palliative care (Soares, Chan, 2007). The complex nature of the many persistent pain conditions indicates the need for appropriate combinations of analgesics to target differing underlying mechanisms (Argoff, Albrecht, Irving, et al., 2009). Broad acceptance of a role in pain management for the adjuvant analgesic drugs is premised on the growing importance of multimodal treatment for persistent pain (see Section V).

Multimodal therapy also is a useful strategy for addressing the common problem of symptom distress related to symptoms other than pain. Patients with acute or chronic pain commonly experience additional symptoms, which may influence the decision to try one analgesic rather than another. More broadly, the experience of multiple symptoms also may guide the use of multiple drugs, some of which are targeted to relieve distressing conditions such as insomnia that accompany pain and may be factors in worsening it (Gan, Meyer, Apfel, et al., 2007; Gartner, Kroman, Callesen, et al., 2008).

Multimodal Therapy versus Polypharmacy

The term *polypharmacy* carries a negative connotation, in contrast to multimodal therapy or combination therapy. Whereas multimodal therapy is based on rational combinations of analgesics with differing underlying mechanisms to achieve the greatest benefit in pain control, polypharmacy suggests the use of drug combinations that are irrational and less effective or less safe than would be a regimen that had fewer or different agents.

Persistent Postsurgical and Posttrauma Pain

As many as 50% of patients undergoing surgical procedures, such as inguinal hernia repair; breast, cardiac, or thoracic surgery; leg amputation; and coronary artery bypass, experience persistent pain; in 2% to 10% of these individuals, the intensity of persistent postsurgical pain is severe (Kehlet, Jensen, Woolf, 2006). A study of 90 women who underwent abdominal hysterectomy pain for noncancer conditions found that 16.7% experienced persistent postoperative pain (Brandsborg, Dueholm, Nikolajsen, et al., 2009). The incidence of persistent postmastectomy pain is reported to be as high as 65% (Smith, Bourne, Squair, et al., 1999).

Pain following traumatic injury is common as well. A multicenter study conducted in 69 hospitals in 14 states in the United States found that 62.7% of patients (N = 3047) reported injury-related pain at 12 months after a traumatic injury (Rivara, MacKenzie, Jurkovich, et al., 2008). A quarter of patients in an earlier study (N = 397) described pain that interfered with daily activity 7 years following limb-threatening lower extremity trauma; 40% reported high pain intensities (Castillo, MacKenzie, Wegener, et al., 2006).

Further research is needed, but multiple factors are thought to contribute to the likelihood of postsurgical pain, including surgical nerve injury, preexisting pain, and genetic susceptibility. For example, severe pre-amputation pain has long been associated with a higher incidence of phantom limb pain (Bach, Noreng, Tjellden, 1988; Katz, 1997; Nikolajsen, Ilkjaer, Kroner, et al., 1997). A 2-year study of 57 patients who underwent lower extremity amputation revealed that high levels of both pre-amputation pain and acute pain after

amputation predicted persistent post-amputation pain (Hanley, Jensen, Smith, et al., 2006). Greater analgesic requirements during the immediate postoperative period following coronary artery bypass surgery predicted persistent pain (at multiple anatomic sites) in a study of 736 patients (Taillefer, Carrier, Belisle, et al., 2006). Older patients tend to have a lower risk of developing persistent postsurgical pain than younger patients (Poobalan, Bruce, Smith, et al., 2003; Smith, Bourne, Squair, et al., 1999). For example, one study showed that patients under the age of 40 years were at increased risk for persistent post-inguinal hernia repair pain (Poobalan, Bruce, King, et al., 2001). Another found that the prevalence of persistent chest and leg pain following cardiac surgery was 55% in patients who were less than 60 years old and 34% in those over 70 years old (Bruce, Drury, Poobalan, et al., 2003). The reader is referred to an excellent review by Perkins and Kehlet (2000) that includes predictive factors, etiology, and progression of postsurgical pain conditions.

The presence of pain at 3 months after injury was a predictive factor for both the presence and the high severity of persistent pain following major trauma (Rivara, MacKenzie, Jurkovich, et al., 2008). Although the presence of persistent pain varied with age, in this study it was more common in women and in those who had untreated depression before the traumatic injury. Another study found that multiple factors influenced the likelihood of persistent pain 7 years after major lower extremity trauma (Castillo, MacKenzie, Wegener, et al., 2006); these factors included having less than a high-school education; having less than a college education; low self-efficacy for return to usual major activities; a high level of alcohol consumption in the month prior to injury; and high pain intensity, high levels of sleep and rest dysfunction, and elevated levels of depression and anxiety at 3 months after hospital discharge. Interestingly, those who were treated with opioid analgesics during the first 3 months after discharge in this study had lower levels of persistent pain at 7 years, underscoring the importance of early initiation of aggressive pain management approaches.

The clinical presentation of persistent postsurgical or posttrauma pain is primarily a patient's report of the features characteristic of neuropathic pain, such as continuous burning pain and pain beyond the expected time of pain resolution (see Section II for assessment of neuropathic pain). Strategies for preventing these persistent pain states are being investigated, but sustained multimodal pharmacologic approaches that target the underlying mechanisms of neuropathic pain (described earlier) are recommended (Kehlet, Jensen, Woolf, 2006). See Sections III, IV, and V for discussion of the role of the various analgesics and techniques in the prevention of persistent postsurgical and posttrauma pain. See Table I-2 for the many other harmful effects of unrelieved Pain.

Table I-2 | Harmful Effects of Unrelieved Pain

Domains Affected	Specific Responses to Pain
Endocrine	↑ Adrenocorticotrophic hormone (ACTH), ↑ cortisol, ↑ antidiuretic hormone (ADH), ↑ epinephrine, ↑ norepinephrine, ↑ growth hormone (GH), ↑ catecholamines, ↑ renin, ↑ angiotensin II, ↑ aldosterone, ↑ glucagon, ↑ interleukin-1; ↓ insulin, ↓ testosterone
Metabolic	Gluconeogenesis, hepatic glycogenolysis, hyperglycemia, glucose intolerance, insulin resistance, muscle protein catabolism, ↑ lipolysis
Cardiovascular	↑ Heart rate, ↑ cardiac workload, ↑ peripheral vascular resistance, ↑ systemic vascular resistance, hypertension, ↑ coronary vascular resistance, ↑ myocardial oxygen consumption, hypercoagulation, deep vein thrombosis
Respiratory	↓ Flows and volumes, atelectasis, shunting, hypoxemia, ↓ cough, sputum retention, infection
Genitourinary	↓ Urinary output, urinary retention, fluid overload, hypokalemia
Gastrointestinal	↓ Gastric and bowel motility
Musculoskeletal	Muscle spasm, impaired muscle function, fatigue, immobility
Cognitive	Reduction in cognitive function, mental confusion
Immune	Depression of immune response
Developmental	↑ Behavioral and physiologic responses to pain, altered temperaments, higher somatization, infant distress behavior; possible altered development of the pain system, ↑ vulnerability to stress disorders, addictive behavior, and anxiety states
Future pain	Debilitating chronic pain syndromes: postmastectomy pain, postthoracotomy pain, phantom pain, postherpetic neuralgia
Quality of life	Sleeplessness, anxiety, fear, hopelessness, ↑ thoughts of suicide

↓, Decreased; ↑, increased.

From Pasero, C., & McCaffery, M. *Pain assessment and pharmacologic management*, p. 11, St. Louis, Mosby. Data from Cousins, M. (1994). Acute postoperative pain. In P. D. & Wall, R. Melzack (Eds.), *Textbook of pain*, ed 3, New York, Churchill Livingstone; Kehlet, H. (1998). Modification of responses to surgery by neural blockade. In M. J. Cousins, & P. O. Bridenbaugh (Eds.), *Neural blockade*, Philadelphia, Lippincott-Raven; Mcintyre, P. E., & Ready, L. B. (1996). *Acute pain management: A practical guide*, Philadelphia, Saunders. © 2011, Pasero C, McCaffery M. May be duplicated for use in clinical practice.

References

Adler, J. E., Nico, L., VandeVord, P., et al. (2009). Modulation of neuropathic pain by a glial-driven factor. *Pain Med, 10*(7), 1229–1236.

Argoff, C. E., Albrecht, P., Irving, G., et al. (2009). Multimodal analgesia for chronic pain: Rationale and future directions. *Pain Med, 10*(Suppl 2), S53–S66.

Ashburn, M. A., Caplan, R. A., Carr, D. B., et al. (2004). Practice guidelines for acute pain management in the perioperative setting: An updated report by the American Society of Anesthesiologists task force on acute pain management. *Anesthesiology, 100*(6), 1573–1581.

Bach, S., Noreng, M. J., & Tjellden, N. U. (1988). Phantom pain in amputees during the first 12 months following limb amputation, after preoperative lumbar epidural blockade. *Pain, 33*(3), 297–301.

Baker, K. (2005). Chronic pain syndromes in the emergency department: Identifying guidelines for management. *Emergency Medicine Australasia: EMA, 17*(1), 57–64.

Beydoun, A., & Backonja, M. M. (2003). Mechanistic stratification of antineuralgic agents. *Journal of Pain and Symptom Management, 25*(Suppl 5), S18–S30.

Botting, R. (2003). COX-2 and COX-3 inhibitors. *Thrombosis Research, 110*(5–6), 269–272.

Brandsborg, B., Dueholm, M., Nikolajsen, L., et al. (2009). A prospective study of risk factors for pain persisting 4 months after hysterectomy. *The Clinical Journal of Pain, 25*(4), 263–268.

Bridges, D., Thompson, S. W. N., & Rice, A. S. C. (2001). Mechanisms of neuropathic pain. *British Journal of Anaesthesia, 87*(1), 12–26.

Brodner, G., Van Aken, H., Hertle, L., et al. (2001). Multimodal perioperative management: Combining thoracic epidural analgesia, forced mobilization, and oral nutrition reduces hormonal and metabolic stress and improves convalescence after major urologic surgery. *Anesthesia and Analgesia, 92*(6), 1594–1600.

Bruce, J., Drury, N., Poobalan, A. S., et al. (2003). The prevalence of chronic chest and leg pain following cardiac surgery: A historical cohort study. *Pain, 104*(1–2), 265–273.

Busch, C. A., Shore, B. J., Bhandari, R., et al. (2006). Efficacy of periarticular multimodal drug injection in total knee arthroplasty. *The Journal of Bone and Joint Surgery, 88a*(5), 959–963.

Butterfield, N. N., Schwarz, S. K., Ries, C. R., et al. (2001). Combined pre- and post-surgical bupivacaine wound infiltrations decrease opioid requirements after knee ligament reconstruction. *Canadian Journal of Anaesthesia = Journal Canadien D'anesthesie, 48*(3), 245–250.

Byers, M. R., & Bonica, J. J. (2001). Peripheral pain mechanisms and nociceptors plasticity. In J. D. Loeser, S. H. Butler, R. C. Chapman, & D. C. Turk (Eds.), *Bonica's management of pain.* (3rd ed., pp. 26–72). Philadelphia: Lippincott, Williams & Wilkins.

Carlton, S. M. (2009). Peripheral NMDA receptors revisted—Hope floats. *Pain, 146*(1–2), 1–2.

Carr, D. B., Reines, H. D., Schaffer, J., et al. (2005). The impact of technology on the analgesic gap and quality of acute pain management. *Regional Anesthesia and Pain Medicine, 30*(3), 286–291.

Cassinelli, E. H., Dean, C. L., Garcia, R. M., et al. (2008). Ketorolac use for postoperative pain management following lumbar decompression surgery: A prospective, randomized, double-blinded, placebo-controlled trial. *Spine, 33*(12), 1313–1317.

Castillo, R. C., MacKenzie, E. J., Wegener, S. T., et al. (2006). Prevalence of chronic pain seven years following limb threatening lower extremity trauma. *Pain, 124*(3), 321–329.

Dahl, J. B., & Moiniche, S. (2004). Pre-emptive analgesia. *British Medical Bulletin, 71*(1), 13–27.

Dib-Hajj, S. D., Black, J. A., Waxman, S. G. (2009). Voltage-gated sodium channels: Targets for pain. *Pain Med, 10*(7), 1260–1269.

Dickenson, A. H., Matthews, E. A., & Suzuki, R. (2002). Neurobiology of neuropathic pain: Mode of action of anticonvulsants. *European Journal of Pain, 6*(Suppl A), 51–60.

Dworkin, R. H., Backonja, M., Rowbotham, M. C., et al. (2003). Advances in neuropathic pain: Diagnosis, mechanisms, and treatment recommendations. *Archives of Neurology, 60*(11), 1524–1534.

Finch, P. M., Knudsen, L., Drummond, P. D. (2009). Reduction of allodynia in patients with complex regional pain syndrome: A double-blind placebo-controlled trial of topical ketamine. *Pain, 146*(1–2), 18–24.

Finnerup, N. B., Biering-Sorensen, F., Johannesen, I. L., et al. (2005). Intravenous lidocaine relieves spinal cord injury pain. *Anesthesiology, 102*(5), 1023–1030.

Fishman, S. (2009). Opioid-based multimodal care of patients with chronic pain: Improving effectiveness and mitigating risks. *Pain Med, 10*(Suppl 2), S49–S52.

Gan, T. J., Meyer, T. A., Apfel, C. C., et al. (2007). Society for ambulatory anesthesia guidelines for the management of postoperative nausea and vomiting. *Anesthesia and Analgesia, 105*(6), 1615–1628.

Gartner, R., Kroman, N., Callesen, T., et al. (2008). Multimodal treatment of pain and nausea in breast cancer surgery. *Ugeskr Laeger, 170*(23), 2035–2038.

Gatchel, R. J., & Okifuji, A. (2006). Evidence-based scientific data documenting the treatment and cost-effectiveness of comprehensive pain programs for chronic nonmalignant pain. *The Journal of Pain, 7*(11), 779–793.

Hains, B. C., Klein, J. P., Saab, C. Y., et al. (2003). Upregulation of sodium channel Na$_v$1.3 and functional involvement in neuronal hyperexcitability associated with central neuropathic pain after spinal cord injury. *The Journal of Neuroscience, 23*(26), 8881–8892.

Huang, Y. M., Wang, C. M., Wang, C. T., et al. (2008). Perioperative Celebrex administration for pain management after total knee arthroplasty: A randomized, controlled study. *BMC Musculoskeletal Disorders, 9,* 77.

Jensen, T. S. (2002). Anticonvulsants in neuropathic pain: Rationale and clinical evidence. *European Journal of Pain, 6*(Suppl A), 61–68.

Katz, J. (1997). Pain begets pain. Predictors of long-term phantom limb pain and post-thoracotomy pain. *Pain Forum, 6*(2), 140–144.

Kehlet, H., Jensen, T. S., & Woolf, C. J. (2006). Persistent postsurgical pain: Risk factors and prevention. *Lancet, 367*(9522), 1618–1625.

Marchand, S. (2008). The physiology of pain mechanisms: From the periphery to the brain. *Rheumatic Diseases Clinics of North America, 34*(2), 285–309.

Muth-Selbach, U. S., Tegeder, I., Brune, K., et al. (1999). Acetaminophen inhibits spinal prostaglandin E$_2$ release after peripheral noxious stimulation. *Anesthesiology, 91*(1), 231–239.

Nikolajsen, L., Ilkjaer, S., Kroner, K., et al. (1997). The influence of preamputation pain on postamputation stump and phantom pain. *Pain, 72*(3), 393–405.

Pasero, C. (2003). Multimodal analgesia in the PACU. *Journal of Perianesthesia Nursing, 18*(4), 265–268.

Pasero, C. (2004). Pathophysiology of neuropathic pain. *Pain Management Nursing, 5*(4), 3–8.

Perkins, F. M., & Kehlet, H. (2000). Chronic pain as an outcome of surgery. *Anesthesiology, 93*(4), 1123–1133.

Polomano, R. C., Rathmell, J. P., Krenzischek, D. A., et al. (2008). Emerging trends and new approaches to acute pain management. *Journal of Perianesthesia Nursing, 23*(Suppl 1), S43–S53.

Poobalan, A. S., Bruce, J., Smith, W. C., et al. (2003). A review of chronic pain after inguinal herniorrhaphy. *The Clinical Journal of Pain, 19*(1), 48–54.

Poobalan, A. S., Bruce, J., King, P. M., et al. (2001). Chronic pain and quality of life following open inguinal hernia repair. *The British Journal of Surgery, 88*(8), 1122–1126.

Rivara, F. P., MacKenzie, E. J., Jurkovich, G. J., et al. (2008). Prevalence of pain in patients 1 year after major trauma. *Archives of Surgery, 143*(3), 282–287.

Smith, W. C. S., Bourne, D., Squair, J., et al. (1999). A retrospective cohort study of post mastectomy pain syndrome. *Pain, 83*(1), 91–95.

Soares, L. G., & Chan, V. W. (2007). The rationale for a multimodal approach in the management of breakthrough cancer pain: A review. *The American Journal of Hospice & Palliative Care, 24*(5), 430–439.

Taillefer, M. C., Carrier, M., Belisle, S., et al. (2006). Prevalence, characteristics, and predictors of chronic nonanginal postoperative pain after a cardiac operation: A cross-sectional study. *The Journal of Thoracic and Cardiovascular Surgery, 1131*(6), 1274–1280.

Tang, R., Evans, H., Chaput, A., et al. (2009). Multimodal analgesia for hip arthroplasty. *The Orthopedic Clinics of North America, 40*(3), 377–387.

Telleria-Diaz, A., Schmidt, M., Kreusch, S., et al. (2010). Spinal antinociceptive effects of cyclooxygenase inhibition during inflammation: Involvement of prostaglandins and endocannabinoids. *Pain, 148*(1), 26–35.

White, P. F. (2005). The changing role of non-opioid analgesic techniques in the management of postoperative pain. *Anesthesia and Analgesia, 101*(Suppl 5), S5–S22.

Assessment

Margo McCaffery, Keela Herr, and Chris Pasero

Terminology

Addiction A chronic neurologic and biologic disease. As defined by pain specialists, it is characterized by behaviors that include one or more of the following: impaired control over drug use, compulsive use, continued use despite harm, and craving. Continued craving for an opioid and the need to use the opioid for effects other than pain relief. Physical dependence and tolerance are not the same as addiction.

Breakthrough pain (BTP) A transitory increase in pain that occurs on a background of otherwise controlled chronic pain.

Comfort-function goal The pain rating identified by the individual patient above which the patient experiences interference with function and quality of life, that is, activities that the patient needs or wishes to perform.

DSM-IV *Diagnostic and Statistical Manual of Mental Disorders*. A guide for clinical practice that identifies mental disorders and lists diagnostic criteria. A revised edition, DSM-5, is in progress. The DSM-IV is most commonly used in the studies cited in this section.

Faces Pain Scale-Revised (FPS-R) A series of 6 faces, numbered 0, 2, 4, 6, 8, and 10, beginning with a bland facial expression and subsequent faces that increase in expression of distress. The patient is asked to point to the face that best reflects the intensity of his/her pain.

Hypoalgesia Decreased sensitivity to pain.

Intellectual disability Type of developmental disability that involves cognitive impairment that is evident in childhood and continues throughout life. Sometimes referred to as *mental retardation*. An intellectual disability may or may not be accompanied by a physical disability.

Malingering Intentionally produced symptom (e.g., pain) motivated by various factors, such as financial gain.

Neuropathic (pathophysiologic) pain Neuropathic (pathologic) pain is distinctly different from physiologic (nociceptive) pain. It is pain sustained by abnormal processing of sensory input by the peripheral or central nervous system, most often as a result of injury or trauma.

Nociceptive (physiologic) pain Normal processing of stimuli that damages normal tissues.

Numerical Rating Scale (NRS) Several types exist. The most commonly used NRS and the one used in this book consists of numbers placed along a horizontal line; the patient is asked to rate pain from 0 to 10, with 0 equaling no pain and 10 equaling the worst possible pain. It is recommended for use in clinical practice. The NRS can be presented verbally, but visual presentation is preferred. This scale may also be presented on a vertical line.

Opioid This term is preferred to *narcotic*. Opioid refers to codeine, morphine, and other natural, semisynthetic, and synthetic drugs that relieve pain by binding to multiple types of opioid receptors.

Placebo Any medication or procedure, including surgery, that produces an effect in a patient because of its implicit or explicit intent and not because of its specific physical or chemical properties.

Reliability Regarding pain measures, it means that the scale consistently measures what it is intended to measure, such as pain intensity or presence of pain, from one time to the next.

Self-report The ability of an individual to give a report, in this case, of pain, especially intensity. This is considered the "gold standard" of pain assessment. Patients may do this by marking on a scale such as the NRS or pointing to a number on a scale or a face. Head nodding and eye blinking can also be used to signal presence of pain and is sometimes used to rate intensity.

Substance abuse In the pain literature, this term is usually used to indicate problematic opioid use that is not as severe a problem as addictive disease. Based on DSM-IV criteria, which were used for most of the research presented in this book.

Substance dependence A term used in the pain literature to indicate addictive disease. Defined by DSM-IV criteria that differ from the criteria used for *addiction* proposed by pain specialists (see **addiction**).

Titration Adjusting the amount (e.g., adjusting the dose of an opioid).

Validity Regarding pain measures, it means that the tool accurately measures what it is intended to measure, such as pain intensity or presence of pain. A fundamental aspect of validity for pain rating scales is that they demonstrate sensitivity to changes in the magnitude of pain.

Verbal Descriptor Scale (VDS) Several types exist. This pain intensity rating scale is a list of adjectives describing different levels of pain intensity. An example that can be placed on a 0 to 10 metric scale is: no pain (0), mild pain (2), moderate pain (4), severe pain (6), very severe pain (8), and most intense pain imaginable (10).

Verbal Numerical Scale (VNS) A verbal presentation of the NRS, often a 0 to 5 scale or 0 to 10 scale; studies suggest that the patient should also be shown a visual of the scale.

Visual Analog Scale (VAS) A horizontal (sometimes vertical) 10-cm line with word anchors at the extremes, such as "no pain" on one end and "pain as bad as it could be" or "worst possible pain" on the other end. The patient is asked to mark the line to indicate intensity of pain, and the length of the mark from "no pain" is measured and recorded in centimeters or millimeters. Impractical for use in daily clinical practice.

The focus of this section is on assessment of the pain report itself, with some attention to how clinicians respond to these assessments. Misconceptions that hamper assessment and subsequent treatment of patients who report that they have pain will be discussed, followed by practical assessment tools for both verbal patients that can self-report and nonverbal patients who cannot self-report such as those with cognitive impairment. These include pain rating scales, pain behavioral scales, initial pain assessment tools, and flow sheets for reassessment of pain. Finally, challenges in pain assessment are addressed and include patients who deny pain or refuse analgesics, patients of different cultural backgrounds, the mentally retarded, and the mentally ill.

Chapter 1 Underlying Complexities of Pain Assessment

FAILURE of clinicians to ask patients about their pain and to accept and act on patients' reports of pain are probably the most common causes of unrelieved pain and unnecessary suffering. Basic pain assessment is a simple but, unfortunately, infrequently performed task. Even when appropriate assessments are made, clinicians do not necessarily accept the findings and might not take appropriate action. Some of the misconceptions that cause this are listed in Table 1-1, and these and others are discussed later in this chapter and in other chapters in Section II.

Failure to Assess Pain and Underestimation of Pain

Some of the problems related to the assessment of pain and decisions about treatment have been studied using vignettes such as the ones in Box 1-1 (p. 18). These vignettes are used to illustrate several problems revealed by research and encountered in clinical practice. Take time now to review Box 1-1 and answer the questions (without previewing the answers presented in the tabulated surveys in Table 2-1, p. 21).

For years, many studies have shown that either the lack of pain assessment or the existence of differences between clinicians' pain ratings and those of patients has been a major cause of inadequate pain management (Grossman, Sheidler, Swedeen, et al., 1991; Von Roenn,

Cleeland, Gonin, et al., 1993). In one study of the skills of resident physicians in assessing chronic cancer pain, only 58% were deemed competent (Sloan, Donelly, Schwartz, et al., 1996). Assessment of simple characteristics of the pain was often omitted. For example, more than half the physicians failed to assess pain intensity.

Approximately 7 years later, research shows that such problems still exist in some cancer centers. In a review in five hospitals of 117 charts of 80 inpatients and 37 outpatients with cancer who had pain documented in their medical records, pain intensity was noted for only 57% of outpatients and 55% of inpatients (Cohen, Easley, Ellis, et al., 2003). In a study of medical patients, 11% who reported unbearable pain had never been assessed, and 14% were never offered analgesics. The authors concluded that one reason for poor analgesia was inadequate pain assessment (Dix, Sandhar, Murdoch, et al., 2004).

Initial efforts to improve pain assessment are not always successful. The Veterans Health Administration launched a study of the impact of a pain initiative requiring that a pain rating be recorded at all clinical encounters (Mularski, White-Chu, Overbay, et al., 2006). The initiative was adopted in 1999 and fully implemented in 2001. In a general medicine outpatient clinic, a retrospective review of 300 charts before 1999 and 300 after 2001 was conducted. The quality of care was unchanged before and after the pain initiative. For example, pain ratings were documented 49.5% of the time prior to the initiative and 48.7% afterwards.

Overall, research shows that when clinicians do not obtain pain ratings from patients, they are likely to underestimate pain, especially moderate to severe pain (Graffam, 1981; Larue, Fontaine, Colleau, 1997; Zalon, 1993). In a study of 103 patients with cancer pain, the pain ratings of the patients were compared with those of nurses, house officers, and oncology fellows. All groups underestimated the patients' pain (Grossman, Sheidler, Swedeen, et al., 1991). When pain was severe, only 7% of nurses, 20% of oncology fellows, and 27% of house officers correctly assessed the pain levels. These caregivers were more accurate in rating moderate pain and even

Table 1-1 | Misconceptions: Barriers to the Assessment and Treatment of Pain

Misconception*	Correction
The best judges of the existence and severity of patients' pain are the physicians and nurses caring for the patients.	Patients are the authorities on their pain. Patients' self-reports are the most reliable indicators of the existence and intensity of pain.
Clinicians should use their personal opinions and beliefs about the truthfulness of patients to determine patients' true pain status.	Allowing each clinician to act on personal beliefs presents the potential for different pain assessments by different clinicians, leading to different interventions by each clinician. This results in inconsistent and often inadequate pain management. It is essential to establish the patients' self-reports of pain as the standard for pain assessment.
Clinicians must believe what patients say about pain.	Clinicians need not believe the patients' reports of pain, but clinicians must accept and respect patients' reports of pain and proceed with appropriate assessment and treatment. Clinicians are always entitled to their personal opinions, but those opinions cannot be allowed to guide professional practice.
Comparable noxious stimuli produce comparable pain in different people. The pain threshold is uniform.	Findings from numerous studies have failed to support the notion of a uniform pain threshold. Comparable stimuli do not result in the same pain in different people. After similar injuries, one person may suffer moderate pain and the other severe pain.
There is no reason for patients to hurt when no physical cause for pain can be found.	Pain is a new and inexact science, and it would be foolish of us to think that we will be able to determine the cause of all the pains that patients report.
Patients should not receive analgesics until the cause of pain is diagnosed.	Pain is no longer clinicians' primary diagnostic tool. Symptomatic relief of pain should be provided while the investigation of cause proceeds. Early use of analgesics is now advocated for patients with acute abdominal pain.
Visible signs, either physiologic or behavioral, accompany pain and can be used to verify its existence and severity.	Even with severe pain, periods of physiologic and behavioral adaptation occur, leading to periods of minimal or no signs of pain. Lack of pain expression does not necessarily mean lack of pain.
When it is time to reassess patients' pain following an analgesic and the patients are sleeping, it is not necessary to awaken them.	Sleep does not mean the absence of pain, and not all patients who appear to be sleeping are actually sleeping. Until patients' responses to analgesics are established as being effective and safe, patients should be awakened to obtain a pain rating. This should be explained to patients. However, if the same analgesic dose has been administered before and has produced effective pain relief, and patients are not aroused by simple stimuli such as calling their names in a normal tone of voice, patients with acceptable respiratory status may be allowed to sleep. If patients' pain is relatively constant and the analgesic effect is known to wear off after a certain time, e.g., 4 hours, consider awakening patients for the next dose before pain awakens the patients. Discuss this option with the patients.
Anxiety makes pain worse.	Anxiety is often associated with pain, but the cause-and-effect relationship has not been established. Pain often causes anxiety, but it is not clear that anxiety necessarily makes pain more intense.
Patients who are knowledgeable about opioid analgesics and who make regular efforts to obtain them are drug seeking (addicted).	Patients with pain should be knowledgeable about their medications; use of opioids for pain relief is not addiction. When patients are accused of drug seeking, it may be helpful to ask, "What else could this behavior mean? Might these patients be in pain?"
When patients report pain relief after a placebo, it means that the patients are malingerers or that the pain is psychogenic.	About one third of patients who have obvious physical stimuli for pain (e.g., surgery) report pain relief after a placebo injection. Therefore, placebos cannot be used to diagnose malingering, psychogenic pain, or any psychologic problem. Sometimes placebos relieve pain, but why this happens remains unclear.
The pain rating scale preferred for use in daily clinical practice is the Visual Analog Scale (VAS).	For patients who are verbal and can count from 0 to 10, the Numeric Rating Scale (NRS) is preferred for adult patients. It is easy to explain, measure, and record, and it provides numbers for setting pain-management goals. The VAS is a straight line with anchors at each end and no numbers or adjectives in between.

Continued

Table 1-1 | Misconceptions: Barriers to the Assessment and Treatment of Pain—cont'd

Misconception*	Correction
Cognitively impaired older patients are unable to use pain rating scales.	When an appropriate pain rating scale (e.g., 0 to 5) is used and patients are given sufficient time to process information and respond, many cognitively impaired elderly people can use a pain rating scale.
Cognitively impaired patients, especially those who are unable to self-report, do not experience as much pain as those who are cognitively intact.	Recent studies examining mechanisms and differences in pain transmission and perception in older adults with dementia document that the pain transmission process is unaltered, but these adults may respond with behaviors that are different from those of cognitively intact adults. In other words, cognitive impairment may result in less pain being reported, but there is no evidence that cognitive impairment reduces the ability to feel painful stimuli.
Critically ill patients, especially those who appear to be unconscious or have received a neuromuscular blocking agent, do not feel pain and do not recall painful episodes in intensive care units (ICUs).	Levels of consciousness are difficult to determine, and patients who are thought to be unconsciousness in the ICU often recall moderate to severe pain. Patients under the influence of neuromuscular blocking agents may still be fairly alert and able to feel pain. Patients with endotracheal tubes are unable to self-report verbally but may be able to provide self-reports if attempts are made, such as establishing head nod, pointing, or eye blink in response to questions about a pain.
Persons with intellectual disabilities (IDs) or mental retardation are either insensitive to pain or have greater tolerance for it.	This perception appears to be based on observations that behavior following a potentially painful event is delayed or unconventional. These observations are often valid but do not necessarily indicate insensitivity to pain or indifference to it. Measurements of sensitivity to pain using heat-pain thresholds indicated greater sensitivity to pain than is experienced by normal controls. Behavioral responses to pain may not occur in some individuals with IDs because of physical disabilities such as cerebral palsy.
Schizophrenic patients' reports of pain are commonly expressions of the mental illness.	For some time, decreased reactivity to pain in some patients with schizophrenia has caused clinicians to believe they were experiencing insensitivity to pain. Some patients with schizophrenia fail to report pain until it becomes severe. As a result, these patients seek medical care at a later stage of the physical disease and may suffer complications as a consequence. Postoperative pain is a risk factor for postoperative confusion and should be treated with analgesics. The appearance of insensitivity to pain by schizophrenic patients is poorly understood but may be the result of abnormal processing of sensory input. In one study of experimental pain, it was noted that individuals with schizophrenia had difficulty focusing on their pain. Furthermore, pain is rarely a hallucination. Recently, studies have suggested that absence of pain reactivity does not mean absence of pain sensitivity.
Patients with posttraumatic stress disorder (PTSD) show low sensitivity to acute pain and rarely have chronic pain.	Although a few studies have shown that patients with PTSD are less sensitive to very brief painful stimuli, chronic pain is commonly present in patients with PTSD and, conversely, patients with chronic pain often have PTSD, although both of these co-occurences are underdiagnosed.

*These misconceptions are discussed in this section, along with appropriate references.

From Pasero, C., & McCaffery, M. *Pain assessment and pharmacologic management*, p. 17, St. Louis, Mosby. © 2011, Pasero C, McCaffery M. May be duplicated for use in clinical practice.

better when identifying mild pain. It is interesting to note that in another study, nurses tended to overestimate mild pain (Zalon, 1993).

Underestimation of pain by caregivers understandably contributes to undertreatment of pain. In a study of more than 1000 outpatients with metastatic cancer, the most powerful predictor of inadequate analgesia was the discrepancy between the physicians' and the patients' estimates of pain severity (Cleeland, Gonin, Hatfield, et al., 1994). For almost half the patients, physicians underestimated the extent to which pain interfered with the patients' activities.

Failure to Accept Patient's Reports of Pain

When clinicians do obtain pain ratings from patients, they do not necessarily accept what the patients say. In a study of 24 surgical patients, the pain ratings by patients

Box 1-1 | Survey: Assessment and Use of Analgesics

Directions: Please select one answer for each question.

PATIENT A

Andrew is 25 years old, and this is his first day after abdominal surgery. As you enter his room, he smiles at you and continues talking and joking with his visitor. Your assessment reveals the following information: BP, 120/80; HR, 80; R, 18; on a scale of 0 to 10 (0 = no pain/discomfort, 10 = worst pain/discomfort), he rates his pain as 8.

1. On the patient's record you must mark his pain on the scale below. Circle the number that represents your assessment of Andrew's pain:

   0   1   2   3   4   5   6   7   8   9   10

   No pain/   Worst pain/
   discomfort   discomfort

2. Your assessment, above, is made 2 hours after the patient received morphine, 2 mg IV. Half-hourly pain ratings after the injection ranged from 6 to 8, and he had no clinically significant respiratory depression, sedation, or other untoward side effects. He has identified 2 as an acceptable level of pain relief. His physician's order for analgesia is "morphine IV 1 to 3 mg q1h PRN for pain relief." Check the action you will take at this time:*
   ___ (a) Administer no morphine at this time.
   ___ (b) Administer morphine, 1 mg IV, now.
   ___ (c) Administer morphine, 2 mg IV, now.
   ___ (d) Administer morphine, 3 mg IV, now.

PATIENT B

Robert is 25 years old, and this is his first day after abdominal surgery. As you enter his room, he is lying quietly in bed and grimaces as he turns in bed. Your assessment reveals the following information: BP, 120/80; HR, 80; R, 18; on a scale of 0 to 10 (0 = no pain/discomfort, 10 = worst pain/discomfort) he rates his pain as 8.

1. On the patient's record you must mark his pain on the scale below. Circle the number that represents your assessment of Robert's pain:

   0   1   2   3   4   5   6   7   8   9   10

   No pain/   Worst pain/
   discomfort   discomfort

2. Your assessment, above, is made 2 hours after the patient received morphine, 2 mg IV. Half-hourly pain ratings after the injection ranged from 6 to 8, and he had no clinically significant respiratory depression, sedation, or other untoward side effects. He has identified 2 as an acceptable level of pain relief. His physician's order for analgesia is "morphine IV, 1 to 3 mg q1h PRN, for pain relief." Check the action you will take at this time:*
   ___ (a) Administer no morphine at this time.
   ___ (b) Administer morphine, 1 mg IV, now.
   ___ (c) Administer morphine, 2 mg IV, now.
   ___ (d) Administer morphine, 3 mg IV, now.

---

*Or what should be given at this time.

As appears in Pasero, C., & McCaffery, M. (2011). *Pain assessment and pharmacologic management*, p. 18, St. Louis, Mosby. © 1999, McCaffery M, Ferrell B. May be duplicated for use in clinical practice.

were compared with those documented on the patient-controlled analgesia record by the nurses (Carey, Turpin, Smith, et al., 1997). The nurses consistently documented lower pain ratings than those reported by patients. Once again, the greatest discrepancies occurred at the highest pain levels. Findings from other research using patient vignettes also reveal that even when patients report pain intensity as a specific number on a pain rating scale, some nurses record a different number in patients' records (McCaffery, Ferrell, 1991a, 1991b, 1992a, 1992b, 1992c, 1997a; McCaffery, Pasero, Ferrell, 2007).

The findings of several studies suggest that clinicians believe that patients exaggerate their pain. In one study, when medical and nursing staff were asked to rate what they believed were patients' pain intensities, they rated the pain levels lower than the patients did (Krivo, Reidenberg, 1995). However, when they were asked what pain rating they thought the patients would report, more than two thirds of the staff stated higher pain ratings that were much closer to those the patients gave, revealing that they thought the pain was really less intense than the patients said it was.

In a comparison of oncology nurses and long-term care facility nurses, the latter were more likely to believe that patients with cancer pain overreport their pain (Ryan, Vortherms, Ward, 1994). Nurses in long-term care facilities believed that about 25% of these patients were exaggerating the severity of their cancer pain. In another study of nurses across the United States, more than one third of them believed that 20% or more of patients with cancer overreport their pain (McCaffery Ferrell, 1995b).

In a study of hospitalized oncology patients, physicians and nurses were asked to have patients rate their pain daily (Au, Loprinzi, Chodapkar, et al., 1994). Compliance with this request was poor, but when they did ask their patients for pain ratings, they tended to downgrade patient pain scores when they reported them verbally to the investigators.

Failure to Act on Patient's Reports of Pain

If clinicians believe that patients overstate their pain, this would help explain why assessment of pain using patients' self-reports does not necessarily result in improved pain management. The clinicians may assess pain accurately but may be planning pain management on the basis of their own beliefs rather than on what the patients say.

This possibility was illustrated in a study of pain ratings by nurses and surgical patients in the critical care setting (Puntillo, Miaskowski, Kehrie, et al., 1997). These nurses consistently, although not significantly, underestimated mild to moderate pain. Most important, the amount of opioid administered was better correlated with the nurses' own pain ratings than those they obtained from the patients.

In a prospective study of patients admitted to the emergency department with long-bone fractures versus those without fracture, clinicians' decisions about pain management were not based primarily on patients' reports of pain intensity (Bijur, Berard, Esses, et al., 2006). Statistical analysis showed that at every level of pain intensity, a consistently higher proportion of patients with fractures received opioid analgesics than did those without fractures. Apparently, clinicians gave more credence to pain ratings when a physical cause such as fracture was documented.

Some improvement has been shown in pain assessment. From 1992 to 2001 data from 20 studies at eight hospitals analyzed pain intensity and pain documentation. There was increased frequency of pain assessment but no significant decrease in pain intensity or in pain's interference with activities (Gordon, Pellino, Miaskowski, et al., 2002). Clearly, pain assessment is not enough. It is essential to tie pain assessment to pain treatment.

A study by the Veterans Health Administration, mentioned earlier, described the results of pain management before and after the implementation of a pain initiative (Mularski, White-Chu, Overbay, et al., 2006). Not only did pain assessment not improve, but also the quality of pain treatment showed no signs of improvement. After the initiative was implemented, 39% of patients reported substantial pain (a rating of 4 or more on a 0-to-10 scale) but often did not receive recommended care; 59% received no new therapy for pain.

Failure to act on patients' reports of pain also is influenced by many other factors, in particular, institutional barriers. For example, many hospitals do not have policies that allow nurses to titrate analgesic doses or to implement analgesics as needed around the clock when pain is present most of the day. And, as mentioned throughout this book, many clinicians lack knowledge about appropriate pain management.

Conclusion

Clearly, many clinicians need instruction about how to conduct even the most basic pain assessments such as pain intensity. Clinicians also need education about the importance of regularly scheduled assessments, the responsibility to accept what the patient says rather than downgrading reports of pain, and the necessity of planning action on the basis of a patient's report of pain, not their own personal judgments. It is essential that clinicians understand their own attitudes and misconceptions about pain so they can assess and treat pain effectively.

Although the subject is not covered in this book, clinicians are reminded that comprehensive initial and ongoing assessments of patients with pain also should include appropriate physical and neurologic examinations as well as inquiries about psychosocial factors related to the pain, such as the patients' and their families' concerns about pain and the financial impact of pain. Every effort should be made to diagnosis the underlying mechanism or cause of pain, not only initially but also at regular intervals when the pain does not subside. Any significant increase in pain or change in the characteristics of pain should signal the need for another comprehensive physical assessment and possibly neurologic, psychosocial, and other examinations. Increases in pain should never be explained solely as drug-seeking behavior or as simply the result of tolerance to opioid analgesia or psychosocial problems.

Chapter 2 Misconceptions that Hamper Assessment and Treatment of Patients Who Report Pain

REGARDLESS of what patients say about their pain, the subjectivity of pain seems to invite speculation from everyone—clinicians, families, and acquaintances—about the "true" nature of patients' pain. Numerous reasons are given by clinicians to explain why they find it difficult to accept some patients' reports of pain and why they fail to respond with appropriate treatment. These reasons include lack of a known cause for the pain or lack of behavioral indicators such as grimacing. Still other reasons remain less obvious, often below the level of awareness, but still cause clinicians to have doubts. For example, the patients' gender or ethnic origins may unknowingly influence clinicians' decisions about pain management.

Subjectivity of Pain

Patient versus Caregivers/Family

Who is the authority on patients' pain? Whose pain is it? Clinicians sometimes believe they know more about the patient's pain than the patient does. No matter how appealing that belief may be, it is false. Nevertheless, privately or among themselves, clinicians may comment about a patient, "He doesn't have as much pain as he thinks he does" or "The pain is not that bad," implying that the clinicians are the true authorities on patients' pain. In research cited earlier, clinicians' tendencies to underestimate patients' pain is noted.

No objective measures of pain exist. The sensation of pain is completely subjective. Pain cannot be proved or disproved. One definition of pain used in clinical practice says "Pain is whatever the experiencing person says it is, existing whenever he says it does" (McCaffery, 1968, p. 95). Statements by the American Pain Society (APS) have echoed the same approach to patients' reports of pain by statements such as:

- "The clinician must accept the patient's report of pain." (APS, 2003, p. 1)
- "Self-report should be the primary source of pain assessment when possible." (APS, 2003, p. 33).
- "...the patient's self-report should be used as the foundation for the pain assessment." (Miaskowski, Cleary, Burney, et al., 2005, p. 19)

The gold standard for assessing the existence and intensity of pain is patients' self-reports. No other source of information has ever been shown to be more accurate or reliable than what a patient says. Patients' behaviors, the opinions of nurses and physicians delivering care, patients' vital signs—none of these is as reliable as patients' reports of pain and should never be used instead of what a patient says.

The Andrew-Robert survey presented in Box 1-1 (p. 18) illustrates what happens when clinicians do not adopt the patient's self-report as the standard for assessment of pain intensity. This survey has been used by many nurse educators in hundreds of educational programs to explain the necessity of accepting the patient's report of pain as the standard for assessment. The survey has become so familiar to staff nurse educators that it is often referred to simply as the Andrew-Robert survey. Several publications have reported the results of studies using this survey and modifications of it (McCaffery, Ferrell, 1991a, 1991b, 1992a, 1992b, 1994a, 1997a; McCaffery, Ferrell, O'Neil-Page, 1992). A summary of survey findings from 1990 to 2006

has been published by the originators of the survey (McCaffery, Pasero, Ferrell, 2007). The results of the Andrew-Robert survey as presented in Table 2-1 are based on the responses of 615 registered nurses who attended pain programs throughout the United States. The survey was administered to registered nurses before the pain conference began. In viewing the nurses' responses to pain assessment (question 1), it is apparent that not all nurses understood that the patient's self-report of pain is the single most reliable indicator of pain. Both of these patients reported their postoperative pain as 8, but 14% of the nurses did not record 8 for the smiling patient and 5% did not record 8 for the grimacing patient. Those nurses who did not record 8 falsified the record and made it impossible for the next nurse to evaluate previous treatment for pain.

The percentages of nurses who recorded what the patients said are high but there is no room for false entries in the chart. If these results were from a single institution, then one would have to say that up to 14% of the nurses were not recording what the patients said, and this is made more complex because we do not know who they are. Thus, all recordings of pain intensity would have to be viewed with some suspicion.

The Andrew-Robert survey is a quick and easy survey to use in small and large populations of nurses. The results of the survey help to generate discussion of common problems that arise in patient care. Another brief and more comprehensive survey of staff knowledge is titled Pain Knowledge and Attitude Survey and is available in Appendix A.

The survey findings illustrate what is sometimes seen in clinical practice—each person caring for a patient may have a different opinion about the intensity of a patient's pain. Without a standard for assessing pain, chaos quickly ensues. For example, four different clinicians caring for the same patient may arrive at four different pain ratings, all of which are different from the patient's own pain

Table 2-1	Nurses' Responses to the Survey: Assessment and Use of Analgesics*		
	Nurses' Correct Responses to Patient A: Smiling Andrew	**Correct Response**	**Nurses' Correct Responses to Patient B: Grimacing Robert**
Question 1: Pain assessment	86%	Pain Rating: 8	94%
Question 2: Choice of opioid dose	51%	Morphine IV: 3 mg	64%

*Data collected in 2006; N = 615.
As appears in Pasero, C., & McCaffery, M. (2011). *Pain assessment and pharmacologic management*, p. 21, St. Louis, Mosby. Data from McCaffery, M., Pasero, C., & Ferrell, B. (2007). Nurses' decisions about opioid dose. *Am J Nurs*, 107, 35-39. © 2011, McCaffery M, Pasero C, Ferrell B. May be duplicated for use in clinical practice.

rating (and usually are underestimations of a patient's pain). How do you resolve five different pain ratings so that intervention can be planned?

The need to establish the patient's self-report as the standard becomes apparent. There appears to be no alternative. It is reassuring to realize that the validity and reliability of patients' self-reports of pain are testified to in the numerous double-blind studies of analgesics, in which the patients' pain ratings always determine the analgesic effect of the drugs being tested. Initial recommended doses of analgesics and equianalgesic charts have relied on the patient's self-report for decades.

When a patient reports pain, the health care professional's responsibility is to accept and respect the report and to proceed with appropriate assessment and treatment based upon the self-report. All reports of pain are taken seriously. When difficulties arise in accepting the patient's report of pain, some of the strategies listed in Box 2-1 may be helpful.

Health Care Conditions that Influence Clinicians' Judgments of Pain

Numerous factors influence clinicians' tendencies to doubt patients' reports of pain. This section discusses the effects of length of time caring for patients with pain, environmental cues that promote suspicion of patients' pain reports, and the effects of the nature of one's clinical practice.

GUIDELINES

Box 2-1 Strategies to Use When the Patient's Report of Pain Is not Accepted

Strategies: What do we do if the health care team does not respond positively to the patient's report of pain?

- Acknowledge that everyone is entitled to a personal opinion, but personal opinion does not form the basis for professional practice.
- Clarify that the sensation of pain is subjective and cannot be proved or disproved.
- Quote recommendations from clinical practice guidelines, especially those published by the APS.
- Ask, "Why is it so difficult to believe that this person hurts?"

From Pasero, C., & McCaffery, M. *Pain assessment and pharmacologic management*, p. 22, St. Louis, Mosby. © 2011, Pasero C, McCaffery M. May be duplicated for use in clinical practice.

Studies report conflicting results about the effects of length of time caring for patients with pain. As reported earlier, clinicians frequently underestimate patients' pain ratings. This has been explained as being a process of habituation. Repeated exposure to patients' pain seems to promote the development of insensitivity to pain (Kappesser, Williams, Prkachin, 2006). Yet other studies have not shown this (Everett, Patterson, Marvin, 1994; Hamers, van den Hout, Halfens, 1997). In a study of 50 registered nurses randomly selected from 2 general surgical units, two general medical units, and a combined intensive care unit/coronary care unit, participants completed an instrument that contained 60 vignettes describing a patient's illness or injury (Dudley, Holm, 1984). Nurses were instructed to rate each patient on the degree of pain and psychologic distress. Nurses inferred significantly less pain than psychologic distress. Correlation analysis revealed a markedly weak and statistically insignificant correlation between years of practice and pain scores.

Other factors that may influence clinicians' estimates of patients' pain may be access to the patients' self-reports and the atmosphere of suspicion surrounding particular patients. In one study, 60 physicians and nurses from the emergency department (ED) and 60 from the oncology setting watched videotapes of facial expressions of patients with shoulder pain undergoing range-of-motion exercises (Kappesser, Williams, Prkachin, 2006). Participants were divided into three groups and given different information: Group 1, videotape only; Group 2, the same videotape plus the patients' reported pain intensity; and Group 3, the same videotape plus being told the patient pain reports and that some of the people were faking pain to obtain opioid drugs. All participants were asked to rate the patients' pain, and participants in groups 2 and 3 were asked to state whether they had the impression that any of the patients had faked pain or hidden pain. Clinicians in all three groups underestimated patient pain intensity. The least discrepancy between clinicians' and patients' pain ratings occurred when the clinicians were given the patients' self-reports but were not told that some patients were faking pain to obtain opioids.

The greatest discrepancy occurred when clinicians were given the patients' pain reports but were told that patients might be faking pain to obtain opioids. This suggests that a clinical atmosphere of suspicion, such as sometimes occurs in trauma units or EDs, may cause an increase in clinicians' doubting patients' reports of pain. In all clinical areas clinicians need to be cognizant of the attitudes they convey when they discuss patient care with their colleagues. Managers and supervisors can be alert to stigmatizing labels and help staff to avoid them. For example, the term *drug-seeking*, which has no universally accepted definition, commonly conveys that a patient is addicted to opioids, abusing pain medicine, or manipulative (McCaffery, Grimm, Pasero, et al., 2005). In fact, the American Society for Pain Management Nurses (ASPMN; 2002) recommends that this term not be used because it creates bias and prejudice that subsequently have negative effects on pain management.

The nature of a particular clinical practice may influence clinician estimates of patient pain intensity. The effect of repeatedly inflicting pain on patients was studied by using brain scans to compare the responses of physicians who practice acupuncture with the responses of naïve participants while watching animated visual stimuli depicting body parts in both a nonpainful situation (being touched by a Q-tip) and a potentially painful situation (acupuncture [being pricked by needles]) (Cheng, Lin, Liu, et al., 2007). The acupuncturists rated these situations as being significantly less painful and unpleasant than did the naïve control participants.

In addition, the brain scans supported the notion that mechanisms are triggered in the areas of the brain that regulate emotions and cognitive control. The authors commented that without some regulatory mechanism, it is likely that clinicians would experience personal distress and anxiety that would interfere with their ability to perform. Acupuncturists know that they may be inflicting pain and seem to have learned throughout their training to inhibit the empathy-pain response.

Many other clinical practices, such as burn care and surgery, involve repeated infliction of pain. A study of burn care found that staff members who had spent more time working with burned patients believed débridement was less painful than did the staff members who had spent less time working with burned patients (Perry, Heidrich, 1982). To continue to manage pain effectively, such clinicians need to be aware of their tendencies to underestimate the painful impacts of what they do and to recognize that doing so may be an essential mechanism that allows them to continue to give care. Rather than be embarrassed or ashamed of this reaction, they can acknowledge it to themselves (and perhaps others) and try to compensate by obtaining and listening carefully to information from their patients.

Other examples are clinicians who perform venipunctures or bone marrow aspirations daily; they may become less sensitive to the amount of pain they are inflicting. Clinicians who work in a pain clinic several days a week may grow weary of and less sensitive to patients who continue to report pain despite their best efforts to relieve the pain. Again, to continue to practice effectively in such conditions it may be necessary to make a conscious personal inventory that honestly admits to having less empathy for patients as time goes by. Once this is acknowledged, the clinician can plan a systematic approach to obtaining information from the patient and ensure that it is acted upon.

Considerations When Doubts Arise

On occasion, accepting and acting on the patient's report of pain are difficult. Because pain cannot be proved, health care professionals are vulnerable to being fooled by the patient who wishes to lie about pain. However, although accepting and responding to the report of pain will undoubtedly result in giving analgesics to some patients who do not have pain, doing so ensures that everyone who does have pain receives attentive responses. Health care professionals do not have the right to deprive a patient of appropriate assessment and treatment simply because they believe a patient is lying.

An important distinction exists between believing the patient's report of pain and accepting the report. Following the recommendations of the clinical practice guidelines does not require that the clinician agree 100% with what the patient says. Clinicians are not required to believe a patient but are required to accept what a patient says, convey acceptance to the patient, and take the appropriate action. Clinicians are entitled to their personal doubts and opinions, but they cannot be allowed to interfere with appropriate patient care. Box 2-1 summarizes some strategies that can be used when the patient's report of pain is not accepted.

Although accepting the patient's report of pain occasionally results in being fooled, no stigma or blame should be attached to being duped. In any relationship, each party has certain responsibilities. Fault is assigned to the parties who fail to meet their responsibilities (Wesson, Smith, 1990). If the clinicians fulfills his or her responsibility to respond to all reports of pain with appropriate assessment and treatment, the clinician will be able to say, "Although I was probably fooled by some patients, I never failed to help those who did have pain. No one can find fault with my behavior or professional conduct."

Furthermore, accepting the patient's report of pain avoids an adversarial relationship. When a clinician conveys to a patient that a report of pain has not been accepted, it amounts to accusing the patient of lying. Understandably, this is upsetting and frightening to a patient who has asked the health care provider for help with pain. Much has been written in the literature about the distinction between suffering and pain. It is worth noting that in his analysis of suffering, Eric Cassell (1982) mentions that one source of suffering is physicians who do not validate a patient's pain but rather ascribe it to psychologic causes or accuse the patient of faking. Clinicians ask patients to trust them. At some point clinicians must return the favor.

The term *malingering* may be encountered when a patient's report of pain is doubted. *Malingering* can be defined as a conscious effort to produce symptoms such as pain for the purpose of deceiving or misrepresenting the facts, usually for monetary or other gains. Malingering seems to be suspected most commonly in patients with persistent pain, especially low back pain. A review of the literature prior to 1999 reveals 68 references to research of persistent pain malingering or disease simulation (Fishbain, Cutler, Rosomoff, et al., 1999). These studies conclude that malingering does occur, perhaps in 1.25% to 10.4% of patients, but these figures are not reliable because of the quality of the studies. This review concludes that there are no reliable methods of identifying malingering. The International Association for the Study of Pain notes that the process of identifying malingering is, in the final analysis, a legal, not a medical, process (Merskey, Bogduk, 1994).

On reflection, one might ask whether it is justifiable to be suspicious of all patients in an attempt to avoid being fooled by the few who lie. It is a burden to the clinician and an insult to the patient to wrestle with potential dishonesty at each encounter.

Pain Threshold: Uniform versus Variable

Pain threshold may be defined as the point at which an increasing intensity of stimuli is felt as painful. Several decades ago, preliminary research erroneously suggested that everyone perceives the same intensity of pain from the same stimuli (Hardy, Wolff, Goodell, 1943). This has been called the uniform pain threshold. However, further research failed to support the uniform pain threshold theory (Beecher, 1956). For half a century it has been known that comparable stimuli in different people do *not* produce the same intensities of pain. A uniform relationship does not exist between tissue damage and pain. A given type of tissue damage may produce more or less pain than one might expect. Not only does pain intensity vary among patients, but duration and other characteristics also vary.

In a small study, healthy volunteer subjects were asked to rate experimental pain consisting of nerve shocks. Given the same intensity of pain stimulus, various persons did not always give the same pain ratings, and the same intensity of pain stimulus given to the same person repeatedly did not always result in the same pain rating (Mader, Blank, Smithline, et al., 2003).

The idea that a particular patient "shouldn't hurt that much" probably is based on the misconception that comparable stimuli produce comparable pain in different people. A more appropriate appraisal might be that a painful event hurts one patient more than it hurts another. Concluding that one patient is exaggerating the pain is judgmental and may result in a number of potentially harmful effects, such as failing to detect a complication or providing inadequate analgesia. When a patient reports pain that is considerably more than expected, it is always wise to reassess that patient.

Pain Tolerance: High versus Low

Pain tolerance is not the same as pain threshold; it may be defined as the duration or intensity of pain that a person is willing to endure. An example of high pain tolerance is the willingness to endure prolonged and severe pain without desiring relief, whereas low pain tolerance might be the desire for relief of brief, mild pain.

Pain tolerance varies from person to person and within the same person depending on numerous factors, such as past experiences with pain, coping skills, motivation to endure pain, and energy level. For example, a patient may be willing to endure intense pain during childbirth to minimize the infant's exposure to medications but may be unwilling to endure mild episiotomy pain later if she is not breast-feeding.

Society places a high value on a high pain tolerance. The findings of one study suggest that nurses do not like patients who have severe pain or who are perceived as coping poorly with their pain (Salmon, Manyande, 1996). When patients were perceived as being unable to cope with pain, they were evaluated by the nurses as demanding and were unpopular with the staff.

Low pain tolerance seems to be regarded as a weakness, a character flaw, a lack of will power, or perhaps even self-indulgence. The implication appears to be that the patient should be stronger and muster the energy to cope with pain more successfully.

The routine use of the phrase *complains of pain* suggests a negative attitude toward patients with pain and may reflect a desire for patients to cope better and talk less about pain. Saying that patients "report pain" is much less evaluative. It is probably worthwhile making a conscious effort to avoid using the word *complain*. The reader may note that throughout this book, the authors never use the word *complain* in reference to patients' reports of pain.

One cannot escape the fact that this society and many others value a stoic response to pain, which is probably very closely aligned with valuing a high pain tolerance. No doubt most readers share this value. However, health care providers must guard against requiring this of patients and certainly must avoid criticizing patients who are unable to meet this expectation. Patients have a right to determine their own pain tolerance.

Expecting a high pain tolerance may translate into deciding that patients ought to be able to tolerate particular painful experiences. There may be procedures; persistent pain conditions, such as arthritis or low back pain; surgeries; wound care; or a variety of other circumstances. In cases of procedural pain, it is not unusual for clinicians to voice their belief that providing sedation/analgesia is unnecessary for very short, but very painful procedures, believing that patients should be able to "tolerate" brief pain.

A common misconception is that increased experience with pain should teach a person to be more tolerant of it and better able to cope with it. However, repeated experience with pain often teaches a person how severe pain can become and how difficult it is to get pain relief. Thus, a person who has repeated experiences with pain may have higher levels of anxiety and lower pain tolerance. In one study of adults, previous surgeries appeared to result in greater pain intensity and emotion during later surgical experiences (Wells, 1989).

Identifying the patient's pain tolerance is a critical part of providing pain relief. Setting pain rating and activity goals (discussed later in this section) is an effort to identify the level of pain a patient can endure without distress and still perform necessary activities easily.

Patients, as well as clinicians, value stoicism. When a patient is unable to meet his or her own expectations of being able to tolerate unavoidable pain or minimize behavioral expressions of pain, the clinician can at least minimize the psychologic trauma to the patient by conveying that the patient's response to pain is fully acceptable. Simply saying, "This is tough. You're doing well," may help reduce the patient's distress.

Behavioral and Physiologic Responses to Pain

Acute Pain Model versus Adaptation

The acute pain model says that if the patient has pain, visible signs of discomfort, behavioral or physiologic, will be present. Examples of behavior usually expected of patients with pain include grimacing, rigid body posture, limping, frowning, or crying. Physiologically, elevated vital signs are commonly expected. Clinicians and laymen alike usually fail to appreciate that both physiologic and behavioral adaptation occurs, leading to periods of minimal or no signs of pain. Absence of behavioral or physiologic signs of pain does not necessarily mean absence of pain.

The acute pain model is of limited value for assessing pain. When pain is sudden or severe, behavioral and physiologic indicators may be present for a brief time. However, very quickly the patient may make an effort to cease behaviors such as crying or moaning. Behavioral adaptation or suppression of pain behaviors may occur because the patient values the stoic response or simply becomes exhausted. Physiologic indicators such as increased blood pressure (BP) or heart rate may also disappear. In a healthy individual, the body seeks homeostasis or equilibrium, returning to the former physiologic state despite severe pain. Or a patient may have a medical condition that causes low BP, such as hypothyroidism or dehydration, which has a much greater impact on vital signs than pain has. In such patients, sudden, severe pain may elevate the vital signs only briefly and minimally.

The APS addresses the misconceptions about the acute pain model by stating the following:

- With regard to acute pain, the APS (2003) says, "Often *but not always* [italics ours], it is associated with objective physical signs of sympathetic branch autonomic nervous system activity, including tachycardia, hypertension. . . ." (p. 2).
- With regard to persistent cancer pain, the APS (2003) says, "The lack of objective signs may prompt the inexperienced clinician to wrongly conclude the patient does not appear to be in pain" (p. 3).

Responses Clinicians Expect of Patients with Pain

Nurses' responses to the Andrew-Robert survey (see Table 2-1, p. 21) reveal that patients' behavioral responses have significant effect on nurses' pain assessments and treatment decisions (McCaffery, Pasero, Ferrell, 2007). The only difference between Andrew and Robert is their behavior—Andrew smiles and laughs with visitors, whereas Robert lies in bed and grimaces. This simple difference has a startling effect on nurses' decisions about opioid doses.

Although the patients were exactly alike except for their behaviors, the nurses were more likely to increase the morphine dose for the grimacing patient. Both patients had received morphine, 2 mg IV, 2 hours before; half-hourly pain ratings had ranged from 6 to 8 out of 10 and were currently 8; and no clinically significant adverse effects such as sedation had occurred. The pain rating goal was 2. Nurses were given a choice of administering no morphine or 1 mg, 2 mg, or 3 mg IV. Morphine, 3 mg IV, was the correct choice for both patients because the previous dose of 2 mg was safe but ineffective. However, only 50.6% of the nurses would increase the dose for the smiling patient, whereas 64.3% would increase the dose for the grimacing patient. Both patients were undertreated, but at least 14% of the nurses knew that it was safe to increase the dose for the smiling patient, but they did not. Over the years since 1990, other similar vignette surveys conducted by these authors have shown similar findings, which show little improvement in nurses' choices of opioid doses (McCaffery, Pasero, Ferrell, 2007).

The same discouraging results were found when the Andrew-Robert survey was adapted to reflect the needs of elderly patients in a long-term care facility (Katsma, Souza, 2000). The participants were 89 licensed nurses working in long-term care facilities. As in the original vignette, one patient was described as smiling and the other as grimacing. After receiving medication, hourly pain ratings were 6 to 8, and the patients showed no serious adverse effects. In response to the question about which analgesic dose they would now give, only 30% correctly selected a higher dose for the smiling patient, but 43% did so for the grimacing patient.

These same biases about behavior also exist in laypersons. The Andrew-Robert survey was revised to be appropriate for a nonnurse audience and was administered to 85 college students who were not enrolled as medical or nursing majors (McCaffery, Ferrell, 1996a). College students' responses to assessment and relief of pain showed trends similar to those of practicing nurses. The smiling patient's pain rating was accepted by 38% of the college students, whereas 55% accepted the grimacing patient's report of pain.

Vital signs also influence nurses' willingness to record a patient's report of pain. A survey using the same format as the original Andrew-Robert survey was constructed; the only difference between the patients was their vital signs (McCaffery, Ferrell, 1992a, 1992b). One patient had low to normal vital signs, and the other patient had elevated vital signs. The responses of 166 nurses revealed that more nurses were willing to accept the report of severe pain from the patient with elevated vital signs than from the patient with low to normal vital signs.

As part of the Missoula Demonstration Project, a 15-year process to study end-of-life issues, surveys about pain knowledge and attitudes were sent to 942 nurses and produced 311 responses (Mayer, Torma, Byock, et al., 2001). The survey revealed that 93% of the nurses knew that vital signs were not reliable indicators of pain, but 75% said that vital signs moderately or greatly influenced their decisions to treat or not to treat pain.

In a small study designed to identify the criteria nurses use to assess postoperative pain, 10 nurses were interviewed about their pain assessments of 30 postoperative patients (Kim, Schwartz-Barcott, Tracy, et al., 2005). The strategy most frequently reported by the nurses relied on the patient's appearance and drew on past experience of which physical signs to look for, such as facial expression, body movement, and heart rate. For example, nurses mentioned frowning or wincing as being indicative of pain and a patient's being able to fall asleep as a sign of little or no pain. The researchers commented on the fact that the predominant strategy of looking for objective signs of pain was in marked contrast to current guidelines that emphasize the patient's self-report of pain.

Expectations that certain behaviors indicate pain also influence the prescribing of analgesics. To identify factors that affect physicians' decisions to prescribe opioids for persistent noncancer patients, the records of 191 patients referred to a pain center were examined to determine pain severity, physical findings, pain duration, age, gender, observed pain behaviors, reported functional limitations, and affective distress (Turk, Okifuji, 1997). Of all these variables, only observed pain behaviors were significantly related to receiving opioid prescriptions. In other words, patients who exhibited pain behaviors were most likely to receive opioids for pain relief. The extent of physical findings and the severity of the pain did not appear to influence the decision to prescribe opioids. Because opioids are prescribed for the purpose of pain relief, it would seem more logical to find that severity of pain determined prescription of opioids, but this was not the case.

Similar findings also were reported regarding patients with low back pain. Decisions about lumbar surgery were not made on the basis of physical pathologic conditions but rather on behaviors demonstrated by patients during their evaluations (Waddell, Main, Morris, et al., 1984). As summarized by Turk and Okifuji (1997), "physicians appear to believe that behavioral demonstrations of pain, such as limping and grimacing, indicate something important about the nature of the patient's pain and the need for prescribing specific treatments such as surgery and opioids" (p. 334).

Patients' Knowledge of Clinicians' Expectations of Pain Behaviors

Interviews with patients who had used intravenous patient-controlled analgesia (IV PCA) for opioid administration after surgery revealed that a major reason for patients' valuing PCA was related to the fact that PCA decreased the need to interact with the nursing staff regarding pain (Hall, Salmon, 1997; Taylor, Hall, Salmon, 1996a, 1996b). Not only did patients see PCA as being better than waiting for a nurse to administer opioids intramuscularly, they also believed it protected them from having to show distress to the nurses.

Apparently many patients with pain are aware of the behaviors expected of them, or they learn them quickly. Patients may learn from early childhood experiences with pain, television, the responses of their clinicians, and a variety of other sources how to behave to signal others that pain exists and that help is needed. It is a common observation that patients with pain change their behavior in the presence of clinicians and in other selected circumstances. Patients may appear to be calm and to read or have lively telephone conversations, but as soon as clinicians enter, patients may replace these activities with a solemn facial expression and may even grimace, moan, and restrict movement—just the behaviors clinicians want to see when patients report pain, but not necessarily the behavior patients prefer.

Consider what might happen if the patients in the Andrew-Robert survey were roommates. It would not take long for smiling Andrew to realize that grimacing Robert was receiving better pain relief, and the reason probably would be quite apparent to smiling Andrew. Andrew might take pride in looking energetic and happy in front of his visitors or may find that such distraction is very helpful as a coping mechanism. But if he wants better pain relief, he may decide to change that behavior, at least during the time clinicians are present. When clinicians see this change occur, they often regard patients as being manipulative, not realizing that it is the expectations that clinicians convey to patients that cause this behavior change.

Taking this hypothetical situation further, by succumbing to expectations of pain behavior to obtain relief, Andrew may begin to jeopardize his recovery. For example, both patients might be told to ambulate. Smiling Andrew may walk the hall until he begins to hurt and then go to the nurses' station and ask for something for relief. The staff may feel that if Andrew can be this active, he could not hurt enough to require an analgesic. Grimacing Robert, on the other hand, may remain in bed grimacing rather than ambulating and may also ask for an analgesic. Robert may very well be more likely to receive the analgesic than Andrew. Andrew may then learn to stay in bed, prolonging his recovery time and increasing the risk of complications, but increasing his chances of receiving pain relief.

Comparable circumstances were observed in a study of cancer patients (Cleeland, Gonin, Hatfield, et al., 1994). The more active patients were more likely to receive inadequate pain management.

Because clinicians differ in how they expect patients to behave in response to pain, patients may have difficulty learning which behaviors will effectively convince which clinicians. An analysis of staff and patient behavior in an orthopedic unit revealed that the staff assessed pain by observing patients' behaviors and that their expectations about how patients should express their pain varied within and between shifts (Wiener, 1975). Some, but not all, patients were adept at reading the explicit and implicit cues given by staff and changed their behaviors accordingly. Patients sometimes felt forced to use tactics that they believed were unacceptable but were expected by the staff and were necessary to obtain pain relief.

Expecting patients to behave in certain ways to verify their pain becomes more confusing when clinicians are especially particular about the intensity or type of behavior that a patient should display. Sometimes clinicians say that a patient does not appear to be in pain, but when a patient exhibits pain behavior, clinicians may say that a patient is making too much fuss about the pain.

Correction of the Misconceptions Concerning the Acute Pain Model

One of the most interesting aspects of the misconception that the patient's behavioral response is more reliable than the patient's self-report of pain is that it is totally illogical. Virtually every human being has had the personal experience of trying to hide pain and to function in spite of it, smiling when appropriate and even deliberately using humor as distraction. One of the oldest maxims in health care is that laughter is the best medicine. Why couldn't the nurses and college students responding to the Andrew-Robert survey use this folk wisdom and their own personal experiences with pain to realize that patients with severe pain most certainly may smile and laugh? Nurses are probably the largest group of clinician advocates for nondrug pain relief measures, of

which distraction and laughter are highly ranked. And no research has ever even suggested that smiling and joking are incompatible with feeling pain. Why clinicians seem to have such difficulty accepting and acting on reports of pain from smiling and active patients remains a mystery, at least to these authors.

A substantial amount of research refutes the value of the acute pain model, showing that neither behavioral indicators nor physiologic responses are dependably related to the intensity of a patient's pain. Physiologic indicators appear to be even less valuable than a patient's behavioral responses to pain.

Most nurses seem to have been taught to use elevated vital signs to assess or verify the presence of pain, especially severe pain. However, in literature reviews, investigators found very little research that supported using physiologic manifestations as specific indicators of pain (Herr, Coyne, Key, et al., 2006; van Cleve, Johnson, Pothier, 1996). In a study of 1063 patients admitted to the ED with conditions that could be verified to be painful, such as fractures and nephrolithiasis, no clinically significant associations were identified between pain scores self-reported on a scale of 0 to 10 and heart rate, BP, or respiratory rate (Marco, Plewa, Buderer, et al., 2006). In a study published in French, investigators found that absence of increased vital signs does not mean absence of pain (reported in Gelinas, Johnston, 2007).

Critical care nurses usually consider vital signs to be relevant indicators of pain, possibly because the signs are readily available, and it is often difficult to obtain pain reports from critically ill patients, whose behavioral responses may be compromised and who may be unconscious, intubated, or otherwise unable to communicate. In a study involving 30 conscious patients in an intensive care unit, no significant relationship was found between physiologic indicators and patients' self-reports of pain, reinforcing the fact that physiologic indicators should not be considered primary indicators for pain assessment (Gelinas, Johnston, 2007). In other words, physiologic indicators were not related to patients' reports of pain.

In another study of 755 patients, primarily in intensive care units, physiologic responses were monitored while the patients were undergoing tracheal suctioning (Arroyo-Novoa, Figueroa-Ramos, Puntillo, et al., 2007). Statistically significantly higher increases were noted in heart rate and systolic and diastolic BP, but these changes were not clinically significant. The authors suggest that methods of measuring these physiologic parameters may not be sensitive enough to capture the response to acute pain. For further discussion of the limited usefulness of physiologic measures in assessing pain, see the discussion of patients who are critically ill in Chapter 4, pp. 143-147.

The usefulness of physiologic measures of pain is further compromised by the presence of dementia in older adults. In a small study of adults 65 years old and older, 50 of whom were cognitively intact and 44 of whom had varying degrees of dementia, heart rate and other physiologic responses were monitored before and during venipuncture (Porter, Malhotra, Wolf, et al., 1996). Increasing severity of dementia was associated with the blunting of physiologic responses as measured by diminished heart rate increase in the preparatory phase and during venipuncture.

Thus, little research supports vital signs as being relevant indicators of pain, although they can be used as indicators of the need for further assessment of pain. A position statement by the ASPMN regarding assessment of pain in nonverbal patients (available at http://www.aspmn.org/Organization/documents/NonverbalJournalFINAL.pdf) suggests that physiologic indicators should not be used alone to assess pain but should be considered cues for further assessment of the possibility of pain (Herr, Coyne, Key, et al., 2006).

Considerable research demonstrates that the behavioral expressions of pain that clinicians expect to see in patients are often absent. In the late 1970s, investigators interviewed 102 adult patients with various types of pain, acute and persistent (Jacox, 1979). Many patients did not report pain and made strong efforts to conceal it. When the patients were asked whether they discussed pain with others, 70% said no or were ambivalent. When they were asked how they responded to pain, 66% said they tried to remain calm and not show pain. More than a decade later a similar finding was reported in a study of 45 patients with pain related to lung cancer (Wilkie, Keefe, 1991). Of the patients, 42% revealed that they coped with pain by trying not to let others know about it (Wilkie, Keefe, 1991).

Some researchers have attempted to use facial movements as a method of studying malingering. A review of the literature found that the results of these studies were inconsistent and concluded that it is unclear whether facial expressions of pain can be used as a reliable method for identifying malingering (Fishbain, Cutler, Rosomoff, et al., 1999). A few years after this literature review, facial expressions were studied in 40 patients with low back pain who were videotaped during rest and painful straight-leg raises (Hill, Craig, 2002). During painful movement they were asked to express their pain genuinely or to pretend that it did not hurt. Without moving, they were asked to fake pain. Although distinctions could be made between faked and genuine painful facial expressions, this research confirmed the difficulty of discriminating between them.

Patients with pain may deliberately engage in certain behaviors that are incompatible with those of the acute pain model but are helpful in coping with pain. In a study of 13 patients with pain related to advanced cancer, the patients reported that behaviors they used to control their pain included watching television (9 patients) or chatting with family and friends (Wilkie, Lovejoy, Dodd, et al., 1988). A questionnaire survey of 53 patients with persistent cancer pain asked them to identify and rate the effectiveness of the self-initiated, noninvasive pain control

measures they used to cope with their pain (Fritz, 1988). Patients rated laughing as being the most effective.

Recently, researchers have identified that patients actually smile during painful situations, yet they did not find one tool for behavioral observation to assess pain that included smiling (Kunz, Prkachin, Lautenbacher, 2009). The facial expression of pain has been studied in both experimental and clinical research, and facial expression is often a part of behavioral observation tools to assess pain in both children and adults who cannot self-report. When these researchers viewed several videotapes of patients undergoing painful stimulation, one of the most unexpected findings in response to pain was the oblique raising of the lip that results in a smile. Their research revealed that the percentage of patients who smile at least once during painful stimulation ranges from 22% to 57%. A satisfactory explanation for this requires more research, but clinicians should not discount pain just because the patient smiles. Among other things, the smile could represent embarrassment over other behavioral responses to pain, an attempt to mask feelings of pain, or a willingness to endure the pain.

Sleep may be mistakenly equated with lack of pain, but even patients with severe pain may sleep. Some patients use sleep to help control their pain (Wilkie, Lovejoy, Dodd, et al., 1988). In one study, 100 patients were interviewed about the experiences of pain and sleep following abdominal surgery (Closs, 1992). Pain was the most common cause of sleep disturbance at night, demonstrating that pain occurs during sleep. Analgesics helped more patients get back to sleep than any other intervention. Also, about half of the patients felt that pain was worse at night.

Further, an appreciation of the fact that sleeping patients may have pain is demonstrated in analgesic research. When the effectiveness of analgesics is studied, trained observers ask patients to rate their pain at specific intervals, such as every hour, after the administration of the analgesic. When the observer finds the patient asleep at the time a pain rating is required, the observer awakens the patient to obtain a pain rating (Forbes, 1991).

This information does not necessarily indicate that in clinical practice sleeping patients should always be awakened to assess pain. If a patient has been given an analgesic and assessment of pain ratings afterward has shown that the analgesic has been effective, when the patient is given further doses, there usually is no need to awaken the patient to assess pain rating following a dose. Pain assessments can be made when the patient awakens. However, it may be wise to awaken the patient for the next analgesic dose if the analgesic lasts only 4 hours and the patient has continuous pain. This option can be discussed with the patient, explaining that if he or she is allowed to sleep beyond 4 hours, the pain may return to awaken him or her. If this happens, pain control is jeopardized. The patient must notify the nurse or obtain the analgesic on his or her own, take the analgesic, and then wait for it to be effective. In this scenario, a patient's sleep is interrupted for longer than it would have been had the patient been awakened at 4 hours and given an analgesic before pain returned. Once this is explained to a patient, he or she may opt to be awakened or to wait to be awakened by pain. If the latter is chosen, a patient should be cautioned to notify the nurse immediately so the analgesic can be given. (If a patient's sedation levels needs to be assessed, then it may be wise to awaken the patient. See the discussion of sedation levels on pp. 510-511.)

Very little research has been done to evaluate pain control using around-the-clock (ATC) dosing of analgesics versus administering them as needed, and the results are often inconclusive. However, one small study compared these two types of dosing schedules in 35 patients following abdominal surgery (De Conno, Ripamonti, Gamba, et al., 1989). Patients who received ATC analgesia had significantly better pain control, slept longer, and spent more time out of bed rather than lying down over the first postoperative week. Another study of medical inpatients compared ATC dosing of opioids to a control group and found that patients with ATC dosing reported lower pain intensity ratings than those reported by the control group yet did not take higher doses than the control group (Paice, Noskin, Vanagunas, et al., 2005).

Sedation is erroneously equated with analgesia. However, in a study of sedation and pain relief in the postanesthesia care unit, researchers found that opioid-induced sedation did not ensure adequate self-reported pain relief (Lentschener, Tostivint, White, et al., 2007). About half of the 26 patients who experienced opioid-induced sedation had persistently high pain scores in the postanesthesia care unit and during the initial 24-hour postoperative period. Further, morphine-induced sedation did not suppress the patients' memories of early postoperative pain. Still another study confirmed that opioid-induced sedation could not arbitrarily be equated with analgesia (Paqueron, Lumbroso, Mergoni, et al., 2002). Of patients receiving intravenous morphine in whom morphine was discontinued because of sedation, 25% still had pain levels on the Visual Analog Scale (VAS) above 50. (In patients receiving morphine whose pain relief is unacceptable, a multimodal approach to analgesia should be considered; see pp. 9-10.)

Many sedating drugs, such as benzodiazepines and phenothiazines, are given to patients who are experiencing pain, but most of them provide no analgesia, and the resulting sedation may limit the amount of opioid that can be given safely to a patient in pain. Except for pain related to muscle spasm, benzodiazapines do not relieve pain. Further, available phenothiazines neither relieve pain nor potentiate opioid analgesia (APS, 2003).

When a patient's report of pain is not accepted and acted on, an effective strategy is to ask, "Why is it so difficult to believe this patient has pain?" When the problem revolves around expecting the acute-pain model to exist, the answer is likely to be "He doesn't look like he's in pain." When you find yourself thinking this or hearing someone say it, try asking, "How would this person have to act for us to believe he has pain?" A clinician might answer that a patient in that much pain would grimace or be less active. Unfortunately, expecting a patient to "act like he is in pain" may lead to those behaviors and contribute to manipulative behavior and physical harm such as disability or complications resulting from decreased function.

Causes of Pain

When a patient reports pain and the cause clearly is established, clinicians are almost always more willing to treat the pain than when the cause of pain is in doubt. Surveys of nurses' responses to hypothetical patients who report pain show that nurses tend to assume less intense pain when no physical pathologic condition is present (Halfens, Evers, Abu-Saad, 1990; Taylor, Skelton, Butcher, 1984) and when pain is persistent rather than acute (Burgess, 1980; Taylor, Skelton, Butcher, 1984). Also, nurses take fewer actions to relieve pain in patients with persistent pain (Burgess, 1980).

Lack of Physical Evidence of Pain

A previously suggested strategy for addressing clinicians' reluctance to accept a patient's report of pain is also useful here. Once again, try asking, "Why is it so difficult to believe this patient has pain?" If lack of a known physical cause is the reason, the answer is likely to be "There's no reason for this patient to hurt." A more accurate and appropriately humble response would be that we are as yet unable to establish the cause of the pain (Teasell, Merskey, 1997).

Statements that may help us reconsider our misconceptions include a reminder that the study of pain is a new and inexact science and that it would be foolish of us to think that we will be able to determine the causes of all the pains that patients report. It also may be helpful to articulate the underlying thought process, which is "We seem to be thinking that if there is pain, there is a cause. If there is a cause, we can find it. If we cannot find the cause, there is no pain." Once it has been stated, we begin to recognize the absurdity of this idea.

Available assessment tools are not infallible and do not exhaust all possible means for determining the causes of pain. This has been especially true of chronic noncancer pain. In a study of 60 patients with persistent pain who had been referred to a diagnostic center, the overall rate of inaccurate or incomplete diagnosis at referral was 66.7% (Hendler, Kozikowski, 1993). In particular, neuropathic pain, which is often severe burning or shooting pain, tends to be underdiagnosed. It is not detectable by ordinary diagnostic tests because nerves, not muscles or other somatic structures, are involved.

Sometimes the physical cause of pain is known, but the pain is more intense or lasts longer than expected. In the 1980s (when hospital stays were longer than they are now), a study examined the belief that postoperative pain subsides rapidly over the first 3 days and is negligible by the fourth day. Research did not support this. Of 88 patients on a general surgical unit, 31% had pain that persisted beyond day 4, often related to being older or to complications such as infection (Melzack, Abbott, Zackon, et al., 1987). These patients typically received inadequate pain control because less effective analgesics were prescribed. Probably the staff believed there was no reason for these patients to hurt that much or for that long.

Clearly, the causes of pain cannot always be determined. This does not mean that the pain is absent or that clinicians are entitled to ignore a patient's report of pain. Pain is subjective, and it seems rather easy to engage in faulty reasoning about it. An analogy that may clarify our responsibility to such patients is our response to patients with objective symptoms that have unknown causes. For example, if a patient vomits, we may not know why it has occurred, but because it is objective (an undeniable symptom), we treat it anyway. The cause of the vomiting is sought, but meanwhile treatment, such as antiemetics, is provided. Pain deserves the same respect as objective symptoms.

Belief that Noncancer Pain Is not as Painful as Cancer Pain

When persistent pain is not associated with a terminal illness, especially when the cause of the pain is unclear, that pain seems to be regarded as being more suspicious, less painful, or less in need of relief. Doubting the trustworthiness of the patient with persistent noncancer pain is thought by some to be at the heart of most treatment problems that arise with these patients (Richeimer, Case, 2004). For example, the patient's motive for seeking care may be under suspicion. The cause of pain may not be identifiable or obvious, and the clinician may be suspicious that a patients is seeking opioids or disability compensation (Victor, Richeimer, 2005). Negative attitudes toward patients with noncancer low back pain have been recognized for many years (Burgess, 1980; Wiener, 1975).

Even when the causes of pain are known, non-life-threatening pain is less likely to be treated than is pain associated with terminal illnesses. In one study of physicians treating patients with cancer, inadequate pain management was more likely when pain was not attributed to cancer (Cleeland, Gonin, Hatfield, et al., 1994). A mail survey responded to by 368 physicians in Michigan asked them to identify their treatment goals for acute pain, cancer pain, pain due to terminal illness, and persistent noncancer pain (Green, Wheeler, Marchant, et al., 2001). Although their goals for pain relief for terminally ill

patients and patients with cancer pain were similar, the goals were significantly lower for patients with persistent noncancer pain.

Surveys of laypeople also reveal differing attitudes toward various types of pain. A telephone survey of 1000 Americans asked whether high doses of analgesics should be prescribed for any of these three conditions: severe persistent pain, cancer pain, and rheumatoid arthritis (RA) (The Mayday Fund, 1998). Approximately 80% supported high doses for cancer pain, approximately 70% supported high doses for severe persistent pain, but only about 50% supported high doses for RA. Perhaps both the public and clinicians tend to believe that some types of pain should be tolerated or are not very painful. In any case, the study reflects the tendency to provide less aggressive analgesia for one type of noncancer pain.

However, non-life-threatening conditions can result in very intense and prolonged pain. In a survey of 204 people with persistent noncancer pain, respondents revealed that their average length of time in pain was 9.5 years, with a range of 6 months to 74 years (Hitchcock, Ferrell, McCaffery, 1994). They were in pain an average of 80% of the time. For 30% the usual intensity of pain was severe, with a rating of 4 to 5 out of 5.

A common temporal classification of pain types is acute, cancer, and nonmalignant. Turk (2002) proposes that the mechanisms underlying cancer pain and nonmalignant pain are no different and that it makes no sense to discriminate between cancer pain and nonmalignant pain. He says that to do so results in paying insufficient attention to knowledge gained about cancer pain, and he suggests that greater effort be made to classify and treat pain according to the underlying mechanisms causing that pain as opposed to basing all treatment of persistent pain on whether the pain is caused by cancer. As a consequence, both cancer pain and persistent nonmalignant pain are now more often grouped together and referred to as persistent or prolonged pain.

Treating noncancer pain in the same way as cancer pain does raise legitimate concerns about the prolonged administration of medications. Certainly the chronic use of opioids remains controversial to some extent because of questions about the occurrence of addictive disease, hyperalgesia, hormonal changes, and other outcomes. (See Addiction on pp. 32-42 and Opioid Analgesics in Section IV for discussions of these conditions.) Prolonged use of nonsteroidal antiinflammatory drugs is of even greater concern than the use of opioids because of the possibility of life-threatening gastrointestinal bleeding or adverse cardiovascular events. (See Nonopioid Analgesics in Section III for a discussion of this subject.) Thus, long-term treatment by pharmacologic measures poses many challenges but cannot be ignored as a possible source of relief for persistent pain.

Implication that Anxiety or Depression Is the Cause

In a previously described study, 50 registered nurses completed an instrument that contained 60 vignettes describing patients' illnesses or injuries (Dudley, Holm, 1984). Nurses were instructed to rate the patients on the degree of their pain and psychologic distress. Nurses inferred significantly less pain than psychologic distress, whereas in actuality, patients were experiencing both. Unfortunately, patients are then likely to receive psychologic support but not the analgesic needed to decrease pain.

When the physical cause of pain is unknown or seems insufficient to account for the severity of pain a patient reports, clinicians may attribute the pain to the patient's emotional state and cease treating the pain. A comment that suggests this is so is, "The patient is just upset." It is interesting that in a survey of the public's attitude toward stress and pain, 95% of respondents agreed with the statement that stress increases pain (The Mayday Fund, 1998). Actually, evidence that stress increases pain is limited.

An erroneous and simplistic view promoted around the middle of the 20th century was that physical and psychologic causes of pain were mutually exclusive; that is, that pain is caused by either organic or psychologic factors (IASP ad hoc Subcommittee for Psychology Curriculum, 1997). Gagliese and Katz (2000) state that Melzack's gate control theory argues against the simplistic thinking that leads to categorizing pain as being either organic or psychogenic. The authors believe that medically unexplained pain is not caused by psychopathology and that thinking that separates mind and body should be abandoned. Trying to differentiate between psychogenic and physical pain is usually fruitless. Pain caused solely by psychologic factors is rare, as is pain caused solely by physical causes. Most pain is a combination of physical and psychologic factors and is best treated as such. The subsequent discussion concerns the as yet unclear relationships between pain and anxiety or depression.

The International Association for the Study of Pain defines pain as "an unpleasant sensory and emotional experience which we primarily associate with tissue damage or describe in terms of such damage, or both" (Mersky, Bogduk, 1994, p. 210). By definition, pain is always unpleasant and always subjective, so pain is always an emotional experience. But what are the relationships between pain and various emotions? A common assumption is that anxiety or depression makes pain worse, but this is not always true.

One review of the literature found that research findings are conflicting and inconsistent regarding the relationship between depression and pain and between anxiety and pain (Zimmerman, Story, Gaston-Johansson, et al., 1996). Another literature review pointed out that a high proportion of patients with persistent pain have some kind of depressive syndrome; however, the depression

may precede, follow, or develop concomitantly with the persistent pain (Dellemijn, Fields, 1994).

For the purposes of discussion, it is helpful to consider how anxiety and depression affect coping with pain as well as how they affect the intensity of pain. Although certain levels of anxiety are actually helpful in mobilizing appropriate coping mechanisms, high levels of anxiety and possibly any level of depression may adversely affect a patient's ability to cope with pain.

Roughly 50% of patients with persistent pain also have depression or an anxiety disorder (Weisberg, Boatwright, 2007). It has been relatively well established that persistent pain is often the precipitating factor for mood disorders and for anxiety disorders, yet the interaction between persistent pain and such disorders is less well understood (Weisberg, Boatwright, 2007). Depression may adversely affect coping by causing a patient to be less motivated to engage in activities and try new ideas for rehabilitation or treatment.

Pain-related anxiety or pain-related fear may also immobilize patients. Such fear or anxiety may cause hypervigilence and avoidance of activities that a patient fears may cause pain. This concern with avoiding painful activities may result in a patient's having difficulty freeing attention to focus on nonpainful activities (Vlaeyen, Crombez, 2007). One approach to helping these patients to improve their functioning has been exercise and graded activity programs in which patients gradually increase their physical activities. Another approach is verbal reassurance, but this can have an opposite effect unless done carefully. Simply telling patients not to worry, that they do not have a severe disease, or that their tests have shown negative results may increase their distress. Fearful patients may become more puzzled because they still hurt and no explanations have been offered. Such patients need credible explanations of why they hurt (Vlaeyen, Crombez, 2007).

How anxiety and depression influence pain intensity is an even more complicated issue. Anxiety certainly is associated with many types of pain, and depression is common in patients with persistent pain. However, the cause-and-effect relationship is unclear. Does anxiety cause pain or is it the result of pain? Is depression the cause or the result of pain? Some studies show a relationship between depression and pain, and some do not. Likewise, anxiety has been correlated with increased pain in some studies but not in others. Anxiety unrelated to pain may actually decrease pain, possibly because the anxiety increases the production of endorphins (Janssen, Arntz, 1996).

In a study of 120 patients with cancer pain, no difference was found in pain intensity measures or functional status between the depressed patients and those who were not depressed (Grossman, Sheidler, Sweeden, et al., 1991). In other words, the depression associated with pain did not alter a patient's report of the intensity of the pain. In another study of patients who had cancer, the presence of depression, hostility, and anxiety did not correlate with the effectiveness of attempts at pain relief (Cleeland, 1984). Cleeland warns us that when patients do not respond to analgesics, clinicians should be wary of blaming this result on the patients' depression rather than on inappropriate analgesic therapy.

The relationship between preoperative-state and postoperative-state anxiety and pain magnitude has been addressed by a few studies. (State anxiety is situational, whereas trait anxiety is a general level of anxiety.) A study of 96 patients after coronary artery bypass graft surgery examined the relationship between postoperative-state anxiety and the perception of postoperative pain. The results showed that even in the range of low to moderate state anxiety, higher anxiety postoperatively was associated with higher pain intensities (Nelson, Zimmerman, Barnason, et al., 1998). The correlations between postoperative-state anxiety and postoperative pain ranged from low to moderate but were nevertheless statistically significant. However, again, the direction of causality has not been established. In other words, although increased pain and increased anxiety may occur together, it is not always clear whether the anxiety causes the pain or the pain causes the anxiety.

An exploratory study of 24 patients undergoing varicose vein surgery examined the relationship between pain ratings and preoperative state anxiety (Terry, Niven, Brodie, et al., 2007). Pre- and postoperative-state anxiety and pain ratings in the postoperative period were significantly positively correlated. However, the actual postoperative pain ratings were relatively low, with a mean VAS rating of 28.1 mm on a 100-mm linear scale. Nevertheless, the authors point out that the findings show the need to decrease anxiety in the clinical setting whenever possible. Suggestions about how to reduce anxiety were not included.

Another small study of women undergoing termination of pregnancy investigated the links between preoperative-state and trait anxiety and pain magnitude (Pud, Amit, 2005). About 1 hour before the procedure the women completed Spielberger's State-Trait Anxiety Inventory. Postoperatively, patients were asked to mark a 100-mm VAS at 50, 30, and 60 minutes. State anxiety was able to predict pain magnitude at 15 minutes, and trait anxiety predicted pain magnitude at 30 minutes. The authors explained this finding on the basis that state anxiety was expected to disappear when patients felt the immediate threat had been removed, whereas patients with trait anxiety needed more time to relax. The authors suggest that patients with high anxiety may require additional information relevant to the impending pain along with effective pain-relief protocols.

The belief that anxiety causes pain is reflected in the common practice of combining anxiolytics and opioids. Based on a literature review, Pud and Amit (2005) found that two methods, information giving and relaxation techniques, were beneficial in relieving anxiety and pain

but that the use of pharmacologic approaches to anxiety such as benzodiazepines was more controversial. In one study, lorazepam (Ativan) preoperatively did not significantly relieve pain (Wiebe, Podhradsky, Dijak, 2003). The findings in a study of postoperative patients who had access to IV PCA morphine and midazolam (Versed) separately revealed that use of midazolam did not influence pain scores or amount of PCA morphine used (Egan, Ready, Nessly, et al., 1992). In another study of postoperative pain, the administration of diazepam (Valium) preoperatively was shown to have an ongoing antianalgesic effect on morphine analgesia (Gear, Miaskowski, Heller, et al., 1997). In a double-blind study, combinations of various doses of midazolam and meperidine were administered to 150 patients with postoperative pain and, once again, midazolam did not significantly enhance the analgesic effect of the opioid (Miller, Eisenkraft, Cohen, et al., 1986).

No doubt exists that pain results in considerable distress for many patients, causing anxiety, depression, and hostility and interfering with all domains of quality of life (e.g., Ferrell, Grant, Funk, et al., 1997; Zimmerman, Story, Gaston-Johansson, et al., 1996). Until the relationships among pain and anxiety, depression, and other emotional states are clarified, the most practical initial approach to patients who are both in pain and anxious or depressed probably is to assume that pain causes these emotional responses rather than to assume that the emotional responses cause or intensify pain. Anxiety and depression appear to be normal responses to pain. When a patient is both in pain and anxious, initial intervention probably should be aimed at reducing the pain. The APS (2003) states, "In anxious patients with pain, opioid titration should precede treatment with benzodiazepines" (p. 46). Pain relief may well reduce the anxiety and minimize the need for a benzodiazepine. Likewise, for patients who are in pain and depressed, the most logical initial approach probably is to relieve the pain, which may then reduce the depression. If anxiety or depression persists following pain relief, other interventions, such as behavioral and pharmacologic approaches, are indicated.

Addiction

Seeking Drugs versus Seeking Pain Relief

Perhaps the most common reason for not accepting and acting on a patient's report of pain is the belief that the patient is or will become addicted to an opioid. A previously suggested strategy for addressing clinicians' reluctance to accept a patient's report of pain is to ask, "Why is it so difficult to believe this patient has pain?" Suspicion of addiction is often the answer. Clinicians may say, "The patient is drug seeking," "He just wants drugs," or "He's getting addicted." At present, in many clinical settings, the term *drug seeking*, though poorly defined, is used to mean addiction to opioids, abuse of opioids, or manipulative behavior (McCaffery, Grimm, Pasero, et al., 2005). Although patients seek drugs for many legitimate purposes, such as treating an infection, diabetes, or heart disease, somehow the term *drug seeking* has become associated with seeking opioids for reasons clinicians believe are inappropriate.

Questions, discussed later, that may be helpful in clarifying the confusion that surrounds beliefs about addiction are:

- What is the definition of addiction?
- What is the likelihood that patients who receive opioids are becoming or will become addicted?

Definitions Related to Addiction

Tolerance to opioids and physical dependence on opioids are not the same as addiction to opioids, but these three terms are often confused. Following are the definitions proposed by the American Academy of Pain Medicine (AAPM), the APS, and the American Society of Addiction Medicine (ASAM) (AAPM, APS, ASAM, 2001; APS, 2003):

- *Physical dependence* is a normal response that occurs with repeated administration of an opioid for more than 2 weeks and cannot be equated with addictive disease. It is a state of adaptation that is manifested by the occurrence of withdrawal symptoms when the opioid is suddenly stopped or rapidly reduced or an antagonist such as naloxone (Narcan) is given. When the opioid is no longer needed for pain relief, withdrawal symptoms usually are easily suppressed by the natural, gradual reduction of the opioid as pain decreases or by gradual, systematic reduction, referred to as tapering (not detoxification, which is a term used when opioids are decreased in a person with addictive disease).
- *Tolerance* is also a normal response that occurs with regular administration of an opioid and consists of a decrease in one or more effects of the opioid (e.g., decreased analgesia, decreased sedation or decreased respiratory depression). It cannot be equated with addictive disease. Tolerance to analgesia usually occurs in the first few days to 2 weeks of opioid therapy but is uncommon after that. It may be treated with increases in dose. However, disease progression, not tolerance to analgesia, appears to be the reason for most dose escalations. Stable pain usually results in stable doses. Fortunately, tolerance to opioid-induced respiratory depression, sedation, and other adverse effects (except for constipation) occur to some degree within a few days of starting regular doses of opioids. So tolerance poses very few clinical problems.
- *Opioid addiction* or *addictive disease* is a chronic neurologic and biologic disease. Its development

and manifestations are influenced by genetic, psychosocial, and environmental factors. No single cause of addiction, such as taking an opioid for pain relief, has been found. It is characterized by behaviors that include one or more of the following: impaired control of drug use, compulsive use, continued use despite harm, and craving. The diagnosis of addictive disease is not based on a single event but is based on a pattern of behavior that is observed over time. Most pain specialists and addiction specialists agree that in patients treated with prolonged opioid therapy, addictive disease is not a predictable drug effect and does not usually occur. The actual risk is not known. The disease of addiction is complex and multicausal and occurs over time, certainly not as a result of one hospital experience.

Each of these conditions—physical dependence, tolerance, and addictive disease—is a separate entity requiring different treatment. One may occur alone, any two together, or all three together. Physical dependence and tolerance are a result of repeated administration of the opioid and should be expected if regular daily doses of opioids are taken for 2 to 4 weeks or longer. Addiction, however, is a rare consequence of using opioids for pain relief.

Pseudoaddiction, as the name implies, is a mistaken diagnosis of addictive disease. The term was first used and the behaviors described by Weissman and Haddox (1989). Patients with undertreated pain may manifest behaviors very similar to those typical of addictive disease, such as escalating demands for more or different medications, repeated requests for opioids before the prescribed interval between doses has elapsed, illicit drug use (such as obtaining opioids from others), and deception (APS, 2003). Pseudoaddiction can be distinguished from true addictive disease in that the behaviors resolve when pain is effectively treated.

Likelihood of Occurrence of Addictive Disease

To address concerns about the likelihood of the occurrence of addictive disease in patients who receive opioids for pain relief, two separate questions must be addressed:

- What is the likelihood that a patient will develop addictive disease as the result of taking opioids for pain relief?
- What is the likelihood that a patient taking opioids for pain relief already has addictive disease?

Inconsistency in Defining Terms Related to Problematic Opioid-Taking Behavior

To attempt to answer either question, one must admit that it is extremely difficult to design studies about addiction and that the findings of studies done to date are certainly open to question. One of the major difficulties in interpreting and comparing these studies is inconsistency in the definitions and criteria used to determine addictive disease, opioid abuse, and other problematic drug-taking behaviors (a term usually used to cover all uses of opioids that are of concern). Many of the studies used the Diagnostic and Statistical Manual of Mental Disorders (DSM-IV; APA, 1994) criteria for *substance dependence*, a term usually equated with addictive disease. This definition of addiction, however, is not the same as that proposed by AAPM, the APS, and the ASAM (2001), cited above. The term *substance abuse*, also used in these studies and defined by DSM-IV, is not the same as substance dependence or addictive disease. Substance abuse as it applies to opioids is generally reserved for behaviors somewhat similar to those of addictive disease but not as severe. The behaviors are destructive to the life of the individual and persist over time. They may include use of opioids in situations in which drug use is physically hazardous such as driving an automobile, or legal problems may occur such as forging prescriptions. The term *substance misuse* as it applies to opioids is generally reserved for behaviors less severe than substance abuse, such as calling for early refills, not taking the opioid as prescribed, giving the medication to someone else, or unauthorized dose escalation.

Since the DSM-IV (1994) does not use the term *addictive disease* but rather the term *substance dependence*, which incorporates symptoms of addiction, this creates confusion. DSM-IV (1994) incorporates symptoms of addiction. To minimize confusion, an effort has been made to resolve this (Heit, Gourlay, 2009). Pain specialists argue that *dependence* is too misleading because it gets confused with *physical dependence*, which is expected, and physical dependence differs from DSM-IV's use of the term *substance dependence*. As the DSM-IV manual is being updated, pain specialists are encouraging the American Psychiatric Association DSM-5 committee to restore the term *addiction* (Heit, Gourlay, 2009). One of the committee's objections to this is that the word *addiction* is too stigmatizing. However, in recognition of the need to clarify terminology and establish addiction as a disease (Heit, Gourlay, 2009), the National Institute on Drug Abuse (NIDA) may be changed to the National Institute on Diseases of Addiction. Another example of the term *addiction* being more commonly used by professionals is the creation of the ASAM. Use of the word *addiction* promotes understanding that it is a disease and should be treated as one. As this book goes to print, the decision of the DSM-5 committee is not known.

Despite this confusion about the meaning of terms used in research when referring to addictive disease, we review some of the studies to identify trends in the currently available information.

Development of Addictive Disease in Patients Who Are Taking Opioids

In response to the first question, the findings of several studies have shown that addiction as a result of using opioids for pain relief occurs in less than 1% of patients. Possibly the most interesting research in this area was conducted in the 1970s during a time when heroin was widely used as an analgesic in England. Heroin was used for a variety of types of pain, such as postoperative pain and pain associated with terminal illness. In fact, the popular "magic" mixture called Brompton's Cocktail, which originated in England, contained heroin, cocaine, gin, and honey. It was modified and used in the United States in the 1970s for pain relief in terminal illness. Many clinicians are unaware that the Brompton's Cocktail initially was used in England as an analgesic for postthoracotomy pain (Kerrane, 1975). Thus the use of heroin as an analgesic was widespread in England in the 1970s. In two studies of more than 500 patients taking regular doses of heroin orally or parenterally for pain relief for weeks or months, no patients could be documented as having become addicted (Twycross, 1974; Twycross, Wald, 1976).

In a frequently quoted study by the Boston Collaborative Drug Surveillance Program (Porter, Jick, 1980), a review of their files to determine the incidence of opioid addiction in hospitalized medical patients identified 11,882 patients of 39,946 patients who received at least one opioid preparation and had no history of addictive disease. Only 4 cases (less than 1%) of reasonably well-documented addictive disease could be identified. The findings of this study can be questioned for several reasons, such as failure to state a working definition of addiction and the difficulty of carefully evaluating such a large number of patients, but it is one attempt to answer the question of how likely it is that persons without a history of addictive disease will develop it as a result of taking opioids for pain relief.

Another large study shows the same trend. Questionnaires about pain management were sent to 151 burns units in the United States, and 181 staff members responded from 93 burn units (Perry, Heidrich, 1982). These respondents had an average experience of more than 6 years on a burn unit and represented the accumulated knowledge of at least 10,000 hospitalized burn patients. Not one case of addictive disease resulting from the use of opioids could be documented in patients with no history of addictive disease.

In a literature review of addiction as a consequence of taking opioid analgesics, findings revealed that more than 24,000 patients had been studied (Friedman, 1990). Yet only 7 (less than 1%) patients could be documented as having become addicted as a result of receiving opioids for pain relief.

In a large prospective study of 15,160 veterans who were chronic users of opioids for persistent noncancer pain, the rate of newly physician-diagnosed opioid abuse or opioid dependence was 2% (Edlund, Steffick, Hudson, et al., 2007). These patients had no diagnosed opioid abuse or opioid dependence in the previous 2 years. The investigators felt that the rate of 2% of opioid abuse or opioid dependence might be lower than the actual occurrence, but it is important to note that this figure includes both opioid abuse (such as unauthorized escalation of dose or obtaining opioids from multiple sources) and opioid dependence (a term more commonly equated with addiction) and therefore may reflect less than a 2% occurrence of addictive disease.

In a metaanalysis of studies of the safety and effectiveness of opioids in patients receiving opioids for 6 months or longer for persistent noncancer pain, 115 studies were identified but only 17 met inclusion criteria (Noble, Tregear, Treadwell, et al., 2008). Of these, only 7 studies specifically mentioned opioid addiction, but the criteria for addiction and methods of monitoring were unclear. Nevertheless, in the 2042 patients in these 7 studies, only 1 patient was reported as having possibly developed opioid addiction (Anderson, Burchiel, 1999), for an overall addiction rate of 0.042%.

In an evidence-based review of all available studies of the development of abuse, addiction, and aberrant drug-related behaviors in patients who had persistent pain and were exposed to chronic opioid analgesic therapy, only four studies preselected patients for no previous or current history of abuse/addiction (Fishbain, Cole, Lewis, et al., 2008). In these studies the percentage of abuse/addiction was calculated to be 0.19%. In other words, in patients with no previous or current history of abuse/addiction, chronic use of opioids resulted in only 0.19% of abuse/addiction.

A more recent and much better designed study examined the likelihood of addiction occurring in patients with no history of addictive disease who received controlled-release oxycodone for as long as 3 years (Portenoy, Farrar, Backonja, et al., 2007). This study was exceptional in that a systematic effort was made to identify problems in each study patient with taking drugs both before and during the study. Patients who self-reported past or present substance or alcohol abuse were excluded. In addition to self-report, some of the patients were also screened by the Drug Abuse Screening Test-20 questionnaire to establish eligibility. At each 3-month visit, physician investigators also completed brief questionnaires indicating whether patients showed any signs of problematic drug-taking behavior. If the response was positive, the physicians answered further questions and, if they were concerned about drug use, their assessments were further evaluated by a panel of experts who rated physicians' reports as positive, possible, alleged, or negative for abuse, misuse, or withdrawal. This study revealed that of 227 patients only 6 cases (2.6%) of possible drug misuse could be identified but none (0) were actual addictive disease. In other words, there were no cases of new addiction after taking controlled-release oxycodone for as along as 3 years.

That study is not meant to reflect the likelihood of drug abuse or addiction already existing in patients with pain who are receiving chronic opioid therapy. Rather, it is, so far, the best controlled study to shed light on the likelihood that addictive disease develops in patients with pain who are treated by chronic opioid therapy and do not have a history of addictive disease or abuse. The finding was that 0 patients without histories of addictive disease developed addictive disease in the course of chronic opioid therapy. This investigation is reassuring and substantiates the findings of previous studies that suggest that the likelihood that addictive disease will develop as a result of the administration of opioids to treat pain in a population of patients with no history of addiction or abuse is likely to be below 1%.

Preexisting Addictive Disease in Patients Who Are Taking Opioids

To address the second question, how many patients being treated with opioids already had addictive disease prior to treatment with opioids, requires examining other types of studies. This question is most often raised in relation to patients with persistent pain. Again, the findings of these studies are open to question because of the recurring problem of the absence of a universally accepted definition of addictive disease.

Based on their review of the literature, Nicholson and Passik (2007) found that some studies indicate that the rate of addiction to illicit drugs, prescribed opioids, and alcohol in the population that has persistent pain is approximately the same as it is in the general population; it ranges from 6% to 10% (Savage, 2002). Other studies report a wide range of prevalence of current substance abuse or dependence in patients receiving opioids for persistent pain. As a reminder, prevalence data cannot be used to establish how many patients became addicted to opioids as a result of receiving them for pain relief.

In a review of the literature in 1992 (Fishbain, Rosomoff, Rosomoff), 24 articles were found that addressed the prevalence of substance dependence, but this information was limited in part by the lack of agreement on how *addictive disease* was defined. Only seven studies used acceptable diagnostic criteria for drug misuse. Six studies found that the prevalence of addictive disease ranged from 3.2 % to 16%, and one study reported 18.9% prevalence of opioid dependence. A study in Denmark revealed similar findings of a 3% to 19% prevalence of addictive disorders in patients with persistent noncancer pain (Breivik, 2005).

In a metaanalysis of five studies examining the prevalence of current substance use disorders in patients receiving opioid therapy for persistent back pain (Martell, O'Connor, Kerns, et al., 2007), only one study was judged to be of good quality (Brown, Patterson, Rounds, et al., 1996). In this study the current prevalence estimate of substance-use disorders was 23% for those receiving opioids for persistent back pain and for those with back pain who were not receiving opioids. Again, adequate definitions were lacking, but this prevalence may be high because it covers both abuse and addictive disease.

In a study of 801 patients receiving daily opioid therapy for persistent noncancer pain, the current prevalence of substance abuse or dependence (based on criteria in the DMS-IV) was 9.7% (Fleming, Balousek, Klessig, et al., 2007). The current prevalence of opioid-use disorder was 3.8%, four times higher than the 0.9% in the general population. Once more, it is important to note that this covers abuse as well as addictive disease.

The prevalence of addictive disease in acute care varies markedly between one population and another. It is estimated that addictive disorders occur in approximately 19% to 25% of hospitalized patients and in 40% to 60% of patients who sustain major trauma (Savage, 2002). Another estimate is that 25% to 40% of hospitalized patients have prior problems related to drug or alcohol addiction (Kissen, 1997).

In summary, it is difficult to determine the likelihood that patients with persistent pain already have addictive disease when they are placed on chronic opioid therapy. Studies to date are helpful but do not use the same definitions of addictive disease, so their findings are in question. Perhaps the best guess is the suggestion by Nicholson and Passik (2007), cited earlier, that the rate of addiction to alcohol and other drugs in the population with persistent pain is approximately the same as it is in the general population, and that ranges from 6% to 10%. In the acute care setting the prevalence is higher because many medical illnesses such as cancer are complications of addictive disease, and alcohol and other drugs are often involved in trauma, burns, and orthopedic injuries.

Addiction as a Stigmatizing Label: Societal versus Medical Views

An understanding of some of the stigma clinicians associate with addiction arises from confusion related to society's general views of addiction (the moral and criminal model), which are at odds with the validated view of addiction as a disease (the disease model; Table 2-2) (Compton, 1999). Taken to its extreme, the moral model of addiction views substance abuse as a shameful behavior in which good and moral persons do not participate.

It is seen as a behavior that is the individual's fault and that an individual can freely choose that behavior or not. Because addicts in this model appear unwilling to adhere to the so-called virtuous path, they are viewed as being at fault for any negative consequences arising from their drug use and commonly are considered less worthy of care and concern than patients suffering a "faultless" disease (Malone, 1996).

Somewhat different, but resulting in the same negative, judgmental view of addiction, is the criminal or criminal justice model. It is illegal in this country and many others around the world to use certain drugs for the purpose of experiencing their psychoactive effects, so persons possessing or ingesting drugs are criminals and are subject to punishment and imprisonment (Compton, 1999). The predominance of the criminal justice view of addiction is reflected in the high percentage of Americans incarcerated in federal (59.5%) and state prisons (22.3%) for drug offenses (Office of National Drug Control Policy [ONDCP], 1997). Although the use of alcohol is legal, laws against drunk driving and public intoxication criminalize excessive alcohol use too. It is interesting that addiction is the only recognized disease for which its sufferers risk arrest rather than medical care when impaired by its symptoms. Thus, in the criminal justice model, like the moral model, persons suffering addictive disease are characterized as bad, unethical, and deserving of criminal justice or social sanctions.

Unlike the moral and criminal justice models, the medical model views addiction as a disease, specifically as a disease acquired by the brain. Like any disease, addiction has identifiable risk factors and a demonstrated pathophysiologic basis, can be diagnosed according to a well-described cluster of signs and symptoms, follows a predictable pattern of progression, and can be managed and treated. Unlike the moral and criminal justice models, the medical model of addiction places no blame or negative social value on the sufferer. The focus is on understanding the factors that result in the disease's development and progression and on evaluating methods of prevention and treatment. Punishing and stigmatizing addicted individuals are not viewed as being effective methods of intervention for addiction in the disease model, whereas treatment approaches, including pharmacotherapy,

Table 2-2	Models of Addiction: Society's Views of Addiction		
	Moral Model	**Criminal Model**	**Disease Model***
Cause	Moral weakness, lack of willpower	Bad or evil character	Acquired brain disease
Treatment goal	Increase moral strength/fortitude	Rehabilitation	Normalize brain disruption
Treatment strategies	Religious conversion	Incarceration	Pharmacotherapy, cognitive-behavioral therapy

* This is the validated medical model to be used in clinical practice.

From Pasero, C., & McCaffery, M. *Pain assessment and pharmacologic management*, p. 36, St. Louis, Mosby. © 2011, McCaffery M, Pasero C, Compton P. May be duplicated for use in clinical practice.

cognitive-behavioral skill training, group support, and lifestyle change are (Compton, 1999).

Unfortunately, drug abuse and addiction often are treated as crimes rather than as public health problems (Cotton, 1994). Consequently, clinicians judgmentally regard addicts as bad people rather than focusing on addiction as a bad disease that requires treatment. So the label of addiction is stigmatizing and should be avoided. The term *addiction* should be used only to refer to a brain disease that requires appropriate treatment.

When a patient is referred to as being addicted or drug seeking, it is helpful to ask, "Has the patient been diagnosed as being an addict? If so, how does this affect our plan for pain relief? How do we plan to treat the addictive disease?" If a patient is addicted, he or she still deserves the best possible pain relief that can be provided safely. The following position is unethical: I can provide safe and effective pain relief for this patient, but I will not because I do not believe the patient deserves it.

Behaviors Mistaken as Indicators of Addiction and What They Could Mean

The following material discusses patients who are labeled, not diagnosed, as being addicted or are referred to as drug seeking. These patients have not been assessed appropriately for the presence of addiction, and a diagnosis of addiction probably is not written in these patients' charts. Yet clinicians may continue to say that these patients are addicted or are drug seeking. These stigmatizing words can adversely influence patients' pain treatment plans and other aspects of care. Clinicians may be reluctant to accept patients' reports of pain and may be opposed to providing pain relief.

To detect and correct this situation, several questions may be explored with the staff:

- Has the patient been diagnosed by qualified clinicians as having addictive disease?
- If this is a label, not a diagnosis, what has the patient done to cause us to believe he or she is drug seeking or addicted?
- Is there another way to explain behaviors that seem to indicate drug seeking or addiction? Acknowledge that the behaviors *may* mean addiction but could be something else.
- Could the patient who is seeking opioids actually be seeking pain relief?

Some clinicians seem to believe that addicted patients are easily identified by the presence of certain behaviors. The list of "aberrant drug-related behaviors that raise concern about the potential for addiction," originated by Portenoy (1994) and subsequently revised (Fine, Portenoy, 2007), is one such list that is often misinterpreted. The list is divided into behaviors more suggestive of addiction (such as prescription forgery or multiple episodes of prescription loss) and those less suggestive of addiction (such as drug hoarding or requesting specific drugs). As

Portenoy (1994; 1996; Fine, Portenoy, 2007) states, the behaviors require differential diagnosis because they may also indicate unrelieved pain or confusion about drug intake; they exist on a continuum, and no single behavior is diagnostic of addictive disease. Table 2-3 includes some of these behaviors.

However, Table 2-3 is based primarily on the findings of a study that attempted to identify behaviors that may cause nurses to refer to a patient as being drug seeking and to identify what nurses think the term *drug seeking* means (McCaffery, Grimm, Pasero, et al., 2005). The nurses believed that when the term *drug seeking* is used, it is very likely to mean that a patient is addicted to opioids, is abusing pain medicine, or is manipulative. The behaviors that would cause the majority of the nurses in this study (N = 369) to refer to patients as being drug seeking were: they went to various EDs to get opioids; they told inconsistent stories about pain or medical history; or they asked for a refill because the prescription had been lost or stolen. The majority of nurses (82% to 85%) agreed that *drug seeking* has a negative meaning, and the majority of nurses (91% to 93%) denied using the term in charting. Thus, the term *drug seeking* should be avoided in clinical practice. A position paper, Pain Management in Patients with Addictive Disease, issued by ASPMN (2002) recommends that the term *drug seeking* not be used because it creates prejudice and barriers to care.

Again, none of the behaviors in the previously mentioned study of drug seeking is diagnostic of addiction. Like the list of aberrant drug-taking behaviors, the drug-seeking behaviors may indicate pseudoaddiction, and improved pain control is recommended as one way to identify this (Passik, Kirsh, 2004; Portenoy, 1994).

The first column in Table 2-3 lists behaviors that seem to cause clinicians, especially nurses, to think that patients have addictive disease. The second column lists comments made about what these behaviors may indicate other than addiction, and suggestions are made for remedying some of the problems.

Some of the behaviors in Table 2-3 can be explained easily by simply looking at other logical options mentioned in the table. In some cases, knowledge about opioid analgesia (discussed in detail in Section IV) is helpful. Other comments in Table 2-3 revolve around some complex issues that are discussed here.

Patient Seeks Pain Relief Persistently, Repeatedly, or from Several Sources. Several of the behaviors listed in Table 2-3 probably reflect inadequate pain management, which causes a patient to make multiple or persistent attempts to obtain analgesia. Research has established that many clinicians lack knowledge of the principles of analgesic use (e.g., McCaffery, Robinson, 2002). No doubt this is a major reason for clinicians' failing to see that a poor pain treatment plan is responsible for certain patient behaviors. Clinicians may believe that the pain relief provided for a patient should be effective. When it is not, clinicians

Table 2-3 | Misconceptions: Behaviors Indicating Addiction

Behaviors that Are Commonly Mistaken as Indicators of Addiction or Drug Seeking	Corrections and Comments (What Else Could it Be?)
Patient is a "frequent flier," often visiting one or more emergency departments (EDs) to obtain opioid analgesics.	This is not desirable behavior, but it may be caused by inadequate pain treatment. If treatment in the ED results in poor pain relief or if staff convey that the patient comes in too often, the patient may go to another ED for additional pain relief or to decrease the frequency of visits to a single ED. The patient may have persistent pain problems that are not being well managed by private prescribers, so the patient is forced to seek help in the ED. If the patient returns often to the ED, a plan should be developed and placed on file to document previous assessments, the effectiveness of treatments, and recommendations for initiating pain relief on subsequent ED visits.
Patient obtains opioids from another prescriber despite being told not to do so.	This is not desirable behavior, but as in the above situation, it may reflect poor pain management. For example, a patient's prescriber may prescribe long-acting opioids plus short-acting opioids at doses that do not relieve the pain. Out of desperation, the patient may try taking additional doses (an unauthorized escalation of dose) and find that doing so successfully controls the pain. When the prescriber refuses to increase the dose, the patient may seek help from other prescribers. Obviously, a solution to this situation is for the original prescriber to increase the dose or try alternative methods of controlling the patient's pain.
Patient tells inconsistent stories about pain or medical history.	It is well recognized that a patient's memories of illnesses and treatments are often inconsistent from one time to another. This includes recall of pain and of its treatment. The patient may forget, combine, or separate incidents or may remember events as having occurred more recently than they did. Recall is influenced by intensity of pain at the time of interview and by emotional state. Cognitive impairment, adverse effects of medications, and psychiatric illness can also influence recall. To minimize the chance of inconsistent stories, a clinician may take several actions: interview the patient about pain in the same manner each time (e.g., using pain rating scales or pain assessment forms) or begin with the most recent episode and work backward in time.
Patient asks for refills because a prescription was lost or stolen.	Patients with cognitive impairment may misplace medications. Other patients may be unaware of the abuse potential of opioids and fail to protect supplies from friends and family members. They need to be cautioned about how to secure their prescriptions carefully. Patients should be told to make a police report when theft is suspected. However, some patients suspect theft because they have taken more than they realize and have run out of medication. The adequacy of the treatment plan then needs to be reassessed.
Patient is manipulative (e.g., changing behavior when clinician arrives).	Undertreatment of pain may lead to manipulative behavior. When patients report pain and clinicians do not respond by providing adequate relief, patients may become less than honest with the clinicians. This may result in behavior changes, such as more grimacing or reporting the pain at a higher intensity.
Patient tells nurse where to give the opioid or how fast (e.g., "Give it fast and close to the port").	This is most likely to occur in a patient who has become familiar with this route of administration and has discovered that giving it faster and closer to the port results in faster pain relief. It is also possible that a patient enjoys some nonanalgesic effects by this method, such as sudden feelings of relaxation and reduced anxiety.
Patient requests analgesics by name, dose, interval between doses, and/or route of administration (e.g., "I'll need two Vicodin every 4 hours," or "Morphine, 10 mg IV, works best for my headaches").	This is likely to be a well-educated patient who probably has had pain previously or has persistent pain. Patients need to be educated about all their medications, including analgesics. If the patient was diabetic and talking about insulin requirements, it would be welcomed information. The patient is providing helpful information for the pain treatment plan.

Continued

Table 2-3	Misconceptions: Behaviors Indicating Addiction—cont'd
Behaviors that Are Commonly Mistaken as Indicators of Addiction or Drug Seeking	**Corrections and Comments (What Else Could it Be?)**
Patient may be a clock watcher and may ask for analgesics in advance of a specified time. The patient may say, "I'll need my next dose in about 30 minutes."	Sometimes analgesics are prescribed at intervals longer than their durations. When the patient asks for a dose before the interval elapses, the clinician often tell the patient how much time he or she must wait. For example, "You can't have your next pill for 2 hours." Because the patient must wait in pain for 2 hours, he or she is likely to note the time and ask for the medication as soon as the 2 hours pass. The patient may then find that it takes the nurse another 30 minutes to deliver the dose. A patient may work with this reality by calculating when the next dose can be given and asking for it 30 minutes in advance. This situation strongly suggests that the patient's opioid prescription should be changed to a longer acting opioid or the interval between doses should be shortened.
Patient enjoys the opioid (e.g., is happy, active, or wants to leave the unit to smoke).	Once pain is relieved, it is natural for a patient to feel happier and engage in more activities, such as talking and ambulating. It may appear that a patient is "high" or euphoric, but it is simply a return to normal mood, perhaps with some elation at being in less pain. Wanting to go to a smoking area for a cigarette is certainly understandable if the patient regularly smokes. Withdrawal symptoms from nicotine can occur rather quickly and may result in a patient feeling irritable and having an intense desire to smoke. Further, nicotine has analgesic properties and may provide additional mild to moderate pain relief. Nicotine also decreases the incidence of PONV.
Patient says he or she is allergic to everything except one particular opioid.	Allergy to opioids is rare, but patients often mistake adverse effects, such as nausea, vomiting, and itching, for allergic reactions. These may have been poorly managed adverse effects, or patients may indeed have more severe adverse effects with some opioids than others, and these should be avoided. If a patient is convinced that he or she experiences greater effectiveness with one opioid than with others, it is possible that he or she will try to avoid the others by saying he or she is allergic to them. Even when an analgesic is not terribly effective, a patient may be afraid to try another analgesic for fear the results will be even worse. If it is not necessary for a patient to change to another opioid, he or she should receive what is preferred. If a change is necessary, perhaps because the preferred opioid has an active metabolite that is accumulating (a potential problem with meperidine), then selection of another opioid should depend on careful assessment to determine whether a patient is allergic or has experienced unmanaged or unmanageable adverse effects resulting from other opioids.

From Pasero, C., & McCaffery, M. *Pain assessment and pharmacologic management*, pp. 38-39, St. Louis, Mosby. © 2011, McCaffery M, Pasero C. May be duplicated for use in clinical practice.

may label the patient or blame him or her rather than the treatment plan. For example, a patient who is a clock watcher probably should receive a longer acting opioid, or the interval between doses should be changed. The patient should not be labeled as an addict for trying to make the best of inadequate analgesia by asking for it in a timely manner.

Patients who receive inadequate analgesia in the ED or from a physician should not be labeled as being addicted or drug seeking if they seek help elsewhere. One study found that one third of patients presenting to EDs with pain did not have their pain resolved (Johnston, Gangon, Pepler, 2005). At follow-up 1 week later, approximately one third of patients still could not return to normal activities. Understandably, these patients might return to the ED or seek relief elsewhere. For many patients, improving their pain-treatment plans would negate the need to return to the ED or to see other physicians.

Recognizing the limits of what can be done to help certain patients may enable clinicians to be less impatient and frustrated. In a study of 46 heavy users of EDs in two West Coast inner-city trauma-center hospitals, findings revealed that many of them were homeless, poor, or disabled (Malone, 1996). Many had no family and most had one or more chronic medical problems. It is not too surprising that these vulnerable populations of patients might not follow up on prescribed treatment or suggestions to obtain additional help or might seek pain relief from clinics or places other than the ED. Further, some patients may not be able to take time off from work to follow up on referrals to pain clinics or may not have the transportation to get there.

Some individuals who come repeatedly to EDs are seeking treatment for pain, and because they visit the ED frequently, it is likely that they have a persistent pain condition. Migraine headache, sickle cell crisis, and flares of low back pain are common. Planning for the next visit is far more practical than feeling angry with the patient or labeling him or her as being addicted when he or she returns. A carefully developed treatment plan greatly facilitates a patient's care and discourages the tendency to label the patient because he or she has a persistent problem.

An example of an innovative approach to the care of "frequent flyers" is the use of a passport document (a small booklet or plasticized card) for patients with frequent sickle cell crises. The booklet summarizes the initial comprehensive clinical assessment and contains a written pain-treatment plan that has been developed and agreed on by patients, families, and caregivers (Beyer, Platt, Kinney, et al., 1994). The ED also may develop and have on file protocols or individualized treatment plans for other patients who are seen regularly (Nichols, 1996).

Such treatment plans help clinicians to realize the vast differences in opioid requirements and to appreciate that the same dose is not effective for everyone. For identical painful problems, some patients require eight or more times the amount required by other patients (APS, 2003). Patients with moderate to severe low back pain of noncancer origin are also frequent users of many EDs. Again, individualized treatment plans or protocols are helpful. In this group of patient, an additional aid is to assess for neuropathic pain, which seems to be commonly overlooked. While patients are waiting to be seen, an assessment tool like the ID Pain tool or the Neuropathic Pain Scale, discussed later in this section (see Forms 3-4 and 3-5, pp. 97 and 99, for copies of these tools), can be completed by the patients to help discriminate between nonneuropathic pain and neuropathic pain (Fishbain, Lewis, Cutler, et al., 2008). Differing treatment approaches must be used for pain of neuropathic origin as opposed to pain that is nociceptive. Opioids are helpful for both types of pain but often are inadequate for neuropathic pain. Adjuvant analgesics, such as certain anticonvulsants and antidepressants (see Section V, Adjuvant Analgesics), have been identified as being effective for many types of neuropathic pain.

An aggressive protocol for rapid titration of fentanyl, a short-acting opioid, is useful for many patients who present with moderate to severe pain. When these patients are discharged from the ED, careful choice of an oral opioid is essential to keep moderate to severe pain under control. The automatic use of a prescription for one to two tablets of oral hydrocodone or oxycodone with acetaminophen (e.g., Vicodin or Percocet) is often inadequate, and the patient then returns to the ED or seeks pain relief elsewhere.

Patient Gives Inconsistent Stories about Pain or Medical Histories. It is well recognized that patients' memories of past symptoms, treatments, illnesses, and episodes of care are inconsistent from one time to another (Barsky, 2002). Yet when patients with pain report inconsistently about their pain, they may be suspected of drug seeking. Unreliability of recall is influenced by many factors, such as psychiatric condition, cognitive impairment, medication adverse effects, current pain intensity, or simple difficulty in recalling details that occurred some time ago or even recently.

Barsky (2002) states that one of the major sources of contradictory information is variance, situations in which patients answer the same question differently on differing occasions. Patient variance takes several forms:

- Patients forget and therefore underreport the incidence of previous symptoms. Memory of dates is particularly problematic, and patients may knowingly resort to guesswork. Forgetting may occur when the information is embarrassing or stigmatizing such as alcohol abuse.
- Patients have a tendency to combine multiple, separate incidents into a single one. This is called *recomposition*.
- Patients may engage in forward telescoping, which means that remote events tend to be displaced forward in time and are remembered as having occurred more recently.

One study looked at a health maintenance organization patients' recall of all outpatient visits made within a 12-month period. This information was compared with their medical records. Patients recalled only 41% of the visits recorded in their medical records, and there was a 28% incidence of false recall in which patients recalled a visit of which there was no record (Means, Nigam, Zarrow, et al., 1989).

In a study of 125 patients with a long history of facial pain, self-reported dates of onset of pain were compared with onset dates that patients had reported 7 years earlier (Raphael, Marbach, 1997). The dates reported differed by more than a year in 74% of the patients. As time went by, patients underestimated how chronic their pain had been. They recalled pain as having begun more recently than had actually been recorded in their records.

A review of the literature revealed that persistent pain that varies in intensity over weeks and months may be especially difficult to remember accurately (Smith, Safer, 1993). In patients experiencing persistent pain, the intensity of present pain affects the recall of their pain and medication use for 1 day to several weeks previously. Pain is recalled as having been less severe when present pain is at relatively low intensity and as having been more severe when present pain is at relatively high intensity. Likewise, medication use is recalled as having been less frequent when a patient's present level of pain is low. In one study, patients with persistent headache noted past pain as having been more intense when they were currently having pain than when asked about pain during a period of less intense pain (Eich, Reeves, Jaeger, et al., 1985). When pain was less intense, they remembered past pain as having been milder than they had rated it when they were actually experiencing it. Therefore, a patient's memory of symptoms since the previous inquiry may actually depend on how severe the symptoms are at the time of the present inquiry.

The patient's emotional state also influences memory. Researchers concluded in one study that patients who had anxiety or depression at the time of the interview were more likely to recall somatic symptoms that they had not remembered to report 1 year earlier (Simon, Gureje, 1999).

Therefore, clinicians should not be surprised that sometimes patients tell inconsistent stories about their pain. Barsky (2002) suggests several ways to minimize this effect.

- Try to interview the patient about pain in the same manner each time. Having a standardized form similar to the Brief Pain Inventory (see Form 3-2, p. 53) may be helpful.
- Interpret the patient's responses consistently, such as clarifying what the patient means by "a lot of pain," by using a pain rating scale such as 0 (no pain) to 10 (worst pain imaginable).
- Note the patient's current state, such as current level of pain, anxiety, or depression, at the time of the interview. As mentioned earlier, this state can influence a patient's report of pain. If a patient is feeling well at the time of the interview, he or she is less likely to remember details.
- Try to establish an anchor point, such as an important event (e.g., new job, graduation), for the information being recalled. Patients remember health events more easily when they have occurred close to a landmark event.
- Begin with the most recent episode and work backward in time.

The fact that patients may tell inconsistent stories about their pain or medical histories should come as no surprise to clinicians. Some techniques can be used to minimize this effect, but when it occurs, patients should not automatically be labeled drug seekers or addicted persons.

Patient is Manipulative. Misconceptions about the acute pain model and expectations clinicians have about how patients with pain should act were discussed on p. 27. That material is relevant here as we discuss why patients may be manipulative. In brief, research shows that clinicians expect patients to act like they are in pain by displaying certain behaviors, such as limping or frowning, and by not displaying other behaviors, such as smiling or being active. The Andrew-Robert vignette research illustrated this by comparing nurses' responses to smiling patients and to grimacing patients. If patients' behaviors do not meet the clinicians' expectations, for example, if they smile while reporting severe pain, the reports of pain might not be accepted and that pain might be undertreated. In an example reported earlier in this chapter, researchers looked at the prescribing practices of physicians in a pain center; they were treating patients with persistent noncancer pain and found that the prescribing of opioids was more likely to be based on whether the patients exhibited pain behaviors than on pain severity or the extent of physical findings (Turk, Okifuji, 1997).

When patients are undertreated for pain, it is understandable that they may begin to change their behaviors in an attempt to find out how to convince clinicians that they need better pain relief. Fisher (2004) has pointed out that undertreatment of pain can easily cause a patient to be less than honest with a prescriber. When a patient is referred to as being manipulative, clinicians may mean that they suspect the patient of lying by rating pain level higher than it actually is or by claiming to be allergic to all opioids except one, so as to obtain the opioid of choice. Clinicians might also observe that a patient sometimes acts differently in the presence of clinicians than when alone or with friends. In fact, these suspicions and observations may be accurate if a patient's pain has been undertreated when the patient acted differently. When manipulation is suspected, the question that should be asked is "Have I ignored the patient's other attempts to get pain relief? Is the patient now changing behavior to convince me to provide better pain relief?"

Patient Enjoys Pain Relief. When some patients receive pain relief, especially relief from moderate to severe pain, their behaviors tend to change. Whereas they were quiet, immobile, or perhaps crying prior to receiving analgesia, afterward they may become active, happy, and talkative. This is normal behavior—it's the way people act when they are not in pain. However, especially when patients have received opioids, some clinicians think this behavior means the patients are getting high on the medication.

One of the behaviors often mentioned by nurses at full-day conferences we (MM, CP) presented and noted in the commentary section of our drug-seeking research (McCaffery, Grimm, Pasero, et al., 2005) is the patient leaving the clinical unit to smoke a cigarette. Why this disturbs some nurses and is viewed as such a negative behavior is unclear. Based on our survey about drug seeking, a few nurses seem to think that going out to smoke indicates opioid addiction or that it is somehow the reason for a patient requesting opioid analgesia.

However, the desire to smoke has other more likely explanations. Regular smokers are probably physically dependent on nicotine. After abrupt cessation, a patient usually begins to crave cigarettes after a few hours. Within

24 hours of nicotine cessation, the patient may experience withdrawal symptoms, such as depression, irritability, anxiety, frustration, anger, or restlessness (Schmitz, Schneider, Jarvik, 1997). These uncomfortable feelings easily explain why the patient wants to obtain enough pain relief to be able to ambulate to an area where smoking is allowed.

Another, less well-known reason for a patient in pain to want to smoke is that some research has shown that nicotine has mild to moderate analgesic properties. In a study of 20 female nonsmoking patients who received one dose of intranasal nicotine at the conclusion of uterine surgery found that pain scores during the first day were significantly lower than those of the control group, and morphine use was less (Flood, Daniel, 2004). No hypertension or tachycardia was noted. The authors speculated that this might have occurred because the patients receiving nicotine were experiencing less pain.

That study included only nonsmokers, who could not have been in withdrawal from nicotine postoperatively. So patients with pain who smoke and want to smoke a cigarette may not simply be relieving their withdrawal symptoms. In a series of three experimental studies using a heat stimulus and nicotine nasal spray, both smokers and nonsmokers were included (Perkins, Grobe, Stiller, et al., 1994). Nicotine decreased pain sensitivity and, overall, no significant differences were noted in relation to whether the subjects were smokers or nonsmokers.

Some studies have found that the analgesic effects of nicotine are almost absent or are much lower in females than in males (e.g., Shapiro, Jarvik, 1998), but the previously mentioned study that included only females does not support this finding. However, Shapiro and Jarvik (1998) found that among men (but not women), smokers had significantly higher pain thresholds and tolerance levels than did nonsmokers. Hence, it appears that whether or not patients are smokers, nicotine is likely to have mild to moderate analgesic effects, especially in males.

One last note about the possible benefits of smoking is related to postoperative nausea and vomiting (PONV). Several studies have found that PONV is likely to be less severe in patients who have a history of smoking (Apfel, Laara, Koivuranta, et al., 1999; Gan, Meyer, Apfel, 2007). This benefit of smoking seems to be conferred on nonsmokers when a nicotine patch is used after surgical procedures. PONV was studied in three groups of patients: (1) nonsmokers who had never smoked; (2) nonsmokers who had previously smoked but had given up smoking for at least 5 years and who had received a nicotine patch (16.6 mg) perioperatively; and (3) current smokers (Ionescu, Badescu, Acalovschi, 2007). The researchers found a significant reduction in the incidence of PONV in groups two (nicotine patch) and three (smokers), and there was no significant difference between these two groups. They concluded that use of a nicotine patch might reduce the incidence of PONV.

Pain Relief from Placebos

A *placebo* may be defined as any medication or procedure, including surgery, that produces an effect in a patient because of its implicit or explicit intent, not because of its specific physical or chemical properties. An example is a saline injection for analgesia. When a patient responds to a placebo in accordance with its intent, it is called a *positive placebo response*. Administration of a medication at a known subtherapeutic dose (e.g., 0.05 mg of morphine in an adult) is also considered a placebo (Sullivan, Terman, Peck, et al., 2005).

Placebos are often appropriately used as controls in preliminary research into the effects of new medications. New drugs are compared with placebos and must demonstrate more favorable effects than placebos to warrant further investigation of or marketing of the drugs. In such studies, patients or volunteers are informed of the nature of the project and are told that placebos may be given, along with other medications. To be included in the study, persons must give informed consent. Unfortunately, placebos also may be used clinically in a deceitful manner and without informed consent.

Misconceptions about the Meaning of Positive Placebo Responses

Occasionally, when the question is asked, "Why is it so difficult to believe this patient has pain?" the answer is that the patient reported satisfactory pain relief after receiving a placebo. Pain relief resulting from a placebo is mistakenly believed to invalidate patients' reports of pain. This may result in the patient being deprived of pain-relief measures.

Common misconceptions about pain relief resulting from a placebo are that patients are malingering (lying about pain) or the pain is psychogenic rather than being physical in origin. The fallacy of this is apparent in the results of research using placebos as controls in the evaluation of potential analgesic drugs. Beginning in the 1950s, numerous placebo-controlled analgesic studies were conducted with postoperative patients. Thus we know the answer to this question: What percentage of patients will report adequate relief of pain after having received a placebo injection the day after abdominal surgery? The answer commonly quoted is 36% (Beecher, 1955; Evans, 1974; Goodwin, Goodwin, Vogel, 1979); however, no fixed percentage of the population responds to placebos (Wall, 1992).

In fact, researchers find that the belief that overall, the positive placebo effects occur approximately one third of the time in any individual circumstance is incorrect (Moerman, Harrington, 2005). Beecher's (1955) study (as reported in Turner, Deyo, Loeser, et al., 1994), which proposed that on average, one third of the time a placebo would relieve pain, was based on a review of 15 studies of patients suffering a variety of painful conditions; and the placebo response rate ranged from 15% to 58%. In trials of antisecretory medications for peptic ulcer disease, one study examined the 4-week endoscopically verified healing rates in 117 control groups and showed that the placebo response ranged from 0% to 100% (Moerman, 2000).

If, on average, one third of patients who have obvious physical stimuli for pain (abdominal surgery) report pain relief after a placebo injection, clearly placebos cannot be used to diagnose malingering, psychogenic pain, or any psychologic problem and cannot be used to justify denying the patient pain relief. Quite simply, all we can conclude is that sometimes placebos are effective in relieving moderate to severe pain of known physical origin.

Although it is well documented that positive placebo responses occur, *why* placebos relieve pain remains poorly understood. Many theories have been proposed, including operant conditioning, faith, anxiety reduction, expectation, and endorphin release (Finniss, Benedetti, 2007; Grevert, Albert, Goldstein, 1983; Levine, Gordon, Fields, 1978; Lidstone, de la Fuente-Fernandez, Stoessl, 2005; Price, Chung, Robinson, 2005; Richardson, 1994). Yet none has been proved, and the mystery remains. It is interesting that in studying the role of endogenous opioids in producing a positive placebo response, researchers have demonstrated that placebo-induced respiratory depression may occur and can be reversed by naloxone (Finniss, Benedetti, 2005).

Misconceptions about Using Placebos for Pain Relief

Because placebos can provide pain relief in a rather large portion of patients, why wouldn't they be a legitimate option for pain relief? One reason placebos are not appropriate as pain treatment is that a positive placebo response cannot be predicted in an individual, and a placebo may be effective for one person at one time and not another (Sullivan, Terman, Peck, 2005). Although deceitful use of placebos is not recommended, efforts to enhance legitimate therapies with positive placebo effects is encouraged (Brody, 1997). This may be as simple as saying to the patient when an injection of morphine is administered, "This medication usually is a very effective way to relieve pain, and we can adjust it as necessary." Placebo effects occur with both inert substances such as saline injections and with proven analgesics such as opioids.

Another reason for not using placebos for pain relief is that they may produce harm as well as benefit. Research shows that placebos may mimic active drugs, may produce adverse effects (such as respiratory depression, as mentioned earlier) and toxic reactions, may worsen symptoms (negative placebo effects), and may directly affect many body organs (Benedetti, Amanzio, Baldi, et al., 1998; Lavin, 1991; Wolf, Pinsky, 1954). Therefore, substituting a placebo for an opioid cannot be justified on the basis of avoiding adverse effects, such as sedation or preventing addiction.

Unfortunately, placebos are most likely to be used in patients the staff regard as being difficult. The most extensive study of placebo use was undertaken in the 1970s (Goodwin, Goodwin, Vogel, 1979). Researchers surveyed placebo knowledge of and use by 60 physicians and 39 nurses in a university teaching hospital. Most of the physicians (78%) had ordered placebos, and most of the nurses (82%) had administered them. The reasons given for administering placebos revolved around proving the patients "wrong" and administering to patients who were disliked, who did not obtain pain relief by standard treatment, or who had frustrated or angered the staff. Not only does this deceitful use of placebos in place of appropriate therapy violate patients' rights to the highest quality of care possible, it clearly poses a moral, ethical, and professional danger to the clinicians.

Perhaps the most important reason for not using placebos in the assessment and treatment of pain is that deception is involved. The clinician lies to the patient. Deceit is harmful to both patients and health care professionals. When discovered (and it usually is), it may permanently damage a patient's trust in health care professionals.

Legal and ethical considerations involved in the deceitful use of placebos in pain management include liability for fraud, malpractice, breach of contract, and medical negligence (Fox, 1994). Nurses should examine their nurse practice acts and the policies of their state boards of nursing for guidance. For example, in 1997, the Board of Registered Nursing in California specifically stated that the use "of placebos for management of pain would not fulfill informed consent parameters" (p. 12).

Placebo use violates the rights of all patients who receive them outside of the context of approved clinical trials in which patients have given informed consent to participate. Even under these circumstances, placebo use may not be justified when the drug being studied could be evaluated by comparing it with an effective medication instead of a placebo (Hampton, 2006; Rothman, Michels, 1994; Sullivan, Terman, Peck, 2005).

There are no individuals for whom and no conditions for which placebos are the recommended treatment. Literature review shows no basis for the assumption that placebo pain medication is useful to patients (Kleinman, Brown, Librach, 1994). Therefore, the use of placebos inevitably deprives patients of more appropriate methods of assessment or treatment. In other words, there is always a better way to assess and treat patients with pain than to administer a placebo.

Recommendations against the Use of Placebos

Avoidance of deceitful use of placebos is recommended in the APS clinical guideline "Principles of Analgesic Use in the Treatment of Acute Pain and Cancer Pain": "Do not use placebos to assess the nature of pain. . . . The deceptive use of placebos and the misinterpretation of the placebo response to discredit patients' pain reports are unethical and should be avoided" (APS, 2003, p. 37).

Nursing organizations have issued placebo policy statements that strongly recommend against the use of placebos in pain management. The Oncology Nursing Society (ONS) (McCaffery, Ferrell, Turner, 1996) developed the first position statement. Soon afterward, 27 or more professional organizations, such as the National Association of Orthopaedic Nurses (NAON), endorsed the statement. The ONS position statement focuses on patients with diagnoses of cancer, but the article accompanying its publication verifies that the facts and ethical issues presented are equally applicable to other patients with pain, regardless of their diagnoses.

The ASPMN (2004) adopted a position statement on placebo use similar to that of ONS, the primary difference being that the opposition to placebo use in pain management applies to all patients, regardless of age or diagnosis. The ASPMN's position statement says, "placebos should not be used by any route of administration in the assessment and/or management of pain in any individual regardless of age or diagnosis" (p. 1). Box 2-2 summarizes the key elements to consider concerning the use of placebos in clinical practice.

Debate about Use of Placebos in n-of-1 Trials

In 2005, the APS issued a position paper about placebo use that was in agreement with the statement by the ASPMN except for one thing—to find the least invasive or damaging treatment for patients. The APS states that "trials involving alternation between active and placebo treatments in a single patient (known as "n-of-1 trials") might provide clinically useful and scientifically valid information" (Sullivan, Terman, Peck, et al., 2005, p. 216). *n of 1* literally means the number of subjects in the trial is 1. In such cases, treatment decisions might be made on the basis of a positive placebo response, and a patient might be denied active treatment. The APS states that ethically, such treatment requires a patient's consent, so a patient should be informed prior to the treatments that a placebo will be used as one of the treatments.

As an example, a patient who is being evaluated for an anesthetic block or injection would be told that a placebo would be used, and then the patient might receive a placebo injection of saline and later an injection of local anesthetic. If the patient responded positively to the placebo, active treatment using a local anesthetic might be denied. This does not seem consistent with other parts of the APS position that include the statement that "placebo response does not prove that pain is not 'real' or unworthy of any real treatment" (Sullivan, Terman, Peck, 2005, p. 216). The APS also states that placebo use might "delay specific treatments, thereby leading to disease or symptom escalation" (Sullivan Terman, Peck, 2005, p. 216).

| **Box 2-2** | Key Points about Placebo Use in Pain Management |

1. Placebos can be effective in relieving pain, but this does not justify their use. On average, one third of patients who have obvious physical stimuli for pain (e.g., surgery) may report pain relief after administration of a placebo. However, a positive response varies between and within individuals and, therefore, cannot be predicted.
2. No medical conditions exist for which placebos are recommended as a method of assessment or treatment. A positive placebo response should not be used to deny the patient any active treatment.
   a. Placebos cannot be used to diagnose malingering, psychogenic pain, or any psychologic problem.
   b. Use of placebos for pain relief does not prevent addiction to opioids.
   c. Placebo use deprives the patient of appropriate treatment or diagnostic measures.
3. Institutional policies that restrict the use of placebos to IRB-approved clinical trials in which informed consent is obtained are necessary not only to protect patients,

but also to protect nurses and other staff from moral, ethical, and legal concerns.
   a. Placebos tend to be used in vulnerable patient populations (e.g., those with substance abuse or with pain that is difficult to diagnose or treat). This constitutes a dual standard of care.
   b. Deceitful placebo use endangers the patient's trust in caregivers and violates the patient's rights.
   c. Deceitful use of placebos violates informed consent and constitutes medical negligence, placing caregivers in the position to be sued.
   d. Resorting to deceitful placebo use prevents caregivers from increasing their knowledge of more effective ways to assess and to treat pain.
   e. Deceit threatens the professional caregiver's own integrity.

From Pasero, C., & McCaffery, M. *Pain assessment and pharmacologic management*, p. 44, St. Louis, Mosby. © 2011, McCaffery M, Pasero C. May be duplicated for use in clinical practice.

Thus, the APS seems to contradict its own statement about making a decision to withhold treatment based on a positive placebo response.

The ASPMN does not agree with the APS's support of the n-of-1 trial for some of the same reasons stated earlier by the APS as well as for other reasons (McCaffery, Arnstein, 2006). The ASPMN's position statement on use of placebos in pain management (2004) says that the ASPMN "supports the use of placebos only in Institutional Review Board (IRB)-approved clinical trials" (p. 1). Further, this policy states that "placebo use for the assessment and/or treatment of pain, including the evaluation of response to pain treatments, constitutes fraud and deception" (p. 4). The ASPMN agrees with the need to identify patients who will not benefit from treatments that are irreversible or invasive, but it does not agree that the n-of-1 trial accomplishes this. There is no research that provides strong support for this method of determining whether to provide a patient with active treatment for pain relief.

N-of-1 trials pose several problems. The sequence of injections (placebo versus local anesthetic) is not random; clinicians are not blinded as to which is being injected; the trials are not done with the oversight of an IRB; and the effects when a placebo is administered might be caused simply by the puncture or the instillation of fluid (McCaffery, Arnstein, 2006). Also, patients may respond positively to placebos once and never do so again. Further, patients who do not get pain relief from the local anesthetic the first time it is administered might respond later after proper dosing and titration. And, finally, the placebo response tends to be more common and more pronounced with highly invasive procedures such as spinal nerve blocks. In one study of seven patients with complex regional pain syndrome who were receiving a nerve block with saline followed by a local anesthetic, significant pain relief occurred after saline in six of the seven patients (Price, Long, Wilsey, et al., 1998). Thus, in n-of-1 trials involving invasive procedures, the positive placebo effect is very likely to occur and would not seem to be an adequate reason for denying patients active treatment.

An even greater danger exists when n-of-1 trials are supported. It opens the door to uses of placebos in situations other than invasive procedures. For example, hospitalized patients with cancer pain caused by widespread metastases might be taking large doses of opioids and, under the conditions of an n-of-1 trial, could be given placebos. If patients reported pain relief, the opioids might be discontinued (McCaffery, Arnstein, 2006).

Institutional Policies Concerning Placebos

For the protection of patients and staff, written institutional policies about placebo use appear to be essential. The current frequency of deceitful or inappropriate placebo use in the assessment and treatment of pain is unknown, but it undoubtedly exists. Articles on this topic have appeared regularly through the years in the professional literature, and misunderstandings persist (Arnstein, 2006; Fox, 1994; Fox, McCaffery, Ferrell, et al., 1995; Grace, 2006; Haddad, 1993; Kleinman, Brown, Librach, 1994; McCaffery, Arnstein, 2006; McCaffery, Ferrell, 1994a; McCaffery, Ferrell, 1997b; McCaffery, Ferrell, Pasero, 1998; McCaffery, Pasero, 1995; Oh, 1994; Wall, 1993).

Surveys of nurses reveal that they are susceptible to becoming participants in deceitful use of placebos. Surveys completed by 601 nurses during 1995 revealed that a significant percentage of these nurses exhibited a high level of readiness to participate in deceitful placebo use (McCaffery, Ferrell, 1996b). About one of five nurses (19%) thought pain was a clinical problem for which placebos could be used. Even more respondents (27%) endorsed placebo use for anxiety; 25% believed placebos were appropriate in patients whose symptoms (pain) were questionable. Clearly, if placebos were suggested or prescribed, many nurses would participate in the action.

All hospitals and other health care agencies should have written policies that address unethical use of placebos. When policies are in place, communication among health care providers is less difficult. If placebos are prescribed, the nurse may use the existing placebo policy as a point of departure for communicating concerns about the patient's quality of care and for explaining why a nurse will not administer placebos, even when a prescription exits.

The ASPMN's (2004) position paper concerning placebos states that a policy is necessary to ensure that no patient receives a placebo unless it is in the context of an IRB-approved clinical trial. This should include mechanisms for reporting a clinician who violates the policy and the actions to be taken to censure such an individual. The policy should also provide a means of protecting any person who reports inappropriate use of placebos or refuses to participate in the use of placebos outside the context of an IRB-approved clinical trial. Other guidelines for developing a policy may be found in the ASPMN (2004) position paper and in Box 2-2.

Other Hidden Biases and Misconceptions

Biases and misconceptions that lead to inadequate pain management are not new. They are evident in recent history. In the late 1800s, many physicians and scientists believed that cultural and intellectual development were accompanied by increased sensitivity to pain (de Moulin, 1979). In 1892, Mitchell said, "The savage does not feel pain as we do." Mitchell suggested that increased capacity for feeling pain began at the end of the 18th century. Van den Berg (1963) was more exact, stating that pain sensitivity increased between 1780 and 1845. Racial and class prejudices were also apparent. In the Old South of the 1700s and 1800s, black people were considered insensitive to pain and underwent limb amputation without anesthesia. However, upper-class white women were believed to have "delicate nerves," and the same surgeon would use ether or chloroform to deliver a baby (Pernick, 1985). No doubt many of these physicians believed that they were practicing medicine in professionally and ethically acceptable ways. Clinicians today probably believe the same thing about their clinical practices, but what will be said of our pain management in the year 2099?

Do we know when our biases are showing? Following is a brief overview of research findings related to some biases that are likely to escape conscious awareness but influence clinical practice:

- *Physical appearance.* Physicians infer more pain in unattractive patients and in those who express pain (e.g., by facial expression); they infer less pain in attractive patients and in those who do not express pain (Hadjistavropoulos, Ross, von Baeyer, 1990).
- *Gender.* Most studies seem to show that women are more likely to be undertreated for pain than are men. Workups by physicians in response to five common types of pain, including back pain, headache, and chest pain, were found to be significantly more extensive in men than in women (Armitage, Schneiderman, Bass, 1979). In a study of cancer patients, inadequate pain management was more likely in females than in males (Cleeland, Gonin, Hatfield, et al., 1994). In a study of differences between patients and physicians in their assessment of pain intensity in an ED, patients and physicians rated pain on arrival and on discharge from the ED (Marquie, Raufaste, Lauque, et al., 2003). Gender played a complex role, but one finding was that male physicians rated the pain of female patients as being less than that of male patients when the cause of pain was obvious. Using vignettes of patients with surgical pain, nurses' medication choices for men and women were compared, revealing that nurses were significantly more likely to undertreat pain in women than in men (Cohen, 1980). In a survey of 368 physicians in Michigan, using vignettes of patients with pain, significantly more physicians chose optimal pain treatment for men than they did for women (Green, Wheeler, 2003). Physicians more frequently chose the optimal pain management response for men undergoing prostatectomy (56.2%) than for women following myomectomy (42%) and following cesarean section (44.5%). They also chose the optimal pain management response more frequently for metastatic prostate cancer (16.3%) than for metastatic breast cancer (10.7%) However, gender biases are not always predictable. In one study of patients with persistent nonmalignant pain, men were no more likely than women to receive opioids (Turk, Okifuji, 1997).

The gender of the clinicians may further complicate assessment. In one laboratory study, men reported significantly less pain to female experimenters than to male experimenters (Levine, De Simone, 1991). In another experimental study, volunteer subjects tolerated pain longer when they were tested by an experimenter of the opposite sex (Kallai, Barke, Voss, 2004).

- *Age.* In a study of 56 men who were 65 or older and undergoing major elective surgery, 16 received no parenteral postoperative analgesics (Short, Burnett, Egbert, et al., 1990). On the basis of vignette research, reports of severe pain are more likely to be accepted from elderly than from young-adult patients, but the elderly are less likely to receive adequate doses of opioid analgesics (McCaffery, Ferrell, 1991b). In a study of 1492 nursing homes, data from 13,625 patients with cancer who were 65 or older revealed that 4003 reported daily pain and more than 25% of them received no analgesic. One of the risk factors for failing to receive any analgesic included being 85 years old or older (Bernabei, Gambassi, Lapane, et al., 1998). In a study of 1360 patients admitted to the ED with documented pain, patients older than 50 years were half as likely to receive analgesia as were younger patients (Heins, Grammas, Heins, et al., 2006). The undertreatment of older patients continued with regard to discharge analgesics.
- *Race/culture.* Racial and ethnic minorities are at high risk for receiving inadequate pain relief. A longitudinal study that took place between 1993 and 2005 analyzed data from the National Hospital Ambulatory Medicine Care Survey and showed that the number of patients who received opioids to manage pain increased steadily and significantly (Pletcher, Kertesz, Kohn, et al., 2008). However, the use of opioids in nonwhites and Hispanics lagged behind that in whites. For the 13-year period, the overall rate of opioid use was 31% for whites, 23% for blacks, 24% for Hispanics, and 28% for Asians and others. In 2005, the rate for whites was 40% but was 32% for all others. In a survey of an ED in a large teaching hospital, Hispanic patients were twice as likely as non-Hispanic whites to receive *no* analgesia (Todd, Samaroo, Hoffman, 1993). In a later study of ED practices, 90 white and 127 black patients with extremity fractures were compared regarding the likelihood of their receiving analgesics, and the findings were similar, with 74% of whites and 57% of blacks receiving analgesics, despite similar reports of pain in their medical records (Todd, Deaton, D'Adamo, et al., 2000). In other words, disparities in the prescription of analgesics could not be attributed to differences in pain assessments. In a study to determine whether differences in waiting times for pain treatment in

EDs existed in adults of ethnic and minority groups suffering from long-bone fractures, 234 European-American, African-American, and Hispanic patients were included (Epps, Ware, Packard, 2008). All reported substantial pain caused by long-bone fractures, but a significant difference in waiting times was found between Hispanic and European-American patients; Hispanic patients waited an average of 102 minutes for the first dose of analgesic, and European-Americans waited an average of 67 minutes, a 35-minute difference. The African-American group was too small for any conclusions to be drawn about that group. These last two studies clearly indicate that assessment is not enough and, indeed, that patients' reports of pain might not be accepted by clinicians. Hence, pain relief is not forthcoming or is delayed. In a study of outpatients with metastatic cancer who were treated at 54 locations, patients seen at centers treating predominantly minorities were three times more likely than those treated elsewhere to have received inadequate pain management (Cleeland, Gonin, Hatfield, et al., 1994). In other words, in centers treating predominantly minorities, cancer patients were found to be three times more likely to have inadequate pain management (Cleeland, Gonin, Hatfield, et al., 1994). In a study of outpatients with cancer pain, 65% of minority patients did not receive appropriate analgesic prescriptions for their pain, compared with 50% of nonminority patients (Cleeland, Gonin, Baez, et al., 1997). Hispanic patients, in particular, were less likely to experience adequate analgesia. In a study of 454 patients with postoperative pain who were receiving IV PCA opioids, the amount of opioid prescribed for Asians, blacks, Hispanics, and whites differed, with blacks and whites being prescribed more analgesic than Hispanics. No differences were found among these groups as to the amount of opioid self-administered (Ng, Dimsdale, Rollnik, et al., 1996).

A review of the literature concerning studies of racial disparities in pain management acknowledged that disparities do exist but that the magnitude of the disparities was, for the most part, small (Ezenwa, Ameringer, Ward, et al., 2006).

- *Personal experience with pain.* In a study of vignette descriptions of patients, nurses who had experienced intense pain inferred higher levels of pain in patients than did nurses who had not experienced intense pain (Holm, Cohen, Dudas, et al., 1989). By contrast, a study of 29 nurses who had not undergone any surgery and 33 who had undergone surgery found that nurses who had not experienced wound pain resulting from surgery estimated the intensity of wound pain to be higher than did those who had experienced surgical wound pain (Ketovuori, 1987).

A study of nurses, physicians, and medical and nursing students in medical centers in Israel were given questionnaires that elicited demographic information along with whether or not they had consumed opioids (Pud, 2004). Those who had consumed opioids considered pain management a lower priority than did the group that had not consumed opioids.

- *"Irresponsible" lifestyle.* In a vignette survey, 452 nurses' answers about assessments and analgesic choices for patients described as risk takers, consumers of alcohol, or unemployed were compared with their responses to patients described as typically middle class (McCaffery, Ferrell, O'Neil-Page, 1992). The nurses said they themselves would provide the same care for both kinds of patients, but they believed their colleagues would treat the patients differently, tending to disbelieve and undertreat the "irresponsible" patients. Nurses revealed that they did not want personal values to interfere with their quality of care, but that they needed assistance (e.g., permission to say they do not like a certain patient and discussion about how to prevent this from interfering with care).

In a study of 167 nurses working in the medical-surgical and critical care units and in EDs, two vignettes were used to determine whether the level of social acceptability of a patient's behavior at the time of injury would affect pain management (Hazelett, Powell, Androulakakis, 2002). In one vignette, the patient injured himself while playing football with his son. In the other vignette, the patient injured himself while driving intoxicated, a less socially acceptable behavior. The vignettes were randomly distributed, and each nurse received one vignette. Significantly more nurses would have correctly increased the dose of morphine for the patient who had injured himself playing football with his son compared with the patient who had injured himself while driving intoxicated.

Conclusion

The preceding discussion of biases, misconceptions, and misunderstandings that cause clinicians to doubt a patient's report of pain and refuse to take action to relieve pain covers only a few of the many misunderstandings that may lead to inadequate pain management. Some of them are well hidden from consciousness and very difficult to correct. It is, therefore, foolish to believe that we provide an equally high quality of care for all of our patients who are experiencing pain, regardless of our personal values, preferences, or painful experiences. No doubt all of us have conscious and unconscious biases and misconceptions that may adversely affect the care we provide for patients with pain.

This sounds like a harsh judgment of humankind, but it may be true. A veritable mountain of literature published during the past three decades attests to the undertreatment of pain. Much of this literature is consistent with the hypothesis that human beings, including health care providers in all societies, have strong tendencies or motivations to deny or discount pain, especially severe pain, and to avoid relieving the pain. Certainly we should struggle to identify and correct personal tendencies that lead to inadequate pain management, but this may not be a battle that can be won. Perhaps it is best to assume that there are far too many biases to overcome and that the best strategy is to establish policies and procedures that protect patients and ourselves from being victims of these influences. The next chapter includes some simple tools that can be made mandatory in clinical practice as some ways to hold clinicians accountable for assessing and treating pain.

Chapter 3 Assessment Tools

T RADITIONALLY, asking patients about pain has been avoided. The fear of causing pain by suggesting the possibility of pain and the fear of increasing pain by focusing the patient's attention on it are but a few of the reasons given for not discussing pain. However, no studies have shown that asking the patient about pain increases pain. A literature review concluded that when patients attend to and rate their pain levels, it usually lowers, not raises, their pain levels (Cruise, Broderick, Porter, et al., 1996). To explore this result, these researchers asked patients with chronic rheumatoid arthritis (RA) to complete pain diaries for 1 week, rating their pain and mood seven times a day. The findings did not indicate that this intense self-assessment of pain increased pain, but pain was not lessened either.

Perhaps questioning the patient about pain also has been avoided because it might identify a pain problem that the clinician did not know how to handle or was fearful of relieving. The clinician might fear that opioids would be necessary and that use of them would cause addiction or death by respiratory depression. "How are you feeling today?" is still about as close as many clinicians get to assessing pain. As one nurse explained, "I find it hard to talk about pain. I think it's the fear of stirring something up. . . . If you're really going to talk about pain, you have to be able to handle things properly" (de Schepper, Francke, Abu-Saad, 1997, p. 425).

Thus, routine assessment of pain is a relatively new idea and is recognized as being essential in the prevention of inadequate pain relief. The following material presents practical tools for initial and ongoing assessments that may be used to facilitate regular pain assessment in a variety of clinical settings.

Tools for Initial Pain Assessment

Nursing Admission Assessment

When patients are admitted to a health care facility, such as a hospital or an outpatient clinic, nurses perform general admission assessments. Along with such information as the patient's self-care abilities and nutritional needs, a section should be included to identify pain problems. Patients may have chronic pain conditions for which they are already receiving treatment, or pain may be the primary reason for admission. Examples of questions that are appropriate for routine admission assessments are shown in Box 3-1.

The purpose of these questions is to identify new or ongoing pain problems. If a pain problem is ongoing and the patient already has an effective pain treatment plan, steps should be taken to ensure that the plan is

Box 3-1 Questions about Pain to Be Included in the Routine Nursing Admission Assessment

1. Do you have any ongoing pain problems? ___ Yes ___ No

2. Do you have pain now? ___ Yes ___ No

If yes to either of the above:

3. Location of pain: 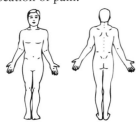 _____ (body figure drawing similar to the one in Form 3-1 may be included on the assessment form to mark the location of pain)

4. Pain intensity on a scale of 0 to 10: Now: _____ On average (usual): _____

5. What, if any, medications do you take for pain relief?

6. What, if any, other treatment do you receive for your pain?

7. Is your pain satisfactorily controlled now?

Note: If a pain problem is identified and is not under satisfactory control, completion of a more comprehensive pain assessment tool, such as Form 3-1 or 3-2, may be indicated.
From Pasero, C., & McCaffery, M. *Pain assessment and pharmacologic management*, p. 50, St. Louis, Mosby. © 2011, McCaffery M, Pasero C. May be duplicated for use in clinical practice.

continued. If a treatment plan must be developed, further assessments using the Initial Pain Assessment Tool (Form 3-1, p. 51) or the Brief Pain Inventory (BPI; Form 3-2, p. 53) may be indicated.

Tools for Initial Overall Pain Assessment

Two tools widely used for overall initial pain assessments are referred to as Initial Pain Assessment Tool (see Form 3-1) and the BPI (see Form 3-2). Both of these were included in the cancer pain clinical guidelines published by the Agency for Health Policy and Research (Jacox, Carr, Payne, et al., 1994a), and the BPI is included in the revised cancer pain guidelines published by APS (Miaskowski, Cleary, Burney, et al., 2005). The patient or the clinician may complete these tools. Another over-

all pain assessment tool often used in research and clinical practice is the short-form McGill Pain Questionnaire (Melzack, 1987).

These pain assessment tools need not be used for all patients with pain. The policies and procedures of a health care agency must identify the criteria necessary for these tools to be considered. Certainly if the patient has chronic pain problems that are not satisfactorily controlled, an overall pain assessment tool should be completed. Hospices and pain treatment centers may need far more extensive initial overall assessment tools than those offered here. For patients with acute pain that is not easily controlled by the usual pain treatments (e.g., intravenous patient-controlled analgesia [IV PCA] following surgery), an overall assessment also is indicated.

Both the Initial Pain Assessment Tool and the BPI, described later, attempt to assess some aspects of suffering. Suffering, like pain, is subjective, but it goes beyond simply feeling pain. Pain may exist without suffering. Suffering eludes definition but has been characterized as an individual's experience of threat to self, a meaning given to events such as pain or loss (Kahn, Steeves, 1996). Suffering involves the person's evaluations of the significance or meaning of pain (Spross, 1993). To some extent, suffering is similar to an impairment in quality of life. Items on the assessment tools directed at the effects of pain on various aspects of living are an attempt to assess some aspects of the patient's suffering.

Initial Pain Assessment Tool

The Initial Pain Assessment Tool (Form 3-1) may be completed by the patient or used to guide the clinician in collecting information about the patient's pain. A discussion of each assessment point follows.

1. *Location of pain.* This is most easily and quickly accomplished by asking the patient to mark the location on the figure drawings. Alternately, the clinician may ask the patient to point to the locations of pain on his or her own bodies, and the clinician can mark figure drawings. If there is more than one site of pain, letters (A, B, C, etc.) may be used to distinguish the various sites. These letters may be used in answering the remainder of the questions.

2. *Intensity.* The pain rating scale used by the patient is identified. The patient is asked to rate pain intensity for present pain, worst pain, the least pain felt, and comfort-function goals (pain rating that will not interfere with necessary or desired functioning, such as ambulation and decreased anxiety). If the patient has more than one site of pain, the letter designations mentioned simplify recording. For example, for present pain intensity, the recording might be A = 4, B = 6. A time period may be specified for answering

Initial Pain Assessment Tool

Date _____

Patient's Name _____ Age _____ Room _____

Diagnosis _____ Physician _____

Nurse _____

1. LOCATION: Patient or nurse mark drawing.

2. INTENSITY: Patient rates the pain. Scale used _____

Present pain: _____   Worst pain gets: _____   Best pain gets: _____   Comfort-Function goal: _____

3. IS THIS PAIN CONSTANT? _____ YES; _____ NO
IF NOT, HOW OFTEN DOES IT OCCUR? _____

4. QUALITY: (For example: ache, deep, sharp, hot, cold, like sensitive skin, sharp, itchy) _____

5. ONSET, DURATION, VARIATIONS, RHYTHMS: _____

6. MANNER OF EXPRESSING PAIN: _____

7. WHAT RELIEVES THE PAIN? _____

8. WHAT CAUSES OR INCREASES THE PAIN? _____

9. EFFECTS OF PAIN: (Note decreased function, decreased quality of life.)
Accompanying symptoms (e.g., nausea) _____
Sleep _____
Appetite _____
Physical activity _____
Relationship with others (e.g., irritability) _____
Emotions (e.g., anger, suicidal, crying) _____
Concentration _____
Other _____

10. OTHER COMMENTS: _____

11. PLAN: _____

Form 3-1 | May be completed by patients or used by clinicians to interview patients.

From Pasero, C., & McCaffery, M. *Pain assessment and pharmacologic management*, p. 51, St. Louis, Mosby. © 2011, Pasero C, McCaffery M. May be duplicated for use in clinical practice.

the next questions about pain intensity. For example, worst pain intensity may be asked in relation to the past 24 hours or the past week.

3. *Is this pain constant? If not, how often does it occur?* These questions help screen for the presence of breakthrough pain (BTP), defined as a transitory increase in pain that occurs on a background of otherwise controlled chronic pain. If the patient says the pain is constant, this rules out BTP. But if the patient say the pain is not constant, further questioning is indicated, specifically asking the patient whether there are temporary flares of pain that are more intense than the constant pain. The Screening Tool for Pain Flares—Breakthrough Pain, Form 3-6 (p. 103), and the Assessment of Pain Flares—Breakthrough Pain, Form 3-7 (p. 104), may be helpful. Roughly 50% or more of patients with chronic, constant pain also have BTP that might be overlooked.

4. *Quality of pain.* This information is helpful in diagnosing the underlying pain mechanism. Soreness is commonly more likely to be indicative of somatic pain, whereas burning or knifelike pain is more likely to be indicative of neuropathic pain. This information may have direct implications for the type of pain treatment chosen. For example, an anticonvulsant (an adjuvant analgesic; see Section V) may be indicated for knifelike pain. One study found that the quality of pain seemed to cluster in three groups: (1) paroxysmal pain sensations, such as shooting, sharp, and radiating pains; (2) superficial pain, such as itchy, cold, sensitive, and tingling pains; and (3) deep pain, such as aching, dull, cramping, and throbbing pain (Victor, Jensen, Gammaitoni, et al., 2008).

   If the patient has difficulty describing pain, the clinician should ask the patient about the appropriateness of possible descriptors, such as throbbing, shooting, sharp, cramping, aching, tender, pricking, burning, or pulling. For the patient who continues to have difficulty, try asking him or her, "What could you do to me to make me feel the pain you have?"

5. *Onset, duration, variations, rhythms.* To detect variations and rhythms, ask the patient, "When did this pain begin?" "Is the pain better or worse at certain times, certain hours of the day or night, or certain times of the month?"

6. *Manner of expressing pain.* Ask the patient if he or she is hesitant or embarrassed to discuss the pain or whether the patient tries to hide it from others. Ask the patient if using the pain rating scale is acceptable.

7. *What relieves the pain?* If the patient has had pain for a while, he or she may know which medications and doses are helpful and may have found some nondrug methods, such as cold packs, helpful. If appropriate, these methods should be continued.

8. *What causes or increases the pain?* A variety of activities, body positions, and other events may increase pain, and efforts can be made to avoid them or to provide additional analgesia at those times.

9. *Effects of pain.* These items help to identify how pain affects the patient's quality of life and how pain interferes with recovery from illness. Information obtained in this section may be useful in developing pain management goals. If pain interferes with sleep, a major goal may be to identify a pain rating that will allow the patient to sleep through the night without being awakened by pain.

10. *Other comments.* No tool is comprehensive. This space simply allows for information the patient may wish to add.

11. *Plan.* Immediate and long-range plans can be mentioned here and developed in greater detail as time passes.

Brief Pain Inventory

The BPI (Form 3-2, p. 53) is a 9-item tool that gathers information about pain severity and rates level of pain interference with seven key areas of function. Regular use of this tool helps track progress in treating pain intensity and degree of pain interference with general activity, mood, walking ability, normal work (both work outside the home and house work), relations with other people, sleep, and enjoyment of life. The BPI is relatively short and easy for patients to complete, taking about 10 to 15 minutes. It has been used successfully with older adults (Ersek, Turner, Cain, et al., 2004; Kemp, Ersek, Turner, 2005).

The BPI assessment tool has been used extensively in research too. It has reasonable validity and reliability (Daut, Cleeland, 1982; Daut, Cleeland, Flanery, 1983) and has proven useful in a variety of clinical settings (Cleeland, Gonin, Hatfield, et al., 1994). The BPI has been translated into other languages, including Japanese (Uki, Mendoza, Cleeland, et al., 1998); Vietnamese (Cleeland, Ladinsky, Serlin, et al., 1988); Chinese (Wang, Mendoza, Gao, et al., 1996); the Philippine language (Cleeland, Nakamura, Mendoza, et al., 1996); Russian (Kalyadina, Ionova, Ivanova, et al., 2008); and French (Serlin, Mendoza, Nakamura, et al., 1995). The BPI has been shown to be reliable and valid in several patient populations, such as patients with cancer pain (Cleeland, Gonin, Hatfield, 1994) and with chronic noncancer pain (Tan, Jensen, Thornby, et al., 2004); in patients 6 months after cardiac surgery (Gjeilo, Stenseth, Wahba, et al., 2007); and in Canadian veterans with pain who are suffering from traumatic stress (Poundja, Fikretoglu, Guay, et al., 2007). A modified version of the BPI has been validated in patients with painful diabetic peripheral neuropathy (Zelman, Gore, Dukes, et al., 2005).

Brief Pain Inventory

Date ____ / ____ / ____   Time: _____

Name: _____ _____ _____
           Last   First   Middle Initial

1) Throughout our lives, most of us have had pain from time to time (such as minor headaches, sprains, and toothaches). Have you had pain other than these everyday kinds of pain today?
   1. Yes   2. No

2) On the diagram, shade in the areas where you feel pain. Put an X on the area that hurts the most.

3) Please rate your pain by circling the one number that best describes your pain at its **worst** in the past 24 hours.

0   1   2   3   4   5   6   7   8   9   10
No   Pain as bad as
pain   you can imagine

4) Please rate your pain by circling the one number that best describes your pain at its **least** in the past 24 hours.

0   1   2   3   4   5   6   7   8   9   10
No   Pain as bad as
pain   you can imagine

5) Please rate your pain by circling the one number that best describes your pain on the **average**.

0   1   2   3   4   5   6   7   8   9   10
No   Pain as bad as
pain   you can imagine

6) Please rate your pain by circling the one number that tells how much pain you have **right now**.

0   1   2   3   4   5   6   7   8   9   10
No   Pain as bad as
pain   you can imagine

7) What treatments or medications are you receiving for your pain?

_____

_____

8) In the past 24 hours, how much **relief** have pain treatments or medications provided? Please circle the one percentage that most shows how much relief you have received.

0% 10 20 30 40 50 60 70 80 90 100%
No   Complete
relief   relief

9) Circle the one number that describes how, during the past 24 hours, pain has **interfered** with your:
   A. General activity

0   1   2   3   4   5   6   7   8   9   10
Does not   Completely
interfere   interferes

   B. Mood

0   1   2   3   4   5   6   7   8   9   10
Does not   Completely
interfere   interferes

   C. Walking ability

0   1   2   3   4   5   6   7   8   9   10
Does not   Completely
interfere   interferes

   D. Normal work (includes both work outside the home and housework)

0   1   2   3   4   5   6   7   8   9   10
Does not   Completely
interfere   interferes

   E. Relations with other people

0   1   2   3   4   5   6   7   8   9   10
Does not   Completely
interfere   interferes

   F. Sleep

0   1   2   3   4   5   6   7   8   9   10
Does not   Completely
interfere   interferes

   G. Enjoyment of life

0   1   2   3   4   5   6   7   8   9   10
Does not   Completely
interfere   interferes

Form 3-2

From Pasero, C., & McCaffery, M. *Pain assessment and pharmacologic management*, p. 53, St. Louis, Mosby. © 2011, Pasero C, McCaffery M. May be duplicated for use in clinical practice.

Questions on the BPI focus on pain during the past 24 hours.

- Question 1 asks if the patient has experienced pain other than common everyday kinds of pain and if the patient has experienced that pain today.
- Question 2 asks the patient to identify the location of that pain in the figure drawing.
- Questions 3 through 6 ask the patient to use a pain rating scale of 0 to 10 to rate pain at its worst and least in the past 24 hours and its intensity on average and right now.
- Question 7 asks about treatment or medication the patient is receiving for pain.
- Question 8 asks the percentage of pain relief provided by these treatments.
- Question 9 has seven parts that attempt to identify how much pain has interfered with the patient's life, including general activity, mood, work, sleep, and enjoyment of life.

Pain Intensity Rating Scales

Pain intensity rating scales used in daily clinical practice deal with how much pain the patient is feeling. When a patient uses the scale to report pain, it is called a self-report scale. Numerous self-report scales for measuring pain intensity exist. They have been referred to by many different names, but often each scale has no standardized title or definition. No "best" scale exists, but some are more practical and more widely used in clinical practice than others. Following is a discussion of criteria for selecting pain rating scales for daily clinical practice and a discussion of the visual analogue scale (VAS) and specific pain rating scales appropriate for clinical use in assessing pain intensity in cognitively intact adolescents, adults, and older persons. Later in this chapter, tools for assessing patients who have difficulty with the commonly used self-report scales or who are unable to self-report are discussed.

Criteria for Selecting Pain Rating Scales for Use in Daily Clinical Practice

Criteria for selecting self-report pain rating scales for use in daily clinical practice are summarized in Box 3-2. Most important, the pain rating scale selected must have been tested and found to be reliable and valid. Reliability means that the scale consistently measures pain intensity from one time to the next, and validity means that the scale accurately measures pain intensity. Probably the most fundamental aspect of validity for pain rating scales is that they demonstrate sensitivity to changes in the magnitude of pain (Herr, Spratt, Garand, et al., 2007). For example, they must be sensitive enough to measure effects of analgesic medication. (For more detailed infor-

GUIDELINES

Box 3-2 Selecting a Pain Rating Scale for Use in Daily Clinical Practice

Research has established that the tool is:
- Reasonably valid and reliable.
- Developmentally appropriate. Some scales commonly used with adults (e.g., 0-to-10 scale) are clearly inappropriate for use with children who cannot count. On the other hand, some scales, such as the Faces Pain Scale-Revised (FPS-R) that are appropriate for young children may be appropriate for any age group, especially cognitively impaired patients.
- Easily and quickly understood by patients who have minimal formal education.
- Well liked by patients.
- Well liked by clinicians.
- Not burdensome on clinicians.
- Quickly explained.
- Easily scored and recorded.
- Easily used with patients to set pain management goals (i.e., comfort-function goals).
- Inexpensive.
- Easily disinfected (or inexpensive enough to discard, e.g., scales that are photocopied).
- Readily available. Multiple copies are easily and inexpensively made for distribution to clinicians, patients, and their families.
- Appropriate for patients of different cultures.
- Available in various languages spoken in the clinical setting (or may be translated easily).

As appears in Pasero, C., & McCaffery, M. (2011). *Pain assessment and pharmacologic management*, p. 54, St. Louis, Mosby. Modified from Hester, N. O. (1995). Integrating pain assessment and management into the care of children with cancer. In D. B. McGuire, C. H. Yarbro, & B. R. Ferrell (Eds). *Cancer pain management*, Boston, Jones and Bartlett. May be duplicated for use in clinical practice.

mation about the reliability and validity of a variety of pain measures, refer to Jensen [2003] and Herr, Spratt, Mobily, et al. [2004]).

Usually the main purpose of using pain rating scales in clinical practice is to identify the intensity of pain over time for the purpose of evaluating the effectiveness of interventions to relieve pain. Scales used to obtain self-reports of pain intensity fail to provide other information that is important to assessing pain and determining pain treatment. This is one of the reasons for remembering to use the Initial Pain Assessment Tool (see Form 3-1) or the Brief Pain Inventory (see Form 3-2).

Certain open-ended questions are also used in addition to the pain rating scale. Research with older adults (N = 312) has shown that an open-ended pain question such as "Tell me about your pain, aches, soreness, or discomfort" when initiating pain assessment discussions provided significantly more pain information than asking the patient to rate his or her pain or simply asking "How are you feeling?" (McDonald, Shea, Rose, et al., 2009). The latter question resulted in the least amount of information about pain. Thus, clinicians should be aware that simply asking a patient to rate the intensity of pain provides useful but not complete information about important aspects of the pain and the implications for treatment.

Unfortunately, pain rating scales seem to invite creativity. Sometimes colors are added to a preexisting scale such that different colors are used to indicate different intensities of pain, or colors are added to a faces scale. Some of the problems with this practice are that some health care facilities do not have copiers that duplicate in color and that research into colors as indicators of pain intensity is limited. Colors are subject to personal preferences and cultural differences and are best avoided. Another change to a preexisting valid and reliable scale is drawing hats on a faces rating scale. When a validated and reliable scale is changed in any of these ways, additional research is required to establish the reliability and validity of the new scale. Sometimes clinicians develop and use an entirely new scale without testing it for reliability and validity. Such energy is better spent on promoting the routine use of a single, simple pain rating scale that has already been established as being valid and reliable.

As stated in Box 3-2, the tool also should be sufficiently graded so it can capture changes in pain intensity and should be easily understood, easy to score, and liked by patients and staff. The tool should place a low burden on staff; that is, it should be quickly explainable and easily scored. It should also be inexpensive and easy to duplicate. The tool should also be appropriate for patients of various cultures and available in several languages.

Visual Analogue Scale

The tool that is probably used most frequently in research but is inappropriate for clinical use is the VAS. It is difficult to say how long pain rating scales have been used, but the VAS has been used for assessment of subjective

phenomena such as loudness of a sound for more than 80 years (Freyd, 1923; Hayes, Patterson, 1921). At some point the VAS began to be used in pain research, and it is a reliable and valid instrument (Huskisson, 1974; Jenson, Karoly, 2001).

Currently, the term *VAS* is used loosely and inaccurately to refer to several different pain intensity scales such as the Numerical Rating Scale (NRS). However, the VAS has a fairly precise definition as a horizontal (sometimes vertical) 10-cm line (100 mm) with word anchors at the extremes, such as "no pain" on one end and "pain as bad as it could be" on the other end (Figure 3-1). The patient is asked to make a mark on the line to represent pain intensity. In this manual, the term *VAS* refers only to a horizontal or vertical straight line with word anchors at the ends.

Probably because the VAS is reliable and valid and is commonly used in research, it is sometimes used in clinical practice. However, it has several disadvantages in that setting. Although the VAS is usually easy to administer (unless the patient has an injury to the arm or hand or is lying down) and easy to reproduce, scoring is time consuming. As mentioned, the patient is asked to mark the line to indicate the level of pain. A number is then obtained by measuring in millimeters up to the point the patient has indicated. Also, without specific numbers being arranged along the VAS line, it is difficult to use the scale to discuss pain rating goals with the patient, especially over the telephone. Further, patients tend to have more difficulty understanding and using a VAS than the other scales such as the NRS (Herr, Spratt, Mobily, et al., 2004; Jensen, Karoly, 1992; Peters, Patijn, Lame, 2007). In research comparing the VAS with the verbal descriptor scale (VDS) and with 11-point and 21-point numeric box scales, patients made more mistakes using the VAS (Peters, Patijn, Lame, 2007). (A box scale shows connected boxes along a vertical or horizontal line with numbers in the boxes, such as 0 to 10 or 0 to 20. Figure 3-2 is an example.)

Recommended Pain Intensity Rating Scales

After we (the authors) considered a wide array of pain intensity rating scales, the self-report scales we now recommend for use in clinical practice with cognitively intact adolescents, adults, and older adults consist of the NRS plus a faces pain rating scale (Box 3-3). This gives the patient a choice of using either the NRS or a faces scale. Some patients are

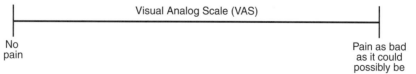

Figure 3-1 | This horizontal visual analog scale (VAS) for rating pain intensity is a 10-cm line with word anchors. Patients are asked to mark the line. Although the VAS is frequently used in research, it is not recommended for clinical practice because scoring is time-consuming.

No pain	0	1	2	3	4	5	6	7	8	9	10	Worst pain

Figure 3-2 | Horizontal 0-to-10 box scale.

From Pasero, C., McCaffery, M. *Pain assessment and pharmacologic management*, p. 56, St. Louis, Mosby. The scale is in the public domain. May be duplicated for use in clinical practice.

Box 3-3 | Recommended Pain Intensity Rating Scales for Clinical Practice

1. Numerical Rating Scale (NRS) using 0 to 10 (0 = no pain; 10 = worst possible pain) presented visually. Patients are asked to report a number or mark the scale. *OR:*
2. The NRS combined with one of the following:
   - Wong-Baker FACES Pain Rating Scale (FACES). *OR:*
   - Faces Pain Scale-Revised (FPS-R), again using 0 to 10 to represent the faces.

From Pasero, C., & McCaffery, M. *Pain assessment and pharmacologic management*, p. 56, St. Louis, Mosby. © 2011, Pasero C, McCaffery M. May be duplicated for use in clinical practice.

---

unable to understand the NRS but are able to use one of the faces scales. Other patients simply do not like the NRS. For example, in a study of 267 hospitalized patients ranging in age from 16 to 91 years, almost half preferred the Wong-Baker FACES Pain Rating Scale (FACES) to the 0 to 10 NRS or the VAS (Carey, Turpin, Smith, et al., 1997).

Specifically, we suggest a horizontal NRS using 0 to 10 (0 = no pain; 10 = worst possible pain) presented visually. The patient is asked to report a number or mark the scale. Or the patient may choose a faces scale. We recommend that the NRS be combined with either (a) the Wong-Baker FACES Pain Rating Scale (FACES), using 0 to 10 to represent the 6 faces; or (b) the Faces Pain Scale-Revised (FPS-R), again using 0 to 10 to represent the 6 faces (Figures 3-3 and 3-4). No single-word anchor has been identified as being the best one for the number 10 on the 0 to 10 scale. Examples of word anchors that have been used fairly frequently are "worst imaginabale pain," "worst possible pain," "most intense pain imaginable," "terrible pain," and "pain as bad as it can be."

Numerical Rating Scale. The NRS is sometimes presented as a 0 to 5 scale or as a vertical line, but in this manual, unless otherwise specified, NRS refers to a 0 to 10 horizontal scale with numbers between 0 and 10. Although occasionally the 0 to 5 scale is appropriate for patients who are unable to comprehend more items on a scale, the 0 to 10 is now widely accepted. In a survey of health care professionals that asked them which scale they preferred for use in clinical practice, the majority (70%) favored 0 to 10 (von Baeyer, Hicks, 2000). Regarding use of the horizontal line, it is worth noting that research indicates that the vertical VAS may be more

Pain Scales Combined: NRS + FACES

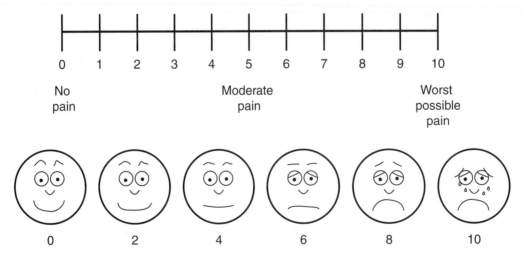

Figure 3-3 | Example of how the Numerical Rating Scale (NRS) can be combined with the Wong-Baker FACES Pain Rating (FACES) in a horizontal format with a 0-to-10 metric and placed on the same paper or card to present to patients. They have a choice of pain rating scales. If the NRS is not easily understood, the FACES scale is an alternative.

From Hockenberry, M. J., Wilson, D., & Winkelstein, M. L. (2005). *Wong's essentials of pediatric nursing*, ed 7, St Louis, Mosby, p. 1259. Used with permission. From Pasero, C., & McCaffery, M. (2011). *Pain assessment and pharmacologic management*, p. 56, St. Louis, Mosby. Permission to use the FACES scale for purposes other than clinical practice can be obtained at http://www.us.elsevierhealth.com/FACES/. The NRS is in the public domain. May be duplicated for use in clinical practice.

Pain Scales Combined: NRS + FPS-R

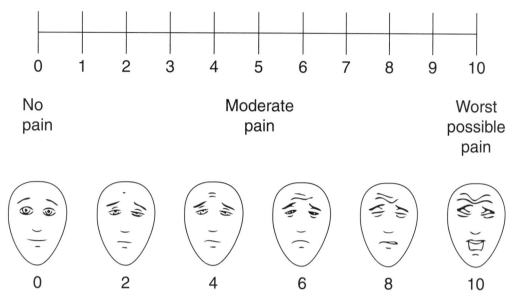

Figure 3-4 | Example of how the Numerical Rating Scale (NRS) can be combined with the FPS-R in a horizontal format with a 0-to-10 metric and placed on the same paper or card to present to patients. Patients have a choice of pain rating scales. If the NRS is not easily understood, the FPS-R scale is an alternative.

sensitive and easier for patients to use, especially patients who are under the stress of having a narrowed visual field (Gift, 1989; Gift, Plaut, Jacox, 1986). Further, some research has found that the vertical format may be more easily understood by older persons (Herr, Garand, 2001; Herr, Mobily, 1993). Therefore, the vertical NRS (Figure 3-5, *A*) may be advisable for some patient populations or may be presented as an alternative to patients who have difficulty with the horizontal scale (Figure 3-5, *B*).

The reliability and validity of the 0 to 10 NRS are well established (Jensen, Karoly, 1992). Other major strengths of the 0 to 10 NRS are that most patients and clinicians are familiar with it, and it is easily administered. The universal adoption of a 0 to 10 NRS has been promoted for some time (Dalton, McNaull, 1998; Paice, Cohen, 1997; von Baeyer, Hicks, 2000). Also, numeric scales are well liked. In a group of younger adults and a group of older adults, one study compared the VAS, a 21-point numeric rating scale, a verbal descriptor scale, the 11-point (0 to 10) verbally presented numeric rating scale, and a faces pain scale (Herr, Spratt, Mobily, et al., 2004). Both the younger and the older groups preferred the 21-point numeric rating scale. Research conducted with younger and older surgical patients suggests that the 0-10 NRS has good psychometric properties and is the preferred scale when compared to a verbal descriptor scale, a horizontal VAS, and a vertical VAS (Gagliese, Weizblit, Ellis, et al., 2005).

Probably the most frequent way the NRS is presented is verbally, without a visual aid. This method is appealing because, unless the patient's ability to speak is compromised, such as in the presence of an endotracheal tube, the patient can provide verbal responses at any time and in any position and regardless of difficulty in using the arms or hands. However, presentation of the NRS without a visual aid is not recommended because of the high error rate. Research has shown that when the NRS is presented verbally, without a written copy of the scale, patients make more mistakes, such as giving a score higher than 10 or a number between whole numbers (Herr, Spratt, Garand, 2007). However, when a 21-point box scale (numbers in boxes from 0 to 100 in increments of 5) and a verbally administered 0 to 10 box scale were compared, the results supported the validity of a verbally administered 0 to 10 point scale while showing a visual of the box scale, strongly suggesting that the NRS should be shown visually along with asking the patient to verbally rate pain on a 0 to 10 scale (Jensen, Miller, Fisher, 1998).

Therefore, when the NRS is used, every effort should be made to show the patient a copy of the scale. Patient reporting-error rates when using the 0 to 10 NRS in the absence of a visual presentation are sufficiently great for some to suggest that hospitals rethink their choice of using 0 to 10 without a visual aid (Feldt, 2007). Rather than abandoning the highly popular verbally presented 0 to 10 scale, a more practical solution is to make multiple copies of the 0 to 10 NRS along with whichever faces

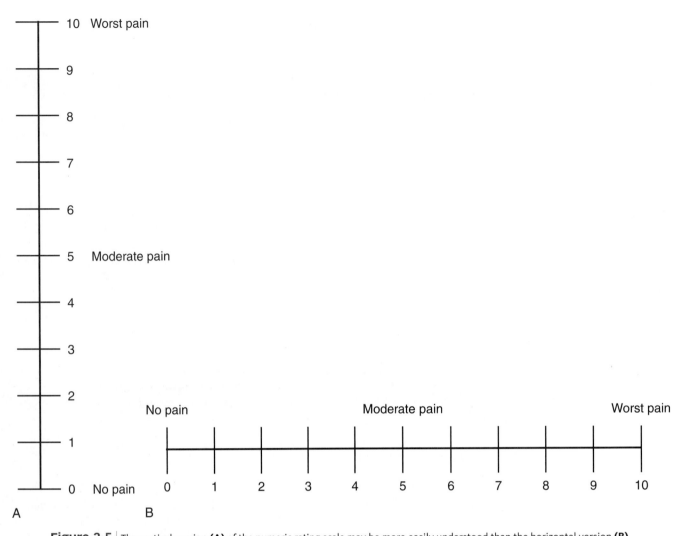

Figure 3-5 | The vertical version **(A)** of the numeric rating scale may be more easily understood than the horizontal version **(B)**.

From Pasero, C., & McCaffery, M. (2011). *Pain assessment and pharmacologic management*, p. 58, St. Louis, Mosby. The scale is in the public domain. May be duplicated for use in clinical practice.

scale is chosen and post them in patients' rooms, clinic areas, treatment rooms and other places where patients and clinicians might discuss pain.

As discussed earlier, pain rating scales seem to invite change and creativity without testing for reliability or validity. One problem with the 0 to 10 self-report scale is that some clinicians try to attach behaviors to each of the numbers. In one study of sedated patients, researchers tried to substitute behaviors for the sedated patients' self-report of pain, overriding the patients' stated pain levels (Salmore, 2002). However, there is no evidence that pain ratings by a sedated patient are less reliable than behaviors. The study in question requires further investigation.

When patients, such as very cognitively impaired patients and unconscious patients, are unable to self-report pain one must begin to rely on known pathology and behavioral indicators (see Box 3-9, p. 123). Otherwise, the gold standard for measuring pain intensity is a self-report, such as a number or word.

Another problem we (the authors) have seen across the United States is clinicians' attaching behaviors to each number on the NRS and asking patients to state a number to indicate their pain levels. These scales are seldom published but are nevertheless used in clinical practice in some institutions. In one example of a 0 to 10 NRS with behaviors attached to each number, the number 5 was accompanied by the statement that pain "can't be ignored for more than 30 minutes." This has not been researched and is negated by the statements of many patients who have practiced learning to ignore pain. This also requires timing how long patients can ignore pain, which is cumbersome, time consuming, and a little on the humorous side. The same scale stated with the number 7 that pain "interferes with sleep," again contradicted by patients who have learned to use sleep as a coping mechanism. (Readers may want to review the section on the acute pain model, presented earlier in this manual, on pp. 28-29). Again, on the humorous side, that same scale stated with the number 10 that "pain makes you pass out." Again, no research substantiates this, and it makes it almost impossible for patients to rate pain as a 10 because they would be unconscious. Patients' behavioral responses vary enormously and cannot be pigeonholed at one particular level of pain. Patients cannot be told how they have to behave in order to rate their pain at a particular level.

A similar problem has arisen with a published functional pain scale (Gloth, Scheve, Stober, et al., 2001). To associate numbers with levels of activity seems like a reasonable way to assess function but not pain. On this scale the number 5 is the highest level of pain, and the behavior listed for 5 is that the pain is so severe that the patient is unable to communicate verbally. Therefore, on this scale, if patients say their pain level is 5, they must reconsider because they are able to communicate that score verbally. Further, it seems somewhat ridiculous to think that patients writhing in pain and rating pain at 5 would not be allowed to do so.

These attempts to assign behaviors to pain levels seem to reflect the desire to make pain levels uniform within and among patients. However, what is a 7 for one patient on a scale of 0 to 10 is not going to be a 7 for all other patients. And a given level of pain that is a 7 for a patient on one day may not be a 7 for that patient the next day. Some patients with chronic pain have commented that as their pain increases over time, what they had considered severe pain is now what they would rate as moderate pain.

One error, mentioned earlier, that is fairly common in research and clinical practice is that some patients select a point between numbers on a 0 to 10 scale, such as 6.5. This deserves some explanation. Although difficult to handle when a computer is programmed to accept only 11 points of scale, a review of research shows that people can actually distinguish among 21 levels of pain (Jensen, Miller, Fisher, 1998). Further, research with older adults that compared a faces scale, a 0 to 5 verbal rating scale, and a vertical and a horizontal 21-point box scale, the horizontal 21-point box scale emerged as the best scale with respect to psychometrics and regardless of mental status (Chibnall, Tait, 2001). But the 0 to 10 scale is well entrenched, and using a 0 to 20 scale in clinical practice does not seem practical at this time. However, even when compared with the VAS, a 21-point box scale may be the instrument of choice for research in mixed populations, such as various levels of cognitive ability (Herr, Spratt, Mobily, et al., 2004; Peters, Patijn, Lame, 2007).

The 0 to 10 NRS has been translated into many languages. A few translations are seen in Figure 3-6 (p. 60). Further, there is preliminary evidence that a 0 to 10 NRS (presented with a visual) has higher reliability in illiterate patients when compared to the VAS or a verbal rating scale (such as no pain, mild, moderate, severe, unbearable) (Ferraz, Quaresma, Aquino, et al., 1990). Results are difficult to generalize because the study was conducted only with Portuguese patients.

Wong-Baker FACES Pain Rating Scale. Work on the Wong-Baker FACES Pain Rating Scale (henceforth referred to as the FACES scale) began in 1981 by Donna

Wong, a nurse consultant, and Connie Morain Baker, a child life specialist, who were working in a burn unit. In 1988, Wong and Baker published a study of 150 children aged 3 to 18 years. The FACES scale was presented in a circular format and was compared to five other scales: (1) a simple descriptive scale with numbers assigned to five adjectives on a horizontal line; (2) a numeric scale with the numbers 0 to 10 on a horizontal line; (3) a five-glasses scale in which the glasses contained varying amounts of water, ranging from no water to a full glass; (4) a chips scale using five white plastic chips; and (5) a color scale that included six colors. This study demonstrated the initial reliability and validity of the FACES scale, and no single scale demonstrated superior validity or reliability. The most preferred scale was the FACES scale. Because the FACES scale was presented in a circular format, the results of this study are difficult to compare with those of the numerous other studies in which these faces and other faces scales are presented to children and adults in a horizontal format. Other information concerning the development of this scale and its use in children is available at http://www.mosbysdrugconsult.com/WOW/faces.html and http://www.mosbysdrugconsult.com/WOW/facesStatisticalAnalysis.html. Unfortunately, several studies of reliability and validity listed at this website are unpublished.

The FACES scale was developed for use with children, but is it appropriate for some adults? Indeed, some studies of adults have revealed that they often prefer the faces scales to other scales. For example, in one study of 267 adults, the FACES, VAS, and NRS were compared, and the FACES was preferred (Carey, Turpin, Smith, et al., 1997). In another study of children and their parents, a comparison of five faces scales revealed that the parents as well as the children preferred the FACES scale (Chambers, Giesbrecht, Craig, et al., 1999). The cartoon-like features of this scale seem to contribute to this preference. The high preference for the FACES scale is one reason for combining the FACES scale with the NRS to give adults a choice in pain rating scales (see Figure 3-3, p. 56). Of the various faces scales, the FACES scale is currently probably the most widely used in both children and adults in the United States.

In a study of 37 older adults in a long-term care facility, some of whom were cognitively impaired and others cognitively intact, pain was assessed using the VAS, VRS, McGill Word Scale (Melzack, 1975), and FACES scale (Wynne, Ling, Remsburg, 2000). The FACES scale was completed by 61% of the participants, the McGill Word Scale by 51%, and the VAS by 57%. Patients with cognitive impairment had more difficulty completing the instruments. Nevertheless, more participants were able to complete the FACES scale than the other scales.

The FACES scale meets many of the criteria for selecting a pain rating scale for use in clinical practice (see Box 3-2, p. 54). The faces do not depict age, gender, or culture. The FACES scale has been translated into several languages (Figure 3-7, pp. 66-67; translations are available at http://www.mosbysdrugconsult.com/WOW/faces Translations.html). It is therefore appropriate

English

Please point to the number that best describes your pain.

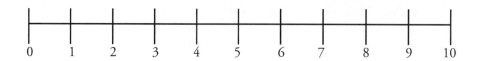

No pain   Terrible pain

Chinese*

請指出那個數字反應你痛的程度.

Please point to the number that best describes your pain.

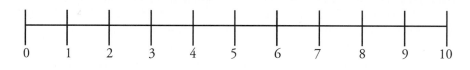

無痛   **劇痛**
No pain   Terrible pain

French†

Veuillez indiquer le chiffre qui décrit le mieux votre douleur.

Please point to the number that best describes your pain.

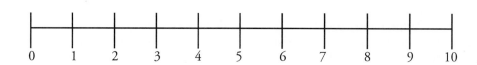

Pas de douleur   **Douleur intense**
No pain   Terrible pain

Continued

Figure 3-6 | Translations of 0-10 numerical rating scale.
*Courtesy of Pain-Management Committee, St. Francis Medical Center, Honolulu, NY.
†Compiled by Josephine Musto, St. Vincent's Hospital and Medical Center, New York, NY.

German[†]

Deuten Sie bitte zu der Zahl, die ihren Schmerzen am besten entspricht.

Please point to the number that best describes your pain.

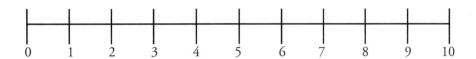

Keine Schmerzen
No pain

Fürchterliche Schmerzen
Terrible pain

Greek (modern)[†]

Παρακαλώ, δείξετε με το δάκτυλό σας τον αριθμό που δείχνει πόσο πόνο έχετε.

Please point to the number that best describes your pain.

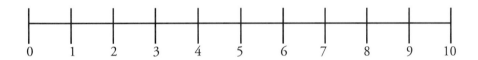

Δεν έχω πόνο
No pain

Ἔχω πολύ πόνο
Terrible pain

Hawaiian*

E ʻoluʻolu e kuhi i ka helu e like me ke ʻano o kou ʻeha.

Please point to the number that best describes your pain.

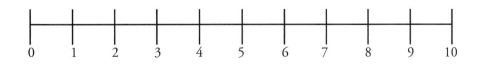

ʻAʻohe ʻeha
No pain

He ʻeha palena ʻole
Terrible pain

Figure 3-6 | Cont'd.

Continued

Hebrew[†]

אנא הצבע על המספר אשר מתאר במדויק- את הכאב.

Please point to the number that best describes your pain.

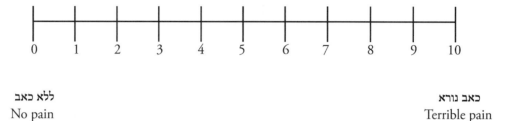

כאב נורא   ללא כאב
Terrible pain   No pain

Ilocano (spoken in the Philippines)[*]

Itudom man iti numero nga mangipakita nu kasano't kasakit iti marikriknam.

Please point to the number that best describes your pain.

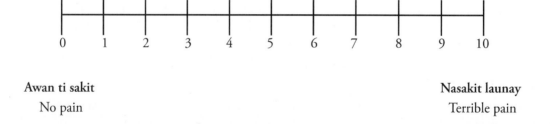

Awan ti sakit   Nasakit launay
No pain   Terrible pain

Italian[*]

Per piacere indica il numero che descrive meglio il tuo dolore.

Please point to the number that best describes your pain.

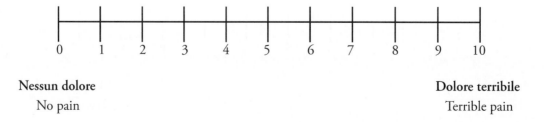

Nessun dolore   Dolore terribile
No pain   Terrible pain

Figure 3-6 | Cont'd.

Continued

Japanese[†]

痛みの強さの度合を0~10までの段階で示して下さい 。

Please point to the number that best describes your pain.

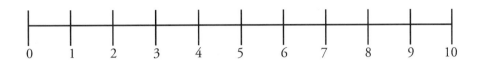

ゼロ　全く痛みがない

No pain

激痛

Terrible pain

Korean

현재 통증의 강도를 가장 잘 나타내는 번호에 표시하십시오.

Please point to the number that best describes your pain.

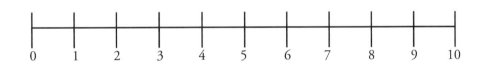

통증이 없음

No pain

통증이 너무 심함

Terrible pain

Urdu (spoken in Pakistan)[†]

برائے مہربانی اس نمبر کی طرف اشارہ کریں جو آپ کے درد کی شدت کو بہتر
طور پر بتلاتا ہے۔

Please point to the number that best describes your pain.

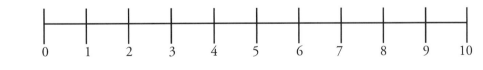

کوئی درد نہیں ہے

No pain

شدید ترین درد ہے

Terrible pain

Figure 3-6 | Cont'd.

Continued

Polish[†]

Proszę wskazać numer, który najlepiej określa jak silny jest ból.

Please point to the number that best describes your pain.

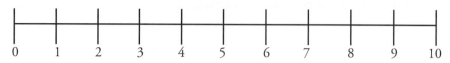

Nie mam bólu

No pain

Straszny ból

Terrible pain

Russian[†]

Пользуясь десятибалльной шкалой, укажите, пожалуйста, насколько сильно Вы чувствуете боль.

Please point to the number that best describes your pain.

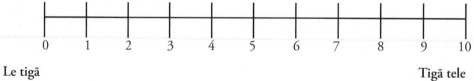

Боли нет совсем

No pain

Очень сильная боль

Terrible pain

Samoan[*]

Faamolemole ta'u mai le numera e faamatala ai le ituaiga tigā o loo e lagonaina.

Please point to the number that best describes your pain.

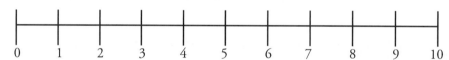

Le tigā

No pain

Tigā tele

Terrible pain

Spanish[†]

Por favor señale el número que mejor describe su dolor.

Please point to the number that best describes your pain.

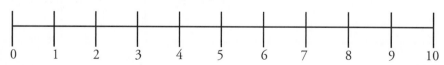

No tiene dolor

No pain

Tiene un terrible dolor

Terrible pain

Figure 3-6 | Cont'd.

Continued

Tagalog (spoken in the Philippines)[†]

Ituro po ninyo ang bilang na nagpapahiwatig ng tindi ng sakit.

Please point to the number that best describes your pain.

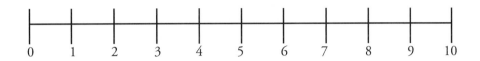

Walang sakit

No pain

Napakasakit

Terrible pain

Tongan (spoken in Tonga, an island in the south Pacific)[†]

I he ngaahi fika koena, fakailongai mai ai e tuunga ho felanga'aki.

Please point to the number that best describes your pain.

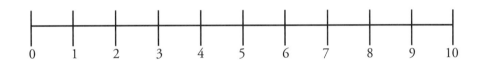

Ikai ha felanga'aki

No pain

Ikai matuuaki'e langa

Terrible pain

Vietnamese

Vui lòng chỉ ra số mô tả tốt nhất cơn đau của quý vị.

Please point to the number that best describes your pain.

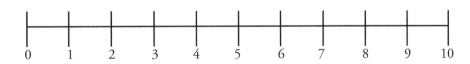

Không đau

No pain

Đau kinh khủng

Terrible pain

Figure 3-6 | Cont'd.

for patients of various cultures. It is often preferred by adults when they compare it to other scales. It is quickly explained and easily scored, easily and quickly understood, well-liked by clinicians and patients, and inexpensive to duplicate.

No pain rating scale is perfect, and several objections have been made regarding the use of the FACES scale. One frequently mentioned concern has been that the presence of tears in the last face, depicting the greatest pain, might cause both children and adults to be reluctant to select that face if they were not crying or if they wanted to appear more stoic. Similarly, tearful patients may avoid selecting a face that shows no tears. The instructions for the scale attempt to avert this problem by telling a patient that a person does not have to cry to select the tearful face or may be crying and select a face without tears. Still, patients have been concerned. In a pilot study of 267 adults conducted in preparation for comparing scales that included the FACES scale, clinicians found that patients who selected the faces with tears said something about the tears, highlighting the need to include the instruction that one does not have to be crying to select the face with tears (Carey, Turpin, Smith, et al., 1997).

Some clinicians have asked about simply eliminating the tears on the FACES scale when they copy it for clinical use. However, this could affect the validity of the scale.

In one study of parents and their children, a similar problem occurred in adults' understanding of the instructions for using the FACES scale (Chambers, Giesbrecht, Craig, et al., 1999). The researchers reported that some parents experienced difficulty understanding how to apply the scale to judge pain in their children when they were given the same verbal instructions as their children received, which included the statement that a person does not have to cry to select the last face with tears. Nevertheless, as an example, one parent commented that the child had a lot of pain but that his face never looked like the face with tears, so the adult selected a face at the lower end of the scale. This requires further investigation but suggests that when the FACES scale is used with adults, directions that are given for children may need to be clarified for the adults.

Another concern arises over the fact that a smiling face rather than a neutral face is placed at the beginning of the scale to denote no pain. In the FACES scale, the second face has a slight smile, and the third face is neutral. Some other faces scales, such as the FPS-R described next, begin with a neutral face to represent no pain. A person with no pain who is not smiling might select the third neutral face on the FACES scale, resulting in falsely high pain ratings. One study comparing five faces scales, two beginning with a smiling face and three beginning with a neutral face, used by children 5 to 12 years old and their parents, found that both the children and their parents gave higher pain scores when the smiling faces scales were used (Chambers, Giesbrecht, Craig, et al., 1999). The implications of these findings have been

Which Face Shows How Much Hurt You Have Now?

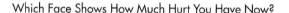

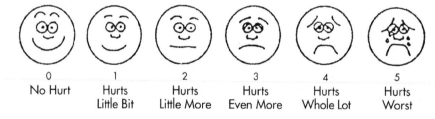

| 0 | 1 | 2 | 3 | 4 | 5 |
| No Hurt | Hurts Little Bit | Hurts Little More | Hurts Even More | Hurts Whole Lot | Hurts Worst |

Explain to the person that each face is for a person who feels happy because he has no pain (hurt) or sad because he has some or a lot of pain. **Face 0** is very happy because he doesn't hurt at all. **Face 1** hurts just a little bit. **Face 2** hurts a little more. **Face 3** hurts even more. **Face 4** hurts a whole lot. **Face 5** hurts as much as you can imagine, although you don't have to be crying to feel this bad. Ask the person to choose the face that best describes how he is feeling.

Rating scale is recommended for persons age 3 years and older.

*The *brief word instructions* under each face can also be used. Point to each face using the words to describe the pain intensity. Ask the child to choose face that best describes own pain and record the appropriate number. *Note:* In a study of 148 children ages 4 to 5 years, there were no differences in pain scores when children used the original or brief word instructions. (In Wong D, Baker C: Reference manual for the Wong-Baker FACES Pain Rating Scale, Duarte, CA, 1996, City of Hope Mayday Pain Resource Center.)

Continued

Figure 3-7 | Translations of Wong-Baker FACES Pain Rating Scale.

From Hockenberry, M. J., Wilson, D., & Winkelstein, M. L. (2005). *Wong's essentials of pediatric nursing,* ed 7, St. Louis, Mosby, p. 1259. Used with permission. From Pasero, C., & McCaffery, M. (2011). *Pain assessment and pharmacologic management,* p. 66-67, St. Louis, Mosby. Permission to use the FACES scale for purposes other than clinical practice can be obtained at http://www1.us.elsevierhealth.com/FACES/. The NRS is in the public domain. May be duplicated for use in clinical practice.

Chinese

　　解釋給人聽用每張臉譜來代表著一個人的感覺是因爲沒有疼痛〔傷痛〕而感快樂或是因爲些許疼痛或者是許多疼痛而感傷心。第零張臉是很快樂的因爲他一點也不覺得疼痛。第一張臉只痛一丁點兒。第二張臉又痛多了一些。第三張臉痛得更多了。第四張臉是非常痛了。第五張臉是爲人們所能想像到的劇痛既使感到這樣難過，卻不一定哭出來。請這人選擇出最能代表他現在感覺的一張臉譜。此量表適用於三歲以上的人。

French

Expliquez à la personne que chaque visage représent un personne qui est heureux parce qu'elle n'a pas point du mal ou triste parce qu'il a un peu ou beaucoup du mal. **Visage 0** est trés heureux parce qu'elle n'a pas point du mal. **Visage 1** a un petit peu de mal. **Visage 2** a plus du mal. **Visage 3** a encore plus du mal. **Visage 4** a beaucoup du mal. **Visage 5** a autant mal que vous pouvez imaginer, bien que ces mauvais sentiments ne finissent pas nécessairement a vous faire pleurer. Demandez à la personne de choisir le visage qui convient le mieux avec ses sentiments.

Ces evaluations sont recommendés pour des personnes de trois ans et davantage.

Italian

Spiegare a la persona che ogni facien è per una persona che si sente felice perchè non tiene dolore oppure triste perchè ha poco o molto dolore. **Faccia O** è molto felice perchè non tiene dolor. **Faccia 1** tiene poco dolore. **Faccia 2** tiene un po più di dolore. **Faccia 3** tiene più dolore. **Faccia 4** tiene molto dolore. **Faccia 5** tiene molto dolore che non puoi immaginare però non devi piangere per tenere dolore. Domandi ala persona di scegliere quale faccia meglio descrive come si sente.

Grado scale è raccomandata a la persona di tre anni in sù.

Japanese

　　3歳以上の患者に望ましい。それぞれの顔は、患者の痛み (pain, hurt) がないのでご機嫌な感じ、または、ある程度の痛み・沢山の痛みがあるので悲しい感じを表現していることを説明して下さい。0＝痛みがまったくないから、とても幸せな顔をしている、1＝ほんの少し痛い、2＝もう少し痛い、3＝もっと痛い、4＝とっても痛い、5＝痛くて涙を流す必要はないけれども、これ以上の痛みは考えられないほど痛い。今、どのように感じているか最もよく表わしている顔を選ぶよう、患者に求めて下さい。

Figure 3-7 | Cont'd.

Portuguese

Explique a pessoa que cada face representa uma pessoa que está feliz porque não têm dor, ou triste por ter um pouco ou muita dor. **Face 0** está muito feliz porque não têm nenhuma dor. **Face 1** tem apenas um pouco de dor. **Face 2** têm um pouco mais de dor. **Face 3** têm ainda mais dor. **Face 4** têm muita dor. **Face 5** têm uma dor máxima, apesar de que nem sempre provoca o choro. Peça a pessoa que escolhe a face que melhor descreve como ele se sente.

Esta escala é aplicável a pessoas de tres anos de idade ou mais.

Romanian

Explică persoanei că fiecare față este specifică diferitelor stări fizice; o persoană este ferioita pentru că nu are nici o durere ori tristă pentru că suferă puțin sau mai mult. **Fața 0** este foarte ferioită pentru că nu are absolut nici o durere. **Fața 1** are un pic de durere. **Fața 2** are ceva mai mult. **Fața 3** suferă și mai mult. **Fața 4** suferă foarte mult. **Fața 5** este greu de imaginat cât de mult suferă, căci nu trebuie neapărat să plângi, oricat de tare te-ar durea. Intreabă persoana să indice figura care-i desorie cel mai bine starea fizică.

Acest **grad de durere** este racomandat pentru persoanele de la 3 ani în sus.

Spanish

Explíquele a la persona que cada cara representa una persona que se siente feliz porque no tiene dolor o triste porque siente un poco o mucho dolor. **Cara 0** se siente muy feliz porque no tiene dolor. **Cara 1** tiene un poco de dolor. **Cara 2** tiene un poquito más de dolor. **Cara 3** tiene más dolor. **Cara 4** tiene mucho dolor. **Cara 5** tiene el dolor más fuerte que usted pueda imaginar, aunque usted no tiene que estar llorando para sentirse asi de mal. Pidale a la persona que escoja la cara que mejor describe su proprio dolor.

Esta escala se puede usar con personas de tres años de edad o más.

Vietnamese

Xin cắt nghĩa cho mỗi người, từng khuôn mặt của một người cảm thấy vui vẻ tại vì không có sự đau đớn hoặc, buồn vì có chút ít hay rất nhiều sự đau đớn.

Cái **mặt** với **số** 0 thì rất là vui tại vì mặt ấy không có sự đau đớn. **Mặt số** 1 chỉ đau một chút thôi. **Mặt số** 2 hơi đau hơn một chút nữa. **Mặt số** 3 đau hơn chút nữa. **Mặt số** 4 đau thật nhiều. **Mặt số** 5 đau không thể tưởng tượng, mặc dù người ta không cần phải khóc mới cảm thấy được sự buồn khổ như thế.

Bạn hỏi từng người tự chọn khuôn mặt nào diễn tả được sự đau đớn của chính mình.

disputed by Wong and Baker (2001). However, another study of children and their parents comparing five faces scales, including the FACES scale and a color scale, found that scales beginning with a smiling face produced significantly higher pain ratings (Chambers, Hardial, Craig, et al., 2005). Children's pain ratings were the highest when the FACES scale was used.

Thus, when adults as well as children use the smiling faces scales, higher pain ratings may result than when faces scales begin with a neutral face. This problem can be circumvented by using a faces scale that begins with a neutral face, and we suggest the FPS-R, presented next.

Another objection to the FACES scale is the difficulty in obtaining studies of reliability and validity. As mentioned earlier, on the website that lists studies of the reliability and validity of the FACES scale, several are unpublished and difficult to obtain.

Faces Pain Scale-Revised. The FPS-R is a modification of a scale with seven faces developed by Bieri, Reeves, Champion, and others (1990). A scale with seven faces does not adapt well to the 0 to 10 metric used by the majority of pain scales. The revised scale has six faces, so it is easily presented with the 0 to 10 metric (see Figure 3-4, p. 57) (Hicks, von Baeyer, Spafford, et al., 2001). Although numbers beneath the faces are not used when the scale is shown to young children, they are developmentally appropriate to use with adults. In fact by the age of eight years most children are able to use a 0 to 10 scale (Spagrud, Piira, von Baeyer, 2003).

The FPS-R was developed for use in preschool and school-age children. Initially, two studies were designed to establish the psychometric properties of the scale in children experiencing nonclinical pain and clinical pain (Hicks, von Baeyer, Spafford, et al., 2001). Comparing the FPS-R and the VAS, the validity of the FPS-R was established in a study of 76 children aged 5 to 12 years old having ear piercing. The next study established validity of the FPS-R in a group of 90 children 4 to 12 years of age experiencing clinical pain associated with hospitalization. The FPS-R was compared with a color analog scale and the VAS.

Studies have also shown that the FPS-R is appropriate for adults. One study compared the FPS-R with a verbal descriptor scale, the NRS and the Iowa Pain Thermometer in 40 cognitively intact and 28 cognitively impaired older minority adults, including African-Americans (74%), Hispanics (16%), and Asians (10%) (Ware, Epps, Herr, et al., 2006). The study was conducted in an acute care facility in the southern United States. The reliability and validity of the FPS-R were supported in this group, and the FPS-R was preferred by African-Americans and Hispanics and those who were cognitively impaired.

Another study of adults in Spain compared the Spanish version of the FPS-R with a pain thermometer (Miro, Huguet, Nieto, et al., 2005). Using five hypothetic painful situations, 177 cognitively intact subjects aged 65 years and older were asked to rate pain. The study provided preliminary evidence of the scale's reliability and validity in this group. Also, subjects preferred the FPS-R. The study established the usefulness of the FPS-R in cognitively intact elderly patients.

In a study conducted in China of 173 Chinese surgical patients, aged 18 to 78 years, reliability, validity, and scale preference were studied by comparing the FPS-R, VAS, NRS, and a verbal descriptor scale (Li, Liu, Herr, 2007). Patients were interviewed preoperatively and asked to rate any vividly recalled pain and anticipated postoperative pain intensity. Then they were asked for pain intensity

ratings on the day of surgery through the sixth postoperative day. On the last day they were asked their scale preference. All four scales had good reliability and validity. The FPS-R had a low error rate, and almost half of the subjects preferred the FPS-R. The researchers concluded that the FPS-R was the best one for Chinese adults.

In summary, the reliability and validity of the FPS-R has been established in the following groups of adults:

- Cognitively impaired and intact older adults who were Asian, African-American, or Hispanic. The last two groups preferred the FPS-R.
- Cognitively intact elderly Spanish patients; most preferred the FPS-R.
- Cognitively intact Chinese adults ranging in age from 18 to 78 years old; almost half preferred the FPS-R; the FPS-R had a low error rate.

These studies ensure that the FPS-R meets some of the criteria for selecting a pain rating scale for use with adults in daily clinical practice (see Box 3-2, p. 54). Research establishes it as being reasonably valid and reliable in children and adults. It is developmentally appropriate not only for children but also for adults as young as 18 years and for cognitively intact and cognitively impaired elderly. It is easily understood and well liked by patients. It has demonstrated appropriateness for patients of various cultures, such as minorities, Chinese, and Spanish. Further, the tool is available in approximately 30 languages (Figure 3-8). It is inexpensive and easily explained, scored, and recorded.

The FPS-R minimizes some concerns associated with the FACES scale. The first face is neutral, not smiling, so it lowers the possibility of artificially high scores. Tears, which might be objectionable to some patients, are not shown on any of the faces of the FPS-R scale, including the one that denotes the most severe pain.

Principles of Using Pain Rating Scales

Whichever pain rating scale is chosen for a patient should be used consistently with that patient. Using the same pain rating scale makes it possible to compare the pain ratings. Also, using the same scale is obviously easier for the patient than switching from one scale to another. Further, using the same pain rating scales and the same metric (that is, 0 to 10) throughout the institution facilitates communication about patients' pain. Standardization is helpful within a given health care system, so that the same scale is used in the emergency department, the hospital, and the outpatient care services. A standard pain rating scale minimizes confusion for both patients and staff.

The primary reason for using pain rating scales is to evaluate the effectiveness of pain treatment plans. Reassessment is essential. The frequency with which pain ratings are obtained depends on the situation.

The Guideline for the Management of Cancer Pain in Adults and Children (Miaskowski, Cleary, Burney, et al., 2005) recommends that at "a minimum pain should be reassessed and documented:

- at regular intervals after a management plan is initiated,
- with each new report of pain; and
- at an appropriate interval after each pharmacologic or nonpharmacologic intervention, such as 15 to 30 minutes after parenteral drug therapy or 1 hour after oral administration of an analgesic" (p. 28).

When pain is out of control, such as a 10 on a scale of 0 to 10, and a rapidly acting analgesic is used, pain ratings every 5 minutes may be appropriate. However, at the beginning of treatment, asking the patient for a pain rating may be entirely inappropriate. When a patient is obviously in pain or is not focused enough to learn to use a pain rating scale, pain treatment should proceed without pain ratings. Once a patient can use a pain rating scale, pain assessment may be necessary as often as every 15 minutes until pain is brought under control, then every 1 to 2 hours for 24 hours, followed by every 4 hours. Once pain has been well controlled, however, in hospitalized patients, obtaining pain ratings every 8 to 12 hours may be sufficient; in nursing homes a daily or even weekly pain assessment may be appropriate. In home care, once pain has been controlled, patients are not ordinarily asked to keep records of pain ratings.

An intricate part of using pain rating scales to evaluate pain management is to set goals for treatment. These may be referred to as comfort-function goals and are discussed later. Basically, it is essential to know what pain rating is necessary for individual patients.

Teaching Patients and Families How to Use a Pain Rating Scale

It is not unusual for clinicians to claim that patients cannot use pain rating scales. However, even in cognitively impaired elderly patients in nursing homes, 83% who report pain are able to use at least one type of pain rating scale (Ferrell, Ferrell, Rivera, 1995). Another study that included older cognitively impaired minority patients used a verbal descriptor scale (no pain, mild pain, moderate pain, severe pain, extreme pain, and most intense pain

Text continued on p. 84

Faces Pain Scale-Revised (FPS-R)

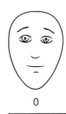 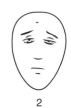 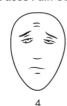 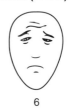 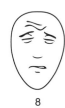 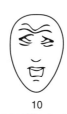

0   2   4   6   8   10

English language instructions

In the following instructions, say "hurt" or "pain," whichever seems right for a particular child.

"These faces show how much something can hurt. This face *[point to left-most face]* **shows <u>no pain</u>. The faces show more and more pain** *[point to each from left to right]* **up to this one** *[point to right-most face]* **- it shows <u>very much pain</u>. Point to the face that shows how much you hurt** [right now]**."**

Score the chosen face 0, 2, 4, 6, 8, or 10, counting left to right, so '0' = 'no pain' and '10' = 'very much pain.' Do not use words like 'happy' and 'sad'. This scale is intended to measure how children feel inside, not how their face looks.

Figure 3-8 | Translations of Faces Pain Scale-Revised. *Continued*

Albanian

Këto figura dëftojnë sa mundet të dhëmbet. Kjo figurë (tregoje e cila është në majsht) dëfton nji person qi nuk i dhimbet asnji sen. Këta figura (dëfto një pas një, pi të majshtës et të gjajtës) e tregojnë një person qi i dhembët sa ma shumë deri sa (dëftoje figurën që është ma në të gjajtë), i dhembet shumë tepër.
Tani dëftoje ty sa të dhembet një ketë moment.

Numrat janë pi të majshtës deri të gjajtës : 0,2,4,6,8,10.
0 domethonë që nuk dhimbet kurse 10 domethonë që shumë dhimbet.

- Duhet të tregohen limitat extreme për shembull : "hiç nuk dhemb" ose "shumë shumë me dhemb"
- Nuk duhet të përdoren fjalat "mërzit" ose "gëzim"
- *Duhet të tregohet mirë se këta vizatime janë, sensasione e mrenshme të trupit e jo vetëm të ftyrës.*
Tregom si e ke trupin në vet vetën.

Translation credit: Pétrit Zekiri, Hôpital Robert Debré, Paris, France
* Sentence in italics has not been verified in back-translation.

Arabic

مقياس الوجوه للألم

حسب التعليمات التالية، استعمل كلمة "ألم" أو "وجع" أيهما يناسب الطفل.

"هذه الوجوه تظهر كم هناك من الألم (الوجع): هذا الوجه (أشر إلى الوجه في أقصى اليسار) يظهر وجه بلا ألم. الوجوه تظهر ألم متزايد: أشر إلى كل الوجوه من (اليسار إلى اليمين) حتى الأخير (الوجه في أقصى اليمين), هذا الوجه يظهر الكثير من الألم (الوجع). أشر إلى الوجه الذي يظهر كم أنت تتألم الآن.

أعطي علامة للوجه المختار 2،4،6،8،10، 0 ،ابدأ بالعد من اليسار إلى اليمين حيث أن 0 =لا ألم و 10 = ألم كثير. لا تستعمل كلمات مثل "سعيد" أو "حزين". هذا المقياس أعد لقياس كيف يشعر الأطفال وليس كيف يظهر وجههم.

Translation credit: Maha Arnaout, King Hussein Cancer Center, Amman, Jordan

---

Bulgarian

"Тези лица показват колко много може да боли. Това лице (посочете лицето най-вляво) показва, че хич не боли. Лицата показват, че повече и повече боли (посочете ги едно по едно отляво надясно), до това лице (посочете лицето най-вдясно) - то показва, че много го боли. Посочи лицето, което показва колко много те боли (точно сега)".Направете скàла отбелязвайки избраното лице с *0, 2, 4, 6, 8* и *10,* отляво надясно, така *'0'* = "*не боли*" и *'10'* = "*много силно боли*". Не употребявайте думи като "*радостен*" и "*тъжен*". Тази скàла е предназначена да се прецени как се чувстват децата вътрешно, а не как изглежда лицето им.

Translation credit: Chiristo Gargov, France

Figure 3-8 | Cont'd.

Continued

Catalan (revised 2004)

En les següents instruccions utilitza el terme 'dolor' o 'mal', considerant la seva idoneïtat en cada cas.

Aquestes cares expressen quant de dolor pots sentir. Aquesta casa [l'avaluador assenyala la cara extrema de la banda esquerra] no expressa dolor. Les cares expressen cada vegada més dolor [l'avaluador assenyala cadascuna de les cares d'esquerra a dreta] fins que aquesta [l'avaluador assenyala la cara extrema de la banda dreta] té molt de dolor. Assenyala la cara que millor em mostri el dolor que sents ara.

La puntuació assignada a la cara seleccionada és 0, 2, 4, 6, 8 o 10, seguint un ordre d'esquerre a dreta, en el que 0 significa 'no dolor' i 10 significa 'molt de dolor'. No utilitzis paraules com 'content' o 'trist'. Aquesta escala pretén mesurar com es sent realment el nen, no pas l'aparença externa del seu rostre.

Translation credit: A. Huguet, J. Miró, University Rovira I Virgili, Spain (revised October 2004)

Chinese

指示: 這些面孔代表痛楚的程度。最左面的面孔代表沒有痛楚(指向最左), 最右面的面孔代表極為痛楚 (指向最右) 。因此, 越近左面的面孔代表越少痛楚, 越近右面的面孔代表痛楚越大(從左到右, 逐一指著面孔)。
請指出哪個面孔最能代表你的痛楚程度。

Translation credit: Emma Wong, Ide Chan, Mary Lee, Josephine Chu, Tony Wong. Working Group on Pain Services Development, Hospital Authority, Hong Kong

Dutch

"Gebruik bij de onderstaande instructie 'au' of 'pijn' al naar gelang het kind waar het om gaat. "Aan deze gezichtjes kun je zien hoe veel pijn je kan hebben. Aan dit gezichtje [wijs het meest linkse gezichtje aan] zie je geen pijn. Je ziet steeds meer pijn aan de gezichtjes [wijs ze aan van links naar rechts] tot aan deze [wijs het meest rechtse gezichtje] - aan deze zie je heel veel pijn. Kun je het gezichtje aanwijzen dat laat zien hoe veel pijn je voelt [op dit moment]?"Scoor het gekozen gezichtje 0, 2, 4, 6, 8, of 10, van links naar rechts rekenend, dus '0' = 'geen pijn'en '10'= 'heel veel pijn' Gebruik geen woorden zoals 'blij'en 'bedroefd'. Deze schaal is bedoeld om te meten hoe kinderen zich van binnen voelen, niet hun gezichtsuitdrukking.

Translation credit: Ko Hagoort and Monique van Dijk, Sophia Children's Hospital Rotterdam, The Netherlands

Figure 3-8 | Cont'd.

Continued

Estonian

Järgnevates juhistes kasuta sõnu "teeb haiget" või "on valus" sõltuvalt lapsest.

Need näod näitavad, kui valus võib olla.
See nägu (osuta kõige vasempoolsele) näitab, et pole üldse valus. Need näod näitavad (osuta eraldi igale näole vasemalt paremale), et on üha rohkem ja rohkem valus kuni selle näoni (osuta kõige parempoolsemale), mis näitab, et on väga valus.
Missugune nägu näitab, kui valus sul praegu on.

Vastavalt valitud näole antakse 0,2,4,6,8 või 10 punkti, loendades vasakult paremale: 0 = pole üldse valus. 10 = on väga valus

Ärge kasutage sõnu "kurb" või "rõõmus".
Täpsustage, et jutt käib sellest, kuidas laps ennast tunneb, mitte aga näo välisest ilmest.

Translation credit: Ursula Koorits and Reet Kikase, Tartu University Clinic, Estonia

French

Ces visages montrent combien on peut avoir mal. Ce visage (montrer celui de gauche) montre quelqu'un qui n'a pas mal du tout. Ces visages (les montrer un à un de gauche à droite) montrent quelqu'un qui a de plus en plus mal, jusqu'à celui-ci (montrer celui de droite), qui montre quelqu'un qui a très très mal. Montre-moi le visage qui montre combien tu as mal en ce moment.
Les scores sont de gauche à droite : 0, 2, 4, 6, 8, 10. 0 correspond donc à "pas mal du tout" et 10 correspond à "très très mal".
Remarques : Exprimez clairement les limites extrêmes : "pas mal du tout" et "très très mal". N'utilisez pas les mots "triste" ou "heureux". Précisez bien qu'il s'agit de la sensation intérieure, pas de l'aspect affiché de leur visage. "Montre-moi comment tu te sens à l'intérieur de toi"

Translation credit: Chantal Wood, Hôpital Robert Debré, Paris, France, and Michel Duval, Université de Montréal, Canada

Figure 3-8 | Cont'd.

Continued

German (Germany) (revised 2004)

Wählen Sie die Formulierung „weh tun" oder „Schmerzen", je nachdem was zu dem jeweiligen Kind am besten zu passen scheint.

Diese Gesichter zeigen, wie weh etwas tun kann (wie sehr etwas schmerzen kann). Dieses Gesicht hier *(auf das Gesicht ganz links zeigen)* zeigt, dass es gar nicht weh tut (schmerzt). Die anderen Gesichter zeigen, dass es mehr und mehr weh tut (schmerzt) *(auf die Gesichter der Reihe nach zeigen)* bis hin zu diesem Gesicht, das zeigt, dass es ganz stark weh tut (schmerzt). Zeig mir mal das Gesicht, dass am besten zeigt, wie sehr es Dir (gerade) weh tut (wie stark deine Schmerzen (gerade) sind).

Vergeben Sie die Punkte 0, 2, 4, 6, 8 oder 10 für die Gesichter von links nach rechts, so dass „0" = „kein Schmerz" und „10" = „sehr starker Schmerz" bedeutet. Vermeiden Sie Worte wie „glücklich" und „traurig". Ziel dieser Skala ist es zu messen, wie die Kinder sich innerlich fühlen, und nicht wie ihr Gesichtsausdruck ist.

Translation credit: Ruth Diehl, Göttingen; Sandra Schürmann, Children's Hospital of Datteln, University Witten/Herdecke, Datteln, Germany

---

German (Switzerland)

Diese Gesichter zeigen, wie fest etwas weh tun kann (wieviel Schmerzen man haben kann). Zeigen Sie auf das Gesicht links aussen: *dieses Gesicht zeigt, dass es nicht weh tut* (oder: *zeigt jemanden der gar kein Weh hat*). Zeigen Sie auf die Gesichter und zwar von links nach rechts: *diese Gesichter zeigen, dass es mehr und mehr weh tut* (Oder: *zeigen jemanden der immer mehr Weh hat*). Zeigen Sie auf das Gesicht rechts aussen: *bis zu diesem da; das zeigt jemand der sehr sehr fest weh hat.* Sagen Sie zum Kind: *Zeige mir das Gesicht das zeigt, wieviel weh Du jetzt gerade hast* (Oder: *zeige mir das Gesicht, dem es genauso weh tut wie Dir*).

Translation Credit: Ketsia Schwab, Universitätskinderkliniken, Inselspital, Bern, Switzerland

---

Figure 3-8 | Cont'd.

Continued

Greek

Αυτά τα προσωπάκια δείχνουν το πόσο μπορεί να πονάς.
Αυτό το πρόσωπο (δείχνουμε το πρόσωπο στα αριστερά) δείχνει κάποιον που δεν πονάει καθόλου.
Αυτά τα πρόσωπα (τα δείχνουμε ένα-ένα από τα αριστερά προς τα δεξιά) δείχνουν κάποιον που πονάει όλο και περισσότερο, μέχρι αυτόν εδώ (δείχνουμε το πρόσωπο στα δεξιά), που πονάει πάρα πολύ.
Δείξε μου το προσωπάκι που δείχνει πόσο πολύ πονάς τώρα.
Οι βαθμοί είναι από τα αριστερά στα δεξιά: 0,2,4,6,8,10. Το Ο αντιστοιχεί λοιπόν στο « δεν πονάω καθόλου » και το 10 αντιστοιχεί στο « πονάω πάρα πάρα πολύ ».
Σημειώσεις: Εξηγήστε σαφώς τα δύο άκρα: « δεν πονάω καθόλου » και « πονάω πάρα πάρα πολύ ». Μην χρησιμοποιείτε λέξεις όπως « λυπημένος » ή « χαρούμενος ». Εξηγήστε σαφώς ότι πρόκειται για την εσωτερική αίσθηση του πόνου, όχι για την εικόνα που βλέπουμε στα πρόσωπα. « Δείξε μου πώς αισθάνεσαι μέσα σου ».

Translation credit: Eleni Panagiotakaki and Malika Benkerrou

Hebrew

הפרצופים האלה מציגים עד כמה משהו יכול לכאוב. הפרצוף הזה (הצבע על הפרצוף השמאלי ביותר) מציג <u>אין כאב</u>. הפרצופים מציגים עוד ועוד כאב (הצבע על כל פרצוף משמאל לימין) עד לזה (הצבע על הפרצוף הימני ביותר) – זה מציג <u>הרבה מאוד כאב</u>. הצבע על הפרצוף שמציג כמה כואב לך (עכשיו).

Translation credit: Bar-Shalita Tami and Parush Shula, School of Occupational Therapy, Hebrew University, Jerusalem and Vatine Jean-Jacques, Reuth Medical Center, Tel Aviv

Hindi

इस काम में , प्रत्येक बच्चे के आधार पर , 'दुख' या 'दर्द' जैसे शब्दों का प्रयोग करे .

ये चेहरें बताते हैं , कितना दर्द हो सकता है . यह चेहरा (*बाएं ओर से पहला चेहरा दिखाओ*) बताता है कि कोई दर्द नहीं है . ये चेहरे ज्यादा से ज्यादा दर्द बताते हैं (*बाएं से दाहिने तरफ एक एक चेहरा दिखाओ*) इस चेहरे तक (*दाहिनी ओर का अंतिम चेहरा दिखाओ*) - यह बहुत दर्द दिखाता है (अभी) .

चुना हुआ चेहरा दिखाओ, 0, 2, 4, 6, 8 या 10 , बाएं से गिनो, 0 = दर्द के बिना और 10 = बहुत बहुत दर्द, 'खुश' या 'उदास' शब्दों का प्रयोग नहीं करें, यह काम आंतरिक दर्द को मापने के लिए है , चेहरे की दिखावट के लिए नहीं .

Translation credit: Roopa Sukthankar, Dileep Bhagwut, Rajan Gulhati, Paris, France

Figure 3-8 | Cont'd.

Continued

Hungarian (Magyar)

Az arcok a fàjdalomérzet fokozatàt mutatjàk.Ezen az arcon még nem làtszik a fàjdalom (mutassa meg a baloldali arcot). Ezeken az arcokon (mutassa meg egyenként balrol jobbra) làthato az egyre jobban erösödö fàjdalomérzet majd az utolson màr az igazàn erös fàjdalom làtszik (a jobboldali arcot mutassa). Vàlaszd ki és mutass rà arra az arcra amelyik a te fàjdalomérzetednek felel meg ebben a pillanatban. A szàmskàla 0-tol 10-ig,balrol jobbra: 0, 2, 4, 6, 8,10-es szàm jegyek. A 0 azt jelenti,hogy "egyàltalàn nem fàj" és a 10-es azt jelenti,hogy nayon -nagyon fàj. Megjegyzés: fejezze ki tisztàn az abszolut,szèlsöséges hatàrokat példàul "egyàltalàn nem fàj" vagy "nagyon -nagyon fàj". Ne hasznàlja a következö kifejezéseket : "szomoru" vagy "boldog". Hivja fel a figyelmét,hogy a sajàt érzéseit hatàrozza meg pontosan és nem az arcoknak a kifejezését. " Mutad meg a te sajàt belsö érzéseidet".

Translation credit: Edith Miklosi, Paris, France

Indonesian

SKALA NYERI WAJAH (REVISI)
Pada Instruksi berikut, katakana "sakit" atau "nyeri", keadaan yang lebih mendekati sebenarnya (yang mana tampaknya tepat) pada anak tertentu.
"GAMBAR WAJAH INI MENUNJUKKAN SEBERAPA JAUH RASA SAKIT YANG DIALAMI. GAMBAR WAJAH INI (*ditunjuk gambar paling kiri*) MENUNJUKKAN <u>TIDAK ADA RASA SAKIT</u>. GAMBAR BERIKUTNYA MENUNJUKKAN RASA SAKIT YANG BERAT (tunjuk satu persatu dari kiri kekanan) SAMPAI GAMBAR INI (tunjuk gambar paling kanan), INI MENUNJUKKAN <u>SANGAT NYERI</u>. TUNJUKKAN PADA GAMBAR INI, SEBERAPA JAUH SAKIT YANG ANDA RASAKAN! (sekarang)"
Skor untuk gambar waja yang dipilih adalah **0, 2, 4, 6, 8,** atau **10**, mulai dari paling kiri ke paling kanan, sehingga "**0**" = tidak nyeri dan "**10**" = sangat nyeri.
Jangan menggunakan istilah atau kata seperti "*senang*" atau "*sedih*". Skala ini dimaksudkan untuk mengukur sejauh mana rasa nyeri yang dialami, dan bukan penampakan wajah yang terlihat.

Translation credit: Indonesian associates of Kaiser Ali, Saskatoon, Canada

Figure 3-8 | Cont'd.

Continued

Italian (revised 2004)

Nelle istruzioni che seguono, parlare di "male" o "dolore", a seconda di ciò che sembra più adatto al bambino in questione.

"Queste facce mostrano quanto una cosa può fare male. Questa faccia (indicare la faccia più a sx) indica nessun DOLORE. Le facce mostrano sempre più dolore (indicare ogni faccia, da sx verso dx) fino a questa (indicare la faccia più a dx) che mostra TANTISSIMO dolore.

Indica la faccia che mostra quanto male hai (in questo momento)."

Calcola il punteggio della faccia scelta 0, 2, 4, 6, 8, oppure 10, contando da sinistra a destra, così che '0' = nessun dolore e '10' = tantissimo dolore.' Non usare parole quali 'felice' e 'triste'. Questa scala misura come i bambini si sentono dentro, non l'espressione sul loro volto.

Translation credit: Manuella Trapanotto, Department of Pediatrics, University of Padova, Italy

Japanese

表情でわかる痛みの程度

説明するときにはその子供に応じて「HURT」と「PAIN」という単語を使い分けてください

これらの表情はどのくらい痛いかをあらわしています。一番左はまったく痛みがない時の表情。一番右はとても痛い時。痛みがひどくなるにつれて表情も左から右へと変わっていきます。今あなたの痛みはこれらの表情の中から選ぶならどれですか？

０、２、４、６、８、１０の番号で選びましょう。一番左の痛みがない時の表情が０、右端の痛いときの表情が１０です。楽しいか悲しいかを聞くのではありません。あくまでも子供たちがどう感じているかを判断するものです。

Translation credit: Heideki Toramatsu

Figure 3-8 | Cont'd.

Continued

Laotian

ໃນຂໍ້ຊີ້ແຈງ ຄັ້ງຕໍ່ໄປນີ້) : ເອົ້າວ່າ "ເຈັບ" ຫລື "ປວດ" ທີ່ເຫັນວ່າ ເຫມາະສົມ ກັບສະພາບ ຂອງ ເດັກນ້ອຍ ແຕ່ລະຄົນ ໂດຍ ສະເພາະ

ໃນບັນດາຮູບ ນີ້ ຂ້ຶໃຫ້ເຫັນ ວ່າ ມີຄວາມເຈັບຂະຫນາດໃດ. ໃນຮູບໃບຫນ້າ (ແຕ່ ຂ້າງ ຊ້າຍ) ຂ້ຶໃຫ້ເຫັນ ຄົນຄົນນີ້ ບໍ່ ມີຄວາມເຈັບ ຈັກຫນ່ອຍເລີຍ. ບັນດາໃບຫນ້າ (ເລີ່ມແຕ່ຂ້າຍຫາຂວາ ຂ້ຶໃຫ້ເຫັນວ່າ ມີ ຄວາມເຈັບປວດ ເພີ່ມຂຶ້ນ ໄປເຖິງ ຮູບ ທີ່ ຢູ່ຂ້າງຂວາສຸດ, ທີ່ຂ້ຶໃຫ້ເຫັນວ່າ ຄົນນີ້ ມີຄວາມເຈັບ ຫລາຍທີ່ສຸດ. ຈຶ່ງ ຂ້ຶຮູບ ໃບ ຫນ້າ ໃຫ້ຂ້ອຍເບິ່ງ ເພື່ອບອກໃຫ້ຂ້ອຍ ຮູ້ ວ່າ ເຈົ້າເຈັບຫລາຍຂະຫນາດໃດ ໃນເວລານີ້.

ໃຫ້ຄະແນນ ເລກເລີ່ມແຕ່ ຊ້າຍ ຫາ ຂວາ : 0, 2, 4, 6, 8, 10. ຄະແນນ 0 ຈຶ່ງ ກົງກັບ ຄຳວ່າ "ບໍ່ເຈັບຈັກຫນ່ອຍເລີຍ" ແລະ 10 ແມ່ນກົງກັບ "ເຈັບຫລາຍທີ່ສຸດ"

ບໍ່ໃຫ້ໃຊ້ ຄຳວ່າ "ດີໃຈ" ຫລື "ເສັຍໃຈ"
ການໃຊ້ຄະແນນ ນີ້ ແມ່ນ ເພື່ອຈຸດປະສົງ ວັດແທກ ຄວາມເຈັບພາຍໃນ ຂອງເດັກນ້ອຍ ແຕ່ບໍ່ແມ່ນ ເພື່ອ ເບິ່ງ ວ່າ ເດັກນ້ອຍ ມີທ່າທ່າແນວໃດ.

Translation credit: Sisamay Luangchandavong, Ambassade de la RDP Lao, Paris, France

Malagasy (Malgache)

Mampiseho hendrik' olona araka ny ambaratongan' ny faharariny ireo sary ireo. Ny farany havia dia mampiseho hendrik' olona salama tsara, tsy marary. Ireo hendrika ireo (tondroy tsirairay avy any ankavia miankavanana) dia mampiseho olona iray miamarary hatrany hatrany, atramin' ilay farany havanana izay mampiseho fa tena marary mafy. Tondroy ho ahy hoe aiza amin' ireo hendrik' olona, marary ireo no mahazo anao amin' izao fotoana izao .
Ny fomba fanisàna dia avy any ankavia miankavanana : 0, 2, 4, 6, 8, 10 . Ny 0 dia milaza hoe "tsy marary mihitsy" ary ny 10 dia "tena marary faran' izay mafy".
Fanamariana : Lazao mazava tsara ny hoe : "tsy mahatsiaro marary mihitsy" sy ny hoe "tena marary mafy".   Aza mampiasa ny teny hoe "malahelo" na "faly".
Hamarino tsara fa fahatsapana anaty no lazaina eto fa tsy ny fiseho hita eo amin' ny hendriny akory. "Tondroy ho ahy hoe inona no tsapanao ao anatinao ao".

Translation credit: Ndrianarivo Ratsaramiafara, Hôpital de Mahanoro, Madagascar

Figure 3-8 | Cont'd.

Continued

Mongolian

"Эдгээр хүмүүсийн царайны илрэл нь хэн нэгэнд хир их өвдөлттэй байж болохыг харуулж байна. Хамгийн зүүн талд байрлаж байгаа хүний царай бол ерөөсөө өвдөхгүй байгаа хүнийг харуулж байна. Зүүнээс баруун тийшлэх тутам /дараа дараагийн хүмүүсийн царайны илрэл нь улам их өвдөлттэй болж байгааг заана. Хамгийн баруун талд байрлаж байгаа хүний царай хамгийн их өвдөлттэй буюу маш их өвдөж байгаа хүнийг харуулж байна. Яг энэ мөчид чамд хир их өвдөлттэй байгааг чи надад энэ дундаас олж заа".

Тооцоолохдоо зүүнээс баруун тал руугаа чиглэж 0, 2, 4, 6, 8, 10 гэсэн байдлаар дүгнэлт өгнө. "0"= "огт өвдөлтгүй", харин "10"=" хамгийн их буюу маш их өвдөлттэй" гэснийг заана. Анхаарах нь : 1/ "огт өвдөлтгүй" ба "маш их өвдөлттэй" гэсэн хоёр заагийг маш тодорхой ялгаж илэрхийлэх хэрэгтэй. 2/ "гунигтай буюу уйтгартай" ба "аз жаргалтай буюу баяр баясгалантай" гэсэн 2 үгийг огт хэрэглэж хэлэхгүй байх. 3/ эдгээр хүмүүсийн царай нь хүүхдийн зөвхөн гадаад царайны төрхийг илэрхийлж байгаа гэдгийг онцлоно. Чиний бие чинь юу мэдэрч байгааг надад энэ зурган дээрээс /царайнууд дотроос/ олж заа.

Translation credit: Enkhzul Erdeneshoo and Nyamjargal Mangalsuren, Mongolia

Norwegian

ANSIKT SMERTE SKALA – Revidert

I følgende instruksjon, si "vondt" eller "smerte", ut fra hva som virker riktig for det enkelte barnet.

"Disse ansiktene viser hvor vondt noe kan gjøre. Dette ansiktet (pek på ansiktet lengst til venstre) viser ingen smerte. Ansiktene viser mer og mer smerte (pek på hvert og et fra venstre mot høyre) helt til dette (pek på ansiktet lengst til høyre) – det viser veldig mye smerte. Pek på det ansiktet som viser hvor vondt du har (akkurat nå)."

Poengsett det valgte ansikt 0, 2, 4, 6, 8 eller 10, telt fra venstre til høyre, slik at '0' = 'ingen smerte' og '10' = 'veldig mye smerte'. Ikke bruk ord som 'glad' og 'trist'. Denne skalaen har til hensikt å måle hvordan barn føler seg, ikke hvordan deres ansikt ser ut.

Translation credit: Kari Sørensen and Lise Tuset Gustad

Figure 3-8 | Cont'd.

Continued

Persian (Farsi)

اين عكس ها نشان مي دهند كه چقدر مي توانيم درد داشته باشيم .

اين تصوير (تصوير سمت چپ را نشان دهيد) كسي را نشان مي دهد كه اصلا درد ندارد.

اين تصاوير (از چپ به راست يكي يكي نشان دهيد) كسي را نشان مي دهد كه بيش از پيش درد مي كشد تا جايي كه (تصوير سمت چپ را نشان دهيد) كسي را نشان مي دهد كه خيلي زياد درد مي كشد .

حالا تصويري را به من نشان بده كه نشان دهد كه در اين لحظه چقدر درد مي كشي درجه درد كشيدن از چپ به راست 0 — 2-4-6-8-10 است . صفر نشان مي دهد كه تو اصلا درد نداري و 10 نشان مي دهد كه تو خيلي خيلي زياد درد داري .

تذكر : دقيقا درد واقعي خودت را بگو و از كلماتي مانند ناراحت ؛ خوشحال و غيره استفاده نكن .

دقيقا احساس داخلي خودت را بگو و نه قيافه تصوير را .

Translation credit: Faezeh Legrand-Izadifar, Hôpital Necker Enfants Malades, Paris, France

Polish

Skala Bólu czytana z twarzy

Przedstawione twarze pokazują jak silny może być ból. Ta twarz [wskaż pierwszą po lewej stronie] pokazuje całkowity brak bólu. Kolejne twarze pokazują nasilanie się bólu [wskazuj kolejno twarze od lewej do prawej aż do tej po prawej stronie] Twarz po prawej stronie wskazuje największe nasilenie bólu [największy ból]. Wskaż teraz twarz która pokazuje jak bardzo cię boli [w tej chwili].

Punktuj wskazane twarze 0,2,4,6,8 lub 10 punktów licząc od lewej strony do prawej. 0 = 'nie boli' i 10 = 'boli bardzo mocno' Nie używaj słów typu 'wesoły' lub 'smutny'. Skala jest stworzona po to aby zmierzyć jak się dzieci czują wewnętrznie a nie jak wyglądają ich twarze.

Translation credit: Tomek Michalski and Anna Michalski

Figure 3-8 | Cont'd.

Continued

Portuguese (Portugal)

Nas instruções que se seguem, diga "magoar" ou "doer", de acordo com o que lhe parece correcto para determinada criança.

"Estas caras mostram o quanto algo pode magoar. Esta cara [aponte para a face mais à esquerda] nao mostra dor. As caras mostram cada vez mais dor [aponte para cada uma das faces da esquerda para a direita] até chegar a esta [aponte para a face mais à direita] – que mostra muita dor. Aponta para a cara que mostra o quanto te dói [neste momento]."

Atribua à face escolhida 0, 2, 4, 6, 8 ou 10, contando da esquerda para a direita, de modo que "0" = sem dor e "10" = muita dor. Não use palavras como "alegre" e "triste". Esta escala destina-se a medir como as crianças se sentem por dentro, não como aparentam estar.

Translation credit: Luís Batalha, Higher Nursing School of Bissaya Barreto, Portugal, and Elizabete Rocha, University of Saskatchewan, Canada

Portuguese (Brazil)

Estas caras mostram o quanto alguma coisa pode doer. Esta cara *[aponte para a face mais à esquerda]* não mostra dor. As caras mostram cada vez mais dor *[aponte para cada uma das faces da esquerda para a direita]* até chegar a esta *[aponte para a face mais à direita]* que mostra muita dor. Aponte para a cara que mostra o quanto te dói *[neste momento]*.

Alternate:

Estas faces mostram o quanto algo pode doer. Esta face (apontar a face mais à esquerda) indica não dor. As faces mostram cada vez mais dor (apontar para cada uma das faces da esquerda para a direita) até chegar a esta face (apontar a face mais à direita) que mostra muita dor. Aponte a face que mostra o quanto você sente dor (neste exato momento)

Pontue a face escolhida como 0, 2, 4, 6, 8 ou 10, contando da esquerda para a direita; sendo 0 = sem dor e 10 = com muita dor. Não use palavras como "alegre" ou "triste". Esta escala tem por objetivo medir como as crianças se sentem internamente e não como aparentam estar.

Translation credit: Cláudia Lígia Esperanza Charry Poveda, José Aparecido Da Silva, Paola Passareli, Joseane dos Santos, Maria Beatriz Martins Linhares, University of São Paulo, Brazil

Figure 3-8 | Cont'd.

Continued

Romanian

Scara imaginilor durerii – Revizuită
« Aceste imagini indică cât de puternică este durerea pe care o avem. Această imagine (arătaţi imaginea din stânga) indică pe cineva care nu are nici o durere. Imaginile (arătaţi-le pe rând de la stânga la dreapta) indică o persoană care are o durere din ce în ce mai puternică, până la aceasta (arătaţi figura din dreapta), care indică pe cineva care are o durere foarte foarte puternică. Arată-mi imaginea care exprimă cât de puternică este durerea ta acum. »

Punctajul este de la stânga la dreapta : 0, 2, 4, 6, 8, 10.
0 corespunde deci la « nici o durere », iar 10 corespunde la « o durere foarte foarte puternică » .

Atenţie : - exprimaţi clar limitele extreme : « nici o durere » şi « o durere foarte foarte puternică ».
-        nu folosiţi cuvintele « trist » sau « vesel »
-        precizaţi bine că este vorba de o senzaţie interioară şi nu de aspectul imaginilor. « Arată-mi cum te simţi în interiorul tău. »

Translation credit: Dr Valentin Calgaru, Protontherapy Centre of Orsay, BP 65 91402 Orsay Cedex, France, and Miss Monica Huidu

Russian

« Эти лица показывают сколько можно иметь боли. Это лицо (покажите самое слева) показывает кого-то, которому совсем не больно. Эти лица (покажите каждое лицо слева направо) показывают кого-то, которому всё больше и больше больно, до этого, (покажите самое направо), которое показывает кого-то, которому очень очень больно. Покажи мне теперь лицо, показывающее на сколько тебе больно сейчас. »
Очки показаны слева направо : 0, 2, 4, 6, 8, 10
0 значит « совсем не больно »
10 значит « очень очень больно »
Примечания :
- Ясно выражайте экстремальные пределы : « совсем не больно », и « очень очень больно »
- Не употребляйте слова "грустный" или "счастливый"
- Хорошо уточняйте, что речь идет о внутреннем чувстве, а не о внешнем виде лица : « Покажи мне, как ты себя чувствушеь внутри себя ».

Translation credit: Dr Laurent Holvoet-Vermaut, Hôpital Robert Debré, Paris

Figure 3-8 | Cont'd.

Continued

Serbian

« Ova lica pokazuju koliko jak bol moze biti. Ovo lice (pokazati lice krajnje levo) pokazuje osobu koja uopste ne oseca bol. Ova lica (pokazati ih s leva na desno) pokazuju osobu koju nesto sve vise i vise boli sve do ove (pokazati lice krajnje desno) koja oseca veoma jak bol. Pokazi mi lice koje pokazuje koliko jak bol sada osecas. »

Stepeni bola s leva na desno : 0,2,4,6,8,10. 0 dakle znaci da osoba uopste ne oseca bol a 10 veoma veoma jak bol.

Dodatna uputstva :
Izrazite jasno krajnje granice : « uopste ne oseca bol » i « veoma jak bol ».
Ne koristite reci « tuzan » ili « srecan »
Objasnite dobro da se radi o unutarnjem osecaju, a ne o trenutnom izrazu njegovog ili njenog lica. « Pokazi mi kako se osecas iznutra »

Translation credit: Olga Ignjatovic-Wood

Spanish (Argentina)

*Por favor, lea las instrucciones completas antes de mostrarle la escala al niño.*Pregúntele al niño qué nombre le da al "dolor" y use ese mismo término a lo largo de esta evaluación.Doble la página por la línea de puntos y dígale al niño (siempre recuerde reemplazar la palabra dolor por aquella elegida por el niño): "Estas caras muestran cuánto algo puede doler. Esta cara *[señale la cara del extremo izquierdo]* indica que <u>no hay nada de dolor</u>. Las caras van mostrando más y más dolor *[señale cada una de izquierda a derecha]* hasta llegar a ésta *[señale la cara del extremo derecho]* – que muestra <u>muchísimo dolor</u>. Señalá la cara que indique cuánto dolor tenés [ahora]."Luego que el niño señala una cara: Asigne un puntaje según la cara seleccionada por el niño: contando de izquierda a derecha asigne 0, 2, 4, 6, 8, o 10, de manera que '0' = 'ausencia de dolor' y '10' = 'muchísimo dolor.' NO use palabras como 'contento' o 'triste'. La intención de esta escala es medir como el niño se siente en su interior, no como luce su rostro.

Translation credit: Verónica Dussel and Silvina Bevilaqua, Hospital Garrahan, Buenos Aires, Argentina

Figure 3-8 | Cont'd.

Continued

Spanish (Spain)

Por favor, lea las instrucciones completas antes de mostrarle la escala al niño. En las instrucciones que siguen, utilice la palabra "daño" o "dolor" según sea la forma más adecuada a cada caso (es decir, según sea la forma que utilice el niño o la niña para referirse a la experiencia de dolor). "Estas caras expresan cuánto dolor puede sentir una persona. Esta cara [señalar la cara del extremo izquierdo] no expresa dolor, es decir, no siente ningún dolor. Las caras expresan más y más dolor [señalar cada una de las caras de izquierda a derecha] hasta llegar a ésta [señalar la cara del extremo derecho] - que tiene muchísimo dolor. Señala la cara que mejor exprese el dolor que tienes ahora." Una vez el niño ha realizado la tarea, asigne una puntuación a la cara que ha seleccionado. Contando de izquierda a derecha sería 0, 2, 4, 6, 8, o 10, de manera que '0' significa 'ausencia de dolor' y '10' significa 'muchísimo dolor.' No se deben usar palabras como 'contento' o 'triste'. El objetivo de esta escala es medir como se siente el niño en su interior, no la apariencia externa de su rostro.

Translation credit: Dr Jordi Miró and Anna Huguet, Universitat Rovira i Virgili, Tarragona, Spain

Swedish (revised 2004)

I följande instruktioner, säg ont eller smärta, utifrån vad som verkar vara mest lämpligt för barnet.

De här ansiktena visar hur ont något kan göra. Det här ansiktet (peka på ansiktet längst till vänster) visar ingen smärta. Ansiktena visar mer och mer smärta (peka på var och en från vänster till höger) ända till den här (peka på ansiktet längst till höger) – det visar väldigt mycket smärta. Peka på det ansikte som visar hur ont du har (just nu).

Poängsätt det valda ansiktet 0, 2, 4, 6, 8, 10 från vänster till höger så att 0 = ingen smärta och 10 = väldigt mycket smärta. Använd ej ord som glad och ledsen. Den här skalan avser att mäta hur barn känner sig, ej hur deras ansikte ser ut.

Translation credit: Gustaf Ljungman, Lena Högberg, Loise von Essen

Figure 3-8 | Cont'd.

Continued

Tamil

இந்த முகங்கள் ஒருவருக்கு எவ்வளவு நோவுகிறது என்று காட்டுகிறது. இந்த முகம் (இது பக்க முகத்தைத் காட்டவும்) ஒருவருக்கு வலி இல்லை என்று காட்டுகிறது. இந்த முகங்கள் (இது பக்கமிருந்து வலது பக்கமாக ஒவ்வொரு முகங்களையும் காட்டவும்) வலி கூடிக்கொண்டு போவதைக் காட்டுகிறது. கடைசியில் (வலது பக்கமுள்ள முகத்தைக் காட்டவும்). ஒருவருக்கு மிகவும் கடும் வலி என்று காட்டுகிறது. இப்போது உங்களுக்கு எவ்வளவு நோவுகிறது என்று இதிலுள்ள எந்த முகம் என்று காட்டவும்.

இடமிருந்து வலமாக இருக்கும் புள்ளிகள் : 0,2,4,6,8,10
« 0 » வலி இல்லை என்றும்   «10 » மிகவும் கடும் வலி என்று குறிக்கிறது.
குறிப்புகள்: விளக்கமாக தெரிவிக்கவும் : «வலி இல்லை » அல்லது «மிகவும் கடும் வலி » « கவலை » அல்லது «மகிழ்ச்சி » என்ற சொற்களை பாவிக்க வேண்டாம். உங்களுக்கு இருக்கும் வலியை உங்களுடைய முகத்தில் காட்டாமல், எப்படி இருக்கிறது என்று எமக்கு சரியாக படத்தில் காட்டவும்.

Translation credit: Mrs Arulappu and Mr Anbazhagam Rajagopalan, Hôpital Robert Debré, Paris

Thai

ในคำชี้แจงต่อไปนี้ ให้ใช้คำว่า "เจ็บ" หรือ "ปวด" ตามความเหมาะสมแก่ผู้ป่วยเด็กแต่ละคน
"รูปหน้าต่อไปนี้จะแสดงให้เห็นว่ามีความปวดมากเท่าไร รูปหน้านี้(ซ้ายสุด)แสดงว่า<u>ไม่ปวดเลย</u>
รูปหน้าถัดมาแสดงว่าปวดมากขึ้น มากขึ้น(ชี้รูปหน้าจากซ้ายมาขวา)
จนถึงรูปหน้านี้ (ชี้รูปขวาสุด)แสดงว่า<u>ปวดมากๆ</u>
ให้หนูชี้รูปหน้าที่แสดงว่าหนูปวดมากแค่ไหน(ตอนนี้)" ให้คะแนนตามรูปหน้าที่เลือก
0,2,4,6,8,10 ตามลำดับจากซ้ายไปขวา คะแนน 0 = ไม่ปวดเลย คะแนน 10 = ปวดมากๆ
ไม่ควรใช้คำว่า "สุข" หรือ "เศร้า"
การให้คะแนนนี้มีจุดประสงค์เพื่อวัดว่าผู้ป่วยเด็กมีความปวดมากแค่ไหน
ไม่ใช่การให้คะแนนจากการดูลักษณะสีหน้าของเด็ก

Translation credit: Wimonrat Krisanaprakornkit and Duenpen Horatanaruang, Department of Anesthesiology, Srinagarind Hospital, Khon Kaen University, Khon Kaen, Thailand

Figure 3-8 | Cont'd.

Continued

imaginable), a 0 to 10 NRS, a FPS-R, and an Iowa Pain Thermometer (Figure 3-9, p. 87) and found that all these scales were relatively easy for these patients to use (Ware, Epps, Herr, et al., 2006). Therefore, most adolescents and adults who are not cognitively impaired should be able to learn to use a pain rating scale. It is simply a matter of having a plan that ensures that when patients are admitted to clinical settings, someone is responsible for teaching all patients about the pain rating scale, having patients demonstrate their understanding of it, and documenting this in the records.

The steps for teaching the 0 to 10 NRS are in Box 3-4 on p. 86. Steps 1, 2, and 3 provide information; steps 4 and 5 ask the patient to demonstrate understanding of the information; and Step 6 focuses on the goals for comfort and function/recovery. Along with each step are specific examples of what may be said to the patient and family. A teaching brochure titled "Understanding Your Pain: Using

Turkish

Bu yüzler ne kadar ağrılı olunabileceğini gösteriyor. Bu yüz [en soldakini işaret et] hiç ağrısı olmayan birisini gösteriyor. Bu yüzler [soldan sağa birer birer işaret ederek] ağrısı giderek artan birisini gösteriyor, [sağdakini gösteriniz] en çok ağrısı olan birine kadar. Bana şu anda ne kadar ağrın olduğunu ifade eden yüzü göster.Sayılar soldan sağadır: 0, 2, 4, 6, 8, 10 ile ölçülendirin. '0', 'ağrısız'a karsılık geliyor, '10' ise 'en çok ağrılı' olmaya.Uyarılar: Aşırı uçları açıkça belirtiniz: 'Ağrısız' ve 'en çok ağrılı'. "Mutlu" veya "üzüntülü" sözcüklerini kullanmayınız. Bu ölçeğin, yüz ifadelerinin nasıl olduğunu değil, hissedilenleri ölçmeyi amaçladığını iyice açıklayın. "Bana kendini nasıl hissettiğini onu göster".

Translation credit: Çiçek Oya Cengiz-Sakiroğlu, Centre Thérapeutique Pédiatrique de Margency and Hôpital Robert Debré, Paris, France

---

Wallisean (Uvean) (Wallis Islands, New Caledonia, Vanuatu)

<<Koteu fofoga aena e ha mai ai teu faahiga mamahi kehekehe. Kote fofoga (ae taupotu i hema) e ha mai ai kohe tahi e mole iai hona mamahi. Koteu fofoga leva ae e hoa mai (mai hema hema ki matan)
e ha mai kohe tahi kua lesili lahi mai tona mamahi, (o au mai kite fofoga faka osi), ena fakaha mai he tahi mole keina faa tall tona mamahi. Faka hinohino mai la koe te fofoga ae ena fakaha mai tou mamahi ite laka nei.>>

Koeni teu faka fuafua numelo mai hema ki matau : selo (0), lua (2), fa (4), ono (6), valu (8), hogofulu (10). Kote numelo selo (0) kotona uhiga kohe tahi << mole mamahi tua tahi >>. Kote numelo hogofulu (10) kohe tahi <<kua lahi fau osi tona mamahi >>.

E tonu keke:
+ Faka mahino lelei mai: <<te mole mamahi >> mote << mamahi kovi osi>>
+ Tuku tau faka aoga te kupui lea ko << loto mamahi >> mo << loto fiafia>>
+ E tonu keke faka mahino lelei mai teu mamahi o tou sino, kae tuku teu faka a'pe otou fofoga. <<Faka ha lelei mai tau logoi teu mamahi ae eke logoi mai tou loto kakano >>.

Translation credit: Mario Frediani and Lenei Falakiko, Noumea, New Caledonia

---

Figure 3-8 | Cont'd.

a Pain Rating Scale" is patterned after the steps in Box 3-4 and is available at www.endo.com.

Patients tend to have a narrow concept of the word *pain*, often restricting its use to excruciating and intolerable sensations. The patient's concepts of pain may be expanded by explaining that pain includes several different uncomfortable sensations, such as tightness and pressure, and by using the words aching and hurting (Step 3). In a study of four different ethnic groups—Hispanics, American Indians, blacks, and whites—participants were asked to describe and rate painful experiences. Findings revealed that in all groups, the word *ache* was used for mild pain, *hurt* for moderate pain, and *pain* for the most intense discomfort (Gaston-Johansson, Albert, Fagan, et al., 1990).

Setting the Comfort-Function Goal

How much pain is too much pain? When clinical practice guidelines first began to be published, the need for

Box 3-4 Teaching Patients and Their Families How to Use a Pain Rating Scale

Step 1. Show the pain rating scale to the patient and family and explain its primary purpose.

Example: "This is a pain rating scale that many of our patients use to help us understand their pain and to set goals for pain relief. We will ask you regularly about pain, but any time you have pain you must let us know. We don't always know when you hurt."

Step 2. Explain the parts of the pain rating scale. If the patient does not like it or understand it, switch to another scale (e.g., vertical scale, FACES).

Example: "On this pain rating scale, 0 means no pain and 10 means the worst possible pain. The middle of the scale, around 5, means moderate pain. A 2 or 3 would be mild pain, but 7 and higher means severe pain."

Step 3. Discuss pain as a broad concept that is not restricted to a severe and intolerable sensation.

Example: "Pain refers to any kind of discomfort anywhere in your body. Pain also means aching and hurting. Pain can include pulling, tightness, burning, knifelike feelings, and other unpleasant sensations."

Step 4. Verify that the patient understands the broad concept of pain.

Ask the patient to mention two examples of pain he or she has experienced.

If the patient is already in pain that requires treatment, use the present situation as the example.

Example: What to say if the patient is not in significant the pain: "I want to be sure that I've explained this clearly, so would you give me two examples of pain you've had recently?"

If the patient's examples include various parts of the body and various pain characteristics, that indicates that he or she understands pain as a fairly broad concept.

Example: The patient might say, "I have a mild, sort of throbbing headache now, and yesterday my back was aching."

Step 5. Ask the patient to practice using the pain rating scale with the present pain or to select one of the examples mentioned.

Examples: "Using the scale, what is your pain right now?" "What is it at its worst?" Or "Using the pain rating scale and one of your examples of pain, what is that pain usually?" "What is it at its worst?"

Step 6. Set goals for comfort and function/recovery. Ask patients what pain rating would be acceptable or satisfactory, considering the activities required for recovery or for maintaining a satisfactory quality of life. (Research strongly suggests that pain rating goals of 4 or more on a 0-to-10 scale are not appropriate.)

Example: For a surgical patient: "I have explained the importance of coughing and deep breathing to prevent pneumonia and other complications. Now we need to determine the pain rating that will not interfere with this so that you may recover quickly. If you're not sure, you can guess, and we can change it later."

Example: For a patient with chronic pain or a terminally ill patient: "What do you want to do that pain keeps you from doing? What pain rating would allow you to do this?"

From Pasero, C., & McCaffery, M. *Pain assessment and pharmacologic management*, p. 86, St. Louis, Mosby. © 2011, McCaffery M, Pasero C. May be duplicated for use in clinical practice.

a goal was recognized. One of the first guidelines stated: "Determine the level of pain above which adjustment of analgesia or other interventions will be considered" (Acute Pain Management Guideline Panel, 1992, p. 7). The primary reason for using pain rating scales is to evaluate the effectiveness of the pain treatment plan. To do this, it is essential to set goals, as described in Box 3-4, Step 6. In a review of studies of primary care physicians' goals for pain treatment, goals for pain relief were the single best predictor of the quality of pain management (Green, Anderson, Baker, et al., 2003).

The purpose of establishing a comfort-function goal is to identify how much pain can exist without interfering with the function and quality of life; that is, activities that the patient needs or wishes to perform. Goals should be as concrete as possible. For example, identifying a pain rating of 3 for accomplishing recovery is too general, whereas identifying a pain rating of 3 for ambulation is much more concrete. The goal is always established by working with the patient and identifying goals that are consistent with what the patient wants. An examination of longitudinal data from quality assurance studies revealed that charted goals for pain relief were often higher than the goals patients reported wanting (Ward, Gordon, 1996). However, clinicians should not establish comfort-function goals in the absence of input from patients.

Comfort-function goals are appropriate for both acute pain and persistent pain, and they encompass physical as well as emotional status and cognitive-behavioral activities. The patient should be assured that reported pain ratings above the goal will result in consideration of additional interventions.

When a clinician works with a patient to set comfort-function goals, the patient must understand that the intent

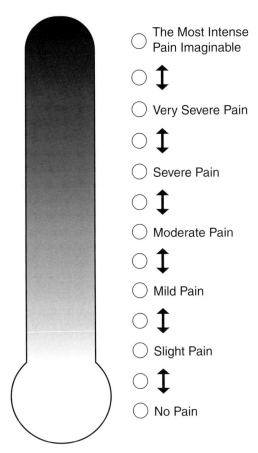

Iowa Pain Thermometer (IPT)

○ The Most Intense Pain Imaginable

↕

○ Very Severe Pain

↕

○ Severe Pain

↕

○ Moderate Pain

↕

○ Mild Pain

↕

○ Slight Pain

↕

○ No Pain

Figure 3-9 | Iowa Pain Thermometer (IPT).

From Herr, K., Spratt, K., Spratt, K. F., et al. (2006). Evaluation of the Iowa Pain Thermometer and other selected pain intensity scales in younger and older adult cohorts using controlled clinical pain: A preliminary study. *Pain Manag Nurs*, 7(2), 44-52. From Pasero, C., & McCaffery, M. (2011). *Pain assessment and pharmacologic management*, p. 87, St. Louis, Mosby. May be duplicated for use in clinical practice.

is not to identify the highest pain level the patient can tolerate, but rather to identify how much pain can exist without interfering with function. In other words, what level of pain may be noticeable but not bothersome?

With some patients, such as those with persistent pain, multiple goals may be appropriate, but for most patients, setting more than one goal can be avoided by identifying the pain levels that would allow the patients to perform the function that is most painful but also of great importance. Following are examples of how this is done in various settings.

Patient Example

In an *acute* pain setting such as postoperative pain, pain may not yet exist but is anticipated. Whenever possible, the comfort-function goal should be identified before pain occurs. In such cases, the clinician may know bet-ter than the patient which recovery activities probably will be the most painful but are of great importance to recovery. So the clinician may explain that using an incentive spirometer may be quite uncomfortable but is essential for avoiding complications postoperatively. The clinician may then ask the patient, "What pain rating would make it easy for you to use your incentive spirometer frequently?" The patient may reply that a pain rating of 2 would be all right. The pain rating would then be documented as "2/10 to use incentive spirometer." This can be renegotiated postoperatively if necessary.

By setting a goal for one of the most painful postoperative activities, the hope is that achieving that goal at all times will suffice to make possible other, less painful activities such as ambulation and sleep. Note that the patient is asked to identify a pain rating that makes it easy to perform the painful activity. Again, the emphasis is not placed on what the patient can tolerate but on a goal that makes important activities easy to perform.

Patient Example

Incident pain may also require setting a goal. A patient with chronic noncancer pain that is well controlled may be unable to participate in physical therapy because of the pain it causes. The patient is then asked, "What level of pain would make it easy for you to fully participate in physical therapy?" The patient may answer that a pain rating of 3 would be sufficient. That becomes the comfort-function goal, 3/10 to participate in physical therapy. The plan may be to provide an oral analgesic 1 hour prior to physical therapy.

Patient Example

A patient with *persistent* pain may be unable to achieve satisfactory quality of life. The patient may be asked, "What is it that you can do and want to do, but pain keeps you from doing?" Answers vary and range from walking the dog around the block to being less depressed or having pain interfere less with concentration. Patients with persistent pain of nonmalignant origin may not have been approached with the idea of setting their own priorities and may not expect pain to be less than a 5 which, as discussed, has been shown to interfere significantly with function.

A study of patients with moderate to severe persistent pain related to osteoarthritis (OA), metastatic cancer, and low back pain were found to prefer the terms *manageable* and *tolerable* when describing a day of pain control to the term *acceptable* (Zelman, Smith, Hoffman, et al., 2004). Many of the participants objected to the phrase "an acceptable day of pain control" because it suggested that it would be possible to have days when their painful situations were acceptable or when they could experience full pain relief, a condition they felt was not possible. On the other hand, interviews with some patients indicated that it may be that patients whose pain is well controlled do not object to the term *acceptable*. Thus, objection to the term *acceptable* may indicate that pain is not well controlled.

The patients in the study identified that a manageable or tolerable day of pain control included (1) taking the edge off pain (note that this phrase may signal that pain should be reduced); (2) performing valued activities; (3) relief from dysphoria and irritability; (4) reduced adverse effects caused by medications; and (5) feeling well enough to socialize. These may be common themes in setting goals with patients who have persistent pain.

When patients are asked what level of pain they desire, some will report zero. The process of setting comfort-function goals helps set realistic goals because zero pain is not always possible. In fact, research involving patients with rheumatic diseases showed that on a 100-mm VAS, patients may interpret scores of less than 10 mm as no pain and that scores less than 25 mm may be considered to be relatively normal (Sokka, 2005). However, once the goal is achieved, such as a pain rating of 2 out of 10, the possibility of even better pain relief can always be considered. Over time or with experience, goals may change. For example, if a patient find that the pain rating goal is too high to facilitate frequent use of the incentive spirometer postoperatively, it should be changed to a lower number.

For some patients, especially those with persistent uncontrolled pain, setting goals may take place in stages. For example a patient, in sickle cell crisis may have had uncontrolled severe pain that has lasted for days and deprived him or her of sleep. The first objective may be to provide enough relief for the patient to get uninterrupted sleep. Once this is achieved, another goal related to activities may be established.

It may be difficult to engage some patients with chronic persistent pain of noncancer origin in pain management plans. They may be depressed and reluctant to participant for fear of failure (Filoramo, 2007). Many have tried multiple methods of pain control that have failed, or they have failed to accomplish their goals in the past. It is especially important in these cases to set goals that are concrete, that incorporate the patient's personal goals, and that occur in stages that are achievable. For example, beginning with a goal that establishes a pain rating of 3 out of 10 when walking for 5 minutes may be relatively easy for a patient to accomplish. After this goal is achieved, the next goal might be to walk for 10 minutes. This approach incorporates the concept of pacing; that is, stopping an activity before it becomes painful. In this way, a patient begins to believe that improvement in function is attainable and becomes more strongly committed to the plan of care.

Not only does setting a comfort-function goal help the entire team, including the patient and family, to know what the pain-treatment plan should achieve, it also helps the patient to see how pain relief contributes to recovery or improves quality of life. Not all patients understand the importance of pain relief or the possible harmful effects of pain. Some patients do not expect to have their pain relieved, are frightened of taking opioid analgesics, or value a stoic response to pain. These patients may be reluctant to set a low pain rating as the goal. By setting pain rating goals that correspond to function, patients learn that pain relief helps them to recover faster from circumstances such as surgery. In cases of persistent pain, patients learn that pain control puts them back in control of their daily lives rather than allowing pain to control their lives.

The patient's comfort-function goal should be visible on all records where pain ratings are recorded, such as bedside flow sheets. Whether the goal has been achieved or not should also be routinely included at change-of-shift hand-off reports. If the pain rating is below the goal, documentation should show which efforts were made to achieve the desired goal. For outpatient pain management, a diary or flow sheet kept by the patient (discussed later; see Form 3-11, p. 116) is one way to document and make visible progress toward goals. Establishing comfort-function goals for individual patients and holding clinicians accountable for attempting to achieve those goals may help clinicians to avoid basing pain-management decisions on their own biases.

Research Related to Setting Comfort-Function Goals

Research helps to guide the process of setting a comfort-function goal by suggesting that certain pain levels are more than a patient should attempt to tolerate. The findings of several studies of different cultures have found that on a 0 to 10 NRS, pain ratings of 5 or more interfere significantly with daily function (Cleeland, 1984; Cleeland, Gonin, Hatfield, et al. 1994; Serlin, Mendoza, Nakamura, et al., 1995). The data from several countries (Philippines, France, China, and the United States) confirmed that pain ratings of 5 or greater were clearly more significant in their functional impact than pain ratings of 4 or less (Cleeland, Serlin, Nakamura, et al., 1997). In a study of 271 patients with AIDS-related pain, ratings on the BPI interference items (see Form 3-2, p. 53) found that patients with pain ratings up to 4 out of 10 reported that pain interfered most with mood and enjoyment of life (Breitbart, McDonald, Rosenfeld, et al., 1996). Patients with pain ratings of 5 or 6 out of 10 reported somewhat higher levels of interference on the BPI items, with pain again interfering most with mood and enjoyment of life. Patients with pain of 7 or more out of 10 reported even greater pain interference on the BPI items, with pain interfering most with walking ability, general activity, and sleep. Another study of 274 patients with AIDS-related pain revealed that higher levels of pain intensity resulted in increased levels of depressive symptoms and psychological distress (Rosenfeld, Brietbart, McDonald, et al., 1996). Thus, as pain intensity increases, it is associated with greater impairment in functional ability and psychologic distress.

Of note, one study using the BPI scales showed that a change in pain intensity from 4 (out of 10) to 5 was associated with a greater increase in interference with activity and enjoyment of life than any other change in pain intensity (Daut, Cleeland, 1982). Another study across four cultures, using the 0 to 10 NRS, also found that both a change in pain intensity from 4 to 5 and also a change from 6 to 7 were more significant than other increases in terms of interference with function (Serlin, Mendoza, Nakamura, et al., 1995). This suggests that preventing pain from increasing from 4 to 5 out of 10 is of great importance.

Other research suggests that 4, rather than 5, is the point at which pain significantly interferes with function. The results using the BPI to assess 111 patients with pain and advanced cancer showed that on a 0 to 10 scale, pain ratings of 4 or greater interfered markedly with activity, and interference with enjoyment increased markedly between scores of 6 and 7 (Twycross, Harcourt, Bergl, 1996). Another study of women during childbirth found that almost all patients (93%) wanted more analgesia when the NRS score was greater than 3 (Berlin, Hossain, Bodian, 2003). In a study of titrating drug doses for patients with neuropathic pain, patients were satisfied with their pain relief and stopped increases of drug doses at an average level of 3 out of 10 (Gilron, Bailey, Tu, et al., 2005). These findings and others, combined with clinical experience, have led many clinicians to the conclusion that pain ratings greater than 3 signal the need to revise the pain treatment plan by higher doses of analgesics or different medications and other interventions (Cleeland, Syrjala, 1992; Syrjala, 1993). In addition, even temporary pain at a level of 6 or more should mandate immediate intervention.

This information helps in guiding patients who select goals of 4, 5, or 6 out of 10. Such patients need to be cautioned that pain ratings this high may significantly interfere with function. Further, clinicians should ask these patients why they do not want better pain relief. In research in patients with persistent pain, mentioned earlier, almost all patients said that they did not expect pain to diminish to below 4 or 5 out of 10 without excessive interference from medications' adverse effects (Zelman, Smith, Hoffman, et al., 2004). Patients felt they were trading pain relief for lower function. Clinicians should pursue this problem with patients

and determine whether the adverse effects can be managed. If the problem is related to opioids, the addition of other medications such as nonopioids or adjuvants for pain relief can be explored. Or the adverse effects may respond to treatment. If the adverse effect of concern is sedation, patients can be informed that increases in opioid dosages may initially cause significant cognitive impairment but that with stable dosages of opioid this effect usually subsides in about a week (Bruera, Macmillan, Hanson, et al., 1989). If the adverse effect is constipation, a more aggressive bowel regime can be put in place to prevent this effect. (See Section IV for additional information about management of opioid-induced adverse effects.)

Minimum Clinically Important Changes. These changes are sometimes referred to as minimal important changes. In the process of adjusting pain treatment plans, such as titrating opioids, to accomplish the comfort-function goal, it is helpful to know how much reduction in pain intensity will be important to patients. A statistically significant decrease in pain intensity may not be meaningful to a patient. Therefore, it is important to look at the degree of reduction in pain that is clinically meaningful from the patient's perspective. Several studies have found that approximately a 30% reduction in pain intensity in cases of acute or persistent pain is minimally clinically meaningful but that it depends on the baseline intensity of pain (Farrar, Young Jr., LaMoreaux, et al., 2001; Jensen, Chen, Brugger, 2003; Ostelo, Devo, Stratford, 2008; Sloman, Wruble, Rosen, et al., 2006). For example, a clinical reduction of 2 points on the 0 to 10 NRS may have clinical relevance for someone with mild pain but is of little or no relevance to someone with severe pain (Cepeda, Aficano, Polo, 2003). Specifically, a 2-point reduction in pain intensity from 4 to 2 on a 0 to 10 NRS (a 50% reduction) is likely to be meaningful to a patient with mild pain, but a 2-point reduction from 10 to 8 (a 20% reduction) may not be meaningful and may provide "only some relief" to a patient with severe pain.

Patients Who Deny Pain or Refuse Pain Relief

When a patient denies pain, clinicians must accept this rating because a patient's self-report is the single most reliable indicator of pain. However, when a patient's behavior, known pathology, or other findings suggest the existence of pain, clinicians are responsible for exploring this seeming contradiction with the patient and family. Sometimes a patient acknowledges the pain but refuses analgesics. Clinicians must respect this decision but, again, the reasons should be discussed with the patient and family. Giving a patient information or considering other approaches to pain management may result in the admission of pain or the acceptance of measures to relieve it.

Reluctance to report pain or to use analgesics obviously results in poor pain relief. The reasons patients may act this way have been shown to be associated with a variety of specific concerns (Ward, Goldberg, Miller-McCauley, et al., 1993); many further reasons are supported by a survey of laymen's attitudes (Mayday Fund, 1993). The relationships between patients' attitudes about pain and its treatment and their willingness to report pain and take analgesics were investigated using the Barriers Questionnaire (BQ), an 8-item tool (Ward, Goldberg, Miller-McCauley, et al., 1993). The patients in the study had chronic cancer pain. The patients' responses to the BQ revealed that poor pain control was related to concerns about addiction (the most problematic misconception), adverse effects, and tolerance (the need to "save" the pain medicine); the belief that increased pain meant increased disease; concern that complaining about pain would distract physicians from curing illness; and the belief that "good" patients do not complain about pain.

The BQ was later revised to reflect changes in pain management, such as patients' believing that pain medicine could weaken the immune system, and the result was the 27-item Barriers Questionnaire-II (BQII), a reliable and valid measure of patient-related barriers to the management of cancer pain (Gunnarsdottir, Donovan, Serlin, et al., 2002). The BQ-II confirmed that inadequate analgesia was related to higher scores than those found in the group that used adequate pain medication. Further study of the BQ-II has resulted in the Barriers Questionnaire Short Form, a 9-item survey shown in Form 3-3 (p. 91) (Ward, personal communication, 2008).

The BQ Short Form is recommended for use with patients and their families to help identify what may be causing a patient with cancer to deny pain or refuse analgesics. For patients newly diagnosed with a disease that may become painful eventually, the BQ Short Form may be administered before pain occurs to identify barriers to pain control before problems arise. Depending on the patient population, clinicians may wish to adapt the BQ Short Form by omitting some items or adding others, such as concerns about finances, hiding pain from the family and others, distrust of caregivers, not being a "sissy," or wanting to avoid highly technologic methods of pain control.

Immediately after the BQ Short Form is administered, clinicians should discuss the results with the patient. The patient and family should be assured that many others have similar concerns, but that the concerns need not be problems. Appropriate patient teaching should follow. However, one session of patient teaching probably will not be sufficient to reassure the patient and family.

Correct information about addiction is almost always needed. One study found that the impact of concern about addiction may be somewhat alleviated by the way the prescriber presents information about the medication (Dawson, Sellers, Spross, 2005). More than half of the patients who received prescriptions for opioids said they would be very likely to take them if the prescribers advised them that it would not be addictive if used according to instructions. However, this statement is not entirely true. Correct use of opioids does not protect patients from developing addictive disease. It is more accurate, as discussed in Chapter 2, to say that that far less than 1% of patients exposed to chronic opioid use will become addicted. Unfortunately, this may not be as reassuring to patients as being told that they simply will not become addicted if they follow instructions. For this reason, another strategy clinicians use is to tell patients to ask themselves a question: If you were not in pain would you want to take this medication? A "no" answer means they have not become addicted. (See Section IV for more information about talking with patients and families about addiction.)

Most literature that teaches patients about pain control covers many of the concerns listed in the BQ Short Form. A teaching brochure concerning taking oral opioids that addresses many of the concerns patients have, including addiction, adverse effects, and tolerance, is titled "Understanding Your Pain: Taking Oral Opioid Analgesics" and is available at www.endo.com. One use of the BQ Short Form is to evaluate patient-education interventions by having the patient or family complete the BQ Short Form before and after information has been provided.

A consistent finding has been that patients who used inadequate analgesics had higher barrier scores on the BQ than did those who used adequate analgesics (Lin, Ward, 1995; Ward, Goldberg, Miller-McCauley, et al., 1993; Ward, Hernandez, 1994). Although misconceptions about pain management exist in patients who do not have pain as well as in those who have cancer-related pain (Yeager, Miaskowski, Dibble, et al., 1997), some research has suggested that these misconceptions may exist because current pain is undertreated (Dawson, Sellers, Spross, 2005). Patients' beliefs about pain management seem to be shaped in part by the fact that their pain management provides less than adequate pain relief. Thus, not only do patients' education about misconceptions require attention, so do patients' pain management regimens.

One of the most frustrating occurrences in pain management is knowing that a patient with pain does not have to suffer, yet the patient refuses help. The BQ Short Form may help clinicians begin the process of exploring why a particular patient has decided to endure pain. Despite receiving accurate information about misconceptions and being given choices regarding methods of pain management, some patients, for cultural or religious reasons, choose to experience pain. These decisions must be respected, and at some point clinicians must refrain from further efforts to change these patients' minds.

It is interesting that denial of pain is not always deliberate or conscious. Sometimes patients have narrow concepts of pain and deny its presence when asked.

Barriers Questionnaire Short Form

We are interested in learning more about your attitudes toward treatment of pain. There are no right or wrong answers. We just want to know what you think. Please answer all the questions. For each of the items below, please check Agree, Disagree, or Don't know. Thank you.

1. Pain medicine cannot really control cancer pain.

    Agree _____   Disagree _____   Don't know _____

2. Pain with cancer is inevitable.

    Agree _____   Disagree _____   Don't know _____

3. People get addicted to pain medicine easily.

    Agree _____   Disagree _____   Don't know _____

4. Good patients avoid talking about pain to their physicians.

    Agree _____   Disagree _____   Don't know _____

5. Side effects from pain medicine are worse than the pain itself.

    Agree _____   Disagree _____   Don't know _____

6. If one uses pain medicine early in one's disease then it won't work well if the pain gets worse.

    Agree _____   Disagree _____   Don't know _____

7. Complaints of pain could distract a doctor from focusing on treating the cancer.

    Agree _____   Disagree _____   Don't know _____

8. Pain medicine weakens the immune system.

    Agree _____   Disagree _____   Don't know _____

9. Pain medicine can hide changes that are happening in one's body.

    Agree _____   Disagree _____   Don't know _____

Form 3-3 |

As appears in Pasero, C., & McCaffery, M. (2011). *Pain assessment and pharmacologic management*, p. 91, St. Louis, Mosby. From Gunnarsdottir, S., Donovan, H., Serlin, R. C., et al. (2002). Patient-related barriers to pain management: The Barriers Questionnaire II (BQ-II). *Pain 99*(3), 385-396; Heidrich, S., Ward, S., Julesberg, K., et al. (2003). Conducting intervention research through the Cancer Information Service: A feasibility study. *Oncology Nurs Forum, 30*(1), 131-134. © Ward S. May be duplicated for use in clinical practice.

Following-up with other terms, such as aching or hurting, may uncover the existence of pain.

Other situations in which pain is denied are related to the energizing effect of visits from physicians or health team members. Before and after such visits, the patient may report pain. But encounters during hospital rounds or clinic visits sometimes have powerful positive placebo effects, and a patient honestly reports feeling fine at that time. Clinicians must remember to question the patient further and to check the patient's record to determine what occurred before the visit.

Some patients who have experienced pain for a long time seem to lose their frame of reference. They may forget what it is like not to have pain. As one patient reported after reluctantly taking an analgesic, "I didn't know I had pain. I guess I had been in pain too long to know the difference."

Sometimes pain is not reported not because of any wish to deny pain, but because the patient believes that the health care provider knows about the pain. The patient may reason that the clinicians knows about his or her disease or surgery and knows that pain is present, so it is unnecessary to tell them. For example, a study comparing adolescents' pain ratings with their perceptions of nurses' evaluations of their pain revealed that adolescents perceived that nurses know how much pain they are experiencing (Favaloro, Touzel, 1990).

Although self-report is considered the gold standard for determining the presence and severity of pain (AGS, 2002; APS, 2003; Hadjistavropoulos, Herr, Turk, et al., 2007), older adults often deny or underreport the presence of pain. A number of misbeliefs or concerns underlie lack of pain reporting by older adults, including the belief that pain is to be expected with aging and should be endured; the desire to avoid bothering clinicians or distracting them from focusing on the primary disease; expecting the health care providers to anticipate pain based on condition and diagnoses; fear of the meaning of pain; and fear that acknowledging pain will lead to unpleasant diagnostic tests, hospitalization, and loss of independence (Gagliese, 2001; Herr, Garand, 2001; McAuliffe, Nay, O'Donnell, et al, 2008). Given the high prevalence of common conditions that can be painful in older adults, clinicians must be proactive in asking about pain and exploring possible reasons for denial. (See the previous section on denial of pain, pp. 89-92).

Older adults may deny the presence of pain but when asked about other sensations, such as aching, hurting, or discomfort, respond positively (Closs, Briggs, 2002; McDonald, Shea, Rose, et al., 2009). In the continuum of pain severity, some older adults consider pain to be the most extreme sensation, so clinicians must ask about pain using additional descriptors. Use of open-ended questions without social desirability (such as "Tell me about your pain, aches, soreness, or discomfort") and use of follow-up questions significantly increased the amount of important pain information obtained from older adults with OA pain (McDonald, Shea, Rose, et al., 2009). If older patients cannot self-report verbally, it may be possible to learn about the presence of pain by establishing communication by using a head nod or eye blink. A variety of approaches can help solicit self-reports of pain in older persons with cognitive impairment.

Many pain conditions may not cause discomfort at rest, but movement or other activity may precipitate a pain response (Husebo, Strand, Moe-Nilssen, et al., 2008; Shega, Rudy, Keefe, et al., 2008). So, a denial of pain at rest should be followed by assessment during activity that is likely to cause pain, such as transferring, range of motion, or ambulation, especially in those who may have difficulty reporting.

Selection of Pain Rating Scales for Patients Who Have Difficulty with the Commonly Used Self-Report Scales

As cognitive impairment advances in the older patient, obtaining a reliable pain report becomes more difficult (Hadjistavropoulos, 2005; Kelley, Siegler, Reid, 2008). Many (Pesonen, Kauppila, Tarkkila, et al, 2009) will be unable to use the 0 to 10 pain rating scale previously described but will be able to self-report using other scales. No clear method has been determined to establish a patient's ability to use a self-report scale reliably, but an attempt should be made. When reliability is an issue, it does not negate the importance of attempting to obtain a self-report in those with cognitive impairment. The MMSE is often used in research but is not readily reproducible for clinical use (Folstein, Folstein, McHugh, 1975). However, another simple tool may be used.

One approach is the Pain Screening Tool (Buffum, Miaskowski, Sands, 2001) (Box 3-5, #5). Focusing on their current pain, patients are asked to rate the intensity on a 0 to 3 scale and to say a word that describes their pain. Following 1 minute of distracting conversation, a patient is asked to recall the number and word. He or she receives 1 point for being able to provide the number and 1 point for providing the word. Half a point is given for recalling the word and half a point for recalling the number. A score of 3 suggests that the patient can use a self-report scale reliably. Most important, a score of less than 3 provides evidence that the patient cannot report pain reliably and that another pain assessment tool is necessary, such as a behavioral observation tool (see p. 126 for a discussion of behavioral tools). Another approach to evaluate whether the patient understands the use of the pain scale is to ask him or her to show on a pain scale where a severe pain would be located and to compare that to where the patient shows a mild pain would be located. This approach is discussed earlier in this chapter in the

Box 3-5 Strategies for Obtaining Pain Intensity Reports from Older Persons with Cognitive Impairment

1. Solicit self-report in all older persons, including those with mild to moderate pain severity. If a patient denies pain, use other descriptors, such as discomfort, aching, or soreness. Assess pain during both rest and movement.
2. Use pain scales that are valid and reliable in older persons, including a numeric rating scale, a verbal descriptor scale, and/or a faces pain scale.
3. Once an appropriate pain scale is identified for a patient, use the same pain scale with each assessment of that patient, and document the assessments.
4. Ensure that approaches to pain assessment address any sensory impairments, including vision and hearing losses:
   a. Hearing aids are in place
   b. Glasses are in place.
   c. Tools have been enlarged (a minimum of a 14-point font) and drawings are bold.
   d. Written and oral instructions are provided.
   e. Adequate lighting is available.
5. Determine the reliability of patient self-reports when using a pain intensity scale if the reports are in question.
   a. Consider using the Pain Screen Test (PST)*
      Step 1: Ask patient to select a word describing current pain. Ask patient to identify intensity on a 0 to 3 scale.
      Step 2: Distract patient with conversation for 1 minute.

Step 3: Ask patient to recall the word and the number.
Step 4: Score 1 point each for word and number given and ½ point for each recalled word and number.
Step 5: A score of 3 is considered reliable reporting.
   b. Ask patient to use the selected pain scale and identify where a very bad pain would be located on the scale and where a mild pain would be located on the scale. Evaluate appropriate placement based on severity of pain.
6. Use a visual of the pain scale, rather than a verbal request for a pain report.
7. Repeat clear, simple instructions for using a pain-intensity scale each time the tool is used.
8. Provide sufficient time for older adults to process the task and respond to the tool.
9. Ask about pain in the present, that is, right now.
10. Use a drawing of a figure to identify the location of pain.

---

*Buffum, M. D., Miaskowski, C., Sands, L., et al. (2001). A pilot study of the relationship between discomfort and agitation in patients with dementia. *Geriatr Nurs,* 22(2), 80-85.
As appears in Pasero, C., & McCaffery, M. (2011). *Pain assessment and pharmacologic management,* p. 93, St. Louis, Mosby. © 2011, Herr K. May be duplicated for use in clinical practice.

section about teaching patients how to use pain rating scales (see Box 3-4, p. 86).

Asking about pain in the present, that is "right now," decreases issues related to memory losses that increase with advancing cognitive impairment. Studies have shown that asking older patients to identify pain severity that is dependent on memory, such as worst pain, least pain, or pain in the past week, may provide unreliable responses. (Bergh, Sjostrom, Oden, et al., 2000; Closs, Barr, Briggs, et al., 2004; Feldt, Ryden, Miles, 1998; Kelly, Siegler, Reid, 2008; Taylor, Herr, 2003). Soliciting reports of current pain and reassessing for change and for response to intervention are recommended. Box 3-5 illustrates strategies that can be used to increase success in soliciting self-report and pain scale use in older adults with cognitive impairment.

For older adults with mild to moderate cognitive impairment, a number of pain intensity scales have adequate reliability and validity (Hadjistavropoulos, Herr, Turk, et al., 2007; Weiner, Herr, 2002). There is wide individual variability in preference for and understanding of

format, so no single tool is recommended for all patients. Organizations should identify several options that can be used when assessing pain severity in older patients with cognitive impairment. Tool formats that are acceptable and clinically useful include NRSs (Chibnall, Tait, 2001; Gagliese, Weizblit, Ellis, et al., 2005; Herr, Spratt, Mobily, et al., 2004); verbal descriptor scales (Closs, Barr, Briggs, et al., 2004; Herr, Spratt, Garand, et al., 2007; Herr, Spratt, Mobily, et al., 2004); and faces pain scales, such as FPS-R (Chibnall, Tait, 2001; Kaasalainen, Crook, 2003; Scherder, Sergeant, Swaab, 2003; Taylor, Herr, 2003). These scales are discussed earlier in the chapter (pp. 55-85) and are addressed here in relation to their use in older patients who have difficulty with commonly used scales such as the 0 to 10. Many older adults who are verbal simply have difficulty with scales that provide too many options, such as a 0 to 10 scale, but may be able to use a simpler scale such as a verbal descriptor scale that includes only four options (none, mild, moderate, severe) (Caraceni, Cherny, Fainsinger, et al., 2002; Closs, Barr, Briggs, et al., 2004; Dworkin, Turk, Farrar, et al., 2005).

Although a 4-point scale is less sensitive to change, a scale with fewer options is preferable to no self-report at all. A substantial number of older adults (with and without cognitive impairment) have difficulty responding to an NRS, particularly if it is administered verbally and without a visual representation (Kaasalainen, Crook, 2003; Wynne, Ling, Remsburg, 2000). Vertical presentation (see Figure 3-5, *A*, p. 58) may be easier for persons with alterations in abstract thinking and often is preferred by older adults (Herr, Spratt, Mobily, et al., 2004).

Verbal descriptor scales (e.g., none, slight, mild, moderate, severe, extreme, most intense pain possible) have good reliability and validity, increased sensitivity to change, and a very low failure rate. Further, the verbal descriptor scale has been identified as the instrument preferred by many older adults, and it has strong clinical utility (Chibnall, Tait, 2001; Gagliese, Katz, 2003; Herr, Spratt, Mobily, et al., 2004; Kaasalainen, Crook, 2003; Pautex, Herrmann, Le Lous, et al., 2005; Pesonen, Kauppila, Tarkkila, et al., 2009; Taylor, Herr, 2003).

A recent quasiexperimental study compared the use of five pain intensity scales, including a novel pain thermometer called the Iowa Pain Thermometer (IPT; Figure 3-9, p. 87), with verbal descriptors in a sample of 61 younger and 36 older adults with osteoarthritic pain (Herr, Spratt, Garand, et al., 2007). The IPT provides a range of adjectives that have been supported in earlier research, including no pain, slight pain, mild pain, moderate pain, severe pain, very severe pain, the most intense pain imaginable (Herr, Spratt, Mobily, et al., 2004), along with a thermometer to assist understanding of the tool by older persons who have difficulties with abstract thinking. The IPT had the lowest failure rate of all pain intensity scales evaluated, was sensitive in detecting changes in pain following intervention, and was most preferred by both younger and older patients, including those with cognitive impairment. This and other studies provide further support for the IPT, as well as for the NRS (a 0 to 20 scale with 5-point intervals); the VDS (same adjectives as the IPT but no thermometer); and the FPS (7 line-drawn faces) in cognitively impaired elders (Taylor, Harris, Epps, et al., 2005; Ware, Epps, Herr, et al., 2006).

A simplified version of the verbal descriptor scale that was evaluated in long-term care includes only the adjectives none, mild, moderate, and severe (Closs, Barr, Briggs, et al., 2004). Treatment decisions are based on level of pain severity, and although this simple tool may be most useful for those with advanced dementia, it may be less sensitive than a verbal descriptor scale to detect changes in pain that move from severe to moderate or moderate to severe.

The FPS (7 faces) (Bieri, Reeves, Champion, et al., 1990) was revised in studies with children and presented in a 6-face version that is scored 0 to 10 (FPS-R), presented earlier in this chapter, p. 69) (Hicks, von Baeyer, Spafford, et al., 2001; Spagrud, Piira, von Baeyer, 2003). Subsequent studies in older populations have shown the FPS-R to be reliable and valid and to be the pain intensity scale preferred by cognitively impaired older African-Americans, Hispanics, and Chinese elders (Li, Liu, Herr, et al., 2007; Ware, Epps, Herr, et al., 2006). Although testing of the FPS-R in older Caucasian adults has not been published, the comparability of the FPS and FPS-R in children and the validity established in minority elders suggest that it would be appropriate in the general older-adult population. It should be noted that the FPS-R tends to correlate less strongly with other pain intensity scales, suggesting it may be capturing other characteristics besides intensity (e.g., pain affect). This does not negate its usefulness, but clinicians should be aware that it may be capturing a broader view of pain.

A consideration in tool selection that has not received much attention in the literature is the impact of a patient's education and literacy on tool use and understanding. Low education level might suggest the need to focus tool selection on the simplest and most concrete options; however, education has not been a significant factor in failure to use pain intensity scales correctly in older adults (Gagliese, Weizblit, Ellis, et al., 2005; Herr, Spratt, Garand, et al., 2007). A study presenting a new scale for patients with low education, the Full Cup Test (FCT), demonstrated a statistically significant correlation between the FCT and the VAS (a 100-mm horizontal line with word anchors at the extremes; see p. 55 for discussion of and an image of VAS) and the ability to complete this alternative tool reliably in a sample of 114 patients with 9.23 years of education (Ergun, Say, Ozer, et al., 2007). Of 14 patients with low education, 3 could not understand the VAS, but all were able to complete the FCT. However, the literature shows that many older persons are unable to complete the VAS regardless of education level (Herr, Spratt, Mobily, et al., 2004). Calculation of a pain score using the FCT is cumbersome, so a copy of the tool is not included here, but it is mentioned and referenced, should the reader need such a tool.

Language challenges impact our ability to evaluate pain and are a consideration in tool selection. These challenges may relate to inability to read or write but also to those whose primary language is not English. A study of Portuguese patients with RA compared those who were literate (N = 66) with those who could not read or write in Portuguese (N = 25) using a VAS, VRS (separate boxes for no pain, mild, moderate, severe, unbearable), and NRS (boxes with 0 to 10) (Ferraz, Quaresma, Aquino, et al., 1990). The NRS that uses numbers rather than the VRS with word descriptors had higher reliability in both groups. Tools that avoid words, such as the FPS-R, may be useful options in older persons who are illiterate, dyslexic, or non-English speaking, although testing in these samples is needed.

In addition to pain intensity scales, the use of a pain map or figure drawing such as an enlargement of the figure in Form 3-1 (p. 51) can be a useful tool in identifying the location of pain. Even those with dementia have been able to use this approach to communicate the location of their pain (Weiner, Peterson, Logue, et al., 1998; Wynne, Ling, Remsburg, 2000). In those with cognitive impairment, information about pain location can guide approaches to care that minimize the activities and movements that precipitate discomfort. Knowledge of pain location can also help clinicians decide when anticipatory pain intervention would be useful (e.g., prior to range of motion exercises or transfer of a patient who located pain in the shoulders and hip joints).

In summary, the goals are to identify a pain assessment tool that older patients with cognitive impairment can use easily, to use the same tool consistently in each assessment, to establish a comfort-function goal, and to document the reports of pain in an accessible location in the medical records. The organization should identify valid and reliable tools from which to select for use with patients having varying levels of cognitive impairment (see Patient Example, below). A reasonable approach would be to have a vertical NRS such as 0 to 5, a VDS, and the FPS-R

as options for this population. Unfortunately, no research has yet tested the 0-to-5 NRS in the cognitively impaired population. Development of documentation strategies that keep pain assessment information in a visible place is needed to monitor changes in pain and response to treatment. Table 3-1 (p. 96) provides a summary of research information on pain-intensity tools recommended for use in older adults with cognitive impairment.

Assessment of Neuropathic Pain

Characteristics of Neuropathic Pain

The International Association for the Study of Pain defines neuropathic pain as "pain initiated or caused by a primary lesion or dysfunction of the nervous system" (Merskey, Bogduk, 1994, p. 212). This remains the current definition and includes neuropathies, postherpetic neuralgia, and radiculopathy. There are, however, a variety of clinical conditions that have neuropathic features but do not exactly fit this definition because they do not seem to involve an injury or dysfunction of the nervous system (Audette, Emenike, Meleger, 2005; Fishbain, Lewis, Cutler, et al., 2008). These conditions include complex regional pain syndrome, fibromyalgia, and others in which whether they represent neuropathic pain is controversial.

Patient Example

This is an example of a scenario for determining an effective method of pain-intensity evaluation in cognitively impaired older patients.

Mrs. H is a 70-year-old African-American admitted from the nursing home to the hospital because of a recent fall resulting in fracture of the right hip. She has diagnoses of OA, spinal stenosis, congestive heart failure, and Alzheimer's disease. The nurse encounters Mrs. H on admission to the orthopedic surgery unit. Mrs. H is disoriented about time and place but able to state her name. She is moaning and rubbing her right hip and exhibits facial grimacing when moved. When asked if she is hurting, Mrs. H responds "a lot." The nurse shows her the unit's standard 0-to-10 NRS and asks her to rate the severity of her pain. She looks at the tool and points at the low end of the scale. Based on the patient's description of having "a lot" of pain and observation of Mrs. H's behaviors, the nurse suspects that she does not understand the NRS. The nurse shows Mrs. H a simple VDS using none, mild, moderate, and severe pain. Mrs. H selects the words "severe pain." The nurse provides her pre-

scribed analgesic and reassesses her pain using the same VDS 1 hour later. Mrs. H selects "mild pain" and is no longer grimacing and moaning.

KEY POINTS

- Attempt to use the clinical unit's standard pain scale first.
- Consider pain what patient's say about their pain and their pain behaviors in judging the reliability of the pain report obtained from the unit's standard scale. Behaviors can support the presence of pain, but the absence of pain behaviors does not negate the presence of pain.
- Select an alternative tool if the reliability of the report obtained from the unit's standard scale is questionable.
- Select a simple pain scale for cognitively impaired patients experiencing pain.
- Use the same pain scale to reassess pain and response to interventions.

Table 3-1 | Pain Intensity Tools Recommended for Use with Older Adults Who Have Difficulty with Commonly Used Self-Report Scales

Name of Measure	Reliability	Validity/Utility
Verbal Descriptor Scales (VDS), such as Iowa Pain Thermometer, or none, mild, moderate, or severe[1-3]	Adequate test-retest reliability in the cognitively intact ($r = 0.67$), and those with cognitive impairment ($r = 0.50$),	Tested in acute care, nursing home, assisted-living facility, and outpatient clinic Strong positive correlation with other pain intensity scales Validated in Caucasian and African American samples Preferred by older adults, with low failure rate even in the cognitively impaired Thermometer adaptation may assist with understanding of tool Easy to explain
Faces Pain Scale-Revised FPS-R[4-6]	Acceptable to high test-retest reliability in the cognitively intact ($r = 0.62$-0.89); decreased in those with cognitive impairment ($r = .26$-$.67$)	FPS-R tested in acute care and community dwelling; FPS tested in subacute care, pain clinic, long-term care, assisted living facility Less strong positive correlation with other pain intensity scales; may represent more than intensity Validated in Caucasian, African American, Spanish, and Chinese FPS-R preferred by many older adults; most preferred by African American, Spanish, and Asian older adults Does not require language or reading ability

As appears in Pasero, C., & McCaffery, M. *Pain assessment and pharmacologic management*, p. 96, St. Louis, Mosby. © 2011, Pasero C, McCaffery M. May be duplicated for use in clinical practice.

[1]Closs, S. J., Barr, B., Briggs, M., et al. (2004). A comparison of five pain assessment scales for nursing home residents with varying degrees of cognitive impairment. *J Pain Symptom Manage* 27, 196-205.

[2]Herr, K., Spratt, K., Garand, L., et al. (2007). Evaluation of the Iowa pain thermometer and other selected pain intensity scales in younger and older adult cohorts using controlled clinical pain: A preliminary study. *Pain Medicine, 8*(7), 585-600.

[3]Taylor, L. J., Harris, J., Epps, C. D., et al. (2005). Psychometric evaluation of selected pain intensity scales for use with cognitively impaired and cognitively intact older adults. *Rehabilitation Nursing, 30*, 55-61.

[4]Ware, L. J., Epps, C., Herr, K., et al. (2006). Evaluation of the Revised Faces Pain Scale, verbal descriptor scale, numeric rating scale, and Iowa Pain Thermometer in older minority adults. *Pain Management Nursing, 7*(3), 117-125.

[5]Li, L., Liu, X, & Herr, K. (2007). Postoperative pain intensity assessment: A comparison of four scales in Chinese adults. *Pain Medicine, 8*(3), 223-234.

[6]Miro, J., Huguet, A., Nieto, R., et al. (2005). Evaluation of reliability, validity, and preference for a pain intensity scale for use with the elderly. *The Journal of Pain, 6*(11), 727-735.

Neuropathic (pathologic) pain is distinctly different from physiologic (nociceptive) pain (see Section I). It is pain sustained by abnormal processing of sensory input by the peripheral or central nervous system, most often as a result of injury. There are numerous causes of nervous system damage that can result in neuropathic pain, including toxins, infection, viruses, metabolic disturbances, nutritional deficiencies, and trauma (Pasero, 2004).

The types of neuropathic pain are commonly divided into categories on the basis of the mechanism thought to be primarily responsible for causing the pain (i.e., peripheral or central nervous system activity) (see Figure I-1, p. 2). Note that in some cases the original injury occurs in the peripheral nerves (e.g., amputation), but the mechanisms that underlie the pain (e.g., phantom pain) seem to be generated primarily in the central nervous system.

Screening Tools and Measurement Tools for Neuropathic Pain

In relation to neuropathic pain, two types of assessment scales may be used: screening tools and measurement tools. Tools have been developed for screening populations of patients with chronic pain to distinguish neuropathic pain from other types of chronic pain (Bennett, Attal, Backonia, et al., 2007). Those that are self-report tools and do not require examination by a clinician are reliable and valid and are easy to score; they include the ID Pain tool (Portenoy, 2006); the Self-Administered Leeds Assessment of Neuropathic Symptoms and Signs (S-LANSS) tool (Bennett, Smith, Torrance, et al., 2005); and the painDETECT tool (Freynhagen, Baron, Gockel, et al., 2006). This type of tool may be especially useful for non-pain specialists in primary care settings. Once neuropathic pain has been identified, the need to refer a patient to a pain specialist can be evaluated, and measurement tools such as the Neuropathic Pain Scale (NPS) (Galer, Jensen, 1997) may be used to measure the qualities of neuropathic pain over time and evaluate the effects of various treatments (see discussion of the NPS below).

Because of its brevity, simplicity, reliability, and validity, the complete ID Pain tool has been selected for inclusion here (Form 3-4). This tool was validated using

Screening Tool for Neuropathic Pain: ID Pain

On the diagram below, shade in the areas where you feel pain. If you have more than one painful area, circle the area that bothers you the most.

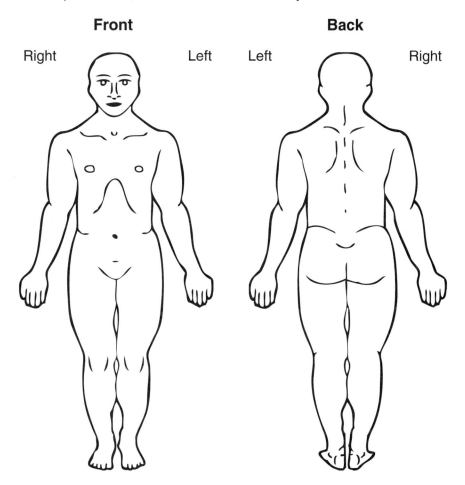

Mark "Yes" to the following items that describe your pain over the past week and "No" to the ones that do not. If you have more than one painful area, answer the questions in relation to the area most bothers you the most.

Question	Score	
	Yes	No
1. Did the pain feel like pins and needles?	1	0
2. Did the pain feel hot/burning?	1	0
3. Did the pain feel numb?	1	0
4. Did the pain feel like electrical shocks?	1	0
5. Is the pain made worse with the touch of clothing or bed sheets?	1	0
6. Is the pain limited to your joints?	−1	0

Form 3-4

As appears in Pasero, C., McCaffery, M. (2011). *Pain assessment and pharmacologic management*, p. 97, St. Louis, Mosby. Used with permission. From Portenoy, R. (2006). Development and testing of a neuropathic pain screening questionnaire: ID Pain. *Curr Med Res Opin*, 22(1), 1555-1565. May be duplicated for use in clinical practice.

data from two independent multicenter study samples (Portenoy, 2006). It is composed of a drawing, five sensory descriptor items requiring a yes or no answer, and one item relating to whether pain is located in the joints, which is used to identify nociceptive pain. The scale is self-administered, is easily scored, and can be used to quickly identify patients who have neuropathic components to their pain. Scores range from –1 to 5, with 3 being identified as the cut-off point for neuropathic pain. Scores of 3 or higher indicate the likely presence of a neuropathic component of the pain and justify a more detailed evaluation.

In the late 1990s a brief yet comprehensive assessment tool, the NPS, was designed specifically to measure the qualities of neuropathic pain (Galer, Jensen, 1997). The complete tool is included here (Form 3-5). Studying 288 patients with peripheral neuropathic pain, the researchers identified eight common qualities: sharp, hot, dull, cold, sensitive (like raw skin or a sunburn), itchy, and deep versus surface pain. These are included on the NPS as items 2 through 7 and item 10. Each item is rated on a 0 to 10 scale (0 = none; 10 = most imaginable). The tool is easy for most patients to learn, takes about 5 minutes to complete, and is sensitive to the effects of treatment. It also has been translated into Italian (Negri, Bettaglio, Demartini, et al., 2002). One limitation of the scale is that it does not include some pain qualities typical of neuropathic pain, such as numbness, tingling (pins and needles), and electric shock (Jensen, Dworkin, Gammaitoni, et al., 2005).

The NPS also appears to be a useful tool in the assessment of patients with central pain caused by multiple sclerosis. In a study of 141 patients with chronic pain related to multiple sclerosis, the NPS was found to be a valid and reliable assessment tool and possibly useful in measuring treatment outcomes (Rog, Nurmikko, Friede, et al., 2007). It was also found to be versatile in that it was reliable and valid when administered face-to-face as well as by postal survey.

In a study of 159 patients with diabetic-related foot pain, the NPS was administered before, during, and after treatment with placebo versus opioid (modified-release oxycodone) (Jensen, Friedman, Bonzo, et al., 2006). More participants receiving opioids responded to the six NPS items than those receiving placebos. The three NPS items that were most responsive to opioid treatment as compared to placebo were pain intensity, unpleasantness, and deep pain. The results support the validity of the NPS for detecting change in neuropathic pain with treatment, and this is probably the first study to show a significant effect of opioid treatment on specific pain sensations.

A study of 470 patients with peripheral neuropathic pain, low back pain, or OA, demonstrated the utility of the NPS for assessing changes in pain after treatment with a lidocaine patch (Jensen, Dworkin, Gammaitoni, et al., 2005).

With the exception of cold, each of the qualities of pain on the NPS showed significant change after treatment in each of the three diagnostic groups, supporting the validity of the NPS for detecting change in pain. Eventually, this type of research might help to identify which qualities of pain respond to which analgesics and to better understand the mechanisms of analgesic effects.

The words used by patients to describe pain may indicate the underlying pain mechanism. For example, postherpetic neuralgia is more likely to be described as sharp, less cold, and more sensitive and itchy than other types of neuropathic pain (Galer, Jensen, 1997). Patients with diabetic neuropathy who described sharp and shooting pain were found in one study to be more likely to respond to clonidine than those who did not use these descriptors (Byas-Smith, Max, Muir, et al., 1995). Although the NPS was not designed to discriminate between neuropathic and nonneuropathic pain, further study of patients with persistent pain has shown that the NPS appears to be able to do this (Fishbain, Lewis, Cutler, et al., 2008).

In summary, the NPS may be a practical tool in the initial assessment of patients suspected of having neuropathic components in their pain, such as low back pain. It may also be useful in evaluating the effects of treatment of patients with neuropathic pain. As the tool is developed further it may become a practical method of distinguishing one type of neuropathic pain from another. As mentioned, the NPS or the ID Pain tool can be provided to patients presenting to the emergency department with conditions such as low back pain so they can complete it while waiting to be evaluated. This will help clinicians to better determine the type of pain patients are having and the appropriate treatment to prescribe.

For patients who do not have neuropathic pain initially, routine pain assessment tools completed at each visit to the clinician might include a list of the eight descriptors on the NPS. The patient could be asked to indicate whether any of these sensations had been noted since the last visit. In that way, a patient who did not originally have neuropathic pain might be identified, and changes in the progression of pain and in underlying pathologic conditions may be assessed and treated more quickly. This method of identifying neuropathic pain has not been tested for reliability and validity as has the ID Pain form, but it may be a practical method to use in some situations.

Along with the NPS, there is another self-report scale that is a reliable and valid instrument for measuring the qualities of neuropathic pain: the Neuropathic Pain Symptom Inventory (NPSI). The reader may wish to compare this scale with the NPS to determine which is preferred. The NPSI tool is available in both English and French (Bouhassira, Attal, Fermanian, et al., 2004).

Measurement Tool for Neuropathic Pain: Neuropathy Pain Scale

Date _____   Name _____

There are several different aspects of pain which we are interested in measuring: pain **sharpness, heat/cold, dullness, intensity,** overall **unpleasantness** and **surface vs. deep** pain.

The distinction between these aspects of pain might be clearer if you think of taste. For example, people might agree on how *sweet* a piece of pie might be (the *intensity* of sweetness), but some might enjoy it more if it were sweeter while others might prefer it to be less sweet. Similarly, people can judge the loudness of music and agree on what is more quiet and what is louder, but disagree on how it makes them feel. Some prefer quiet music and some prefer it louder. In short, the *intensity* of a sensation is not the same as how it makes you feel. A sound might be unpleasant and still be quiet (think of someone grating their fingernails along a chalkboard). A sound can be quiet and "dull" or loud and "dull."

Pain is the same. Many people are able to tell the difference between many aspects of their pain: for example, *how much* it hurts and *how unpleasant* or annoying it is. Although often the intensity of pain has a strong influence on how unpleasant the experience of pain is, some people are able to experience more pain than others before they feel very bad about it.

There are scales for measuring different aspects of pain. For one patient, a pain might feel extremely hot, but not at all dull, while another patient may not experience any heat, but feel like their pain is very dull. We expect you to rate very high on some of the scales below and very low on others. We want you to use the measures that follow to tell us exactly what your experience of pain has been, on average, *during the past week.*

Instructions: Please think about each sensation listed below and rate that sensation as the *average* you have experienced *during the past week.* Place an "X" through the number that best describes this.

1. Please use the scale below to tell us how **intense** your pain has been on average during the past week.

| No pain | 0 | 1 | 2 | 3 | 4 | 5 | 6 | 7 | 8 | 9 | 10 | The most **intense** pain sensation imaginable |

2. Please use the scale below to tell us how **sharp** your pain has felt on average during the past week. Words used to describe "sharp" feelings include: "like a knife," "like a spike," "jabbing" or "like jolts."

| No pain | 0 | 1 | 2 | 3 | 4 | 5 | 6 | 7 | 8 | 9 | 10 | The most **sharp** sensation imaginable ("like a knife") |

3. Please use the scale below to tell us how **hot** your pain has felt on average during the past week. Words used to describe very hot pain include: "burning" and "on fire."

| Not hot | 0 | 1 | 2 | 3 | 4 | 5 | 6 | 7 | 8 | 9 | 10 | The most **hot** sensation imaginable ("on fire") |

4. Please use the scale below to tell us how **dull** your pain has felt on average during the past week. Words used to describe very dull pain include: "like a dull toothache," "dull pain," "aching" and "like a bruise."

| Not dull | 0 | 1 | 2 | 3 | 4 | 5 | 6 | 7 | 8 | 9 | 10 | The most **dull** sensation imaginable |

Form 3-5 |

Continued

From Pasero, C., McCaffery, M. (2011). *Pain assessment and pharmacologic management*, pp. 99-100, St. Louis, Mosby. From Galer, B. S., & Jensen, M. P. (1997). Development and preliminary validation of a pain measure specific to neuropathic pain: The neuropathic pain scale. *Neurology*, 48, 337-338. © Jensen MP, Galer BS. Permission for all use in research activities is required and must be obtained by contacting the MAPI Research Trust (http://www.mapiresearch.fr).

Measurement Tool for Neuropathic Pain: Neuropathy Pain Scale–cont'd

5. Please use the scale below to tell us how **cold** your pain has felt on average during the past week. Words used to describe very cold pain include: "like ice" and "freezing."

| Not cold | 0 | 1 | 2 | 3 | 4 | 5 | 6 | 7 | 8 | 9 | 10 | The most **cold** sensation imaginable ("freezing") |

6. Please use the scale below to tell us how **sensitive** your skin has been to light touch or clothing on average during the past week. Words used to describe sensitive skin include "like sunburned skin" and "raw skin."

| Not sensitive | 0 | 1 | 2 | 3 | 4 | 5 | 6 | 7 | 8 | 9 | 10 | The most **sensitive** sensation imaginable ("raw skin") |

7. Please use the scale below to tell us how **itchy** your pain has felt on average during the past week. Words used to describe itchy pain include: "like poison oak" and "like a mosquito bite."

| Not itchy | 0 | 1 | 2 | 3 | 4 | 5 | 6 | 7 | 8 | 9 | 10 | The most **itchy** sensation imaginable ("like poison oak") |

8. Which ot the following best describes the **time** quality of your pain on average during the past week?
   Please check only one: a, b, or c.
   a. ❑ I felt background pain <u>all of the time</u> **and** occasional flare-ups (breakthrough pain) <u>some of the time</u>.

   Describe the background pain: _____
   Describe the flare-up (breakthrough pain): _____

   b. ❑ I felt a single type of pain <u>all of the time</u>. Describe this pain: _____

   c. ❑ I felt a single type of pain <u>only sometimes</u>. Describe this pain: _____

9. Now that you have told us the different physical aspects of your pain, the different types of sensations, we want you to tell us overall how **unpleasant** your pain has been. Words used to describe very unpleasant pain include: "miserable" and "intolerable." Remember, pain can have a low intensity, but still feel extremely unpleasant, and some kinds of pain can have a high intensity but be very tolerable. Please use the scale below to tell us how **unpleasant** your pain has felt on average during the past week.

| Not unpleasant | 0 | 1 | 2 | 3 | 4 | 5 | 6 | 7 | 8 | 9 | 10 | The most **unpleasant** sensation imaginable ("intolerable") |

10. Lastly, we want you to give us an estimate of the severity of your deep versus surface pain. We want you to rate each location of pain separately. We realize that it can be difficult to make these estimates, and most likely it will be a "best guess," but please give us your best estimate.

HOW INTENSE HAS YOUR **DEEP** PAIN BEEN ON AVERAGE DURING THE PAST WEEK?

| No **deep** pain | 0 | 1 | 2 | 3 | 4 | 5 | 6 | 7 | 8 | 9 | 10 | The most **intense** **deep** pain sensation imaginable |

HOW INTENSE HAS YOUR **SURFACE** PAIN BEEN ON AVERAGE DURING THE PAST WEEK?

| No **surface** pain | 0 | 1 | 2 | 3 | 4 | 5 | 6 | 7 | 8 | 9 | 10 | The most **intense** **surface** pain sensation imaginable |

Form 3-5 | Cont'd.

Assessment of Breakthrough Pain

No universally accepted definition of BTP exists. It is defined differently in different countries and in different specialties, and definitions have varied over the years (Payne, 2007). Probably the first comprehensive definition of BTP was developed in relation to research involving patients with persistent cancer-related pain and was defined as "a transitory increase in pain to greater than moderate intensity (that is, to an intensity of 'severe' or 'excruciating') which occurred on a baseline pain of moderate intensity or less (that is, no pain or pain of 'mild' or 'moderate' intensity)" (Portenoy, Hagen, 1990, p. 274). It is pain that breaks through other pain that is well controlled. BTP has also been studied in relation to persistent noncancer pain. A definition that is commonly used now in clinical practice is that BTP is a transitory increase in pain that occurs on a background of otherwise controlled persistent pain (Portenoy, Bennett, Rauck, et al., 2006).

Characteristics of Breakthrough Pain

BTP is divided into three subtypes: incident, idiopathic, and end-of-dose. Incident BTP is further divided into two types: predictable and unpredictable (Box 3-6). Idiopathic pain is not associated with any known cause.

Box 3-6	Subtypes of Breakthrough Pain

Breakthrough pain (BTP) is a transitory increase in pain that occurs against a background of otherwise controlled persistent pain. Subtypes of BTP are as follows:

1. Incident pain: Cause of pain is generally identifiable but occurrence may be unpredictable.
   a. Predictable incident pain: Something identifiable, such as movement, predictably causes the pain.
   b. Unpredictable incident pain: Occurrence of pain is unpredictable, and may be caused by events such as bladder spasm. Occurs spontaneously.
2. Idiopathic: Cause is not readily identifiable.
3. End-of-dose: An increase in baseline pain that occurs prior to a scheduled dose of around-the-clock analgesic. Onset is usually gradual, and duration may be longer than that of incident or idiopathic pain.

From Pasero, C., & McCaffery, M. *Pain assessment and pharmacologic management*, p. 101, St. Louis, Mosby. Data from Bennett, D., Burton, A. W., Fishman, S., et al. (2005). Consensus panel recommendations for the assessment and management of breakthrough pain: Part I: Assessment. *Pharmacol Ther*, 30(5), 296-301. © 2011, Pasero C, McCaffery M. May be duplicated for use in clinical practice.

End-of-dose pain refers to pain returning before the interval between doses elapses. Defining these types of BTP may assist with selecting a form of treatment. Use of a short-acting opioid is commonly the treatment for incident pain and idiopathic pain, whereas an increase in the dosage of around-the-clock analgesic or a decrease in the interval between doses is usually the treatment for end-of-dose BTP.

In a review of 5 studies of cancer populations, BTP was found to occur in 50% to 90% of patients with persistent pain, confirming that BTP is a significant problem for patients with cancer-related pain (Portenoy, Bennett, Rauck, et al., 2006). In one study of BTP in 164 patients with persistent cancer pain, the median number of episodes was 6 per day, and the median interval from onset to peak was 3 minutes (Portenoy, Payne, Jacobsen, 1999). Almost two thirds (61.7%) could identify precipitants such as movement, but almost half (48.2%) stated that BTP was never predictable. Patients with BTP experienced more functional impairment and psychologic distress than did patients with controlled background pain and no BTP. BTP has not been as well studied in patients with persistent noncancer pain, but in a survey of 228 patients with noncancer pain, 74% had BTP (Portenoy, Bennett, Rauck, et al., 2006). The most common cause for their persistent pain was low back pain (52%). The median number of episodes of BTP per day was 2, median time to maximum intensity was 10 minutes, and median duration was 60 minutes. Patients identified a precipitant for 69% of the occurrences of BTP, and it was almost always activity related. Onset could not be predicted in 45% of bouts of BTP and could be predicted only sometimes in 31%.

A study of 43 patients with persistent noncancer pain assessed for impact of BTP on quality of life (Taylor, Webster, Chun, et al., 2007). In response to questions about how BTP affected patients' lives, the two questions that 93% of the patients found affected their lives the most ("quite a bit or very much") were related to general activity levels and the ability to work both outside the home and in the home doing housework. The next category most commonly rated (86%) as affecting their lives the most was enjoyment of life.

Tools for Assessment of Breakthrough Pain

Only a few tools have been developed for use in clinical practice to screen for or to assess BTP. Some have been used only for research purposes, and others are meant only for clinician assessment; that is, they guide a clinician's interview of a patient. A list of questions that clinicians can use to interview patients about BTP has been published by a multidisciplinary panel (Bennett, Burton, Fishman, et al., 2005). A pain assessment algorithm has been published; it begins with the clinician asking a patient questions that screen for BTP and then follows up with specific questions about the BTP (Portenoy, Bennett, Rauck, et al., 2006). This was used in a research study of BTP in opioid-treated patients with noncancer pain and was modified from one originally developed for patients with cancer-related pain, neither of which has been validated (Portenoy, Payne, Jacobsen, 1999). Another published tool for assessing BTP, the Alberta Breakthrough Pain Assessment Tool, was developed for research with cancer patients (Hagen, Stiles, Nekolaichuk, et al., 2008). Some of the questions must be completed by the clinician as they interview the patient, and one section of the tool is suitable for completion by the patient. Evidence suggests that this tool is understandable by patients and clinicians, so further validation of the tool is warranted.

A screening tool for BTP is difficult to develop because BTP is not easily characterized when baseline pain has not been controlled. Baseline pain can be defined as almost always being present, continuous, steady, or constant or would be if medication did not control the pain. Thus, a screening tool for BTP in clinical practice is best designed to be used after baseline pain has been determined to exist and has been well managed.

Most patients with persistent pain who have controlled baseline pain experience only one type of BTP. In a study of 228 patients with persistent noncancer pain and controlled baseline pain, 74% had one or more types of BTP (Portenoy, Bennett, Rauck, et al., 2006). Of these patients, 88.7% had one type of BTP, and the remainder of the patients had up to three types of BTP. Precipitants were identified for 69% of the BTP episodes, and 92% of them were activity related. In a study of 164 patients with chronic cancer pain and controlled baseline pain, 51.2% experienced one or more types of BTP (Portenoy, Payne, Jacobsen, 1999). Of these patients, 83.1% experienced only one type of BTP, and the remainder experienced as many as three types of BTP. Precipitants of BTP could be identified by 61.7% of patients, with movement being the most common, 20.4%. However, almost half of the patients said that precipitants were never predictable.

Forms 3-6 (p. 103) and 3-7 (pp. 104-105) have been developed to provide simple, short forms to screen for and assess BTP. These forms have not been tested for reliability and validity, but they have been created in the absence of such forms in the hope that they will encourage assessment of BTP until simple, reliable, and valid forms are available. The short screening tool may be included in an already existing initial pain assessment tool, as is done with Form 3-1 (p. 51), or may be included in the clinician's interview with the patient. The purpose of this form is to identify patients with persistent, constant, controlled baseline pain who also have pain that breaks through the controlled pain; that is, BTP. When such a patient is identified, he or she may complete the assessment form, or the clinician may use the form to ask the patient about BTP.

A detailed pain diary is commonly recommended as being the best account of the occurrence, predictability, severity, and duration of BTP (Payne, 2007). The Pain Control Diary, Form 3-11 (p. 116), may be used for this purpose and perhaps modified to include columns for noting physical activity at the time pain started and the time pain ended. A daily pain diary that may be more suitable for assessing BTP can be found at http://www.healthinaging.org/public_education/pain/my_pain_diary.pdf.

Reassessment

Once the initial assessments of the patient is complete and treatment for pain relief has begun, reassessment of the patient is essential to determine the effects of treatment. This is facilitated by using a variety of types of flow sheets. Flow sheets for pain management are work sheets that document progress toward achieving and maintaining pain-management goals. They are used for ongoing evaluation of pain treatments.

Following is a discussion of paper-based flow sheets for analgesic infusions in acute care, pain control diaries for outpatient care, and a standardized record for reassessing patients with chronic pain who are taking opioids. The current focus on patient safety as well as efficient administration of care has brought about the introduction of the electronic health record to patient care. Also called the *electronic medical record*, the electronic health record is a comprehensive patient-centered clinical information system that contains data from multiple care settings as well as from the patient. (See Appendix C [pp. 837-857] for an overview of the electronic medical record, including its implementation in the clinical setting and examples of screens, such as pain management order sets and flow sheets, medication administration records, and assessment alerts.)

Flow Sheets for Analgesic Infusions in Acute Care

Obtaining pain ratings before and after the administration of analgesics is especially important because clinicians tend to assume that analgesics are safe and effective. Research has verified that the use of pain flow sheets, compared with the routine narrative charting in nursing notes, is effective in improving pain management (e.g., decreasing pain intensity and sedation) (Brown, 1992; Faries, Mills, Goldsmith, et al., 1991; McMillan, Williams, Chatfield, et al., 1988).

Flow sheets must be tailored to the patient population, clinical setting, and type of pain being managed. For example, some are designed for staff to complete for hospitalized patients using IV PCA for severe pain. Typically, flow sheets include, at a minimum, columns for time, pain ratings, facts about the analgesic administered (e.g., dose, route) or other pain treatment, and

Screening Tool for Pain Flares — Breakthrough Pain (BTP)*

Instructions: We are interested in a particular type of pain you may have. Please answer the following questions:

1. Do you have pain that is:

a. constant, almost always present, or would be present if not for the treatment you are receiving?

_____ yes   _____no

b. or, do you have constant pain that is usually:

_____ moderate pain   _____ severe pain

2. Do you have temporary flares of pain that are more intense than your constant pain?

_____ yes   _____no

*Note to clinician: The above questions may be placed with an existing initial pain assessment tool, such as Form 3-1 on p. 51, or the patient may complete the above form. If the patient has constant pain that is usually moderate to severe, then this needs to be controlled before addressing flares of pain. If the patient has constant pain that is usually controlled and answers yes to question 2, consider having the patient complete the form on "Assessment of Pain Flares — Breakthrough Pain (BTP)," on pp.104-105.

Form 3-6

From Pasero, C., & McCaffery, M. *Pain assessment and pharmacologic management*, p. 103, St. Louis, Mosby. © 2011, Pasero C, McCaffery M. May be duplicated for use in clinical practice.

adverse effects pertinent to the situation. Adverse effects pertinent to the use of opioids for severe pain in opioid-naive patients (those not taking regular daily doses of opioids) include sedation level and respiratory status. Information about pain ratings should be obtained and recorded near the time of the event, whenever possible. For example, in a study of 60 patients being discharged from the postanesthesia care unit, many were unable to recall the pain ratings they gave when they were admitted to the unit (DeLoach, Higgins, Caplan, et al., 1998).

Frustration about the failure of staff nurses to reassess and document the effects of analgesics in acute care inpatient settings is frequently reported by nurses attending programs on pain management and is often a topic discussed on the nursing issues LISTSERV provided by the American Pain Society (APS) and the American Society for Pain Management Nursing. Research reflects this problem as well. In an Australian study of 52 nurses caring for 364 postoperative patients, 316 pain-related activities occurred in 74 observation periods (2 hours each), but only 4.4% were reassessments after analgesic

administration (Bucknall, Manias, Botti, 2007). Before or during the observation period, 147 patients received analgesics but in only 13.6% was the pain reassessed. Most of these reassessments were opportunistic in that they were performed when the nurse was in the patient's room carrying out other nursing activities such as administering other medications. Some have argued that reassessment following analgesic administration occurs but is not documented. However, this study was of actual nursing activity at the patient's bedside, not documentation, and still reassessment of administered analgesics was substantially lacking.

In the United States, abstracts of the medical records of 709 older patients hospitalized for hip fracture were made for the purpose of determining nurses' documentation of their pain assessments, including reassessments following administration of non-PCA analgesics (Herr, Titler, Schilling, et al., 2004). For the first 24-hour period following admission, 2965 analgesics were administered, and only 21.8% (646) were followed by reassessment of pain within 60 minutes. For the entire 72-hour period,

Assessment of Pain Flares — Breakthrough Pain (BTP)

Instructions: The following questions are about your flares of pain, that is, pains that are more intense than your constant pain. These flares are often referred to as breakthrough pain (BTP).

Begin now with the type of pain flare that bothers you the most.

1. On the figure drawing below, please mark the location of your pain flare.

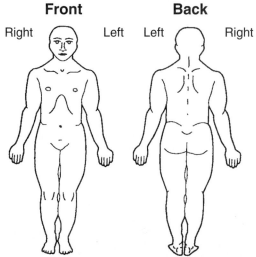

2. About how many times does this pain flare occur? _____ per day _____ per week

3. How long is it from the time the pain starts to when the pain is at its worst?
   _____ less than 1 minute _____1-5 minutes _____6-15 minutes _____15-60 minutes

4. How intense is this pain at its worst?
   _____ mild pain _____moderate pain _____ severe pain _____ very severe

5. How long does each pain flare usually last?
   _____ seconds _____ minutes _____ hours

6. Does your pain flare usually start a certain amount of time before your next scheduled pain medicine? _____ yes _____ no

7. Is your pain flare an increase in your constant, ongoing pain?
   _____ yes _____ no

8. What does your pain flare feel like? For example, aching, sharp, burning, tight, crampy, radiating)?_____

9. Do you know what causes your pain flare? _____ yes _____ no
   If so, please describe._____

10. Can you predict when your pain flare is going to occur?
    _____never _____ sometimes _____ usually

11. Do you know how to relieve your pain flare? _____ yes _____ no
    If yes, how? _____

12. How does your pain flare affect your daily life, for example, keeps you from walking, sleeping, concentrating, enjoying life? _____

For legend, see p. 105

Form 3-7 | This form may be used for clinicians to interview patients or may be completed by the patients themselves. It is appropriate for patients with chronic pain who have controlled baseline pain and breakthrough pain. This form should not be used unless baseline pain is usually controlled. These questions should be answered in relation to the type of pain flare that bothers the patient the most. Determine whether the patient has more than one type of pain flare, and consider using this assessment tool for each one.

only 15.3% (1497) of 9782 analgesic administrations were following by reassessments of pain within 60 minutes. In a study of frail elderly patients postoperatively who received analgesics, only 4% were reassessed following the analgesic (MacDonald, Hilton, 2001).

The medical records were reviewed for reassessment of 52 critically ill intubated patients who had had 183 pain episodes (Gelinas, Fortier, Viens, 2004). Pharmacologic interventions were used 89% of the time, and nonpharmacologic interventions were used less than 25% of the time. However, almost 40% of the time, pain was not reassessed after an intervention. Self-report was recorded for only 1 patient. Reassessment of patients consisted primarily of recorded behavioral and physiologic manifestations. Some of the physiologic indicators are questionable signs of pain, and although they were recorded within 1 hour of an intervention, it is not clear that they were done to reassess pain.

Another study of 117 charts of 80 inpatients and 37 outpatients with cancer whose pain had been documented in their charts revealed that reassessment after analgesic treatment was reported in 34% of the outpatient charts and 44% of the inpatient charts (Cohen, Easley, Ellis, et al., 2003). The more favorable results shown in this study may have occurred because charts that did not document pain at all were excluded from the sample, meaning that pain may have existed, and treatment may have been provided but not documented. For example, the researchers found one outpatient setting with no charts that documented pain at all, and the staff said they simply did not document pain.

Reassessment of pain after administration of an opioid is not just a documentation issue, it is also an issue of patient safety following administration of a drug that could lead to death. Reassessment should be the basis of planning for further intervention, in particular knowing when change in the treatment plan is needed. For example, measures such as decreasing the opioid dosage in a patient who is excessively sedated can be implemented to prevent life-threatening respiratory depression. Range orders for opioid analgesics simply cannot be effectively implemented unless the previous dose of analgesic is followed by reassessment of pain intensity and adverse effects. (See Section IV for additional information about opioid-range orders and treatment of opioid-induced adverse effects.)

Most health care facilities have incorporated guidelines for pain documentation into their policies and procedures and have provided space for documentation of basic pain assessments in standard nursing care forms; flow sheets are often used for analgesic infusions and IV bolus administration. Unit-specific quality improvement activities and ongoing education initiatives routinely include documentation of pain assessment following interventions for pain relief. In cases in which compliance is exceptionally low, management may decide to implement disciplinary measures such as linking documentation compliance to the nurses' annual performance reviews.

In the initial treatment of moderate to severe pain with opioids, the patient's pain rating is usually recorded every 1 to 2 hours during the first 24 hours, then every 4 hours if pain is controlled and other observations, such as sedation level, show the opioid is safe. When the patient appears to be sleeping at the time a pain rating should be obtained, it is often questioned whether to awaken the patient. Several factors should be considered. Not all patients who appear to be sleeping are actually sleeping. Further, sleep does not mean pain has been relieved. When a patient appears to be sleeping, his or her name may be called in a normal tone of voice. If the patient does not rouse and has acceptable respiratory status, pain assessment could be delayed until the patient awakens, and "appears to be sleeping" could be charted. However, even this approach has its limits, because sleep does not mean absence of pain. Therefore, if the medication has been given previously and the patient has rated relief as satisfactory, when that same medication is given again it is not necessary to awaken the patient after administration. However, if the patient has pain that is still out of control, discuss the situation with the patient and tell him or her that he or she may be awakened to determine whether the medication is providing effective pain relief.

Creative ways of reminding nurses to obtain and document pain ratings are often implemented as well. For example, hospital-wide competitions for prizes to be awarded to the unit demonstrating the highest compliance record can be good incentives for improving documentation. Some hospitals have installed, outside of patients' rooms, colored flags (similar to those seen in clinics or office-based practices) that can be moved to a position perpendicular to the wall after an analgesic has been given so as to provide visual reminders to nurses of the need for reassessments. Enlisting the help of other staff members (e.g., nursing technicians or even patients can remind nurses of the need for reassessment at a specific time). (See the discussion of pain diaries on pp. 110-119 and oral PCA in Chapter 12.)

As health care facilities move toward the use of electronic health records, computer software has the potential to become an excellent tool for improving the documentation of pain. Carefully placed prompts and alerts can remind and even force clinicians to document pain assessment before moving on to the next computer screen. (See Appendix C for additional information about electronic health records.)

Following is a discussion of a flow sheet for use in acute care settings in which patients with severe pain are being treated with opioids. Examples are provided.

Characteristics of the Flow Sheet for Analgesic Infusions in Acute Care

The flow sheet for analgesic infusions, such as IV PCA, epidural analgesia, and continuous perineural blockade, provides a quick and easy assessment and evaluation tool (Form 3-8). Because the flow sheet provides a comprehensive snapshot of how well a patient is tolerating therapy, it is often used for documentation of single or intermittent clinician-administered bolus doses as well. Flow sheets are used primarily in hospital settings where nurses are responsible for recording the information.

Most flow sheets are designed to prevent duplicate documentation. Space can be provided on the back of the flow sheet for documenting detailed information (e.g., description of how severe pain or an adverse effect was brought under control; see Forms 3-9 and 3-10 as examples). A mechanism such as an asterisk can be incorporated into the flow sheet for referring other members of the health care team to this detailed information. For ease in using the flow sheet, the type of information and the order in which it is recorded in the columns of the flow sheet should correspond with the type and order of the information displayed on the screens of the institution's infusion pump. This explains why there is such wide variability from one institution to another in terms of the information found on flow sheets and the way it is presented.

The example of the flow sheet for analgesic infusions shown in Form 3-8 has numbered spaces and columns that match the numbered explanations that follow.

1. *Date.* A new flow sheet can be started at 12 midnight (2400) every 24 hours or when space for documentation runs out. The day, month, and year are entered.
2. *Route of administration.* Analgesic therapies documented on flow sheets are usually given by the IV, subcutaneous (SC), epidural, spinal (or intrathecal), intrapleural, or perineural route of administration.

3. *Location.* Examples of locations include the extremity in which an IV is inserted for IV PCA, the targeted nerve or nerve plexus for continuous perineural blockade, and lumbar or thoracic epidural catheter placement.
4. *PCA.* A checkmark is made if the therapy is patient controlled (PCA).
5. *Comfort-function goal.* The comfort-function goal is a pain level that enables the patient to participate in specific recovery activities with relative ease (e.g., 2/10 to 3/10, discussed on pp. 85-88). The patients is encouraged to set a comfort-function goal, which is recorded in the space provided at the top right-hand corner of the flow sheet. Pain ratings greater than the patient's comfort-function goals should trigger further assessment and possible intervention. This information can also be used for quality-improvement purposes to help ensure unrelieved pain is being addressed appropriately.
6. *Time.* At various times during therapy, patient assessment and infusion data are recorded in the column spaces provided (see following numbers 7 through 23 for detailed descriptions of these entries). The analgesic prescription (also called *pump parameter*), which include, a the drug(s) and concentration(s), PCA doses, delay (or lockout) intervals, basal rate, and hour limit, are recorded typically only every 4 to 8 hours. Double-checks of pump programming are performed as safeguards against errors and require two clinicians or pharmacists to confirm that the drug(s) and concentration(s) listed on the reservoir label and the pump programming match the prescription. Practices vary among institutions as to when double-checks must be performed, but they are usually performed when therapy is initiated, when a prescription is changed, and when a patient's care is transferred from one care area to another (e.g., from postanesthetia care unit to clinical unit). Other data found in most pumps are the number of successful injections (INJ) and attempts (ATT) the patient makes to obtain a PCA dose during therapy and the administration of clinician boluses. Pain ratings, nurse-monitored respiratory status and sedation level (LOS), oxygen saturation, and carbon dioxide concentration if mechanical monitoring is prescribed, and presence of adverse effects (AE) usually are recorded every 1 to 2 hours for the first 24 hours of analgesic infusion therapies in opioid-naive patients. After that time, these parameters usually can be monitored every 4 hours, and mechanical monitoring, if prescribed, often is discontinued or performed PRN in stable patients. Motor and sensory assessments in patients receiving local anesthetic are usually recorded every 4 to 8 hours. Site and system assessments are documented at least every 8 hours.

24-Hour Pain Management Flow Sheet for Analgesic Infusions (start new sheet at 12 midnight daily)   Date _____ (1)

Check (√) therapy: IV (2) SC (2) Epidural (2) Spinal (2) Perineural (2) PCA (4) Comfort-Function Goal _____ (5)

Time (6)	Drug(s) (7)	Drug Conc(s) (8)	Vol Infus (9)	# INJ (10)	# ATT (11)	PCA Dose (12)	Delay (13)	Basal Rate (14)	Hour Limit (15)	Clin Bolus (16)	Pain Rating (17)	Resp Rate / LOS (18)	O₂ Sat (19)	ETCO₂ (20)	AE (21)	Motor / Sensory (22)	Site / System (23)	Initials (24)

(25) Ask patient to rate pain with one of these scales

0   1   2   3   4   5   6   7   8   9   10
No pain   Moderate pain   Worst possible

0   2   4   6   8   10 (faces scale)

LOS = LEVEL OF SEDATION (26)
S - Sleep, easy to arouse (no action necessary)
1 - Alert, easy to arouse (no action necessary)
2 - Occasionally drowsy, easy to arouse (no action necessary)
3 - Frequently drowsy, falls asleep mid-sentence (decrease opioid dose)
4 - Somnolent, difficult to arouse (stop opioid, consider naloxone, notify primary)

ADVERSE EFFECTS* (27)
M - Medicated
N - Nausea
V - Vomiting
C - Constipation
P - Pruritus
UR - Urinary retention
MT - Metallic taste
ER - Ear ringing
PN - Perioral numbness
*See orders for treatment, when to notify primary

MOTOR ASSESSMENT* (28)
0 - Flexes hip/knee/ankle; able to raise leg
1 - Flexes ankle/knee; unable to raise leg
2 - Flexes ankle; unable to flex knee or raise leg
3 - Unable to flex ankle/knee or raise leg
SENSORY ASSESSMENT*
0 - Full sensation; no numbness/tingling
1 - Reduced response to touch; no numbness or tingling
2 - Moderate numbness or tingling
3 - Full block (no sensation or response to touch)
*See orders for when to notify anesthesia

SITE/INFUSION SYSTEM √ = agree, * = see reverse
Site: Clean, dry, no redness, no edema, no tenderness; no back soreness (intraspinal)
System: Securely taped, tubings patent, reservoir has volume
PCA: Patient-only use, pendant within patient's reach
TUBING CHANGE: Time _____ Initials _____ (32)

SIGNATURE (32)   SIGNATURE (32)

CATHETER REMOVAL (29)
Catheter removed without difficulty, tip intact, site clean, dry, no redness
√ = agree, * = see reverse
Time _____ Initials _____ (32)

SIGNATURE (32)

DRUG WASTED (30)
Amount _____
Date _____ Time _____ (31)
Signature _____
Witness _____

SIGNATURE (32)

Continued

Form 3-8 | The back of the 24-hour pain management flow sheet provides space for comments when patients or infusion systems are outside of the norm. Comments can be made at any time by any member of the health care team and do not necessarily coincide with the flow sheet.

From Pasero, C., & McCaffery, M. Pain assessment and pharmacologic management, pp. 107-108, St. Louis, Mosby. © 2011, Pasero C, McCaffery M. May be duplicated for use in clinical practice.

24-Hour Pain Management Flow Sheet for Analgesic Infusions–cont'd

DATE	TIME	COMMENTS

Form 3-8 | Cont'd.

7. and 8. *Drug(s) and concentration(s).* After checking the drug reservoir labels against the prescriptions, the name of the drug(s) and the concentration(s) in the drug reservoir are recorded in this column every 4 to 8 hours and when prescriptions are changed, new reservoirs are added, or clinicians' boluses are administered. The drug concentrations, which are the amounts of drug per 1 milliliter of solution (X mg/mL, X mcg/mL) programmed into the pump are also checked for accuracy against the drug concentrations recorded on the drug reservoir labels.

9. *Volume infused (sometimes called "given" volume).* The amount of solution delivered since the start of therapy or since the last time the amount was cleared from the pump is recorded every 4 to 8 hours. (This feature is not available on all pumps; some pumps have volume remaining rather than volume infused, and some have both.) Some institutions record a running total of volume infused; others require pumps to be cleared at the end of every shift.

10. and 11. *Injections and attempts.* The term *injections* means the number of times patients self-administer a dose of PCA. *Attempts* are the number of times a patient presses the PCA button (pendant), whether a dose is delivered or not. If this information is available (some disposable pumps do not offer this information), these amounts can be recorded for patients receiving PCA. Most PCA pumps store in memory the number of injections and attempts every hour. This information is used to help determine the type of interventions that would most benefit the patient (e.g., patient teaching, increase dosage) (see Section IV).

12. *PCA dose.* The amount patients receive each time a PCA bolus dose is self-administered is recorded every 4 to 8 hours.

13. *Delay (or lockout) interval.* The number of minutes that must elapse between doses of PCA is recorded every 4 to 8 hours.

14. *Basal rate.* The amount of the continuous infusion is recorded every 4 to 8 hours. Many pumps bypass this display screen if a basal rate has not been programmed.

15. *Hour limit.* The total amount the patient can receive in 1 or 4 hours by PCA dose, and basal rate is recorded every 4 to 8 hours. Some pumps are programmed to bypass this display screen (see Section IV for more about hour limits).

16. *Clinician bolus.* Clinician-administered bolus doses (supplemental, breakthrough doses) are recorded when administered.

17. *Pain rating.* The patient's pain rating is usually recorded every 1 to 2 hours during the first 24 hours, then every 4 hours if pain is controlled. The pain rating scales are provided in a box in the lower left side of the flow sheet. A pain rating higher than patient's comfort-function goal (upper right-hand corner of flow sheet) should trigger further assessment and action (see item 5).

18. *Respiratory rate and level of sedation (LOS).* Two of the most important assessments in the opioid-naive patient are that of respiratory status (nurse monitored), which includes respiratory rate, depth, regularity, and noisiness, and level of sedation. These two parameters are recorded every 1 to 2 hours during the first 24 hours, then every 4 hours if the they are stable; respiratory rate and LOS are recorded on the face of the flow sheet, and any excessive sedation or abnormalities or trends and changes from baseline in respiratory rate, depth, regularity, or noisiness (e.g., snoring) require an asterisk notation (*) on the front of the flow sheet and detailed information on the back. After the first 24 hours, significant increases in opioid dose warrant the return to respiratory and sedation monitoring every 1 to 2 hours until stable patterns are observed. Depending on the respiratory status and sedation levels, further action may be necessary. The Pasero Opioid-Induced Sedation Scale (POSS) is used to assess LOS and is shown on the bottom half of the flow sheet (see item 26). On this scale, sedation levels 3 and 4 require action; a sedation level of 3 should trigger further assessment and a decrease in the opioid dose; a sedation level of 4 requires a clinician to stop opioid administration, consider naloxone administration, and notify the prescriber. (See Section IV for additional information about opioid-induced sedation and respiratory depression.)

19. *Oxygen (O_2) saturation.* When continuous or intermittent oxygen saturation monitoring (pulse oximetry) is prescribed, readings should be recorded with the same frequency as those of respiratory status and level of sedation.

20. *End tidal carbon dioxide ($ETCO_2$) concentration.* When continuous or intermittent $ETCO_2$ monitoring (capnography) is prescribed, readings should be recorded with the same frequency as respiratory status and level of sedation.

21. *Adverse effects (AE).* Using the code for adverse effects (bottom of flow sheet; see item 27), the presence of adverse effects is recorded every 1 to 2 hours during the first 24 hours, then every 4 hours if the patient has no adverse effects. The letter *M* recorded above or next to an adverse effect signifies that the patient was given medication to treat the adverse effects. Depending on the adverse effects, further action may be warranted and noted in the comment section on the back of the flow sheet (see also Section IV).

22. *Motor/sensory.* Assessment for detection of motor or sensory deficits in patients receiving local anesthetic is usually performed every 4 to 8 hours. Modified versions of the Bromage Scale and the Inova Sensory Assessment Scale (Nisbet, personal

communication, 2008), both shown in the bottom half of the flow sheet (see item 28), are used for motor and sensory assessment, respectively. The level at which the anesthesia provider should be notified depends on the therapy and individual provider practice; orders or protocol should stipulate this information (see Section IV for more about regional analgesia techniques).

23. *Site/system.* This column is used to document that the infusion sites and systems, from a patient's access to the infusion pumps, have been assessed and are functioning properly. Usually, this information is documented as often as IV site assessment is documented in the institution (e.g., every 8 hours or every shift) and whenever patients are experiencing inadequate pain control. A check mark ($\sqrt{}$) in the space provided signifies acceptable assessment findings (agreement with the statement at the bottom of the flow sheet; see item 29). If a patient is receiving PCA, the check mark also signifies patient-only use and that the PCA pendant is within the patient's reach. An asterisk in this space means that detailed information is provided on the back of the flow sheet.

24. *Initials.* The initials of the clinician who performs the assessment, pump programming, clinician-administered boluses, or double checks (see item 26) are recorded in the box in the last column. All initials on the flow sheet should have a matching signature at the bottom of the flow sheet (see item 32).

25. *Pain rating scale.* The first section, at the bottom of the flow sheet, provides an example of the 0-to-10 NRS and the 0-to-10 FPS-R for clinicians' reference.

26. *Level of sedation.* The second section, at the bottom half of the flow sheet, contains the POSS for clinicians' reference to guide documentation of LOS. (See item 18 and Section IV for more about this scale.)

27. *Adverse effects.* The third section at the bottom half of the flow sheet, contains the codes for recording various adverse effects (see item 21).

28. *Motor and sensory assessment.* The third section, at the bottom half of the flow sheet, contains the modified version of the Bromage Scale for motor assessment and the Inova Sensory Assessment Scale (Nisbet, personal communication, 2008) for sensory assessment to help clinicians in documentation (see item 22 and Section IV for more about regional analgesia techniques).

29. *Site/infusion system*: A description of acceptable infusion sites, systems, and PCA setups for clinicians' reference, as well as space to record infusion tubing changes, are provided at the bottom of the flow sheet (see item 23).

30. *Catheter removal.* Space is provided for documentation of catheter removal. A check mark ($\checkmark$) signifies agreement with the description; an asterisk (*) means that detailed information is recorded on the back of the flow sheet.

31. *Drug waste.* Space is provided for documentation of drug waste, including the signature of the clinician wasting the drug and the clinician witnessing the waste.

32. *Signature.* The signatures of the clinicians who perform the assessments, tubing changes, double checks, and catheter removal are recorded at the bottom of the flow sheet. All initials on the flow sheet should have a matching signature.

The medication administration record (MAR) is used to document analgesic use when patients are switched from analgesic infusions to oral pain medication. Then, wherever vital signs are recorded is the most logical place to document pain ratings. Space should be provided for recording the institution's minimum standards for pain assessment (e.g., pain rating at least every 8 hours) and to record pain ratings at the time analgesics are administered and at the time of reassessment after administration. When pain is difficult to control, the Pain Control Record (Form 3-8) can be kept at the bedside for closer monitoring.

Examples of the use of the analgesic infusion flow sheet for patients receiving IV PCA (Form 3-9) and patients receiving epidural analgesia (Form 3-10) are shown on pp. 111-114.

Pain Diaries for Outpatient Care

A pain control diary is a type of flow sheet for a patient to use in the outpatient setting, although there may be instances when it is appropriate to use it in inpatient settings too. Increasing numbers of patients with pain are being cared for on an outpatient basis. Patients with severe and sometimes escalating pain related to cancer are often cared for at home by family caregivers. Patients with moderate to severe pain related to surgical procedures are discharged from the hospital quickly, sometimes on the same day of the surgery. Both types of patients might benefit from the use of a pain diary.

Because the flow sheets or diaries of patients at home are kept by patients or their families, they must be particularly easy to use. Form 3-11 (p. 116) presents a paper pain diary designed for these circumstances. A patient teaching brochure titled "Understanding Your Pain: Using a Pain Rating Scale" contains an almost identical diary and is available at www.endo.com. It is similar to the diary presented in our previous book (McCaffery, Pasero, 1999). A nurse with chronic pain reported that she modified the diary for the purpose of clarifying for her physicians her pain intensity and the effectiveness of treatments (Aguirre, Nevidjon, Clemens, 2008). It helped her to identify trends in her pain and what worsened her pain. This adaptation of the diary is available at http://download.lww.com/wolterskluwer_vitalstream_com/PermaLink/NAJ_108_6_Aguirre_1059_SDC1.pdf.

As illustrated in Form 3-11, a paper diary for outpatients usually includes, at the minimum, columns or

Text continued on p. 115

24-Hour Pain Management Flow Sheet for Analgesic Infusions: Patient Example (start new sheet at 12 midnight daily)   Date ___ 4/10

Check (√) therapy: IV √   SC ___   Epidural ___   Spinal ___   Perineural ___   Location _Right arm_   PCA √   Comfort-Function Goal _3_

Time	Drug(s)	Drug Conc(s)	Vol Infus	# INJ	# ATT	PCA Dose	Delay	Basal Rate	Hour Limit	Clin Bolus	Pain Rating	Resp Rate / LOS	O₂ Sat	ETCO₂	AE	Motor / Sensory	Site / System	Initials
2400	morphine	1 mg/1 mL	20	4	4	1 mg	8 min	0	7 mg		3	18/1			0		√	NN
0200												16/S						NN
0400												16/S						NN
0500	morphine	1 mg/1 mL		1	1	1 mg	8 min	add 0.5 mg	7 mg	2 mg	8	18/1			0		√	NN/JN
0515	morphine	1 mg/1 mL		1	1					2 mg	6	18/1			0			NN
0530				1	1						4	18/1			0			NN
0600				2	2						2	16/1			0			NN
0800	morphine	1 mg/1 mL	34	3	3	1 mg	8 min	0.5 mg	7 mg		2	18/1			0		√	VN
1000												18/S						VN
1200												20/S						VN
1600	morphine	1 mg/1 mL	48	10	12	1 mg	8 min	0.5 mg	7 mg		3	18/1			0		√	CN
2000											2	20/1			0		√	CN

Ask patient to rate pain with one of these scales

0 1 2 3 4 5 6 7 8 9 10
No pain — Moderate pain — Worst possible

(faces scale: 0   2   4   6   8   10)

LOS = LEVEL OF SEDATION
S - Sleep, easy to arouse *(no action necessary)*
1 - Alert, easy to arouse *(no action necessary)*
2 - Occasionally drowsy, easy to arouse *(no action necessary)*
3 - Frequently drowsy, falls asleep mid-sentence *(decrease opioid dose)*
4 - Somnolent, difficult to arouse *(stop opioid, consider naloxone, notify primary)*

ADVERSE EFFECTS*
M - Medicated
N - Nausea
V - Vomiting
C - Constipation
P - Pruritus
UR - Urinary retention
MT - Metallic taste
ER - Ear ringing
PN - Perioral numbness
See orders for treatment, when to notify primary

MOTOR ASSESSMENT*
0 - Flexes hip/knee/ankle; able to raise leg
1 - Flexes ankle/knee; unable to raise leg
2 - Flexes ankle; unable to flex knee or raise leg
3 - Unable to flex ankle/knee or raise leg
SENSORY ASSESSMENT*
0 - Full sensation; no numbness/tingling
1 - Reduced response to touch; no numbness or tingling
2 - Moderate numbness or tingling
3 - Full block (no sensation or response to touch)
See orders for when to notify anesthesia

SITE/INFUSION SYSTEM √ = agree, * = see reverse
Site: Clean, dry, no redness, no edema, no tenderness; no back soreness (intraspinal)
System: Securely taped, tubings patent, reservoir has volume
PCA: Patient-only use, pendant within patient's reach
TUBING CHANGE: Time ___   Initials ___

SIGNATURE	SIGNATURE
N. Nurse	J. Nurse

CATHETER REMOVAL
Catheter removed without difficulty, tip intact, site clean, dry, no redness
√ = agree, * = see reverse
Time ___   Initials ___

SIGNATURE
V. Nurse

DRUG WASTED
Amount ___
Date ___   Time ___
Signature ___
Witness ___

SIGNATURE
C. Nurse

Continued

Form 3-9 | Back of 24-hour pain management flow sheet provides space for comments when patient or infusion system is outside of the norm. Comments can be made at any time by any member of the health care team and do not necessarily coincide with the flow sheet. Patient assessment columns on the front of the flow sheet show that the patient had satisfactory pain control while awake, but after sleeping and 5 hours of no self-administered PCA doses, the patient was awakened by pain. Pain was brought under control with two clinician-administered bolus doses and the addition of a low-dose basal rate. The patient's pain, respiratory status, LOS, and adverse effects are recorded every 2 hours during the first 24 hours after surgery. Site assessment and pump parameters are recorded only every 8 hours.

From Pasero, C., & McCaffery, M. *Pain assessment and pharmacologic management*, pp. 111-112, St. Louis, Mosby. © 2011, Pasero C, McCaffery M. May be duplicated for use in clinical practice.

24-Hour Pain Management Flow Sheet for Analgesic Infusions: Patient Example–cont'd

DATE	TIME	COMMENTS
4/10	0500	Called to room by patient who reported he was awakened by severe
		pain. No PCA doses last 5 hours while asleep. Given bolus dose and
		basal rate added. N. Nurse
	0515	Improved but still uncomfortable. Bolus repeated. N. Nurse
	0530	Patient reports "I feel much better." States he will use PCA to reduce
		pain further. LOS and respiratory status stable. Told to call me
		whenever needed. N. Nurse
	0600	Patient reports good pain control and is pleased with addition of basal
		rate. N. Nurse
	1200	Stable at 24 h post op. Switched to q 4 h resp. status, LOS, pain rating
		and adverse effects. C. Nurse

Form 3-9 | Cont'd.

24-Hour Pain Management Flow Sheet for Analgesic Infusions: Patient Example (start new sheet at 12 midnight daily)   Date ___4/10___

Check (√) therapy: IV ___ SC ___ Epidural ✓ Spinal ___ Perineural ___ Location ___T-10___ PCA ✓ Comfort-Function Goal ___3___

Time	Drug(s)	Drug Conc(s)	Vol Infus	# INJ	# ATT	PCA Dose	Delay	Basal Rate	Hour Limit	Clin Bolus	Pain Rating	Resp Rate / LOS	O₂ Sat	ETCO₂	AE	Motor / Sensory	Site / System	Initials
2400	Fentanyl + Ropivacaine	5 mcg/1 mL 0.0625%	40	1	1	10 mcg	15 min	30 mcg	70 mcg		1	18 / 2			0	0 / 0	✓ /	NN
0200												16 / S				/ ✓		NN
0400 *	Fentanyl + Ropivacaine	5 mcg/1 mL 0.0625%		0	0	10 mcg	15 min	↓20 mcg	60 mcg		0	18 / 2			ᵐP	0 / 0	/	NN/JN
0600											0	16 / 2			0			NN
0800 *	Fentanyl + Ropivacaine	5 mcg/1 mL 0.0625%	82	1	1	10 mcg	15 min	↓10 mcg	50 mcg		0	16 / 2			ᵐP	0 / 0	✓ /	VN/LN
1000											2	18 / 2			0			VN
1200											2	18 / 1			0	0 / 0		VN
1400												20 / S						VN
1600 *	Fentanyl + Ropivacaine	5 mcg/1 mL 0.0625%		4	4	10 mcg	15 min	10 mcg	50 mcg		2	18 / 1			0	0 / 0	✓ /	CN
2000											2	20 / 1						

Ask patient to rate pain with one of these scales

[Faces pain scale]   0   2   4   6   8   10
No pain — Moderate pain — Worst possible

0 1 2 3 4 5 6 7 8 9 10

LOS = LEVEL OF SEDATION
S - Sleep, easy to arouse *(no action necessary)*
1 - Alert, easy to arouse *(no action necessary)*
2 - Occasionally drowsy, easy to arouse *(no action necessary)*
3 - Frequently drowsy, falls asleep mid-sentence *(decrease opioid dose)*
4 - Somnolent, difficult to arouse *(stop opioid, consider naloxone, notify primary)*

ADVERSE EFFECTS*
M - Medicated
N - Nausea
V - Vomiting
C - Constipation
P - Pruritus
UR - Urinary retention
MT - Metallic taste
ER - Ear ringing
PN - Perioral numbness
See orders for treatment, when to notify primary

MOTOR ASSESSMENT*
0 - Flexes hip/knee/ankle; able to raise leg
1 - Flexes ankle/knee; unable to raise leg
2 - Flexes ankle; unable to flex knee or raise leg
3 - Unable to flex ankle/knee or raise leg
SENSORY ASSESSMENT*
0 - Full sensation; no numbness/tingling
1 - Reduced response to touch; no numbness or tingling
2 - Moderate numbness or tingling
3 - Full block (no sensation or response to touch)
See orders for when to notify anesthesia

CATHETER REMOVAL
Catheter removed without difficulty, tip intact, site clean, dry, no redness
√ = agree, * = see reverse
Time ___   Initials ___

DRUG WASTED
Amount ___
Date ___   Time ___
Signature ___
Witness ___

SITE/INFUSION SYSTEM √ = agree, * = see reverse
Site: Clean, dry, no redness, no edema, no tenderness; no back soreness (intraspinal)
System: Securely taped, tubings patent, reservoir has volume
PCA: Patient-only use, pendant within patient's reach
TUBING CHANGE: Time ___ Initials ___ Time ___ Initials ___

SIGNATURE	SIGNATURE	SIGNATURE	SIGNATURE	SIGNATURE
N. Nurse	J. Nurse	V. Nurse	L. Nurse	C. Nurse

Form 3-10 | See legend on p. 114.

Continued

DATE	TIME	COMMENTS
4/10	0400	Patient reports discomfort from facial and neck itching. No rash or
		redness. Given Benadryl and basal rate decreased. N. Nurse
	0800	Patient reports return of facial "itchiness". No rash or redness. Given
		Benadryl and basal rate decreased. V. Nurse
	1600	24 h post op. To q 4 h pain rating, resp. status, LOS, and adverse
		effects. Stable in all these aspects. C. Nurse

Form 3-10 | Back of 24-hour pain management flow sheet provides space for comments when patient or infusion system is outside of the norm. Comments can be made at any time by any member of the health care team and do not necessarily coincide with the flow sheet. Patient assessment columns on the front of the flow sheet show that the patient had adequate pain control with ratings of 0-1, which are less than the patient's comfort-function goal of 3, and that the analgesic dose was safe with LOS of 2 or 1-2. Itching (pruritus) is the only adverse effect and was handled by decreasing the basal rate. Note that the patient's pain, respiratory status, LOS, and adverse effects are recorded every 2 hours during the first 24 hours after surgery. Site assessment and pump parameters are recorded only every 8 hours.

From Pasero, C., & McCaffery, M. *Pain assessment and pharmacologic management*, pp. 113-114, St. Louis, Mosby. © 2011, Pasero C, McCaffery M. May be duplicated for use in clinical practice.

spaces for time, pain rating, medication taken or pain treatment, effect of the pain treatment on the pain rating, and comments, such as related activities or adverse effects. To avoid burdening patients and their families, certain criteria should be established regarding when to keep the record and for how long. The instructions for the pain diary in Form 3-11 stipulate that the record is to be kept only until an effective pain management plan has been developed. The example shown in Form 3-12 concerns a patient with chronic, progressive, cancer-related pain whose pain has escalated.

A paper diary may also be helpful for patients having ambulatory surgery. In a study of 20,817 patients who underwent same-day surgery, pain was the most common reason for unanticipated return to the hospital, occurring in 38% of the patients whose return was not anticipated (Coley, Williams, DaPos, et al., 2002). In ambulatory surgery, patients are usually discharged before there is time to establish the effectiveness of the oral analgesics they will be taking at home. Patients known to be at risk for moderate to severe pain, such as those having certain orthopedic procedures, may be asked to complete this diary about every 2 hours for the remainder of the day. The patients then have records that can be referred to when the clinicians contact them or the patients call with unrelieved pain or unmanageable adverse effects. Information from the pain control diary will be helpful in correcting the problem. For example, unrelieved pain may be due to failure to take the analgesic, or the analgesic prescription may be inadequate. Ideally, clinicians contact high risk patients the evening of discharge rather than the next day. Attempts to manage problems can be initiated before patients spend an uncomfortable night and develop complications.

In a hospitalized patient for whom the switch from parenteral or spinal analgesia to oral analgesia is not going smoothly, this paper pain diary may be modified and kept by the patients at the bedside. The information may be summarized in the nursing notes. Pain ratings every 2 hours may expedite identification of effective oral analgesic plans.

For certain periods of time, weeks or months, a daily pain diary may be indicated for a patient with chronic noncancer pain, such as headaches or low back pain. This type of record is especially important when medications or other treatments are being evaluated for continued use or are being adjusted to improve their effectiveness.

Poor recall of pain underscores the importance of asking some patients to keep records of pain management in the outpatient setting. The patient's recall of pain often influences both the diagnosis and the treatment of pain. In one study of patients with chronic headache, pain ratings recorded in daily pain diaries kept over approximately 1 week were compared with patients' memories of pain felt during that time (Eich, Reeves, Jaeger et al., 1985). Recall of pain intensity for maximum, usual, and minimum levels was influenced by the intensity of the pain felt at the time of the interview. The patients recalled their previous levels of pain as being more severe than they actually had been when the intensity of their present pain was high but recalled them as being less severe when their present pain intensity was low. In another study of patients with persistent pain, results with regard to recall of pain were similar (Smith, Safer, 1993). In addition, findings revealed that patients with lower present pain ratings also recalled their use of medication as having been less than it actually was.

In a study of patients receiving nerve blocks for pain, pain ratings were obtained before and after the blocks as well as 2 days and 2 weeks after the procedure (Porzelius, 1995). Findings revealed that memory distortions were common. At 2 days and 2 weeks after the nerve block, many patients recalled that the pain they had felt immediately after receiving the block was higher than they had reported at the time.

In outpatient care of patients with chronic pain, it is common to ask them, at each clinic visit, about their average or usual pain over the past week. Clinicians must realize that when precise information about pain ratings is needed so as to determine further treatment, daily records are more accurate than recall. Under these circumstances, a daily pain control diary is indicated.

Some patients will be asked to complete paper pain diaries only when problems are encountered, as in the example in Form 3-12. That patient was awakened by moderate to severe pain, and several supplemental doses were taken. Had the patient and family member not kept a diary, variations in pain ratings and the times breakthrough doses were taken, especially during the night, may not have been recalled accurately.

One of the limitations of paper diaries, when patients are asked to keep them over weeks or longer in the outpatient setting, is that some patients complete diaries immediately before they are to be turned in, or a week's diary may be completed in advance (Gendreau, Hufford, Strone, 2003). Others have found that patients completing paper diaries are frequently noncompliant, tending to fabricate data if they have not completed the requested information at the times requested (Litt, Cooney, Morse, 1998). The use of electronic diaries that are programmed to prohibit invalid entries are helpful with respect to compliance (Hadjistravropoulos, Herr, Turk, et al., 2007). Momentary data are less likely to be falsified (Schwartz, Stone, 1998). The advantages of using electronic diaries are portability, low cost, ease of sharing data, and the availability of numerous software applications (Smith, Sheplock, 1999). Nevertheless their use is still limited by the much lower cost of paper dairies.

To study compliance with keeping paper diaries versus electronic diaries, 80 patients with chronic pain were asked to complete diaries; 40 patients kept paper diaries, and 40 patients kept electronic diaries (on palmtop computers) for 21 days, making entries three times a day (Stone, Shiffman, Schwartz, et al., 2002). Unknown to the patients, the paper diary was equipped with photosensors that identified the times at which entries were

Pain Control Diary

This is a record of how your pain medicines are working. Please keep this record until you and your nurse/doctor find the dose and frequency of medicine that provides satisfactory pain relief for you most of the time. After that, you only need to keep this record when you have problems related to your pain medicines.

Name: _____ Date: _____

GOALS Satisfactory pain rating: _____ Activities: _____

Analgesics: _____

_____

My pain rating scale:

```
|----|----|----|----|----|----|----|----|----|----|
0    1    2    3    4    5    6    7    8    9    10
```

No pain   Moderate pain   Worst possible pain

Directions: Rate your pain before you take pain medicine and 1 to 2 hours later.

Time	Pain Rating	Pain Medicine I Took	Side Effects (drowsy? upset stomach?)	Other

If pain is greater than _____, or if you have other problems with your pain medicine, call:

Nurse: Name/phone   _____

Doctor: Name/phone   _____

Form 3-11

From Pasero, C., & McCaffery M. *Pain assessment and pharmacologic management*, p. 116, St. Louis, Mosby. © 2011, Pasero C, McCaffery M. May be duplicated for use in clinical practice.

Pain Control Diary: Patient Example

This is a record of how your pain medicines are working. Please keep this record until you and your nurse/doctor find the dose and frequency of medicine that provides satisfactory pain relief for you most of the time. After that, you only need to keep this record when you have problems related to your pain medicines.

Name: _____ *Martin* _____ Date: _____ *Friday* _____

GOALS Satisfactory pain rating: ____*3*____   Activities: _*Sleep through the night; walk around the house*_

Analgesics: _*ibuprofen 400 mg 8 am, 2 pm, 8 pm; duloxetine 30 mg 8 am,*_

*8 pm; MS Contin 100 mg 8 am, 8 pm; MSIR 30 mg every 2 hours if needed.*

My pain rating scale:

| 0 | 1 | 2 | 3 | 4 | 5 | 6 | 7 | 8 | 9 | 10 |

No pain — Moderate pain — Worst possible pain

Directions: Rate your pain before you take pain medicine and 1 to 2 hours later.

Time	Pain Rating	Pain Medicine I Took	Side Effects (drowsy? upset stomach?)	Other
12:15 am	6	30 MSIR	No	
3	6	30 MSIR		can't sleep
5:15	5	30 MSIR		
8	6	30 MSIR + ibuprofen + MS Contin 100 mg + duloxetine		staying in bed
10	5			talk with nurse
10:30	6	MSIR 45 mg MS Contin 30 mg		
12:30 pm	3			planning to nap

If pain is greater than ____*5*____ , or if you have other problems with your pain medicine, call:

Nurse: Name/phone ____*C. Adams*_____*555-1234*____

Doctor: Name/phone ____*Jones*_____*555-4321*____

For legend, see p. 118

Form 3-12 | Patient example. This patient has increasing pain resulting from metastasizing cancer. He has been receiving the following analgesics around the clock every day: ibuprofen 400 mg tid (8 AM, 2 PM, 8 PM); duloxetine 30 mg bid (8 AM and 8 PM); modified-release morphine (MS Contin) 100 mg q12h (8 AM and 8 PM). His breakthrough dose (BTD) is short-acting morphine (MS IR) 30 mg PO q2h as needed. Until 2 days ago he was taking BTDs twice a day. That relieved his pain to the level of 3 or less and met his goals of walking around his home and sleeping through the night uninterrupted by pain. This record reveals that his pain is no longer controlled. As indicated at the top of the diary, he needs to complete this diary when he has problems related to his pain medicines. The diary reveals that his pain ratings are now greater than 3, that pain awakens him at night, and that he stays in bed. The patient talks with the nurse at 10 AM, reads the diary to the nurse, and says that this is approximately what had happened during the past 2 days. The nurse contacts the physician and the decision is made to increase his morphine doses by approximately 30% to 50% to 45 mg of short-acting MS q2h and to 130 mg of modified-release morphine q12h. (When a dose of opioid is safe but ineffective, an increase of 25% usually produces a small increase in pain relief.) From previous prescription, the patient has modified-release morphine tablets 30 mg on hand, and the nurse instructs the patient to take one 30 mg tablet now along with short-acting MS 45 mg (½ 30 mg MS IR), which he does at 10:30 AM. The entry at 12:30 PM shows that pain is reduced to the goal of 3, and the patient can sleep. Because of the increase in pain over 3 days, the patient is instructed to make an appointment to see the physician the next day.

made so as to compare actual compliance with reported compliance. Among those who kept the paper diaries, reported compliance was 90%, but actual compliance was 11% to 20%. Actual compliance with the electronic diaries was 94%. The low compliance by those keeping the paper diaries is all the more remarkable considering the subjects were given $150 to participate in the study.

No other study has yet reported a comparison between compliance with electronic diary entries versus compliance with paper diary entries. The relatively higher compliance with paper diaries reported in the following studies may not be as high as actual compliance; that is, entries may not actually have been made at the times indicated in the paper diaries. In one study, 36 patients with chronic low back pain were asked to monitor their pain for 1 year (Jamison, Raymond, Levine, et al., 2001). Of the 36, 20 used both electronic diaries and paper diaries, and 16 used paper diaries alone. Two-way messaging available with the electronic diaries seemed to encourage the patients to use them, and they preferred them to the paper diaries. Further, patients were much more compliant with the monitoring of pain when using the electronic diaries (89.9%) than when using the paper diaries (55.9%). However, noncompliance resulted primarily from failure to return the paper diaries. Analysis of the data gathered by telephone calls and paper diaries suggested that the data in the electronic diaries were reliable and valid.

In another study, 155 cancer patients with metastasized bone pain were asked to complete daily paper pain diaries to determine the usefulness for themselves of doing so (Schumacher, Koresawa, West, et al., 2002). These were simple diaries that the patients were asked to complete once a day. (A copy of the diary is published in the Schumacher citation.) The pain diary was reported by 74% of the patients to be useful, and 10% felt it clearly was not. Very few patients and caregivers found the diary to be burdensome. No compliance data were reported. A group of 159 patients with cancer-related pain were asked to record their pain twice daily in a paper pain diary for 2 months at home (de Wit, van Dam, Hanneman, et al., 1999). Even in seriously ill patients, compliance was high

(85.9%). High compliance may have been due in part to the guidance given by specially trained nurses and to the practice in completing the diaries before discharge. Although 37% of the patients reported that the diaries were of no benefit, 60% found that they helped them to cope with pain, giving them a sense of control over their pain. However, for patients with stable pain, the use of pain diaries may not be beneficial.

In a study of 91 patients with persistent noncancer pain, the patients used electronic diaries to monitor their pain during 2 weeks (Stone, Broderick, Schwartz, et al., 2003). Patients were divided into three groups and asked to monitor their pain 3, 6, or 12 times per day. Compliance was 94% or higher. Patients did not feel this was a burden and were willing to participate again in a similar study. One purpose of this study was to determine whether completing momentary diaries of pain would cause a shift in levels of pain over time (referred to as reactivity), and little support was found for such an occurrence.

In a crossover trial, 36 patients with persistent pain were asked to monitor their pain, mood, activity interference, medical use, and pain location in either paper or electronic diaries for 2 weeks (Marceau, Link, Jamison, et al., 2007). Patients reported that the electronic diary was easier to use than the paper diary, and 61% said that they would continue using it if given the choice. No compliance data were reported in this study. A serendipitous finding was that the patients using the electronic diary more frequently reported that their providers suggested medication changes based on information in the electronic diaries.

An emerging type of pain diary is an ordinary paper diary together with a digital pen and wireless mobile Internet technology. The digital pen looks, feels, and functions like an ordinary ballpoint pen. The strokes made by the pen are recorded and transferred by the Internet. In a small study of 12 palliative care patients using this technology, the patients reported that they found it easy to use despite severe illness and difficulties in comprehending the technology (Lind, Karlsson, Fridlund, 2008). The patients were asked to record immediate pain ratings three times a day and to complete a question about consumed doses. The patients could transmit their assessments at any time of any day. Caregivers gave the patients feedback on received assessments. It was this aspect of the methodology that the patients seemed to like the most. In postinterviews it was discovered that the patients believed that the transferred assessments were monitored by the caregivers around the clock, although the patients were not told that. Although the patients always recorded their pain at the requested times, initially they had difficulty using the VAS, and none of the patients understood how to mark the boxes to indicate the times at which they had taken their extra doses. Clearly, better directions should have been given. Nonetheless, the medical records indicated that the information from the assessments was useful and resulted in quick medical responses to changes in the patients' statuses.

Research thus far suggests that electronic diaries and possibly digital pens are preferable to paper diaries when data are needed for 1 week or longer. Patients prefer electronic diaries to paper diaries, and compliance is better with electronic diaries. Based on the one study involving digital pens, it seems that this technology may be even better. Perhaps most important, it appears likely that data from electronic diaries or digital pens are most useful to physicians in making medication adjustments for patients.

When paper diaries, digital pens, or electronic diaries are used, the patient and family should receive explanations of the purpose of using them, along with information about how and when to complete the diaries and practice sessions with the diaries. Electronic diaries and digital pens are not always available in clinical practice, so paper diaries will serve as an alternative.

The low actual compliance with the use of paper diaries reported in one study (Stone, Shiffman, Schwartz, et al., 2002) suggests that when patients are asked to use paper diaries, it may be wise to caution them about the tendency to record information much later than it actually occurred, about the fact that recall is often inaccurate, and about the need to be honest about the times at which they actually make their entries. The most effective way to encourage compliance may be frequent feedback between clinician and patient. Calling the patient, perhaps every day or two, to remind him or her to complete the diary may help the patient to feel that the entries are of value. Perhaps the most important encouragement to complete the diaries lies in clinicians' use of diary information to adjust care. Doing so gives the patient a reason to use the diary. In the studies mentioned, the patients responded very positively to having regular contact with clinicians and to feeling that their data were being used. Compliance may also be increased by decreasing the number of entries expected per day, although some patients did not feel overburdened by making as many as 12 entries per day (Stone, Broderick, Schwartz, et al., 2003).

Clinic Record for Reassessment of Patients with Persistent Pain Who Are Taking Opioids

A standardized tool for assessing patients with persistent pain who are receiving opioid therapy is almost essential to determine the effects of opioid management and to identify problems, such as undertreatment of pain, adverse effects, or problematic patient behaviors. Relevant domains for monitoring are often referred to as the Four As: Analgesia, Activities of daily living, Adverse effects, and Aberrant drug-related behaviors (Nicholson, Passik, 2007). The Pain Assessment and Documentation Tool (PADT), which assesses these four domains, has been published (Passik, Kirsh, Whitcomb, et al., 2004). The original, longer tool was field-tested by 27 clinicians who applied it to the assessments of 388 patients receiving long-term opioid therapy for persistent noncancer pain. The result is the PADT, a brief, two-sided chart note that can be included in a patient's medical records (Form 3-13). It should require only a few minutes of a clinician's time to complete.

The PADT assesses the four As in four sections of the tool. In the first section, Analgesia is assessed using the 0 to 10 scale. The second section, Activities of daily living, includes physical functioning, social relationships, and sleep patterns. The third section, Adverse effects, includes the effects that sometimes accompany chronic opioid use, such as nausea, constipation, and mental cloudiness. The fourth section assesses Aberrant drug-related behaviors, including those that may indicate undertreatment of pain, or abuse, or addictive disease, and they require differential diagnoses.

Aberrant drug-related behavior is too often interpreted as being indicative of abuse or addictive disease, and little thought may be given to the fact that the behavior may be caused by undertreatment of pain. The term *aberrant drug-related behavior* refers to behavior that is inconsistent with the expressed intentions of the prescriber, such as taking the drug for sleep when it was intended for pain relief (Fine, Portenoy, 2007). Another example of aberrant behavior is hoarding opioids during periods of reduced symptoms for later use when pain is worse or for occasions when the opioid is unexpectedly unavailable, such as a mail-order pharmacy's being late in filling the prescription or the local pharmacy's being temporarily out of the medication. Clearly, the presence of aberrant drug taking behavior should not automatically result in denying a patient opioid therapy.

The ultimate goals of using the PADT are to optimize analgesia, to improve activities of daily living, to minimize adverse analgesic effects, and to minimize aberrant drug behaviors. Further validation of the PADT is under way. The published tool is presented along with a survey of 19 clinicians who participated in the development of the PADT, revealing that 63.2% felt the tool would also be helpful in documenting behaviors or concerns for legal purposes (Passik, Kirsh, Whitcomb, et al., 2004).

Communication Strategies

Pain is best managed by using a team approach. Seldom does any one clinician possess the time, knowledge, and skill to provide all the care required by a patient with

PROGRESS NOTE
Pain Assessment and Documentation Tool (PADT™)

Patient Name: _____ Record #: _____

Assessment Date: _____

Current Analgesic Regimen

Drug name	Strength (e.g., mg)	Frequency	Maximum Total Daily Dose
_____	_____	_____	_____
_____	_____	_____	_____
_____	_____	_____	_____

The PADT is a clinician-directed interview; that is, the clinician asks the questions, and the clinician records the responses. The Analgesia, Activities of Daily Living, and Adverse Events sections may be completed by the physician, nurse practitioner, physician assistant, or nurse. The Potential Aberrant Drug-Related Behavior and Assessment sections must be completed by the <u>physician</u>. Ask the patient the questions below, except as noted.

Analgesia

If 0 indicates "no pain" and 10 indicates "pain as bad as it can be," on a scale of 0 to 10, what is your level of pain for the following questions?

1. What was your pain level on average during the past week? (Please circle the appropriate number)

No Pain 0 1 2 3 4 5 6 7 8 9 10 **Pain as bad as it can be**

2. What was your pain level at its worst during the past week?

No Pain 0 1 2 3 4 5 6 7 8 9 10 **Pain as bad as it can be**

3. What percentage of your pain has been relieved during the past week? (Write in a percentage between 0% and 100%.) _____

4. Is the amount of pain relief you are now obtaining from your current pain reliever(s) enough to make a real difference in your life?

☐ Yes   ☐ No

5. Query to clinician: Is the patient's pain relief clinically significant?

☐ Yes   ☐ No   ☐ Unsure

Activities of Daily Living

Please indicate whether the patient's functioning with the current pain reliever(s) is Better, the Same, or Worse since the patient's last assessment with the PADT.* (Please check the box for Better, Same, or Worse for each item below.)

	Better	Same	Worse
1. Physical functioning	☐	☐	☐
2. Family relationships	☐	☐	☐
3. Social relationships	☐	☐	☐
4. Mood	☐	☐	☐
5. Sleep patterns	☐	☐	☐
6. Overall functioning	☐	☐	☐

*If the patient is receiving his or her first PADT assessment, the clinician should compare the patient's functional status with other reports from the last office visit.

Form 3-13 | The revised pain assessment and documentation tool shown as a two-sided chart note.

Continued

PROGRESS NOTE
Pain Assessment and Documentation Tool (PADT™)

Adverse Events

1. Is patient experiencing any side effects from current pain reliever(s)? ☐ Yes ☐ No

Ask patient about potential side effects:

	None	Mild	Moderate	Severe
a. Nausea	☐	☐	☐	☐
b. Vomiting	☐	☐	☐	☐
c. Constipation	☐	☐	☐	☐
d. Itching	☐	☐	☐	☐
e. Mental cloudiness	☐	☐	☐	☐
f. Sweating	☐	☐	☐	☐
g. Fatigue	☐	☐	☐	☐
h. Drowsiness	☐	☐	☐	☐
i. Other _____		☐	☐	☐
j. Other _____		☐	☐	☐

2. Patient's overall severity of side effects?
☐ None   ☐ Mild   ☐ Moderate   ☐ Severe

Potential Aberrant Drug-Related Behavior
This section must be completed by the <u>physician</u>.

*Please **check** any of the following items that you discovered during your interactions with the patient. Please note that some of these are directly observable (e.g., appears intoxicated), while others may require more active listening and/or probing. Use the "Assessment" section below to note additional details.*

☐ Purposeful over-sedation
☐ Negative mood change
☐ Appears intoxicated
☐ Increasingly unkempt or impaired
☐ Involvement in car or other accident
☐ Requests frequent early renewals
☐ Increased dose without authorization
☐ Reports lost or stolen prescriptions
☐ Attempts to obtain prescriptions from other doctors
☐ Changes route of administration
☐ Uses pain medication in response to situational stressor
☐ Insists on certain medications by name
☐ Contact with street drug culture
☐ Abusing alcohol or illicit drugs
☐ Hoarding (i.e., stockpiling) of medication
☐ Arrested by police
☐ Victim of abuse
Other: _____
_____
_____

Assessment: (This section must be completed by the <u>physician</u>.)
Is your overall impression that this patient is benefiting (e.g., benefits, such as pain relief, outweigh side effects) from opioid therapy? ☐ Yes   ☐ No   ☐ Unsure

Comments:_____

_____

Specific Analgesic Plan:

☐ Continue present regimen   Comments: _____
☐ Adjust dose of present analgesic   _____
☐ Switch analgesics   _____
☐ Add/Adjust concomitant therapy   _____
☐ Discontinue/taper off opioid therapy _____

Date: _____   Physician's signature: _____

Form 3-13 | Cont'd.

pain. Usually the care of a single patient requires at least the involvement of a prescriber, nurse, and pharmacist, and sometimes many other health care professionals representing various disciplines.

Nurses have emerged as pivotal members of the pain management team. As has been known in the palliative care setting for decades, the nurse is the cornerstone of the team approach to caring for patients with pain. The nurse uses, as necessary, the expertise of all team members, applies their recommendations to the care of individual patients, and reports to team members regarding the success of the plan or the problems that emerge and require revision of the plan.

The assessment tools previously discussed are important methods of fostering a team approach. Standardization of these tools and other communication formats facilitates communication and minimizes delays in making appropriate changes in pain treatment plans.

A team approach requires collaboration among the clinicians and the patients and their families. In simple terms, collaborative practice means working together, not against each other. Following are some basic requirements for a team/collaborative approach to pain management, many of which have already been incorporated in the assessment tools presented in this chapter. The numbers correspond to those in Box 3-7.

1. *Common goals.* In each specific situation, the prescriber, nurse, patient, and others involved in the care must agree on a common goal, referred to as the comfort-function goals (discussed on pp. 85-88). This is often a simple matter of identifying activities, emotional states, or cognitive

abilities that a patient values or needs to perform and determining the pain ratings that would be necessary for achieving the goal of performing. Simply put, if the team does not know where it is going, it will not know when it gets there or whether it has not yet arrived.

2. *Common language.* Obviously, communication is facilitated when all people involved are using the same words to refer to important elements of the situation. Pain rating scales are an example of using a common language. One of the most essential components of pain management is assessment of pain intensity. Pain rating scales that are valid, reliable, and easy to understand and use have been discussed in this chapter. For each individual patient, a single pain rating scale appropriate for that patient should be chosen and should be used by all team members when they discuss pain management among themselves and with the patient and family.

Among clinicians, another component of a common language is using standardized assessment tools and formats for written communication and documentation. Examples of these, already discussed in this chapter, are the flow sheets.

3. *Common knowledge.* Because pain is a relatively new scientific discipline, lack of education about pain management is to be expected. Knowledge of pain management varies widely among clinicians and in various clinical situations. For this reason, clinical practice guidelines have been developed by professional organizations such as the APS. They may be used to provide clinicians with a quick summary of current recommendations for pain management. One or more of them can be distributed to clinicians and referred to for guidance each time a question arises about the assessment and treatment of pain. An example of a brief guideline that applies to many clinical areas is published by the APS and is titled "Principles of Analgesic Use in the Treatment of Acute Pain and Cancer Pain" (2003). This guideline might be given to prescribers, nurses, and pharmacists during orientation. Home care agencies might mail this guideline to referring physicians with a cover letter explaining that the agency is aiming to implement these recommendations.

Other guidelines published by the APS include those that focus on pain management in sickle cell disease (Benjamin, Dampier, Jacox, et al., 1999), cancer in adults and children (Miaskowski, Cleary, Burney, et al., 2005), and various types of arthritis (2002). Although a considerable amount of essential information is contained in the clinical practice guidelines, the single most important directive is that clinicians must accept a patient's report of pain. Repeated reference to this recommendation may well be necessary.

4. *Regular communication.* Common goals, language and knowledge must be shared by team members on a regular and predictable basis. In some instances, such

---

GUIDELINES

Box 3-7 Establishing a Team/ Collaborative Approach to Pain Management

1. Common goals: Agreement on comfort-function goals for pain relief (e.g., pain rating needed for certain activities)
2. Common language: Pain rating scales, standardized assessment tools
3. Common knowledge base: Refer to clinical practice guidelines (e.g., those of the APS); agreement on patient education, e.g., pain rating scale, comfort-function goals
4. Regular communication: Regular contact within the team (e.g., daily progress reports, weekly e-mails, notes); standardized report format

- What is the pain rating now? Over the past period of time?
- What pain rating are we aiming for? Why?
- How do you recommend the patient's treatment be changed to reduce the pain rating?
- What professional reference can be used, if needed, to support this recommendation?

as the care of patients with persistent pain, regular communication takes place at a weekly team meeting. In other situations, such as the care of surgical patients, communication make take the form of pain ratings recorded every 4 hours on a flow sheet and included at the change-of-shift or hand-off report. Home health care agencies may use a standardized format to fax or e-mail updates to referring prescribers and may follow up with telephone calls when there are problems. Care should be taken, however, to report the positive too, not just the problems.

Box 3-8 lists some very simple and basic reminders to prepare clinicians for communicating unrelieved pain to colleagues. It is not a comprehensive list, but it includes the essential information needed in a conversation about improving the patients' pain management.

Pain Assessment in Patients Who Cannot Self-Report

Before discussing strategies for assessing pain in patients who cannot self-report, it is important to correct a common misconception—that patients who are cognitively impaired do not experience as much pain as those who are cognitively intact. Recent studies examining mechanisms and differences in pain transmission and perception in older adults with dementia document that the pain transmission process is unaltered, although cognitive processing and interpretation of the pain stimulus may be impaired, resulting in different presentations or responses to painful stimuli (Gibson, Voukelatos, Amers, et al., 2001; Karp, Shega, Morone, et al., 2008; Kunz, Mykius, Scharmann, et al, 2009; Scherder, Oosterman, Swaab, et al., 2005; Scherder, Sergeant, Swaab, 2003; Schuler, Njoo, Hestermann, et al., 2004). Cognitive impairment

often results in less pain reported, even though there is no evidence that cognitive impairment reduces the ability to feel painful stimuli (Benedetti, Arduino, Vighetti, et al., 2004; Reynolds, Hanson, DeVellis, et al., 2008; Scherder, Herr, Pickering, 2009). Lower reporting and recognition of pain in cognitively impaired patients add to the vulnerability of these older adults and to the smaller likelihood of their receiving treatment that can mediate the profound consequences of untreated pain. Proactive recognition of pain is important and requires understanding the likelihood of underreporting of pain and using methods recommended to recognize pain in those who cannot self-report.

As cognitive impairment advances, obtaining self-reports may not be possible so other approaches are necessary to recognize presence of pain. A hierarchical approach to identifying the presence of pain in nonverbal patients has been recommended and provides a comprehensive strategy for assessing pain in the vulnerable older adults unable to self-report (Buffum, Hutt, Chang, et al., 2007; Herr, Bjoro, Decker, 2006; McCaffery, Pasero, 1999; Pasero, McCaffery, 2005) (Box 3-9). This approach includes the following steps: (1) determine ability to

1. Attempt first to elicit a self-report of pain from patient. If patient is unable to give a self-report, explain why and proceed with the following steps.
2. Identify pathologic conditions and common problems or procedures that may cause pain.
3. Observe for behaviors recognized as pain-related in older persons with dementia. A behavioral assessment tool may be used.
4. Solicit information from caregivers and family members familiar with the older adult about possible indicators of pain.
5. Attempt an analgesic trial and observe changes in the patient's behavior.

self-report, and if unable to obtain self-report, document why and continue with the following steps; (2) investigate for possible pathologies and procedures that might produce pain; (3) observe for possible behaviors that may signal pain; (4) incorporate surrogate reporting; and (5) attempt a trial of analgesic even if only suspicious of pain; and evaluate whether this causes a reduction in the behavioral indicators thought to be related to pain. If a patient is unable to self-report, evidence indicative of pain in any of items 2 through 5 is sufficient to assume pain present (APP) (Pasero, McCaffery, 2002).

Strategies for obtaining self-reports in the cognitively impaired were presented earlier, and efforts should be made to secure self-reports. For those unable to report, searching for potential causes of pain or discomfort is an important approach to identifying pain. Becoming familiar with common diagnoses, conditions, and procedures known to be painful can increase awareness of the possibility of pain in those who cannot report. Box 3-10 provides a list of potential causes of pain that guide review of a patient's medical history and physical examinations and the search for potentially painful conditions.

Behavioral observation is a key strategy for recognizing the presence of pain and can include direct observation of behaviors or obtaining reports from proxies or surrogates, including certified nursing assistants (CNAs), family members, or other caregivers. For patients with dementia, the scope of potential pain indicators is much broader than common pain behaviors, such as grimacing, moaning, groaning, bracing, rubbing, and guarding. Clinicians should be familiar with typical and atypical behavioral presentations (e.g., agitation, restlessness, irritability, combativeness, resisting care, changes in appetite or sleep, or usual activities) that are potential pain indicators and warrant evaluation.

The American Geriatrics Society (AGS) provided a list of pain indicators that may represent pain in cognitively impaired older adults (AGS, 2002) (Table 3-2). The framework is a list of potential pain indicators that can guide observation. Behaviors that are most frequently observed during direct observation are being identified through ongoing study. Shega, Rudy, Keefe, and others (2008) recently found that grimacing was the most common behavior observed, during a guided movement protocol, in both cognitively impaired and cognitively intact older persons with persistent low back pain. They also noted that the frequency of other behaviors differed based on cognitive status, with more rubbing and guarding and less bracing in the cognitively impaired. Facial expression is emerging as a reliable and prominent behavior that can detect and judge severity of pain in both those with and without dementia (Chapman, 2008; Kunz, Scaharmann, Hemmeter, et al., 2007). Studies are needed to examine the frequency of less typical pain behaviors occurring in natural circumstances to guide behavioral tool refinement and pain recognition.

Clinicians should solicit information about pain presence, typical patterns of behavior, and judgment of cur-

---

Box 3-10 | Potential Causes of Pain in Nonverbal Older Adults

PROCEDURAL

- Surgery
- Wound care
- Rehabilitation activities
- Positioning/turning
- Blood draws

CONDITIONS/DIAGNOSES

- History of persistent pain
- OA
- RA
- Low back pain
- Osteoporosis and fractures
- Degenerative disk disease
- Peripheral neuropathies
- Postherpetic neuralgia
- Trigeminal neuralgia
- Diabetic neuropathy
- Peripheral vascular disease
- Myofascial pain
- Fibromyalgia
- Gout
- Bone pain
- Cancer
- Recent fall
- Urinary tract infection
- Pneumonia
- Skin tear
- Constipation

As appears in Pasero, C., & McCaffery, M. (2011). *Pain assessment and pharmacologic management*, p. 124, St. Louis, Mosby. From Herr, K., Coyne, P., Key, T., et al. (2006). Pain assessment in the nonverbal patient: Position statement with clinical practice recommendations. *Pain Manag Nurs*, 7(2), 44-52. May be duplicated for use in clinical practice.

---

rent pain severity from surrogates or proxies who have knowledge about the patients (e.g., family, CNA). In the long-term care setting, the CNA plays an important role and has been shown to be effective in recognizing presence of pain (Mentes, Teer, Cadogan, 2004; Nygaard, Jarland, 2006), whereas in the acute care setting, family members may be most familiar with typical pain behaviors or changes in usual activities that might suggest presence of pain (Nygaard, Jarland, 2006; Shega, Hougham, Stocking, et al., 2004).

Although observation of behavior occurs commonly in clinical practice, a standardized approach to regular observation and documentation that facilitates consistency and more effective communication across provider and setting

Table 3-2 | Common Pain Behaviors in Cognitively Impaired Older Persons

Behavior	Examples
Facial expressions	• Slight frown; sad, frightened face • Grimacing, wrinkled forehead, closed or tightened eyes • Any distorted expression • Rapid blinking
Verbalizations, vocalizations	• Sighing, moaning, groaning • Grunting, chanting, calling out • Noisy breathing • Asking for help • Verbal abusiveness
Body movements	• Rigid, tense body posture, guarding • Fidgeting • Increased pacing, rocking • Restricted movement • Gait or mobility changes
Changes in interpersonal interactions	• Aggressiveness, combativeness, resisting care • Decreased social interactions • Socially inappropriate, disruptive behaviors • Acting withdrawn
Changes in activity patterns or routines	• Refusing food; appetite changes • Increase in rest periods • Changes in sleep and rest patterns • Sudden cessation of common routines • Increased wandering
Changes in mental status	• Crying or tears • Increased confusion • Irritability or distress

Note: Some patients demonstrate little or no specific behaviors in association with severe pain.
As appears in Pasero, C., & McCaffery, M. (2011). *Pain assessment and pharmacologic management*, p. 125, St. Louis, Mosby. Used with permission from American Geriatrics Society Panel on Persistent Pain in Older Adults. (2002). The management of persistent pain in older persons. *J Am Geriatr Soc, 50,* S211. May be duplicated for use in clinical practice.

is needed. Use of a behavioral pain assessment tool is one part of this template (see Step 3, Box 3-9, p. 123) and requires careful selection and use to ensure that vulnerable older patients with pain are recognized and treated. A discussion of behavioral pain assessment tools follows.

The final step in the hierarchical approach to pain assessment in those unable to self-report involves the use of a trial of analgesic to validate whether the suspicion of pain based on information obtained from the previously mentioned steps, such as observation of behavior, is valid. This is especially important when considering atypical presentations of pain by patients when the causes are uncertain. Blinded trials comparing analgesic and placebo

interventions on pain-related outcomes are few, and the findings are mixed. Two randomized controlled trials focused on the use of acetaminophen and its effect on agitation and function. The first trial found no effect on agitation among nursing home residents, although the acetaminophen dosing of 1500 mg per day may not have provided a therapeutic level of analgesia (Buffum, Sands, Miaskowski, et al., 2004), whereas the second trial demonstrated increased levels of social activity and interaction after a therapeutic dose of acetaminophen (3000 mg/day), although no significant change in agitation was noted (Chibnall, Tait, Harman, et al., 2005). A study of low-dose opioid treatment (20 milliequivalent morphine/24 h) compared with placebo showed significant effect on agitation in the over-85 age group only (Manfredi, Breuer, Wallenstein, et al., 2003).

Kovach and colleagues evaluated a systematic method of assessing and treating behaviors that may be pain-related in patients with severe dementia in a clinical protocol called the Serial Trial Intervention, which incorporates an analgesic trial (Kovach, Noonan, Schlidt, et al., 2006). In a randomized controlled trial involving 114 subjects residing in 14 nursing homes, those who received the intervention had significantly less discomfort and more frequent return of behavioral symptoms to baseline than those who did not.

An analgesic trial can be used to confirm suspicion that a nonverbal older person is experiencing pain. It also serves as the foundation for developing a pain treatment plan when the trial confirms the presence of pain. Box 3-11 provides a guide for use of an analgesic trial and development of a treatment plan for suspected pain in cognitively impaired older adults. Because many of the potential pain indicators could also be caused by other conditions related to the dementia diagnosis, it is useful to understand the rationale for attempting an analgesic trial before psychiatric management. Compared with psychotropic intervention, response to an analgesic intervention is more rapid, the adverse reactions are usually less severe, and pain will not be obscured by the sedative properties of psychotropic agents (Herr, Bjoro, Decker, 2006). Psychiatric intervention can be considered if behaviors do not improve with an analgesic trial. The limited studies suggest that analgesic trials to validate pain in persons with behavioral manifestations of potential pain hold promise, although algorithms for this approach need further development and testing.

At any step in the process described, pain may be suspected but difficult to confirm. However, when any information indicating pain is obtained in any of items 2 through 5 in Box 3-9 (p. 123), the clinician may *assume pain is present* and document it with the abbreviation *APP* if that acronym is approved by the institution (Pasero, McCaffery, 2002). For example, if a patient shows no behavioral signs of pain, the presence of pathology or procedures that are normally painful is sufficient to assume pain is present (Pasero, McCaffery, 2002).

| Box 3-11 | Analgesic Trial for Suspected Pain in Cognitively Impaired Older Adults |

Initiate an analgesic trial if:

- Pathologic conditions likely to cause pain exist.
- Procedures likely to cause pain are scheduled.
- Pain behaviors continue after attention to cause of pain.
- Pain behaviors continue after attention to basic needs and comfort measures.
- Behaviors suggest pain.
- Surrogate reports previous chronic pain or behaviors indicative of pain.

Provide an analgesic trial and titration appropriate to the estimated intensity of the pain based on the above information, analgesic history, and prior assessment:

- Mild to moderate pain—A nonopioid analgesic may be given initially (e.g., acetaminophen 500 to 1000 mg every 6 hours for 24 hours). If the oral or rectal route is not an option, low-dose ketorolac* (e.g., 7.5 mg) IV every 6 hours if not contraindicated, or low-dose opioid (e.g., morphine 1 to 2 mg) IV every 2 to 4 hours for 24 hours may be given initially.
- If behaviors improve, assume pain was the cause; continue analgesic, and add appropriate nonpharmacologic interventions.
- If behaviors continue, consider a single low-dose, short-acting opioid (e.g., hydrocodone, oxycodone, or morphine) and observe the effect.
- If no change in behavior, titrate dose upward by 25% to 50% and observe effect.
- Continue to titrate upward until a therapeutic effect is seen, bothersome adverse effects occur, or no benefit is determined.
- Explore other potential causes if behaviors continue after reasonable analgesic trial.

---

*Ketorolac is recommended for short-term management of no longer than 5 days.

As appears in Pasero, C., & McCaffery, M. (2011). *Pain assessment and pharmacologic management*, p. 126, St. Louis, Mosby. Data from Herr, K., Coyne, P., Key, T., et al. (2006). Pain assessment in the nonverbal patient: Position statement with clinical practice recommendations. *Pain Manag Nurs*, 7(2), 44-52. © 2011, Herr K. May be duplicated for use in clinical practice.

Physiologic measures are not included in the hierarchy of pain assessment techniques because of their limited sensitivity to pain. It is a misconception that elevated vital signs can be used to verify severe pain, and autonomic responses to pain, including vital signs, are often decreased in persons with dementia and thus not accurate indicators of pain presence (Kunz, Mykius, Scharmann, et al., 2009). Details related to this are discussed earlier (p. 26). For example, in the critical care unit, vital signs are readily observable but they are influenced by many factors other than pain (Gelinas, Johnston, 2007). Elevated vital signs in patients with moderate to severe chronic pain are usually not evident. Thus, absence of elevated vital signs does not mean absence of pain.

Types of Behavioral Pain Assessment Tools

Tools for the observation of pain behaviors have been developed to assist in the recognition of pain in those unable to self-report. A number of reviews have critiqued existing behavioral tools and similarly concluded that no tool is currently recommended for general use across all populations and settings (Hadjistavropoulos, 2005; Herr, Bjoro, Decker, 2006; Stolee, Hillier, Esbaugh, et al., 2005; van Herk, van Dijk, Baar, et al., 2007; Zwakhalen, Hamers, Abu-Saad, et al., 2006). However, additional research into some existing tools and the development of new tools continue to broaden the selection of instruments for consideration. When selecting a standard observation tool for implementation, it is important for clinicians to consider the psychometric properties of a tool and its clinical utility and appropriateness for the setting and population. The next section provides information about existing tools that can guide clinicians in determining which tool to incorporate into a comprehensive approach to pain assessment in persons unable to self-report. Because of rapid changes in the field and ongoing research, monitoring for new developments is recommended.

The Mayday Fund provided support for the development of resources to assist clinicians in behavioral pain assessment tool selection, available in the resource section at the Pain Resource Center at the City of Hope (http://.prc.coh.org/PAIN-NOA.htm). A detailed critique of existing pain tools, a brief summary of tool strengths and challenges, information regarding tool access and permission, and a comparison across tools are available at the website.

There are a variety of ways to categorize the pain behavior assessment tools available for use with nonverbal older patients. One approach is to organize them as pain behavior checklists, pain behavior intensity scales, and a combination of both. Alternatively, tools can be organized by whether they are direct-observation tools or informant-based tools. Direct-observation tools can usually be completed by those without prior knowledge of the patients as they gather information about specific behaviors observed during a specified period or activity. They identify the presence or absence of the behavior and may include a rating of the behavior's intensity or frequency (Feldt, 2000; Snow, Weber, O'Malley, et al., 2004; Warden, Hurley, Volicer, 2003). Informant-based tools (also called surrogate/proxy tools) rely on information from family members, caregivers, and health care providers familiar with the individuals' baseline behaviors and they can detect changes in activities and behaviors from usual presentation. There also may be overlap in direct observation and informant report. Regardless of the categorization of tools, several considerations are necessary in determining the best approach for given populations and settings.

A key consideration is tool specificity versus sensitivity. Because of individual variability in behavioral presentation related to pain, short, direct observation tools that focus on key common pain behaviors (e.g., grimacing, moaning, bracing) may recognize pain in those who present with these common pain behaviors (specificity) but may fail to detect pain in those who present with more atypical changes in activity or behavior (sensitivity) (e.g., decreased appetite, increased sleeping, greater agitation, acting withdrawn, or increased irritability). Longer comprehensive tools that include more potential pain indicators may be more sensitive but less specific. This means that more patients who present with less common pain behaviors will be identified, but in some of those, pain may not be the cause of their behaviors. Follow-up evaluation is necessary to determine the causes of the behaviors observed.

One factor influencing tool use is whether behavior is observed at rest, during or following some activity, or during an activity intended to evoke pain. Studies have illustrated that observation at rest is misleading and can lead to incorrect judgment about the presence of pain (Feldt, 2000; Hadjistavropoulos, LaChapelle, MacLeod, et al., 2000; Husebo, Strand, Moe-Nilssen, et al., 2008). Thus, observation during movement or activity is recommended. The timing of the observation should be consistent and should be part of the assessment procedure in persons requiring behavioral observation (e.g., during morning care, transfers, or ambulation).

In patients with severe dementia, studies support the ability of surrogates to recognize pain's presence, but not accurately rate its severity (Manfredi, Breuer, Wallenstein, et al., 2003; Pautex, Herrmann, Michon, et al., 2007; Shega, Hougham, Stocking, et a., 2004). This may be related to individual variability in patients' behavioral presentations. For example, one patient with severe dementia may present with agitation and aggressive behavior, whereas another may become withdrawn and quiet. Their behavioral presentations are quite different, but they both could be experiencing moderate pain; this indicates that it is unreliable to determine the severity of pain on the basis of the severity of restlessness and agitation. Some authors have attempted to establish a direct relationship between behavior scores and pain intensity, such as adding up the score on a behavioral tool and equating it with pain intensity. Given current knowledge about this topic, number or intensity of behaviors cannot be added up to equal a pain score. We emphasize that no self-report means no pain-intensity rating (Pasero, McCaffery, 2005). The low correlations shown in most studies between surrogate judgment of pain severity and patient reports of severity

contribute to concern about using behavioral scores as pain-intensity ratings (vanHerk, vanDijk, Biemold, 2009). Further, if clinicians could reliably determine the intensity of pain in patients who cannot self-report, there would be no need for behavioral assessment tools (Zwakhalen, Hamers, Abu-Saad, et al., 2006).

Certain studies that have focused on direct observation of typical pain behaviors (such as grimacing, vocalizations, and guarding) show stronger correlations between pain behaviors and pain severity (Horgas, Nichols, Schapson, et al., 2007; Husebo, Strand, Moe-Nilssen, et al., 2007). However, the behaviors observed were typical pain behaviors, and the circumstances were controlled, so the results might not apply to assessments involving broader circumstances and less typical behaviors. Future research may reveal approaches that guide judgments of pain's severity on the basis of behaviors. However, until there is stronger evidence to support this relationship, the score on a pain behavior assessment tool is not the same as a pain-intensity rating scale, and the two should not be directly compared (Herr, Coyne, Key, et al., 2006). However, for an individual patient, an increasing score on a behavioral pain assessment tool usually indicates increasing pain, and a decreasing score probably represents a decrease in pain.

Selection of a tool is determined by the tool's reliability and validity, the setting of the care and the population to be assessed, the availability of knowledgeable caregivers, and the clinical utility. Foremost, a pain assessment tool must have at least moderate reliability and validity. A tool that is not reliable and valid is not useful for supporting clinical judgments. It is very tempting to develop a new tool or adapt an existing tool to meet a clinical need. For example, a tool such as the Face, Legs, Activity, Cry, and Consolability (FLACC) may seem like a good tool to use with older persons. However, the FLACC was based on children's development and has not yet been demonstrated to be reliable and valid for older persons (Baiardi, Parzuchowski, Kosik, et al., 2002). A recent study of the FLACC in citically ill patients who could not self-report included older adults, but it was not clear how many of the population were 65 to 70 years and older (Voepel-Lewis, Zanotti, Dammeyer, 2010). Therefore, further study of the FLACC in older patients is warranted. Considerable time and effort are required to establish a tool's validity and reliability, which are essential before integrating a tool into clinical use.

One key aspect of a tool's validity is its sensitivity to change—a critical aspect of a tool's utility that has received limited attention in the research to date. Several of the existing tools have been evaluated for their abilities to detect responses to intervention (e.g., analgesia) (Cohen-Mansfield, Lipson, 2008; Morello, Jean, Alix, et al., 2007). Ensuring that tools can detect response to treatment is part of the development of a tool's validity.

The setting of care is important in evaluating the appropriateness of a tool. For example, a number of tools that have been developed require observation over time and knowledge of patients' usual behaviors, so they would not be useful in acute care settings to look for procedural pain or postoperative pain. In acute care settings, a short, direct-observation tool may be well suited for use with patients who have acute pain problems and are unknown to the nursing staff. In the long-term care setting, a short, direct-observation tool that can be used on a regular basis by CNAs during usual care combined with a more comprehensive screening tool that is completed at regular intervals may work well. Finally, a pain assessment tool that requires excessive training, is perceived as being too complex, or requires too much time to administer will not be helpful in promoting regular clinical use of the tool. Careful consideration of these characteristics can guide the selection of an appropriate tool. Detailed critiques and summaries of tools are available at http://pcr.coh.org/PAIN-NOA.htm.

Tools for Assessing Pain in Cognitively Impaired Patients and Others Who Cannot Self-Report

For those caring for older adults in long-term care facilities, the minimum data set (MDS) may be considered a source of assessment data. The MDS is a federally mandated system for the assessment of residents of long-term care nursing facilities. It systematizes the assessment of each resident's functional, mental, psychosocial, and medical status at admission and at regular intervals thereafter (Kovach, Noonan, Griffie, et al., 2002). However, concerns have been raised regarding the underreporting of pain in cognitively impaired residents when reports are based on MDSs (Chu, Schnelle, Cadogan, et al., 2004; Cohen-Mansfield, 2004). A revised MDS 3.0 has been under development and evaluation and includes additional pain assessment content, including documentation of behaviors related to pain. Once implemented, the value of the revised MDS may be improved although evaluation of its ability to detect pain in nonverbal patients and to demonstrate response to intervention will be needed.

A number of standardized tools for pain assessment have been developed and are at various stages of testing and refinement. Following is a description of selected tools that merit consideration, depending on the setting and population. We have chosen not to include discussions of tools that do not have support for use with older adults with cognitive impairment or that focus primarily on the detection of discomfort rather than pain. Information about other tools can be obtained at http://prc.coh.org/PAIN-NOA.htm.

Recommended Tools for Patients Who Cannot Self-Report

No perfect behavioral assessment tool exists, but based on current research and clinical utility, the three tools we recommend for use in clinical practice with patients who cannot self-report are (1) Checklist of Nonverbal Pain Indicators (CNPI); (2) The Pain Assessment in Advanced Dementia (PAINAD); and (3) Pain Assessment Checklist for Seniors with Severe Dementia (PACSLAC). These tools are described, and an overview of them is provided in Table 3-3. Other tools are also described.

The tools presented here are in varying stages of development, and further testing may establish greater reliability and validity; however, considerable detail is presented regarding the current stages of the research that establishes their psychometric properties. Research terminology unfamiliar to some readers has been used. To facilitate understanding of the research findings, Table 3-4 provides definitions of selected research-related terms.

The Checklist of Nonverbal Pain Indicators (CNPI) (Feldt, 2000) is a brief, clinically useful observation list of six behavior items that are scored as being present or absent at rest and during movement in cognitively impaired older adults. (Form 3-14 on p. 131 shows the tool as it is used in clinical practice.) The tool includes only the common behaviors that reveal pain, thus limiting the measure's ability to capture the full range of possible pain behaviors. Preliminary testing provided initial support for use of the tool with older adults in acute care settings, although internal consistency was low. Recent evaluation in long-term care (Jones, Fink, Hutt, et al., 2005) demonstrated support of the CNPI as a measure of pain's severity; increases in CNPI scores were associated with increases in self-reports of pain (Jones, Fink, Hutt, et al., 2005). However, 50% of residents reporting pain had no visible indicators of pain, which raises concerns about the tool's sensitivity and its ability to detect persistent pain in those unable to report. Cutoff scores for determining the presence and severity of pain are not available. Another study, conducted in a group of Norwegian nursing homes, provides evidence of acceptable test-retest and inter-rater reliabilities and concurrent validity, as well as the tool's practicality when administered by various categories of nursing personnel (Nygaard, Jarland, 2006). Further testing in acute care and long-term care settings in the United States is recommended.

The Pain Assessment in Advanced Dementia (PAINAD) Scale (Warden, Hurley, Volicer, 2003) was developed as a short, easy-to-use observation tool for assessing pain in individuals with advanced dementia. (Form 3-15 on pp. 132-134 shows the tool as it is used in clinical practice.) The PAINAD is an adaptation of the Discomfort Scale for Dementia of the Alzheimer Type (DS-DAT) (Hurley, Volicer, Hanrahan, et al., 1992) and the FLACC (Merkel, Voepel-Lewis, Shayevitz, et al., 1997) and includes five items: breathing, negative vocalization, facial expression, body language, and consolability. These items are not comprehensive, and the ability to detect pain in those with less obvious changes in behavior may be compromised. No data attach level of pain severity (mild, moderate, or

Table 3-3 | Overview of Selected Behavioral Pain Assessment Scales for Older Adults Unable to Self-Report

Nonverbal Pain Behavior Scale	Description	Compre-hensiveness	Validity	Reliability	Feasibility/Clinical Utility	Summary
Checklist of Nonverbal Pain Indicators (CNPI)[1]	6 items, including nonverbal vocalizations, facial grimacing or wincing, bracing, rubbing, restlessness, vocal complaints Items scored present or absent at rest and on movement Total score range from 0 to 12	Limited Addresses 3 of 6 AGS pain behavior categories	Moderate construct and discriminant validity differentiating pain at rest vs. on movement Moderate correlations with verbal descriptor scale on movement, but low at rest	Low to moderate internal consistency reliability Good inter-rater reliability Moderate to good intra-rater reliability	Easy to use Time to complete not specified, but likely 5 minutes or less Scoring instructions provided Interpretation of score not clear Tested in acute and long-term care	Concern regarding sensitivity in detecting persistent pain Further testing is needed
The Pain Assessment in Advanced Dementia Scale (PAINAD)[2]	5 categorical items: breathing, negative vocalizations, facial expressions, body language, consolability Scoring range 0 to 10 0 to 2 scale	Limited Addresses 3 of 6 AGS pain behavior categories	Ability to differentiate between pleasant and unpleasant activities Ability to detect change before and after pain medication in some studies Convergent validity with other pain scales	Moderate to strong internal consistency reliability Good inter-rater reliability Strong test-retest reliability	Easy to use Scoring instructions provided Time to complete: 1 to 3 minutes Limited training required Tested in long-term and acute care	Usefulness of breathing and consolability items for pain detection are questioned Further study of tool sensitivity needed
The Pain Assessment Scale for Seniors with Limited Ability to Communicate (PACSLAC)[3]	60 items in four dimensions: facial expression (N = 13); activity/body movements (N = 20); social/personality/mood (N = 12); physiologic/eating/ sleeping/vocal (N = 15) Rates present or absent Scoring range 0 to 60 PACSLAC-D (Dutch version with 24 items; Zwakhalen, Hamers, Berger, 2007)	Good Addresses all 6 AGS pain behavior categories	Congruent and discriminant validity demonstrated Ability to detect differences in levels of pain Moderate correlation with global rating of pain	Moderate to good internal consistency Excellent inter-rater reliability Strong intra-rater reliability Good internal consistency	Long list of items Easy to use 5 minute estimated completion time Preliminary cutoffs for pain presence determined Tested in long-term care	Further testing in larger English-speaking samples with increased diversity are needed

Note: The tools selected for inclusion were those with the highest scores based on overall evaluation of psychometric properties and utility.

[1]Feldt, 2000; Jones et al., 2005; Nygaard, Jarland, 2006.

[2]Warden, Hurley, Volicer, 2003; DeWaters et al., 2008; Leong, Chong, Gibson, 2006; Zwakhalen, Hamers, Bergen, 2006; Cohen-Mansfield, Lipson, 2008.

[3]Fuchs-Lacelle, Hadjistavropoulos, 2004; Fuchs-Lacelle, Hadjistavropoulos, 2005; Zwakhalen, Hamers, Bergen, 2006. From Pasero, C., & McCaffery, M. (2011). *Pain assessment and pharmacologic management*, p. 129, St. Louis, Mosby. Adapted and used with permission from Hadjistavropoulos, T., Herr, K., Turk, D., et al. (2007). An interdisciplinary expert consensus statement on assessment of pain in older persons. *Clin J Pain* 23(1), S1-S43. May be duplicated for use in clinical practice.

Table 3-4 | Definitions of Selected Research-Related Terms

Term	Definition
Content or face validity	The examination of tool items to determine whether the items look like they are measuring the concept of interest (i.e., pain)
Construct validity	The ability of a tool to measure what it is intended to measure. Concurrent, convergent, and discriminant validity are forms of construct validity.
Concurrent validity	The ability of a tool to differentiate among individuals in performance or behavior by comparing performance against a similar tool. For example, a numeric rating scale should be strongly related to scores reported on a verbal descriptor scale.
Convergent validity	The relationship of a tool to other tools measuring the same concept. For example, in comparing a new tool measuring ability to perform ADLs to a standardized ADL tool, a strong relationship supports convergent validity.
Discriminant validity	The relationship of a tool to other tools measuring different concepts. For example, a tool measuring pain intensity and a tool measuring hostility would not be expected to be strongly related to each other and support divergent validity.
Internal consistency	The extent to which the items in a tool measure the same concept. For example, in the Brief Pain Inventory the pain interference items all examine the impact of pain on function and thus has high internal consistency.
Inter-rater reliability	The degree of agreement among different raters independently scoring the same data in the same way. For example, two raters observe 10 patients and record their observations on the PAINAD. The more their scorings agree, the higher the inter-rater reliability.
Normative data and cutoffs	The normal or average scores to be expected on a given measure for a representative sample. Cutoffs are the scores on a scale that determine whether the subject meets or does not meet the criteria. For example, normative data from a number of studies were used to establish cutoffs for mild, moderate, and severe pain on the numeric rating scale.

ADL, Activities of daily living.
As appears in Pasero, C., & McCaffery, M. (2011). *Pain assessment and pharmacologic management,* p. 130, St. Louis, © 2011, Herr K. May be duplicated for use in clinical practice.

severe) to the number obtained in the tool, although higher scores do represent greater reports of pain.

The PAINAD has been translated into four languages and tested, and three additional English studies have provided additional information about the tool's psychometrics and utility. Subsequent studies have provided support for its construct and its concurrent validity and ability to detect pain and to differentiate between groups with and without pain in both long-term and acute care settings (Costardi, Rozzini, Costanzi, et al., 2007; DeWaters, Faut-Callahan, McCann, et al., 2008; Leong, Chong, Gibson, 2006; Schuler, Becker, Kaspar, et al., 2007; van Iersel, Timmerman, Mullie, 2006; Zwakhalen, Hamers, Abu-Saad, et al., 2006).

One study that compared the PAINAD to other tools in terms of their abilities to detect change resulting from treatment raises questions regarding the tool's sensitivity (Cohen-Mansfield, Lipson, 2008). Follow-up studies demonstrate good internal consistency, inter-rater reliability, and test-retest reliability. Several studies question the utility of including the items *breathing* and *consolability*, but removal of these items did not demonstrate

improved internal consistency. Further study is needed to investigate the tool's sensitivity to change in behavior in response to treatment.

The Pain Assessment Checklist for Seniors with Limited Ability to Communicate (PACSLAC) (Fuchs-Lacelle, Hadjistavropoulos, 2004), developed by a Canadian team, is an observational tool that uses direct observation and familiar caregiver information to assess both common and uncommon pain behaviors. (Form 3-16, pp. 135-136, shows the tool as it is used in clinical practice.) The PACSLAC is potentially a clinically useful behavior checklist that appears to be simple to use for assessing and monitoring changes in persons with dementia and diverse presentations of pain-related behavior. The tool is comprehensive; 60 indicators address all six pain behavior categories included in the AGS guidelines. Prospective evaluation has supported the tool's reliability and validity (Fuchs-Lacelle, Hadjistavropoulos, 2005; Zwakhalen, Hamers, Berger, 2006; Zwakhalen, Hamers, Berger, 2007) and has done a factor analysis to determine the most efficient and useful indicator set for clinical use. Because of the length of the tool, it may not be suitable

Checklist of Nonverbal Pain Indicators (CNPI)

(Write a 0 if the behavior was not observed, and a 1 if the behavior occurred even briefly during activity or rest.)

	With Movement	Rest
1. Vocal Complaints: Non-Verbal (Expression of pain, not in words, moans, groans, grunts, cries, gasps, sighs)	_____	_____
2. Facial Grimaces/Winces (Furrowed brow, narrowed eyes, tightened lips, jaw drop, clenched teeth, distorted expressions)	_____	_____
3. Bracing (Clutching or holding onto side rails, bed, tray table, or affected area during movement)	_____	_____
4. Restlessness (Constant or intermittent shifting of position, rocking, intermittent or constant hand motions, inability to keep still)	_____	_____
5. Rubbing (Massaging affected area)	_____	_____

In addition, record verbal complaints.

	With Movement	Rest
6. Vocal Complaints: Verbal (Words expressing discomfort or pain, "ouch" "that hurts"; cursing during movement, or exclamations of protest: "stop", "that's enough")	_____	_____
Subtotal Scores	_____	_____
Total Score		_____

Form 3-14

As appears in Pasero, C., McCaffery, M. (2011). *Pain assessment and pharmacologic management*, p. 131, St. Louis, Mosby. From Feldt, K. S. (1996). Treatment of pain in cognitively impaired versus cognitively intact post-hip-fractured elders. Doctoral dissertation, University of Minnesota *Dissertation Abstracts International, 57-09B*, 5574; Feldt, K. S. (2000). Checklist of nonverbal pain indicators. *Pain Manag Nurs, 1*(1). 13-21. May be duplicated for use in clinical practice.

for acute care settings. However, clinicians report that it actually takes very little time to complete the form once they are familiar with it. Even if the tool is not formally used in the acute care setting, it can be posted in the clinical units as a resource for identifying behaviors.

A study was conducted to determine whether systematic pain assessment of older adults with severe dementia in a nursing home, using the PACSLAC, would improve pain management and decrease nursing stress in comparison with a control group (Fuchs-Lacelle, Hadjistavropoulos,

Pain Assessment IN Advanced Dementia — PAINAD

	0	1	2	Score
Breathing Independent of vocalization	Normal	Occasional labored breathing. Short period of hyperventilation	Noisy labored breathing. Long period of hyperventilation. Cheyne-Stokes respirations.	
Negative Vocalization	None	Occasional moan or groan. Low level speech with a negative or disapproving quality.	Repeated troubled calling out. Loud moaning or groaning. Crying.	
Facial Expression	Smiling, or inexpressive	Sad. Frightened. Frown.	Facial grimacing.	
Body Language	Relaxed	Tense. Distressed pacing. Fidgeting.	Rigid. Fists clenched, Knees pulled up. Pulling or pushing away. Striking out.	
Consolability	No need to console	Distracted or reassured by voice or touch.	Unable to console, distract, or reassure.	
				TOTAL:

Continued

Form 3-15

As appears in Pasero, C., & McCaffery, M. (2011). *Pain assessment and Pharmacologic management*, pp. 132-134, St. Louis, Mosby. From Warden, V., Hurley, A. C., & Volicer, L. (2003). Development and psychometric evaluation of the pain assessment in advanced dementia (PAINAD) scale. *JAMA, 4*(1), 9-15. May be duplicated for use in clinical practice.

Pain Assessment IN Advanced Dementia — PAINAD

Item Definitions

Breathing

1. <u>Normal breathing</u>. DESCRIPTION: Normal breathing is characterized by effortless, quiet, rhythmic (smooth) respirations.

2. <u>Occasional labored breathing</u>. DESCRIPTION: Occasional labored breathing is characterized by episodic bursts of harsh, difficult, or wearing respirations.

3. <u>Short period of hyperventilation</u>. DESCRIPTION: Short period of hyperventilation is characterized by intervals of rapid, deep breaths lasting a short period of time.

4. <u>Noisy labored breathing</u>. DESCRIPTION: Noisy labored breathing is characterized by negative sounding respirations on inspiration or expiration. They may be loud, gurgling, wheezing. They appear strenuous or wearing.

5. <u>Long period of hyperventilation</u>. DESCRIPTION: Long period of hyperventilation is characterized by an excessive rate and depth of respirations lasting a considerable time.

6. <u>Cheyne-Stokes respirations</u>. DESCRIPTION: Cheyne-Stokes respirations are characterized by rhythmic waxing and waning of breathing from very deep to shallow respirations with periods of apnea (cessation of breathing).

Negative Vocalization

1. <u>None</u>. DESCRIPTION: None is characterized by speech or vocalization that has a neutral or pleasant quality.

2. <u>Occasional moan or groan</u>. DESCRIPTION: Occasional moaning is characterized by mournful or murmuring sounds, wails or laments. Groaning is characterized by louder than usual inarticulate involuntary sounds, often abruptly beginning and ending.

3. <u>Low level speech with a negative or disapproving quality</u>. DESCRIPTION: Low level speech with a negative or disapproving quality is characterized by muttering, mumbling, whining, grumbling, or swearing in a low volume with a complaining, sarcastic, or caustic tone.

4. <u>Repeated troubled calling out</u>. DESCRIPTION: Repeated trouble calling out is characterized by phrases or words being used over and over in a tone that suggests anxiety, uneasiness, or distress.

5. <u>Loud moaning or groaning</u>. DESCRIPTION: Loud moaning is characterized by mournful or murmuring sounds, wails or laments in much louder than usual volume. Loud groaning is characterized by louder than usual inarticulate involuntary sounds, often abruptly beginning and ending.

6. <u>Crying</u>. DESCRIPTION: Crying is characterized by an utterance of emotion accompanied by tears. There may be sobbing or quiet weeping.

Facial Expression

1. <u>Smiling or inexpressive</u>. DESCRIPTION: Smiling is characterized by upturned corners of the mouth, brightening of the eyes and a look of pleasure or contentment. Inexpressive refers to a neutral, at ease, relaxed, or blank look.

2. <u>Sad</u>. DESCRIPTION: Sad is characterized by an unhappy, lonesome, sorrowful, or dejected look. There may be tears in the eyes.

3. <u>Frightened</u>. DESCRIPTION: Frightened is characterized by a look of fear, alarm, or heightened anxiety. Eyes appear wide open.

4. <u>Frown</u>. DESCRIPTION: Frown is characterized by a downward turn of the corners of the mouth. Increased facial wrinkling in the forehead and around the mouth may appear.

5. <u>Facial grimacing</u>. DESCRIPTION: Facial grimacing is characterized by a distorted, distressed look. The brow is more wrinkled as is the area around the mouth. Eyes may be squeezed shut.

Body Language

1. <u>Relaxed</u>. DESCRIPTION: Relaxed is characterized by a calm, restful, mellow appearance. The person seems to be taking it easy.

2. <u>Tense</u>. DESCRIPTION: Tense is characterized by a strained, apprehensive, or worried appearance. The jaw may be clenched. (Exclude any contractures.)

3. <u>Distressed pacing</u>. DESCRIPTION: Distressed pacing is characterized by activity that seems unsettled. There may be a fearful, worried, or disturbed element present. The rate may by faster or slower.

4. <u>Fidgeting</u>. DESCRIPTION: Fidgeting is characterized by restless movement. Squirming about or wiggling in the chair may occur. The person might be hitching a chair across the room. Repetitive touching, tugging, or rubbing body parts can also be observed.

5. <u>Rigid.</u> DESCRIPTION: Rigid is characterized by stiffening of the body. The arms and/or legs are tight and inflexible. The trunk may appear straight and unyielding. (Exclude any contractures.)

6. <u>Fists clenched.</u> DESCRIPTION: Fists clenched is characterized by tightly closed hands. They may be opened and closed repeatedly or held tightly shut.

7. <u>Knees pulled up.</u> DESCRIPTION: Knees pulled up is characterized by flexing the legs and drawing the knees up toward the chest. An overall troubled appearance. (Exclude any contractures.)

8. <u>Pulling or pushing away.</u> DESCRIPTION: Pulling or pushing away is characterized by resistiveness upon approach or to care. The person is trying to escape by yanking or wrenching him or herself free or shoving you away.

9. <u>Striking out.</u> DESCRIPTION: Striking out is characterized by hitting, kicking, grabbing, punching, biting, or other form of personal assault.

Consolability

1. <u>No need to console.</u> DESCRIPTION: No need to console is characterized by a sense of well being. The person appears content.

2. <u>Distracted or reassured by voice or touch.</u> DESCRIPTION: Distracted or reassured by voice or touch is characterized by a disruption in the behavior when the person is spoken to or touched. The behavior stops during the period of interaction with no indication that the person is at all distressed.

3. <u>Unable to console, distract, or reassure.</u> DESCRIPTION: Unable to console, distract or reassure is characterized by the inability to sooth the person or stop a behavior with words or actions. No amount of comforting, verbal or physical, will alleviate the behavior.

Form 3-15 | Cont'd.

Lix, 2008). The most common pain-related diagnosis was arthritis. The experimental group of nurses was asked to complete the PACSLAC regularly, that is, at least three times a week. The use of PRN medications by the experimental group increased more over time than it did in the control group. Further, the nurses in the experimental group reported a decrease in work-related emotional exhaustion over time; the control group did not. Rather than increasing stress in the experimental group, the addition of a 60-item assessment tool to their workload led them to find that regular use of the assessment tool reduced their stress. One explanation for this result is that pain caused disruptive and aggressive behavior, and assessment identified this pain and led to increased analgesic medication. This reduced patients' pain and hence decreased disruptive behaviors, which in turn decreased the nurses' stress.

The revised PACSLAC-D (Zwakhalen, Hamers, Berger, 2006) is a 24-item tool but does not include items based on changes in behavior or activity. Because of this revision, the PACLSAC and PACSLAC-D psychometric properties should be considered independently. The PACSLAC has good internal consistency, inter-rater reliability, and intra-rater reliability. The PACSLAC-D also shows good reliability estimates in preliminary testing. Preliminary normative data and cutoffs are provided but require validation in larger, more diverse samples. Further refinement of the PACSLAC has been reported, with a shorter tool including 18 valid and reliable indicators confirmed (van Nispen tot Pannerdan, Candel, Zwakhalen, et al., 2009). Additional factor analysis in English-speaking samples and evaluation of sensitivity in detecting treatment effects are recommended.

Pain Screens and Patient Examples

The development and use of pain screens and flow sheets or other methods of documentation, including electronic medical records, are important to ensure consistency in the practice and communication of relevant assessment information. Forms 3-17 through 3-20, pp. 137-140, provide examples of a pain screen for use with older patients unable to self-report and a flow sheet for monitoring pain behaviors.

Other Tools in Development

Several other tools are in development for use in clinical practice. Some of them are discussed briefly; however, new tools and further evaluation of existing tools occur

Pain Assessment Checklist for Seniors with Limited Ability to Communicate—PACSLAC

DATE: _____   TIME ASSESSED: _____

NAME OF PATIENT/RESIDENT: _____

PURPOSE:

This checklist is used to assess pain in patients/residents who have dementia and have limited ability to communicate.

INSTRUCTIONS:

Indicate with a checkmark which of the items on the PACSLAC occurred during the period of interest.

Scoring the Sub-Scales is derived by counting the checkmarks in each column.

To generate a Total Pain Score, sum all four Sub-Scale totals.

Comments:
_____
_____
_____
_____
_____
_____
_____
_____
_____

Form 3-16   *Continued*

regularly in the literature. Readers are encouraged to study the literature so as to stay abreast of new research findings.

The Abbey Pain Scale (ABBEY) (Abbey, Piller, DeBellis, et al., 2004) is an Australian informant-based tool that measures pain intensity in people with late-stage dementia. The tool attempts to measure acute pain, chronic pain, and acute-on-chronic pain and produces ranges of scores to determine pain intensity. The rationale for mixing and differentiating pain types, pain behaviors, and pain causes is not clear nor is the justification for the pain intensity ranges. Although a recent evaluation of the

Facial Expressions	Present
Grimacing	
Sad look	
Tighter face	
Dirty look	
Change in eyes (squinting, dull, bright, increased movement)	
Frowning	
Pain expression	
Grim face	
Clenching teeth	
Wincing	
Opening mouth	
Creasing forehead	
Screwing up nose	
Activity/Body Movement	
Fidgeting	
Pulling away	
Flinching	
Restless	
Pacing	
Wandering	
Trying to leave	
Refusing to move	
Thrashing	
Decreased activity	
Refusing medications	
Moving slow	
Impulsive behavior (e.g., repetitive movements)	
Uncooperative/resistant to care	
Guarding sore area	
Touching/holding sore area	
Limping	
Clenched fist	
Going into foetal position	
Stiff/rigid	

Social/Personality/Mood Indicators	Present
Physical aggression (e.g., pushing people and/or objects, scratching others, hitting others, striking, kicking)	
Verbal aggression	
Not wanting to be touched	
Not allowing people near	
Anygry/mad	
Throwing things	
Increased confusion	
Anxious	
Upset	
Agitated	
Cranky/irritable	
Frustrated	
Physiologic indicators/Eating/ Sleeping Changes/Vocal Behaviors	
Pale face	
Flushed, red face	
Teary eyed	
Sweating	
Shaking/trembling	
Cold & clammy	
Changes in sleep (please circle): Decreased sleep or Increased sleep during day	
Changes in Appetite (please circle): Decreased appetite or Increased appetite	
Screaming/yelling	
Calling out (i.e., for help)	
Crying	
A specific sound or vocalization for pain 'ow', 'ouch'	
Moaning and groaning	
Mumbling	
Grunting	

Sub-Scale Scores:

Facial Expressions _____

Activity/Body Movement _____

Social/Personality Mood _____

Other _____

Total Checklist Score _____

This version of the scale does not include the items "sitting and rocking", "quiet/withdrawn", and "vacant blank stare" as these were not found to be useful in discriminating pain from non-pain states.

Form 3-16 | Cont'd.

Pain Screen for Use with Older Patients Unable to Self-Report

1. Patient self–report: Unable:_____   Occasionally:_____   Inconsistent:_____

2. Conditions/diagnoses painful: _____

3. Pain Behavior Scale (select one scale)

    PACSLAC (Pain Assessment Checklist for Seniors with Limited Ability to Communicate)

    PAINAD (Pain Assessment IN Advanced Dementia)

	Breathing _____
Facial Expressions _____	Negative Vocalization _____
Activity/Body Movement _____	Facial Expression _____
Social/Personality Mood _____	Body Language _____
Other _____	Consolability _____
Total Checklist Score _____	**Total Checklist Score** _____

4. Other behaviors indicative of pain: _____

    _____

    _____

5. Family (caregiver) assessment: 0 to 10 and why: _____

    _____

    _____

6. Assessment: ❑ Assume Pain Present   ❑ Assume Pain Absent   ❑ Unable to Determine

Form 3-17 | This form coordinates information that may be used in the initial assessment of pain in patients who are unable to provide self-report. Both the PACSLAC and the PAINAD are included in the flow sheet because they are both good options for monitoring pain behavior changes depending on patients' circumstances. The PACSLAC may be used on a less frequent basis as a comprehensive screen for potential pain indicators, whereas the PAINAD may be used on a regular basis for patients with observable pain behaviors and the need for frequent reassessment.

From Pasero, C., & McCaffery, M. (2011). *Pain assessment and pharmacologic management*, p. 137, St. Louis, Mosby. May be duplicated for use in clinical practice.

Pain Screen for Use with Older Patients Unable to Self-Report: Patient Example

1. Patient self–report: Unable:__X__   Occasionally:_____   Inconsistent:_____

   Other:_____

2. Conditions/diagnoses painful: _post-stroke neuropathy, history of osteoarthritic and chronic low back pain,_
   immobile, skin tear over left hip _____

3. Behavior Scale (select one scale)

PACSLAC (Pain Assessment Checklist for Seniors with Limited Ability to Communicate)		**PAINAD** (Pain Assessment IN Advanced Dementia)	
		Breathing	_____1_____
Facial Expressions	_____	Negative Vocalization	_____1_____
Activity/Body Movement	_____	Facial Expression	_____2_____
Social/Personality Mood	_____	Body Language	_____2_____
Other	_____	Consolability	_____0_____
Total Checklist Score	_____	**Total Checklist Score**	_____6_____

4. Other behaviors indicative of pain: _Ongoing pain suggested by lack of movement, resists getting out of bed._
   With dressing change pt. groans, frowns and attempts to pull leg away. Resist nurse attempting ROM and
   turning _____

5. Family (caregiver) assessment: 0 to 10 and why: _Wife states patient appears to have moderate pain, rates_
   as a 5 out of 10. She observed dressing change and believed pain was 7 during procedure

6. Assessment: ☒ Assume Pain Present   ❏ Assume Pain Absent   ❏ Unable to Determine

Form 3-18 | The patient described above is in a long-term care facility. He is 78 years old and has been nonverbal since a cerebrovascular accident 6 months ago. He does not appear to be oriented to his environment, but he seems to recognize his wife, who visits several times a week. The PAINAD was used for this patient because he presents with observable behaviors indicative of pain and requires regular reassessment. The score of 6 (out of 10) on the PAINAD and the specific behaviors noted by the nurse and the family's reports of pain severity strongly support the conclusion that pain is present in this patient unable to self-report.

From Pasero, C., & McCaffery, M. (2011). *Pain assessment and pharmacologic management*, p. 138, St. Louis, Mosby. May be duplicated for use in clinical practice.

Flow Sheet: Ongoing Pain Assessment in the Absence of Self-Report

Patient:_____ Date:_____

Analgesics:_____

Behavior Tool Used: ❑ PACSLAC   ❑ PAINAD

Time	Behavior Tool Score	Comments	Analgesics	Plan

Form 3-19 | Ongoing pain assessment in the absence of a self-report. This form is used after completion of the Pain Screen, Forms 3-17 and 3-18.

Flow Sheet: Ongoing Pain Assessment in the Absence of Self-Report: Patient Example

Patient: John Smith   Date:

Analgesics: *acetaminophen 1000mg q 6 hr PRN; hydrocodone 2.5 mg po 1-2 PRN 1 h prior to*

dressing change

Behavior Tool Used: ☐ PACSLAC   ☒ PAINAD

Time	Behavior Tool Score	Comments	Analgesics	Plan
0800	PAINAD=7	Resisting care, hitting at nurses	Acetaminophen 1000 mg	
0900	PAINAD=4	Allowing nurses to do AM care		Continue acetaminophen q 6 h ATC
1300	PAINAD=6		Hydrocodone 2.5 mg PO	
1400	PAINAD=2	Dressing change completed without resistance, combat		Continue current plan with premedication before dressings

Form 3-20 | This form shows observation of Mr. Smith using the PAINAD. His scores suggest a high level of pain along with aggressive behavior. Treatment is initiated, and reassessment shows improvement in his pain behavior score. A low-dose opioid is added to his regimen for use prior to dressing changes, and his pain behavior score, based on the PAINAD, suggests effective pain management with current treatment plan.

ATC, Around the clock.
From Pasero, C., & McCaffery, M. *Pain assessment and pharmacologic management,* p. 140, St. Louis, Mosby. © 2011, Pasero C, McCaffery M. May be duplicated for use in clinical practice.

use of the ABBEY with palliative care patients found that the staff perceived the tool to be helpful in judging pain (van Iersel, Timmerman, Mullie, 2006), facial expressions, vocalizations, and body language were identified as being the best and easiest pain indicators to observe. Information about the tool's reliability and validity is limited, and tool revision and additional testing in well-designed studies are recommended.

The Doloplus 2 (Lefebvre-Chapiro, 2001; http:// www.doloplus.com) is a French tool developed for the multidimensional assessment of pain in nonverbal older adults. It has been translated into several languages, including English, although none of the studies available were conducted using the English-translated tool. The Doloplus 2 is a comprehensive tool based on behavior change that addresses many key indicators noted in the literature and in the AGS persistent pain guidelines and that includes three subscales with 10 items focusing on somatic reactions, psychomotor reactions, and psychosocial reactions. The items are rated according to increasing severity of pain, and the result is a total score that ranges from 0 to 30, with 5 being identified as the threshold for pain. Justification of the cutoff score is not available in the English literature. Recent studies conducted in French, Norwegian, and Dutch samples have been published in English and provide strong support of the tool's reliability, validity, and clinical utility (Holen, Saltvedt, Fayers, et al., 2005; Pautex, Herrmann, Michon, et al., 2007; Pautex, Michon, Guedira, et al., 2006; Zwakhalen, Hamers, Berger, 2006). Translation issues are evident, and further study or description regarding the use of Doloplus 2 in English-speaking populations is needed.

Elderly Pain Caring Assessment 2 (EPCA-2) (Morello, Jean, Alix, et al., 2007) was developed by a team of French physicians in long-term care facilities to evaluate both persistent and acute pain in non-verbal older adults. The tool relies on caregiver familiarity with a patient to report changes in behavior. The tool has eight items that comprise five of the six categories of nonverbal pain behaviors noted in the AGS persistent pain guidelines. The items are observed prior to and during caregiving; the time needed for observation and completion of the tool is 15 minutes. The hierarchy of pain behaviors according to pain intensity appears logical, but no conceptual basis for the ordering is offered. In other words, in the fifth subscale item ("Observations during caregiver intervention"), "restless" is rated lower than is "aggressive," and this seems a logical order. However, validation of the ordering of items in each subscale of the tool has not been provided.

Preliminary internal consistency and inter-rater reliabilities are moderate to strong. There was high convergent and discriminant validity and strong responsiveness to treatment. The tool requires training and time for proper administration and has not been validated in English-speaking samples, limiting its clinical utility in the United States.

The **CNA Pain Assessment Tool (CPAT)** (Cervo, Raggi, Bright-Long, et al., 2007) is an informant-based assessment tool for use by certified nursing assistants (CNAs) for the assessment of pain in patients who have been diagnosed with severe dementia. The tool uses 12 items and collapses them into 5 categories, including 3 of the 6 categories of pain indicators consistent with AGS pain guidelines: facial expressions, body movements, and verbalizations. The tool requires approximately 1 minute to administer, with an uncomplicated forced choice numeric scoring of 0 to 5 and a score of 1 or greater requiring further action by the CNAs. Initial validity was established comparing ratings between patients with and without pain.

Subsequent evaluation of the CPAT (Cervo, Bruckenthal, Chen, et al., 2009; Cervo, Raggi, Bright-Long, et al., 2007) noted acceptable levels of both interrater reliability and test-retest reliability. Construct validity was established comparing ratings before and after a known painful or uncomfortable event and criterion validity established by comparing to another established pain scale, the DS-DAT. Based on a practicality survey, the CPAT was shown to be clinically useful and feasible. The CPAT requires further evaluation of ability to measure severity of pain and response to treatment.

The **Mobilization-Observation-Behavior-Intensity-Dementia Pain Scale (MOBID)** (Cervo, Raggi, Bright-Long, et al., 2007; Husebo, Strand, Moe-Nilssen, et al., 2007) is a nurse-administered instrument used to observe pain behaviors and infer pain intensity at rest and with standardized guided activity. It is intended for use with patients who have severe cognitive impairment and chronic musculoskeletal pain and are living in long-term care settings. A patient is guided through five structured activities (mobilization of both hands, both arms, and both legs; turning in bed; sitting at bedside) and the presence and intensity of pain are rated by nurses on an 11-point NRS for sounds, facial expressions, and defense, with increased behaviors indicating increased pain (e.g., combative behaviors when moved). The tool does not include subtle cues or changes in behavior and may limit recognition of pain in those presenting atypically. The MOBID has good internal consistency. There was a wide range of inter-rater reliability for the presence of pain behaviors, but reliability was better for pain intensity. The MOBID was able to detect increased pain with movement, and there was a linear trend among external raters toward more pain behaviors being associated with higher pain intensity. Recent follow-up evaluation supports reliability of MOBID scoring during video evaluation of behaviors in older persons with severe dementia (Huesebo, Strand, Moe-Nilssen, et al., 2009). More evidence is needed to support the validity of the tool for both the presence of pain behaviors and inferred pain intensity.

The **Non-Communicative Patient's Pain Assessment Instrument (NOPPAIN)** (Snow, Weber, O'Malley, et al., 2004) is an instrument that focuses on nursing assistants' (nursing technicians') observations and assessments of pain in patients with dementia at rest and with movement. Nursing assistants observe for pain-related behaviors as they perform common caregiving tasks. The NOPPAIN contains common pain behaviors, not subtle cues or changes in behavior. Because the NOPPAIN is based on proxy reports of pain intensity, evidence is needed to support the validity of the judgments of intensity of pain behaviors as indicators of pain severity. Preliminary support for the tool's reliability and validity was reported based on responses to video simulations, rather than on actual observation of patients. One follow-up study provides support for the convergent validity of proxy reports by means of detailed behavioral coding in patient videos (Horgas, Nichols, Schapson, et al., 2007). The tool's reliability and validity have been established by means of video coding by nursing assistants and patient videos scored by nursing students in a laboratory setting. Although ease of administration by nursing assistants is a strength of the tool, evaluation of nursing assistants' abilities to use the scale in actual patient care situations is needed.

Pain Assessment in Noncommunicative Elderly Persons (PAINE) (Cohen-Mansfield, 2006) is an informant-based assessment tool developed to assess pain in noncommunicative elders. The tool includes a comprehensive list of 22 behaviors representing 4 of the 6 pain behavior categories consistent with the AGS persistent pain guidelines. The tool has been administered only by research assistants and has not been studied for feasibility in the clinical setting. No information about the time or skill level needed to complete the PAINE is reported. Preliminary evaluation suggests good internal consistency and good inter-rater reliability, even among staff members who have varying familiarity with patients. Although procedures are unclear and difficult to follow, it appears that the PAINE has construct validity and

good correlation with other tools testing responsiveness to intervention (Cohen-Mansfield, Lipson, 2008). However, PAINE is weakly correlated with other observational and self-report assessment tools. Further evaluation of reliability and validity when used by nursing assistants directly is needed.

Two newer instruments that warrant consideration are the Rotterdam Elderly Pain Observation Scale (REPOS) (van Herk, van Dijk, Tibboel, et al., 2009) and the Mahoney Pain Scale (Mahoney, Peters, 2008). These tools were not available to include in the critical review completed in 2008 on the City of Hope Pain Resource Center website and discussed in this chapter. However, the reader is encouraged to access the most recent information when reviewing possible tools for consideration.

Conclusion

Clinicians should carefully review the tools in light of the particular population and setting so as to determine which tools are good matches. As noted earlier, considerable ongoing research has the goals of revising existing tools so as to maximize their reliability, validity, and clinical usefulness; providing additional information about tools' psychometrics; and developing new approaches to pain assessment in this vulnerable population. Readers should monitor the literature for updates on progress in this area.

A pain policy that addresses comprehensive and appropriate assessment of pain in all patients must include procedures for identifying and monitoring pain in older persons who are cognitively impaired or nonverbal. The process should be comprehensive and should incorporate procedures that address the issues discussed here.

Chapter 4 Other Challenges in Pain Assessment

SOME patients with pain are simply incapable of providing self-reports of pain. They may be cognitively impaired or unconscious. Such circumstances necessitate using other, less reliable indicators of pain, always being mindful that in the absence of self-reports all else is an educated guess.

This group includes patients who have a wide range of communication difficulties, from those who are conscious but unable to speak to those who are unconscious and, of course, unable to speak. Examples are adults who have cognitive impairment, as discussed in the previous chapter; who have severe emotional disturbances; who are intubated; who are developmentally delayed; who speak a language other than English; or whose educational or cultural backgrounds are significantly different from those of the health care team (APS, 2003). Such patients pose assessment challenges and are at risk for undertreatment.

Patients who are critically ill, intellectually disabled, mentally ill, or unconscious are discussed in this chapter. Cultural considerations are also included.

Patients Who Are Critically Ill

Some critically ill patients are mistakenly believed to be unconscious or pain-free, but pain in critically ill patients has been well documented for some time. For example, patients with endotracheal tubes and those who have received neuromuscular blocking agents such as pancuronium (which does not alter sensitivity to pain) may be fairly alert, and some are fully capable of feeling pain and are able to self-report pain if given the appropriate opportunity. In a sample of 24 patients in an intensive care unit (ICU), interviews after transfer from the ICU revealed that all but 1 patient recalled their ICU stays, and 63% recalled moderate to severe pain (Puntillo, 1990). The patients described pain caused by surgical incisions, movement, coughing, endotracheal suctioning, and chest tube removal. Those who could not talk (80% had endotracheal tubes) described numerous behaviors they used in attempts to tell staff they were in pain, such as signaling with their eyes and moving their legs up and down. These patients are actually capable of giving self-reports of pain. Some can use writing materials and can be taught to use a pain rating scale. Some can use the call button, which should be placed within easy reach. Others can be asked questions and be taught to signal with their eyes that pain is present. For example, the clinician can establish with the patient that when asked about pain, squeezing the eyes once means *yes* and twice means *no*.

Clinicians are prone to overlook pain at rest as well as pain resulting from common procedures such as turning and suctioning. In a study of 30 critically ill, traumatically injured patients, pain was measured at rest in a supine position and after being turned onto their sides (Stanik-Hutt, Soeken, Belcher, 2001). On a visual analog scale (VAS) (0 to 100 mm), mean at-rest scores were 34.5, which indicates mild pain bordering on moderate pain. Immediately after the turns, the mean scores were 48.1 on the VAS, indicating moderate pain. Terms commonly used to describe pain at rest included throbbing, sharp, sore, hurting, and annoying. After turning, the pain was often described with the same words used for pain at rest (except for hurting) plus pressing, pulling, tender, tiring, and miserable. Of these patients, 13 were not included in the study because they refused to be turned, giving as the reason severe pain at rest or anticipated pain with turning. Their pain at rest was 47.1 on the VAS. Based on their review of the literature, the researchers concluded that pain intensity at rest in this study was in the same range as that in other studies of critically ill patients.

Endotracheal suctioning also causes considerable pain. In a study of 45 adults having cardiovascular (CV) surgery, patients rated their pain during endotracheal suctioning on a 0-to-10 scale (Puntillo, 1994). The mean pain intensity score was 4.5, and more than one third of the patients reported a pain intensity of 7 or greater, indicating severe pain. Patients described the pain as tiring-exhausting, stabbing, tender, sharp, and heavy.

The results of the Thunder Project II, a multisite study, provide extensive information about procedural pain in acute and critically ill patients (Puntillo, White, Morris, et al., 2001). In a total of 153 clinical sites, information was collected from 6201 patients, 5957 of whom were 18 years or older. Patients were alert and able to answer questions. Data were obtained about pain related to six procedures: turning, wound drain removal, tracheal suctioning, femoral catheter removal, placement of a central venous catheter, and nonburn-wound dressing change. Adults rated their procedural pain intensity as 2.65 to 4.93 on a 0-to-10 numerical rating scale (NRS). The most painful and distressing procedure for adults was turning; the mean pain intensity was 4.93 and the mean distress score was 3.47 on a scale of 0 to 10. After turning, the most painful procedures in adults, in descending order, with mean pain intensity in parentheses, were wound drain removal (4.67); wound care (4.42); tracheal suctioning (3.94); central line placement (2.72); and femoral sheath removal (2.65). Pain at rest was usually described as aching, and procedural pain was often described as sharp.

Thus, critically ill patients experience mild to moderate pain throughout the day. At rest, the pain is commonly mild, but turning, which usually occurs at least every 2 hours, is associated with moderate pain and, compared to other painful procedures, is the most distressing.

In a follow-up to the study just described, Puntillo, Wild, Morris, and others (2002) examined analgesic and local anesthetic administration in the 5957 adults they assessed prior to and during the six procedures. Undertreatment of procedural pain was apparent. More than 63% of the patients received no analgesics before or during the procedures, and less than 20% received opioids. The patients most likely to receive opioids were those undergoing femoral sheath removal (28.6%), and those least likely to were undergoing tracheal suctioning (3.7%). A total of 18.4% of patients received local anesthetics, and 89.5% of them were undergoing placement of a central venous catheter. Part of this undertreatment may be the result of failure to assess pain or anticipate pain. All of these patients were alert, and pain could have been assessed at least during the procedure or prior to the procedure for those who had already experienced the procedure, such as turning or tracheal suctioning.

Further analysis of data available from the previously mentioned study of 5957 critically ill adults revealed information about behavioral responses associated with the six procedures being studied (Puntillo, Morris, Thompson,

et al., 2004). All the patients in this study were alert and able to self-report, but many critical care patients are unable to provide self-reports of pain because of intubation, motor impairments, cultural or language barriers, or altered levels of consciousness. Behavioral responses to pain may then become one of the most valuable contributions to pain assessment. A 30-item behavioral tool was used to observe patients' behaviors before and during the procedures. Significantly more behaviors were exhibited by patients with procedural pain than by those without that pain. Behaviors specific to procedural pain were grimacing, rigidity, wincing, shutting of eyes, verbalizations, moaning, and clenching of fists.

The FLACC (Face, Legs, Activity, Cry, Consolability) Behavioral Scale has recently been studied in 29 critically ill adults and children who could not self-report pain (Voepel-Lewis, Zanotti, Dammeyer, 2010). This is the first study to provide support of the FLACC in this population, but further study is warranted.

Several behavioral scales for use with adult patients in critical care and unable to self-report are being developed, and the psychometric properties of six of these scales have been compared (Li, Puntillo, Miaskowski, 2008). They are listed here with references that include the actual tool:

- The Behavioral Pain Rating Scale (BPRS) (Mateo, Krenzischek, 1992)
- The Behavioral Pain Scale (BPS) (Payen, Bru, Bosson, et al., 2001)
- Pain Behavior Assessment Tool (PBAT) (Puntillo, Morris, Thompson, et al., 2004)
- Critical-Care Pain Observation Tool (CPOT) (Gelinas, Fillion, Puntillo, et al., 2006)
- Pain Assessment and Intervention Notation (PAIN Algorithm) (Puntillo, Miaskowski, Kehrie, et al., 1997)
- Nonverbal Pain Scale (NVPS) (Odhner, Wegman, Freeland, et al., 2003).

Review of these assessment tools revealed that none had undergone vigorous validation or had been accepted as standardized measures, but two showed good evidence of validity and reliability—the BPS and the CPOT (Li, Puntillo, Miaskowski, 2008). Both are described here, and both are easy to use. However, we feel that the CPOT is a slightly better choice for clinical practice because it includes four behavioral domains instead of the three that are in the BPS, and because the CPOT divides the domain of patients on ventilators into two groups, patients who are intubated and patients who are not; whereas the BPS addresses only ventilated patients. Therefore, the actual tool for the CPOT is included (Form 4-1).

The CPOT evaluates four behavioral domains: facial expressions, movements, muscle tension, and ventilator compliance (Gelinas, Fillion, Puntillo, et al., 2006) . Each domain has three behaviors, which are scored from 0 to 2.

The Critical-Care Pain Observation Tool (CPOT)

Indicator	Score		Description
Facial expression	Relaxed, neutral	0	No muscle tension observed
Relaxed, neutral 0 Tender 1 Grimacing 2	Tense	1	Presence of frowning, brow lowering, orbit tightening and levator contraction, or any other change (e.g., opening eyes or tearing during nociceptive procedures)
	Grimacing	2	All previous facial movements plus eyelid tightly closed (the patient may present with mouth open or biting the endotracheal tube)
Body movements[1]	Absence of movements or normal position	0	Does not move at all (doesn't necessarily mean absence of pain) or normal position (movements not aimed toward the pain site or not made for the purpose of protection)
	Protection	1	Slow, cautious movements, touching or rubbing the pain site, seeking attention through movements
	Restlessness	2	Pulling tube, attempting to sit up, moving limbs/thrashing, not following commands, striking at staff, trying to climb out of bed
Compliance with the ventilator (intubated patients)[2]	Tolerating ventilator or movement	0	Alarms not activated, easy ventilation
	Coughing but tolerating	1	Coughing, alarms may be activated but stop spontaneously
	Fighting ventilator	2	Asynchrony: blocking ventilation, alarms frequently activated
OR			
Vocalization (extubated patients)[3]	Talking in normal tone or no sound	0	Talking in normal tone or no sound
	Sighing, moaning	1	Sighing, moaning
	Crying out, sobbing	2	Crying out, sobbing
Muscle tension	Relaxed	0	No resistance to passive movements
Evaluation by passive flexion and extension of upper limbs when patient is at rest[4] or evaluation when patient is being turned	Tense, rigid	1	Resistance to passive movements
	Very tense or rigid	2	Strong resistance to passive movements, incapacity to complete them
TOTAL	___ /8		

Form 4-1

Continued

As appears in Pasero, C., & McCaffery, M. (2011). *Pain assessment and pharmacologic management*, p. 145, St. Louis, Mosby. Instructions © 2011, Gélinas C. Form modified from Gélinas, C., Fillion, L., Puntillo, K. A., et al. (2006). Validation of the Critical-Care Pain Observation Tool (CPOT) in adult patients. *Am J Crit Care*, 15(4), 420-427.

[1]Puntillo, K. A., Miaskowski, C., Kehrle, K., et al. (1997). Relationship between behavioral and physiological indicators of pain, critical care self-reports of pain, and opioid administration. *Crit Care Med*, 25(7), 1159-1166; [2]Devlin, J. W., Boleski, G., Mlynarek, M., et al. (1999). Motor activity assessment scale: A valid and reliable sedation scale for use with mechanically ventilated patients in an adult surgical intensive care unit. *Crit Care Med*, 27(7), 1271-1275; [3]Harris, C. E., O'Donnell, C. MacMillan, R. R., et al. (1991). Use of propofol by infusion for sedation of patients undergoing haemofiltration: Assessment of the effect of haemofiltration on the level of sedation and on blood propofol concentration. *J. Drug Dev, 4*(Suppl 3), 37-39; [4]Payen, J. F., Bru, O., Bosson, J. L., et al. (2001), Assessing pain in the critically ill sedated patients by using a behavioral pain scale. *Crit Care Med, 29*(12), 2258-2263; [5]Mateo, O. M., Krenzischek, D. A. (1992). A pilot study to assess the relationship between behavioral manifestations and self-report of pain in postanesthesia care unit patients. *J Post Anes Nurs, 7*(1), 15-21; [6]Ambuel, B., Hamlett, K. W., Marx, C. M., et al. (1992). Assessing distress in pediatric intensive care environments: The COMFORT scale. *J Pediat Pscych, 17*(1), 95-109.

Directions for Use of the CPOT

1. The patient must be observed at rest for one minute to obtain a baseline value of the CPOT.
2. Then, the patient should be observed during nociceptive procedures (e.g., turning, endotracheal suctioning, wound dressing) to detect any changes in the patient's behaviors to pain.
3. The patient should be evaluated before and at the peak effect of an analgesic agent to assess if the treatment was effective in relieving pain.
4. For the rating of the CPOT, the patient should be attributed the highest score observed during the observation period.
5. The patient should be attributed a score for each behavior included in the CPOT and muscle tension should be evaluated the last, especially when the patient is at rest because just the stimulation of touch (passive flexion and extension of the arm) may lead to behavioral reactions.

CPOT — Facial Expressions

0	1*	2
Relaxed, neutral	**Tense**	**Grimacing**
(no muscle tension)	(frowning, brow lowering, orbit tightening, little levator contraction)	(contraction of the whole face: frowning, brow lowering, eyes tightly closed, levator contraction – mouth may be opened or the patient may be biting the endotracheal tube)

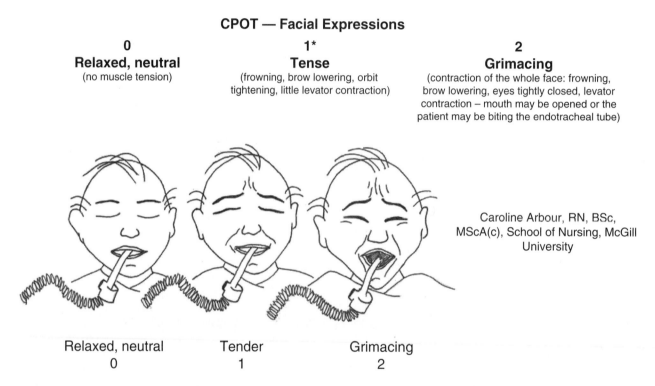

Caroline Arbour, RN, BSc, MScA(c), School of Nursing, McGill University

Relaxed, neutral	Tender	Grimacing
0	1	2

A score of 1 may be attributed when a change in the patient's facial expression is observed compared with rest assessment (e.g., open eyes, tearing).

Form 4-1 | Cont'd.

The critical review of assessment tools used with seriously ill patients points out that a weakness of the CPOT is that generally low scores were reported in all patients during painful procedures (Li, Puntillo, Miaskowski, 2008). This should be kept in mind when using the tool, and clinicians should remember that pain behaviors are merely indicators of pain and that the number of behaviors do not equate with pain intensity (Pasero, McCaffery, 2005).

The sensitivity and specificity of the CPOT was studied in a sample of 105 adults in an ICU following cardiac surgery (Gelinas, Harel, Fillion, et al., 2009). Pain was evaluated during the painful procedure of turning. Sensitivity was high during turning, meaning that the tool could detect when pain was not present. The specificity of the CPOT was also high; that is, it correctly identified the patients who did have pain. This reduces the likelihood of administering an analgesic to a patient who does not have pain.

The BPS consists of three behavioral domains: facial expression, movements of upper limbs, and compliance with ventilation. Each domain contains four behaviors, each rated from 1 to 4 (Payen, Bru, Bosson, et al., 2001). In the critical review of assessment tools used with critically ill patients, the point is made that the observation of no body movement is equated with a pain-free state in the BPS (Li, Puntillo, Miaskowski, 2008). However, no body movement may simply reflect sedation, restraints, or other restrictions of movement. Another criticism concerns the numbering system, which starts with 1, meaning no pain behavior. It is suggested that starting with 0 more readily reflects no pain behaviors.

The American Society for Pain Management Nursing (ASPMN) published a position statement on pain assessment in the nonverbal patient (available at http://www.aspmn.org/Organization/documents/NonverbalJournalFINAL.pdf) that includes a section about intubated and unconscious patients (Herr, Coyne, Key, et al., 2006). Recommendations for assessment utilize the template for the hierarchy of pain measures, as presented previously (see Box 3-9, p. 123):

- The hierarchy begins with an attempt to obtain a self-report. If that fails, the following indicators should be assessed, and one can assume pain is present (APP) if any of the measures indicates pain. Again, the abbreviation *APP* may be used for documentation if approved by institutional policy and procedure.
- Potential causes of pain, such as procedures or existing painful conditions, are next on the hierarchy. These should include noting that pain at rest can cause aching and that the following procedures have been found to be painful: turning (the most painful of this group), wound drain removal, tracheal suctioning, femoral catheter removal, placement of a central venous catheter, and nonburn wound dressing change.
- Following assessment for causes of pain, clinicians look for patient behaviors that may indicate pain. This is the point at which a behavioral pain assessment tool is used, and we recommend using the CPOT for critically ill patients.
- Next, reports of pain or observations of behaviors that might indicate pain are elicited, when possible, from people who know the patient well, such as caregivers and family members. They may know of previously existing painful conditions such as arthritis that have been causing pain.
- Finally, when in doubt about the presence of pain or when wanting to confirm the suspicion of pain, an analgesic trial may be helpful. The analgesic trial is used as the basis for developing the pain treatment plan once pain has been confirmed. (See Boxes 3-9 and 3-11, pp. 123 and 126, for more ideas about using the analgesic trial.)

Physiologic indicators of pain such as changes in blood pressure are omitted from the hierarchy of pain assessment techniques. Their limited usefulness in assessing pain is discussed in Chapter 2, pp. 27-28. They are occasionally helpful but, especially in critically ill patients, these measures are often influenced by factors other than pain, such as medications, mechanical ventilation, change in level of consciousness, and patients' illnesses or surgeries. In critically ill patients, behavioral indicators have been found to provide more valid information for pain assessment than physiologic indicators (Arbour, Gelinas, 2009; Gelinas, Arbour, 2009; Gelinas, Johnston, 2007).

For example, a study of 254 critically ill patients in intensive care units who were mechanically ventilated (144 conscious and 114 unconscious) examined potential behavioral and physiologic indicators of pain and their association with self-reports of pain (Gelinas, Arbour, 2009). These patients were observed at rest, during a nociceptive procedure (such as endotracheal suctioning), and 20 minutes postprocedure. Behaviors were measured with the CPOT, and physiologic indicators were obtained from the available monitoring. Patients able to self-report pain were asked if they had pain or not immediately after being scored with the CPOT. This prevented bias in the raters because the CPOT was used before requesting a self-report. Based on the patient's self-report, only the CPOT score, not changes in vital signs, could predict the presence or absence of pain; consequently, only behavioral observation was recommended for pain assessment in unconscious patients. The researchers noted that changes in vital signs could be used as a cue to begin further assessment of pain.

Probably because the physiologic changes are so readily able to be observed in the ICU, critical care nurses are tempted to use them as indicators of pain, especially in patients who are unable to self-report. However, as mentioned above, many patients actually are able to self-report pain if the right approaches are used, such as eye blinking and the CPOT. Research strongly recommends use of behaviors to assess pain in unconscious patients and warns that vital signs should be used with caution (Gelinas, Arbour, 2009).

Patients Who Are Unconscious

Some critically ill patients appear to be unconscious due to injury such as brain trauma or disease, sedating medications, or neuromuscular blocking agents. But unconscious patients also exist outside the critical care setting. For example, patients in vegetative states may be found in long-term care facilities. Terminally ill patients may become unconscious as death approaches.

If *unconsciousness* is defined as no awareness of self or environment, how is it possible that an unconscious patient could feel pain and suffer from it? The problem is that unconsciousness is not easily determined, and there are varying levels of unconsciousness. A minimally conscious state is described as one in which there is some evidence of awareness of self and environment, and a persistent vegetative state is defined as wakefulness without awareness of self or environment (Boly, Faymonville, Schnakers, et al., 2008). Anecdotal evidence and some research strongly suggest that quite a few patients who appear to be unconscious and unresponsive to painful stimuli actually feel and recall pain. Thus, clinicians should assume that the unconscious patient may feel pain and should provide analgesia if anything known to be painful is present.

In a study of 100 critically ill patients whose records indicated that they were unconscious, interviews with the patients revealed that only about one quarter of them were actually unaware of themselves and their surroundings (Lawrence, 1995). The remaining three quarters had some awareness of themselves and their environments, and about 25% were able to hear and to feel pain.

During general anesthesia, some patients experience periods of awareness that they recall postoperatively. In a study of 26 patients who had experienced awareness during general anesthesia, hearing sounds and feeling paralyzed were reported by 89% and 85%, respectively (Moerman, Bonke, Oosting, 1993). Of those patients, 10% reported feeling pain. Aftereffects such as sleep disturbances, nightmares, and flashbacks occurred in 70%, and pain was recalled by one half of these patients. In another study of 45 patients who experienced awareness during general anesthesia, 8 patients reported feeling severe pain (Schwender, Kunze-Kronawitter, Dietrich, et al., 1998). A large study of 3921 patients undergoing general anesthesia identified an incidence of 1% (39 patients) who experienced awareness with recall (Errando, Sigl, Robles, et al., 2008). Pain was felt by 11 patients.

An anecdotal report illustrates the tragedy of assuming an unconscious patient does not feel pain. A terminally ill patient was receiving intravenous morphine for cancer-related pain; as her disease progressed, she gradually became unresponsive to voices and no longer grimaced during position changes, which previously had been painful for her. Because she appeared to be unconscious and unresponsive to painful stimuli, morphine was no longer administered. After 3 days the patient regained consciousness and immediately asked for morphine. The patient reported that during the apparent "coma," she had heard voices and felt intense pain (Stephens, 1994).

Regarding pain in terminally ill patients who appear to be unconscious, a recommendation made almost 3 decades ago is worth repeating: "When patients are no longer able to verbally communicate whether they are in pain or not, the best approach is to assume that their cancer is still painful and to continue them on their regular medications…. a therapeutic narcotic level should be maintained…. continued narcotics simply ensure that the death will be as peaceful and painless as possible" (Levy, 1985, pp. 397-398).

Whether patients in persistent vegetative states feel pain remains controversial. This state is defined as complete unawareness of self and environment, including lack of the cortical capacity to feel pain. However, some have voiced reservations about assuming that patients in vegetative states do not feel pain and have suggested that, until it can be proved otherwise, clinicians should assume that such patients feel pain and should treat that pain (Bushnell, 1997; Klein, 1997).

This position is also advocated by researchers who studied brain activation during noxious stimulation consisting of electrical stimulation of the median nerve, comparing 5 patients in minimally conscious states, 15 normal controls, and 15 patients in persistent vegetative states (Boly, Faymonville, Schnakers, et al., 2008). No brain area was less activated in patients in minimally conscious states than in the controls. All areas of the cortical pain matrix showed greater activation in these patients than in patients in persistent vegetative states. The researchers concluded that this evidence confirmed the need for analgesic treatment for patients in minimally conscious states. They pointed out, however, that misdiagnosis of patients in persistent vegetative states and minimally conscious states is common and concluded that analgesic treatment is indicated in both groups. Analgesics for patients in persistent vegetative states are indicated also to prevent potentially damaging defensive hormonal reactions such as the production of adrenal stress hormones, despite the possible absence of feelings of pain.

For some unconscious patients the CPOT, discussed earlier (see Form 4-1, pp. 145-146), may be appropriate if they are capable of responding in the four behavioral domains: facial expressions, movements, muscle tension, and ventilator compliance (Gelinas, Fillion, Puntillo, et al., 2006). If these behaviors are absent, documenting procedures or pathologies that probably cause pain may be relied upon to assume pain is present (APP), as is suggested in Box 3-9 (p. 123). A behavioral tool is appropriate only with patients who are able to respond with the tool's requisite behaviors.

Clinicians often wonder which dose of opioid to administer on an ongoing basis to a patient who cannot respond with any behaviors to indicate the effectiveness of a dose one way or another. In such cases, opioid therapy should be initiated and maintained at the recommended starting dose (e.g., 2.5 mg/hr morphine IV for adults in possibly severe pain). However, clinicians should not hesitate to increase doses if there are any behaviors whatsoever that might indicate pain (see Chapter 27 for more about analgesic administration in the ICU).

Patients Who Are Intellectually Disabled

The term *developmental disabilities* encompasses mental or physical disabilities that are evident in childhood and continue throughout life (Craig, 2006). Intellectual disability (ID), as defined for this chapter, is a type of developmental disability in which some form of intellectual disability or cognitive impairment is noted in childhood. The ID may or may not be accompanied by physical disability. Conversely, physical disabilities such as cerebral palsy are not always accompanied by mental disabilities.

IDs are commonly defined by IQ scores. An IQ score of 50 to 70 indicates mild cognitive impairment, a score of 35 to 49 indicates moderate impairment, a score of 20 to 34 indicates severe impairment, and profound impairment is an IQ score below 20 (Bottos, Chambers, 2006; Grossman, 1983). Individuals with mild cognitive impairment make up 85% of those with IDs and usually acquire about a sixth grade level of academic skills (American Psychiatric Association [APA], 1994). Moderate cognitive impairment occurs in about 10% of cases of ID, and severe and profound impairment constitute 1% to 4% of cases of ID.

This chapter focuses on adults with IDs, that is, adults who have been cognitively impaired since birth or early childhood. This state is not to be confused with that of adults who have been cognitively intact for most of their lives but become cognitively impaired in their later years. Dementia is an example of a cognitive impairment that occurs late in life in individuals who were cognitively intact previously. The literature can be confusing because the publications that use the term *cognitive impairment* in their titles may be focusing on adults who have become impaired as they have grown older or on adults who have been cognitively impaired since childhood. Pain assessment strategies previously discussed in the section on cognitively impaired older patients probably are not useful in assessing pain in adults with mental retardation. Adults who have been cognitively impaired since childhood require assessment tools that have been specially designed for them because these individuals do not have the same understandings and experiences as adults who have been cognitively intact for many years and become cognitively impaired in later life.

Most of the research on pain and ID has been conducted in infants and children, but many of the issues raised in those studies, such as assessment, are regarded as being relevant to the care of adults with IDs (Symons, Shinde, Gilles, 2008). Consequently, some studies of children are reviewed here even though this book focuses on adults. Some pain assessment tools used with children with IDs have been adapted and studied in adults with IDs.

A long-standing misconception is that persons with IDs, or mental retardation, are insensitive or indifferent to pain (Symons, Shinde, Gilles, 2008). After reviewing several studies of children with IDs, Symons and others (2008) concluded that caregivers of children with IDs frequently underestimated pain intensity. Consequently, these individuals are undertreated. This conclusion appears to be based on observations of behavior, not measurements of sensitivity to pain. It is hypothesized that what may be confusing about behavioral observations of these patients is that behavioral indicators of pain may be delayed or unconventional, contributing to the belief that this population has a lowered sensitivity to pain or a greater tolerance. However, testing of patients with mild intellectual disabilities by measuring heat-pain

thresholds showed that their pain threshold was significantly lower than that of normal controls (Defrin, Pick, Peretz, et al., 2004). Thus, these individuals not only are sensitive to pain but also may be more sensitive to some types of pain than persons without IDs.

Along the same lines, children with autism have also been thought to be insensitive to pain, but this is not supported by research. In a study comparing 21 children with autism with 22 without autism, all of them undergoing venipuncture, the children with autism manifested significant facial reactions quite similar to those in the unimpaired group but characterized by more facial activity (Nader, Oberlander, Chambers, et al., 2004). A perplexing finding was that the children who were the most reactive during the venipuncture had been identified by the parents as being less sensitive and less reactive to pain.

Understanding the misconceptions of caregivers of children with disabilities may be helpful in recognizing the possibility that the same misconceptions may occur in reference to adults with IDs. The degree of agreement between parent and child regarding pain intensity was examined in 68 children with spina bifida who were able to communicate (Clancy, McGrath, Oddson, 2005). Children rated their pain, and their parents completed a proxy report of the pain. Parents tended to underestimate the intensity of the pain their children felt. In another study, 65 caregivers of children with IDs completed questionnaires about their beliefs regarding pain in this population and revealed complex beliefs (Breau, MacLaren, McGrath, et al., 2003). Caregivers believed that children's sensations of pain increased as the severity of the ID increased. They also believed that children with mild cognitive impairment might overreact to pain. Perhaps most alarming was the finding that the more caregivers had learned about ID, the more they believed that those with IDs experienced less pain than those without IDs. The authors suggested several reasons for this finding, including the possibility that the information that was being taught was inaccurate or misunderstood.

Educational materials for caregivers of individuals with IDs should be carefully examined. Caregivers may enter the learning situation already harboring misconceptions. If these are not addressed, they may persist. Underestimation of pain by caregivers of individuals with IDs may result in underreporting of pain to clinicians, leading to undertreatment.

In a literature review, Bottos and Chambers (2006) identified types of pain likely to occur in individuals with IDs. Pain in children with IDs, particularly cerebral palsy, includes gastrointestinal discomfort, such as gastroesophageal reflux and constipation, and musculoskeletal pain. Children with autism also tend to experience gastrointestinal disorders. Individuals with Down syndrome are prone to developing leukemia, hence experiencing all the usual pain associated with the disease, diagnostic tests, and treatment. They also tend to have hip abnormalities and oral health problems such as periodontal disease. In adults with severe to profound mental retardation, pain is more often chronic than acute. An extensive review of the literature about this population revealed that a significant percentage of these people experience significant intensities of pain on a daily basis (Bodfish, Harper, Deacon, et al., 2006).

A review of the literature found that in the adult population of individuals with cerebral palsy, as much as 84% reported one or more types of chronic pain; 56% experienced pain daily and 53% reported moderate to severe pain (Bottos, Chambers, 2006). In one study of 63 women with cerebral palsy, of the 53 who had pain, the most common sites were the head (28%), back (26%), and arms (23%) (Turk, Geremski, Rosenbaum, et al., 1997). Activities of daily living, such as assisted sitting, walking, stretching, toileting, and standing, are especially painful and common, being reported by 35% to 93% of individuals with cerebral palsy (Bottos, Chambers, 2006). Some of the musculoskeletal pain may worsen with aging. It is important to note that studies of the prevalence of pain in adults with cerebral palsy have usually been restricted to those with mild or no cognitive impairment, although those with greater cognitive impairment are not known to be less sensitive to pain or to have fewer types of pain. In fact, the prevalence of pain in children with IDs is higher than in healthy children, and children with greater cognitive impairment tend to experience the most intense and most frequent pain but are least able to communicate their pain (Bottos, Chambers, 2006). Thus, studies suggest that the prevalence of pain in adults with IDs is higher than in adults without IDs.

Assessment of individuals with IDs is extremely challenging and, although considerable research has gone into creating assessment tools for children with IDs, few studies have included adults with IDs. A large majority of adults with IDs achieve a sixth grade level of functioning, so many may be able to provide self-reports of pain, and others with greater cognitive impairment may also be able to self-report. The greatest challenge is the assessment of those without verbal ability. The following studies suggest what to look for as indicators of pain in adults with IDs who cannot self-report.

To identify differences in the pain indicators used by nurses to assess pain in children and adults with severe versus profound IDs, a questionnaire consisting of 158 possible indicators of pain was completed by 109 nurses (Zwakhalen, van Dongen, Hamers, et al., 2004). More than 50% of the nurses found the following seven indicators to be very important: moaning during manipulation, crying during manipulation, painful facial expression during manipulation, swelling, screaming during manipulation, not using the affected body part, and moving the body in "a specific way of behaving." Pain appeared to be assessed differently in those with severe versus profound IDs. Physiologic indicators, such as gasping for breath,

vomiting, and turning red in the face, were scored somewhat higher by the group of nurses specializing in individuals with profound IDs (N = 47). Nurses specializing in the care of persons with severe IDs (N = 42) gave the highest score to "unusual way of crying." Other indicators used by nurses specializing in the care of those with severe IDs included seeking comfort and being grouchy. (The remaining 53 nurses were taking care of both groups of patients.)

Interviews with eight nurses caring for patients with learning disabilities, who might be in pain but who could not communicate their feelings verbally, identified numerous behaviors they used as indicators of pain (Donovan, 2002). The ages of the patients were not given but some were probably adults because mention was made of nurses' developing close relationships with patients over a long period of time. Change in facial expression was the most frequently cited nonverbal behavior indicative of pain or distress. Crying was also mentioned frequently. Other behaviors the nurses thought were possible indicators of pain were pacing, out-stretched arms, self-harm such as picking at the skin, aggressive behaviors such as biting or kicking others, pallor, altered rates of breathing, wincing, clenching teeth, and changes in activities such as avoiding weight bearing. One nurse described a patient with limited verbal ability that used the word *arm* for pain in any part of the body. These nurses emphasized the importance of caring for patients over time so that changes in behavior could be noted. Because changes in usual daily activities are often mentioned as clues to the presence of pain, it is noteworthy that these nurses mentioned that the patients were often determined to carry out normal activities even when seriously injured.

In one study, 40 adults with IDs who were undergoing intramuscular injections were studied to identify the usefulness of facial expressions in detecting pain (LaChapelle, Hadjistavropoulos, Craig, 1999). Only 65% of the subjects were able to provide self-reports. Observing the intensity of facial expressions, specifically brow lowering and chin raising, proved to be useful for assessing pain in these adults. Further, the frequency and intensity of facial expressions did not vary with level of cognitive functioning. In other words, persons with levels of ID that prevented self-report of pain showed facial expressions similar to those shown by persons with less intellectual impairment, providing further evidence against pain insensitivity in persons with IDs.

Somewhat contrary to that study, which found that facial expression did not vary with level of cognitive functioning, another study of adults with IDs found that facial expressions differed in individuals with mild to moderate cognitive impairment compared to those with severe to profound ID (Defrin, Lotan, Pick, 2006). In a study of 159 adults with varying levels of mental retardation and a control group of 38 with normal cognition, behavior was observed before and during the painful stimulus of a vaccination. During the vaccination, facial expression increased in those with mild to moderate IDs and in those without impairment. However, in those with severe to profound impairment, 47% to 50% exhibited stillness, or a "freezing reaction" (face and body not moving for several seconds), suggesting that pain assessment tools based only on facial expressions might contribute to the misconception that these patients are insensitive to pain. An increase in cognitive impairment was associated with a significant increase in freezing. In a few patients, freezing was accompanied by a full-blown smile, and some laughed, reactions that could easily be misinterpreted as insensitivity to pain. Freezing was exhibited by only 8% to 13% of individuals with mild to moderate IDs.

One reason for the differing conclusions in the studies described may be related to the sizes of the samples. It is possible that the study of 40 adults (LaChapelle, Hadjistavropoulos, Craig, 1999) did not include a large enough sample to allow for the detection of differences in behavior among the levels of ID, whereas the study of 159 adults with IDs (Defrin, Lotan, Pick, 2006) did allow for such detection.

Two behavioral pain scales were used in the study of 159 adults with ID: the Non-Communicating Children's Pain Checklist-Revised (NCCPC-R) and the Facial Action Coding System (FACS) (Defrin, Lotan, Pick, 2006). The FACS is impractical to use in daily clinical practice because it involves coding video tapes. The NCCPC-R involves observing and rating behaviors (over a 2-hour period) and was found to be more sensitive to changes occurring in individuals at all levels of cognitive functioning, whereas the FACS was more sensitive to those with mild to moderate IDs. The NCCPC-R consists of 30 behaviors divided into seven categories: vocal, eating/sleeping, social, facial, activity, body/limb, and physiologic signs (Breau, McGrath, Camfield, et al., 2002). An observer scores the frequency of occurrence of the behaviors on a scale of 0 to 3: not at all, just a little, fairly often, and very often. The NCCPC-R was found to be reliable for measuring acute pain in adults with IDs.

One problem with the NCCPC-R is that it was validated by using a 2-hour observation period, which is impractical in many clinical settings. For that reason Breau, McGrath, and Zabalia (2006) recommend using the Non-Communicating Children's Pain Checklist-Postoperative Version (NCCPC-PV) over a 10-minute period when a 2-hour period is not feasible. Research using the NCCPC-PV in adults with IDs and acute pain is needed. A variety of versions of the NCCPC are currently being researched in various populations with IDs. So far, the NCCPC-R and the NCCPC-PV have the greatest support for use with children because of their psychometric properties.

Assessment of location of pain may be difficult, especially in those with Down syndrome. In a study involving cold stimuli applied to the wrists and the temples of 26 individuals with Down syndrome, all were able to express themselves verbally but had some difficulty locat-

ing the site of the cold stimuli (Hennequin, Morin, Feine, 2000). In a later study of parents' perceptions of pain in their children with Down syndrome (ages 1 to 39 years), the parents reported having greater difficulty in identifying locations of pain in their children with Down syndrome than in their children without Down syndrome (Hennequin, Faulks, Allison, 2003). Their abilities improved as the children grew older.

Two of the pain assessment tools that have been researched in adults with severe to profound mental retardation are the Pain and Discomfort Scale (PADS) (developed from the NCCPC-R) and the Pain Examination Procedure (PEP), and it is recommended that they be used together (Bodfish, Harper, Deacon, et al., 2006). These tools have acceptable levels of reliability and validity. The research into the development of these tools is extensive and is summarized in the chapter by Bodfish and others (2006) cited earlier. Studies indicate that the PADS is sensitive to nonverbal signs of pain in adults with severe IDs and is sensitive to everyday pain, acute pain responses, chronic pain, and effects of treatments to relieve pain. The authors found that administering the PADS plus the PEP takes trained personnel approximately 10 minutes. However, training for administering the PADS and PEP is extensive. A CD-ROM that includes a manual and workbook for the PADS and a DVD training video are available by calling 919-966-4896.

Other researchers disagree with the soundness of using the PADS in adults with IDs (Burkitt, Breau, Salsman, et al., 2009). They state that research to date is insufficient to support the general use of the PADS with adults with IDs. Indeed, further research is needed to identify pain assessment tools for this population. Meanwhile, the PADS plus the PEP may be a good alternative to using no tool at all.

Another potential tool, the Chronic Pain Scale for Nonverbal Adults with Intellectual Disabilities (CPS-NAID) (Form 4-2), is being researched (Burkitt, Breau, Salsman, et al., in press; reported in Breau, Burkett, 2009). This scale was arrived at by having two observers use the NCCPC-R to observe 16 nonverbal adults with IDs and chronic or recurrent pain conditions for a period of 5 minutes under conditions of pain and no pain. The observers also rated the pain using a VAS. Analyses indicated that six items should be removed from the NCCPC-R, resulting in a 24-item scale. This yielded 94% sensitivity to pain and 87% specificity for the presence of pain. These researchers concluded that the CPS-NAID has sound psychometric properties and can be used to assess chronic pain in adults with IDs. They think that this tool is superior to the original NCCPC-R, but further studies are needed to compare the two.

An attempt was made to establish cutoff points for pain on the basis of the total score of the CPS-NAID. However, it was based on proxy pain reports. As mentioned previously, in the section on behavioral scales for cognitively impaired adults, given current knowledge,

Chronic Pain Scale for Nonverbal Adults with Intellectual Disabilities (CPS-NAID)

Please indicate how often this person has shown the signs referred to in *items 1-24* in the <u>last 5 minutes</u>. Please circle a number for each item. If an item does not apply to this person (for example, this person cannot reach with his/her hands), then indicate "not applicable" for that item.

0	=	Not present at all during the observation period. (Note if the item is not present because the person is not capable of performing that act, it should be scored as "NA").
1	=	Seen or heard rarely (hardly at all), but is present.
2	=	Seen or heard a number of times, but not continuous (not all the time).
3	=	Seen or heard often, almost continuous (almost all the time); anyone would easily notice this if they saw the person for a few moments during the observation time.
NA	=	Not applicable. This person is not capable of performing this action.

0 = NOT AT ALL   1 = JUST A LITTLE   2 = FAIRLY OFTEN   3 = VERY OFTEN   NA = NOT APPLICABLE

1. Moaning, whining, whimpering (fairly soft)	0	1	2	3	NA
2. Crying (moderately loud)	0	1	2	3	NA
3. A specific sound or word for pain (e.g., a word, cry, or type of laugh)	0	1	2	3	NA
4. Not cooperating, cranky, irritable, unhappy	0	1	2	3	NA
5. Less interaction with others, withdrawn	0	1	2	3	NA
6. Seeking comfort or physical closeness	0	1	2	3	NA
7. Being difficult to distract, not able to satisfy or pacify	0	1	2	3	NA
8. A furrowed brow	0	1	2	3	NA
9. A change in eyes, including: squinching of eyes, eyes opened wide, eyes frowning	0	1	2	3	NA
10. Turning down of mouth, not smiling	0	1	2	3	NA
11. Lips puckering up, tight, pouting, or quivering	0	1	2	3	NA
12. Clenching or grinding teeth, chewing or thrusting tongue out	0	1	2	3	NA
13. Not moving, less active, quiet	0	1	2	3	NA
14. Stiff, spastic, tense, rigid	0	1	2	3	NA
15. Gesturing to or touching part of the body that hurts	0	1	2	3	NA
16. Protecting, favoring or guarding part of the body that hurts	0	1	2	3	NA
17. Flinching or moving the body part away, being sensitive to touch	0	1	2	3	NA
18. Moving the body in a specific way to show pain (e.g., head back, arms down, curls up, etc.)	0	1	2	3	NA
19. Shivering	0	1	2	3	NA
20. Change in color, pallor	0	1	2	3	NA
21. Sweating, perspiring	0	1	2	3	NA
22. Tears	0	1	2	3	NA
23. Sharp intake of breath, gasping	0	1	2	3	NA
24. Breath holding	0	1	2	3	NA

TOTAL SCORE: _____

SCORING:

1. Add up the scores for each item to compute the Total Score. Items marked "NA" are scored as "0" (zero).
2. Check whether the score is greater than the cut-off score.
   A score of <u>10 or greater</u> means that there is a 94% chance that the person <u>has pain</u>.
   A score of 9 or lower means that there is an 87% chance that the person does not have pain.

Form 4-2

As appears in Pasero, C., & McCaffery M. (2011). *Pain assessment and pharmacologic management*, p. 152, St. Louis, Mosby. From Burkitt, J. C., Breau, L. M., Salsman, S., et al. (2009). Pilot study of the feasibility of the non-communicating children's pain checklist revised for pain assessment for adults with intellectual disabilities. *J Pain Manage, 2*(1).

scores on behavioral pain scales do not equate with pain-intensity scores (Pasero, McCaffery, 2005). In most studies of pain assessment tools, there are low correlations between proxy judgments of pain severity and patients reports of severity. This raises concern about comparing pain-behavior scores with pain-intensity scores. If clinicians could reliably determine the intensity of pain in patients who cannot self-report, there would be no need for a behavioral assessment tool (Zwakhalen, Hamers, Abu-Saad, et al., 2006).

The hierarchy of pain assessment techniques (see Box 3-9, p. 123) is helpful in the assessment of patients with IDs. Following are the steps in that hierarchy, with comments related to assessing adults with IDs, starting with attempts to obtain self-reports.

- Try to obtain a self-report. A large majority of adults with IDs achieve a sixth grade level of academic skill and may be able to use some of the self-report scales mentioned in the section on self-report tools for adults who have difficulty with the commonly used tools such as the 0 to 10 NRS (pp. 92-95).
- Identify pathologic conditions and procedures that commonly cause pain, paying particular attention to those sources of pain characteristic of the type of ID. For example, individuals with cerebral palsy or autism often experience gastrointestinal discomfort such as gastroesophageal reflux. Individuals with Down syndrome are prone to developing leukemia, with all the usual pain associated with the disease and its treatment. Chronic pain is very common, one source being musculoskeletal pain in cerebral palsy.
- Observe behaviors indicative of pain. Changes in facial expression, especially brow lowering and chin raising, are probably the most frequently cited indicators of pain in persons with IDs, and they do not seem to vary with the level of cognitive functioning. Numerous other behaviors are cited in research into pain in adults with IDs. Some behaviors indicative of pain are unconventional, such as kicking others, picking at own skin, or freezing. Consider using the CPS-NAID (see Form 4-2) to assess chronic pain in adults with IDs.
- Physiologic indicators such as vital signs are not usually very helpful in assessing pain, but in the ID literature physiologic indicators often refer to the following behaviors, which may be helpful in assessing individuals with severe or profound IDs: gasping for breath, vomiting, and becoming red in the face.
- Obtaining information from caregivers who know the patient well, sometimes over a period of years, is a common way of assessing pain in individuals with IDs and is high on the hierarchy of pain assessment.
- Finally, when in doubt about the presence of pain or when wanting to confirm the suspicion of pain, an analgesic trial may be helpful. Assess for changes in behavior following use of an analgesic. (See Box 3-11, p. 126, for suggestions concerning analgesic trials.)

Patients Who Are Mentally Ill

Most of this part of the chapter focuses on assessment of pain in patients who have one of two mental disorders: (1) schizophrenia, in which decreased sensitivity to pain (hyppoalgesia) or impaired pain responsiveness has been documented in some patients (Singh, Giles, Nasrallah, 2006); and (2) posttraumatic stress disorder (PTSD), in which both decreased and increased sensitivity to pain have been reported(Geuze, Westenberg, Jochims, et al., 2007). The occurrence and the perception of pain in persons who have these two mental disorders are examined. Depression and anxiety in relation to pain are discussed briefly in Chapter 2 (pp. 31-32).

Schizophrenia

The extent of apparent insensitivity to pain in patients with schizophrenia can be extreme, as revealed in some clinical case reports. One such example is a patient with diagnosed schizophrenia for 20 years who burned his arm so severely it had to be amputated (Virit, Savas, Altindag, 2008). The patient explained, "I put my hand on the burning flames of the LPG (liquefied petroleum gas) cylinder in order to get warm…. I did not feel any pain" (p. 384).

Insensitivity to pain by schizophrenic patients has been suggested for more than 100 years, and failure to respond to pain is clearly associated with increased morbidity and mortality rates. A literature review of physical diseases in patients with schizophrenia documented the long-held observation that many types of physical illness, such as CV diseases, HIV infections, and dental problems, are more common in these patients than in the general population (Leucht, Burkard, Henderson, et al., 2007). This is thought to be caused in part by the stigma attached to patients with schizophrenia; it leads to undertreatment. Further, the tendency to ascribe patients' expressions of physical illness to the mental illness sometimes leads to missing a medical diagnosis. In addition, patients themselves simply fail to report symptoms of physical illness. It appears that patients with schizophrenia who fail to respond to pain also seek medical care at later stages of disease. For example, in a small study of 55 patients with schizophrenia undergoing appendectomy, 34 appendixes were perforated and 9 were gangrenous (Cooke, Magas, Virgo, et al., 2007).

In a literature search for studies of postoperative complications in seriously mentally ill patients, 10 studies relating to patients with schizophrenia were identified (Copeland, Zeber, Pugh, et al., 2008). Of the studies, 9 had fewer than 100 patients, but one large retrospective study included 466 patients with schizophrenia and 338,257 patients without schizophrenia (Daumit, Pronovost, Anthony, et al., 2006). Those with schizophrenia had higher rates of postoperative complications, such as respiratory failure and deep-vein thrombosis, than did patients without schizophrenia. Again, it appears that patients with schizophrenia are insensitive to pain and seek medical care at later stages of disease.

One small study of 50 schizophrenic patients and 25 controls found that those with schizophrenia reported significantly lower pain intensity postoperatively and consumed 60% less analgesic medication (Kudoh, Ishihara, Matsuki, 2000). This shows that schizophrenic patients seem to be less responsive to postoperative pain. Nevertheless, postoperative pain in schizophrenic patients is a risk factor for postoperative confusion (Kudoh, Takahira, Katagal, et al., 2002), which occurs more commonly in schizophrenic patients than in those without schizophrenia. Although pain scores do not reflect very much conscious awareness of pain, adequate postoperative pain relief is necessary to prevent postoperative confusion (Kudoh, 2005).

The lack of responsiveness to pain of schizophrenic patients is poorly understood. One way of comprehending the denial of pain and the low pain ratings in the presence of noxious stimuli that ordinarily cause severe pain is that the mental illness overwhelms the patient's thought processes (e.g., hallucinations, intrusive thoughts), and the patient simply does not focus on pain. Patients with schizophrenia also may be preoccupied with their psychotic symptoms and may suffer from fatigue and a lack of drive, consequently failing to seek help for physical symptoms (Leucht, Burkard, Henderson, et al., 2007). Some studies find that patients with schizophrenia, when compared to healthy controls, have higher sensory perception thresholds, such as the perception of warmth and the onset of thermal pain. This trait seems to be caused by abnormalities in information processing (Jochum, Letzsch, Greiner, et al., 2006). The tests for these sensations required sustained attention, and the researchers noted that the patients had difficulty focusing. A review of 12 studies of individuals with schizophrenia revealed that their responses to experimental pain were diminished (Potvin, Marchand, 2008).

Antipsychotic medications have sometimes been thought to have analgesic effects, and that could help explain seeming decreased sensitivity to pain in individuals with schizophrenia. However, in the previously mentioned study, antipsychotic medications did not alter the finding of high sensory thresholds. Drug-free patients also had hypoalgesic responses. Therefore, hypoalgesia could not be explained solely by the effects of antipsychotic drugs (Potvin, Marchand, 2008).

Another explanation for hypoalgesia is derived from a review of the literature that suggests that seeming pain insensitivity may be a familial trait rather than a function of the psychotic state (Singh, Giles, Nasrallah, 2006). One study compared the responses to finger pressure by college students who did not have diagnoses of schizophrenia, but who had relatives who did, with the responses of students with no family history of schizophrenia (Hooley, Delgado, 2001). Pain threshold and tolerance were higher in the healthy adults who had relatives diagnosed with schizophrenia, suggesting that pain insensitivity may be a familial trait.

To summarize, apparent insensitivity to pain in patients with schizophrenia may reflect a true lack of pain sensitivity or may be caused by other factors such as failure to focus on pain or respond to pain in the presence of a psychotic state. Unfortunately, a review of the literature did not produce sufficient evidence of whether hypoalgesia is present in schizophrenic patients when they are stable as well as during acute phases of psychosis (Potvin, Marchand, 2008).

More recently, researchers have questioned whether some patients with schizophrenia are insensitive to pain or just seem insensitive to pain because of communication impairments that accompany schizophrenia (Bonnot, Anderson, Cohen, et al., 2009). A review of the scientific literature on pain in patients with schizophrenia yielded 431 articles, of which 57 were considered relevant to examining sensitivity to pain. These included 9 case reports, 23 clinical studies, 20 experimental research, and 5 review articles. Only 1 experimental study used a neurophysiologic measure of pain reactivity, and it showed a normal pain threshold in schizophrenia. Misconceptions about patients with schizophrenia being insensitive to pain are probably derived from observations that many of these patients show reduced pain reactivity in the form of decreased behavioral responses and self-reported pain.

How can pain be assessed in patients who do not report pain or report low intensities of pain? A survey was conducted of 74 staff members of a geriatric psychiatry service to explore pain assessment and management issues in that population (Stolee, Hillier, Esbaugh, et al., 2007). Part of the survey consisted of a list of 37 potential indicators of pain, and staff were asked to rate the extent to which they agreed or disagreed that these could be indicators of pain. Those pain indicators that were endorsed most often were facial grimacing or wincing, verbal pain complaints, diagnoses of painful conditions (such as arthritis), body positioning, and groaning or moaning. The accuracy of these indicators of pain was not assessed. Also, in this population of patients both mental illness and cognitive impairment existed, so the extent to which each condition influenced the perception of pain is unknown. However, the majority of respondents (more than 80%) were not so much interested in specific behaviors but rather in identifying changes in usual behaviors as indicators of pain in patients with mental illness. This preliminary research provides a clue to the assessment of pain in patients with schizophrenia, namely, notation of changes in the patients' usual behaviors.

Many behaviors, such as personality changes, sleep disturbances, and fatigue, may occur as the result of either pain or exacerbations in mental illness (McCaffery, Pasero, 2001; Rutledge, Donaldson, 1998). Because apparent insensitivity to pain and impaired pain responsiveness are common in mental illness, it is recommended that such behaviors be interpreted as potential indicators of pain and that the pain be treated first, before attempting to determine whether the behaviors are a result of a mental disorder.

The finding of the appearance of insensitivity to pain in many, but not all, patients with schizophrenia presents clinicians with assessment challenges. In some ways assessment is comparable to that in previous recommendations that pain in nonverbal patients and those unable to respond with behavioral indicators should be assumed and treated when usually painful underlying pathologies or procedures are present. Because pain is rarely experienced as a hallucination (Watson, Chandarana, Merskey, 1981), any report of pain should always be taken seriously.

The assessment of pain in patients with schizophrenia should not differ from the assessment of pain in mentally healthy individuals. For example, if an institution's policy recommends assessment of pain during every shift, it should also be done on units caring for patients with mental illness, bearing in mind that a patient with schizophrenia may deny pain, even in the presence of a disease known to be painful such as an infected appendix.

For the assessment of pain in adult patients with schizophrenia, information from the previous discussion can be applied to the hierarchy-of-pain assessment techniques, Box 3-9 (p. 123), as follows:

- As in all patients, give priority to obtaining self-reports of pain. Beware of ascribing reports of pain to the mental illness. If reports of pain are ignored, diagnosis of physical illness may be delayed, subjecting a patient to complications such as a ruptured appendix. Pain is rarely a hallucination. In fact, clinicians should maintain a high index of suspicion of pain in these patients because they are known for late reporting of the symptoms of physical illnesses.

  In schizophrenic patients with the intellectual capacity for self-reporting of pain, reports of no pain or mild pain may indicate lack of responsiveness to pain, not lack of pain. However, each patient should be assessed for a history of lack of responsiveness to pain.
- Identify pathologic conditions and procedures that commonly cause pain such as surgery. Consider obtaining a consultation for assistance in diagnosing a physical illness. Clinicians skilled in the care of patients with mental illness may not be as skilled in the detection of physical illness.
- Observe behaviors indicative of pain. Consider the possibility that pain is present when changes in patients' usual behaviors occur, such as increased fatigue, sleep disturbances, postoperative confusion, or personality changes. In one study, clinicians identified facial grimacing or wincing and groaning or moaning as common indicators of pain. Studies have shown that clinicians value changes in usual behavior as the most important indicators of pain. "Absence of pain reactivity does not mean absence of pain sensitivity" (Bonnot, Anderson, Cohen, 2009, p. 246).

- Obtain information from caregivers and medical records regarding past or current pain, potential causes of pain, and any indications of lack of responsiveness to pain.
- Finally, when in doubt about the presence of pain or when wanting to confirm the suspicion of pain, an analgesic trial may be helpful. Behavior changes that could be caused by either pain or exacerbation of mental illness should first be treated as pain before initiating treatment for the mental illness. Assessment of behavior after a trial use of analgesic may help to determine whether changes in behavior are due to a physical illness or to the mental illness.

In conclusion, when addressing the problem of pain in patients with serious mental illness, two important considerations are (1) patients with chronic pain who also have mental disorders have a poorer quality of life than those without mental disorders; and (2) better treatment outcomes are likely when both pain and the mental illness are treated than when only one or the other is treated (Nicholas, 2007). Thus, whether the mental illness causes pain or is a consequence of pain, both pain and the mental illness should be treated.

Posttraumatic Stress Disorder

Posttraumatic stress disorder (PTSD) is an anxiety disorder that can occur following an extremely traumatic event that involves being threatened by or witness to a situation that involves death or injury (APA, 1994). Traumatic events may include military combat, physical attacks, torture, or severe automobile accidents. The prevalence rates of individuals' at risk for developing PTSD, such as combat veterans and victims of criminal violence, range from 3% to 58%.

Soldiers returning from the Iraqi war report very high levels of combat exposure, with 90% describing being shot at and a high percentage report handling dead bodies, knowing someone who was injured or killed, or killing an enemy combatant (Hoge, Castro, Messer, et al., 2004) Research has shown that soldiers with extensive combat exposure are four times more likely to develop PTSD than those with low combat exposure (Kulka, Schlenger, Fairbank, et al., 1990). In a convenience sample of Iraqi veterans, 71% had pain, 57% had PTSD, and 64% had mild traumatic brain injury; 36% had all three (Tan, Fink, Dao, et al., 2009). This population also displayed compromised autonomic nervous system function, suggesting that autonomic abnormality may contribute to, result from, or be a useful marker of symptoms of pain in traumatic brain injury and PTSD.

Soon after a traumatic event, "psychic numbing" or "emotional anesthesia" occurs; it is a symptom of decreased responsiveness to the external world (APA, 1994). Symptoms of PTSD usually begin within the first 3 months of the precipitating event, and approximately half of patients experiencing such symptoms completely recover within 3 months, whereas many others have persistent symptoms for longer than 12 months. PTSD is characterized by distress or impairment in functioning, socially or occupationally; persistent anxiety; sleep disturbances; and recurrent nightmares about the traumatic event. The patient may develop hypervigilence, irritability, exaggerated startle responses; and difficulty concentrating. When persons are exposed to events that are reminders of the original traumatic event, extreme psychologic distress or physiologic reactions commonly occur. Usually, they make deliberate efforts to avoid all reminders.

The prevalence of PTSD has been estimated to be between 6% and 9% or more in the general population of the United States (Breslau, 2001). Unfortunately, PTSD is much more common and is often underdiagnosed in primary care and mental health settings. For example, in a study of 295 psychiatric outpatients, 46% had PTSD but only 7% were diagnosed as such by physicians (Villano, Rosenblum, Magura, et al., 2007).

The presence of high levels of pain during the peritrauma period has been associated with increased risk for the development of PTSD (Norman, Stein, Dimsdale, et al., 2008). Related to this finding is a study of 24 children admitted to the hospital for acute burns (Saxe, Stoddard, Courtney, et al., 2001). The children were assessed for PTSD while in the hospital and 6 months after discharge. All children received morphine, but those who received higher doses of morphine showed greater reduction in PTSD symptoms over 6 months. It is interesting that in another study, of 147 soldiers in Iraq who were treated in a military treatment center for burns and had had at least one surgery, 119 who had received ketamine during surgery were compared with 28 who had not (McGhee, Maani, Garza, et al., 2008). The prevalence of PTSD was 27% in those who had received ketamine and 46% in those who had not received ketamine despite the fact that their burns were larger and their injury severity scores higher. A pilot study of placebo versus 40 mg of propranolol (Inderal) four times a day following acute, psychologically traumatic events found that propranolol had a preventive effect on subsequent PTSD (Pitman, Sanders, Zusman, et al., 2002). This offers the hope that ketamine, propranolol, morphine, or perhaps some other medications can be used soon after trauma or injury to prevent or reduce the symptoms of PTSD.

When PTSD involves a physically painful injury, it has been suggested that pain may be a flashback to the original traumatic injury (Asmundson, Coons, Taylor, et al., 2002). Therefore, it may be possible to prevent or minimize the development of pain-related PTSD flashbacks by assessing pain and treating it with analgesics at an early stage. Another small study (N = 6) of veterans with both chronic pain and PTSD examined the effects of using components of cognitive processing therapy for PTSD and cognitive behavioral therapy for chronic pain (Otis, Keane, Kerns, et al., 2009). A 12-session integrated treatment for veterans with both chronic pain and PTSD was developed

and used by the participants. Although half the participants withdrew from the study, participants appeared to benefit from the treatment, and further research is being conducted to evaluate the efficacy of this approach.

PTSD and chronic pain often occur together and are frequently observed within the Department of Veterans Affairs health care system (Otis, Keane, Kerns, 2003). When patients with PTSD are being assessed, chronic pain is commonly identified, regardless of the nature of the traumatic experience, and vice versa; when patients with chronic pain are being assessed, PTSD is commonly found too (Asmundson, Coons, Taylor, et al., 2002; Schwartz, Bradley, Penza, et al., 2006). In a study of 295 psychiatric outpatients, 24% had both PTSD and chronic severe pain (Villano, Rosenblum, Magura, et al., 2007). In another study of 85 veterans seeking treatment for PTSD, 66% had chronic pain diagnoses (Shipherd, Keyes, Jovanovic, et al., 2007).

Unfortunately, because of the stigma placed on seeking psychiatric help, most veterans do not seek help from this source. If they develop painful conditions, they are more likely to seek help from pain clinics (DeCarvalho, Whealin, 2006). Because PTSD may hamper treatment for chronic pain, pain specialists should know about the possibility that PTSD can coexist with chronic pain and should watch for symptoms, such as being easily startled, hypervigilence, isolation, and use of alcohol or other substances to deal with PTSD or pain. An appropriate screening tool for PTSD should be used.

Studies have reported both increased and decreased sensitivity to pain in individuals with PTSD (Geuze, Westenberg, Jochims, et al., 2007). Decreased sensitivity to pain in patients with PTSD has been documented in only a few experimental studies. In a small study of 12 veterans with PTSD and 12 without PTSD, neuroimaging was done while each group was exposed to heat stimuli (Geuze, Westenberg, Jochims, et al., 2007). Subjects rated pain using an NRS of 0 to 100. Compared to controls, individuals with PTSD rated the heat stimuli as being significantly less painful, and neuroimaging revealed an analgesic response and altered pain processing in certain brain areas.

In another small, double-blind, crossover study, eight Vietnam veterans with PTSD and a control group of eight veterans without PTSD, matched for combat severity, watched a videotape of dramatized combat (Pitman, van der Kolk, Orr, et al., 1990). None were receiving opioid analgesics. The tape was viewed by each group while under the effects of naloxone hydrochloride or placebo. In the placebo condition, those with PTSD experienced a 30% decrease in pain ratings, but no decreases in pain ratings occurred in the naloxone condition, which suggests that naloxone blocked endogenous opioid analgesia. The veterans without PTSD showed no decrease in pain ratings under either condition. It appeared that veterans with PTSD had opioid-mediated analgesic responses (endogenous opioids). Thus, decreased sensitivity to pain in patients with PTSD appears to occur briefly when a patient is exposed to acute pain or something that triggers memories of or reminds the patient of the original trauma.

Patients with PSTD and chronic pain tend to have increased sensitivity to pain. The mechanisms most often proposed to understand the cooccurrence of chronic pain and PTSD are shared vulnerability and mutual maintenance (Asmundson, Coons, Taylor, et al., 2002). For example, in terms of the concept of shared vulnerability, it seems possible that anxiety sensitivity is shared by patients with both PTSD and chronic pain. With respect to the concept of mutual maintenance, it seems possible that certain cognitive or affective components of chronic pain exacerbate symptoms associated with PTSD and that certain affective and behavioral components of PTSD exacerbate symptoms associated with chronic pain.

Analysis of pain intensity was compared in three groups, all members of which had chronic pain; but one group had accident-related pain and high PTSD symptoms, one group had accident-related pain and few or no symptoms of PTSD, and the third group had pain that was not accident related and had no symptoms of PTSD (Geisser, Roth, Bachman, et al., 1996). Patients with accident-related pain and strong PTSD symptoms reported higher levels of pain than did the other two groups.

To examine sensitivity to pain, three groups of subjects—32 outpatients with combat- and terror-related PTSD, 29 outpatients with anxiety disorder, and 20 healthy individuals—were compared (Defrin, Ginzburg, Solomon, et al., 2008). The first two groups were randomly selected from an outpatient psychiatric clinic and contacted by telephone to request participation in the study. Higher rates of chronic pain, more intense chronic pain, and more painful body regions were found in the subjects with PTSD than in the other two groups. Further, the greater the severity of PTSD, the greater the severity of chronic pain.

A review of the literature also confirms this finding (Smith, Egert, Winkel, et al., 2002). In addition to being at high risk for PTSD, individuals with persistent pain who do develop PTSD are also likely to experience more intense and pervasive pain than those who do not develop PTSD.

In the study by Defrin and others (2008), differences emerged when the groups were tested for measurement of warmth, cold, light touch, and heat-pain thresholds and for responses to acute suprathreshold heat and mechanical stimuli. Although the patients with PTSD were less sensitive to thresholds for warmth, cold, touch, and heat-pain than the other two groups, they found the suprathreshold heat and mechanical stimuli much more intense than did the other groups. The researchers offered several possible explanations for this paradoxical finding, such as altered sensory processing in subjects with PTSD, and recommended further research. Other researchers suggest that the increased sensitivity to suprathreshold pain may reflect in part that the subjects were exposed to this type of pain for a longer time (repeated painful stimuli) in the experimental situation than when tested for the heat-pain threshold in which they were simply asked to identify the point at which the heat stimulus became painful (Asmundson, Katz, 2008).

A study of 145 individuals with diagnoses of HIV/AIDS who also had persistent pain was conducted to examine the relationship between PTSD and pain (Smith, Egert, Winkel, et al., 2002). In this sample, approximately half (51.8%) had diagnoses of PTSD. Individuals with PTSD reported higher levels of pain at its worst, worse physical and mental health, and higher levels of pain that interfered with daily activities and mood than did those without PTSD. One obvious implication of the study is that individuals with HIV should be assessed for symptoms of PTSD.

A study of 93 patients diagnosed with the chronic pain condition of fibromyalgia syndrome (FMS) was undertaken to determine the prevalence of PTSD-like symptoms (not the diagnostic category of PTSD) and to evaluate the relationship between PTSD symptoms, FMS symptoms, and disability (Sherman, Turk, Okifuji, 2000). More than half (56%) of the sample reported significant levels of PTSD-like symptoms, and this group reported significantly greater levels of pain, interference with life, emotional distress, difficulty adapting to FMS, depressive symptoms, and disability than did individuals without clinically significant levels of PTSD symptoms. Another study of PTSD and FMS yielded similar results. The frequency of occurrence of PTSD was examined in 77 patients with FMS, and 57% were found to have significant levels of PTSD symptoms (Cohen, Neumann, Haiman, et al., 2002). The most frequently reported traumatic event associated with PTSD was the unexpected death of a loved one (as is true for the other patients with PTSD). These patients did not regard their FMS as a traumatic event.

Clearly PTSD symptomatology is prevalent in individuals with FMS and probably has a negative impact on coping with FMS, suggesting that interventions for the treatment of PTSD, such as stress management, may be helpful for patients with FMS. These interventions overlap with interventions for persistent pain and probably can be incorporated easily in a pain management program for patients with FMS.

The relationship between analgesic use and PTSD was studied in 173 African-Americans who were outpatients at a mental health center (Schwartz, Bradley, Penza, et al., 2006). Those with PTSD, 43.5% of the sample, used significantly more opioid and nonopioid analgesic medications than did those who did not have PTSD. Of the patients with PTSD, 68% were prescribed analgesics, and 59% received opioids, whereas only 51% of patients without PTSD received analgesics, 42% of them receiving opioids. (Pain ratings were not reported in this article.) Patients receiving opioids had the highest severity of PTSD symptoms. PTSD was notably underdiagnosed in this group of patients; only 6.5% of the total sample had documented diagnoses of PTSD.

Chronic pain and PTSD often coexist, and PTSD exacerbates chronic pain but is frequently underdiagnosed. It is therefore critical to assess patients with chronic pain for the symptoms of PTSD and to assess patients with PTSD for chronic pain. This makes it possible to recognize and arrange for both the pain and the PTSD to be addressed. A convenient screening tool for PTSD in the primary care setting is the Primary Care PTSD (PC-PTSD) screen shown in Form 4-3 (Prins, Quimette, Kimerling, et al., 2003). It is psychometrically sound, identifying PTSD in 78% of 188 men and women in a primary care setting at the Veterans Administration. It is brief, written at an eighth grade reading level, and easy to score. It consists of four yes/no questions, and a positive answer to two or more items suggests the need for further assessment of PTSD.

Based on the previous discussion of PTSD, suggestions for assessment of pain and PTSD, along with possible prevention of or decrease in symptoms of PTSD are as follows:

- Obtain self-reports of pain as indicated in the hierarchy of pain assessment techniques (see Box 3-9, p. 123). PTSD itself does not seem to hinder the ability to provide a self-report of pain, but chronic pain is often underdiagnosed, although it is common in patients with PTSD. Other steps in the hierarchy of pain assessment should be followed if self-report is hampered by some other condition such as brain injury.
- At times of extremely traumatic events, assess for pain and, if present, treat it aggressively in the hope of preventing or decreasing the symptoms of PTSD. If individuals are unable to respond at the time of the traumatic event and physical stimuli suggest that pain is present, assume that pain is present and treat it aggressively as a prophylactic measure
- Clinicians treating patients with PTSD should assess for the cooccurrence of chronic pain.
- Clinicians treating patients with chronic pain, especially soldiers with long exposure to combat, should assess for the cooccurrence of PTSD or PTSD symptomatology. Watch for symptoms such as hypervigilence, isolation, being easily startled, and use of alcohol and other drugs to cope with pain or PTSD. A useful screening tool is PC-PTSD (Form 4-3).
- If a patient with PTSD also has pain, recognize the possibility of increased sensitivity to pain, higher pain ratings, and the need for more analgesia than required by other patients with comparable injuries but no PTSD.
- Be alert to diagnoses such as the HIV and advanced cancer that expose individuals to a number of psychologically traumatic events, such as receiving the diagnosis, disclosing the diagnosis to others and, in some cases such as infection by HIV, infecting significant others. Assess for symptoms of PTSD and chronic pain.

To summarize the implications of these assessment suggestions, when PTSD or PTSD symptomatology and pain cooccur, a cognitive-behavioral therapy program is appropriate but will have to be modified to address both problems (Asmundson, Coons, Taylor, et al., 2002). No

---

Primary Care PTSD Screen (PC-PTSD)

Instructions: The patient completes this form. A positive answer to two or more items suggests the need for further assessment of PTSD.

In your life, have you ever had an experience that was so frightening, horrible, or upsetting that, <u>in the past month</u>, you...

1. Have had nightmares about it or thought about it when you did not want to?

    YES   NO

2. Tried hard not to think about it or went out of your way to avoid situations that reminded you of it?

    YES   NO

3. Were constantly on guard, watchful, or easily startled?

    YES   NO

4. Felt numb or detached from others, activities, or your surroundings?

    YES   NO

Form 4-3 |

As appears in Pasero, C., & McCaffery, M. (2011). *Pain assessment and pharmacologic management*, p. 158, St. Louis, Mosby. Used with permission. From Prins, A., Ouimette, P., Kimerling, R., et al. (2003). The primary care PTSD screen (PC-PTSD): Development and operating characteristics. *Prim Care Psychiat*, 9(1), 9-14. May be duplicated for use in clinical practice.

data yet exist to suggest that either PTSD or chronic pain should be treated first when they cooccur. Thus, treating the conditions simultaneously seems indicated.

Specific treatment of coexisting pain and PTSD is beyond the scope of this chapter, but DeCarvalho and Whealin (2006) suggest additional practical ideas that can be quickly initiated after PTSD is suspected. Educate the patient about the symptoms of PTSD, and provide written materials when possible. One short patient education sheet about chronic pain and PTSD can be obtained from http://www.ncptsd.va.gov/ncmain/ncdocs/fact_shts/ fs_chronic_pain_and_patients.html?opm=1&rr=rr102& srt=d&echorr=true. When possible, give returning service members with pain and possible PTSD the option of attending a military or a civilian pain clinic. This may reduce their fear of stigmatization. Relaxation therapy may be helpful, although some patients find that it allows for disturbing intrusive thoughts.

Cultural Considerations

As racial and cultural diversity increases in the United States, clinicians are increasingly likely to care for patients from backgrounds quite different from their own. There is little doubt that various ethnic groups express pain and suffering differently. The same can be said of people in general. Fortunately, many of the pain assessment tools used in English in the United States can be used successfully in other cultures if they are translated into the appropriate languages. Culture affects behavioral responses to pain and treatment preferences. However, patients of many different cultures may be assessed using similar pain assessment tools, and the findings will have similar meanings across cultures. Following is a reminder of some of the assessment tools discussed in this section that have been used in other cultures.

This section provides translations of the horizontal 0 to 10 NRS (see Figure 3-6, pp. 60-65); the Wong-Baker FACES Pain Rating Scale (see Figure 3-7, pp. 66-67); and the Faces Pain Scale-Revised (FPS-R) (see Figure 3-8, pp. 69-85) into numerous languages. However, some minor changes may be made when necessary. For example, a study of Chinese patients' responses to a VAS revealed that it was a suitable method for assessing pain intensity but that the vertical presentation was more quickly understood than the horizontal line, probably because traditionally, the Chinese read vertically downward and from right to left, not left to right (Aun, Lam Collett, 1986). If difficulties are encountered with the horizontal Chinese translation in Figure 3-6 (pp. 60-65), readers are encouraged to make a vertical presentation with 10 at the top.

The reliability and validity of the FPS-R has been established in several different cultural groups. In one study, the reliability and validity of the FPS-R was established in cognitively impaired and cognitively intact older adults who were Asian, African-American, and Hispanic (Ware, Epps, Herr, et al., 2006). The last two groups preferred the FPS-R. This pain rating scale has also been found to be reliable and valid in cognitively intact elderly Spanish patients (Miro, Huguet, Nieto, et al., 2005) and in cognitively intact Chinese adults ranging in age from 18 to 78 years (Li, Liu, Herr, 2007). In the latter group almost half preferred the FPS-R, and the FPS-R had a low error rate. The FPS-R is available in approximately 30 languages (see Figure 3-8, pp. 69-85).

The Brief Pain Inventory (BPI) (see Form 3-2, p. 53) has also consistently demonstrated a high degree of reliability and validity when administered to cancer patients from countries other than the United States. The BPI has been translated into a number of languages, including Japanese (Uki, Mendoza, Cleeland, et al., 1998); Vietnamese (Cleeland, Ladinsky, Serlin et al., 1988); Chinese (Wang, Mendoza, Gao, et al., 1996); the Philippine language (Cleeland, Nakamura, Mendoza, et al., 1996); Russian (Kalyadina, Ionova, Ivanova, et al., 2008); and French (Serlin, Mendoza, Nakamura, et al., 1995). Using the BPI, several studies of various cultures (e.g., Kalyadina, Ionova, Ivanova, et al., 2008) have found that on a 0 to 10 pain rating scale, pain ratings of 5 or more interfere significantly with daily function (Cleeland, 1984; Cleeland, Gonin, Hatfield, 1994; Serlin, Mendoza, Nakamura, et al., 1995). Although behavioral expression of pain may differ considerably among cultures, pain ratings and the impact of pain on quality of life appear to be very similar.

Some of the behavioral tools developed for assessment of pain in nonverbal patients with dementia have been translated into other languages and used in other countries, suggesting that many behaviors indicative of pain are similar in different cultures. The Pain Assessment in Advanced Dementia (PAINAD) (see Form 3-15, pp. 132-134) has been translated and tested in five languages: English (DeWaters, Faut-Callahan, McCann, et al., 2008); Italian (Costardi, Rozzini, Costanzi, et al., 2007); Belgian (Dutch translation) (van Iersel, Timmerman, Mullie, 2006); the Netherlands (Dutch translation) (Zwakhalen, Hamers, Abu-Saad, et al., 2006); and German (Schuler, Becker, Kaspar, et al., 2007). The Doloplus 2 was developed in the French language and later translated into English for further testing (Lefebvre-Chapiro, The Doloplus Group, 2001). The Elderly Pain Caring Assessment 2 (EPCA-2) was developed by a French team and is being validated in English-translated samples (Morello, Jean, Alix, et al., 2007).

The usefulness of basic pain assessment tools across cultures is not sufficient to ensure a high quality of care for patients of various cultural backgrounds. Clinicians must be particularly mindful of the fact that the more difference there is between a patient and a clinician, the more difficult it is for the clinician to assess and treat the patient. As an example, in a study of 50 hospitalized patients who spoke Arabic, a comparison of the patients' pain ratings with those of nurses who shared the mother tongue and those who did not revealed that nurses sharing the mother tongue with patients were much more likely to provide pain ratings similar to those of their patients than were the other nurses (Harrison, Busabir, Al-Kaabi, et al., 1996).

Another study of 32 nurses' responses to 60 patients with cholecystectomy pain compared the nurses' estimates of pain to those of each of two ethnic groups, Anglo-American women and Mexican-American women (Calvillo, Flaskerud, 1993). The majority of nurses (45.8%) were Anglo-American and the remainder were a mix of ethnicities. Although there were no significant differences between the two ethnic groups' self-reports of pain, nurses assigned more pain to Anglo-Americans than to Mexican-Americans. Clearly, clinicians must recognize the possibility of this problem and guard against it by always obtaining and acting on a patient's self-report of pain, not their own beliefs about a patient's pain.

In discussing pain it is helpful to know that three terms—pain, hurt, and ache—seem to be used similarly across cultures to describe pain intensity. The term *pain* is usually used for the most intense pain, followed by *hurt*; *ache* means the least pain. This was shown to be true in a study of Hispanics, American Indians, blacks, and whites (Gaston-Johansson, Albert, Fagan, et al., 1990). These terms are also basic words used in the Swedish language to describe pain intensity (Gaston-Johansson, 1984), as well as in the Dutch language (Francke, Theeuwen, 1994). So it is clear that people of diverse ethnic, cultural, and educational backgrounds use similar words to describe the intensity of pain.

The Chinese population has been studied with regard to concepts of pain, and some information is applicable to pain assessment in that group (Chen, Miaskowski, Dodd, et al., 2008). The Chinese culture includes Confucianism, which maintains that pain is an essential element of life and is a trial or a sacrifice that must be endured. A Confucian would rather endure pain and not report it to a clinician. Confucians tend to report pain only when it is unbearable. However, sometimes a patient will report pain to a close family member and ask him or her to report the pain to the clinician. Note that on the hierarchy of pain assessment, one of the steps is to ask people familiar with a patient whether they think the patient has pain. Their reports of pain may be more accurate than a patient's denial of pain. A clinician should also explore the beliefs of a Chinese patient and, when a patient wishes to bear pain, explain the harmful effects of pain. Ultimately, a clinician may have to support a patient's wish to endure pain. A clinician should also assess how a patient wishes to handle pain. A patient may desire Chinese medicines or acupuncture instead of analgesics. However, care must be taken to realize that not all Chinese patients share the beliefs described. Believing that individuals within the same cultural group are alike is a misconception.

The Chinese culture is not the only one in which enduring pain may be regarded as valuable (Mazanee,

Tyler, 2003). In fact, many clinicians reading this probably have also noted in some white Americans the same desire to bear pain and not report it until it is severe. Overall, patients of various cultures may share more similarities than differences. To enhance cultural sensitivity, clinicians must work closely with patients and their families to identify mutual goals of care that take into account different preferences, such as the relative values placed on being free of pain versus being fully alert. Whenever possible, health care practices that are desired by a patient or are specific to the patient's cultural group should be included in patient care if he or she wishes. Teaching materials in patients' own languages may be secured or developed, and cultural resources such as interpreters may be useful (McGuire, Sheidler, 1993).

Some have urged nurses to become "culturally competent," but we share the belief of others who maintain that it is really a matter of nursing competence—that is, encouraging nurses to be sensitive to the differences among all individuals (Dreher, MacNaughton, 2002). Understanding the characteristics of a culture may be helpful in understanding some of the behaviors seen in patients, but that knowledge does not tell us what to expect of individual patients.

Far too many cultures are represented in the patient population to allow consideration of all of them in this section. Further, pain assessment has not been studied in all cultures. Nevertheless, clinicians are encouraged to seek information about the specific cultural backgrounds of their patients through exploration with the patients and through publications. Information about the beliefs concerning health and illness of 17 different cultures is available in Giger and Davidhizar (2008). Care of oncology patients of Hispanic and Japanese-American backgrounds is discussed by Kagawa-Singer (1987). Other articles address pain in Arab-Americans (Reizien, Meleis, 1986); Chinese-Americans (Louie, 1985); and African-Americans (Capers, 1985).

As discussed previously in this chapter, clinicians must realize that despite their assessments of pain, those assessments might not be acted upon appropriately because of hidden biases such as patients' ethnicities. A few salient points are worth emphasizing. One example that represents several similar studies showed that in 217 patients, black patients, as compared with white patients, were undertreated for pain in the emergency department, despite similar notations of pain reports in the medical records (Todd, Deaton, D'Adamo, et al., 2000). A few years later, in a much larger study of patients with pain (N = 374,891) admitted to the emergency department, white patients were more likely to receive opioids than were black, Hispanic, Asians, and other patients (Pletcher, Kertesz, Kohn, et al., 2008). These are probably "hidden" biases; that is, ones that we are not aware of consciously. Those are the ones that are most difficult to recognize and stop before we undertreat patients.

Section II | Conclusion

SECTION II is the most important section in this book. The essential message about pain assessment is easy to summarize: Ask patients about their pain; accept and respect what they say; intervene to relieve their pain according to their pain management goals; and, once intervention has been implemented, ask them again about their pain to evaluate the intervention. It is a circle of assessment, intervention, and reassessment.

It would be unfair to lead the reader to believe that pain assessment will automatically result in improved pain care. Studies described in previous chapters have given examples of how assessment results in better pain management, but this is not always true. Unfortunately, even when seemingly appropriate assessment is performed and appropriate steps are initiated, the outcome for pain care may not be improved. For example, to determine whether systematic pain assessment information would alter a physician's clinical practice, a group of case coordinators used a pain assessment battery to assess a group of elderly patients and reported the results to physicians in the experimental group (Hadjistavropoulos, MacNab, Lints-Martindale, et al., 2009). Physician action in the experimental group was compared to a control group of 56. There were no significant differences between experimental and control groups with respect to medications prescribed or overall pain intensity.

On the other hand, sometimes assessment seems to improve patient care. In a study of mechanically ventilated patients who received analgesia on day 2 of their stay in the ICU, investigators compared those who were assessed for pain (513 patients) with those who were not assessed for pain (631 patients) (Payen, Bosson, Chanques, et al., 2009). Those who were assessed for pain were more likely to receive sedation level assessment, nonopioids, dedicated analgesia during pain procedures, fewer hypnotics, and lower daily doses of midazolam. Patients who were assessed for pain also had a shorter duration of mechanical ventilation and a reduced duration of stay in the ICU. This study suggests a possible link between pain assessment and clinical practices, but it does not establish a cause and effect relationship between pain assessment and improved outcomes in this group. Further study is needed to determine if pain assessment is truly linked to improved length of stay in the ICU, and if not, why not.

Although some improvement has been shown in pain assessment, there may be little progress in alleviating pain. From 1992 to 2001, data from 20 studies at 8 hospitals analyzed pain intensity and pain documentation. There was an increased frequency of pain assessments but no significant decrease in pain intensity or in pain interference with activities (Gordon, Pellino, Miaskowski, et al., 2002). Even with appropriate assessment, many patients continue to suffer pain needlessly.

Nevertheless, without assessment and reassessment of the patient with pain, none of the pain relief measures presented in the following chapters will be useful. If assessment is not used to formulate and implement appropriate pain relief measures, assessment will be largely useless. Even if pain assessment results in appropriate pain relief measures, reassessment is essential. Seemingly appropriate pain relief measures may fail to relieve pain or be harmful to the patient. As essential as assessment is, it is wasted without follow up.

Research tells us that we have a long way to go in improving the care of patients with pain. We can assess patients with pain fairly well, but we need to learn how to teach all members of the health care team to use them. No doubt many of our biases stop us from taking the next step—formulating appropriate intervention for pain relief. It took us 15 to 20 years to develop pain assessment tools, and even today we have not yet established their routine use in many clinical areas, including ICUs and long-term care areas. It is not a hopeless process, but it is a long and difficult one. Numerous pain assessment tools are now available for many patient populations, but assessment alone is not enough. Efforts must be made to act upon that assessment. One approach is to identify comfort-function goals and hold ourselves accountable for intervening until these goals are achieved.

References

Abbey, J., Piller, N., De Bellis, A., et al. (2004). The Abbey pain scale: A 1-minute numerical indicator for people with end-stage dementia. *International Journal of Palliative Nursing*, 10(1), 6–13.

Acute Pain Management Guideline Panel. (1992). *Acute pain management in adults: Operative procedures. Quick reference guide for clinicians.* AHCPR Pub. No. 92-0019, Rockville, MD, Agency for Health Care and Research, Public Health Service, U.S. Department of Health and Human Services.

Aguirre, L. L., Nevidjon, B. M., & Clemens, A. E. (2008). Pain diaries. *The American Journal of Nursing*, 108(6), 36–39.

American Academy of Pain Medicine (AAPM), American Pain Society (APS), American Society of Addiction Medicine (ASAM). (2001). Definitions related to the use of opioids for the treatment of pain. Available at http://www.ampainsoc. org/advocacy/opioids2.htm.

American Geriatrics Society (AGS) Panel on Persistent Pain in Older Persons. (2002). Clinical practice guidelines: The management of persistent pain in older persons. *Journal of the American Geriatrics Society*, 50(6 Suppl), S205–S224.

American Pain Society (APS). (1999). *Guideline for the management of acute and chronic pain in sickle cell disease.* Glenview, IL: APS.

American Pain Society (APS). (2003). *Principles of analgesic use in the treatment of acute pain and cancer pain* (5th ed.). Glenview, IL: APS.

American Psychiatric Association. (1994). *Diagnostic and Statistical Manual of Mental Disorders (DSM-IV)* (4th ed.). Washington, DC: American Psychiatric Association.

American Society for Pain Management Nurses (ASPMN). (2002). *ASPMN position statement: pain management in patients with addictive disease.* Pensacola, FL: ASPMN. Available at http://www.aspmn.org/Organization/documents/addictions_9pt.pdf. Accessed February 3, 2008.

American Society for Pain Management Nurses (ASPMN). (2004). Position statement on use of placebos in pain management. Available at http://www.aspmn.org/pdfs/Use%20of%20Placebos.pdf. Accessed April 3, 2008.

American Society for Pain Management Nurses (ASPMN). (2006). Authorized and unauthorized ("PCA by proxy") dosing of analgesic infusion pumps. Available at http://www.aspmn.org/Organization/documents/PCAbyProxy-final-EW_004.pdf. Accessed February 3, 2008.

Anderson, J. V. C., & Burchiel, K. J. (1999). A prospective study of long-term intrathecal morphine in the management of chronic nonmalignant pain. *Neurosurgery, 44*(2), 289–300; discussion 300–301.

Apfel, C. C., Laara, E., Koivuranta, M., et al. (1999). A simplified risk score for predicting postoperative nausea and vomiting: conclusions from cross-validations between two centers. *Anesthesiology, 91*(3), 693–700.

Arbour, C., & Gelinas, C. (2009). Are vital signs valid indicators of pain in postoperative cardiac surgery ICU adults? *Intens Crit Care Nurs,* doi: 10.1016/j.iccn.2009.11.003.

Armitage, K. J., Schneiderman, L. J., & Bass, R. A. (1979). Response of physicians to medical complaints in men and women. *JAMA: The Journal of the American Medical Association, 241*(20), 2186–2187.

Arnstein, P. (2006). Placebo: no relief for Ms. Mahoney's pain. *The American Journal of Nursing, 106*(2), 54–57.

Arroyo-Novoa, C. M., Figueroa-Ramos, M. I., Puntillo, K. A., et al. (2007). Pain related to tracheal suctioning in awake acutely and critically ill adults: a descriptive study. *Intensive & Critical Care Nursing, 24*(1), 20–27.

Asmundson, G. J. G., Coons, M. J., Taylor, S., et al. (2002). PTSD and the experience of pain: research and clinical implications of shared vulnerability and mutual maintenance models. *Canadian Journal of Psychiatry. Revue Canadienne de Psychiatrie, 47*(10), 930–937.

Asmundson, G. J. G., & Katz, J. (2008). Understanding pain and posttraumatic stress disorder comorbidity: Do pathological responses to trauma alter the perception of pain? *Pain, 138,* 247–249.

ASP ad hoc Subcommittee for Psychology Curriculum. (1997). *Curriculum on pain for students in psychology.* Seattle: International Association for the Study of Pain.

Au, E., Loprinzi, C., Chodapkar, M., et al. (1994). Regular use of a verbal pain scale improves the understanding of oncology inpatient pain intensity. *Journal of Clinical Oncology, 12,* 2751–2755.

Audette, J. F., Emenike, E., & Meleger, A. L. (2005). Neuropathic low back pain. *Current Pain and Headache Reports, 9,* 168–177.

Aun, C., Lam, Y. M., & Collett, B. (1986). Evaluation of the use of visual analogue scale in Chinese patients. *Pain, 25,* 215–221.

Baiardi, J., Parzuchowski, J., Kosik, C., et al. (2002). *Examination of the reliability of the FLACC Pain Assessment Tool with cognitively impaired elderly.* Paper presented at the Annual National Conference of Gerontological Nurse Practitioners, Chicago.

Barsky, A. J. (2002). Forgetting, fabricating, and telescoping. *A.M.A. Archives of Internal Medicine, 162,* 981–984.

Beecher, H. K. (1956). Limiting factors in experimental pain. *Journal of Chronic Diseases, 4,* 11–21.

Beecher, H. K. (1955). The powerful placebo. *JAMA: The Journal of the American Medical Association, 159,* 1602–1606.

Benedetti, F., Amanzio, M., Baldi, S., et al. (1998). The specific effects of prior opioid exposure on placebo analgesia and placebo respiratory depression. *Pain, 75,* 313–319.

Benedetti, F., Arduino, C., Vighetti, S., et al. (2004). Pain reactivity in Alzheimer patients with different degrees of cognitive impairment and brain electrical activity deterioration. *Pain, 111*(1–2), 22–29.

Benjamin, L. J., Dampier, C. D., Jacox, A. K., et al. (1999). *Guideline for the management of acute and chronic pain in sickle cell disease.* APS Clinical Practice Guidelines, Series No. 1 Glenview, IL: American Pain Society.

Bennett, D., Burton, A. W., Fishman, S., et al. (2005). Consensus panel recommendations for the assessment and management of breakthrough pain. *Pharmacology & Therapeutics, 30*(5), 296–301.

Bennett, M. I., Attal, N., Backonia, M. M., et al. (2007). Using screening tools to identify neuropathic pain. *Pain, 127,* 199–203.

Bennett, M. I., Smith, B. H., Torrance, N., et al. (2005). The S-LANSS score for identifying pain of predominantly neuropathic origin: validation for use in clinical and postal research. *The Journal of Pain, 6*(3), 149–158.

Bergh, I., Sjostrom, B., Oden, A., et al. (2000). An application of pain rating scales in geriatric patients. *Aging (Milano), 12,* 380–387.

Berlin, Y., Hossain, S. J., & Bodian, C. A. (2003). The numeric rating scale and labor epidural analgesia. *Anesthesia and Analgesia, 96,* 1794–1798.

Bernabei, R., Gambassi, G., Lapane, K., et al. (1998). Management of pain in elderly patients with cancer. SAGE study group. Systematic assessment of geriatric drug use via epidemiology. *JAMA: The Journal of the American Medical Association, 279,* 1877–1882.

Beydoun, A., & Backonja, M. M. (2003). Mechanistic stratification of antineuralgic agents. *Journal of Pain and Symptom Management, 25,* S18–S35.

Beyer, J. E., Denyes, M. J., & Villarruel, A. M. (1992). The creation, validation, and continuing development of the oucher: A measure of pain intensity in children. *Journal of Pediatric Nursing, 7*(5), 335–346.

Beyer, J. E., Platt, A., Kinney, T., et al. (1994). Assessment of pain in adults and children with sickle cell disease. In B. S. Shapiro, N. L. Schechter, & K. Ohene-Frempong (Eds.), *Sickle cell disease related pain assessment and management: Conference proceedings.* Mt. Desert, ME: New England Regional Genetics.

Bieri, D., Reeves, R., Champion, G., et al. (1990). The Faces Pain Scale for the self-assessment of the severity of pain experienced by children: development, initial validation, and preliminary investigation for ratio scale properties. *Pain, 41*(2), 139–150.

Bijur, P. E., Berard, A., Esses, D. J., et al. (2006). Lack of influence of patient self-report of pain intensity on administration of opioids for suspected long-bone fractures. *The Journal of Pain*, 7(6), 438–444.

Bodfish, J. W., Harper, V. N., Deacon, J. M., et al. (2006). Issues in pain assessment for adults with severe to profound mental retardation. In T. F. Oberlander, & F. J. Symons (Eds.), *Pain in children and adults with developmental disabilities*. Baltimore: Paul H. Brookes.

Boly, M., Faymonville, M. E., Schnakers, C., et al. (2008). Perception of pain in the minimally conscious state with PET activation: An observational study. *Lancet Neurology*, 7(11), 1013–1020.

Bonnot, O., Anderson, G. M., Cohen, D., et al. (2009). Are patients with schizophrenia insensitive to pain? A reconsidertion of the question. *The Clinical Journal of Pain*, 25(3), 244–252.

Bottos, S., & Chambers, C. T. (2006). The epidemiology of pain in developmental disabilities. In T. F. Oberlander, & F. J. Symons (Eds.), *Pain in children and adults with developmental disabilities*. Baltimore: Paul H. Brookes.

Bouhassira, D., Attal, N., Fermanian, J., et al. (2004). Development and validation of the Neuropathic Pain Symptom Inventory. *Pain*, 108(3), 248–257.

Breau, L. M., MacLaren, J., McGrath, P. J., et al. (2003). Caregivers' beliefs regarding pain in children with cognitive impairment: relation between pain sensation and reaction increases with severity of impairment. *The Clinical Journal of Pain*, 19(6), 335–344.

Breau, L. M., McGrath, P. J., Camfield, C. S., et al. (2002). Psychometric properties of the non-communicating children's pain checklist-revised. *Pain*, 99(1–2), 349–357.

Breau, L. M., McGrath, P. J., & Zabalia, M. (2006). Assessing pediatric pain and developmental disabilities. In T. F. Oberlander, & F. J. Symons (Eds.), *Pain in children and adults with developmental disabilities*. Baltimore: Paul H. Brookes.

Breitbart, W., McDonald, M. V., Rosenfeld, B., et al. (1996). Pain in ambulatory AIDS patients. I: pain characteristics and medical correlates. *Pain*, 68(2–3), 315–321.

Breivik, H. (2005). Opioids in chronic non-cancer pain, indications and controversies. *European Journal of Pain (London, England)*, 9(2), 127–130.

Breslau, N. (2001). The epidemiology of posttraumatic stress disorder: what is the extent of the problem? *The Journal of Clinical Psychiatry*, 62(Suppl. 17), 16–22.

Bridge, D., Thompson, S. W. N., & Rice, A. S. C. (2001). Mechanisms of neuropathic pain. *British Journal of Anaesthesia*, 87(1), 12–26.

Brody, H. (1997). The doctor as therapeutic agent: a placebo effect research agenda. In A. Harrington (Ed.), *The placebo effect: An interdisciplinary exploration*. Cambridge, MA: Harvard University Press.

Brown, J. (1992). Nurses' analgesic choices and postoperative patients' perceived pain: the effect of a pain flow sheet. *Am J Pain Manage*, 2, 192–197.

Brown, R. L., Patterson, J. J., Rounds, L. A., et al. (1996). Substance abuse among patients with chronic low back pain. *The Journal of Family Practice*, 43(2), 152–160.

Bruera, E., Macmillan, K., Hanson, J., et al. (1989). The cognitive effects of the administration of narcotic analgesics in patients with cancer pain. *Pain*, 39(1), 13–16.

Bucknall, T., Manias, E., & Botti, M. (2007). Nurses' reassessment of postoperative pain after analgesic administration. *The Clinical Journal of Pain*, 23(1), 1–7.

Buffum, M. D., Hutt, E., Chang, V. T., et al. (2007). Cognitive impairment and pain management: Review of issues and challenges. *Journal of Rehabilitation Research and Development*, 44(2), 315–330.

Buffum, M. D., Miaskowski, C., & Sands, L. (2001). A pilot study of the relationship between discomfort and agitation in patients with dementia. *Geriatric Nursing*, 22(2), 80–85.

Buffum, M. D., Sands, L., Miaskowski, C., et al. (2004). A clinical trial of the effectiveness of regularly scheduled versus as-need administration of acetaminophen in the management of discomfort in older adults with dementia. *Journal of the American Geriatrics Society*, 52(7), 1093–1097.

Burgess, M. M. (1980). *Nurses' pain ratings of patients with acute and chronic low back pain*. Unpublished master's thesis. Charlottesville, VA: University of Virginia School of Nursing.

Burkitt, J. C., Breau, L. M., Salsman, S., et al. (2009). Pilot study of the feasibility of the non-communicating children's pain checklist revised for pain assessment for adults with intellectual disabilities. *J Pain Manage*, 2(1).

Bushnell, M. C. (1997). Commentaries. *European Journal of Pain (London, England)*, 1, 167.

Byas-Smith, M. G., Max, M. B., Muir, J., et al. (1995). Transdermal clonidine compared to placebo in painful diabetic neuropathy using a two-stage "enriched enrollment design." *Pain*, 60(3), 267–274.

California Board of Registered Nursing (BRN). (1997). BRN focuses on pain management. *BRN Report*, 10(1), 12.

Calvillo, E. R., & Flaskerud, J. H. (1993). Evaluation of the pain response by Mexican American and Anglo American women and their nurses. *Journal of Advanced Nursing*, 18(3), 451–459.

Capers, C. F. (1985). Nursing and the Afro-American client. *Topics in Clinical Nursing*, 7(3), 11–17.

Caraceni, A., Cherny, N., Fainsinger, R., et al. (2002). Pain measurement tools and methods in clinical research in palliative care: Recommendations of an Expert Working Group of the European Association of Palliative Care. *Journal of Pain and Symptom Management*, 23(3), 239–255.

Carey, S. J., Turpin, C., Smith, J., et al. (1997). Improving pain management in an acute care setting. *Orthopaedic Nursing/National Association of Orthopaedic Nurses*, 16(4), 29–36.

Carpenter, J. S., & Brockopp, D. (1995). Comparison of patients' ratings and examination of nurses' responses to pain intensity rating scales. *Cancer Nursing*, 18(4), 292–298.

Cassell, E. J. (1982). The nature of suffering and the goals of medicine. *The New England Journal of Medicine*, 306, 639–645.

Cepeda, M. S., Aficano, J. M., & Polo, R. (2003). What decline in pain intensity is meaningful to patients with acute pain? In J. O. Dostrovsky, D. B. Carr, & M. Kolzenburg (Eds.), *Proceedings of the 10th World Congress on Pain. Prog Pain Res Management*. 24, 601–609. Seattle: IASP Press .

Cervo, F., Bruckenthal, P., Bright-Long, L., et al. (2009). Pain assessment in nursing home residents with dementia: Psychometric properties and clinical utility of the CAN Pain Assessment Tool (CPAT). *JAMDA*, 10(7), 505–510.

Cervo, F. A., Raggi, R. P., Bright-Long, L. E., et al. (2007). Use of the certified nursing assistant pain assessment tool (CPAT) in nursing home residents with dementia. *American Journal of Alzheimer's Disease and Other Dementias*, 22(2), 112–119.

Chambers, C. T., & Craig, K. D. (1998). An intrusive impact of anchors in children's faces pain scales. *Pain*, 78, 27–37.

Chambers, C. T., Giesbrecht, K., Craig, et al. (1999). A comparison of faces scales for the measurement of pediatric pain: children's and parents' ratings. *Pain*, 83, 25–35.

Chambers, C. T., Hardial, J., Craig, K. D., et al. (2005). Faces scales for the measurement of postoperative pain intensity in children following minor surgery. *The Clinical Journal of Pain*, 21(3), 277–285.

Chapman, C. R. (2008). Progress in pain assessment: The cognitively compromised patient. *Current Opinion in Anesthesiology*, 21, 610–616.

Chen, L. M., Miaskowski, C., Dodd, M., et al. (2008). Concepts within the Chinese culture that influence the cancer pain experience. *Cancer Nursing*, 31(2), 103–108.

Cheng, Y., Lin, C. P., Liu, H. L., et al. (2007). Expertise modulates the perception of pain in others. *Current Biology: CB*, 17, 1706–1713.

Chibnall, J. T., & Tait, R. C. (2001). Pain assessment in cognitively impaired and unimpaired older adults: a comparison of four scales. *Pain*, 92, 173–186.

Chibnall, J. T., Tait, R. C., Harman, B., et al. (2005). Effect of acetaminophen on behavior, well-being, and psychotropic medication use in nursing home residents with moderate-to-severe dementia. *Journal of the American Geriatrics Society*, 53, 1921–1929.

Chu, L., Schnelle, J., Cadogan, M., et al. (2004). Using the minimum data set to select nursing home residents for interview about pain. *Journal of the American Geriatrics Society*, 52(12), 2057–2061.

Clancy, A. C., McGrath, P. F., & Oddson, B. E. (2005). Pain in children and adolescents with spina bifida. *Developmental Medicine and Child Neurology*, 47, 27–34.

Cleeland, C. S. (1984). The impact of pain on the patient with cancer. *Cancer*, 54, 2635–2641.

Cleeland, C. S., Gonin, R., Baez, L., et al. (1997). Pain and treatment of pain in minority patients with cancer: The Eastern Cooperative Oncology Group Minority Outpatient Pain Study. *Annals of Internal Medicine*, 127, 813–816.

Cleeland, C. S., Gonin, R., Hatfield, A. K., et al. (1994). Pain and its treatment in out-patients with metastatic cancer: The Eastern cooperative oncology group's outpatient study. *The New England Journal of Medicine*, 330, 592–596.

Cleeland, C. S., Ladinsky, J. L., Serlin, J. R. D., et al. (1988). Multidimensional measurement of cancer pain: comparisons of US and Vietnamese patients. *Journal of Pain and Symptom Management*, 3, 23–27.

Cleeland, C. S., Nakamura, Y., Mendoza, T. R., et al. (1996). Dimensions of the impact of cancer in a four country sample: New information from multidimensional scaling. *Pain*, 67, 267–273.

Cleeland, C. S., & Ryan, K. M. (1994). Pain assessment: global use of the brief pain inventory. *Annals of the Academy of Medicine*, 23, 129–138.

Cleeland, C. S., Serlin, R., Nakamura, Y., et al. (1997). Effects of culture and language on ratings of cancer pain and patterns of functional interference. In T. S. Jensen, J. A. Turner, & Z. Wiesenfeld-Hallin (Eds.), *Proceedings of the 8th World Congress on Pain. Pain Research & Management*. 8. 35–51.

Cleeland, C. S., & Syrjala, K. L. (1992). How to assess cancer pain. In D. C. Turk, & R. Melzack (Eds.), *Handbook of pain assessment*. New York: Guilford Press.

Closs, S. J. (1992). Patients' night-time pain, analgesic provision and sleep after surgery. *International Journal of Nursing Studies*, 29(4), 381–392.

Closs, S. J., Barr, B., Briggs, M., et al. (2004). A comparison of five pain assessment scales for nursing home residents with varying degrees of cognitive impairment. *Journal of Pain and Symptom Management*, 27(3), 196–205.

Closs, S. J., & Briggs, M. (2002). Patients' verbal descriptions of pain and discomfort following orthopedic surgery. *International Journal of Nursing Studies*, 39(5), 563–572.

Cohen, F. L. (1980). Postsurgical pain relief: Patients' status and nurses' medication choices. *Pain*, 9, 265–274.

Cohen, H., Neumann, L., Haiman, Y., et al. (2002). Prevalence of post-traumatic stress disorder in fibromyalgia patients: Overlapping symptoms or post-traumatic fibromyalgia syndrome? *Seminars in Arthritis and Rheumatism*, 32(1), 38–50.

Cohen, M. Z., Easley, M. K., Ellis, C., et al. (2003). Cancer pain management and the Joint Commission on Accreditation of Healthcare Organizations's (JACHO's) pain standards: an institutional challenge. *Journal of Pain and Symptom Management*, 25(6), 519–527.

Cohen-Mansfield, J., & Lipson, S. (2008). The utility of pain assessment for analgesic use in persons with dementia. *Pain*, 134(1–2), 16–23.

Cohen-Mansfield, J. (2006). Pain assessment in noncommunicative elderly persons: PAINE. *The Clinical Journal of Pain*, 22(6), 569–575.

Cohen-Mansfield, J. (2004). The adequacy of the minimum data set assessment of pain in cognitively impaired nursing home residents. *Journal of Pain and Symptom Management*, 27(4), 343–351.

Coley, K. C., Williams, B. A., DaPos, S. V., et al. (2002). Retrospective evaluation of unanticipated admissions and readmissions after same-day surgery and associated costs. *Journal of Clinical Anesthesia*, 14, 349–353.

Compton, P. (1999). Substance abuse. In M. McCaffery, & C. Pasero (Eds.), *Pain: Clinical manual*. (2nd ed.). St. Louis, MO: Mosby.

Cooke, B. K., Magas, L. T., Virgo, K. S., et al. (2007). Appendectomy for appendicitis in patients with schizophrenia. *American Journal of Surgery*, 193, 41–48.

Copeland, L. A., Zeber, J. E., Pugh, M. J., et al. (2008). Postoperative complications in the seriously mentally ill: A systematic review of the literature. *Annals of Surgery*, 248(1), 31–38.

Costardi, D., Rozzini, L., Costanzi, C., et al. (2007). The Italian version of the pain assessment in advanced dementia (PAINAD) scale. *Archives of Gerontology and Geriatrics*, 44(2), 175–180.

Cotton, P. (1994). "Harm reduction" approach may be middle ground. *JAMA: The Journal of the American Medical Association*, 271(21), 1641–1645.

Craig, K. (2006). The construct and definition of pain in developmental disability. In T. F. Oberlander, & F. J. Symons (Eds.), *Pain in children and adults with developmental disabilities*. Baltimore: Paul H. Brookes.

Cruise, C. E., Broderick, J., Porter, L., et al. (1996). Reactive effects of diary self-assessment in chronic pain patients. *Pain*, 67, 253–258.

Dalton, J. A., & McNaull, F. (1998). A call for standardizing the clinical rating of pain intensity using a 0 to 10 rating scale. *Cancer Nursing*, 21, 46–69.

Daumit, G. L., Pronovost, P. J., Anthony, C. B., et al. (2006). Adverse events during medical and surgical hospitalizations for persons with schizophrenia. *Archives of General Psychiatry*, *63*, 267–272.

Daut, R. L., & Cleeland, C. S. (1982). The prevalence and severity of pain in cancer. *Cancer, 50*, 1913–1918.

Daut, R. L., Cleeland, C. S., & Flanery, R. C. (1983). Development of the Wisconsin Brief Pain Questionnaire to assess pain in cancer and other diseases. *Pain, 17*, 197–210.

Dawson, R., Sellers, D. E., & Spross, J. A. (2005). Do patients' beliefs act as barriers to effective pain management behaviors and outcomes in patients with cancer-related or non-cancer-related pain? *Oncology Nursing Forum, 32*(2), 363–374.

De Conno, F., Ripamonti, C., Gamba, A., et al. (1989). Treatment of post-operative pain: comparison between administration at fixed hours and "on demand" with intra-muscular analgesics. *European Journal of Surgical Oncology: The Journal of the European Society of Surgical Oncology and the British Association of Surgical Oncology, 15*, 242–246.

de Moulin, D. (1979). A historical-phenomenological study of bodily pain in western man. *Bulletin of the History of Medicine, 48*(4), 540–570.

de Schepper, A. M. E., Francke, A. L., & Abu-Saad, H. H. (1997). Feelings of powerlessness in relation to pain: Ascribed causes and reported strategies. *Cancer Nursing, 20*, 422–429.

de Wit, R., van Dam, F., Hanneman, M., et al. (1999). Evaluation of the use of a pain diary in chronic cancer pain patients at home. *Pain, 79*, 89–99.

DeCarvalho, L. T., & Whealin, J. M. (2006). What pain specialists need to know about posttraumatic stress disorder in operation Iraqi freedom and operation enduring freedom returnees. *J Musculoskel Pain, 14*(3), 37–45.

Defrin, R., Ginzburg, K., Solomon, Z., et al. (2008). Quantitative testing of pain perception in subjects with PTSD: Implications for the mechanism of the coexistence between PTSD and chronic pain. *Pain, 138*, 450–459.

Defrin, R., Lotan, M., & Pick, C. G. (2006). The evaluation of acute pain in individuals with cognitive impairment: A differential effect of level of impairment. *Pain, 124*, 312–320.

Defrin, R., Pick, C. G., Peretz, C., et al. (2004). A quantitative somatosensory testing of pain threshold in individuals with mental retardation. *Pain, 108*, 58–66.

Dellemijn, P. L. I., & Fields, H. L. (1994). Do benzodiazepines have a role in chronic pain management? *Pain, 57*, 137–152.

DeLoach, L. J., Higgins, M. S., Caplan, A. B., et al. (1998). The visual analog scale in the immediate postoperative period: Intrasubject variability and correlation with a numeric scale. *Anesthesia and Analgesia, 56*, 102–106.

DeWaters, T., Faut-Callahan, M., McCann, J. J., et al. (2008). Comparison of self-reported pain and the PAINAD scale in hospitalized cognitively impaired and intact older adults after hip fracture surgery. *Orthopedic Nursing, 27*(1), 21–28.

Dix, P., Sandhar, B., Murdoch, J., et al. (2004). Pain on medical wards in a district general hospital. *British Journal of Anaesthesia, 92*(2), 235–237.

Donovan, J. (2002). Learning disability nurses' experiences of being with clients who may be in pain. *Journal of Advanced Nursing, 38*(5), 458–466.

Dreher, M., & MacNaughton, N. (2002). Cultural competence in nursing: Foundation or fallacy? *Nursing Outlook, 50*(5), 181–186.

Dudley, S. R., & Holm, K. (1984). Assessment of the pain experience in relation to selected nurse characteristics. *Pain, 18*(2), 179–186.

Dworkin, R. H., Turk, D. C., Farrar, J. T., et al. (2005). Core outcome measures for chronic pain clinical trials: IMMPACT recommendations. *Pain, 113*(1–2), 9–19.

Edlund, M. J., Steffick, D., Hudson, T., et al. (2007). Rick factors for clinically recognized opioid abuse and dependence among veterans using opioids for chronic non-cancer pain. *Pain, 129*(3), 355–362.

Egan, K. J., Ready, L. B., Nessly, M., et al. (1992). Self-administration of midazolam for postoperative anxiety: A double-blinded study. *Pain, 49*, 3–8.

Eich, E., Reeves, J. L., Jaeger, B., et al. (1985). Memory for pain: Relation between past and present pain intensity. *Pain, 23*, 375–379.

Epps, C. D., Ware, L. J., & Packard, A. (2008). Ethnic wait time differences in analgesic administration in the emergency department. *Pain Management Nursing, 9*(1), 26–32.

Ergun, U., Say, B., Ozer, G., et al. (2007). Trial of a new pain assessment tool in patients with low education: The full cup test. *International Journal of Clinical Practice, 61*(10), 1692–1696.

Errando, C. L., Sigl, J. C., Robles, M., et al. (2008). Awareness with recall during general anaesthesia: A prospective observational evaluation of 4001 patients. *British Journal of Anaesthesia, 101*(2), 178–185.

Ersek, M., Turner, J. A., Cain, K. C., et al. (2004). Chronic pain self-management for older adults: A randomized controlled trial. *BMC Geriatrics, 4*, 7. Available at http://www.biomed-central.com/1471-2318/4/7. Accessed August 18, 2009.

Evans, F. J. (1974). The placebo response in pain reduction. In *Advances in neurology*. (Vol. 4). New York: Raven Press.

Everett, J. J., Patterson, D. R., & Marvin, J. A. (1994). Pain assessment from patients with burns and their nurses. *The Journal of Burn Care & Rehabilitation, 15*, 194–198.

Ezenwa, M. O., Ameringer, S., Ward, S. E., et al. (2006). Racial and ethnic disparities in pain management in the United States. *Journal of Nursing Scholarship, 38*(3), 225–233.

Faries, J. E., Mills, D. S., Goldsmith, K. W., et al. (1991). Systematic pain records and their impact on pain control: A pilot study. *Cancer Nursing, 14*, 306–313.

Farrar, J. I., Young, J.P., Jr., LaMoreaux, L., et al. (2001). Clinical importance of changes in chronic pain intensity measured on an 11-point numerical pain rating scale. *Pain, 94*, 149–158.

Favaloro, R., & Touzel, B. (1990). A comparison of adolescents' and nurses' postoperative pain ratings and perceptions. *Pediatric Nursing, 16*, 414–417.

Feldt, K. (2007). Pain measurement: present concerns and future directions. *Pain Medicine (Malden, Mass.), 8*(7), 541–542.

Feldt, K. S. (2000). The checklist of nonverbal pain indicators (CNPI). *Pain Management Nursing, 1*(1), 13–21.

Feldt, K. S., Ryden, M. B., & Miles, S. (1998). Treatment of pain in cognitively impaired compared with cognitively intact older patients with hip-fracture. *Journal of the American Geriatrics Society, 46*(9), 1079–1085.

Ferraz, M. B., Quaresma, M. R., Aquino, L. R., et al. (1990). Reliability of pain scales in the assessment of literate and illiterate patients with rheumatoid arthritis. *The Journal of Rheumatology, 17*(8), 1022–1024.

Ferrell, B. A., Ferrell, B. R., & Rivera, L. (1995). Pain in cognitively impaired nursing home patients. *Journal of Pain and Symptom Management, 10,* 591–598.

Ferrell, B. R., Grant, M., Funk, B., et al. (1997). Quality of life in breast cancer. Part I: Physical and social well-being. *Cancer Nursing, 20,* 398–408.

Filoramo, M. A. (2007). Improving goal setting and goal attainment in patients with chronic noncancer pain. *Pain Management Nursing, 8*(2), 96–101.

Fine, B.G, & Portenoy, R. K. (2007). *A clinical guide to opioid analgesia.* Vendome Group.

Finniss, D. G., & Benedetti, F. (2005). Mechanisms of the placebo response and their impact on clinical trials and clinical practice. *Pain, 114*(1–2), 3–6.

Finniss, D. G., & Benedetti, F. (2007). Placebo analgesia, nocebo hyperalgesia. *Pain Clin Updates, 15*(1), 4.

Fishbain, D. A., Cole, B., Lewis, J., et al. (2008). What percentage of chronic nonmalignant pain patients exposed to chronic opioid analgesic therapy develop abuse/addiction and/or aberrant drug-related behaviors? A structured evidence-based review. *Pain Medicine (Malden, Mass.), 9*(4), 444–459.

Fishbain, D. A., Cutler, R., Rosomoff, H. L., et al. (1999). Chronic pain disability exaggeration/malingering and subamaximal effort research. *The Clinical Journal of Pain, 15,* 244–274.

Fishbain, D. A., Lewis, J. E., Cutler, R., et al. (2008). Can the neuropathic pain scale discriminate between non-neuropathic and neuropathic pain? *Pain Medicine (Malden, Mass.), 9*(2), 149–160.

Fishbain, D. A., Rosomoff, H. L., & Rosomoff, R. S. (1992). Drug abuse, dependence, and addiction in chronic pain patients. *The Clinical Journal of Pain, 8,* 77–85.

Fisher, F. B. (2004). Interpretation of "aberrant" drug behaviors. *J Am Phys Surg, 9*(1), 25–28.

Fleming, M. F., Balousek, S. L., Klessig, C. L., et al. (2007). Substance use disorders in a primary care sample receiving daily opioid therapy. *The Journal of Pain, 8*(7), 573–582.

Flood, P., & Daniel, D. (2004). Intranasal nicotine for postoperative pain treatment. *Anesthesiology, 101,* 1417–1421.

Folstein, M. L., Folstein, S. E. M., & McHugh, P. R. (1975). Mini-mental state: A practical method for grading the cognitive status of patients for the clinician. *Journal of Psychiatric Research, 12,* 189–198.

Fong, C. M. (1985). Ethnicity and nursing practice. *Topics in Clinical Nursing, 7,* 1–10.

Forbes, J. A. (1991). The nurse-observer: observation methods and training. In M. B. Max, R. K. Portenoy, & E. M. Laska (Eds.), *Adv Pain Res Therapy,* 18: 607–620.

Fox, A. E. (pseudonym). (1994). Confronting the use of placebos for pain. *The American Journal of Nursing, 94*(9), 42–46.

Fox, A. E. (pseudonym), McCaffery, M., Ferrell, B., et al. (1995). A place for placebos? Reply. *The American Journal of Nursing, 95*(2), 18.

Francke, A. L., & Theeuwen, I. (1994). Inhibition in expressing pain: A qualitative study among Dutch surgical breast cancer patients. *Cancer Nursing, 17,* 193–199.

Freyd, M. J. (1923). The graphic rating scale. *Journal of Educational Psychology, 14,* 83.

Freynhagen, R., Baron, R., Gockel, J., et al. (2006). painDE-TECT: A new screening questionnaire to detect neuropathic components in patients with back pain. *Current Medical Research and Opinion, 22*(10), 1911–1920.

Friedman, D. P. (1990). Perspectives on the medical use of drugs of abuse. *Journal of Pain and Symptom Management, 5,* S2–S5.

Fritz, D. J. (1988). Noninvasive pain control methods used by cancer outpatients. *Oncology Nursing Forum,* (Suppl.), 108.

Fuchs-Lacelle, S., & Hadjistavropoulos, T. (2004). Development and preliminary validation of the pain assessment checklist for seniors with limited ability to communicate (PACSLAC). *Pain Management Nursing, 5*(1), 37–49.

Fuchs-Lacelle, S., & Hadjistavropoulos, T. (2005). A checklist for pain assessment in LTC-PACSLAC: Pain assessment checklist for seniors with limited ability to communicate. *Can Nurs Home, 16*(4), 4–7.

Fuchs-Lacelle, S., Hadjistavropoulos, T., & Lix, L. (2008). Pain assessment as intervention: A study of older adults with severe dementia. *The Clinical Journal of Pain, 24*(8), 697–707.

Gagliese, L. (2001). Assessment of pain in the elderly. In D. C. Turk, & R. Melzack (Eds.), *Handbook of pain assessment.* New York: Guilford Press.

Gagliese, L., & Katz, J. (2000). Medically unexplained pain is not caused by psychopathology. *Pain Research & Management, 5*(4), 251–257.

Gagliese, L., & Katz, J. (2003). Age differences in postoperative pain are scale dependent: A comparison of measures of pain intensity and quality in younger and older surgical patients. *Pain, 103,* 11–20.

Gagliese, L., Weizblit, N., Ellis, W., et al. (2005). The measurement of postoperative pain: A comparison of intensity scales in younger and older surgical patients. *Pain, 117,* 412–420.

Galer, B. S., & Jensen, M. P. (1997). Development and preliminary validation of a pain measure specific to neuropathic pain: The neuropathic pain scale. *Neurology, 48,* 332–338.

Gan, T. J., Meyer, T. A., & Apfel, C. C. (2007). Society for ambulatory anesthesia guidelines for the management of postoperative nausea and vomiting. *Anesthesia and Analgesia, 105,* 1615–1628.

Gaston-Johansson, F. (1984). Pain assessment: differences in quality and intensity of the words pain, ache, and hurt. *Pain, 20,* 69–76.

Gaston-Johansson, F., Albert, M., Fagan, E., et al. (1990). Similarities in pain descriptions of four different ethnic-culture groups. *Journal of Pain and Symptom Management, 5,* 94–100.

Gear, R. W., Miaskowski, C., Heller, P. H., et al. (1997). Benzodiazepine mediated antagonism of opioid analgesia. *Pain, 71,* 25–29.

Geisser, M. E., Roth, R. S., Bachman, J. E., et al. (1996). The relationship between symptoms of post-traumatic stress disorder and pain, affective disturbance and disability among patients with accident and non-accident related pain. *Pain, 66*(2–3), 207–214.

Gelinas, C., & Arbour, C. (2009). Behavioral and physiologic indicators during a nociceptive procedure in conscious and unconscious mechanically ventilated adults: Similar or different? *Journal of Critical Care, 24,* 628e7–628e17.

Gelinas, C., Fillion, L., Puntillo, K. A., et al. (2006). Validation of the critical-care pain observation tool in adult patients. *American Journal of Critical Care, 15*(4), 420–427.

Gelinas, C., Fortier, M., Viens, C., et al. (2004). Pain assessment and management in critically ill intubated patients: A retrospective study. *American Journal of Critical Care, 13*(2), 126–135.

Gelinas, C., Harel, F., Fillion, L., et al. (2009). Sensitivity and specificity of the critical-care pain observation tool for the detection of pain in intubated adults after cardiac surgery. *Journal of Pain and Symptom Management*, 37(1), 58–67.

Gelinas, C., & Johnston, C. (2007). Pain assessment in the critically ill ventilated adult: Validation of the critical-care pain observation tool and physiologic indicators. *The Clinical Journal of Pain*, 23(6), 497–505.

Gendreau, M., Hufford, M. R., & Stone, A. A. (2003). Measuring clinical pain in chronic widespread pain: Selected methodological issues. *Best Practice & Research. Clinical Rheumatology*, 17, 575–592.

Geuze, E., Westenberg, G. M., Jochims, A., et al. (2007). Altered pain perception in veterans with posttraumatic stress disorder. *Archives of General Psychiatry*, 64, 76–85.

Gibson, S. J., Voukelatos, X., Amers, D., et al. (2001). An examination of pain perception and cerebral event-related potentials following carbon dioxide laser stimulation in patients with Alzheimer's disease and age-matched control volunteers. *Pain Research & Management*, 6(3), 126–132.

Gift, A. (1989). Visual analogue scales: Measurement of subjective phenomena. *Nursing Research*, 38, 286–288.

Gift, A. G., Plaut, D. M., & Jacox, A. K. (1986). Psychologic and physiologic factors related to dyspnea in subjects with chronic obstructive pulmonary disease. *Heart and Lung*, 15, 595–601.

Giger, J. N., & Davidhizar, R. E. (2008). *Transcultural nursing: Assessment and intervention* (5th ed.). St. Louis, MO: Mosby.

Gilron, J., Bailey, J. M., Tu, D., et al. (2005). Morphine, gabapentin, or their combination for neuropathic pain. *The New England Journal of Medicine*, 352, 1324–1334.

Gjeilo, K. H., Stenseth, R., Wahba, A., et al. (2007). Validation of the brief pain inventory in patients six months after cardiac surgery. *Journal of Pain and Symptom Management*, 34(6), 648–656.

Gloth, F. M., Scheve, A. A., Stober, C. V., et al. (2001). The Functional Pain Scale: Reliability, validity, and responsiveness in an elderly population. *Journal of the American Medical Directors Association*, 2, 110–114.

Goodwin, J. S., Goodwin, J. M., & Vogel, A. A. (1979). Knowledge and use of placebos by house officers and nurses. *Annals of Internal Medicine*, 91, 106–110.

Gordon, D. B., Pellino, T. A., Miaskowski, C., et al. (2002). A 10-year review of quality improvement monitoring in pain management: Recommendations for standardized outcome measures. *Pain Management Nursing*, 3(4), 116–130.

Gordon, D. B., & Ward, S. E. (1995). Correcting patient misconceptions about pain. *The American Journal of Nursing*, 95(7), 43–45.

Grace, P. J. (2006). The clinical use of placebos. *The American Journal of Nursing*, 106(2), 58–61.

Graffam, S. (1981). Congruence of nurse-patient expectations regarding nursing intervention in pain. *Nursing Leadership*, 4(2), 12–15.

Green, C. R., Anderson, K. O., Baker, T. A., et al. (2003). The unequal burden of pain: Confronting racial and ethnic disparities in pain. *Pain Medicine (Malden, Mass.)*, 4(3), 277–294.

Green, C. R., & Wheeler, J. R. C. (2003). Physician variability in the management of acute postoperative and cancer pain: A quantitative analysis of the Michigan experience. *Pain Medicine (Malden, Mass.)*, 4(1), 8–20.

Green, C. R., Wheeler, J. R. C., Marchant, B., et al. (2001). Analysis of the physician variable in pain management. *Pain Medicine (Malden, Mass.)*, 2(4), 317–327.

Grevert, P., Albert, L. H., & Goldstein, A. (1983). Partial antagonism of placebo analgesia by naloxone. *Pain*, 16, 129–143.

Grossman, H. J. (1983). *Classification in mental retardation*. Washington, DC: American Association on Mental Deficiency.

Grossman, S. A., Sheidler, V. R., Swedeen, K., et al. (1991). Correlation of patient and caregiver ratings of cancer pain. *Journal of Pain and Symptom Management*, 6, 53–57.

Gunnarsdottir, S., Donovan, H. S., Serlin, R. C., et al. (2002). Patient-related barriers to pain management: The barriers questionnaire II (BQ-II). *Pain*, 99, 385–396.

Haddad, A. (1993). Ethics in action: What would you do? *RN*, 56(3), 21–24.

Hadjistavropoulos, H. D., Ross, M. A., & von Baeyer, C. L. (1990). Are physicians' ratings of pain affected by patients' physical attractiveness? *Social Science & Medicine*, 31(1), 69–72.

Hadjistavropoulos, T. (2005). Assessing pain in older persons with severe limitations in ability to communicate. In S. Gibson, & D. Weiner (Eds.), *Pain in the elderly*. Seattle: IASP Press.

Hadjistavropoulos, T., Herr, K., Turk, D. C., et al. (2007). An interdisciplinary expert consensus statement on assessment of pain in older persons. *The Clinical Journal of Pain*, 23(1), S1–S43.

Hadjistavropoulos, T., LaChapelle, D., MacLeod, F., et al. (2000). Measuring movement-exacerbated pain in cognitively impaired frail elders. *The Clinical Journal of Pain*, 16(1), 54–63.

Hadjistavropoulos, T., MacNab, Y. C., Lints-Martindale, A., et al. (2009). Does routine pain assessment result in better care? *Pain Research & Management*, 14(3), 211–216.

Hagen, N. A., Stiles, C., Nekolaichuk, C., et al. (2008). The Alberta breakthrough pain assessment tool for cancer patients: A validation study using a Delphi process and patient think-aloud interviews. *Journal of Pain and Symptom Management*, 35(2), 136–152.

Halfens, R., Evers, G., & Abu-Saad, H. (1990). Determinants of pain assessment by nurses. *International Journal of Nursing Studies*, 27(1), 43–49.

Hall, G. M., & Salmon, P. (1997). Patient-controlled analgesia: Who benefits? *Anaesthesia*, 52, 401–402.

Hamers, J. P. H., van den Hout, M. A., & Halfens, R. J. G. (1997). Differences in pain assessment and decisions regarding the administration of analgesics between novices, intermediates and experts in pediatric nursing. *International Journal of Nursing Studies*, 34, 325–334.

Hampton, T. (2006). Are placebos in advanced cancer trials ethically justified? *Journal of American Medical Association*, 296(3), 265–266.

Hardy, J. D., Wolff, H. G., & Goodell, H. (1943). Pain threshold in man. *Proc Assoc Res Nerv Ment Dis*, 23, 1.

Harrison, A., Busabir, A. A., Al-Kaabi, A. O., et al. (1996). Does sharing a mother tongue affect how closely patients and nurses agree when rating the patient's pain, worry and knowledge? *Journal of Advanced Nursing*, 24, 229–235.

Hayes, M. H. S., & Patterson, D. G. (1921). Experiment development of the graphic rating scale. *Psychological Bulletin*, 18, 98–99.

Hazelett, S., Powell, C., & Androulakakis, V. (2002). Patients' behavior at the time of injury: Effect on nurses' perception of pain level and subsequent treatment. *Pain Management Nursing, 3*(1), 28–35.

Heins, A., Grammas, M., Heins, J. K., et al. (2006). Determinants of variation in analgesic and opioid prescribing practice in an emergency department. *Journal of Opioid Management, 2*(6), 335–340.

Heit, H. A., & Gourlay, D. L. (2009). DSM-V and the definitions: Time to get it right. *Pain Medicine (Malden, Mass.), 10*(5), 784–786.

Hendler, N. H., & Kozikowski, J. G. (1993). Overlooked diagnoses in chronic pain patients involved in litigation. *Psychosomatics, 34*(6), 494–504.

Hennequin, M., Faulks, D., & Allison, P. J. (2003). Parents' ability to perceive pain experienced by their child with Down syndrome. *Journal of Orofacial Pain, 17,* 347–353.

Hennequin, M., Morin, C., & Feine, J. S. (2000). Pain expression and stimulus localisation in individuals with Down syndrome. *Lancet, 356,* 1882–1887.

Herr, K., Bjoro, K., & Decker, S. (2006). Tools for assessment of pain in nonverbal older adults with dementia: A state-of-the-science review. *Journal of Pain and Symptom Management, 31*(2), 170–192.

Herr, K., Coyne, P. F., Key, T., et al. (2006). Pain assessment in the nonverbal patient: Position statement with clinical practice recommendation. *Pain Management Nursing, 7*(2), 44–52. Available at http://www.aspmn.org/Organization/documents/NonverbalJournalFINAL.pdf. Accessed August 18, 2009.

Herr, K., Spratt, K. F., Garand, L., et al. (2007). Evaluation of the Iowa Pain Thermometer and other selected pain intensity scales in younger and older adult cohorts using controlled clinical pain: A preliminary study. *Pain Medicine (Malden, Mass.), 8*(7), 585–600.

Herr, K., Titler, M. G., Schilling, M. L., et al. (2004). Evidence-based assessment of acute pain in older adults: Current nursing practices and perceived barriers. *The Clinical Journal of Pain, 20,* 331–340.

Herr, K. A., & Garand, L. (2001). Assessment and measurement of pain in older adults. *Clinics in Geriatric Medicine, 17,* 457–478.

Herr, K. A., & Mobily, P. R. (1993). Comparison of selected pain assessment tools for use with the elderly. *Applied Nursing Research: ANR, 6,* 39–46.

Herr, K. A., Spratt, K. S., Mobily, P. R., et al. (2004). Pain intensity assessment in older adults: Use of experimental pain to compare psychometric properties and usability of selected pain scales with younger adults. *The Clinical Journal of Pain, 20*(4), 207–219.

Hester, N. O. (1995). Integrating pain assessment and management into the care of children with cancer. In D. B. McGuire, C. H. Yarbro, & B. R. Ferrell (Eds.), *Cancer pain management.* Boston: Jones and Bartlett.

Hicks, C. L., von Baeyer, C. L., Spafford, P. A., et al. (2001). The Faces Pain Scale-Revised: Toward a common metric in pediatric pain measurement. *Pain, 93,* 173–183.

Hill, M. L., & Craig, K. D. (2002). Detecting deception in pain expressions: The structure of genuine and deceptive facial displays. *Pain, 98,* 135–144.

Hitchcock, L. S., Ferrell, B. R., & McCaffery, M. (1994). The experience of "chronic nonmalignant pain." *Journal of Pain and Symptom Management, 9*(5), 312–318.

Hoge, C. W., Castro, C. A., Messer, S. C., et al. (2004). Combat duty in Iraq and Afghanistan, mental health problems, and barriers to care. *The New England Journal of Medicine, 351*(Suppl. 1), 13–22.

Holen, J. C., Saltvedt, I., Fayers, P. M., et al. (2005). The Norwegian Doloplus-2, a tool for behavioral pain assessment: Translation and pilot-validation in nursing home patients with cognitive impairment. *Palliative Medicine, 19*(5), 411–417.

Holm, K., Cohen, F., Dudas, S., et al. (1989). Effect of personal pain experience on pain assessment. *Image–Journal of Nursing Scholarship, 21,* 72–75.

Hooley, J., & Delgado, M. (2001). Pain insensitivity in the relatives of schizophrenia patients. *Schizophrenia Research, 47,* 265–273.

Horgas, A. L., Nichols, A. L., Schapson, C. A., et al. (2007). Assessing pain in persons with dementia: Relationships among the non-communicative patient's pain assessment instrument, self-report, and behavioral observations. *Pain Management Nursing, 8*(2), 77–85.

Hurley, A. C., Volicer, B. J., Hanrahan, P. A., et al. (1992). Assessment of discomfort in advanced Alzheimer patients. *Research in Nursing & Health, 15*(5), 369–377.

Husebo, B., Strand, L., Moe-Nilssen, R., et al. (2009). Pain behavior and pain intensity in older persons with severe dementia: Reliability of the MOBID pain scale by video uptake. *Scandinavian Journal of Caring Sciences, 23*(1), 180–189.

Husebo, B. S., Strand, L. I., Moe-Nilssen, R., et al. (2007). Mobilization-observation-behavior-intensity-dementia pain scale (MOBID): Development and validation of a nurse-administered pain assessment tool for use in dementia. *Journal of Pain and Symptom Management, 34*(1), 67–80.

Husebo, B. S., Strand, L. I., Moe-Nilssen, R., et al. (2008). Who suffers most? Dementia and pain in nursing home patients: A cross-sectional study. *Journal of the American Medical Directors Association, 9*(6), 427–433.

Husskisson, E. C. (1974). Measurement of pain. *Lancet, 1,* 1127–1131.

IASP ad hoc Committee for Psychology Curriculum. (1997). *Curriculum on pain for students in psychology.* Seattle: International Association for the Study of Pain.

Ionescu, D., Badescu, C., & Acalovschi, I. (2007). Nicotine patch for the prevention of postoperative nausea and vomiting. *Clinical Drug Investigation, 27*(8), 559–564.

Jacox, A. (1979). Assessing pain. *The American Journal of Nursing, 79,* 895–900.

Jacox, A., Carr, D. B., Payne, R., et al. (1994a). *Management of cancer pain: Clinical practice guideline No. 9,* AHCPR Pub. No. 94-0592. Rockville, MD: Agency for Healthcare Policy and Research, U.S. Department of Health and Human Services, Public Health Service.

Jacox, A., Carr, D. B., Payne, R., et al. (1994b). *Management of cancer pain: Adults. Quick reference for clinicians. Clinical practice guideline No. 9,* AHCPR Pub. No. 94-0593. Rockville, MD: Agency for Healthcare Policy and Research, U.S. Department of Health and Human Services, Public Health Service.

Jamison, R. N., Raymond, S. A., Levine, J. G., et al. (2001). Electronic diaries for monitoring chronic pain: 1-year validation study. *Pain, 91,* 277–285.

Janssen, S. A., & Arntz, A. (1996). Anxiety and pain: Attentional and endorphinergic influences. *Pain, 56,* 145–150.

Jensen, M. P. (2003). The validity and reliability of pain measures in adults with cancer. *The Journal of Pain*, 4(7), 2–21.

Jensen, M. P., Chen, C., & Brugger, A. M. (2003). Interpretation of visual analog scale ratings and change scores: An .analysis of two clinical trials of postoperative pain. *The Journal of Pain*, 4(7), 407–414.

Jensen, M. P., Dworkin, R. H., Gammaitoni, A. R., et al. (2005). Assessment of pain quality in chronic neuropathic and nociceptive pain clinical trials with Neuropathic Pain Scale. *The Journal of Pain*, 6(2), 98–106.

Jensen, M. P., Friedman, M., Bonzo, D., et al. (2006). The validity of the Neuropathic Pain Scale for assessing diabetic neuropathic pain in a clinical trial. *The Clinical Journal of Pain*, 22(1), 97–103.

Jensen, M. P., & Karoly, P. (1992). Self-report scales and procedures for assessing pain in adults. In D. C. Turk, & R. Melzack (Eds.), *Handbook of pain assessment*. New York: Guilford Press.

Jensen, M. P., Miller, L., & Fisher, L. D. (1998). Assessment of pain during medical procedures: A comparison of three scales. *The Clinical Journal of Pain*, 14, 343–349.

Jensen, M. P., Turner, J. A., & Romano, J. M. (1994). What is the maximum number of levels needed in pain intensity measurement? *Pain*, 58, 387–392.

Jenson, M. P., & Karoly, P. (2001). Self-report scales and procedures for assessing pain in adults. In R. Melzack, & D. C. Turk (Eds.), *Handbook of pain assessment* (2nd ed.). New York: Guilford Press.

Jochum, T., Letzsch, A., Greiner, W., et al. (2006). Influence of antipsychotic medication on pain perception in schizophrenia. *Psychiatry Research*, 142, 151–156.

Johnston, C. C., Gangon, A. J., Pepler, C. J., et al. (2005). Pain in the emergency department with one-week follow-up of pain resolution. *Pain Research & Management*, 10, 67–70.

Joint Commission on Accreditation of Healthcare Organizations. (1994). *Accreditation manual for hospitals*. Oakbrook Terrace, IL: The Commission.

Jones, K. R., Fink, R., Hutt, E., Vojir, C., et al. (2005). Measuring pain intensity in nursing home residents. *Journal of Pain and Symptom Management*, 30(6), 519–527.

Kaasalainen, S., & Crook, J. (2003). A comparison of pain-assessment tools for use with elderly long-term-care residents. *The Canadian Journal of Nursing Research*, 35(4), 58–71.

Kagawa-Singer, M. (1987). Ethnic perspectives of cancer nursing: Hispanics and Japanese-Americans. *Oncology Nursing Forum*, 14, 59–65.

Kahn, D. L., & Steeves, R. H. (1996). The experience of suffering. In B. R. Ferrell (Ed.), *Suffering*. Boston: Jones and Bartlett.

Kallai, I., Barke, A., & Voss, U. (2004). The effects of experimenter characteristics on pain reports in women and men. *Pain*, 112, 142–147.

Kalyadina, S. A., Ionova, T. I., Ivanova, M. O., et al. (2008). Russian brief pain inventory: Validation and application in cancer pain. *Journal of Pain and Symptom Management*, 35(1), 95–102.

Kappesser, J., Williams, A. C., & Prkachin, K. M. (2006). Testing two accounts of pain underestimation. *Pain*, 124, 109–116.

Karp, J., Shega, J., Morone, N., et al. (2008). Advances in understanding the mechanisms and management of persistent pain in older adults. *British Journal of Anaesthesia*, 101(1), 111–120.

Katsma, D. L., & Souza, C. H. (2000). Elderly pain assessment and pain management knowledge of long-term care nurses. *Pain Management Nursing*, 1(3), 88–95.

Katz, E. R., Sharp, B., Kellerman, J., et al. (1982). Beta-endorphin immunoreactivity and acute behavioral distress in children with leukemia. *The Journal of Nervous and Mental Disease*, 170, 72–77.

Kelley, A., Siegler, E., & Reid, C. (2008). Pitfalls and recommendations regarding the management of acute pain among hospitalized patients with dementia. *Pain Medicine*, 9(5), 581–586.

Kemp, C. A., Ersek, M., & Turner, J. A. (2005). A descriptive study of older adults with persistent pain: Use and perceived effectiveness of pain management strategies. *BMC Geriatrics*, 5, 12. Available at http://www.biomedcentral.com/1471-2318/5/12. Accessed August 18, 2009.

Kerrane, T. A. (1975). The Brompton Cocktail. *Nursing Mirror*, 140, 59.

Ketovuori, H. (1987). Nurses' and patients' conceptions of wound pain and the administration of analgesics. *Journal of Pain and Symptom Management*, 2(4), 213–218.

Kim, H. S., Schwartz-Barcott, D., Tracy, S. M., et al. (2005). Strategies of pain assessment used by nurses on surgical units. *Pain Management Nursing*, 6(1), 3–9.

Kissen, B. (1997). Medical management of alcoholic patients. In B. Kissen, & H. Begleiter (Eds.), *The biology of alcoholism, vol. 5, Treatment and rehabilitation of the chronic alcoholic*. New York: Plenum.

Klein, M. (1997). Perception of pain in the persistent vegetative state? *European Journal of Pain (London, England)*, 1, 165–167.

Kleinman, I., Brown, P., & Librach, L. (1994). Placebo pain medication. *Archives of Family Medicine*, 3, 453–457.

Kovach, C. R., Noonan, P. E., Griffie, J., et al. (2002). The assessment of discomfort in dementia protocol. *Pain Management Nursing*, 3(1), 16–27.

Kovach, C. R., Noonan, P. E., Schlidt, A. M., et al. (2006). The Serial Trial Intervention: An innovative approach to meeting needs of individuals with dementia. *Journal of Gerontological Nursing*, 32(4), 18–25.

Krivo, S., & Reidenberg, M. M. (1995). Assessment of patient's pain. *The New England Journal of Medicine*, 334, 59.

Kudoh, A. (2005). Perioperative management for chronic schizophrenic patients. *Anesthesia and Analgesia*, 101, 1867–1872.

Kudoh, A., Ishihara, H., & Matsuki, A. (2000). Current perception thresholds and postoperative pain in schizophrenic patients. *Regional Anesthesia and Pain Medicine*, 25, 475–479.

Kudoh, A., Takahira, Y., Katagal, H., et al. (2002). Schizophrenic patients who developed postoperative confusion have increased nor-epinephrine and cortisol secretion. *Neuropsychobiol*, 46, 7–12.

Kulka, R. A., Schlenger, W., Fairbank, J., et al. (1990). *Trauma and the Vietnam War generation*. New York: Bruner/Mazel.

Kunz, M., Mykius, V., Scharmann, S., et al. (2009). Influence of dementia on multiple components of pain. *European Journal of Pain*, 13, 317–325.

Kunz, M., Prkachin, K., & Lautenbacher, S. (2009). The smile of pain. *Pain*, 145, 273–275.

Kunz, M., Scharmann, S., Hemmeter, U., et al. (2007). The facial expression of pain in patients with dementia. *Pain*, 133(1-3), 221–228.

LaChapelle, D. L., Hadjistavropoulos, T., & Craig, K. D. (1999). Pain measurement in persons with intellectual disabilities. *The Clinical Journal of Pain, 15*(1), 13–23.

Larue, F., Fontaine, A., & Colleau, S. M. (1997). Underestimation and undertreatment of pain in HIV disease: Multicentre study. *BMJ (Clinical Research Ed.), 3144*, 23–28.

Lavin, M. R. (1991). Placebo effects on mind and body. *JAMA: The Journal of the American Medical Association, 265*, 1753–1754.

Lawrence, M. (1995). The unconscious experience. *American Journal of Critical Care, 4*, 227.

Leavitt, F., & Sweet, J. J. (1986). Characteristics and frequency of malingering among patients with low back pain. *Pain, 25*, 357–364.

Lefebvre-Chapiro, S. (2001). The Doloplus 2 scale: Evaluating pain in the elderly. *Eur J Palliat Care, 8*(5), 191–194.

Lentschener, C., Tostivint, P., White, P. F., et al. (2007). Opioid-induced sedation in the postanesthesia care unit does not ensure adequate pain relief: A case-control study. *Anesthesia and Analgesia, 105*(4), 1143–1147.

Leong, I. Y., Chong, M. S., & Gibson, S. J. (2006). The use of a self-reported pain measure, a nurse-reported pain measure and the PAINAD in nursing home residents with moderate and severe dementia: A validation study. *Age and Ageing, 35*(3), 252–256.

Leucht, S., Burkard, T., Henderson, J., et al. (2007). Physical illness and schizophrenia: A review of the literature. *Acta Psychiatrica Scandinavica, 116*, 317–333.

Levine, F. M., & De Simone, L. L. (1991). The effects of experimenter gender on pain report in male and female subjects. *Pain, 44*, 69–72.

Levine, J. D., Gordon, N. C., & Fields, H. (1978). The mechanism of placebo analgesia. *Lancet, 2*, 654–657.

Levy, M. (1985). Pain management in advanced cancer. *Seminars in Oncology, 12*, 394–410.

Li, L., Liu, X., & Herr, K. (2007). Postoperative pain intensity assessment: A comparison of four scales in Chinese adults. *Pain Medicine (Malden, Mass.), 8*(3), 223–234.

Li, D., Puntillo, K., & Miaskowski, C. (2008). A review of objective pain measures for use with critical care adult patients unable to self-report. *The Journal of Pain, 9*(1), 2–10.

Lidstone, S. C., de la Fuente-Fernandez, R., & Stoessl, J. A. (2005). The placebo response as a reward mechanism. *Semin Pain Med, 3*, 37–42.

Lin, C., & Ward, S. (1995). Patient-related barriers to cancer pain management in Taiwan. *Cancer Nursing, 18*(1), 16–22.

Lind, L., Karlsson, D., & Fridlund, B. (2008). Patients' use of digital pens for pain assessment in advanced palliative home healthcare. *International Jorunal of Medical Informatics, 77*, 129–136.

Litt, M. D., Cooney, N. L., & Morse, P. (1998). Ecological momentary assessment (EMA) with treated alcoholics: Methodological problems and potential solutions. *Health Psychology, 17*, 48–52.

Louie, K. B. (1985). Providing health care to Chinese clients. *Topics in Clinical Nursing, 7*, 18–25.

MacDonald, V., & Hilton, B. (2001). Postoperative pain management in frail elderly adults. *Orthopaedic Nursing/National Association of Orthopaedic Nurses, 20*, 63–76.

Mader, T. F., Blank, F. S. J., Smithline, H. A., et al. (2003). How reliable are the pain scores? A pilot study of 20 healthy volunteers. *Journal of Emergency Nursing, 29*(4), 322–325.

Mahoney, A., & Peters, L. (2008). The Mahoney Pain Scale: Examining pain and agitation in advanced dementia. *American Journal of Alzheimer's Disease & Other Dementias, 23*(3), 250–261.

Malone, R. E. (1996). Almost like family: Emergency nurses and frequent flyers. *Journal of Emergency Nursing, 22*(3), 176–183.

Manfredi, P. L., Breuer, B., Wallenstein, S., et al. (2003). Opioid treatment for agitation in patients with advanced dementia. *International Journal of Geriatric Psychiatry, 18*(8), 700–705.

Marceau, L. D., Link, C., Jamison, R. N., et al. (2007). Electronic diaries as a tool to improve pain management: Is there any evidence? *Pain Medicine (Malden, Mass.), 6*(S3), S101–S109.

Marco, C. A., Plewa, M. C., Buderer, N., et al. (2006). Self-reported pain scores in the emergency department: Lack of association with vital signs. *Academic Emergency Medicine, 13*, 974–979.

Marquie, L., Raufaste, E., Lauque, D., et al. (2003). Pain rating by patients and physicians: evidence of systematic pain miscalibration. *Pain, 102*, 289–296.

Martell, B. A., O'Connor, P. G., Kerns, R. D., et al. (2007). Systematic review: Opioid treatment for chronic back pain: Prevalence, efficacy, and association with addiction. *Annals of Internal Medicine, 146*, 116–127.

Mateo, O., & Krenzischek, D. (1992). A pilot study to assess the relationship between behavioral manifestations and self-report of pain in postanesthesia care unit patients. *Journal of Post Anesthesia Nursing, 7*, 15–21.

Maxwell, C. (1978). Sensitivity and accuracy of the visual analogue scale: A psycho-physical classroom experiment. *British Journal of Clinical Pharmacology, 6*, 17–24.

Mayday Fund. (1993). *1993 Pain Survey*. New York: The Mayday Fund.

Mayday Fund. (1998). *Pain in America: A survey of American attitudes toward pain*. New York: The Mayday Fund.

Mayer, D. D. M., Torma, L., Byock, I., et al. (2001). Speaking the language of pain. *The American Journal of Nursing, 101*(2), 44–49.

Mazanee, P., & Tyler, M. K. (2003). Cultural considerations in end-of-life care. *The American Journal of Nursing, 103*(3), 50–58.

McAuliffe, L., Nay, R., O'Donnell, M., et al. (2008). Pain assessment in older people with dementia: Literature review. *Journal of Advanced Nursing, 65*(1), 2–10.

McCaffery, M. (1968). *Nursing practice theories related to cognition, bodily pain, and man-environment interactions*. Los Angeles: University of California at Los Angeles Students' Store.

McCaffery, M., & Arnstein, P. (2006). The debate over placebos in pain management. *The American Journal of Nursing, 106*(2), 62–65.

McCaffery, M., & Ferrell, B. (1991a). How would you respond to these patients in pain? *Nursing, 21*(6), 34–37.

McCaffery, M., & Ferrell, B. (1992c). Opioid analgesics: Addiction. *Age Conc, 1*(5), 1,4.

McCaffery, M., & Ferrell, B. (1995a). Are nurses' analgesic choices influenced by the pain rating scale used? 0-5 versus 0-10. *ASPMN Pathways, 4*(1), 3, 6.

McCaffery, M., Ferrell, B. R., & O'Neil-Page, E. (1992). Does life-style affect your pain-control decisions? *Nursing, 22*(4), 58–61.

McCaffery, M., Ferrell, B. R., & Pasero, C. L. (1998). When the physician prescribes a placebo. *The American Journal of Nursing*, 98(1), 52–53.

McCaffery, M., Ferrell, B. R., & Turner, M. (1996). Ethical issues in the use of placebos in cancer pain management. *Oncology Nursing Forum*, 23, 1587–1593.

McCaffery, M., & Ferrell, B. R. (1991b). Patient age: Does it affect your pain-control decisions? *Nurs*, 21(9), 44–48.

McCaffery, M., & Ferrell, B. R. (1992a). Does the gender gap affect your pain-control decisions? *Nurs*, 22(8), 48–51.

McCaffery, M., & Ferrell, B. R. (1992b). How vital are vital signs? *Nurs*, 22(1), 42–46.

McCaffery, M., & Ferrell, B. R. (1992d). Opioid analgesics: Nurses' knowledge of doses and psychological dependence. *Journal of Nursing Staff Development*, 8(2), 77–84.

McCaffery, M., & Ferrell, B. R. (1994). Say no to placebos. *The American Journal of Nursing*, 94(11), 20.

McCaffery, M., & Ferrell, B. R. (1995b). Nurses' knowledge about cancer pain: A survey of five countries. *Journal of Pain and Symptom Management*, 10(5), 356–369.

McCaffery, M., & Ferrell, B. R. (1996a). Correcting misconceptions about pain assessment and use of opioid analgesics: Educational strategies aimed at public concerns. *Nursing Outlook*, 44(4), 184–190.

McCaffery, M., & Ferrell, B. R. (1996b). Current placebo practice and policy. *ASPMN Pathways*, 5(4), 12–14 1.

McCaffery, M., & Ferrell, B. R. (1997a). Nurses' knowledge of pain assessment and management: How much progress have we made? *Journal of Pain and Symptom Management*, 14(3), 175–188.

McCaffery, M., & Ferrell, B. R. (1997b). Pain and placebos: Ethical and professional issues. *Orthopaedic Nursing/ National Association of Orthopaedic Nurses*, 16(5), 8–11.

McCaffery, M., Grimm, M. A., Pasero, C., et al. (2005). On the meaning of "drug seeking." *Pain Management Nursing*, 6(4), 122–136.

McCaffery, M., Pasero, C., & Ferrell, B. R. (2007). Nurses' decisions about opioid dose. *The American Journal of Nursing*, 107(12), 35–39.

McCaffery, M., & Pasero, C. (2001). Assessment and treatment of patients with mental illness. *The American Journal of Nursing*, 101(7), 69–70.

McCaffery, M., & Pasero, C. (1999). *Pain: Clinical manual.* (2nd ed.). St. Louis, MO: Mosby.

McCaffery, M., & Pasero, C. (1995). Are there circumstances that justify deceitful placebo use? *Pediatric Nursing* 21(6), 588.

McCaffery, M., & Robinson, E. S. (2002). Your patient is in pain: Here's how you respond. *Nursing*, 32(10), 36–45.

McCaffery, M., & Vourakis, C. (1992). Assessment and relief of pain in chemically dependent patients. *Orthopaedic Nursing/ National Association of Orthopaedic Nurses*, 11(2), 13–27.

McDonald, D. D., Shea, M., Rose, L., et al. (2009). The effect of pain question phrasing on older adult pain information. *Journal of Pain and Symptom Management*, 37(6), 1050–1060.

McGhee, L. L., Maani, C. V., Garza, T. H., et al. (2008). The correlation between ketamine and posttraumatic stress disorder in burned severe members. *The Journal of Trauma*, 64(2 Suppl.), S195–S198.

McGrath, P. J., Beyer, J., Cleeland, C., et al. (1990). Report of the subcommittee on assessment and methodological issues in the management of pain in childhood cancer. *Pediatrics*, 86(Suppl. 5), 814–817.

McGuire, D.B, & Sheidler, V. R. (1993). Pain. In S. L. Groenwald, M. H. Frogge, & M. Goodman, et al. (Eds.), *Cancer nursing: principles and practice.* (8th ed.). Chicago, Jones and Bartlett.

McIlveen, K. H., & Morse, J. M. (1995). The role of comfort in nursing care: 1900-1980. *Clinical Nursing Research*, 4, 127–148.

McMillan, S. C., Williams, F. A., Chatfield, R., et al. (1988). A validity and reliability study of two tools for assessing and managing pain. *Oncology Nursing Forum*, 15, 735–741.

Means, B., Nigam, A., Zarrow, M., et al. (1989). Autobiographical memory for health-related events. *Vital and Health Statistics*, 6, 1–37.

Melzack, R. (1975). The McGill Pain Questionnaire: Major properties and scoring methods. *Pain*, 1(3), 277–299.

Melzack, R. (1987). The short-form McGill Pain Questionnaire. *Pain*, 30, 191–197.

Melzack, R., Abbott, F. V., Zackon, W., et al. (1987). Pain on a surgical ward: A survey of the duration and intensity of pain and the effectiveness of medication. *Pain*, 29, 67–72.

Mentes, J. C., Teer, J., & Cadogan, M. P. (2004). The pain experience of cognitively impaired nursing home residents: Perceptions of family members and certified nursing assistants. *Pain Management Nursing*, 5(3), 118–125.

Merkel, S. I., Voepel-Lewis, T., Shayevitz, J. R., et al. (1997). The FLACC: A behavioral scale for scoring postoperative pain in young children. *Pediatric Nursing*, 23(3), 293–297.

Merskey, H., & Bogduk, N. (Eds.). (1994). *Classification of chronic pain* (2nd ed.). Seattle: IASP Press.

Miaskowski, C., Cleary, J., Burney, R., et al. (2005). *Guideline for the management of cancer pain in adults and children.* APS Clinical practice Guidelines Series, No. 3. Glenview, IL: American Pain Society.

Miller, R., Eisenkraft, J. B., Cohen, M., et al. (1986). Midazolam as an adjunct to meperidine analgesia for postoperative pain. *The Clinical Journal of Pain*, 2, 37–43.

Miro, J., Huguet, A., Nieto, R., et al. (2005). Evaluation of reliability, validity, and preference for a pain intensity scale for use with the elderly. *The Journal of Pain*, 6(11), 727–735.

Mitchel, S. W. (1982). Civilization and pain. *JAMA: The Journal of the American Medical Association*, 18, 108.

Moerman, D. E. (2000). Cultural variations in the placebo effect: Ulcers, anxiety, and blood pressure. *Medical Anthropology Quarterly*, 14, 1–22.

Moerman, D. E., & Harrington, A. (2005). Making space for the placebo effect in pain medicine. *Semin Pain Med*, 3, 2–6.

Moerman, H., Bonke, B., & Oosting, J. (1993). Awareness and recall during general anesthesia. *Anesthesiology*, 76(3), 454–464.

Morello, R., Jean, A., Alix, M., et al. (2007). A scale to measure pain in non-verbally communicating older patients: The EPCA-2 study of its psychometric properties. *Pain*, 133(1–3), 87–98.

Mularski, R. A., White-Chu, F., Overbay, D., et al. (2006). Measuring pain as the fifth vital sign does not improve quality of pain management. *J Gen Int Med*, 2(6), 607–612.

Nader, R., Oberlander, T. F., Chambers, C. T., et al. (2004). Expression of pain in children with autism. *The Clinical Journal of Pain*, 20(2), 88–97.

Negri, E., Bettaglio, R., Demartini, L., et al. (2002). Validation of the Italian version of the Neuropathic Pain Scale and its clinical applications. *Minerva Anestesiologica*, 68, 95–104.

Nelson, F. V., Zimmerman, L., Barnason, S., et al. (1998). The relationship and influence of anxiety on postoperative pain in the coronary artery bypass graft patent. *Journal of Pain and Symptom Management, 15*, 102–109.

Ng, B., Dimsdale, J. E., Rollnik, J. D., et al. (1996). The effect of ethnicity on prescriptions for patient-controlled analgesia for post-operative pain. *Pain, 66*, 9–12.

Nicholas, M. K. (2007). Mental disorders in people with chronic pain: An international perspective. *Pain, 129*, 231–232.

Nichols, R. (1996). Pain during sickle-cell crises. *The American Journal of Nursing, 96*, 59–60.

Nicholson, B., & Passik, S. D. (2007). Management of chronic noncancer pain in the primary care setting. *Southern Medical Journal, 100*(10), 1028–1036.

Nisbet, A. (2008). *Inova Sensory Assessment Scale* (Personal e-mail communication). Falls Church, VA: Inova Fairfax Hospital.

Noble, M., Tregear, S. J., Treadwell, J. R., et al. (2008). Long-term opioid therapy for chronic noncancer pain: A systematic review and meta-analysis of efficacy and safety. *Journal of Pain and Symptom Management, 35*(2), 214–228.

Norman, S. B., Stein, M. B., Dimsdale, J. E., et al. (2008). Pain in the aftermath of trauma is a risk factor for post-traumatic stress disorder. *Psychological Medicine, 38*, 533–542.

Nygaard, H. A., & Jarland, M. (2006). The checklist of nonverbal pain indicators (CNPI): Testing of reliability and validity in Norwegian nursing homes. *Age and Ageing, 35*(1), 79–81.

Odhner, M., Wegman, D., Freeland, N., et al. (2003). Assessing pain control in nonverbal critically ill adults. *Dimensions of Critical Care Nursing: DCCN, 22*(6), 260–267.

Office of National Drug Control Policy. (1997). *The national drug control strategy*. Washington, DC: GPO.

Oh, V.M.S (1994). The placebo effect: Can we use it better?. *BMJ (Clinical Research Ed.), 309*, 69–70.

Ostelo, R.W.J.G., Devo, R. A., & Stratford, P. (2008). Interpreting change scores for pain and functional status in low back pain. *Spine, 33*(1), 90–94.

Otis, J. D., Keane, T. M., & Kerns, R. D. (2003). An examination of the relationship between chronic pain and post-traumatic stress disorder. *Journal of Rehabilitation Research and Development, 40*(5), 397–406.

Otis, J. D., Keane, T. M., Kerns, R., et al. (2009). The development of an integrated treatment for veterans with comorbid chronic pain and posttraumatic stress disorder. *Pain Medicine (Malden, Mass.), 10*(7), 1300–3011.

Paice, J. A., & Cohen, F. L. (1997). Validity of a verbally administered numeric rating scale to measure cancer pain intensity. *Cancer Nursing, 20*, 88–93.

Paice, J. A., Noskin, G. A., Vanagunas, A., et al. (2005). Efficacy and safety of scheduled dosing of opioid analgesics: A quality improvement study. *The Journal of Pain, 6*(10), 639–643.

Paqueron, X., Lumbroso, A., Mergoni, P., et al. (2002). Is morphine-induced sedation synonymous with analgesia during intravenous morphine titration? *British Journal of Anaesthesia, 89*, 697–701.

Parmelee, P. A., Smith, B. D., & Katz, I. R. (1993). Pain complaints and cognitive status among elderly institution residents. *Journal of the American Geriatrics Society, 41*, 517–522.

Pasero, C. (2004). Pathophysiology of neuropathic pain. *Pain Management Nursing, 5*(4 Suppl. 1), 3–8.

Pasero, C., & McCaffery, M. (2002). Pain in the critically ill: New information reveals that one of the simplest procedures—turning—can be the most painful one. *The American Journal of Nursing, 102*(1), 59–60.

Pasero, C., & McCaffery, M. (2005). No self-report means no pain-intensity rating. *The American Journal of Nursing, 105*(10), 50–53.

Passik, S. D., Kirsh, K. L., Whitcomb, L., et al. (2004). A new tool to assess and document pain outcomes in chronic pain patients receiving opioid therapy. *Clinical Therapeutics, 26*(4), 552–561.

Passik, S. D., & Kirsh, K. L. (2004). Opioid therapy in patients with a history of substance abuse. *CNS Drugs, 18*(1), 13–25.

Pautex, S., Herrmann, F., Le Lous, P., et al. (2005). Feasibility and reliability of four pain self-assessment scales and correlation with an observational rating scale in hospitalized elderly demented patients. *The Journals of Gerontology. Series A, Biological Sciences and Medical Sciences, 60*(4), 524–529.

Pautex, S., Herrmann, F. R., Michon, A., et al. (2007). Psychometric properties of the Doloplus-2 observational pain assessment scale and comparison to self-assessment in hospitalized elderly. *The Clinical Journal of Pain, 23*(9), 774–779.

Pautex, S., Michon, A., Guedira, M., et al. (2006). Pain in severe dementia: Self-assessment or observational scales? *Journal of the American Geriatrics Society, 54*(7), 1040–1045.

Payen, J. F., Bosson, J. L., Chanques, G., et al. (2009). Pain assessment is associated with decreased duration of mechanical ventilation in the intensive care. *Anesthesiology, 111*(6), 1308–1316.

Payen, J. F., Bru, O., Bosson, J. L., et al. (2001). Assessing pain in critically ill sedated patients by using a behavioral pain scale. *Critical Care Medicine, 29*(12), 2258–2263.

Payne, R. (2007). Recognition and diagnosis of breakthrough pain. *Pain Medicine (Malden, Mass.), 8*(Suppl. 1), S3–S7.

Perkins, K. A., Grobe, J. E., Stiller, R. L., et al. (1994). Effects of nicotine on thermal pain detection in humans. *Experimental and Clinical Psychopharmacology, 2*(1), 95–106.

Pernick, M. S. (1985). *A calculus of suffering*. New York: Columbia University Press.

Perry, S., & Heidrich, G. (1982). Management of pain during débridement: A survey of U.S. burn units. *Pain, 13*, 267–280.

Pesonen, A., Kauppila, T., Tarkkila, P., et al. (2009). Evaluation of easily applicable pain measurement tools for the assessment of pain in demented patients. *Acta Anaesthesiologica Scandinaviac, 53*, 657–664.

Peters, M. L., Patijn, J., & Lame, I. (2007). Pain assessment in younger and older pain patients: psychometric properties and patient preference of five commonly used measures of pain intensity. *Pain Medicine (Malden, Mass.), 8*(7), 601–610.

Pitman, R. K., Sanders, K. M., Zusman, R. M., et al. (2002). Pilot study of secondary prevention of posttraumatic stress disorder with propranolol. *Biological Psychiatry, 51*(2), 189–192.

Pitman, R. K., van der Kolk, S. P., et al. (1990). Naloxone-reversible analgesic response to combat-related stimuli in posttraumatic stress disorder: A pilot study. *Archives of General Psychiatry, 47*(6), 541–544.

Pletcher, M. J., Kertesz, S. G., Kohn, M. A., et al. (2008). Trends in opioid prescribing by race/ethnicity for patients seeking care in US emergency departments. *JAMA: The Journal of the American Medical Association, 299,* 70–78.

Portenoy, R., for the ID Pain Steering Committee. (2006). Development and testing of a neuropathic pain screening questionnaire: ID Pain. *Current Medical Research and Opinion, 22*(1), 1555–1565.

Portenoy, R. K. (1994). Opioid therapy for chronic nonmalignant pain: Current status. In H. L. Fields, & J. C. Liebeskind (Eds.), *Progress in pain research and management, Vol. 1: Pharmacological approaches to the treatment of chronic pain: New concepts and critical issues.* Seattle: IASP Press.

Portenoy, R. K. (1996). Opioid analgesics. In R. K. Portenoy, & R. M. Kanner (Eds.), *Pain management theory and practice.* Philadelphia: FA Davis.

Portenoy, R. K., Bennett, D. S., Rauck, R., et al. (2006). Prevalence and characteristics of breakthrough pain in opioid-treated patients with chronic noncancer pain. *The Journal of Pain, 7*(8), 583–591.

Portenoy, R. K., Farrar, J. T., Backonja, M. M., et al. (2007). Long-term use of controlled-release oxycodone for noncancer pain: Results of a 3-year registry study. *The Clinical Journal of Pain, 23*(4), 287–299.

Portenoy, R. K., & Hagen, N. A. (1990). Breakthrough pain: Definition, prevalence and characteristics. *Pain, 41,* 273–281.

Portenoy, R.K, Payne, D., Jacobsen, P. (1999). Breakthrough pain: Characteristics and impact in patients with cancer pain. *Pain, 81,* 128–134.

Porter, F. L., Malhotra, K. M., Wolf, C. M., et al. (1996). Dementia and response to pain in the elderly. *Pain, 68,* 413–421.

Porter, J., & Jick, H. (1980). Addiction rare in patients treated with narcotics. *The New England Journal of Medicine, 302*(2), 123.

Porzelius, J. (1995). Memory for pain after nerve-block injections. *The Clinical Journal of Pain, 11,* 112–120.

Potvin, S., & Marchand, S. (2008). Hypoalgesia in schizophrenia is independent of antipsychotic drugs: A systematic quantitative review of experimental studies. *Pain, 138,* 70–78.

Poundja, J., Fikretoglu, D., Guay, S., et al. (2007). Validation of the French version of the brief pain inventory in Canadian veterans suffering from traumatic stress. *Journal of Pain and Symptom Management, 33*(6), 720–726.

Price, D. D., Chung, K. C., & Robinson, M. E. (2005). Conditioning, expectation, and desire for relief in placebo analgesia. *Semin Pain Med, 3,* 15–21.

Price, D. D., Long, S., Wilsey, B., et al. (1998). Analysis of peak magnitude and duration of analgesia produced by local anesthetics injected into sympathetic ganglia of complex regional pain syndrome patients. *The Clinical Journal of Pain, 14,* 216–226.

Prins, A., Quimette, P., Kimerling, R., et al. (2003). The primary care PTSD screen (PC-PDST): development and operating characteristics. *Prim Care Psychiat, 9*(1), 9–14.

Pud, D. (2004). Personal past experience with opioid consumption affects attitudes and knowledge related to pain management. *Pain Management Nursing, 5*(4), 153–159.

Pud, D., & Amit, A. (2005). Anxiety as a predictor of pain magnitude following termination of first-trimester pregnancy. *Pain Medicine (Malden, Mass.), 6*(2), 143–148.

Puntillo, K. A. (1990). Pain experiences of intensive care unit patients. *Heart and Lung, 19*(5), 526–533.

Puntillo, K. A. (1994). Dimensions of procedural pain and its analgesic management in critically ill surgical patients. *American Journal of Critical Care, 3,* 116–122.

Puntillo, K. A., Miaskowski, C., Kehrie, K., et al. (1997). Relationship between behavioral and physiological indicators of pain, critical care patients' self-reports of pain, and opioid administration. *Critical Care Medicine, 25,* 1159–1166.

Puntillo, K. A., Morris, A. B., Thompson, C. L., et al. (2004). Pain behaviors observed during six common procedures: Results from Thunder Project II. *Critical Care Medicine, 32*(2), 421–427.

Puntillo, K. A., White, C., Morris, A. B., et al. (2001). Patients' perceptions and responses to procedural pain: Results from Thunder Project II. *American Journal of Critical Care, 10*(4), 238–251.

Puntillo, K. A., Wild, L. R., Morris, A. B., et al. (2002). Practices and predictors of analgesic interventions for adults undergoing painful procedures. *American Journal of Critical Care, 11*(5), 315–429.

Raphael, K. G., & Marbach, J. J. (1997). When did your pain start? Reliability of self-reported age of onset of facial pain. *Pain, 13,* 352–359.

Reizien, A., & Meleis, A. (1986). Arab-Americans' perceptions of and responses to pain. *Critcial Care Nurse, 6,* 30–37.

Reynolds, K., Hanson, L., DeVellis, R., et al. (2008). Disparities in pain management between cognitively intact and cognitively impaired nursing home residents. *Journal of Pain and Symptom Management, 35*(4), 388–396.

Richardson, P. H. (1994). Placebo effects in pain management. *Pain Reviews, 1,* 15–32.

Richeimer, S. H., & Case, G. A. (2004). Ethical issues and problems of trust in the management of chronic pain. In C. A. Warfield, & Z. H. Bajwa (Eds.), *Principles and practice of pain management* (2nd ed.). New York: McGraw-Hill.

Rog, D. J., Nurmikko, T. J., Friede, T., et al. (2007). Validation and reliability of the neuropathic pain scale (NPS) in multiple sclerosis. *The Clinical Journal of Pain, 23*(6), 473–481.

Rosenfeld, B., Brietbart, W., McDonald, M. V., et al. (1996). Pain in ambulatory AIDS patients. II: Impact of pain on psychological functioning and quality of life. *Pain, 68,* 323–328.

Ross, R. S., Bush, J. P., & Crummette, B. D. (1991). Factors affecting nurses' decisions to administer prn analgesic medication to children after surgery: An analog investigation. *Journal of Pediatric Psychology, 16,* 151–167.

Rothman, K. J., & Michels, K. B. (1994). The continuing unethical use of placebo controls. *The New England Journal of Medicine, 331,* 394–397.

Rutledge, D. R., & Donaldson, N. E. (1998). Pain assessment and documentation. Part II: Special populations of adults. *Online J Clin Innov, 1*(6), 1–29.

Ryan, P., Vortherms, R., & Ward, S. (1994). Cancer pain: knowledge, attitudes of pharmacologic management. *Journal of Gerontological Nursing, 20*(1), 7–16.

Salmon, P., & Manyande, A. (1996). Good patients cope with their pain: Postoperative analgesia and nurses' perceptions of their patients' pain. *Pain, 68,* 63–68.

Salmore, R. (2002). Development of a new pain scale: Colorado behavioral numerical pain scale for sedated adult patients undergoing gastrointestinal procedures. *Gastroenterology Nursing*, 25(6), 257–264.

Savage, S. R. (2002). Assessment for addiction in pain-treatment settings. *The Clinical Journal of Pain*, 18, S28–S38.

Saxe, G., Stoddard, F., Courtney, D., et al. (2001). Relationship between acute morphine and the course of PTSD in children with burns. *Journal of the American Academy of Child and Adolescent Psychiatry*, 40(8), 915–921.

Scherder, E., Herr, K., Pickering, G., et al. (2009). Pain in dementia. *Pain*, 145, 276–278.

Scherder, E., Oosterman, J., Swaab, D., et al. (2005). Recent developments in pain in dementia. *BMJ (Clinical Research Ed.)*, 330(7489), 461–464.

Scherder, E. J., Sergeant, J. A., & Swaab, D. F. (2003). Pain processing in dementia and its relation to neuropathology. *Lancet Neurology*, 2(11), 677–686.

Schmitz Schneider, M. E., Jarvik, N. G. (1997). Nicotine. In J. H. Lowinson, P. Ruiz, & R. B. Millman, et al. (Eds.), *Substance abuse: A comprehensive textbook* (3rd ed.). Baltimore: Lippincott Williams & Wilkins.

Schuler, M., Njoo, N., Hestermann, M., et al. (2004). Acute and chronic pain in geriatrics: Clinical characteristics of pain and the influence of cognition. *Pain Medicine (Malden, Mass.)*, 5(3), 253–262.

Schuler, M. S., Becker, S., Kaspar, R., et al. (2007). Psychometric properties of the German Pain Assessment in Advanced Dementia Scale (PAINAD-G) in nursing home residents. *Journal of the American Medical Directors Association*, 8(6), 388–395.

Schumacher, K. L., Koresawa, S., West, C., et al. (2002). The usefulness of a daily pain management diary for outpatients with cancer-related pain. *Oncology Nursing Forum*, 29(9), 1304–1313.

Schwartz, A. C., Bradley, R., Penza, K. M., et al. (2006). Pain medication use among patients with posttraumatic stress disorder. *Psychosomatics*, 47(2), 136–142.

Schwartz, J. E., & Stone, A. A. (1998). Strategies for analyzing ecological momentary assessment data. *Health Psychology*, 17, 6–16.

Schwender, D., Kunze-Kronawitter, H., Dietrich, P., et al. (1998). Conscious awareness during general anaesthesia: Patients' perceptions, emotions, cognition and reactions. *British Journal of Anaesthesia*, 80, 133–139.

Serlin, R. C., Mendoza, T. R., Nakamura, Y., et al. (1995). When is cancer pain mild, moderate or severe? Grading pain severity by its interference with function. *Pain*, 61, 277–284.

Shapiro, D., & Jarvik, M. E. (1998). Pain inhibition, nicotine, and gender. *Experimental and Clinical Psychopharmacology*, 6(1), 96–106.

Shega, J. W., Hougham, G. W., Stocking, C. B., et al. (2004). Pain in community-dwelling persons with dementia: Frequency, intensity, and congruence between patient and caregiver report. *Journal of Pain and Symptom Management*, 28(6), 585–592.

Shega, J. W., Rudy, T., Keefe, F. J., et al. (2008). Validity of pain behaviors in persons with mild to moderate cognitive impairment. *J Am Geriatri Soc*, 56(9), 1631–1637.

Sherman, J. J., Turk, D. C., & Okifuji, A. (2000). Prevalence and impact of posttraumatic stress disorder-like symptoms on patients with fibromyalgia syndrome. *The Clinical Journal of Pain*, 16, 127–134.

Shipherd, J. C., Keyes, M., Jovanovic, T., et al. (2007). Veterans seeking treatment for posttraumatic stress disorder: What about comorbid chronic pain? *Journal of Rehabilitation Research and Development*, 44(2), 153–166.

Short, L. M., Burnett, M. L., Egbert, A. M., et al. (1990). Medicating the postoperative elderly: How do nurses make their decisions? *Journal of Gerontological Nursing*, 16(7), 12–17.

Simon, G. E., & Gureje, O. (1999). Stability of somatization disorder and somatization symptoms among primary care patients. *Archives of General Psychiatry*, 56, 90–95.

Singh, M. K., Giles, L. L., & Nasrallah, H. A. (2006). Pain insensitivity in schizophrenia: Trait or state marker? *Journal of Psychiatric Practice*, 12, 90–102.

Sloan, P. A., Donelly, M. B., Schwartz, R. W., et al. (1996). Cancer pain assessment and management by house staff. *Pain*, 67, 475–481.

Sloman, R., Wruble, A. W., Rosen, G., et al. (2006). Determination of clinically meaningful levels of pain reduction in patients experiencing acute postoperative pain. *Pain Management Nursing*, 7(4), 153–158.

Smith, M. P., & Sheplock, G. J. (1999). The anesthesiologist's guide to pain computing. *Regional Anesthesia and Pain Medicine*, 24, 458–462.

Smith, M. V., Egert, J., Winkel, G., et al. (2002). The impact of PTSD on pain experience in persons with HIV/AIDS. *Pain*, 98, 9–17.

Smith, W. B., & Safer, M. A. (1993). Effects of present pain level on recall of chronic pain and medication use. *Pain*, 55, 355–361.

Snow, A. L., Weber, J. B., O'Malley, K. J., et al. (2004). NOPPAIN: A nursing assistant-administered pain assessment instrument for use in dementia. *Dementia and Geriatric Cognitive Disorders*, 17(3), 240–246.

Sokka, T. (2005). Assessment of pain in rheumatic diseases. *Clinical and Experimental Rheumatology*, 23, S77–S84.

Spagrud, L. J., Piirao, T., & von Baeyer, C. L. (2003). Children's self-report of pain intensity. *The American Journal of Nursing*, 103(12), 62–64.

Spross, J. A. (1993). Pain, suffering, spiritual well-being: assessment and interventions. *Qual Life*, 2, 71–79.

Stanik-Hutt, J. A., Soeken, K. L., Belcher, A. E., et al. (2001). Pain experiences of traumatically injured patients in a critical care setting. *American Journal of Critical Care*, 10(4), 252–259.

Stephens, S. T. (1994). A promise to Billie. *Nursing*, 24(4), 96.

Stolee, P., Hillier, L. M., Esbaugh, J., et al. (2005). Instruments for the assessment of pain in older persons with cognitive impairment. *Journal of the American Geriatrics Society*, 53(2), 319–326.

Stolee, P., Hillier, L. M., Esbaugh, J., et al. (2007). Pain assessment in a geriatric psychiatry program. *Pain Research & Management*, 12(4), 273–280.

Stone, A. A., Broderick, J. E., Schwartz, J. E., et al. (2003). Intensive momentary reporting of pain with an electronic diary: Reactivity, compliance, and patient satisfaction. *Pain*, 104, 343–351.

Stone, A. A., Shiffman, S., Schwartz, J. E., et al. (2002). Patient non-compliance with paper diaries. *British Medical Journal*, 324, 1193–1194.

Sullivan, M., Terman, G. W., Peck, B., et al. (2005). APS position statement on the use of placebos in pain management. *The Journal of Pain*, 6(4), 215–217.

Symons, F. J., Shinde, S. K., & Gilles, E. (2008). Perspectives on pain and intelleactual disability. *Journal of Intellectual Disability Research, 52*(4), 275–286.

Syrjala, K. L. (1987). The measurement of pain. In C. H. Yarbo, & D. B. McGuire (Eds.), *Cancer pain: Nursing management.* Orlando, FL: Grune & Stratton.

Syrjala, K. L. (1993). Integrating medical and psychological treatments for cancer pain. In C. R. Chapman, & K. M. Foley (Eds.), *Current and emerging issues in cancer pain: Research and practice.* New York: Raven Press.

Tan, T., Fink, B., Dao, T. K., et al. (2009). Associations among pain, PTSD, and heart rate. variability in veterans of operation enduring and Iraqi freedom: A pilot study. *Pain Medicine (Malden, Mass.), 10*(7), 1237–1245.

Tan, G., Jensen, M. P., Thornby, J. I., et al. (2004). Validation of the brief pain inventory for chronic nonmalignant pain. *The Journal of Pain, 5*(2), 133–137.

Taylor, A. G., Skelton, J. A., & Butcher, J. (1984). Duration of pain condition and physical pathology as determinants of nurses' assessments of patients in pain. *Nursing Research, 33*, 4–8.

Taylor, D. R., Webster, L. R., Chun, S. Y., et al. (2007). Impact of breakthrough pain on quality of life in patients with chronic, noncancer pain: Patient perceptions and effect of treatment with oral transmucosal fentanyl citrate (OTFC, ACTIQ). *Pain Medicine (Malden, Mass.), 8*(3), 281–288.

Taylor, L. J., Harris, J., Epps, C. D., et al. (2005). Psychometric evaluation of selected pain intensity scales for use with cognitively impaired and cognitively intact older adults. *Rehabilitation Nursing, 30*(2), 55–61.

Taylor, L. J., & Herr, K. (2003). Pain intensity assessment: A comparison of selected pain intensity scales for use in cognitively intact and cognitively impaired African American older adults. *Pain Management Nursing, 4*(2), 87–95.

Taylor, N. M., Hall, G. M., & Salmon, P. (1996a). Is patient-controlled analgesia controlled by the patient? *Social Science & Medicine, 43*, 1137–1143.

Taylor, N. M., Hall, G. M., & Salmon, P. (1996b). Patients' experiences of patient-controlled analgesia. *Anaesthesia, 51*, 525–528.

Teasell, R. W., & Merskey, H. (1997). Chronic pain disability in the workplace. *Pain Research & Management, 2*(4), 197–204.

Terry, R., Niven, C., Brodie, E., et al. (2007). An exploration of the relationship between anxiety; expectations and memory for postoperative pain. *Acute Pain, 9*, 135–143.

Todd, K. H., Deaton, C., d'Adamo, A. P., et al. (2000). Ethnicity and analgesic practice. *Annals of Emergency Medicine, 35*(1), 11–16.

Todd, K. H., Samaroo, N., & Hoffman, J. R. (1993). Ethnicity as a risk factor for inadequate emergency department analgesia. *JAMA: The Journal of the American Medical Association, 269*(12), 1537–1539.

Turk, D. C. (2002). Remember the distinction between malignant and benign pain? Well, forget it. *The Clinical Journal of Pain, 18*(2), 75–76.

Turk, D. C., & Okifuji, A. (1997). What factors affect physicians' decisions to prescribe opioids for chronic noncancer pain patients? *The Clinical Journal of Pain, 13*, 330–336.

Turk, M. A., Geremski, C. A., Rosenbaum, P. F., et al. (1997). The health status of women with cerebral palsy. *Archives of Physical Medicine and Rehabilitation, 78*, S10–S17.

Turner, J. A., Deyo, R. A., Loeser, J. D., et al. (1994). The importance of placebo effects in pain treatment and research. *Journal of American Medical Association, 271*(20), 1609–1614.

Twycross, R. G. (1974). Clinical experience with diamorphine in advanced malignant disease. *International Journal of Clinical Pharmacology, Therapy and Toxicology, 9*, 184–198.

Twycross, R., Harcourt, J., & Bergl, S. (1996). A survey of pain in patients with advanced cancer. *Journal of Pain and Symptom Management, 12*, 273–282.

Twycross, R. G., & Wald, S. J. (1976). Long-term use of diamorphine in advanced cancer. In J. J. Bonica, & D. Albe-Fessard (Eds.), *Advances in pain research and therapy* (Vol. 1). New York: Raven Press.

Uki, J., Mendoza, T., Cleeland, C., et al. (1998). A brief cancer pain assessment tool in Japanese: The utility of the Japanese brief pain inventory—BPI-J. *Journal of Pain and Symptom Management, 16*(6), 364–373.

van Cleve, L., Johnson, L., & Pothier, P. (1996). Pain responses of hospitalized infants and children to venipuncture and intravenous cannulation. *Journal of Pediatric Nursing, 11*, 161–168.

van den Berg, J. H. (1963). *Leven in meervoud.* Nijkerk, GF: Callenback.

van Herk, R., van Dijk, M., Baar, F. P., et al. (2007). Observation scales for pain assessment in older adults with cognitive impairments or communication difficulties. *Nursing Research, 56*(1), 34–43.

van Herk, R., van Dijk, M., Biemold, N., et al. (2009). Assessment of pain: Can caregivers or relatives rate pain in nursing home residents? *Journal of Clinical Nursing, 18*, 2478–2485.

van Herk, R., van Dijk, M., Tibboel, D., et al. (2009). The Rotterdam Elderly Pain Observation Scale (REPOS): A New Behavioral Pain Scale for Non-Communicative Adults and Cognitively Impaired Elderly Persons. *J Pain Manage, 1*(4), 367–378.

van Iersel, T., Timmerman, D., & Mullie, A. (2006). Introduction of a pain scale for palliative care patients with cognitive impairment. *International Journal of Palliative Nursing, 12*(2), 54–59.

van Nispen tot Pannerden, S., Candel, M., Zwakhalen, S., et al. (2009). An item response theory-based assessment of the Pain Assessment Checklist for Seniors with Limited Ability to Communicate (PACSLAC). *The Journal of Pain, 10*(8), 844–853.

Victor, L., & Richeimer, S. H. (2005). Trustworthiness as a clinical variable: The problem of trust in the management of chronic, nonmalignant pain. *Pain Medicine (Malden, Mass.), 6*(5), 385–391.

Victor, T. W., Jensen, M. P., Gammaitoni, A. R., et al. (2008). The dimensions of pain quality: Factor analysis of the pain quality assessment scale. *The Clinical Journal of Pain, 24*(6), 550–555.

Villano, C. L., Rosenblum, A., Magura, S., et al. (2007). Prevalence and correlates of posttraumatic stress disorder and chronic severe pain in psychiatric outpatients. *Journal of Rehabilitation Research and Development, 44*(2), 167–178.

Virit, O., Savas, H. A., & Altindag, A. (2008). Lack of pain in schizophrenia: A patient whose arm was burned and amputated. *General Hospital Psychiatry, 30*, 384–385.

Vlaeyen, J. W. S., & Crombez, G. (2007). Fear and pain. *Pain Clin Updates, 15*(6), 104.

Voepel-Lewis, T., Zanotti, J., & Dammeyer, J. A. (2010). Reliability and validity of the face, legs, activity, cry, consolability behavioral tool in assessing acute pain in critically ill patients. *American Journal of Critical Care, 19*(1), 55–62.

von Baeyer, C. L., & Hicks, C. L. (2000). Support for a common metric for pediatric pain intensity scales. *Pain Research & Management, 5*(2), 157–160.

Von Roenn, J. H., Cleeland, C. S., Gonin, R., et al. (1993). Physician attitudes and practice in cancer pain management: A survey from the Eastern Cooperative Oncology Group. *Annals of Internal Medicine, 119*, 121–126.

Waddell, G., Main, C. J., Morris, E. W., et al. (1984). Chronic low-back pain, psychological distress, and illness behavior. *Spine, 9*, 209–213.

Wall, P. D. (1992). The placebo effect: An unpopular topic. *Pain, 51*(1), 1–3.

Wall, P. D. (1993). Reply to E. Leskowitz. *Pain, 53*(1), 115.

Wang, X. S., Mendoza, T. R., Gao, S. Z., et al. (1996). The Chinese version of the Brief Pain Inventory (BPI-C): Its development and use in a study of cancer pain. *Pain, 67*, 407–416.

Ward, S. (2008). (Personal communication.) Madison, WI: University of Wisconsin School of Medicine and Public Health.

Ward, S. E., Goldberg, N., Miller-McCauley, V., et al. (1993). Patient-related barriers to management of cancer pain. *Pain, 52*, 319–324.

Ward, S. E., & Gordon, D. B. (1996). Patient satisfaction and pain severity as outcomes in pain management: A longitudinal view of one setting's experience. *Journal of Pain and Symptom Management, 11*(4), 242–251.

Ward, S. E., & Hernandez, L. (1994). Patient related barriers to management of cancer pain in Puerto Rico. *Pain, 58*, 233–238.

Warden, V., Hurley, A. C., & Volicer, L. (2003). Development and psychometric evaluation of the pain assessment in advanced dementia (PAINAD) scale. *Journal of the American Medical Directors Association, 4*(1), 9–15.

Ware, L., Epps, D. F., Herr, K., et al. (2006). Evaluation of the revised faces pain scale, verbal descriptor scale, numeric rating scale, and Iowa pain thermometer in older minority adults. *Pain Management Nursing, 7*(3), 117–125.

Watson, G. D., Chandarana, P. C., & Merskey, H. (1981). Relationships between pain and schizophrenia. *The British Journal of Psychiatry, 138*, 33–36.

Weibe, E., Pudhradsky, L., & Dijak, V. (2003). The effect of lorazepam on pain and anxiety in abortion. *Contraception, 67*, 219–221.

Weiner, D. K., & Herr, K. (2002). Comprehensive interdisciplinary assessment and treatment planning: An integrative overview. In D. Weiner, K. Herr, & T. Rudy (Eds.), *Persistent pain in older adults: An interdisciplinary guide for treatment*. New York: Springer.

Weiner, D. K., Peterson, B. L., Logue, P., et al. (1998). Predictors of pain self-report in nursing home residents. *Aging, 10*, 411–420.

Weisberg, J. N., & Boatwright, B. A. (2007). Mood, anxiety and personality traits and states in chronic pain. *Pain, 133*(1–3), 1–2.

Weissman, D. E., & Haddox, J. D. (1989). Opioid pseudoaddiction—an iatrogenic syndrome. *Pain, 36*(3), 363–366.

Wells, N. (1989). Management of pain during abortion. *Journal of Advanced Nursing, 14*, 56–62.

Wesson, D. R., & Smith, D. E. (1990). Prescription drug abuse: patients, physician, and cultural responsibilities. *The Western Journal of Medicine, 152*(5), 613–616.

Whipple, B., & Komisaruk, B. R. (1985). Elevation of pain threshold by vaginal stimulation in women. *Pain, 21*, 357–367.

Wiener, C. L. (1975). Pain assessment on an orthopedic ward. *Nursing Outlook, 23*, 508–516.

Wilkie, D., Lovejoy, N., Dodd, M., et al. (1988). Cancer pain control behaviors: Description and correlation with pain intensity. *Oncology Nursing Forum, 15*(6), 723–731.

Wilkie, D. F., & Keefe, F. J. (1991). Coping strategies of patients with lung cancer-related pain. *The Clinical Journal of Pain, 7*, 292–299.

Wolf, S., & Pinsky, R. H. (1954). Effects of placebo administration and occurrence of toxic reactions. *JAMA: The Journal of the American Medical Association, 155*, 339–341.

Wong, D., & Baker, C. (1988). Pain in children: Comparison of assessment scales. *Pediatric Nursing, 14*, 9–17.

Wong, D., & Baker, C. (1995). *Reference manual for the Wong-Baker FACES pain rating scale*. Tulsa, OK: Wong & Baker.

Wong, D., & Baker, C. M. (2001). Smiling face as anchor for pain intensity scales. *Pain, 89*, 295–297.

Wynne, C. F., Ling, S. M., & Remsburg, R. (2000). Comparison of pain assessment instruments in cognitively intact and cognitively impaired nursing home residents. *Geriatric Nursing (New York, N. Y.), 21*(1), 20–23.

Yeager, K. A., Miaskowski, C., Dibble, S., et al. (1997). Differences in pain knowledge in cancer patients with and without pain. *Cancer Practice, 5*(1), 39–45.

Zalon, M. L. (1993). Nurses' assessment of postoperative patients' pain. *Pain, 54*, 329–334.

Zelman, D. C., Gore, M., Dukes, E., et al. (2005). Validation of a modified version of the brief pain inventory for painful diabetic peripheral neuropathy. *Journal of Pain and Symptom Management, 29*(4), 401–410.

Zelman, D. C., Smith, M. Y., Hoffman, D., et al. (2004). Acceptable, manageable, and tolerable days: Patient daily goals for medication management of persistent pain. *Journal of Pain and Symptom Management, 28*(5), 474–487.

Zimmerman, L., Story, K. T., Gaston-Johansson, F., et al. (1996). Psychological variables and cancer pain. *Cancer Nursing, 19*, 44–53.

Zwakhalen, S. M., Hamers, J. P., Abu-Saad, H. H., et al. (2006). Pain in elderly people with severe dementia: A systematic review of behavioural pain assessment tools. *BMC Geriatrics, 6*, 3.

Zwakhalen, S. M., Hamers, J. P., & Berger, M. P. (2007). Improving the clinical usefulness of a behavioural pain scale for older people with dementia. *Journal of Advanced Nursing, 58*(5), 493–502.

Zwakhalen, S. M. G., Hamers, J. P. H., & Berger, M. P. F. (2006). The psychometric quality and clinical usefulness of three pain assessment tools for elderly people with dementia. *Pain, 126*(1–3), 210–220.

Zwakhalen, S. M. G., van Dongen, K. A. J., Hamers, J. P. H., et al. (2004). Pain assessment in intellectually disabled people: Non-verbal indicators. *Journal of Advanced Nursing, 45*(3), 236–245.

Nonopioid Analgesics

Chris Pasero, Russell K. Portenoy,
and Margo McCaffery

Terminology

Acetaminophen Other generic names include *paracetamol* and *acetylparaaminophenol* (APAP). Also referred to as "aspirin-free."

Addiction A chronic neurologic and biologic disease. As defined by pain specialists, it is characterized by behaviors that include one or more of the following: impaired control over drug use, compulsive use, continued use despite harm, and craving. Continued craving for an opioid and the need to use the opioid for effects other than pain relief. Physical dependence and tolerance are not the same as addiction.

Adjuvant analgesic A drug that has a primary indication other than pain (e.g., anticonvulsant, antidepressant, sodium channel blocker, and muscle relaxant) but is analgesic for some painful conditions.

Analgesic ceiling A dose beyond which further increases in dose do not provide additional analgesia.

Bioavailability The extent to which a dose of a drug reaches its site of action.

Breakthrough dose (BTD) Also referred to as *supplemental dose* or *rescue dose;* the dose of analgesic taken to treat breakthrough pain.

Breakthrough pain (BTP) A transitory increase in pain that occurs on a background of otherwise controlled persistent pain.

Ceiling effect A dose above which further dose increments produce no change in effect.

Comfort-function goal This consists of the pain rating identified by the individual patient above which the patient experiences interference with function and quality of life, that is, activities that the patient needs or wishes to perform.

Distribution half-life The time it takes a drug to move from the blood and plasma to other tissues. Distribution half-life differs from half-life (terminal) (see **half-life**).

Efficacy The extent to which a drug or another treatment "works" and can produce the effect in question—analgesia in this context. To determine whether this is the case, the treatment must be compared to another, typically a placebo, but sometime an active comparator. Maximal efficacy refers to the maximum effect that can be produced by a drug, and comparative efficacy refers to the relative effects of two or more treatments compared at comparable treatment intensities.

Half-life The time it takes for the plasma concentration (amount of drug in the body) to be reduced by 50%. After starting a drug or increasing its dose, four to five half-lives are required to approach a steady-state level in the blood, irrespective of the dose, dosing interval, or route of administration; after four to five half-lives, a drug that has been discontinued generally is considered to be mostly eliminated from the body.

Hydrophilic Readily absorbed in aqueous solution.

Hyperalgesia Increased pain response to noxious stimuli.

Intractable In reference to pain that is unresponsive to all other recommended therapeutic options (e.g., first-line and second-line analgesics).

Lipophilic Readily absorbed in fatty tissues.

Medically ill patients Patients with existing debilitating pathologic condition/illness that may be progressive or stable, as opposed to those who have only the symptom of pain and are otherwise healthy.

Metabolite The product of biochemical reactions during drug metabolism.

Narcotic See Opioid. Obsolete term for *opioid*, in part because the government and media use the term loosely to refer to a variety of substances of potential abuse. Legally, controlled substances classified as narcotics include opioids, cocaine, and various other substances.

Neuropathic pain Neuropathic pain is pain sustained by injury or dysfunction of the peripheral or central nervous systems.

Nociceptive pain Pain that is sustained by ongoing activation of the sensory system that subserves the perception of noxious stimuli;
implies the existence of damage to somatic or visceral tissues sufficient to activate the nociceptive system.

Nociceptor A primary afferent nerve that has the ability to respond to a noxious stimulus or to a stimulus that would be noxious if prolonged.

Nonopioid Used instead of "nonnarcotic." Refers to acetaminophen and nonsteroidal antiinflammatory drugs (NSAIDs).

NSAID: An acronym for nonsteroidal antiinflammatory drug. (Pronounced "in said.") Also referred to as "aspirin-like" drugs.

Opioid This term is preferred to *narcotic*. Opioid refers to codeine, morphine, and other natural, semisynthetic, and synthetic drugs that relieve pain by binding to multiple types of opioid receptors.

Opioid dose-sparing effect The dose of opioid may be lowered when another analgesic, such as a nonopioid, is added.

Opioid-induced hyperalgesia (OIH) A phenomenon clearly demonstrated in experimental models, but of uncertain significance in humans, by which exposure to the opioid induces increased sensitivity, or a lowered threshold, to the neural activity subserving pain perception; it is the "flip side" of analgesic tolerance, which is defined by the loss of analgesic activity due to exposure to the drug.

Opioid-naïve An opioid-naïve person has not recently taken enough opioid on a regular enough basis to become tolerant to the effects of an opioid.

Opioid-tolerant An opioid-tolerant person has taken opioids long enough at doses high enough to develop tolerance to many of the effects of the opioid, including analgesia and sedation, but there is no timeframe for developing tolerance.

Physical dependence Potential for withdrawal symptoms if the opioid is abruptly stopped or an antagonist is administered.

Potency The dose required to produce a specified effect; relative potency is the ratio of the doses of two or more analgesics required to produce the same analgesic effect.

Preemptive analgesia Preinjury pain treatments (e.g., preoperative epidural analgesia and preincision local anesthetic infiltration) to prevent the establishment of peripheral and central sensitization of pain.

Primary afferent neuron See definition of **nociceptor**.

Prodrug An inactive precursor of a drug, converted into its active form in the body by normal metabolic processes.

Protective analgesia An aggressive, sustained multimodal intervention administered perioperatively (e.g., local anesthetic block, acetaminophen, NSAID, and anticonvulsant initiated preoperatively and continued throughout the intraoperative and postoperative periods) and directed toward prevention of pathologic pain (e.g., persistent neuropathic postsurgical pain syndromes).

Refractory Nonresponsive or resistant to therapeutic interventions such as analgesics.

Rescue dose Also referred to as *supplemental dose* or *breakthrough dose*. Administered on a PRN basis (as needed) in combination with the regularly scheduled analgesic to relieve pain that exceeds, or breaks through, the ongoing pain.

Systemic drug treatment; systemic administration Administration of a drug by a given route that allows absorption into the systemic circulation. Routes include oral, parenteral (IV, IM, SC), rectal, vaginal, topical application, transdermal, and transmucosal. By contrast, the spinal route of administration deposits the drug directly into the central nervous system, minimizing the amount of drug that reaches the systemic circulation.

Titration Adjusting the amount (e.g., adjusting the dose of opioid).

Tolerance A process characterized by decreasing effects of a drug at its previous dose, or the need for a higher dose of drug to maintain an effect.

Terminology Related to Research

Anecdotal evidence Evidence derived from clinical observations, clinical experience, or published case reports.

Case reports Published reports of one or more patient cases describing patient experiences, circumstances, or situations that infer specific outcomes that are not based on any scientific method of study.

Case-control study A retrospective observational study used most often to evaluate risk factors that may help explain the appearance or presentation of a disease or condition. Subjects with a known disease or condition are matched with similar individuals who do not possess it. Various potential risk factors, such as age or sex, or lifestyle factors, are then statistically evaluated to determine their levels of association with the disease or condition.

Cohort study A retrospective or prospective study in which a group of subjects who have a specific condition or receive a particular treatment are evaluated over time for a defined period. Data may be compared with another group of subjects who do not have the same condition or receive the same treatment, or subgroups within the cohort may be compared.

Controlled studies/trials Research studies that exert some or total control over the various treatment effects by using a comparison group (placebo group or comparator treatment group) and may use a single- or double-blind design, or random assignment of subjects.

Double-blind study Neither the investigator nor the subject know the critical aspects of the study (e.g., in a placebo-controlled trial, neither the person administering the intervention nor the subject receiving the intervention know if the intervention is experimental or placebo); used to reduce investigator and subject bias.

Meta-analysis Data analysis in which the results of several studies that address related research are combined and analyzed to arrive at one overall measurement of treatment effect.

Number needed to treat (NNT) A parameter that is often used in reporting the results of epidemiologic studies, clinical trials, systematic reviews, and meta-analyses. It is an estimate of how many people would need to receive an intervention to prevent one undesirable outcome or how many people need to receive a treatment in order that one derives a well-defined benefit (e.g., a 50% reduction in pain). NNT is calculated by using a formula that involves a known risk reduction or benefit analysis. Investigators typically determine and define the outcome that is used to compute the NNT for their study.

Open-label Both the investigators and the subjects know what treatment subjects are receiving. An investigator studies the response to an analgesic in a sample of patients and follows them through the treatment phase, observing and recording the effects. A disadvantage of this study design is potential bias for patient selection, observations, and conclusions.

Placebo-controlled trial A study that compares a treatment to a placebo, which is a treatment with no known therapeutic value. The placebo typically resembles the active intervention and is used as the control to determine the active intervention's efficacy.

Randomized controlled trial (RCT) A study in which subjects are randomly assigned (by chance alone) to receive the various interventions in a study. Randomization increases the likelihood that factors that could influence the effects produced by a treatment are distributed evenly across treatment groups, thereby limiting the risk of bias.

Relative risk (RR) A measure of the risk of a certain event happening in one group compared with the risk of the same event happening in another group. For example, in cancer research, relative risk is used in prospective (forward looking) studies, such as cohort studies and clinical trials. A relative risk of 1 means there is no difference between groups in terms of their risk of cancer, based on whether or not they were exposed to a certain substance or factor, or how they responded to two treatments being compared. A relative risk of greater than 1 or less than 1 means that being exposed to a certain substance or factor either increases (relative risk greater than 1) or decreases (relative risk less than 1) the risk of cancer, or that the treatments being compared do not have the same effects (e.g., a relative risk of 2 would mean that those exposed to a certain substance or factor have twice the risk of cancer compared with those who are not exposed to a certain substance or factor). Relative risk is also often called *relative ratio*.

Sequential trials One drug is tried and if the results are unfavorable, it is discontinued and another drug is tried. A trial-and-error approach in which one drug after another is tried until the desired effects occur.

Single-blind study The investigators know what treatment conditions subjects are assigned to, but subjects are "blinded" (not aware) of what they are receiving.

In clinical practice, analgesics may be divided into three groups: nonopioids, opioids, and the so-called "adjuvant" analgesics. This section focuses on the nonopioid analgesics, specifically acetaminophen and the nonsteroidal antiinflammatory drugs (NSAIDs) (see Section IV for opioid analgesics and Section V for adjuvant analgesics). These drugs all are both analgesic and antipyretic, and the NSAIDs are antiinflammatory. They share many of the same effects, but they are a mixed group and contain drugs that differ in chemical structure and adverse effect profiles.

Although all nonopioids sometimes are loosely referred to as NSAIDs, acetaminophen should not be classified this way. Acetaminophen should be distinguished from NSAIDs because it seems to relieve pain by different mechanisms and has minimal antiinflammatory effect. Acetaminophen may be referred to as an *aspirin-free* drug, whereas NSAIDs may be termed *aspirin-like* drugs. Other generic names for acetaminophen are APAP (acetylparaaminophenol) and paracetamol. You may wish to review some of the misconceptions about nonopioids on the next page.

Misconceptions about Nonopioids

Misconception	Correction
Regular daily use of nonopioids is much safer than taking opioids long-term.	Adverse effects from long-term use of NSAIDs are considerably more severe and life threatening than the adverse effects of daily doses of opioids. The most common adverse effect of long-term use of opioids is constipation, whereas NSAIDs can cause gastric ulcers, increased bleeding time, and cardiovascular adverse events. Acetaminophen can cause hepatotoxicity.
Nonopioids are not useful analgesics for severe pain.	Nonopioids alone are rarely sufficient to relieve severe pain, but they are an important part of a multimodal analgesic plan. One of the basic principles of analgesic therapy is: Whenever pain is severe enough to require an opioid, adding nonopioids (acetaminophen and NSAID) should be considered.
It is unacceptable polypharmacy to administer an NSAID, opioid, and one or more adjuvant analgesics (e.g., local anesthetic, anticonvulsant, antidepressant) for pain control.	Analgesics within each of the three analgesic groups relieve pain by different mechanisms. It is acceptable and, in most cases, recommended rational polypharmacy to administer more than one drug if each one is for a specific purpose.
A nonopioid should not be given at the same time as an opioid.	It is safe to administer a nonopioid and opioid at the same time. Giving a dose of nonopioid at the same time as a dose of opioid poses no more danger than giving the doses at different times. In fact, many opioids are compounded with a nonopioid (e.g., Percocet [oxycodone and acetaminophen]).
Administering NSAIDs rectally or parenterally prevents gastric ulcers.	Regardless of the route of administration, NSAIDs inhibit prostaglandins (PGs) that are necessary to maintain the protective barrier in the GI tract. Rectal or parenteral administration will only avoid the local irritation that can occur with oral administration.
Topical nonopioids are not effective analgesics.	Topical nonopioids have been shown to produce effective analgesia for mild to moderate acute or persistent (chronic) pain with a lower incidence of GI adverse effects.
Administering antacids with NSAIDs is an effective method of reducing gastric distress.	Administering antacids with NSAIDs can lessen distress but may be counterproductive. Antacids reduce the absorption and therefore the effectiveness of the NSAID by releasing the drug in the stomach rather than in the small intestine where absorption occurs.
For patients receiving long-term treatment with NSAIDs, H_2 blockers such as cimetidine (Tagamet) provide effective protection against gastric and duodenal ulcers.	H_2 blockers at higher than standard doses may be helpful, but misoprostol (Cytotec) and proton pump inhibitors (PPIs) such as esomeprazole (Nexium), lansoprazole (Prevacid), and omeprazole (Prilosec), are more effective and the only proven methods to reduce the occurrence of gastric and duodenal ulcers.
Gastric distress (e.g., abdominal pain) is indicative of NSAID-induced gastric ulceration.	Most patients with gastric lesions have no symptoms until bleeding or perforation occurs.
NSAIDs affect bone healing and should not be taken following orthopedic surgery.	Withdrawal of COX-2 inhibition when NSAIDs are discontinued after a short-term course (10 to 14 days) restores normal bone healing with no discernible effects on fracture healing (see text for exceptions and references).

From Pasero, C., & McCaffery, M. *Pain assessment and pharmacologic management*, p. 180, St. Louis, Mosby. © 2011, Pasero C, McCaffery M. May be duplicated for use in clinical practice.

Chapter 5 Indications for Administration of Acetaminophen or NSAIDs

NONOPIOIDS are flexible analgesics and may be used for a wide spectrum of painful conditions. Box 5-1 provides a summary of indications for nonopioids based on the discussion that follows. They typically are first-line analgesics for pain of mild to moderate intensity related to tissue injury (so-called *nociceptive pain*). This includes inflammatory pain following trauma or surgery, and pain caused by damage to bone, joint, or soft tissue. Given a relatively rapid onset of analgesia and the ability to initiate administration at a dose that is usually effective, it is reasonable to consider this class for both acute and persistent (chronic) pain. (See Patient Medication Information Forms III-1 through III-5 on pp. 250-259.)

Acetaminophen and aspirin are equi-effective at conventionally-used doses and have long been recognized as multipurpose analgesics (Toms, McQuay, Derry, et al., 2008). As shown in Table 5-1, 650 mg of aspirin or acetaminophen may relieve as much pain as 3 to 5 mg of oral oxycodone or 5 mg of hydrocodone. Single doses of these drugs may be effective. Acetaminophen has a very low incidence of adverse effects. Aspirin is used less today because its adverse effect liability, particularly GI toxicity, is greater than most of the newer NSAIDs, and it must be taken multiple times per day to provide continuous effects.

Although NSAIDs other than aspirin were originally marketed for inflammatory conditions such as rheumatoid arthritis (RA), they too are increasingly used as multipurpose analgesics. Based largely on anecdotal observation, there is a strong likelihood that aspirin and other NSAIDs are relatively more effective for somatic (e.g., musculoskeletal) nociceptive pains, particularly those that involve local inflammation, than they are for other types of pain. Note that, despite having very little peripheral antiinflammatory effect, acetaminophen still may be an effective analgesic for inflammatory conditions, such as RA (Simon, Lipman, Caudill-Slosberg, et al., 2002) and postoperative pain (Schug, Manopas, 2007). As described in Chapter 7, however, there also is evidence that the non-aspirin NSAIDs are more effective than acetaminophen for the pain of osteoarthritis (OA). This has also been shown to be true for postoperative pain. A randomized controlled study demonstrated that oral ibuprofen 800 mg taken three times daily provided better pain relief than 1000 mg of oral acetaminophen taken twice daily after anterior cruciate ligament repair (Dahl, Dybvik, Steen, et al., 2004).

An initial trial of a nonopioid is typical if pain is mild or moderate in severity. Patients usually present to health professionals after having tried acetaminophen, aspirin, and/or an over-the-counter (OTC) NSAID without success.

In some situations, such as the pain associated with serious medical illnesses such as cancer, NSAIDs may be overlooked in the context of moderate to severe pain, while treatment with an opioid is initiated. In other situations, such as neuropathic pain, the likelihood that NSAIDs are relatively less effective may justify the decision to forego trials in lieu of selected drugs in the category of the so-called adjuvant analgesics (see Section V). Moderate to severe somatic pain, such as the pain associated with joint disease, usually is treated first with one of the NSAIDs.

The response to an NSAID, like other analgesics, varies. As noted, some of this variation may be related to the pathophysiologies that sustain the pain. In other cases, it seems to be associated with intensity. Severe pain associated with somatic injury may not decline adequately in response to an NSAID at a maximally safe or effective (ceiling) dose (Schug, Manopas, 2007). Finally, some of the variation in response is related to ill-defined individual patient factors that lead to different levels of response to

GUIDELINES

Box 5-1 | Indications for Nonopioid Analgesics

Mild pain: Start with a nonopioid. Acetaminophen or an NSAID alone often provides adequate relief.

Moderate to severe pain: Pain of any severity may be at least partially relieved by a nonopioid. For some types of moderate pain, especially muscle and joint pain, NSAIDs alone or in combination with acetaminophen may provide adequate relief. However, an NSAID alone usually does not relieve severe pain.

Postoperative pain: Perioperative use of acetaminophen and an NSAID, especially parenteral ketorolac (Toradol) when not contraindicated, should be part of a multimodal analgesic plan begun preoperatively and continued throughout the postoperative course.

Persistent (Chronic) pain: Various types of persistent pain, including cancer-related bone pain, OA, and RA, are appropriate indications for an NSAID.

Pain that requires an opioid: Whenever pain is severe enough to require an opioid, always consider adding a nonopioid for the following reasons:

- Opioid dose-sparing effect (i.e., opioid dose may be lowered without decreasing pain relief. A decreased opioid dose can result in a reduction in opioid-induced adverse effects). A common example is oral or rectal acetaminophen and IV ibuprofen or IV ketorolac plus an opioid postoperatively.
- Opioids and nonopioids relieve pain by different mechanisms.

From Pasero, C., & McCaffery, M. *Pain assessment and pharmacologic management*, p. 182, St. Louis, Mosby. © 2011, Pasero C, McCaffery M. May be duplicated for use in clinical practice.

Table 5-1 | Equianalgesic Chart: Approximate Equivalent Doses of Nonopioids and Opioids for Mild to Moderate Pain

Analgesic	PO Dosage (mg)
Nonopioids	
Acetaminophen	650
Aspirin (ASA)	650
Choline salicylate	870
Diflunisal	500 is superior to 650 of aspirin
Etodolac	100
Ibuprofen	200-400
Indomethacin	25
Ketoprofen	25 is superior to 650 of aspirin
Magnesium salicylate	1000
Meclofenamate	50-100
Mefanamic acid	50-100
Naproxen sodium	275
Sodium salicylate	1000
Sulindac	150-200
Opioids	
Codeine	32-60
Hydrocodone	5
Meperidine (Demerol)	50
Oxycodone	3-5
Pentazocine (Talwin)	30-50
Propoxyphene hydrochloride (Darvon)	65
Propoxyphene napsylate (Darvon-N)	100

From Pasero, C., & McCaffery, M. (2011). *Pain assessment and pharmacologic management*, p. 182, St. Louis, Mosby. Data from American Pain Society. (2003). *Principles of analgesic use in the treatment of acute pain and cancer pain*, ed 5, Glenview, IL, APS; Bradley, R. L., Ellis, P. E., Thomas, P., et al. (2007). A randomized clinical trial comparing the efficacy of ibuprofen and paracetamol in the control of orthodontic pain. *Am J Orthod Dentofacial Ortho*, 132, 511-517; Burke, A., Smyth, E., & FitzGerald, G. A. (2006). Analgesic-anti-pyretic agents: Pharmacotherapy of gout. In L. L. Brunton, J. S. Lazo, & K. L. Parke (Eds.), *Goodman & Gilman's the pharmacological basis of therapeutics*, ed 11, New York, McGraw-Hill; Friday, J. H., Kanegaye, J.T., McCaslin I., et al. (2009). Ibuprofen provides analgesia equivalent to acetaminophen-codein in the treatment of acute pain in children with extremity injuries: A randomized clinical trial. *Acad Emerg Med*, 16(8), 711-716; McCaffery, M., & Portenoy, R. K. (1999). Nonopioid analgesics. In M. McCaffery, & C. Pasero C: *Pain: Clinical manual*, ed 2, St Louis, Mosby; Raeder, J. C., Stein, S., & Vatsgar, T. T. (2001). Oral ibuprofen versus paracetamol plus codeine for analgesia after ambulatory surgery. *Anesth Analg*, 92(6), 1470-1472. © 2011, Pasero C, McCaffery M. May be duplicated for use in clinical practice.

different drugs in the same category. Moderate to severe pain that does not respond to an NSAID, therefore, may be addressed by a trial of another NSAID, or by the addition or substitution of another drug, such as an opioid. All of the nonopioids are compatible with opioid and adjuvant analgesics.

It is wise to avoid combining NSAIDs. This approach may lead to an increase in adverse effects, particularly GI bleeding, and has not been shown to produce better analgesia than a trial with a single NSAID (Kovac, Mikuls, Mudano, et al., 2006). Studies have shown that the combination of acetaminophen and an NSAID produces an additive analgesic effect, however, and concomitant administration may be recommended (Altman, 2004; Bradley, Ellis, Thomas et al., 2007; Hyllested,

Jones, Pedersen, et al., 2002; Miranda, Puig, Prieto, et al., 2006; Pasero, McCaffery, 2007; Schug, Manopas, 2007). An oral formulation of 500 mg acetaminophen combined with 150 mg ibuprofen per tablet (Maxigesic) is available outside of the United States for treatment of pain and fever. A randomized controlled trial of 135 adults undergoing removal of 1 to 4 wisdom teeth under local anesthetic found that the combination formulation provided superior postprocedure pain relief compared with acetaminophen or ibuprofen alone (Merry, Gibbs,

Edwards, et al., 2009). Patients in this study took 2 tablets immediately before surgery and then 2 more tablets 4 times/day for 48 hours following surgery. Most adverse effects were mild, and there were no changes in the adverse event profile when the two drugs were combined.

Acute Pain

Acetaminophen and the NSAIDs are first-line analgesics for acute pain treatment and are often effective alone for mild pain and able to provide additive analgesia when combined with other analgesics for moderate to severe pain (American Pain Society, 2003; Scheiman, Fendrick, 2005; Schug, Manopas, 2007). Among the types of pain that commonly respond to a nonopioid alone are a wide variety of headaches, dental pain, and pain related to trauma or surgery. A Cochrane Collaboration Review concluded that NSAIDs and acetaminophen were similarly effective for treatment of dysmenorrhea pain, with little evidence of superiority of any of the individual NSAIDs (Marjoribanks, Proctor, Farquhar, 2003). A more recent study found that diclofenac more effectively relieved menstrual pain and improved exercise performance than placebo in healthy volunteers (Chantler, Mitchell, Fuller, 2009). The parenteral NSAID, ketorolac (Toradol), is relatively effective and often is tried for acute severe pain in the emergency department or surgical settings (see Chapters 7 and 8 for more on ketorolac).

Multimodal Analgesia

All nonopioids are conventionally used in a relatively narrow dose range, with upper titration limited either by concern about toxicity or because of pharmacologic "ceiling effect." In the effective dose range, NSAIDs may not be adequate for severe pain but may still contribute analgesia as part of a multimodal regimen that combines drugs with different underlying mechanisms, such as nonopioids, opioids, local anesthetics, and anticonvulsants. This approach allows lower doses of each of the drugs in the treatment plan, which lowers the potential for each to produce adverse effects (Ashburn, Caplan, Carr, et al., 2004; Kim, Kim, Nam, et al., 2008; Marret, Kurdi, Zufferey, et al., 2005; Schug, 2006; Schug, Manopas, 2007; White, 2005). Further, multimodal analgesia can result in comparable or greater pain relief than can be achieved with any single analgesic (Busch, Shore, Bhandari, et al., 2006; Cassinelli, Dean, Garcia, et al., 2008; Huang, Wang, Wang, et al., 2008). (See Chapter 8 for a discussion of perioperative multimodal analgesia.)

It is important to note that a successful multimodal approach relies on administration of optimal nonopioid doses. A randomized, placebo-controlled study of 300 patients admitted to the emergency department with acute musculoskeletal injury pain failed to show superior pain relief with combinations of NSAIDs and acetaminophen;

however, this may have been due to the administration of the lowest recommended starting dose of diclofenac and indomethacin (25 mg each) (Woo, Man, Lam, et al., 2005).

Persistent (Chronic) Pain

Persistent (also called chronic) pain is one of the most common reasons people seek health care (Manek, MacGregor, 2005; Shi, Langer, Cohen, et al., 2007). It is sustained by multiple underlying mechanisms and, as such, usually requires consideration of a variety of pharmacologic approaches. As noted, extensive clinical experience suggests that the nonopioid drugs usually play a major role when the pain is related to somatic pathology (particularly musculoskeletal or joint disease), chronic inflammation, or headache. An analysis of data from 10,291 respondents to the National Health and Nutrition Examination Survey (NHANES) revealed a chronic pain prevalence of 10.1% for back pain, 7.1% for pain in the legs or feet, 4.1% for pain in the arms or hands, and 3.5% for headache (Hardt, Jacobsen, Goldberg, et al., 2008).

Persistent pain is common in older adults, affecting as many as 80% of them (Pickering, 2005). Furthermore, many live with severe pain as was demonstrated in an open-label, multicenter, observational trial that found that 67.3% of the enrolled patients (average age 78 years) suffered persistent pain with an intensity of 4 or more (0 to 10 scale) (Gianni, Madaio, D Cioccio, et al., 2009). The American Geriatrics Society (AGS) recommends acetaminophen as a first-choice analgesic for mild to moderate persistent musculoskeletal pain (AGS, 2009). All of the major guidelines on the treatment of OA recommend acetaminophen as the first-line analgesic as well (Altman, Hochberg, Moskowitz, et al., 2000; Roddy, Doherty, 2003; Simon, Lipman, Caudill-Slosberg, et al., 2002; Zhang, Moskowitz, Nuki, et al., 2008) (see Chapter 7 for more on OA). The effectiveness of acetaminophen for persistent musculoskeletal pain was demonstrated in a randomized controlled trial in which nursing home residents with moderate-to-severe dementia were given acetaminophen or placebo 3 times daily (Chibnall, Tait, Harman, et al., 2005). Those who received acetaminophen showed more positive behaviors, such as increased social interaction, compared with those who received placebo.

NSAID therapy should be considered when acetaminophen fails to provide acceptable pain relief (Altman, Hochberg, Moskowitz, et al., 2000; Roddy, Doherty, 2003; Simon, Lipman, Caudill-Slosberg, et al., 2002; Zhang, Moskowitz, Nuki, et al., 2008). This recommendation is supported by a Cochrane Collaboration Review of 15 randomized controlled trials involving nearly 6000 patients, which concluded that NSAIDs were superior to acetaminophen in reduction of pain, global assessments, and improvements in functional status for both knee and hip OA pain (Towheed, Maxwell, Judd, et al., 2006). The Agency for Healthcare Research and Quality (AHRQ) executive summary on the best evidence comparing the various common OA pain treatments also noted that acetaminophen has been shown to be less effective than NSAIDs (AHRQ, 2006).

A trial of NSAIDs should be considered for all types of persistent pain. This includes neuropathic pain (Celiker, Arslan, Inanici, 2002), notwithstanding the consensus view that these drugs are not first-line analgesics for neuropathic pain (Dworkin, O'Connor, Backonja, et al., 2007; Moulin, Clark, Gilron, et al., 2007) (see Section V). NSAIDs should be considered for cancer pain, particularly cancer-related bone pain (Miaskowski, Cleary, Burney, et al., 2005). A Cochrane Collaboration Review of 42 trials (3084 patients) concluded that NSAIDs are more effective than placebo for cancer pain. A 5- to 7-day treatment course of ketorolac has been suggested as a reasonable alternative for neuropathic cancer pain that is unresponsive to first-line analgesics for neuropathic pain, such as anticonvulsants and antidepressants (Kauser, Davis, 2006).

Numerous studies have failed to show efficacy of acetaminophen and NSAIDs for treatment of fibromyalgia. However, patients may experience enhanced analgesia when these agents are combined with other first-line analgesics, such as antidepressants or anticonvulsants, particularly if the fibromyalgia is accompanied by a painful condition such as OA (Rao, Bennett, 2003).

There is no clear distinction among the various NSAIDs in terms of safety and efficacy (McNicol, Strassels, Goudas, et al., 2005). Given the individual variation in the response to the different nonopioids, a reasonable approach is to consider a trial of an alternative NSAID if the initial one does not provide relief.

The characteristic ability of some of the NSAIDs to treat acute pain suggests that some patients receiving a long-term, fixed dose opioid regimen could use an NSAID to treat breakthrough pain. There are no data in support of this practice, however, and most clinicians use a short-acting opioid as the so-called rescue dose for the treatment of breakthrough pain. There also are no studies of breakthrough pain among patients receiving an NSAID regimen. In this situation, acetaminophen may be an appropriate drug to try (Hyllested, Jones, Pedersen, et al., 2002; Miranda, Puig, Prieto, et al., 2006). See Chapter 12 for management of breakthrough pain.

Nonopioid Plus Opioid

Additive analgesia may occur when a nonopioid is added to an opioid, and this may enhance pain relief or result in "opioid sparing." Opioid sparing is clinically valuable if it leads to a reduction of opioid-related adverse effects send thereby improves the tolerability of therapy. Recognition that the addition of a nonopioid to an opioid

potentially can improve outcomes by improving maximal analgesia, reducing opioid adverse effects, or both supports consideration of drug combination therapy in the setting of chronic pain management. This is comparable to the multimodal analgesia described previously.

The possible benefits of combination therapy have been the driver for the development of commercially-available formulations containing acetaminophen, aspirin, or an NSAID plus an opioid. These drugs are very popular for acute pain, but have limited utility for chronic pain because the maximum daily dose of acetaminophen (or other nonopioid) limits the escalation of the opioid dose. Common examples of opioid/nonopioid fixed combinations are (see inside cover for more examples):

- Lortab 5/500 (hydrocodone, 5 mg, and acetaminophen, 500 mg)
- Loracet 10/650 (hydrocodone, 10 mg, and acetaminophen, 650 mg)
- Percocet (oxycodone, 5 mg, and acetaminophen, 325 mg)
- Tylenol No. 3 (codeine, 30 mg, and acetaminophen, 300 mg)
- Tylox (oxycodone, 5 mg, and acetaminophen, 500 mg)
- Vicodin (hydrocodone, 5 mg, and acetaminophen, 500 mg)
- Vicoprofen (hydrocodone, 7.5 mg, and ibuprofen, 200 mg)

With all of these products, patients must be warned to restrict daily use to a level providing a safe dose of the nonopioid constituent. For example, to avoid exceeding the recommended maximum daily dose of 4 g of acetaminophen, the patient cannot take more than 8 tablets per day of those containing 500 mg of acetaminophen or 12 tablets per day of those containing 325 mg of acetaminophen.

When providing an opioid/nonopioid combination product to a patient with acute or recurrent pain, clinicians must assess pain relief and other outcomes regularly. If the ceiling dose of the nonopioid is reached and the patient's pain is not adequately controlled, the drug should be discontinued or supplemented with another agent. One strategy suggests giving the nonopioid separately at a fixed dose while prescribing an opioid as a single entity drug, the dose of which may then be increased without concern about exceeding the recommended dose of nonopioid.

Conclusion

Clinical decisions about the use of nonopioids should be based on a careful assessment of the individual patient and a working knowledge of the indications, administration, and adverse effects of the drugs under consideration. This process should support treatment in terms of a benefit vs. burden analysis.

Chapter 6 Adverse Effects of Acetaminophen and NSAIDs

WITH few adverse effects at doses less than the recommended maximum adult dose of 4 gm per day, acetaminophen is widely considered one of the safest and best tolerated analgesics (Burke, Smyth, Fitzgerald, 2006; Schug, Manopas, 2007). Like other nonopioids, chronic use does not result in tolerance or physical dependence, and carries no risk of respiratory depression. The risk of adverse effects associated with conventional doses of acetaminophen is less than that associated with the other nonopioids (Box 6-1).

Although numerous studies have established the potential for acetaminophen toxicity on diverse systems, the likelihood of clinically-relevant adverse effects when this drug is used in appropriate doses is very low. Overall, the risk of adverse effects is greater during treatment with NSAIDs. The positive aspects of NSAID therapy—good effectiveness in many types of common pain syndromes, lack of tolerance or physical dependence, no risk of respiratory depression, and very low risk of typical CNS adverse effects such as somnolence—must be balanced by the potential for serious adverse effects. (See Chapter 8 for a discussion of adverse effects associated specifically with perioperative acetaminophen and NSAID use.)

Adverse Effects of Acetaminophen

Hepatic Effects

The most serious complication associated with acetaminophen use is hepatotoxicity (liver damage) as a result of overdose. In the healthy adult, a maximum daily dose below 4 gm is only rarely associated with liver toxicity (American Pain Society [APS], 2003; Bolesta, Haber, 2002; Laine, White, Rostom, et al., 2008; Rumack, 2002; Watkins, Kaplowitz, Slattery, et al., 2006). However, repeated doses exceeding this amount can result in hepatotoxicity (Daly, O'Malley, Heard, et al., 2004; United States Food and Drug Administration [U.S. FDA], 2009), and very large single doses can lead to fulminant hepatic failure.

Acetaminophen should be administered cautiously, at lower maximum doses, or not at all in situations that pose an increased risk of acetaminophen-associated hepatic injury. Factors that increase this risk include preexisting liver disease, the concurrent use of potentially hepatotoxic medications, fasting or poor nutrition, and regular consumption of alcohol (AGS, 2009; APS, 2003; Burke, Smyth, Fitzgerald, 2006; Larson, Polson, Fontana, et al., 2005; Miaskowski, Cleary, Burney, et al., 2005). Although some research shows that 4 gm per day can be safely taken in individuals who regularly drink alcohol (Graham, Scott, Day, 2005; Kuffner, Dart, 2001), the APS recommends no more than 2.5 gm per day in individuals who consume more than 2 ounces of alcohol daily because of the elevated risk of hepatotoxicity (Simon, Lipman, Caudill-Slosberg, et al., 2002). The U.S. FDA requires acetaminophen product labeling to

ACETAMINOPHEN

Hepatic effects: Hepatotoxicity occurs with overdose. At recommended doses, certain individuals are also at risk. Preventive strategy is to avoid or use with caution in patients with the following:

- Malnourishment, recent fasting
- Alcoholism, regular and heavy use of alcohol
- Preexisting liver disease
- Concomitant use of other potentially hepatotoxic drugs

Renal effects: Long-term use associated with declines in GFR and chronic renal failure; dose-dependent increases in renal insufficiency.

Cardiovascular effects: Long-term use associated with elevated risk; dose-dependent increases in blood pressure (BP).

Hematologic effects: May interfere with platelet aggregation and interact to potentiate the anticoagulant effect of warfarin (Coumadin).

Gastric effects: more than 500 mg/24 h may diminish gastric mucosal protection, and more than 2000 mg/24 h may produce increased risk of upper GI adverse effects.

NSAIDS

Gastric effects: Acute local irritation from orally administered NSAIDs can produce uncomfortable symptoms (e.g., dyspepsia) but rarely indicative of serious injury. May resolve with continued use. Treatment options:

- Lower the dose.
- Switch to another NSAID.
- Though enteric-coated NSAIDs do not reduce the risk of upper GI adverse events, they may help to relieve dyspepsia.

- Use a topical NSAID.
- Take the NSAID with food or a large glass of water.
- Antacids may reduce symptoms, but they also reduce absorption of the NSAID.
- H_2 antagonists (e.g., cimetidine [Tagamet], famotidine [Pepcid], ranitidine [Zantac]) are less effective than misoprostol and PPIs; all can be expensive.

Systemic gastrointestinal effects: Can occur regardless of route of administration. NSAIDs interfere with PG synthesis throughout the body. PG reduction impairs the protective barrier in the GI tract and allows injury to occur. Patient may be asymptomatic until bleeding or perforation occurs. See Table 6-1 on p. 192 for a complete list of risk factors for NSAID-induced GI adverse events and Table 6-2 on p. 194 for NSAID treatment strategies for all risk levels.

- Risk factors for NSAID-induced GI adverse effects:
  - Presence of prior ulcer disease or ulcer complications
  - Advanced age (older than 60 years)
  - CV disease and other co-morbidities
  - RA
  - Concomitant treatment with corticosteroids or anticoagulants (or other antiplatelet drugs)
  - Use of more than one NSAID, including cardioprotective aspirin
  - High NSAID doses
  - Long-term NSAID use
  - Use of NSAID with high risk of GI toxicity (e.g., indomethacin [Indocin], piroxicam [Feldene], sulindac [Clinoril]) (see Table 6-3 on p. 195 for individual NSAIDs and associated GI risk)
  - Patient unlikely to survive a GI complication

Continued

warn consumers of the increased risk of liver damage when acetaminophen is taken by those who consume three or more alcoholic drinks per day (U.S. FDA, 2009). Acetaminophen at doses less than the maximum recommended amount may be problematic with alcohol intake as well. One study showed 65% of the subjects with acute liver failure who reported taking less than 4 gm per day were alcohol abusers (Larson, Polson, Fontana, et al., 2005). The American Geriatrics Society (AGS) lists chronic alcohol abuse/dependence as a relative contraindication to using acetaminophen (AGS, 2009).

Most experts recommend a reduction in daily dose in individuals who are at high risk for hepatotoxicity (Burke, Smyth, FitzGerald, 2006). For example, the AGS recommends a 50% to 75% reduction in dose in older individuals with hepatic insufficiency (AGS, 2009).

Recommendations vary, however. Some authors recommend avoiding acetaminophen entirely in patients with hepatic insufficiency (Bannwarth, Pehourcq, 2003), whereas others suggest that it should be used as the optimal analgesic for patients with stable chronic liver disease (Graham, Scott, Day, 2005). Liver function tests should be performed every 6 to 12 months in any individual at high risk for hepatotoxicity who is taking acetaminophen (Bannwarth, 2006; Miaskowski, Cleary, Burney, et al., 2005; Simon, Lipman, Caudill-Slosberg, et al., 2002) (see Chapter 7 for more on acetaminophen dosing).

Acetaminophen overdose is a common cause of liver failure. A 6-year prospective study of 662 patients with acute liver failure showed that 42% of the cases resulted from acetaminophen hepatotoxicity, and 48% of those were from unintentional acetaminophen overdose

- Gastroprotective therapies:
  - Misoprostol (Cytotec). Reduces the occurrence of gastric and duodenal ulcers.
  - For patients who cannot afford or tolerate misoprostol, use a proton pump inhibitor (e.g., esomeprazole [Nexium], lansoprazole [Prevacid], and omeprazole [Prilosec])
  - H_2 blockers (e.g., cimetidine [Tagamet], famotidine [Pepcid], ranitidine [Zantac]) are less effective than misoprostol and PPIs.
  - A single strategy such as antacids, buffered tablets, or enteric-coated tablets does not provide sufficient protection.

Cardiovascular effects: All NSAIDs carry a risk of CV adverse effects through prostaglandin inhibition; an increased risk of CV events is associated with COX-2 inhibition, whether it is produced by those drugs labeled COX-2 selective (e.g., celecoxib) or those that are nonselective inhibitors of both COX-1 and COX-2 (e.g., ibuprofen, naproxen, ketorolac), and the risk varies across drugs, even within classes. See Table 6-4 on p. XX for risk factors for NSAID-induced CV event.

Hematologic effects: Most nonselective NSAIDs increase bleeding time. Ibuprofen can interfere with the cardioprotective effect of aspirin, so it should be taken 30 minutes to 2 hours after aspirin intake or at least 8 hours before. Preventive strategies when bleeding is a concern:

- Use NSAIDs that have minimal or no effect on bleeding time, such as COX-2 selective NSAIDs (e.g., celecoxib) or the nonselective NSAIDs choline magnesium trisalicylate (Trilisate), salsalate (Disalcid), and nabumetone (Relafen).

- Use acetaminophen instead of an NSAID (see discussion of concomitant acetaminophen and warfarin use).
- Use an opioid analgesic.
- To decrease bleeding associated with operative procedures, stop aspirin therapy 1 week before surgery (see the text for exceptions), and stop most other NSAIDs 3 days before surgery. Aspirin has an irreversible effect on platelets, but other NSAIDs do not.

Renal effects: Renal insufficiency is uncommon, and acute renal failure is rare, but long-term NSAID use at high doses may cause end-stage renal disease. Preventive strategies in patients with impaired renal function:

- Avoid indomethacin.
- Consider aspirin, celecoxib, or opioid analgesia.
- Use the lowest effective dose for the shortest time needed.
- Monitor kidney function.

Cognitive effects: Mild to moderate sedation and dysfunction can occur (CNS effect). Treatment options:

- Lower the dose.
- Discontinue the NSAID.
- Switch to another NSAID.

CNS, Central nervous system; *COX,* cyclooxygenase; *CV,* cardiovascular; *GFR,* glomerular filtration rate; *h,* hour; *H$_2$,* histamine receptor type-2; *MI,* myocardial infarction; *mg,* milligram; *NSAID,* nonsteroidal antiinflammatory drug; *PG,* prostaglandin; *PPI,* proton pump inhibitor; *RA,* rheumatoid arthritis.
From Pasero, C., & McCaffery, M. *Pain assessment and pharmacologic management,* pp. 186-187, St. Louis, Mosby. © 2011, Pasero C, McCaffery M. May be duplicated for use in clinical practice.

(Larson, Polson, Fontana, et al., 2005). A review of the United Network for Organ Sharing data revealed acetaminophen alone or in combination with other drugs accounted for 49% of the drug-related liver transplants performed in the United States between 1990 and 2002 (Russo, Galanko, Shrestha, et al., 2004).

A retrospective review of 1543 patients hospitalized for acetaminophen overdose revealed that 4.5% developed hepatotoxicity despite antidote treatment (n-acetylcysteine) in 38% (Myers, Shaheen, Li, et al., 2008) (see Chapter 10 for more on overdose treatment). While the occurrence of hepatotoxicity was low in this review, the patients who did develop it were 2.5 times more likely to be admitted to the intensive care unit (ICU) and 40 times more likely to die in the hospital than those without liver damage. This led researchers to conclude that the nature of most acetamin-

ophen overdoses is relatively benign, but the clinical impact for those who do develop hepatotoxicity is significant. This review also reinforced the impact of known risk factors—34% were alcohol abusers, 13% overdosed accidentally, and 3% had underlying liver disease (Myers, Shaheen, Li, et al., 2008). A significant finding was that the 13% who accidentally overdosed represented 49% of the cases of hepatotoxicity in this study. Co-morbidities were common (82%) in the individuals who overdosed; in addition to liver disease and alcohol abuse, 55% suffered depression. Older age was also identified as a risk factor.

The wide availability of formulations that combine acetaminophen with other ingredients for the treatment of a variety of conditions, ranging from the common cold to pain, increases the chances of exceeding recommended daily doses (Myers, Shaheen, Li, et al.,

2008). For example, one of the aforementioned studies (Larson, Polson, Fontana, et al., 2005) noted that, of the 48% who had acute liver failure following unintentional overdose, 38% had taken two or more acetaminophen products simultaneously and 63% had taken opioid-acetaminophen formulations.

The risk of unintentional overdose from acetaminophen mandates that patient teaching be done when prescribing an acetaminophen-containing drug and that this discussion describes safe maximum doses and the types of OTC analgesics and medications, such as cold remedies and sleep aids, that should be avoided (Bataller, 2007; Scharbert, Gebhardt, Sow, et al., 2007) (see Patient Medication Information Form III-4 on pp. 256-257; see Form III-5 on pp. 258-259 for aspirin). In 2009, the U.S. FDA required label changes for acetaminophen and products containing acetaminophen to reflect an increased risk of liver damage under certain circumstances (e.g., maximum daily dose is exceeded, daily intake of three or more alcoholic drinks, preexisting liver disease, concomitant use of other drugs containing acetaminophen) (U.S. FDA, 2009). In addition to product labeling changes, reformulation of acetaminophen-containing opioid analgesics has been proposed to reduce the rising incidence of this preventable form of liver injury (Fontana, 2008).

There may be racial or ethnic differences in the pharmacokinetics of acetaminophen and the development of hepatotoxicity following overdose. A small study comparing acetaminophen in Chinese (N = 11) and Caucasian (N = 9) subjects showed the Chinese more rapidly absorbed a single dose of acetaminophen and tended to produce reduced amounts of cysteine and mercapturic acid conjugates, compounds that may help protect against hepatotoxicity following acetaminophen overdose (Critchley, Critchley, Anderson, et al., 2005). Further research is needed to describe these and other sources of individual variation in the risks associated with this drug.

Renal Effects

The risk of chronic renal failure also has been linked to long-term acetaminophen use (Bannwarth, 2006) (see Chapter 8 for renal effects in the perioperative setting). The Nurses' Health Study, established in 1976, utilized questionnaires to evaluate 121,700 female registered nurses for a wide variety of health-related conditions (Colditz, 1995). A cohort (N = 1697) of this study was evaluated later for the effect of acetaminophen, aspirin, or other NSAID use on renal function, as measured by glomerular filtration rate (GFR) (Curhan, Knight, Rosner, et al., 2004). High acetaminophen, but not NSAID or aspirin use, was associated with an increased risk of decline in renal function. Women who used more than 100 gm of acetaminophen over the 11-year collection period had a GFR decline of at least 30%.

Other epidemiologic studies also have shown an association between acetaminophen use and chronic renal failure. For example, a study of nearly 1000 individuals with newly diagnosed early-stage chronic renal failure and nearly 1000 individuals without renal failure observed that aspirin and acetaminophen were used regularly by 37% and 25%, respectively, of the patients with renal failure, and by 19% and 12%, respectively, of the control group (Fored, Ejerblad, Lindblad, et al., 2001). Regular use (twice weekly for 2 months) of either drug alone was associated with a 2.5 increase in risk of chronic renal failure, and the relative risk rose more with increasing cumulative lifetime doses of acetaminophen than aspirin.

None of these epidemiologic studies confirm causality. Although the renal disease may be directly related to long-term acetaminophen use, it is possible that renal insufficiency caused by other disorders leads to pain and self-medication with acetaminophen, or that both renal dysfunction and acetaminophen use are related to a third factor. It is prudent to consider chronic renal failure as a potential complication of this drug, but recognize the need for additional research to define the relationship better.

Although acetaminophen may cause kidney disease, it usually is preferred over NSAIDs as a treatment for mild to moderate pain in patients with preexisting renal insufficiency (Bannwarth, 2006; Bannwarth, Pehourcq, 2003). This conventional view has been justified by the perceived lack of effect on platelet aggregation (which may be overstated; see discussion later in the chapter) and the low incidence of GI adverse effects (Kurella, Bennett, Chertow, 2003; Launay-Vacher, Karie, Fau, et al., 2005). Dose adjustment also is not necessary in the presence of preexisting renal failure, as it is when acetaminophen is prescribed to those with liver disease.

Cardiovascular (CV) Effects

Although CV adverse effects may be increased by acetaminophen, studies of this phenomenon are minimal and the underlying mechanisms are unclear (Chan, Manson, Albert, et al., 2006). Phenacetin, the precursor to acetaminophen, is associated with increased CV morbidity and mortality (Chan, Manson, Albert, et al., 2006), and there are data suggesting a relationship between acetaminophen dose and CV risk. A prospective study that evaluated the incidence of nonfatal and fatal coronary heart disease, and nonfatal and fatal stroke in nearly 71,000 female NSAID or acetaminophen users found that the relative risk of these outcomes was 1.38 in women who regularly (22 days or more/month) consumed acetaminophen, compared with 1.44 in those with frequent use of NSAIDs (Chan, Manson, Albert, et al., 2006). A dose-dependent risk was evident with a relative risk of 1.86 and 1.68 for those who took 15 tablets or more/week of NSAIDs or acetaminophen, respectively, compared with those who took lower doses.

Acetaminophen use may also contribute to the incidence of hypertension. Curhan and colleagues conducted a prospective study of 80,020 women who participated in the Nurses' Health Study (Colditz, 1995) and had no previous history of hypertension to examine the effect of acetaminophen, aspirin, or other NSAID use on BP (Curhan, Willett, Rosner, et al., 2002). Compared with nonusers, the relative risk of hypertension was 1.2 and 2.0 for those taking acetaminophen for 1 to 4 days/month and 22 days/month, respectively. This means that those taking acetaminophen 22 days/month were twice as likely to develop hypertension as those who did not use acetaminophen. Other analysis has yielded similar elevated risk (Dedier, Stampfer, Hankinson, et al., 2002). An analysis of younger (N = 3220) and older (N = 1903) age cohorts of the Nurses' Health Study revealed a correlation between relative risk of hypertension and dose of acetaminophen (Forman, Stampfer, Curhan, 2005). Dose but not age was associated with increased risk in those who took more than 500 mg/day; relative risk was 1.99 and 1.93 for younger and older women, respectively.

A later study of analgesic use in 16,031 nonhypertensive male health care professionals had similar results (Forman, Rimm, Curhan, 2007). A review of detailed information about the use of acetaminophen, aspirin, and other NSAIDs by these men revealed a relative risk of 1.34 in those who took acetaminophen 6 to 7 days per week compared with those who used no acetaminophen. The relative risk was 1.38 for NSAIDs and 1.26 for aspirin.

In contrast, a large prospective cohort study of 8229 males without hypertension at the start of a 5.8 year (mean) follow-up period found that, compared with those who never used acetaminophen, NSAIDs, or aspirin, there was no significant increase in risk of subsequent hypertension in the men who took at least 2500 pills of any of the analgesics. A small to moderately increased risk cannot be excluded from observational studies (Kurth, Hennekens, Sturmer, et al., 2005), and all observational studies must be interpreted cautiously given the potential for recall and other sources of bias (Vardeny, Solomon, 2008).

Hematologic Effects and Anticoagulant Therapy

Acetaminophen has long been used as an analgesic in patients receiving anticoagulation therapy because it was thought to have no effect on platelet aggregation (Thijssen, Soute, Vervoort, et al., 2004). Nonetheless, there are conflicting observations, which together suggest that acetaminophen may in fact interfere with platelet aggregation and potentiate the anticoagulant effect of warfarin (Coumadin) (Gebauer, Nyfort-Hansen, Henschke, et al., 2003; Mahe, Bertrand Drouet, et al., 2006; Munsterhjelm, Munsterhjelm, Niemi, et al., 2005; Ornetti, Ciappuccini, Tavernier, et al., 2005; Parra, Beckey, Stevens, 2007; Thijssen, Soute, Vervoort, et al., 2004). If indeed this is a clinically relevant effect, it may be related to the weak inhibition of COX-1 produced by acetaminophen (Munsterhjelm, Munsterhjelm, Niemi, et al., 2005)

and the production of metabolites that may interfere with the enzymes involved in vitamin K–dependent coagulation factor synthesis (Mahe, Bertrand, Drouet, et al., 2005, 2006; Thijssen, Soute, Vervoort, et al., 2004).

A small double-blind, crossover study of 13 healthy male volunteers with normal platelet function was conducted to evaluate the dose-dependent effect of acetaminophen on platelet function (Munsterhjelm, Munsterhjelm, Niemi, et al., 2005). Compared with those who received placebo, the men who received IV acetaminophen demonstrated a dose-dependent increase in concentration of arachidonic acid, which was thought to cause the anticoagulant effect seen in the volunteers. In addition, acetaminophen inhibited the release of thromboxane B_2, the stable metabolite of thromboxane A_2, released during platelet aggregation. This effect was also dose dependent. Another small (N = 11) double-blind, crossover study randomized patients to receive 14-day regimens of acetaminophen (4 gm) or placebo with a 14-day wash-out period between (Mahe, Bertrand, Drouet, et al., 2005). The International Normalized Ratio (INR), a measure of coagulation, was significantly elevated in patients who received acetaminophen compared with those who received placebo.

The effect of 2 to 4 gm/day of acetaminophen on patients receiving warfarin anticoagulation therapy was evaluated in a randomized, placebo-controlled trial of 36 adults at an anticoagulation clinic (Parra, Beckey, Stevens, 2007). The patients were receiving warfarin and had stable INRs at the start of the study. The study was terminated after 15 patients demonstrated a significant dose-dependent increase in INR. There was also a significant increase in mean serum alanine aminotransferase (ALT) level (liver function indicator) in the patients who received 4 g/day of acetaminophen compared with those who received placebo. Another randomized, placebo-controlled study (N = 20) showed similar results (Mahe, Bertrand, Drouet, et al., 2006). Again, patients were stabilized on warfarin anticoagulation therapy. The mean INR increased quickly and significantly within 1 week of acetaminophen (4 gm/day) use. There were also significant reductions in vitamin K–dependent clotting factors.

These studies support the view that acetaminophen can have clinically relevant hematologic effects. It also is true, however, that acetaminophen inhibition of thromboxane A_2 is less than that of the nonselective NSAIDs (Munsterhjelm, Niemi, Syrjala, et al., 2003), and studies have shown that surgical bleeding as a result of perioperative acetaminophen intake is low (Ashraf, Wong, Ronayne, et al., 2004; Munsterhjelm, Munsterhjelm, Niemi, et al., 2005) (see Chapter 8 for effect of perioperative nonopioid use on surgical site bleeding). It is probable that the risk of bleeding associated with acetaminophen use is low, but given the extant data, close monitoring of patients receiving acetaminophen and anticoagulation therapy is prudent (Mahe, Bertrand Drouet, et al., 2005, 2006; Ornetti, Ciappuccini, Tavernier, et al., 2005; Parra, Beckey, Stevens, 2007). In 2009, the U.S. FDA required label changes for acetaminophen to advise those who are taking warfarin to discuss the use of acetaminophen with a pharmacist or physician prior to taking acetaminophen (U.S. FDA, 2009).

Gastrointestinal (GI) Effects

The most common adult daily dose of acetaminophen is 1000 mg, a dose that is thought to produce less GI toxicity than most NSAIDs (Burke, Smyth, Fitzgerald, 2006). However, daily doses of more than 500 mg have been shown to diminish gastric mucosal protection (Rahme, Pettitt, LeLorier, 2002), and epidemiologic studies show doses of more than 2000 mg/24 h produce increased risk of severe upper GI adverse effects (Bannwarth, 2006). A study of analgesic overdose by patients with suicidal intent reported endoscopic gastric damage (lesions) from acute high-dose acetaminophen to be similar to that caused by acute high-dose NSAID ingestion (Soylu, Dolapcioglu, Dolay, et al., 2008). This is likely due, at least in part, to peripheral COX-1 inhibition (associated with poorer gastric safety). Indeed, acetaminophen has been shown to be more COX-1 selective than several NSAIDs, including naproxen (Naprosyn, Aleve), diclofenac (Voltaren), and ibuprofen (Advil, Motrin), but less than piroxicam (Feldene) and tolmetin (Tolectin) (Rahme, Pettitt, LeLorier, 2002).

A large cohort study of individuals aged 65 and older was undertaken to compare the rates of GI adverse events occurring with higher versus lower doses of acetaminophen (Rahme, Pettitt, LeLorier, 2002). Data from patients who had received a prescription for acetaminophen (N = 21,000) or a nonaspirin NSAID (N = 27,000) were examined. Unadjusted rates of hospitalization, ulcer, and dyspepsia were higher for patients taking acetaminophen compared with those taking NSAIDs, and the acetaminophen GI adverse events were dose related. After adjustment of risk susceptibility, patients receiving higher acetaminophen doses (more than 3250 mg/day) had higher rates of GI events compared with those receiving lower doses (650 mg or less/day).

Adverse Effects of NSAIDs

Gastrointestinal (GI) Effects

The most common adverse effects of the NSAIDs involve the GI system. The associated clinical conditions are heterogeneous, and the most serious concern involves GI ulceration. Ulcers and their complications, including hemorrhage and perforation, can occur in both the upper and lower GI tract (Hayashi, Yamamoto, Kita, et al., 2005). These serious events may be difficult to detect and can be fatal (Simon, 2007).

NSAID-induced GI events are blamed for an estimated 100,000 hospitalizations and 16,500 deaths annually in the United States (Bombardier, Laine, Reicin, et al.,

2000). Studies have demonstrated that the risk for serious GI complications is 3- to 5-fold higher in those who take NSAIDs than in those who do not (Wilcox, Allison, Benzuly, et al., 2006) and that gastric or duodenal ulceration may occur in 15% to 30% of patients receiving long-term therapy with NSAIDs classified as nonselective COX-1/COX-2 inhibitors (Bombardier, Laine, Reicin, et al., 2000; Cryer, 2004; Laine, 2001). A review of 361 patients with peptic ulcer bleeding revealed that one-half of the cases was associated with NSAID use (Ramsoekh, Van Leerdam, Rauws, et al., 2005). An autopsy study of 713 individuals revealed gastric and duodenum ulceration in 22% of nonselective NSAID users compared with 12% of NSAID nonusers; small bowel ulcers were found in 8.4% of nonselective NSAID users compared with 0.6% of NSAID nonusers (Simon, 2007).

The primary underlying mechanism of NSAID-induced ulceration is thought to be inhibition of COX-1, which leads to reduction in GI-protective prostaglandins (Burke, Smyth, Fitzgerald, 2006; Simon, Weaver, Graham, et al., 1999). This is a systemic effect and can occur regardless of the route of administration of the NSAID (Laine, 2001). This means that GI adverse effects resulting from prostaglandin inhibition are possible when NSAIDs are taken orally, rectally, or parenterally. Systemic effects may be compounded by local processes produced by direct contact between GI mucosa and the drug. With the exception of nabumetone (Relafen), all of the nonselective NSAIDs are highly lipophilic and can easily penetrate the gastric mucosal barrier, which is a hydrophobic mucous layer along the stomach lining (Simon, 2007). This penetration is thought to result in oxidative uncoupling of cellular metabolism, producing cell death and localized tissue injury (Simon, 2007).

NSAID-induced adverse GI effects manifest as distressing symptoms alone, asymptomatic ulceration, or the more serious complications of GI bleeding, perforation, or obstruction (Cryer, 2004; Laine, 2001). Even though dyspepsia and other upper GI symptoms are commonly associated with the use of NSAIDs and often a reason for discontinuing NSAID therapy (Goldstein, Eisen, Burke, et al., 2002), these symptoms do not appear to predict the development of a more serious GI event in patients with no or low GI risk (Laine, 2001; Lanas, Bajador, Serrano, et al., 2000; Mellemkjaer, Biot, Sorensen, 2002; Simon, Fox, 2005). However, endoscopic evaluation is recommended in patients with high GI risk who experience significant NSAID treatment-induced dyspepsia (Chan, Hung, Suen, et al., 2004).

NSAID-induced adverse effects are related to the dose and duration of treatment. The higher the NSAID dose and the longer the duration of NSAID use, the higher the risk of cumulative GI toxicity (Chan, Graham, 2004). This cumulative toxicity also includes a period of relatively higher risk at the start of treatment (Wilcox, Allison, Benzuly, et al., 2006). Serious complications are most frequent during the first 3 months of NSAID administration

(Gabriel, Jaakkimainen, Bombardier, 1991), and there is an 8% incidence of ulcer development within 1 week of regular NSAID use (Laine, 2001).

GI Risk Factors

The greatest risk factor for NSAID-associated GI events is the presence of prior ulcer disease with ulcer complications (Chan, Graham, 2004). The AGS lists current peptic ulcer disease as an absolute contraindication and history of peptic ulcer disease as a relative contraindication to the use of NSAIDs in older adults (AGS, 2009). Other risk factors include age at or older than 60 years, CV disease and other co-morbidities, severe rheumatoid arthritis (RA), and concomitant treatment with corticosteroids or anticoagulants (Bhatt, Scheiman, Abraham, et al., 2008; Chan, Graham, 2004; Laine, 2001; Simon, 2007; Wilcox, Allison, Benzuly, et al., 2006). *Helicobactor pylori (H. pylori)* infection, excessive alcohol consumption, and cigarette smoking generally are considered independent and modifiable risk factors, though the magnitude of their effects is unclear (Burke, Smyth, Fitzgerald, 2006; Wilcox, Allison, Benzuly, et al., 2006). In 2009, the U.S. FDA required label changes for NSAIDs to reflect an increased risk of gastric bleeding, particularly in certain populations, including older adults and individuals taking anticoagulants, steroids, or other NSAID-containing products, or those consuming three or more alcoholic drinks daily (U.S. FDA, 2009). Table 6-1 provides a summary of risk factors for the development of NSAID-induced GI adverse events.

The First International Working Party on GI and CV Effects of NSAIDs and Anti-platelet Agents used a comprehensive series of clinical vignettes and possible scenarios to rate the appropriateness of NSAIDs. This group predefined high GI risk as age at or older than 70 years, prior upper GI event, and concomitant use of aspirin, corticosteroids, anticoagulants, or other antiplatelet drugs (Chan, Abraham, Scheiman, et al., 2008). In addition, risk was determined to be higher with specific NSAIDs and with the combination of an NSAID and low-dose aspirin (Laine, 2001; Simon, 2007; Silverstein, Faich, Goldstein, et al., 2000; Vardeny, Solomon, 2008). In a consensus guideline, the American College of Cardiology Foundation (ACCF), American College of Gastroenterology (ACG), and the American Heart Association (AHA) stated that the use of cardioprotective aspirin (81 mg) is associated with a 2- to 4-fold increase in upper GI adverse events (Bhatt, Scheiman, Abraham, et al., 2008) (see pp. 204-205 for more on cardioprotective aspirin). It is also important to note that any dose of aspirin can cause upper GI adverse events, and because the primary mechanism underlying GI toxicity is systemic rather than local, buffered and enteric-coated formulations do not decrease the incidence (Bhatt, Scheiman, Abraham, et al., 2008; Laine, 2001).

The risk of GI toxicity and death from a GI bleed increases with age at a rate of about 4% per year, and age is an extremely important consideration when starting NSAID therapy (APS, 2003; Wilcox, Allison, Benzuly, et al., 2006). At age 45 to 64 years, 15 in 10,000 individuals will have a serious GI bleed during long-term therapy, and 2 in 10,000 will die from a GI bleed; however, at age 65 to 74 years, 17 in 10,000 will have a serious GI bleed and 3 in 10,000 will die. The highest risk is in individuals age 75 and older; at this age, 91 in 10,000 will experience a GI bleed and 15 in 10,000 will die (AHRQ, 2007). This increased risk may be due to the combined effect of other risk factors associated with aging, such as medical comorbidities and concomitant use of drugs such as aspirin or anticoagulants, as well as an age-related decrease in protective GI prostaglandin concentrations (Wilcox, Allison, Benzuly, et al., 2006).

H. pylori is a gram-negative bacterium that can reside chronically in the stomach and elicit a local inflammatory response. NSAIDs produce a similar destructive effect on the gastric mucosa through COX-1 inhibition of prostaglandins in the protective lining of the gut. Although the data are conflicting, there is growing evidence of an interaction between the presence of *H. pylori* infection and risk of GI complications in NSAID users (Chan, To, Wu, et al., 2002; Huang, Sridhar, Hunt, 2002; Laine, 2001; Wilcox, Allison, Benzuly, et al., 2006). This interaction was suggested in a meta-analysis of 463 studies, which revealed that one-third of patients receiving long-term NSAID therapy had gastric or duodenal ulcers irrespective of the presence of *H. pylori* infection, but peptic ulcer disease was more common in *H. pylori*-infected NSAID users than in noninfected NSAID users (Huang, Sridhar, Hunt, 2002). A 2- to 4-fold increase in risk of upper GI complications in regular NSAID users who are *H. pylori* infected has been reported elsewhere (Chan, Graham, 2004). Eradication of *H. pylori* with antibiotic therapy decreases the incidence of peptic ulcers in patients who begin taking NSAIDs, but this does not seem to extend to patients with a previous history of ulceration (Wilcox, Allison, Benzuly, et al., 2006).

These data support the conclusion that *H. pylori* infection is an independent and modifiable risk factor for GI complications in long-term NSAID users (Chan, To, Wu, et al., 2002; Huang, Sridhar, Hunt, 2002; Kurata, Nogawa, 1997; Laine, 2001; Wilcox, Allison, Benzuly, et al., 2006). Although it may be difficult to justify routinely ruling out *H. pylori* infection prior to initiating NSAID therapy in patients with low risk, testing should be done routinely in patients with high GI risk (Chan, To, Wu, et al., 2002; Chan, Graham, 2004; Wilcox, Allison, Benzuly, et al., 2006). If *H. pylori* infection is present, it should be eradicated prior to initiating NSAID therapy (Chan, Graham, 2004; Wilcox, Allison, Benzuly, et al., 2006) (see Table 6-1).

NSAID Selection with Consideration of GI Risk

The expert panel of the First International Working Party on GI and CV Effects of NSAIDs and Anti-platelet Agents endorsed risk stratification based on a thorough patient

Table 6-1 | Risk Factors for NSAID-Induced Adverse GI Events

Risk Factor	Comments
History of ulcers or GI events; use of anti-ulcer therapy for any reason	Patients with this risk factor are considered at high to very high risk for an adverse GI event.
Age or older 65 years	Risk increases with age. At age 45 to 64 years, 15 in 10,000 individuals will have a serious GI bleed and 2 in 10,000 will die from a GI bleed; at age 65 to 74 years, 17 in 10,000 will have a serious GI bleed and 3 in 10,000 will die from a GI bleed. The highest risk is in individuals age 75 and older when 91 in 10,000 will experience a GI bleed and 15 in 10,000 will die from a GI bleed.
Co-morbidity, e.g., CV disease, CHF, COPD	Individuals with CV disease are likely to take low-dose aspirin, which places them at higher risk for GI complications when NSAIDs are taken concomitantly.
Extensive or severe RA	Individuals with RA are 2 times more likely to develop GI complications than the general population. Pain relief from NSAIDs may be misinterpreted as disease regression; therefore, NSAID use should be in conjunction with disease-modifying therapy.
Concomitant glucocorticoid therapy, particularly in patients with RA	No increased risk of GI complications when glucocorticoids are used alone, however, used with NSAIDs may increase risk by as much as 4-fold; warn patients to avoid NSAIDs during glucocorticoid therapy.
Concomitant anticoagulant therapy	Not strictly prohibited but may predispose to increased risk for GI mucosal break and hemorrhage; increase in INR may occur. INR should be monitored frequently if acetaminophen or NSAID is taken with warfarin. COX-2 selective NSAIDs, which have no effect on platelet aggregation, are best choices in such patients, if not contraindicated (see Tables 6-2 and 6-4).
Type of NSAID	Lower risk = salsalate, magnesium choline trisalicylate, low doses of ibuprofen, naproxen[1], etodolac, meloxicam, nabumetone, or COX-2 selective NSAIDs Higher risk = piroxicam[1], sulindac, indomethacin, ketoprofen, ketorolac (see Table 6-3)
Use of high-dose singular NSAIDs	Effects are dose-related; regardless of NSAID, the higher the dose, the higher the GI risk.
Use of combinations of NSAIDs, including low-dose aspirin co-therapy	Combinations of NSAIDs, including aspirin at any dose, increase GI risk, e.g., combination cardioprotective aspirin and NSAID therapies increase relative GI risk 2 to 4 times that of NSAIDs or aspirin alone. Combination COX-2 selective NSAID plus cardioprotective aspirin provides some GI protection but substantially less than a COX-2 selective NSAID alone.
Helicobacter pylori (H. pylori) infection	Independent and modifiable risk factor; may increase risk by 2- to 4-fold in regular NSAID users. Routinely test for presence in patients with high GI risk. Treat, if present, prior to NSAID therapy (see Table 6-2).
Excessive alcohol intake	Independent risk factor; magnitude unclear.
Cigarette smoking	Independent risk factor; magnitude unclear.

CHF, Congestive heart failure; *COPD*, chronic obstructive pulmonary disease; *COX*, cyclooxygenase; *CV*, cardiovascular; *GI*, gastrointestinal; *INR*, International Normalized Ratio; *NSAID*, nonsteroidal antiinflammatory drug; *RA*, rheumatoid arthritis.
[1]Avoid full-dose naproxen, piroxicam, and oxaprozin in older adults because of long half-life and increased risk of GI toxicity.
From Pasero, C., & McCaffery, M. *Pain assessment and pharmacologic management*, p. 192, St. Louis, Mosby. Data from Agency for Healthcare Research and Quality (AHRQ). (2007). *Choosing non-opioid analgesics for osteoarthritis. Clinician's guide.* Available at *http://effectivehealthcare.ahrq.gov/.* Accessed July 24, 2008; American Geriatrics Society (AGS) Panel on Pharmacological Management of Persistent Pain in the Older Persons. (2009). The pharmacological management of persistent pain in older persons. *J Am Geriatr Soc,* 57(8), 1331-1346; Chan, F. K. L., & Graham, D. Y. (2004). Prevention of non-steroidal anti-inflammatory drug gastrointestinal complications—Review and recommendations based on risk assessment. *Aliment Pharmacol Ther,* 19(10), 1051-1061; Chan, F. K. L., Hung, L. C. T., Suen, B.Y., et al. (2004). Celecoxib versus diclofenac plus omeprazole in high-risk arthritis patients: Results of a randomized double-blind trial. *Gastroenterology,* 127(4), 1038-1043; Fick, D. M., Cooper, J. W., Wade, W. E., et al. (2003). Updating the Beers criteria fo potentially inappropriate medication use in older adults. *Arch Intern Med,* 163(22), 2716-2724; Gabriel, S. E., Jaakkimainen, L., Bombardier, C. (1991). Risk for serious gastrointestinal complications related to use of nonsteroidal anti-inflammatory drugs. A meta-analysis.

Ann Intern Med, 115(10), 787-796; Hanlon, J. T., Backonja, M., Weiner, D., et al. (2009). Evolving pharmacological management of persistent pain in older persons. *Pain Med,* 10(6), 959-961; Kurata, J. H., & Nogawa, A. N. (1997). Meta-analysis of risk factors for peptic ulcer: Nonsteroidal anti-inflammatory drugs, Helicobacter pylori, and smoking. *J Clin Gastroenterol,* 24(1), 2-17; Kuritzky, L., & Weaver, A. (2003). Advances in rheumatology: Coxibs and beyond. *J Pain Symptom Manage,* 25(2S), S6-S20; Laine, L. (2001). Approaches to nonsteroidal anti-inflammatory drug use in the high-risk patient. *Gastroenterology,* 120(3), 594-606; Laine, L., White, W. B., Rostom, A., et al. (2008). COX-2 selective inhibitors in the treatment of osteoarthritis. *Semin Arthritis Rheum,* 38(3), 165-187; Simon, L. S. (2007). Risks and benefits of COX-2 selective inhibitors. Available at *http://www.medscape.com/viewprogram/6872/.* Accessed April 5, 2007; Simon, L. S., & Fox, R. I. (2005). What are the options available for anti-inflammatory drugs in the aftermath of rofecoxib's withdrawal? *Medscape Rheumatology,* 6(1). Available at *http://www.medscape.com/viewarticle/500056.* Accessed April 16, 2005; Solomon, D. H., Glynn, R. J., Rothman, K. J., et al. (2008). Subgroup analyses to determine cardiovascular risk associated with non-steroidal anti-inflammatory drugs and coxibs in specific patient groups. *Arthritis Care Res,* 59(8), 1097-1104; Wilcox, C. M., Allison, J., Benzuly, K., et al. (2006). Consensus development conference on the use of nonsteroidal anti-inflammatory agents, including cyclooxygenase-2 enzyme inhibitors and aspirin. *Clin Gastroenterol Hepatol,* 4(9), 1082-1089. © 2011, Pasero C, McCaffery M. May be duplicated for use in clinical practice.

assessment as a key step in the selection of NSAID therapy. This panel viewed the selection of a nonselective NSAID as appropriate in patients with average GI risk, including those younger than 70 years of age with no prior GI event and no concurrent use of corticosteroids, antithrombotic agents, or anticoagulants (Chan, Abraham, Scheiman, et al., 2008). The American Gastroenterological Association (AGA) (Wilcox, Allison, Benzuly, et al., 2006) and other researchers (Chan, Graham, 2004) also have provided recommendations that guide decision making with regard to NSAID selection and patient management during NSAID therapy. Table 6-2 provides a summary of NSAID treatment strategies correlated with GI risk.

Avoiding NSAIDs altogether is the best way to prevent an NSAID-related complication (Chan, Graham, 2004), and when NSAID therapy is indicated, the lowest effective NSAID should be used for the shortest time needed (APS, 2003; U.S. FDA, 2007). If pain is mild to moderate, a trial of acetaminophen should be tried. Patients with more severe pain who are at relatively high risk for NSAID complications should be considered for a trial of an opioid or another centrally-acting analgesic. The AGS specifically noted that opioids may be safer than NSAIDs in some older patients (e.g., those with high GI and CV risk factors) (AGS, 2002; AGS, 2009), an observation that may be underappreciated by clinicians.

NSAID-induced GI toxicity, like antiinflammatory activity, is believed to correlate with COX-1 inhibition (Chan, Graham, 2004; Simon, 2007). Some NSAIDs (e.g., piroxicam [Feldene], indomethacin [Indocin]) achieve adequate analgesia at doses associated with high antiinflammatory activity, and appear to have a relatively greater risk of GI toxicity (Chan, Graham, 2004). These drugs generally are not first-line for this reason. In addition, NSAIDs with longer half-lives (e.g., sulindac [Clinoril], piroxicam,, indomethacin) may expose GI mucosa to the drug for longer periods at a higher concentration and also have been linked to greater GI toxicity (Wilcox, Allison, Benzuly, et al., 2006). These are the reasons cited for avoiding full-dose piroxicam, oxaprozin, and naproxen in older adults (Fick, Cooper, Wade, et al., 2003; Hanlon, Backonja, Weiner, et al., 2009)

Some of the nonselective NSAIDs exhibit relatively selective COX-2 inhibition and less COX-1 inhibition, particularly at lower doses; these drugs are considered safer in terms of GI toxicity and often are preferred as a result (Simon, 2007). For example, ibuprofen, which is one of the most commonly used NSAIDs in the United States, is considered a relatively safe choice from a GI perspective when doses are kept below full antiinflammatory effect (less than 2.4 gm/day) (Chan, Graham, 2004).

In general, a lower risk of GI toxicity characterizes all nonacetylated salicylates, including salsalate (Disalcid) and magnesium choline trisalicylate (Trilisate), and several of the nonselective, nonsalicylate NSAIDs. The latter group includes etodolac (Lodine), meloxicam (Mobic), nabumetone, and low doses of ibuprofen or naproxen

(Laine, 2001; Simon, 2007; Wilcox, Allison, Benzuly, et al., 2006). It is reasonable to consider these drugs as first-line options for NSAID therapy, although, as mentioned, full-dose naproxen is not recommended in older adults because of its long half-life (Fick, Cooper, Wade, et al., 2003; Hanlon, Backonja, Weiner, et al., 2009). As mentioned, nabumetone also has the advantage of relatively low lipophilicity, leading to less penetration of the gastric mucosal barrier (Bannwarth, 2008; Hedner, Samulesson, Wahrborg, et al., 2004; Simon, 2007). Table 6-3 shows the various NSAIDs and their associated risk for GI events.

The so-called COX-2 selective NSAIDs (e.g., celecoxib [Celebrex]) also carry a relatively lower risk of GI adverse effects, at least when taken by patients who are not also using cardioprotective aspirin therapy (Chan, Graham, 2004; Dajani, Islam, 2008; Jacobsen, Phillips, 2004; Laine, White, Rostom, et al., 2008; Silverstein, Faich, Goldstein, et al., 2000; Simon, 2007; Singh, Fort, Goldstein, et al., 2006). The COX-2 selective NSAIDS, like all NSAIDs, vary in the degree to which they affect COX-2 over COX-1. The ratio of inhibition associated with the best safety profile overall is not known. At the present time, only one drug in this category is available in the United States—celecoxib.

According to one review (Laine, White, Rostom, et al., 2008), COX-2 selective NSAIDs are associated with a 75% relative risk reduction for gastroduodenal ulcers and a 61% relative risk reduction for ulcer complications compared with nonselective NSAIDs. These benefits decline or disappear during concurrent therapy with cardioprotective aspirin (Vardeny, Solomon, 2008). Although the combination of a COX-2 selective NSAID with cardioprotective aspirin may be somewhat safer than the combination of aspirin and a nonselective NSAID, the risks are still substantially higher than during treatment with a COX-2 selective NSAID alone (Simon, Fox, 2005). Nevertheless, a cohort study using government databases of patients age 65 and older concluded that celecoxib may be safer from a GI perspective than other NSAIDs in older patients receiving cardioprotective aspirin (Rahme, Bardou, Dasgupta, et al., 2007).

Although the results have not been uniform, most randomized trials support a relatively better GI risk profile for the COX-2 selective NSAIDs. One study showed no significant difference in gastroduodenal ulcers between celecoxib and naproxen (Simon, Weaver, Graham, et al., 1999), but another showed celecoxib produced a lower incidence of upper GI ulcers and adverse effects compared with diclofenac (Emery, Zeidler, Kvien, et al., 1999). The Celecoxib Long-term Arthritis Safety Study (CLASS), which compared high-dose celecoxib (400 mg twice daily), ibuprofen (800 mg 3 times daily), and diclofenac (75 mg twice daily) in patients with osteoarthritis (OA) or RA observed that celecoxib caused significantly fewer symptomatic ulcers and ulcer complications (Silverstein, Faich, Goldstein, et al., 2000).

Table 6-2 | NSAID Treatment Strategies Correlated with Gastrointestinal (GI) Risk Levels

Risk Level (See Table 6-1 for Risk Factors)	Strategy
All risk levels	1. Assess the indications for NSAID treatment; consider the use of acetaminophen; for persistent musculoskeletal pain treatment, try weight reduction, physical therapy, and orthotics if appropriate. 2. If NSAID therapy is indicated, review individual risk factors for GI and CV complications when selecting the appropriate NSAID; weigh risk vs. benefit. 3. Administer the least ulcerogenic nonselective NSAID, e.g., salsalate, magnesium choline trisalicylate; low doses of ibuprofen, naproxen[1], etodolac, meloxicam, and nabumetone; or COX-2 selective NSAID (see Table 6-3). 4. Consider a topical NSAID. 5. Always give the lowest effective dose for the shortest time possible; periodically evaluate need. 6. Do not combine NSAIDs; be aware of increased risk associated with concomitant low-dose aspirin. 7. Treat *H. pylori* infection if known to be present prior to initiation of NSAID. 8. Assess regularly for NSAID-induced GI and CV adverse effects.
Low (no risk factors)	• Administer the least ulcerogenic NSAID at lowest effective dose (see #3 above).
Moderate (age ≥65 years or 1-2 risk factors)	• Administer least ulcerogenic NSAID at lowest effective dose (see #3 above) + PPI or misoprostol.
High (≥3 risk factors or concomitant aspirin, steroids, or warfarin or clopidogrel)[2,3]	• Routinely test for *H. pylori* prior to NSAID therapy. • Administer COX-2 selective NSAID + PPI or misoprostol. • If COX-2 selective NSAID is contraindicated due to CV risk, consider nonselective NSAID with low CV risk (e.g., naproxen) + PPI or misoprostol; monitor very closely • Consider alternative analgesia, such as acetaminophen, tramadol, or opioid analgesia.
Very high (prior ulcer or ulcer complications)[2,3]	• Routinely test for *H. pylori*. • Avoid NSAIDs if possible, and administer alternative analgesia, such as acetaminophen, tramadol, or opioid analgesia. • If short-term antiinflammatory therapy is required (e.g., gout), use steroids. • If regular antiinflammatory therapy is required, use COX-2 selective NSAID + PPI or misoprostol; if COX-2 selective NSAID is contraindicated due to CV risk, consider nonselective NSAID with low CV risk (e.g., naproxen[3]) + PPI or misoprostol; monitor very closely.

COX, Cyclooxygenase; *CV*, cardiovascular; *GI*, gastrointestinal; *H. pylori*, helicobacter pylori; *NSAID*, nonsteroidal antiinflammatory drug; *PPI*, proton pump inhibitor

[1]Avoid full-dose naproxen, piroxicam, and oxaprozin in older adults because of long half-life and increased risk of GI toxicity.

[2]Routinely test for and eradicate *H. pylori* infection, if present, prior to NSAID therapy.

[3]Further research is needed for consensus recommendations in this risk group. Carefully evaluate safety of COX-2 selective NSAIDs, particularly in patients taking concomitant aspirin or warfarin therapy as they may also have CV conditions in which COX-2 selective NSAIDs are contraindicated.

From Pasero, C., & McCaffery, M. *Pain assessment and pharmacologic management*, p. 194, St. Louis, Mosby. Data from American Geriatrics Society (AGS) Panel on Pharmacological Management of Persistent Pain in the Older Persons. (2009). The pharmacological management of persistent pain in older persons. *J Am Geriatr Soc*, 57(8), 1331-1346; Bhatt, D. L., Scheiman, J., Abraham, N. S., et al. (2008). ACCF/ACG/AHA 2008 expert consensus document on reducing the gastrointestinal risks of anti-platelet therapy and NSAID use. *Am J Gastroenterol*, 103(18), 2890-2907; Chan, F. K. L., & Graham, D. Y. (2004). Prevention of non-steroidal anti-inflammatory drug gastrointestinal complications—Review and recommendations based on risk assessment. *Aliment Pharmacol Ther*, 19(10), 1051-1061; Chan, F. K. L., To, K. F., Wu, J. C. Y., et al. (2002). Eradication of helicobacter pylori and risk of peptic ulcers in patients starting long-term treatment with non-steroidal anti-inflammatory drugs: A randomised trial. *Lancet*, 359(9300), 9-13; Chan, F. K. L., Wong, V. W., Suen, B. Y., et al. (2007). Combination of a cyclo-oxygenase-2 inhibitor and a proton-pump inhibitor for prevention of recurrent ulcer bleeding in patients at very high risk: A double-blind, randomised trial. *Lancet*, 369(9573), 1621-1626; Cryer, B., Hochberg, M. C., Hennekens, C. H., et al. (February 15, 2006). Changing patterns of coxibs/NSAIDs prescribing: Balancing CV and GI risks. CME program. Available at *http://www.medscape.com/viewprogram/5060*. Accessed August 8, 2008; Fick, D. M., Cooper, J. W., Wade, W. E., et al. (2003); Updating the Beers criteria for potentially inappropriate medication use in older adults. *Arch Intern Med*, 163(22), 2716-2724; Hanlon, J. T., Backonja, M., Weiner, D., et al. (2009). Evolving pharmacological management of persistent pain in older persons. *Pain Med* 10(6), 959-961; Laine, L. (2001). Approaches to nonsteroidal anti-inflammatory drug use in the high-risk patient. *Gastroenterology*, 120(3), 594-606; Simon, L. S. (2007). Risks and benefits of COX-2 selective inhibitors. Available at *http://www.medscape.com/viewprogram/6872/*. Accessed August 5, 2007; Simon, L. S., & Fox, R. I. (2005). What are the options available for anti-inflammatory drugs in the aftermath of rofecoxib's withdrawal? *Medscape Rheumatology* 6(1). Available at *http://www.medscape.com/viewarticle/500056*. Accessed April 16, 2005; Vonkeman, H. E., & van de Laar, M. A. F. J. (2008). NSAIDs: Adverse effects and their prevention. *Semin Arthritis Rheum*. Advanced access published on September 29, 2008; Wilcox, C. M., Allison, J., Benzuly, K., et al. (2006). Consensus development conference on the use of nonsteroidal anti-inflammatory agents, including cyclooxygenase-2 enzyme inhibitors and aspirin. *Clin Gastroenterol Hepatol*, 4(9), 1082-1089. © 2011, Pasero C, McCaffery M. May be duplicated for use in clinical practice.

Table 6-3 | NSAID Agents and Associated Risk for GI Events

Drug	Mild GI Events[a] (% of Patients)	Serious Events[b] (% of Patients)	Relative GI Toxicity[c]
Acetic Acids			
Diclofenac	3%-9%	< 2%	++
Etodolac	10%	<1%	+
Indomethacin	3%-9%	<1%	+++
Ketorolac	12%	0.4%-4.6%	+++
Sulindac	3%-9%	<1%	+
Tolmetin	3%-9%	<1%	++
COX-2 Selective NSAIDs			
Celecoxib	0.1%-8.8%[d]	<0.1%	+
Fenamates			
Meclofenamate	1%-3%	<1%	+
Mefenamic acid	1%-3%	<1%	+
Naphthylalkanones			
Nabumetone	13%	<1%	+
Oxicams			
Meloxicam	4.5%	<1%	+
Piroxicam[d]	1%-10%	1%-10%	+++
Proprionic Acids			
Fenoprofen	3%-9%	<1%	+++
Flurbiprofen	1%-9%	1%-3%	+++
Ibuprofen	1%-9%	<1%	++
Ketoprofen	11%	1%-2%	++
Naproxen[d]	1%-3%	<1%	++
Oxaprozin[d]	>1%	>1%	+++
Salicylates Acetylated			
Aspirin	2%-30%	<1%	+++
Salicylates Non-Acetylated			
Choline salicylate	>10%	1%-10%	+
Choline magnesium trisalicylate	<20%	<1%	+
Diflunisal	3%-9%	1%-7%	+++
Salsalate	>10%	1%-10%	+

[a]Dyspepsia, nausea, abdominal pain
[b]Ulceration, perforation, obstruction, bleeding ulcer
[c]+ = low risk; ++ = moderate risk; +++ = high risk
[d]Avoid full doses in older adults because of long half-life.
Note: Incidence may be much lower since many of the patients selected had previous history of GI risk.
From Pasero, C., & McCaffery, M. *Pain assessment and pharmacologic management*, p. 195, St. Louis, Mosby. Data from Clinical Pharmacology Online; Fick, D. M., Cooper, J. W., Wade, W. E., et al. (2003); Updating the Beers criteria for potentially inappropriate medication use in older adults. *Arch Intern Med, 163*(22), 2716-2724; Hanlon, J. T., Backonja, M., Weiner, D., et al. (2009). Evolving pharmacological management of persistent pain in older persons. *Pain Med, 10*(6), 959-961; Gold Standard, Inc. Available at *http://clinicalpharmacology.com.* Accessed August 10, 2008. © 2011, Pasero C, McCaffery M. May be duplicated for use in clinical practice.

As expected, newly developed COX-2 selective NSAIDs, such as lumiracoxib (Prexige) and etoricoxib (Arcoxia), also have a relatively lower risk of GI toxicity. The Therapeutic Arthritis Research and Gastrointestinal Event Trial (TARGET), which evaluated over 18,000 patients, showed a 3- to 4-fold reduction in ulcer complications with the use of lumiracoxib compared with naproxen or ibuprofen (Schnitzer, Burmester, Mysler, et al., 2004). A later study of healthy volunteers who were randomized to receive lumiracoxib, naproxen plus omeprazole (Prilosec), or placebo revealed that lumiracoxib yielded an incidence of small bowel mucosal breaks that was lower than naproxen plus omeprazole and similar to placebo (Hawkey, Ell, Simon, et al., 2008).

The Multinational Etoricoxib and Diclofenac Arthritis Long-term (MEDAL) program demonstrated fewer uncomplicated upper GI adverse events with etoricoxib than diclofenac; however, there was no difference in complicated events (perforation, obstruction, and complicated bleeding) (Laine, Curtis, Cryer, et al., 2007; Laine, Curtis, Langman, et al., 2008). Prior GI event and age 65 years and older were identified as significant risk factors for GI complications. Another study showed similar efficacy and lower GI adverse effects with etoricoxib compared with diclofenac in patients with OA over a 52-week evaluation period (Curtis, Bockow, Fisher, et al., 2005). An international multicenter study of 997 patients with OA compared long-term use of etoricoxib and naproxen and found the drugs had similarly satisfactory efficacy and tolerability, but there was a lower incidence of GI adverse effects and higher incidence of CV adverse effects in patients who took etoricoxib compared with those who took naproxen (Reginster, Malmstrom, Mehta, et al., 2007).

The latter study highlights the observation that diminished GI risk should not be interpreted as lower risk overall; CV risk remains a concern and continues to be evaluated in the newer COX-2 selective NSAIDs (Medscape Medical News, 2005; Topol, Falk, 2004; Wood, 2007) (see pp. 197-204 this chapter for discussion of CV risk). An assessment of risk factors (risk-benefit analysis) prior to NSAID therapy must include factors that go beyond GI risk (Tannenbaum, Bombardier, Davis, et al., 2006; Wilcox, Allison, Benzuly, et al., 2006). If the primary concern is GI risk, selection of an NSAID should focus either on a COX-2 selective drug or a nonselective drug with low GI risk (Wilcox, Allison, Benzuly, 2006) (see p. 204 for discussion of NSAID selection in the presence of both CV and GI risk).

Gastroprotective Co-Therapy

Gastroprotective co-therapy can reduce GI risk during NSAID therapy (Steen, Nurmohamed, Visman, et al., 2008; Wilcox, Allison, Benzuly, et al., 2006). The ACCF/ACG/AHA consensus guideline recommends gastroprotective co-therapy, preferably proton pump inhibitors (PPPs), in individuals who are taking a nonselective or COX-2 selective NSAID in conjunction with low-dose aspirin (Bhatt, Scheiman, Abraham, et al., 2008). The

expert panel of the First International Working Party on GI and CV Effects of NSAIDs and Anti-platelet Agents also recommended co-therapy when NSAIDs are used in individuals with increased GI risk (Chan, Abraham, Scheiman, et al., 2008).

Three classes of gastroprotective agents are suggested as options for co-therapy: (1) the prostaglandin analogues such as misoprostol (Cytotec); (2) histamine receptor type-2 (H_2) antagonists such as cimetidine (Tagamet), famotidine (Pepcid), and ranitidine (Zantac); and (3) PPIs such as esomeprazole (Nexium), lansoprazole (Prevacid), and omeprazole (Prilosec). A Cochrane Collaboration Review of 33 clinical trials concluded that all three classes of drugs reduced the incidence of both gastric and duodenal NSAID-induced ulcers (Rostom, Dube, Wells, et al., 2002); however, their effectiveness varies. Following is an overview of key research related to the three classes of gastroprotective agents.

Misoprostol is a synthetic prostaglandin that has been studied extensively in trials of ulcer prevention (Wilcox, Allison, Benzuly, et al., 2006). A Cochrane Collaboration Review concluded that doses of 800 mcg/day of misoprostol were superior to 400 mcg/day for prevention of gastric ulcers; however, no dose-related response was noted for duodenal ulcers (Rostom, Dube, Wells, et al., 2002). A prospective, double-blind study of long-term NSAID users with a history of gastric ulcer found patients who received 800 mcg/day of misoprostol remained ulcer free longer than those who received placebo or 15 or 30 mg of the PPI lansoprazole; however, a higher number of patients in the misoprostol group reported adverse effects and withdrew early from the study (Graham, Agrawal, Campbell, et al., 2002). The high incidence of adverse effects and study withdrawals led the researchers to conclude that misoprostol is clinically equivalent to PPIs. All doses of misoprostol can produce a high incidence of adverse effects, such as nausea, abdominal cramps, and diarrhea, and may not be well tolerated, particularly by the older patient (Chan, Graham, 2004; Rostom, Dube, Wells, et al., 2002; Wilcox, Allison, Benzuly, et al., 2006). Adherence to the regimen can be another barrier due to misoprostol dosing requirements that include taking the drug 4 times daily with food.

Whereas standard doses of H_2-antagonists are reported to be effective in prevention of duodenal but not gastric ulcers in patients taking NSAIDs, double doses have been shown to be effective against both types of ulcers (Rostom, Dube, Wells, et al., 2002). However, a review of nearly 40 years of randomized controlled trials revealed that misoprostol and PPIs were more effective than H_2-antagonists in reducing the risk of clinically significant GI adverse effects associated with NSAID use (Jacobsen, Phillips, 2004). Further, it has been suggested that any major benefit from H_2-antagonists may be limited to patients with *H. pylori* infection (Chan, Graham, 2004).

The ASTRONAUT study of 541 NSAID users showed that the PPI omeprazole prevented and healed all types of ulcers more effectively than the H_2-antagonist ranitidine

(Yeomans, Tulassay, Juhasz, et al., 1998). A larger double-blind study (N = 935), called the OMNIUM study, randomly assigned NSAID users with a history of ulcers (gastric or duodenal or both) to receive omeprazole or misoprostol for 4 weeks or, in the absence of healing, 8 weeks (Hawkey, Karrasch, Szczepanski, et al., 1998). Rates of successful ulcer treatment were similar between the two drugs; however, omeprazole was associated with a lower relapse rate and was better tolerated than misoprostol. Other PPIs have shown similar results. A prospective, double-blind study of 353 chronic NSAID users with active gastric ulcers found better healing rates after 8 weeks of treatment with lansoprazole than with the H_2-antagonist ranitidine (Agrawal, Campbell, Safdi, et al., 2000). AGA consensus guidelines recommend misoprostol if tolerated or a PPI in patients at high risk for GI complications (Wilcox, Allison, Benzuly, et al., 2006) (see Table 6-2). The AGS recommends a PPI or misoprostol in older adults taking either a nonselective NSAID or a COX-2 selective NSAID with low-dose aspirin (AGS, 2009).

The use of a COX-2 selective NSAID may be as effective as gastroprotective co-therapy in some populations (Chan, Graham, 2004; Jacobsen, Phillips, 2004; Schnitzer, Burmester, Mysler, et al., 2004; Laine, White, Rostom, et al., 2008; Silverstein, Faich, Goldstein, et al., 2000; Simon, 2007; Simon, Fox, 2005). Healthy, lesion-free subjects were randomized to receive celecoxib 200 mg twice daily or naproxen 500 mg twice daily plus omeprazole 20 mg once daily, or placebo for 2 weeks (Goldstein, Eisen, Lewis, et al., 2005). Those taking celecoxib exhibited significantly fewer small bowel mucosal breaks than those who took naproxen plus omeprazole as determined by video capsule endoscopy; those taking placebo had the fewest breaks. A later study by these researchers reported similar findings—celecoxib 200 mg twice daily was associated with significantly fewer small bowel mucosal breaks than ibuprofen 800 mg three times daily plus omeprazole 20 mg once daily, or placebo for 2 weeks (Goldstein, Eisen, Lewis, et al., 2007). There were no significant differences between celecoxib and placebo in this study.

A COX-2 selective NSAID with gastroprotective co-therapy may be most beneficial to patients with a high or very high risk for GI complications. A prospective, double-blind trial (N = 441) recruited long-term nonselective NSAID users with arthritis admitted to the hospital with upper GI bleeding. After ulcer healing, all patients were given 200 mg of celecoxib twice daily and were randomly assigned to receive the PPI esomeprazole or placebo twice daily for 12 months. Combination therapy with the PPI was found to be more effective in preventing GI adverse effects than celecoxib alone, leading the researchers to recommend a COX-2 selective NSAID and a PPI in patients at high risk for recurrent GI bleeding who need to take an NSAID (Chan, Wong, Suen, et al., 2007).

Greater attention to identification of those who might benefit from gastroprotective therapy and surveillance of patient adherence to gastroprotective therapy are warranted. A review of good-quality meta-analyses and large observational studies found that patients with GI risk factors often do not receive a prescription for gastroprotection and that those who do are often nonadherent to the treatment plan (Moore, Derry, Phillips, et al., 2006).

Cardiovascular (CV) Effects

CV homeostasis is among the key processes influenced by the effects of COX-1 and COX-2 on arachidonic acid (Rodriguez, 2001) (see Section I and Figure I-3 on p. 6). COX-1, which is present (constitutive) in most tissues, mediates the production of thromboxane A_2 which in turn *promotes* platelet aggregation, vasoconstriction, and smooth muscle proliferation (Bennett, Daugherty, Herrington, et al., 2005; Segev, Katz, 2004; Vardeny, Solomon, 2008). Conversely, COX-2 is induced at sites of inflammation where it is involved in the production of the prostaglandin prostacyclin from endothelial cells; prostacyclin is a potent vasodilator and *antagonizes* platelet aggregation, counteracting the effects of thromboxane A_2 (Bennett, Daugherty, Herrington, et al., 2005; Rodriguez, 2001; Segev, Katz, 2004; Vardeny, Solomon, 2008).

Presumably, any drug that inhibits COX-2 (thereby reducing levels of prostacyclin) will have prothrombotic effects, and those that inhibit COX-2 to a much greater extent than COX-1 will promote thrombosis more than others because of a disturbance in the physiologic balance between prostacyclin and thromboxane A_2 (Rodriguez, 2001; Scheiman, 2006; Segev, Katz, 2004). Because all NSAIDs inhibit COX-2 to some extent (Antman, DeMets, Loscalzo, 2005; Rodriguez, Patrignani, 2006; Vane, Warner, 2000; Warner, Mitchell, 2004, 2008; Vardeny, Solomon, 2008; Zhang, Ding, Song, 2006), all have prothrombotic effects; those classified as COX-2 selective NSAIDs and those nonselective NSAIDs with relatively greater effects at COX-2 probably have more intense prothrombotic effects than others (Bennett, Daugherty, Herrington, et al., 2005; FitzGerald, 2004; Pratico, Dogne, 2005; Scheiman, 2006; Segev, Katz, 2004; Vardeny, Solomon, 2008). The variability of COX-1 and COX-2 selectivity of a given NSAID is known as the selectivity index or the ratio of COX-1 selectivity to COX-2 selectivity (Patrono, Patrignani, Garcia, 2001; Warner, Mitchell, 2004) (Figure 6-1), and it is possible that this index provides a guide to the CV risk profile of the various NSAIDs. This hypothesis summarizes the so-called Mechanism-Based FitzGerald Hypothesis (Figure 6-2).

This disruption in the balance between platelet thromboxane A_2 and endothelial prostacyclin may explain, at least in part, the relatively high rate of CV adverse events that occurred with the COX-2 selective NSAIDs rofecoxib and valdecoxib. This toxicity led to their eventual withdrawal from the U.S. market (Linton, Fazio, 2002; FitzGerald, 2004; Segev, Katz, 2004).

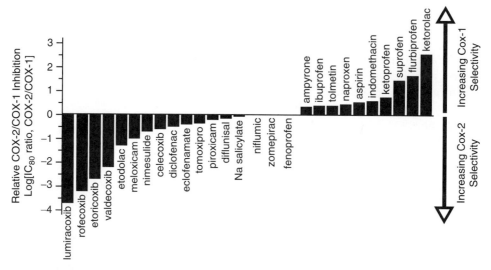

Figure 6-1 | NSAID COX-1 and COX-2 selectivity. From Antman, E. M., DeMets, D., & Loscalzo, J. (2005). Cyclooxygenase inhibition and cardiovascular risk. *Circulation, 112*(5), 759-770. Modified from Warner, T. D., & Mitchell, J. A. (2004). Cyclooxygenases: New forms, new inhibitors, and lessons from the clinic. *FASEB J, 18,* 790-804.

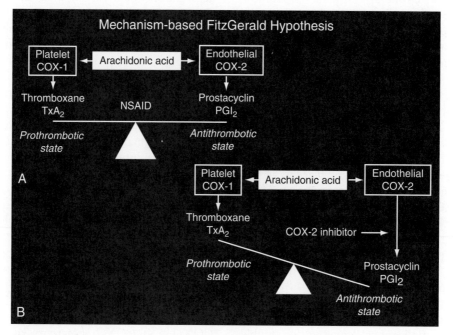

Figure 6-2 | Mechanism-Based Fitzgerald Hypothesis. From Scheiman, J. M., Goldstein, J. L., Sung, J. J. Y, et al. (2006). The power of a new perspective on nonsteroidal anti-inflammatory drug-related gastrointestinal complications: Strategies for endoscopic and medical therapy. *Medscape* Sep 15. Data from FitzGerald, G. A. (2004). Coxibs and cardiovascular disease. *N Engl J Med, 351*(17), 1709-1711; FitzGerald, G. A., & Patrono, C. (2001). The coxibs, selective inhibitors of cyclooxygenase-2. *N Engl J Med, 345*(6), 433-442; Rodriguez, L. A. (2001). The effect of NSAIDs on the risk of coronary heart disease: Fusion of clinical pharmacology and pharmacoepidemiologic data. *Clin Exp Rheumatol, 19*(6 Suppl 25), S41-S44.

Although the hypothesis linking the CV effects of COX isoenzymes to their varied effects on thromboxane A_2 and prostacyclin provides a strong mechanism-based explanation for the observed toxicities, it is likely that other mechanisms also are involved (Joshi, Gertler, Fricker, 2007). For example, inhibition of prostacyclin by COX-2 also reduces the ability of the epithelium to defend against hypertension and atherosclerosis (FitzGerald, 2004; Psaty, Furberg, 2005) and may increase the risk of CV adverse effects on this basis.

The selectivity index also may explain some other differences in the incidences of adverse effects associated with each of the NSAIDs. For example, as Figure 6-1 shows, most of the nonselective NSAIDs have a tendency toward greater COX-1 than COX-2 selectivity, which accounts for their associated greater risk of GI toxicity and increased bleeding times. Presumably, additional studies of newer, highly selective COX-2 NSAIDs will demonstrate that these drugs reduce the risk of GI toxicity while simultaneously having a relatively higher risk of prothrombotic effects. Again, however, it must be emphasized that all NSAIDs, including those classified as nonselective NSAIDs (COX-1/COX-2 inhibitors), have some degree of COX-2 inhibition and associated risk of adverse CV events (Antman, DeMets, Loscalzo, 2005).

CV Risk Factors

All patients who are being considered for ongoing NSAID therapy should be carefully assessed for preexisting risk factors for vascular disease and closely monitored for CV adverse events during NSAID use, regardless of the type of NSAID administered (Andersohn, Suissa, Garbe, 2006; Brophy, Levesque, Zhang 2007; Crofford, Oates, McCune, et al., 2000; FitzGerald, Patrono, 2001; Gislason, Jacobsen, Rasmussen, et al., 2006). For example, Solomon and colleagues (2008) found that individuals with prior CV disease, hypertension, RA, chronic renal disease, chronic obstructive pulmonary disease, and those ≥ 80 years old all are at increased risk of CV events when taking NSAIDs. Assessment of these and other factors, and interventions to reduce risk and monitor over time, are important recommendations for NSAID therapy (Antman, Bennett, Daugherty, et al., 2007; Chan, Abraham, Scheiman, et al., 2008).

The First International Working Party on GI and CV Effects of NSAIDs and Anti-platelet Agents predefined high CV risk as the presence of established CV disease (e.g., prior myocardial infarction (MI), stroke, or angina) or an estimated 10-year CV risk of greater than 20% in patients without CV disease (Chan, Abraham, Scheiman, et al., 2008). The AHA and the American Stroke Association categorize CV risk factors as nonmodifiable, modifiable, or potentially modifiable (Goldstein, Adams, Alberts, et al., 2006). This provides a good format for consideration of CV risk prior to initiating NSAID therapy (see Table 6-4).

Nonmodifiable risks are those beyond the person's ability to change, such as age, sex, and race. Advanced age is a major contributor, with the risk of stroke doubling with each decade after the age of 55 years. It is expected that the aging of the "baby boomer" population will become the biggest factor boosting the prevalence of heart failure (Schoken, Benjamin, Fonarow, et al., 2008). The aging process also brings other conditions that increase CV risk, including hypertension, diabetes, and renal insufficiency (McDermott, Fried, Simonsick, et al., 2000; Schoken, Benjamin, Fonarow, et al., 2008) (see renal effects later in

Table 6-4	Risk Factors for NSAID-Induced Adverse Cardiovascular Events	
Risk Level	**Examples**
Non-modifiable[1]	Advanced age; sex; low birth weight; race/ethnicity; genetic factors[4]
Modifiable[2]	Noncerebrovascular atherosclerotic vascular disease (e.g., coronary heart disease, cardiac failure, symptomatic peripheral arterial disease)[4]; other cardiac conditions (e.g., previous MI, valvular heart disease, cardiomyopathy) [4]; hypertension[4]; diabetes[4]; obesity[4]; cigarette smoke[4]; atrial fibrillation; dyslipidemia; asymptomatic carotid stenosis; sickle cell disease; rheumatoid arthritis; postmenopausal hormone replacement therapy; diet; nutrition; physical inactivity
Potentially modifiable[3]	Metabolic syndrome; oral contraceptive use; sleep disordered breathing; migraine; hyperhomocysteinemia; elevated lipoproteins; inflammation; infection; toxins (alcohol or drug abuse, chemotherapy, some medications including NSAIDs)[1]

MI, myocardial infarction; *NSAID*, nonsteroidal antiinflammatory drug.
[1]Risk factors that are beyond the person's ability to change
[2]Risk factors that are well documented as contributing to adverse CV events and within the individual's ability to change or control effectively enough to significantly reduce risk
[3]Risk factors that can be changed or controlled but are less well documented in terms of their association with adverse CV events
[4]Major clinical risk factor

From Pasero, C., & McCaffery, M. *Pain assessment and pharmacologic management*, p. 199, St. Louis, Mosby. Data from Bhatt, D. L., Scheiman, J., Abraham, N. S., et al. (2008). ACCF/ACG/AHA 2008 expert consensus document on reducing the gastrointestinal risks of anti-platelet therapy and NSAID use. *Am J Gastroenterol*, 103(18), 2890-2907; Goldstein, L. B., Adams, R., Alberts, M. J., et al. (2006). Primary prevention of ischemic stroke. A guideline from the American Heart Association/American Stroke Association Stroke Council: Cosponsored by the Atherosclerotic Peripheral Nursing Council; Clinical Cardiology Council; Nutrition, Physical Activity, and Metabolism Council; and the Quality of Care and Outcomes Research Interdisciplinary Working Group. *Circulation*, 113(24), e873-e923; Pearson, T. A., Blair, S. N., Daniels, S. R., et al. (2002). AHA guidelines for primary prevention of cardiovascular disease and stroke: 2002 update. *Circulation*, 106(4), 388-391; Schoken, D. D., Benjamin, E. J., Fonarow, G. C., et al. (2008). Prevention of heart failure. A scientific statement from the American Heart Association Councils on Epidemiology and Prevention, Clinical Cardiology, Cardiovascular Nursing, and High Blood Pressure Research; Quality of Care and Outcomes Research Interdisciplinary Working Group; and Functional Genomics and Translational Biology Interdisciplinary Working Group. *Circulation*, 117(19), 2544-2565; Solomon, D. H., Glynn, R. J., Rothman, K. J., et al. (2008). Subgroup analyses to determine cardiovascular risk associated with nonsteroidal anti-inflammatory drugs and coxibs in specific patient groups. *Arthritis Rheum* 59(6):1097-1104; Solomon, D. H., Karlson, E. W., Rimm, E. B., et al. (2003). Cardiovascular morbidity and mortality in women diagnosed with rheumatoid arthritis. *Circulation*, 107(9), 1303-1307. © 2011, Pasero C, McCaffery M. May be duplicated for use in clinical practice.

this chapter). The AGS lists heart failure as an absolute contraindication and hypertension as a relative contraindication to the use of NSAIDs in older adults (AGS, 2009).

Other nonmodifiable risk factors, like age, are strongly influenced by related conditions and type of CV event. For example, stroke is more common in men than in women (Goldstein, Adams, Alberts, et al., 2006), whereas mortality from coronary heart disease is higher among women (Jousilahti, Vartiainen, Tuomilehto, et al., 1999). Genetic factors, including genetic disorders such as sickle cell anemia (James, 2000) also are important, both in terms of risk factors and CV events themselves. Although nonmodifiable risk factors cannot be changed, they help identify individuals who are at highest risk and who might benefit from aggressive disease prevention or treatment, as well as close monitoring during NSAID therapy (Goldstein, Adams, Alberts, et al., 2006).

Modifiable risk factors are those that are well documented as contributing to adverse CV events and are within the individual's ability to change or control effectively enough to significantly reduce risk. Preexisting CV disease, hypertension, diabetes, and dyslipidemia are among the modifiable factors (Goldstein, Adams, Alberts, et al., 2006). Obesity, sedentary lifestyle, and diet interact with other physiologic abnormalities such as insulin resistance and a pro-inflammatory state to produce the metabolic syndrome, which has been separately identified as an important risk factor for CV events (Goldstein, Adams, Alberts, et al., 2006). Frank diabetes with poorly controlled glycemia is a potentially major factor (Fox, Coady, Sorlie, et al., 2007), as is hypertension alone (Schoken, Benjamin, Fonarow, et al., 2008). Hypertension, for example, causes a 2- to 3-fold increase in risk of heart failure, as well as an increased risk of coronary artery disease, and early detection and control of BP is perceived to be a key strategy for prevention of CV disease and catastrophic CV events (Pearson, Blair, Daniels, et al., 2002).

The role of hypertension as a mediator of both heart failure and coronary artery disease underscores the need for a careful assessment of CV risk factors in those considered for NSAID therapy. NSAIDs increase the risk of hypertension or worsen preexisting hypertension (Bombardier, Laine, Reicin, et al., 2000; Curhan, Willett, Rosner, et al., 2002; Dedier, Stampfer, Hankinson, et al., 2002; Simon, 2007; Whelton, Lefkowith, West, et al., 2006; Whelton, White, Bello, et al., 2002; White, Kent, Taylor, et al., 2002), and BP monitoring, with adjustment of antihypertensive therapy if needed, is essential to reduce NSAID-associated CV risk that is mediated through BP abnormalities (see pp. 205-206 for more discussion about NSAIDs and hypertension).

Cigarette smoking is another extremely well-documented, potent modifiable CV risk factor; both first-hand and second-hand smoke increase risk (Goldstein, Adams, Alberts, et al., 2006; Hermann, Krum, Ruschitzka, 2005; McAdam, Byrne, Morrow, et al., 2005). NSAID users who smoke have a higher incidence of CV adverse events than NSAID users who do not smoke (Chan, Manson, Albert, et al., 2006).

Some potentially modifiable factors are less well documented in terms of their association with adverse CV events, including obstructive sleep apnea and migraine headache (Goldstein, Adams, Alberts, et al., 2006). In addition to NSAIDs, several drugs have been implicated in heart disease, such as some chemotherapies and hormonal agents, including oral contraceptives; IV drug abuse and alcohol abuse also may predispose to heart disease (Schoken, Benjamin, Fonarow, et al., 2008).

Unfortunately, diseases with an inflammatory component that may benefit from NSAID therapy, such as RA and systemic lupus erythematosus (SLE), have also been shown to produce elevated CV risk (D'Cruz, 2006; de Carvalho, Bonfa, Borba, 2008; Solomon, Karlson, Rimm, et al., 2003). A large cohort study of over 114,000 women who participated in the Nurses' Health Study (Colditz, 1995) found that those with RA had an increased risk for MI (Solomon, Karlson, Rimm, et al., 2003). This led the researchers to recommend aggressive CV disease-prevention strategies in individuals with RA. CV risk factors for individuals with SLE are many and include dyslipoproteinemia with low HDL (high-density lipoprotein) cholesterol and increased triglycerides (de Carvalho, Bonfa, Borba, 2008; Thiagarajan, 2001) as well as an association with autoantibodies to oxidized LDL (low-density lipoprotein) cholesterol (Svenungsson, Jensen-Urstad, Heimburger, et al., 2001).

The link between CV risk and inflammatory diseases is explained, at least in part, by evidence that shows inflammation is a prominent feature of atherosclerotic plaque formation (Solomon, Karlson, Rimm, et al., 2003; Svenungsson, Jensen-Urstad, Heimburger, et al., 2001; Vasan, Sullivan, Roubenoff, et al., 2003), such that atherosclerosis has been called an inflammatory condition of the vessel wall (Thiagarajan, 2001). A variety of inflammatory factors associated with increased CV risk, such as elevated C-reactive protein concentration, are also elevated in RA and SLE (Svenungsson, Jensen-Urstad, Heimburger, et al., 2001).

Potentially modifiable CV risk factors commonly co-exist and may potentiate each other, further highlighting the need to have a comprehensive medical assessment as part of safe NSAID prescribing. For example, women who smoke and use oral contraceptives are at 1.3 times greater CV risk than nonsmoking women who use oral contraceptives (Goldstein, Adams, Alberts, et al., 2006). Alcohol intake may increase CV risk by increasing BP (Schoken, Benjamin, Fonarow, et al., 2008). Obese individuals often experience multiple comorbidities that represent elevated risk including sleep-disordered breathing, physical inactivity, and diabetes (Schoken, Benjamin, Fonarow, et al., 2008).

CV Effects of COX-2 Selective NSAIDs

Shortly after the release of rofecoxib in 1999, the 12-month Vioxx Gastrointestinal Outcomes Research (VIGOR) trial, which was designed to compare GI adverse effects associated with naproxen and rofecoxib, showed a 50% reduction in serious GI events in the subjects who were given rofecoxib (Bombardier, Laine, Reicin, et al., 2000). However, an unexpected and disturbing finding was a 5-fold increase in thromboembolic events, such as acute MI, in the rofecoxib group. The VIGOR trial did not have a placebo control group, which lent plausibility to the frequently-offered explanation that naproxen, a nonselective NSAID, was cardioprotective and thus produced fewer CV events than rofecoxib (Graham, 2006; Graham, Campen, Hui, et al., 2005). Later analysis, however, suggested that naproxen is not cardioprotective (Graham, Campen, Hui, et al., 2005; McGettigan, Henry, 2006; Ray, Stein, Hall, et al., 2002; Salpeter, Gregor, Ormiston, et al., 2006), at least at typical doses (Chan, Abraham, Scheiman, et al., 2008). Graham (2006) proposed that a more accurate interpretation of the VIGOR findings would have been that rofecoxib increased CV risk by 5-fold rather than that the CV risk associated with naproxen was one-fifth that of rofecoxib.

The Adenomatous Polyp Prevention On Vioxx (APPROVe) study was undertaken to determine if long-term (3 years) rofecoxib treatment would reduce the risk of recurrent adenomatous polyps in patients with a history of colorectal adenomas (Bresalier, Sandler, Quan, et al., 2005). Over 2500 patients were randomized to receive either rofecoxib or placebo. During the first 18 months of treatment, the CV adverse event rates were similar among the two groups; however, after 18 months, data suggested a greater number of MIs and ischemic cerebrovascular events occurred in the rofecoxib group. A later systematic review contradicted the suggestion that vascular risk with rofecoxib occurred only after months of treatment (McGettigan, Henry, 2006). Increasing evidence of elevated CV risk prompted the withdrawal of rofecoxib from the worldwide market in September 2004 (Graham, 2006).

Valdecoxib, which is the active metabolite of the parenteral COX-2 selective NSAID parecoxib (Dynastat) available in Europe, was withdrawn from the U.S. market in 2005 following research showing CV events similar to rofecoxib (Vardeny, Solomon, 2008). Studies showing an increase in CV events in patients who were given parecoxib and valdecoxib perioperatively (Nussmeier, Whelton, Brown, et al., 2005; Ott, Nussmeier, Duke, et al., 2003) led to recommendations against the use of any COX-2 selective NSAIDs following high-risk open heart surgery (U.S. FDA, 2007). (See Chapter 8 for a discussion of perioperative NSAID use.) Valecoxib was withdrawn from the market on the basis of the CV risk as well as reported cases of cutaneous hypersensitivity (see pp. 207-208 for discussion of nonopioid hypersensitivity).

Celecoxib currently is the only COX-2 selective NSAID in the United States. The so-called CLASS study randomized 8059 patients with OA or RA to receive a 6-month trial of celecoxib, ibuprofen, or diclofenac (Silverstein, Faich, Goldstein, et al., 2000). Patients were allowed to continue cardioprotective therapy

during the study period. No difference in CV events was found among the three NSAIDs, and new-onset or aggravation of preexisting hypertension was lowest in the celecoxib-treated group. Other studies have shown similar results (Hudson, Rahme, Richard, et al., 2007; Solomon, Schneeweiss, Glynn, et al., 2004; Steinbach, Lynch, Phillips, et al., 2000; Whelton, White, Bello, et al., 2002). These data questioned whether the risk of CV toxicity identified during rofecoxib and valdecoxib therapy, which suggested a class effect (i.e., associated with the so-called COX-2 selective drugs), was indeed this, or rather a risk that attended some drugs and not others.

Numerous other studies followed the early efficacy trials and were intended to clarify the risk of CV events for individual drugs and the classes they occupy. Although some of the data are conflicting, a broad picture of the CV risk associated with NSAID therapy has emerged.

Studies of insurance claims data provide one source of evidence pertaining to this issue. An examination of data of Medicare beneficiaries, which consisted of new users of COX-2 selective NSAIDs (N = 76,082), new users of nonselective NSAIDs (N = 53,014), and non-users of any NSAIDs (N = 46,558), suggested that most NSAIDs, when taken at standard doses, do not significantly increase the risk of CV events (Solomon, Glynn, Rothman, et al., 2008). These data showed that rofecoxib was associated with the highest CV event rates and that naproxen was associated with the lowest—even lower than nonusers. Certain patient characteristics (prior CV disease, hypertension, RA, chronic renal disease, chronic obstructive pulmonary disease, and age 80 years or older) were associated with elevated risk as well. Other large database studies (Ray, Stein, Hall, et al., 2002; Solomon, Schneeweiss, Glynn, et al., 2004; Graham, Campen, Hui, et al., 2005) suggested that the incidence of acute MI with celecoxib use was actually lower than that of other NSAIDs (Simon, 2007).

An extensive systematic review of observational studies that investigated CV events associated with a variety of NSAIDs found that celecoxib at doses of 200 mg/day or less was not associated with CV increased risk and that naproxen was not associated with any reduced CV risk (McGettigan, Henry, 2006). The highest risk among the nonselective NSAIDs was with commonly used doses of diclofenac (e.g., 150 mg daily). This finding may be notable in light of data indicating a relatively higher COX-2 selectivity of this drug than other nonselective NSAIDs (Graham, 2006; McGettigan, Henry, 2006; Vardeny, Solomon, 2008) (see Figure 6-1). Meloxicam, another long-acting nonselective NSAID that preferentially inhibits COX-2, at least in lower prescribed doses, has shown similar efficacy and a better GI profile than the comparable nonselective NSAIDs piroxicam and diclofenac and less peripheral edema and weight gain when compared with diclofenac (Smith, Baird, 2003). Studies are needed to evaluate this and other nonselective NSAIDs that possess relatively higher levels of COX-2 inhibitory activity.

Data from randomized controlled trials of celecoxib and other NSAIDs have yielded mixed results. A meta-analysis of randomized clinical trials evaluated the incidence of CV events in nearly 7500 patients exposed to celecoxib 200 to 800 mg daily; nearly 14,000 patients treated with diclofenac, ibuprofen, naproxen, ketoprofen (Orudis), or loxoprofen (available outside of the United States); and over 4000 patients who were given placebo (White, West, Borer, et al., 2007). The analysis failed to demonstrate a difference in the incidence of CV events associated with celecoxib compared with other NSAIDs or compared with placebo for up to 1 year of treatment exposure. Use of aspirin or presence of CV risk factors did not alter the findings.

In contrast, placebo-controlled trials designed to study a potential role for celecoxib in the prevention of colorectal adenoma revealed an increased CV risk in patients who received celecoxib. The Prevention of Colorectal Sporadic Adenomatous Polyps (PreSAP) trial demonstrated a reduced recurrence of colorectal adenomas in patients who received a single 400-mg dose of celecoxib daily; however, CV events occurred more often in patients who received celecoxib (2.5%) than in those who received placebo (1.9%) (Arber, Eagle, Spicak, et al., 2006). More concerning was the Adenoma Prevention with Celecoxib (APC) trial, which randomized patients to receive celecoxib 200 mg or 400 mg twice daily or placebo (Bertagnolli, Eagle, Zauber, et al., 2006). As in the PreSAP trial, a reduction in the recurrence of colorectal adenomas was noted; however, serious adverse CV events occurred in 18.8%, 20.4%, and 23% of those who received placebo, 200 mg of celecoxib twice daily, and 400 mg of celecoxib twice daily. This increase in CV events led the researchers to caution against the routine use of celecoxib for prevention of colorectal adenomas. Celecoxib administration in several long-term trials, including the APC and PreSAP trials, was halted as a result of CV events (Solomon, Wittes, Finn, et al., 2008). (See Chapter 7 for more on NSAIDs and prevention of cancer.)

The PreSAP and APC trials elucidated interesting findings related to the impact of both dose and dosing regimens on the level of CV risk associated with celecoxib (Solomon, Pfeffer, McMurray, et al., 2006; Solomon, Wittes, Finn, et al., 2008; Vardeny, Solomon, 2008). Vardeny and Solomon (2008) pointed out that the evidence for CV risk in the PreSAP trial, which administered a single 400-mg celecoxib dose daily, was less compelling than that of the APC trial, which showed significant risk associated with a 200-mg or 400-mg twice-daily dosing regimen. This was demonstrated in an independent review of combined data from the APC and PreSAP trials that found a hazard ratio (estimate of relative risk) for death from MI, stroke, or heart failure of 1.3 in patients taking 400 mg once daily (PreSAP), 2.6 in those taking 200 mg twice daily (APC), and 3.4 in

those taking 400 mg twice daily (Solomon, McMurray, Pfeffer, et al., 2005). Similarly, an analysis of pooled data from nearly 8000 patients in six placebo-controlled trials, which included the APC and PreSAP data, assessed CV risk associated with three dosing regimens of celecoxib and found the lowest, intermediate, and highest risk associated with dosing regimens of 400 mg daily, 200 mg twice daily, and 400 mg twice daily, respectively (Solomon, Wittes, Finn, et al., 2008). Patients with highest baseline risk had an increased relative risk for CV events.

Notwithstanding the conflicting data, these studies suggest that there is some CV risk associated with celecoxib treatment, as there is with other NSAIDs. The finding of dose-dependency is relatively strong evidence of a pharmacologic effect. It is curious, however, that two studies observe that lower risk is associated with once-daily dosing compared with twice-daily dosing at the same overall daily dose (400 mg). This also may have a pharmacologic explanation in that the maximum plasma concentration of celecoxib is reached in 90 minutes and the half-life is just 1.5 hours (Paulson, Hribar, Liu, et al., 2000). Because prostacyclin levels require approximately 12 hours to recover following a single oral dose of celecoxib (McAdam, Catella-Lawson, Mardini, et al., 1999), it has been proposed that once-daily dosing (but not twice-daily dosing) of celecoxib may allow enough prostacyclin recovery and normalization to attenuate the prothrombotic effect (Grosser, Fries, FitzGerald, 2006; Vardeny, Solomon, 2008). Although further research is needed, the findings in other studies that utilized once-daily dosing support this theory (Sowers, White, Pitt, et al., 2005; Whelton, Fort, Puma, et al., 2001).

The evidence overall suggests that there is CV risk during all NSAID therapies, however the link with COX-2 inhibition suggests that drugs with COX-2 selectivity must be particularly scrutinized for this effect. This has been done with newer COX-2 selective NSAIDs, such as etoricoxib and lumiracoxib (Andersohn, Suissa, Garbe, 2006; Cannon, Curtis, FitzGerald, et al., 2006; Farkouh, Kirshner, Harrington, et al., 2004; Laine, Curtis, Cryer, et al., 2007; Schnitzer, Burmester, Mysler, et al., 2004). These drugs were not available in the United States at the time of publication (Medscape Medical News, 2005; Wood, 2007).

The TARGET study randomized over 18,000 patients with OA to receive lumiracoxib, naproxen, or ibuprofen (Farkouh, Kirshner, Harrington, et al., 2004). Patients were allowed to take low-dose aspirin during the study. The incidence of adverse CV events was low and did not differ among the NSAID groups, irrespective of aspirin use. Though not statistically significant, there were more nonfatal MIs in the lumiracoxib group than in the naproxen nonaspirin group. The lack of a placebo arm in this study makes it difficult to ascertain actual CV risk associated with lumiracoxib.

The MEDAL program evaluated pooled data from three trials involving 34,701 patients with OA and 9787 with RA who were given etoricoxib or diclofenac at recommended doses for a mean duration of 18 months (Cannon, Curtis, FitzGerald, et al., 2006). Patients in the two groups were reported to have almost identical rates of thrombotic CV events (320 patients in the etoricoxib group; 323 patients in the diclofenac group). This study has been criticized for the lack of a placebo arm and the use of diclofenac as the comparator NSAID (Graham, 2006; Hughes 2006; Rodriquez, Patrignani, 2006). Given the suggestion that diclofenac has a relatively high CV risk (Hernandez-Diaz, Varas-Lorenzo, Rodriguez, 2006; Kearney, Baigent, Godwin, et al., 2006; McGettigan, Henry, 2006), comparability between this drug and etoricoxib does not establish the safety of the latter drug (Graham, 2006). Although diclofenac is widely prescribed and does not appear to interfere with the antiplatelet effects of low-dose aspirin (Cannon, Curtis, FitzGerald, et al., 2006) (see later discussion regarding NSAID interference with cardioprotective aspirin), its use in this study complicates interpretation of the results.

Class Effect. As noted, an important controversy surrounding the emerging data on NSAID CV risk relates to the most useful way to categorize the findings in terms of drug effects vs. drug class effects (Helstrom, Rosow, 2006; Porter, 2005; Pratico, Dogne, 2005). Some researchers claim there is enough evidence showing a "cardiovascular hazard" with three of the COX-2 selective NSAIDs—rofecoxib, celecoxib, and parecoxib—to support the hypothesis that the adverse CV events associated with these drugs are related to a class effect (Pratico, Dogne, 2005). Others view this as problematic given the conflicting data about celecoxib and the evidence that at least some of the drugs classified as nonselective NSAIDs have risk.

In an effort to address this controversy, a meta-analysis was performed that included data from 114 trials involving 116,094 patients who received the COX-2 selective NSAIDs rofecoxib, celecoxib, etoricoxib, lumiracoxib, or valdecoxib plus parecoxib. This analysis yielded insufficient evidence to claim a COX-2 selective class effect (Zhang, Ding, Song, 2006), a conclusion supported by others (Hudson, Rahme, Richard, et al., 2007). Despite some conflicting data that suggest minimal to no risk among the nonselective NSAIDs (NIH, 2004; Salpeter, Gregor, Ormiston, et al., 2006), a recent meta-analysis of randomized trials again showed that COX-2 selective NSAIDs, which as a group impose a 2-fold increased risk of MI compared with placebo and naproxen, did not increase risk compared with non-naproxen NSAIDs (Laine, White, Rostom A, et al., 2008).

Despite these meta-analyses and large epidemiologic studies, the debate surrounding CV risk as drug effect vs. COX-2 selective class effect continues. More head-to-head comparisons between the various NSAIDs are required to better address this ongoing controversy (Porter, 2005). At the present time, the most prudent conclusion continues to be that CV risk is inherent in the capacity to inhibit COX-2, and thereby reduce tissue levels of prostacyclin. Because both nonselective NSAIDs and COX-2 selective NSAIDs have COX-2 effects, and because the various so-called COX-2 selective drugs vary in the extent to which COX-2 is blocked relative to COX-1, it is best to assume that all NSAIDs have CV risk and that the risk varies across drugs, even within classes. The evidence of elevated risk prompted the U.S. FDA to issue almost identical product label warnings for all NSAIDs, irrespective of class (Dajani, Islam, 2008).

NSAID Selection with Consideration of CV Risk

This conclusion obligates clinicians to be aware of evidence that supports different risk profiles for different NSAIDs and to consider relative risks when recommending a specific drug in clinical practice. The First International Working Party on GI and CV Effects of NSAIDs and Anti-platelet Agents suggested that either nonselective NSAIDs or COX-2 selective NSAIDs could be appropriate in patients with no evidence of elevated GI risk and average CV risk; naproxen was preferred in patients with no GI risk but high CV risk (Chan, Abraham, Scheiman, et al., 2008). The panel rated the use of COX-2 selective NSAIDs in patients with high CV risk as uncertain or inappropriate (see later discussion of NSAID selection in the presence of both GI and CV risk). As mentioned, an extensive review of Medicare beneficiary data confirmed the safety of naproxen from a CV perspective as well (Solomon, Glynn, Rothman, et al., 2008).

The AHA proposes a "stepped care" approach for the treatment of musculoskeletal pain in individuals with known CV disease or risk factors for ischemic heart disease (Antman, Bennett, Daugherty, et al., 2007). Others have incorporated similar recommendations into their guidelines for the management of high-risk cardiac patients (Anderson, Adams, Antman, et al., 2007). The first step of the AHA approach recommends acetaminophen, aspirin, tramadol, or short-term opioid analgesics. Nonacetylated salicylates, such as choline magnesium trisalicylate or salsalate (Disalcid), are a second-step option. If this does not control pain, a nonselective NSAID with low COX-2 selectivity such as naproxen or ibuprofen is recommended. The use of a COX-2 selective NSAID is suggested as a last choice. Of note is a review of the literature that suggested the use of a COX-2 selective NSAID with cardioprotective aspirin in patients with CV risk is preferential to nonselective NSAIDs (Strand, 2007). However, some experts have questioned the rationale of using a COX-2 selective NSAID with aspirin at all in patients with high CV risk citing a lack of research showing aspirin can sufficiently mitigate the absolute CV risk imposed by COX-2 selective NSAIDs (Hughes, 2007).

Other general AHA recommendations when NSAIDs are used are to select patients at low risk for thrombotic events, prescribe the lowest dose required to control symptoms, add cardioprotective aspirin (with a PPI) to patients at increased risk of thrombotic events, and regularly monitor for sustained hypertension, edema, worsening renal function, and GI bleeding. The AHA cautions that effective pain relief with the use of NSAIDs may come at the cost of an increase in risk for CV or cerebrovascular complications (Antman, Bennett, Daugherty, et al., 2007).

NSAID Selection in Presence of Both CV and GI Risk

Patients who are at risk for both GI and CV adverse effects present special challenges in determining how to proceed with NSAID therapy. Although the use of naproxen or ibuprofen combined with nonaspirin antiplatelet therapy (e.g., clopidogrel [Plavix]) has been suggested (Hughes, 2006), there are few data that support this approach.

The expert panel of the First International Working Party on GI and CV Effects of NSAIDs and Anti-platelet Agents suggests that the initial choice of an NSAID should depend on the patient's CV risk, whereas the addition of gastroprotective therapy depends on the number and severity of GI risk factors (Chan, Abraham, Scheiman, et al., 2008). The panel rated naproxen plus a PPI or misoprostol as appropriate, regardless of patient age, in patients with both CV and GI risks. Non-naproxen NSAIDs and COX-2 selective NSAIDs, with or without gastroprotective therapy, were rated as uncertain or inappropriate in such patients. Some researchers recommend avoiding full doses of NSAIDs with a long half-life, such as naproxen (Fick, Cooper, Wade, et al., 2003).

A retrospective cohort study using government databases including patients 65 years and older concluded that celecoxib may be safer from a GI perspective than other NSAIDs in older adults receiving cardioprotective aspirin to minimize CV risk (Rahme, Bardou, Dasgupta, et al., 2007). Others have suggested a low-dose COX-2 selective NSAID plus low-dose aspirin plus a PPI if NSAID therapy is used in patients with major GI and CV risk factors (Laine, White, Rostom, et al., 2008).

It is important to remember that avoiding NSAIDs altogether may be the best approach for high-risk patients (Laine, White, Rostom, et al., 2008). In fact, the expert panel of the First International Working Party on GI and CV Effects of NSAIDs and Anti-platelet Agents recommends avoidance of NSAID therapy entirely in patients with high CV risk and multiple GI risk factors (e.g., patients older than age 70 who are receiving concomitant corticosteroids, low-dose aspirin, and other antiplatelet agents or anticoagulants) (Chan, Abraham, Scheiman, et al., 2008). Opioid analgesics are among the safest analgesics from a GI and CV perspective and should be considered in patients with pain who present with significant risk for NSAID-induced adverse effects.

Hematologic Effects and Cardioprotective Aspirin

NSAIDs have the potential to produce cardioprotection through COX-1 inhibition of thromboxane; however, 95% suppression of COX-1 is required to inhibit thromboxane-induced platelet aggregation (Salpeter, Gregor, Ormiston, et al., 2006). Aspirin reaches this level of suppression, producing an irreversible effect on platelets and a reported increase in bleeding time for up to 7 days after the last dose (i.e., until the platelets are replaced with new) (Sun, Crowther, Warkentin, et al., 2005). Nonselective NSAIDs inhibit thromboxane within a range of 59% to 95%, and their inhibition is reversible and not maintained over the dosing interval (Salpeter, Gregor, Ormiston, et al., 2006). As a result, these drugs should not be used in an effort to provide a therapeutic antiplatelet effect. The AHA recommends immediate-release, nonenteric coated aspirin at cardioprotective doses (i.e., 81 mg) for patients at increased risk of thrombotic events (Antman, Bennett, Daugherty, et al., 2007).

Ibuprofen (400-mg doses) competes with aspirin's binding site on the platelet and has been found to interfere with aspirin's cardioprotective (antiplatelet) effect; therefore, patients taking ibuprofen concomitantly with cardioprotective aspirin should be instructed to take the ibuprofen 30 minutes to 2 hours after aspirin intake (Catella-Lawson, Reilly, Kapoor, et al., 2001; Cryer, Berlin, Cooper, et al., 2005; Hong, Gengo, Rainka, et al., 2008) or at least 8 hours before (U.S. FDA, 2006). The AGS recommends that older adults taking cardioprotective aspirin avoid ibuprofen (AGS, 2009).

Although acetaminophen, diclofenac (Antman, Bennett, Daugherty, et al., 2007; Catella-Lawson, Reilly, Kapoor, et al., 2001), and celecoxib (Wilner, Rushing, Walden, et al., 2002) have been shown not to interfere with platelet aggregation induced by low-dose aspirin, a subgroup analysis from a 5-year randomized, placebo-controlled trial (N = 22,071 males) indicated that regular NSAID use (more than 60 days/year), but not intermittent NSAID use (1-59 days/year), interfered with the clinical benefits of aspirin (325 mg every other day) in the prevention of first MI (Kurth, Glynn, Walker, et al., 2003. One study of naproxen found that this drug interfered with the inhibitory effect of aspirin on platelet COX-1 activity (Capone, Sciulli, Tacconelli, et al., 2005), but another did not (Rauscher, 2007). Further studies are needed to determine if other NSAIDs interact with cardioprotective aspirin. See Chapter 8 for a discussion of preoperative discontinuation of aspirin therapy.

NSAIDs with Minimal Effect on Platelet Aggregation

Although NSAIDs do not block platelet function sufficiently to be useful as antithrombotic agents, most of the nonselective NSAIDs do interfere enough to increase bleeding time. For this reason, these drugs may carry relatively higher risk for patients with bleeding disorders, such as hemophilia. In such populations, the least risky drugs classified as nonselective NSAIDs are presumably those that are least likely to exert a COX-1-mediated inhibition of platelet function, such as nabumetone, meloxicam, choline magnesium trisalicylate, magnesium salicylate (Arthriten, Backache, Doan's), and salsalate (Disalcid). The COX-2 selective NSAIDs (e.g., celecoxib) have no effect on bleeding time and should be considered as well if not contraindicated (Visser, Goucke, 2008) (see Chapter 8 for perioperative NSAID use).

Renal Effects and Hypertension

The COX isoenzymes play an important role in renal function through their effects on prostaglandin formation (Barkin, Buvanendran, 2004; Brater, 2002; DeMaria, Weir, 2003). COX-2, the isoenzyme that is largely inducible in response to inflammation, is constitutively expressed in the human kidney (Brune, 2003; Zhang, Ding, Song, 2006). It is present in the ascending limb of the loop of Henle, macula densa, and afferent arteriole and produces prostaglandins that inhibit sodium reabsorption and have diuretic effects (DeMaria, Weir, 2003). COX-1 is located in the glomerulus and afferent arteriole where it produces prostaglandins that affect renal homeostasis and promote dilation of the renal vascular bed (DeMaria, Weir, 2003).

The four categories of NSAID-induced renal toxicity are acute ischemic renal insufficiency (most commonly associated with perioperative use of NSAIDs), acute interstitial nephritis, analgesic associated nephropathy, and progressive hypertensive nephropathy (Forrest, Camu, Greer, et al., 2002). The most common adverse physiologic effects are reduced renal blood flow, glomerular filtration rate (GFR), and sodium and potassium excretion. These changes potentially can result in fluid retention, edema, hypertension, and hyperkalemia (DeMaria, Weir, 2003; Laine, White, Rostom, et al., 2008).

Endogenous renal prostaglandin synthesis does not have a significant role in maintaining optimal GFR and renal blood flow in individuals with normal CV, hepatic, endocrine, and renal function, as long as adequate volume and sodium stores exist (Helstrom, Rosow, 2006; Launay-Vacher, Karie, Fau, et al., 2005). In these healthy individuals, NSAID-induced renal effects are usually minor and transient (Forrest, Camu, Greer, et al., 2002; Helstrom, Rosow, 2006; Lee, Cooper, Craig, et al., 2007). There appears to be no difference in these effects between nonselective and COX-2 selective NSAIDs (Helstrom, Rosow, 2006).

Overall, NSAID-induced adverse renal effects occur in approximately 1% to 5% of NSAID users (DeMaria, Weir, 2003). Large epidemiologic studies provide some detail. For example, a cohort study of data from the 14-year Physicians' Health Study (N = 11,032) revealed no increased risk of renal dysfunction with long-term moderate use (3 to 4 pills/week) of acetaminophen, aspirin, or NSAIDs in men who had no preexisting renal impairment (Rexrode, Buring, Glynn, et al., 2001). In contrast,

a large case-control study of 72,114 men age 45 and older (Verhamme, Dieleman, Van Wijk, et al., 2005) showed that current use of NSAIDs was associated with a 2-fold increased risk of acute urinary retention. The latter study used the primary health care database in the Netherlands to compare cases with 10 age- and time-matched controls and found that the highest risk was in men who had recently started taking NSAIDs and in those who were taking a dose equal to or higher than the recommended daily dose; past use of NSAIDs and low-dose aspirin use were not associated with risk, and potential confounding factors, such as concomitant medication use (including opioids) and history of urinary tract infection, did not modify the results.

A variety of conditions may increase the risk of nephrotoxicity associated with NSAID use. In the setting of acute or chronic volume depletion, prostaglandin synthesis is necessary to maintain adequate renal blood flow ("prostaglandin dependence") (Helstrom, Rosow, 2006). NSAID inhibition of prostaglandin synthesis in such patients can cause acute renal ischemia and acute renal failure (ARF) (Helstrom, Rosow, 2006). It is important to remember that, although NSAID-induced ARF is most often discussed in the literature as a perioperative adverse event, it can develop from both short- and long-term NSAID administration (McQuay, Moore, 2004) (see Chapter 8 for discussion of ARF).

Adverse renal effects also are more likely to occur in patients who have co-morbidities, such as diabetes, hypertension, cirrhosis, ascites, or congestive heart failure (Brater, 2002; Brune, 2003; Launay-Vacher, Karie, Fau, et al., 2005; Solomon, Schneeweiss, Levin, et al., 2004). Some experts have suggested NSAIDs be avoided entirely in patients with cirrhosis, congestive heart failure, or renal insufficiency (Laine, White, Rostom, et al., 2008). The AGS lists heart failure and chronic kidney disease as absolute contraindications and hypertension as a relative contraindication to the use of NSAIDs in older adults (AGS, Panel on Pharmacological Management, 2009). Because NSAIDs do not adversely affect GFR in individuals with normal renal function (Baker, Cotter, Gerrard, et al., 2005), including older adults, age alone is not a risk factor for NSAID-induced renal impairment (Brater, 2002); however, older adults are more likely to have risk factors such as volume depletion and chronic medical illness, and those who are prescribed NSAIDs should be regularly assessed for adverse renal effects (Barkin, Buvanendran, 2004).

Studies have evaluated class-selective and drug-selective risk of NSAID-induced renal toxicity. Although a small placebo-controlled study (N = 67) of older adults showed no significant differences between the nonselective NSAID naproxen and the COX-2 selective NSAIDs rofecoxib and celecoxib in terms of renal adverse effects (Schwartz, Vandormael, Malice, et al., 2002), most research has shown a higher risk for adverse renal effects with rofecoxib than other NSAIDs (Solomon, Schneeweiss, Levin, et al., 2004). Shortly after the release of the first COX-2 selective NSAIDs, an analysis of a safety database found that celecoxib, ibuprofen, and diclofenac had similar cardiorenal safety profiles, but rofecoxib possessed significantly greater renal toxicity (water retention, abnormal renal function, renal failure, cardiac failure, and hypertension) (Zhao, Reynolds, Lejkowith, et al., 2001). Similar findings were revealed in a case-controlled (4:1) study of 3914 patients with preexisting hypertension (Solomon, Schneeweiss, Levin, et al., 2004). Rofecoxib was associated with a significant risk of new hypertension, but there was no association between celecoxib use and the development of hypertension. In addition, relative risk was twice as high in patients with co-morbidities and advanced age taking rofecoxib compared with celecoxib. A nested, case-control study of individuals hospitalized for ARF found that the risk of ARF for all NSAIDs was highest during the first 30 days of NSAID use and was comparable for rofecoxib, naproxen, and nonselective, non-naproxen NSAIDs but was borderline lower for celecoxib (Schneider, Levesque, Zhang, et al., 2006).

Other research of patients with preexisting hypertension further suggests that celecoxib is associated with a relatively low risk of renal adverse effects. A study was conducted to evaluate the cardiorenal effects of COX-2 selective NSAIDs in 810 older patients ($\geq$ 65 years old) with OA who had well-controlled hypertension and were taking antihypertensive medication (Whelton, Fort, Puma, et al., 2001). The patients were randomized to receive either celecoxib (200 mg once daily) or rofecoxib (25 mg once daily). Both groups exhibited significant peripheral edema, but twice as many of the rofecoxib-treated patients than celecoxib-treated patients did so, and 17% and 11% of those receiving rofecoxib and celecoxib, respectively, experienced a significant increase in systolic BP. Another study showed new-onset or worsening edema with weight gain occurring in 7.7% and 4.7% of individuals taking antihypertensive medications who received rofecoxib and celecoxib, respectively (Whelton, White, Bello, et al., 2002). Neither celecoxib nor rofecoxib caused significant increases in BP in patients receiving calcium channel antagonists or diuretic monotherapy; however, rofecoxib caused the greatest increase in systolic BP in patients receiving angiotensin-converting enzyme (ACE) inhibitors or beta blockers. A randomized, placebo-controlled study found celecoxib (200 mg twice daily) was not associated with statistically or clinically significant destabilization of BP in patients treated with the ACE inhibitor lisinopril (Zestril) (White, Kent, Taylor, et al., 2002). Similarly, a randomized-controlled study of patients with medication-stabilized hypertension, OA, and type-2 diabetes demonstrated that rofecoxib but not celecoxib or naproxen induced a significant increase in BP (Sowers, White, Pitt, et al., 2005). Although destabilization of existing hypertension occurred to some extent in all three groups, it was most prominent in those taking

rofecoxib. These studies underscore the likelihood of drug-selective differences and the importance of careful monitoring of BP and renal function in patients receiving NSAIDs while being treated for hypertension (Barkin, Buvanendran, 2004).

Other studies have shown that celecoxib has a relatively low risk of cardiorenal adverse effects. A meta-analysis of 114 randomized trials involving 116,094 patients compared the cardiorenal adverse effects among the various COX-2 selective NSAIDs rofecoxib, celecoxib, etoricoxib, lumiracoxib, and valdecoxib plus parecoxib (Zhang, Ding, Song, 2006). Rofecoxib was associated with all of the adverse renal endpoints in a time- and dose-related manner with increased risk of peripheral edema and renal dysfunction. Celecoxib, on the other hand, was associated with a lower risk of cardiorenal dysfunction than the controls in this analysis. A study evaluating patients with arthritis showed a higher incidence of adverse renal effects in patients taking diclofenac (34.8%) than in those taking celecoxib (24.3%) (Chan, Hung, Suen, et al., 2004). The COX-2 selectivity of diclofenac is similar to celecoxib, notwithstanding its labeling as a nonselective NSAID (see Figure 6-1). The database from the previously mentioned CLASS study (Silverstein, Faich, Goldstein, et al., 2000) (N = 8059) was analyzed to assess the cardiorenal effects of higher-than-clinically-indicated doses of celecoxib (400 mg twice daily) and standard doses of ibuprofen (800 mg 3 times daily) and diclofenac (75 mg twice daily) (Whelton, Lefkowith, West, et al., 2006). The incidence of serious cardiorenal complications was reported to be low in all groups, and the celecoxib-treated patients experienced the lowest risk of cardiorenal adverse effects, particularly those with prerenal compromise.

The previously discussed APC and PreSAP trials underscore that both dose and dosing regimens of celecoxib influence BP (Solomon, Pfeffer, McMurray, et al., 2006). Whereas there were no significant BP changes in patients who took a single 400-mg dose of celecoxib once daily in the PreSAP trial, the twice-daily treatment groups in the APC trial demonstrated a pattern of BP elevation. Patients in the APC treatment group who received celecoxib in doses of 200 mg twice daily experienced an increase in BP of 2.0 mm Hg and 2.6 mm Hg at 1 and 3 years, respectively, and those in the group that received 400 mg twice daily experienced BP elevations of 2.9 mm Hg and 5.2 mm Hg at 1 and 3 years, respectively (see pp. 200-203 for explanation of lower risk associated with once-daily dosing compared with twice-daily dosing of the same overall total daily dose of celecoxib). Solomon and colleagues (2008) reinforce that the timing of BP measurements may be important for interpretation of study results since once-daily dosing may result in less sustained BP elevations than twice-daily dosing (Solomon, Wittes, Finn, et al., 2008).

Hepatic Effects

NSAID-related liver injury is much less common than other adverse effects. NSAIDs were implicated in approximately 10% of the cases of drug-induced liver injury and 1% of the liver transplants reported in European and United States literature (Andrade, Lucena, Fernandez, et al., 2005; Bjornsson, Olsson, 2005; Laine, White, Rostom, et al., 2008). In comparison, acetaminophen alone or in combination with other drugs was associated with 49% of the drug-related liver transplants performed in the United States between 1990 and 2002 (Russo, Galanko, Shrestha, et al., 2004) (see earlier in this chapter for more on acetaminophen-induced hepatotoxicity). Mortality from NSAID-related hepatotoxicity is less than 1 per 100,000 (Laine, White, Rostom, et al., 2008).

A systematic review concluded there is a possibility of a small increase in the risk of hepatotoxicity with NSAID use, and many experts do not recommend NSAID use in individuals with cirrhosis (Laine, White, Rostom, et al., 2008). Large-population epidemiologic studies are required to confirm that such a risk exists (Rubenstein, Laine, 2004). Significant increases in clinical liver events have not been noted with the introduction of the COX-2 selective NSAIDs, although a trend in increased episodes of liver injury with lumiracoxib led to its removal from the Australian market (Laine, White, Rostom, et al., 2008). A review of randomized-controlled trials on a variety of NSAIDs revealed that diclofenac and rofecoxib were associated with elevated aminotransferase levels, but no elevations were noted with naproxen, ibuprofen, celecoxib, valdecoxib, or meloxicam (Rostom, Goldkind, Laine, 2005).

Cognitive Effects

Mild dizziness and drowsiness are relatively common and transient effects of both acetaminophen and NSAIDs (Burke, Smyth, FitzGerald, 2006; McQuay, Moore, 2004). Cognitive dysfunction with symptoms of decreased attention span and loss of short-term memory may also be an adverse effect of NSAIDs. This has been noted in older individuals in response to naproxen and ibuprofen, even when doses are within the accepted range. Other CNS adverse effects are headache, lowered seizure threshold, and adverse mood effects (Burke, Smyth, FitzGerald, 2006; Drug Facts and Comparisons, 2006).

Hypersensitivity to Nonopioids: Respiratory and Cutaneous Reactions

Allergy or (more accurately) hypersensitivity to nonopioids is fairly common (Leimgruber, 2008). Patients may erroneously report an allergy to a nonopioid simply because they have experienced adverse effects such as heartburn or nausea after NSAID use. However, true hypersensitivity involves far more serious symptoms. Most of the research on the incidence of nonopioid hypersensitivity is found in the pediatric literature, where hypersensitivity to aspirin, ibuprofen, and acetaminophen was found to be 60%, 76.5%, and 23.2%, respectively (Hassani, Ponvert, Karila, et al., 2008).

The pathogenesis of NSAID hypersensitivity may be nonimmunologic and related to altered arachidonic acid metabolism and excessive production of leukotriene (inflammatory response mediator) (Babu, Salvi, 2000; Forster, Olze, 2008; Leimgruber, 2008). This is thought to lead to a decrease in PGE_2 (the antiinflammatory prostaglandin) synthesis, tilting the balance in favor of inflammation (Babu, Salvi, 2000). When hypersensitivity to one NSAID occurs, cross-sensitivity to others frequently occurs, further supporting the logic that most reactions result from a nonallergy hypersensitivity to the pharmacologic properties of the drug (Hassani, Ponvert, Karila, et al., 2008).

Although the COX-2 selective NSAIDs theoretically should be a safer alternative to nonselective NSAIDs in terms of hypersensitivity reactions because they preserve PGE_2 (Babu, Salvi, 2000), both nonselective and COX-2 selective NSAIDs are known to produce various skin reactions, including the rare but potentially fatal Stevens-Johnson Syndrome (SJS) and toxic epidermal necrolysis (TEN) (Simon, 2007). SJS produces inflammatory eruptions on the skin and mucous membranes; TEN presents with large areas of bloody-looking lesions and can advance to epidermal detachment.

One study showed the highest risk of skin reactions from nonselective NSAIDs to be with piroxicam and tenoxicam and the lowest with ibuprofen, diclofenac, and ketoprofen (Simon, 2007). A retrospective review of prescription-event monitoring data in England revealed that the incidence of cases of SJS related to the use of the COX-2 selective NSAIDs rofecoxib, celecoxib, etoricoxib, and valdecoxib was very low at 0.08% for all four combined (Layton, Marshall, Boshier, et al., 2006).

Nevertheless, all of the COX-2 selective NSAIDS have been associated with cutaneous adverse reactions of some sort, and a class effect for skin reactions has been suggested (Atzori, Pinna, Pau, et al., 2006). The COX-2 selective NSAID valdecoxib was implicated in several case reports of serious cutaneous adverse reactions (Glasser, Burroughs, 2003; Knowles, Phillips, Wong, et al., 2004; Ziemer, Wiesend, Vetter, et al., 2007), which contributed to the manufacturer's voluntary withdrawal of valdecoxib from the U.S. market in 2005 (U.S. FDA, 2005). The presentation of severe cutaneous reactions associated with COX-2 selective NSAIDs has been described as different from that of SJS and TEN, specifically in terms of a "widespread, erythematous, to some extent target-like, or purpuric skin eruption" (Ziemer, Wiesend, Vetter, et al., 2007, p. 715). Adverse cutaneous reactions, including a case of fatal vasculitis (Schneider, Meziani, Chartier, et al., 2002), have been reported following administration of celecoxib (Atzor, Pinna, Pau, et al., 2006; Drago, Brusati, Desirello, et al., 2004).

Sodium lauryl sulfa is an inactive ingredient of both celecoxib and valdecoxib, and although sulfa allergy is not always identified as the cause of reported cutaneous reactions, it is important to remember that sulfa-based drugs like celecoxib should not be given to individuals who are hypersensitive to sulfonamides. Although no evidence of cross-reactivity between celecoxib and sulfonamide antimicrobials was found in 28 patients with a history of allergy to sulfonamide antimicrobials (Shapiro, Knowles, Weber, et al., 2003), the risk of cross-sensitivity is presumed to exist, and all patients should be routinely asked about previous allergic reactions, and specifically about past reactions to sulfa-based drugs, prior to treatment (Schneider, Meziani, Chartier, et al., 2002).

Respiratory reactions also signal NSAID hypersensitivity and are the second most common NSAID adverse effect (Bannwarth, 2006). Individuals with asthma and chronic urticaria are especially vulnerable to these reactions (Leimgruber, 2008) and must be watched closely during NSAID therapy. As many as 20% of asthmatics are sensitive to aspirin and other NSAIDs and may develop rhinoconjunctivitis, sinusitis, nasal polyps, and asthma symptoms that can progress to bronchoconstriction following ingestion of even small amounts of aspirin or NSAID (Babu, Salvi, 2000).

Cross-sensitivity between the various NSAIDs is common in patients who are hypersensitive to NSAIDs, but only 7% of these individuals experience cross-sensitivity to acetaminophen (Bannwarth, 2006), and cross-sensitivity between NSAIDs may not extend to the COX-2 selective NSAIDs in all cases. A study of 36 adults showed a high incidence of urticaria with naproxen but none

with celecoxib in aspirin-sensitive patients with chronic idiopathic urticaria (Zembowicz, Mastalerz, Setkowicz, et al., 2003). Other research and case reports also describe safe use of celecoxib and other COX-2 selective NSAIDs in asthma patients who are hypersensitive to nonselective NSAIDs (Andri, Falagiani, 2007; Dahlen, Szczeklik, Murray, 2001; Marks, Harrell, Fischer, 2001; El Miedany, Youssef, Ahmed, et al., 2006; Szczeklik, Nizankowska, Bochenek, et al., 2001). Just 1 hypersensitivity reaction to celecoxib occurred in a study of 29 patients who were hypersensitive to acetaminophen and nonselective NSAIDs (Liccardi, Cazzola, De Giglio, et al., 2005). The authors proposed celecoxib as a safe alternative in individuals who cannot tolerate acetaminophen. Following an extensive literature review, researchers recommended that NSAID treatment in individuals with aspirin/NSAID sensitivity should include avoidance of aspirin and other nonselective NSAIDs, use instead of COX-2 selective NSAIDs, acetaminophen in adult doses less than 1000 mg, and desensitization techniques (Knowles, Drucker, Weber, et al., 2007). Daily doses of 300 mg of aspirin are recommended for optimal desensitization (Rozsasi, Polzehl, Deutschle, et al., 2008). The use of other antiplatelet agents, such as clopidogrel (Plavix) or ticlopidine (Ticlid), is recommended in patients with true aspirin hypersensitivity who require cardioprotection (Ramanuja, Breall, Kalaria, 2004).

Conclusion

There is an abundance of evidence to support the use of nonopioid analgesics for a wide variety of acute and persistent (chronic) pain states. Prevention of the adverse effects of acetaminophen and NSAIDs whenever possible is a basic pain management principle. This is accomplished by individualizing the choice of nonopioid and taking into consideration the type of pain and the patient's previous nonopioid use and risk factors.

Chapter 7 Individualizing the Selection of Nonopioid Analgesics

THE POTENTIAL risks and benefits of nonopioid analgesic therapy should be considered in developing a plan of care for all patients with pain. Most clinicians will consider trying a nonopioid unless there is clear evidence of nonefficacy or increased risk. Once the decision is made to try one of these drugs, the goal is to select an agent and a dose that offers satisfactory pain relief with a low risk of adverse effects. Decisions about drug and dose may be influenced by the patient's past experience, pain syndrome, and the assessed risk factors for adverse effects. The patient's ability to pay for nonopioid therapy also should be evaluated. Table 7-1 is a guide to generic and brand names of nonopioids and may be used in conjunction with Table 7-2, which details dosing information and other characteristics for acetaminophen and NSAIDs. See Chapter 6 regarding individualizing the selection of nonopioid analgesics based on GI risk and cardiovascular (CV) risk. See patient medication information in Forms III-1 through III-5 on pp. 250-259.

General Considerations

Acute versus Persistent (Chronic) Pain

When a nonopioid is expected to be used with relatively infrequent dosing, or at low doses, or for only a short period of time (e.g., postoperatively), adverse effects are less problematic than with long-term use. Adverse effects increase dramatically with regular dosing for a period of days or more. Therefore, the importance of the risk:benefits analysis increases over time, and administration of the lowest effective dose for the shortest time needed is a key principle of nonopioid use (American Pain Society [APS], 2003).

Analgesic History

Talking with the patient about previous use of nonopioid analgesics for pain can provide valuable information as to which nonopioid to recommend. Whichever nonopioid has worked well for the patient and has caused minimal or no adverse effects is often the best place to begin with drug selection.

Pain Intensity

Several Cochrane Collaboration Reviews underscore the importance of evaluating the patient's pain intensity when determining the appropriate nonopioid to

Table 7-1 | Nonopioids Listed Alphabetically by Generic Name Followed by Brand Name

Generic Name(s)	Brand Name(s)
Acetaminophen	Tylenol, many other brand names
Aspirin	Bayer, many other brand names
Celecoxib	Celebrex
Choline magnesium trisalicylate	Choline magnesium trisalicylate
Choline salicylate	Arthropan
Diclofenac	Cataflam (short acting for acute pain), Voltaren Delayed Release, Voltaren-XR (extended release for chronic pain therapy), Pennsaid (topical drops); Voltaren topical gel, Arthrotec (combined with misoprostol), Flector (topical patch)
Diflunisal	Dolobid
Etodolac	Lodine, Lodine XL
Etoricoxib	Arcoxia
Fenoprofen calcium	Nalfon, Nalfon 200
Flurbiprofen	Ansaid
Ibuprofen	Advil, Motrin, Tab-Profen, Vicoprofen (combined with hydrocodone), Combunox (combined with oxycodone)
Indomethacin	Indocin, Indocin SR, Indo-Lemmon, Indomethagan
Ketoprofen	Orudis, Oruvail Extended-Release
Ketorolac	Toradol
Lumiracoxib	Prexige
Magnesium salicylate	Arthriten, Doan's, Doan's Extra Strength, Momentum
Meclofenamate sodium	Meclomen
Mefenamic acid	Ponstel
Meloxicam	Mobic
Nabumetone	Relafen
Naproxen	Aleve, Anaprox, Anaprox DS, Naprosyn, EC-Naproxyn, Naprelan, Naprapac (co-packaged with lansoprazole)
Oxaprozin	Daypro
Piroxicam	Feldene
Salsalate	Disalcid
Sulindac	Clinoril
Tolmetin	Tolectin, Tolectin DS, Tolectin 600

From Pasero, C., & McCaffery, M. *Pain assessment and pharmacologic management*, p. 210, St. Louis, Mosby. © 2011, Pasero C, McCaffery M. May be duplicated for use in clinical practice.

administer. As mentioned earlier, acetaminophen has been shown to produce better pain relief than placebo, but NSAIDs were superior for osteoarthritis (OA) pain (Towheed, Maxwell, Judd, et al., 2006) (see pp. 220-221 for more on OA). Another Cochrane Collaboration review evaluating 51 studies and 5762 patients with moderate to severe postoper- ative pain concluded that acetaminophen provided effective analgesia for just half of the patients for 4 to 6 hours (Toms, McQuay, Derry, et al., 2008). These reviews support the appropriateness of acetaminophen as a first-line choice for mild pain and NSAIDs alone or in combination with other analgesics, including acetaminophen, for more severe pain.

Table 7-2 | Acetaminophen and NSAIDs: Adult Dosing Information

Chemical Class	Generic Name[1]	Half-Life (hours)	Dosing Schedule	Recommended Starting Dose (mg)[1]	Maximum Recommended Dose (mg/day)[1]	Comments
P-Aminophenol derivatives	Acetaminophen	2	q4-6h	650	4000	Reduce dose or avoid in presence of chronic alcohol abuse/ dependence and in those with hepatic dysfunction (see text); overdose produces hepatic toxicity; long-term high-dose associated with renal insufficiency and GI toxicity; frequent use, long-term associated with hypertension and elevated CV risk. May produce dose-dependent increase in INR when taken concomitantly with warfarin. Available in liquid and rectal formulations; IV formulation in development.
Salicylates	Aspirin	2-12	q4-6h	650	4000	Standard for comparison. May not be as well tolerated as some of the newer NSAIDs. Available in rectal formulation.
	Diflunisal	8-12	q8-12h	250-500	1500	Less GI toxicity than aspirin.
	Choline magnesium trisalicylate	9-17	q 8-12h	500-1000	4000	Minimal GI toxicity. No effect on platelet aggregation. Available in liquid formulation.
	Choline salicylate	2-3	q4-6h	435-870	5352	Minimal GI toxicity and minimal effect on platelet aggregation. Available in liquid formulation.
	Magnesium salicylate	2-3	q4-6h	500-1000	3500	Half-life varies with dose. Can be as high as 30 hours after high doses.
	Salsalate	16	q 8-12h	500-1000	4000	Minimal effect on platelet aggregation.
Proprionic acids	Ibuprofen, PO	2-4	q4-6h	400-800	3200	Available in liquid and cream formulations.
	Ibuprofen, IV	2-3	q 6 h	400-800	3200	400 mg should be diluted in 100 mL or more (800 mg in 200 mL or more) 5% dextrose or normal saline and infused IV over a 30-minute period.

Continued

Table 7-2 | Acetaminophen and NSAIDs: Adult Dosing Information—cont'd

Chemical Class	Generic Name[1]	Half-Life (hours)	Dosing Schedule	Recommended Starting Dose (mg)[1]	Maximum Recommended Dose (mg/day)[1]	Comments
	Naproxen[2]	14	q12h	250-500	1500	Peak antiinflammatory effect may not be seen until 2-4 weeks of use. Available in liquid formulation. Sodium naproxen doses differ from plain naproxen doses based on milligram amount of added sodium.
	Fenoprofen	2-3	q6-8h	400-600	3200	High GI toxicity.
	Ketoprofen (short acting)	2-3	q6-8h	50-75	300	Available in topical gel formulation.
	Ketoprofen (modified release)	2-3	q24h	200	200	Reduce dose in older patients.
	Flurbiprofen	5-6	q8-12h	100 (do not exceed 100/dose)	300	High GI toxicity.
	Oxaprozin[2]	40-60	q24h	600	1800	High GI toxicity. Inappropriate for acute pain or fever because of slow onset of action.
Acetic acids	Indomethacin	2.5	q8-12h	25-75	200	Higher incidence of GI and CNS adverse effects than proprionic acids. Available in slow-release and rectal formulations.
	Tolmetin	5	q8h	400-600	1800	Food delays and decreases peak concentration.
	Sulindac	7	q12h	150-200	400	Not recommended for prolonged use because of increased risk for GI toxicity.
	Diclofenac	1-2	q8-12h	25-75	150	High COX-2 selectivity. Available in gel, patch, and ophthalmic drop formulations and in combination with misoprostol.
	Ketorolac, PO	4-6	q4-6h	10	40	Use limited to 5 days. Food decreases rate but not extent of absorption. Also available in ophthalmic drop formulation.
	Ketorolac, parenteral	4-6	q 6h	≤30; ≤15 in adults >65 years old	≤120; ≤60 in adults >65 years old	Use limited to 5 days. Single-dose treatment: 30 mg IV or 60 mg IM; 15 mg IV or 30 mg IM in adults >65 years old.

Continued

| Table 7-2 | Acetaminophen and NSAIDs: Adult Dosing Information—cont'd |

Chemical Class	Generic Name[1]	Half-Life (hours)	Dosing Schedule	Recommended Starting Dose (mg)[1]	Maximum Recommended Dose (mg/day)[1]	Comments
Enolic acid derivatives	Piroxicam[2]	45-50	q24h	20	40	5% discontinue treatment due to high incidence of adverse effects, particularly GI effects.
	Meloxicam	15-20	q24h	7.5-15	15	High COX-2 selectivity but better GI profile than piroxicam and diclofenac.
	Nabumetone	24	q12-24h	1000	2000	Minimal effect on platelet aggregation; minimal GI toxicity.
Fenamates	Mefenamic acid	3-4	q6h	250	1000	Use limited to 7 days. Not recommended for analgesia; 25% incidence of GI adverse effects.
	Meclofenamate	2-3	q4-6h	50-100	400	
Pyranocarboxylic acids	Etodolac	6-8	q6-8h	200-400	1200	Better tolerated than aspirin; minimal GI toxicity.
COX-2 selective NSAIDs	Celecoxib	6-12	q12-24h	100-200	400	Low risk of GI adverse effects; avoid in those with high CV risk. Once daily dosing may be safer from a CV perspective than twice daily dosing (see text).

CV, Cardiovascular; *GI*, gastrointestinal; *h*, hour; *IM*, intramuscular; *IV*, intravenous; *mg*, milligram; *PO*, oral; *q*, every

[1]All of the drugs in Table 7.2 are oral formulations and all doses are oral doses unless specified otherwise.

[2]Avoid full doses in older adults due to long half-life and increased risk of GI toxicity.

Clinical Relevance of Information Presented in Table 7-2:

Half-life. Half-life is the time required for 50% of the dose to be eliminated from the body. A short half-life (approximately 2 to 7 hours) is recommended for some patients, such as older adults. Drugs with a short half-life are usually preferred for occasional or unexpected pain because they tend to have a quicker onset of analgesia than drugs with a long half-life.

Dosing schedule. Dosing intervals may range from every 4 hours to once a day. Drugs with short half-lives have shorter dosing intervals than those with long half-lives. If patients can tolerate a drug with a long half-life, dosing once or twice a day is usually preferred. The fewer the doses, the more likely the patient will remember to take the drug.

Recommended starting dose. This dose should be reduced by one half to two thirds in older adults, those taking multiple drugs, or those with renal insufficiency.

Maximum dose recommended. Data are lacking, but the dose listed is thought to be the maximum needed by most patients for analgesia and the dose beyond which adverse effects are more likely. However, in some patients careful dose titration may identify patients who need and tolerate 50% to 100% more than the maximum dose recommended. Others may require or tolerate less. For some patients at risk for adverse effects, the maximum daily dose may be one half or less than recommended.

From Pasero, C., & McCaffery, M. *Pain assessment and pharmacologic management*, pp. 211-213, St. Louis, Mosby. Data based on the clinical experience of the authors and a variety of published sources, including: American Geriatrics Society (AGS) Panel on Pharmacological Management of Persistent Pain in the Older Persons. (2009). The pharmacological management of persistent pain in older persons. *J Am Geriatr Soc*, in press; American Pain Society (APS). (2003). *Principles of analgesic use in the treatment of acute pain and cancer pain*, ed 5, Glenview, IL, APS; Burke, A., Smyth, E., FitzGerald, G. A. (2006). Analgesic-anti-pyretic agents: Pharmacotherapy of gout. In L. L. Brunton, J. S. Lazo, & K. L. (Eds.), *Goodman, Gilman's the pharmacological basis of therapeutics*, ed 11, New York, McGraw-Hill; *Drug facts and comparisons*. (2006). St. Louis, Wolters Kluwer Health; Fick, D. M., Cooper, J. W., Wade, W. E., et al. (2003); Updating the Beers criteria for potentially inappropriate medication use in older adults. *Arch Intern Med* 163(22):2716-2724; Gold Standard, Inc. Available at *http://clinicalpharmacology.com*. Accessed August 20, 2008; Hanlon, J. T., Backonja, M., Weiner, D., et al. (2009). Evolving pharmacological management of persistent pain in older persons. *Pain Med*, 10(6), 959-961; Motov, S. M., & Ast, T. D. (2008). Is there a limit to the analgesic effect of pain medications? Medscape Emergency Medicine. Available at *http://www.medscape.com/viewarticle/574279*. Accessed July 18, 2008; Simon, L. S., Lipman, A. G., Caudill-Slosberg, M., et al. (2002). *Guideline for the management of pain in osteoarthritis, rheumatoid arthritis, and juvenile chronic arthritis*. Glenview, IL, American Pain Society; Smith, H. S., & Baird, W. (2003). Meloxicam and selective COX-2 inhibitors in the management of pain in the palliative care population. *Am J Hosp Palliat Care*, 20(4), 297-306; Vardeny, O., & Solomon, S. D. (2008). Cyclooxygenase-2-inhibitors, nonsteroidal anti-inflammatory drugs, and cardiovascular risk. *Cardiol Clin*, 26(4), 589-601. © 2011, Pasero C, McCaffery M. May be duplicated for use in clinical practice.

Current Analgesic Response

Patients vary in response to nonopioids. If one nonopioid is ineffective after appropriate dose adjustment, it is worthwhile to try another. There is very little evidence to guide these so-called sequential trials, and assessment of risk and benefit should precede each decision about a new drug and dose.

A nonopioid should not be considered ineffective until the dose-response relationship has been explored and the clinician is certain that the dose has been increased either to (1) the highest dose conventionally accepted with the drug in question, (2) the dose associated with adverse effects, or (3) the dose that confirms that no additional analgesia is occurring with increases (i.e., a dose above the ceiling dose for analgesia). Many clinicians believe that it takes a few days to a week to evaluate the analgesia produced at a specific dose of an NSAID (Burke, Smyth, Fitzgerald, 2006), and a trial of at least 2 to 3 gm of acetaminophen per day for several weeks is recommended to evaluate the effectiveness of this drug (Simon, Lipman, Caudill-Slosberg, et al., 2002). Obviously, if severe adverse effects occur, the nonopioid should be stopped and another tried or the appropriateness of non-opioid therapy reconsidered.

Frequency of Dosing

Acetaminophen and NSAIDs may be given PRN for occasional pain or around the clock (ATC) for ongoing pain. Acetaminophen has a short half-life and usually must be given every 4 hours for ongoing pain. The half-lives of NSAIDs differ, and dosing intervals range from every 4 hours to once a day (see Table 7-2). For persistent pain, the use of once or twice a day dosing usually is more convenient and more likely to result in the patient taking all prescribed doses, which will lead to better pain control. This requires an NSAID with a long half-life or one that is formulated for modified release. However, it is recommended that full doses of naproxen, piroxicam, and oxaprozin be avoided in older adults because of their long half-life and an increased risk of GI toxicity (Fick, Cooper, Wade, et al., 2003; Hanlon, Backonja, Weiner, et al., 2009) (see Chapter 6 and later discussion about half-life in this chapter). When patients are taking other analgesics or medications, consideration should be given to NSAIDs that allow for scheduling as many doses as possible at the same time.

Research has shown that once-daily dosing of celecoxib may be safer from a CV perspective than twice-daily dosing, even of the same total daily dose (Vardeny, Solomon, 2008). The maximum plasma concentration of celecoxib is reached in 90 minutes after intake, and the drug has a short half-life of just 1.5 hours (Paulson, Hribar, Liu, et al., 2000). The COX-2 effect of celecoxib (and other NSAIDs) inhibits prostacyclin, a vasodilator that antagonizes platelet aggregation, and prostacyclin levels require approximately 12 hours to recover following a single oral dose of cele-coxib (McAdam, Catella-Lawson, Mardini, et al., 1999). Once-daily dosing may allow enough prostacyclin recovery and normalization to attenuate any thrombotic effect (Grosser, Fries, FitzGerald, 2006; Vardeny, Solomon, 2008). Although further research is needed, the findings in other studies that utilized once-daily dosing support this theory (Sowers, White, Pitt, et al., 2005; Whelton, Fort, Puma, et al., 2001). See Chapter 6 for an extensive discussion of this and the other CV effects of NSAIDs.

Routes of Administration

NSAIDs are taken most often by the oral route of administration. All NSAIDs are available orally, and a few are available parenterally, rectally, and topically. Currently in the United States the only NSAIDs available for parenteral administration are ketorolac (Toradol), ibuprofen (Caldolor), and indomethacin (Indocin). Ketorolac is widely used parenterally as an analgesic for short-term pain (e.g., postoperative), and IV ibuprofen is approved for treatment of acute pain and fever; paren-tal indomethacin is used primarily in infants for closure of patent ductus arteriosus (Burke, Smyth, Fitzgerald, 2006). Other countries have many nonopioids available parenterally, including acetaminophen, aspirin, keto-profen, parecoxib, and diclofenac. At the time of publication, IV acetaminophen (Acetavance) *(http://www.cadencepharm.com/products/apap.html)* and injectable diclofenac (Dyloject) were in development for approval in the United States (Colucci, Wright, Mermelstein, et al., 2009). An intranasal formulation of ketorolac in a disposable, metered spray device for ambulatory patients with acute pain was also in development in the United States (Brown, Moodie, Bisley, et al., 2009; Moodie, Brown, Bisley, et al., 2008). See Chapter 8 for more on these nonopioid formulations.

Rectal Nonopioid Administration

Rectal NSAIDs are used far more often in countries other than the United States. Relatively few are available commercially for rectal administration in the United States, but most pharmacies can compound them as rectal suppositories. Oral formulations can also be administered rectally, either by using the intact tablet or by placing the intact or crushed tablet in a gelatin capsule and inserting the capsule into the rectum (Pasero, McCaffery, 1999). (Note that modified-release nonopioids should not be crushed.) Because rectal NSAIDs have an 80% to 90% oral bio-availability, higher rectal than oral doses may be required to achieve similar effects (Beck, Schenk, Hagemann, et al., 2000). (See Chapter 8 for discussion of rectal admin-istration of perioperative nonopioids and Chapter 14 for rectal administration technique.)

Topical NSAIDs

Of all of the drugs administered topically, the largest amount of clinical evidence exists for NSAIDs (Stanos, 2007). They are used and researched more extensively in Europe than in the United States. The NSAIDs that are administered topically most often are diclofenac, ibuprofen, ketoprofen, piroxicam, and naproxen, but not all are available commercially in topical formulation in the United States (Moore, Derry, McQuay, 2008). Diclofenac is available in both gel and patch formula-tions. Other topical NSAIDs, such as ketoprofen and naproxen, are in development and are likely to become commercially available in the United States (McCleane, 2008). Compounding pharmacies sometimes prepare topical mixtures that contain NSAIDs when they are not available commercially (Coyne, Hansen, Watson, 2003).

Although cyclooxygenase (COX) inhibition is a primary mediator of NSAID analgesia by any route of administration, research is ongoing to elucidate all of the underlying mechanisms of action of topical NSAIDs. For example, in addition to COX inhibition, animal research has demonstrated that topical diclofenac inhibits peripheral NMDA (N-methyl-D-aspartate) receptors (Dong, Svensson, Cairns, 2009), and high tissue concentrations of diclofenac are capable of blocking sodium channels to mediate local anesthetic-like effects (Cairns, Mann, Mok, et al., 2008) (see Section I for more on the role of sodium channels and NMDA receptor antagonism in analgesia). The therapeutic effect of topical NSAIDs is the result of high concentrations of drug in the tissue rather than the systemic circulation (Galer, Rowbotham, Perander, et al., 2000; Mazieres, 2005; Sawynok, 2003; Stanos, 2007). The best use of topical NSAIDs, therefore, is for well-localized pain, such as arthritic joint or soft-tissue injury pain (Galer, Rowbotham, Perander, et al., 2000; McCleane, 2008). The effectiveness of a topical NSAID depends on its ability to reach the tissue generating nociception (Moore, Derry, McQuay, 2008). (See Chapter 24 for discussion of topical vs. transdermal drug delivery and Figure 24-1 on p. 685)

The bioavailability of an NSAID after topical application is 5% to 10% compared with equivalent oral administration (Heyneman, Lawless-Liday, Wall, 2000; Mazieres, 2005). For comparison, oral NSAIDs have a 50% to 70% oral bioavailability after first-pass effect (Wilbeck, Schorn, Daley, 2008). Thus, compared with other routes of administration, topical NSAIDs provide the benefits of a low incidence of systemic adverse effects and the potential for fewer drug-drug interactions (Bannwarth, 2006; Galer, Rowbotham, Perander, et al., 2000; Heyneman, Lawless-Liday, Wall, 2000; McCleane, 2008; Rainsford, Kean, Ehrlich, 2008).

Given their low systemic distribution, topical NSAIDs may be particularly advantageous in patients who have well-localized painful conditions that may respond to NSAID therapy but are at high risk for NSAID adverse effects, such as older adults with OA (McCleane, 2008) (see pp. 220-221 for more on OA). Patients should be advised that they may take acetaminophen concurrently but should avoid other NSAIDs while taking topical NSAIDs because this can increase the incidence of adverse effects (Galer, Rowbotham, Perander, et al., 2000; McCleane, 2008).

Although topical NSAIDs have a lower risk of adverse effects than systemically-administered NSAIDs, it is important to understand that some drug is absorbed and the risk of serious toxicity is not nil. GI adverse effects from a topical NSAID are more likely in individuals who have experienced a previous GI adverse effect, in a manner similar to orally-administered drugs (McCleane, 2008; Sawynok, 2003). Therefore, tolerability should be regularly assessed during topical NSAID use, particularly in patients with a history of GI adverse

effects. Postmarketing surveillance identified reports of hepatotoxicity during the first months of treatment with diclofenac gel (Voltaren), prompting the revision of prescribing information for the drug to state that liver enzyme testing should be done within the first 4 to 8 weeks of treatment initiation (Dawson, 2010).

Topical NSAIDs are used for both acute and persistent (chronic) pain, but their effectiveness has been questioned over the years (McCleane, 2008; Moore, Derry, McQuay, 2008; Simon, 2008). A systematic review of the use of rubefacients (counterirritants) containing salicylates concluded that there is a lack of well-designed and controlled research regarding their use and adverse effects and reported poor efficacy for persistent pain and limited evidence of efficacy for acute pain treatment (Mason, Moore, Edwards, et al., 2004b). One major drawback is that many of the currently available or compounded topical NSAIDs are in short-acting gel or cream formulations only, which have a relatively brief duration of action (McCleane, 2008). This limits their usefulness, particularly for persistent pain. Gels and creams can also be messy and result in inexact dosing and disruption if the preparation is rubbed off. Gels are reported to be more effective than creams (Moore, Derry, McQuay, 2008).

Topical patch formulations seem to be a better option because they allow uniform application, which results in more controlled delivery than is possible with gels or creams (Rainsford, Kean, Ehrlich, 2008; Stanos, 2007). Steady state maximum plasma concentration of the diclofenac epolamine 1.3% patch (Flector) is reached in 5.4 hours following application of the patch, and it has a half-life of 26.4 hours. Significant accumulation of topical diclofenac occurs in the synovial fluid and musculature (Moore, Derry, McQuay, 2008). There are no clinically relevant metabolites, and mild GI symptoms and dermal reactions occur in 2% and 10% of patients, respectively (Rainsford, Kean, Ehrlich, 2008). Patches must be changed every 12 hours for continuous relief.

Patients often like the idea of applying medication directly to a painful area (Underwood, Ashby, Cross, et al., 2008); however, not all pain is responsive to topical NSAIDs; if pain relief is not apparent within a few hours, sustained use is not justified and alternative methods of pain control should be implemented (McCleane, 2008). As with all NSAIDs, the lowest effective dose for the shortest time necessary should be used.

Topical NSAIDs for Acute Pain

A systematic review of 26 double-blind, placebo-controlled trials analyzed data from 2853 patients to evaluate the efficacy and safety of a variety of topical NSAIDs for acute pain conditions, such as sprains and strains (Mason, Moore, Edwards, et al., 2004c). Compared with oral NSAIDs, topical NSAIDs provided better pain relief and similar adverse effects and treatment success. Withdrawals due to an adverse event were rare.

Ketoprofen was more effective than topical ibuprofen, piroxicam, and indomethacin; there was no comparison data on diclofenac.

Zacher and colleagues (2008) performed a review of 19 double-blind, randomized, placebo- or active-controlled trials (> 3000 patients) of topical diclofenac. They concluded that this formulation is effective in reducing pain and inflammation associated with acute soft-tissue injury; benefits included functional improvement, a low incidence of mild dermal adverse effects, and fewer adverse effects than other topical and oral NSAIDs. Banning (2008) found that topical diclofenac in a variety of formulations was either superior or equivalent to oral diclofenac or placebo for orthopedic soft-tissue injury pain. Topical diclofenac produced significant reductions in pain and morning stiffness, and improved physical function. Again, minor dermatitis-type adverse effects were reported. Randomized, placebo-controlled trials that have focused specifically on the diclofenac 1.3% patch formulation have reported similar positive results for sports-related soft-tissue injuries (Galer, Rowbotham, Perander, et al., 2000; Predel, Koll, Pabst, et al., 2004).

At the time of publication, a topical patch containing 100 mg of ketoprofen was in development in the United States. Phase III trials in patients with traumatic soft-tissue injuries and other musculoskeletal pains have shown the patch to be more effective than placebo and similar to the diclofenac patch, to produce minor dermal adverse reactions, and to be associated with a low incidence of GI adverse effects (Mazieres, 2005). For example, a randomized, double-blind, 14-day study of 172 patients showed that the ketoprofen patch was safe and effective in relieving tendonitis (Mazieres, Rouanet, Guillon, et al., 2005). Other research has suggested that the ketoprofen patch may yield slightly better pain relief during activity and higher patient satisfaction than the diclofenac gel (Esparza, Cobian, Jimenez, et al., 2007).

Ibuprofen cream also has been used as a topical analgesic for acute pain. One study found no significant differences in pain relief at rest and with movement between oral ibuprofen 400 mg and ibuprofen 5% gel, both administered 3 times daily, for acute soft-tissue injuries (Whitefield, O'Kane, Anderson, 2002). A placebo-controlled study found that application of 5% ibuprofen cream 2 hours before elective external direct current cardioversion safely and effectively reduced pain and inflammation (Ambler, Zidema, Deakin, 2005); the researchers concluded that it should be used routinely prior to this procedure.

A foam dressing permeated with ibuprofen (Biatain Ibu) is used outside of the United States for the care of painful wounds. One randomized, controlled study showed that the use of ibuprofen foam dressings reduced pain and improved quality of life with minimal adverse effects in patients with painful exuding wounds (Palao, Domenech, Romanelli, et al., 2008). Another study found similar results with the combined use of the ibuprofen-releasing foam dressing and silver-releasing contact layer on locally infected, exuding venous leg ulcers (Jorgensen, Gottrup, Karlsmark, et al., 2008). Pain during dressing change was reduced, and persistent pain decreased from 6.2 to 3.0 (0 to 10 scale) with minimal adverse effects.

Topical NSAIDs for Persistent (Chronic) Pain

Numerous high-quality studies have shown the superiority of topical NSAIDs compared with placebo for persistent pain (McCleane, 2008; Moore, Derry, McQuay, 2008). An extensive, systematic literature review that included 14 randomized, double-blind trials with data on over 1500 patients comparing topical NSAIDs with either placebo or other active treatment concluded that topical NSAIDs were safe and effective for persistent musculoskeletal pain (Mason, Moore, Edwards, et al., 2004c). Local and systemic effects were minimal and similar to placebo.

Topical NSAIDs are presented as first-line analgesic options in a variety of clinical guidelines (Hunter, Lo, 2008). The United Kingdom's National Collaborating Centre for Chronic Conditions recommends that topical NSAIDs be the core treatment for knee and hand OA and, with acetaminophen, should be tried before oral NSAIDs (NCC-CC, 2008). Others have supported this recommendation (Moore, Derry, McQuay, 2008). However, an extensive literature review on the use of topical NSAIDs for the treatment of OA pain concluded that topical NSAIDs produced better pain relief than placebo but inferior pain relief compared with oral NSAIDs (Lin, Zhang, Jones, et al., 2004). A controversial finding of this study was that the pain relief from topical NSAIDs did not extend beyond 2 weeks. This review has been criticized for many reasons, primarily design flaws, and the finding that topical NSAIDs work for only 2 weeks has not been supported by other research (Moore, Derry, McQuay, 2008).

Topical diclofenac has been extensively evaluated in placebo-controlled trials of longer duration. A 4-week randomized, placebo-controlled trial (N = 248) evaluating the effect of topical 1.5% diclofenac solution on OA knee pain found that patients taking diclofenac experienced significantly less pain on walking and improved physical function, and that patient global assessments were superior (Bookman, Williams, Shainhouse, 2004). Adverse effects, such as localized dry skin, were minor. Active drug and placebo groups had similar rates of GI and renal adverse events, suggesting that the topical drug had minimal systemic absorption. A randomized placebo-controlled 8-week trial (N = 385) of 1% diclofenac gel use for hand osteoarthritis (OA) demonstrated significant improvements in pain and global rating of disease; treatment was well tolerated with mild adverse effects, such as application-site paresthesia (Altman, Dreiser, Fisher, et al., 2009). Placebo-controlled studies of 6-week (Baer, Thomas, Shainhouse, 2005) and 12-week (Roth, Shainhouse, 2004) durations evaluated 1.5% diclofenac solution in 216 and 326 patients with knee OA, respectively, and found similarly positive results on pain, function, and patient satisfaction, with no systemic adverse effects. A randomized, placebo-controlled study (N = 153) established that the diclofenac (60 mg) patch produced effective pain control, improved function, and minimal adverse effects for myofascial pain syndrome (Hsieh, Hong, Chern, et al., 2010).

Similar findings were obtained when topical diclofenac was compared with other NSAIDs. The previously mentioned review by Zacher and colleagues (2008) of 19 double-blind, randomized trials (more than 3000 patients) concluded that topical diclofenac produced outcomes in OA pain that were better than other topical NSAIDs and oral diclofenac, ibuprofen, or naproxen. Topical diclofenac has also been shown to be as effective as oral diclofenac in reducing morning stiffness (Banning, 2008). In contrast, another systematic review found no significant differences in effectiveness or systemic effects between topical diclofenac and oral diclofenac, ibuprofen, and indomethacin (Moore, Derry, McQuay, 2008), and a study of a gel formulation of topical 1.16% diclofenac produced comparable findings (Niethard, Gold, Solomon, et al., 2005). More head-to-head research is needed to better compare the effectiveness of topical and oral NSAIDs.

Longer trials of other topical NSAIDs are very limited, and there are no clear conclusions. A randomized, controlled study found that 200 mg of ibuprofen cream (5%) applied to the knee in a 10-cm strip 3 times daily for 1 week provided better pain relief at rest, and overall, than placebo in patients with knee OA (Trnavsky, Fischer, Vogtle-Junkert, et al., 2004). This study confirmed earlier placebo-controlled research on ibuprofen cream (Rovensky, Micekova, Gubzova, et al., 2001). An interesting randomized 1-year study required researchers to advise patients with knee OA to use either oral or topical ibuprofen depending on the patient's preferred route of administration (Underwood, Ashby, Cross, et al., 2008); although patients preferred topical ibuprofen, and both oral and topical ibuprofen were safe, neither were particularly effective, presumably because of relatively poor adherence. The latter study suggests that the outcomes of controlled trials with high adherence may overestimate the benefits actually obtained in clinical practice.

Piroxicam 0.5% gel was found to produce similar effectiveness and tolerability when compared with a gel containing a variety of homeopathic ingredients (van Haselen, Fisher, 2000). The authors recommended concomitant PRN administration of other "simple" analgesics but offered no specific suggestions. Piroxicam is noted to be theoretically inferior in terms of penetration compared with other more commonly used NSAIDs, such as ibuprofen and ketoprofen (Moore, Derry, McQuay, 2008).

Cost

The cost of treatment with a nonopioid analgesic may be an important consideration, particularly when nonopioids are used for persistent pain. Nonprescription generic brands of nonopioids are almost always less expensive than brand names and prescription nonopioids. Further, the APS points out that equianalgesic doses of nonprescription NSAIDs are as effective as prescription NSAIDs (Simon, Lipman, Caudill-Slosberg, et al., 2002).

Analgesics often have wide ranges in cost. The cost of prescription NSAIDs varies from one pharmacy to another, but the newer NSAIDs without generic equivalents tend to be more expensive. There are numerous web sites, such as PharmacyChecker.com (http://www.pharmacychecker.com/), that compare drug costs worldwide. Some pain guidelines include tables displaying the costs of analgesics at the time of publication. Although listed prices are likely to be different from current prices, they provide an idea of relative cost. Based on the 2002 APS *Guideline for the Management of Pain in Osteoarthritis, Rheumatoid Arthritis, and Juvenile Chronic Arthritis* data, aspirin, ibuprofen, and salsalate were among the least expensive nonopioids (Simon, Lipman, Caudill-Slosberg, et al., 2002).

Many pharmaceutical companies have financial assistance programs that allow reduced purchase prices for patients who qualify. Prescribers can find information about this in the *Physician's Desk Reference* and at most pharmaceutical company websites. If drug costs are a significant issue, prices should be checked with the pharmacy.

Gastroprotective co-therapy will increase the cost of NSAID therapy and must be considered as well. The cost of a COX-2 selective NSAID that produces less GI toxicity may be less than an NSAID plus a PPI (Simon, Lipman, Caudill-Slosberg, et al., 2002). Unfortunately, research comparing the gastroprotective strategies in patients receiving long-term NSAID therapy is sparse (Brown, Hooper, Elliott, et al., 2006) (see Chapter 6). More studies also are needed that compare the cost of the various gastroprotective therapies with the cost of treating a serious adverse GI event that could have been prevented had gastroprotective therapy been initiated.

Choice of Starting Dose and Dose Titration

Regardless of which nonopioid analgesic is selected, a principle of pain management that has been reinforced throughout this section is to give the lowest effective nonopioid dose for the shortest time needed. Following is a discussion of starting doses and titration for acetaminophen, followed by NSAIDs (Box 7-1; also see Box 6-1). See patient medication information in Forms III-1 through III-5 on pp. 250-259.

Acetaminophen

The recommended starting dose of acetaminophen is 650 mg every 4 hours, not to exceed 4000 mg in a 24-hour period (APS, 2003). The American Geriatrics Society

Box 7-1 | Selection and Dosing of Nonopioids for Analgesia

After identifying the patient's risk factors for adverse effects (see Chapter 6), the following are relevant to drug selection and dosing.

DRUG SELECTION

- *Acute versus persistent (chronic) pain.* Importance of careful drug selection increases over time.
- *Analgesic history.* Whenever possible, select an NSAID that has worked well and been safe in the past for the patient.
- *Pain intensity.* Acetaminophen is recommended for mild pain and in combination with an NSAID for more moderate pain. Both can be combined with other analgesics, such as opioids, for more severe pain.
- *Current analgesic response.* If one NSAID is ineffective, try another.
- *Frequency of dosing.* For PRN use, 4-6 hourly dosing of a short-acting formulation is acceptable. For ATC use, dosing once or twice a day is preferred. Once-daily is preferable to twice-daily dosing of celecoxib to prevent increased risk of CV adverse effects.
- *Routes.* All are available orally, most can be formulated for rectal administration, NSAIDs are available or can be formulated for topical administration, and ketorolac (Toradol) and ibuprofen are available for IV administration. (Ketorolac may be given IM.)
- *Cost.* Certain NSAIDs are considerably more expensive than others. Those that tend to be the least expensive are aspirin, choline magnesium trisalicylate, diflunisal (Dolobid), ibuprofen, indomethacin (Indocin), naproxen (Naprosyn), and salsalate (Disalcid).

STARTING DOSE AND DOSE TITRATION

(NOTE: Nonopioids have an analgesic ceiling that varies from one individual to another.)

- *Acetaminophen.* Usual recommended dose is 650 mg every 4 hours, not to exceed 4000 mg/24 hr.
- *NSAID for acute pain.* Use the recommended starting dose for analgesia. For rapid onset of oral analgesia, use a short half-life drug and/or a loading dose (50% to 100% higher than recommended dose).
- *NSAID for frail older patients, others at risk for adverse effects, and long-term therapy.* Start with 50% or less of the usual recommended dose.
- *NSAID dose titration.* For patients who are started on a low dose, increase the dose in 50% increments at least weekly until analgesia is satisfactory or a ceiling dose is identified. Do not exceed 200% of the recommended daily dose. Avoid full dose of NSAIDs with a long half-life in older adults (see text).

EVALUATION OF ANALGESIA

- *Acetaminophen.* Pain relief may be evaluated within 2 hours.
- *NSAIDs.* Initial pain relief may be evaluated within 3 hours. Maximum pain relief with repeated dosing may be evaluated in 2 to 7 days, depending on the half-life of the drug.

EVALUATION OF ADVERSE EFFECTS (SEE CHAPTER 6)

- Decrease the nonopioid dose 25% to 50% if adverse effects occur.
- Discontinue nonopioid if significant adverse effects occur, e.g., GI bleeding.

ATC, Around the clock; GI, gastrointestinal; h, hour; mg, milligram; NSAID, nonsteroidal antiinflammatory drug; PRN, as needed.
From Pasero, C., & McCaffery, M. *Pain assessment and pharmacologic management*, p. 218, St. Louis, Mosby. © 2011, Pasero C, McCaffery M. May be duplicated for use in clinical practice.

(AGS) (2009) recommends a daily dose range of 2000 mg to 4000 mg for persistent pain in older adults. The most common adult daily dose of acetaminophen is 1000 mg (Burke, Smyth, Fitzgerald, 2006; Toms, McQuay, Derry, et al., 2008). This is also suggested as the optimal dose with a gradual decline in analgesic activity over a 6-hour period (Bannwarth, Pehourcq, 2003).

Doses of 1000 mg of acetaminophen 4 times a day have been reported to be as effective as ibuprofen at 1200 or 2400 mg per day doses for OA pain (Simon, Lipman, Caudill-Slosberg, et al., 2002) (see pp. 220-221 for more on OA). A systematic review of randomized, controlled trials comparing higher and lower doses of nonopioids concluded 1000 mg of acetaminophen provided statistically

superior analgesia compared with 500 mg (McQuay, Moore, 2006). There is a ceiling on the analgesia of acetaminophen, and increasing each dose greater than 1000 mg will result in very little added analgesia (Motov, Ast, 2008). If pain cannot be controlled with recommended doses, an NSAID or an opioid analgesic should be considered.

Caution is recommended with long-term acetaminophen use, even at therapeutic doses (Bolesta, Haber, 2002) (see Chapter 6 for hepatic effects). Most experts recommend a reduction in daily dose in individuals who are at high risk for hepatotoxicity (Burke, Smyth, FitzGerald, 2006). For example, the AGS (2009) recommends a 50% to 75% reduction in dose in older adults with hepatic dysfunction. Others recommend avoiding acetaminophen entirely in patients with liver disease (Bannwarth, Pehourcq, 2003; Laine, White, Rostom, et al., 2008). Still others suggest it as the optimal analgesic for patients with stable chronic liver disease (Graham, Scott, Day, 2005).

Though some research shows that 4000 mg/24 h can be safely taken in individuals who regularly drink alcohol (Graham, Scott, Day, 2005; Kuffner, Dart, 2001), the APS recommends no more than 2500 mg/24 h in individuals who consume more than 2 ounces of alcohol daily because of the elevated risk of hepatotoxicity (Simon, Lipman, Caudill-Slosberg, et al., 2002). The United States Food and Drug Administration (U.S. FDA) requires acetaminophen product labeling to warn consumers of the increased risk of liver damage when acetaminophen is taken by those who consume three or more alcoholic drinks per day (U.S. FDA, 2009). The AGS lists chronic alcohol abuse/dependence as a relative contraindication to using acetaminophen (AGS, 2009). Liver function tests should be performed every 6 to 12 months in any individual at high risk for hepatotoxicity who is taking long-term acetaminophen (Bannwarth, 2006; Miaskowski, Cleary, Burney, et al., 2005; Simon, Lipman, Caudill-Slosberg, et al., 2002).

Daily acetaminophen doses of greater than 500 mg have been shown to diminish gastric mucosal protection (Rahme, Pettitt, LeLorier, 2002), and epidemiologic studies show doses of greater than 2000 mg/24 h produce increased risk of upper GI adverse effects (Bannwarth, 2006). This risk of GI events is underappreciated. Acetaminophen also has been associated with dose-dependent renal adverse effects, and chronic use should incorporate appropriate precautions and monitoring for renal toxicity (Curhan, Knight, Rosner, et al., 2004; Forman, Stampfer, Curhan, 2005) (see Chapter 6 for GI effects and for renal effects).

NSAIDs

If the target of therapy is pain (and not inflammation), and in the absence of significant co-morbid hepatic disease, NSAID therapy should be considered when pain cannot be controlled by acetaminophen. For most patients, the initial dose is consistent with the lower effective dose suggested by the manufacturer. Pain may not respond until a higher dose is given, however, and the analgesic dose is usually less than the antiinflammatory dose. Dose escalation may be undertaken, therefore, either to explore the dose-response for pain or to gain better control over inflammation. For example, 400 mg of ibuprofen is usually recommended for analgesia, but doses as high as 800 mg 4 times a day may be necessary for an antiinflammatory effect.

There is a ceiling on the analgesia of each NSAID, but it varies from one person to another. Single ibuprofen doses greater than 400 mg and daily doses greater than 1200 mg have been shown to produce little analgesic advantage, leading some researchers to recommend a dosing regimen of 400 mg every 8 hours rather than the customary

600 mg to 800 mg every 6 to 8 hours (Motov, Ast, 2008). Individual patients, however, may demonstrate a clear-cut benefit at relatively higher doses. Higher doses are associated with a higher incidence of adverse effects (Antman, Bennett, Daugherty, 2007; Bertagnolli, Eagle, Zauber, et al., 2006; Wilcox, Allison, Benzuly, et al., 2006), and for this reason, most clinicians explore the dose-response of an NSAID only until the highest dose recommended by the manufacturer or modestly higher is reached.

There is no certainty about the minimal effective analgesic dose, the ceiling dose, or the toxic dose for the individual patient. To avoid giving a patient a higher dose than is needed, dose titration should be considered and may be especially important in those with increased risk of NSAID toxicity (e.g., older adults) and those who are treated with the intention of long-term therapy.

If the NSAID dose is titrated from a relatively low starting dose, it typically requires a period of 5 to 7 days to evaluate the response at each dose level. The occurrence of increased analgesia after a dose increase implies that the ceiling dose has not been reached. Titration can be continued until a further dose increase provides no additional pain relief, adverse effects occur, or a dose conventionally considered the ceiling dose for the specific drug in question is reached. The lowest dose that provides satisfactory pain relief should be maintained.

The potential value of different dosing regimens for pains of different types has not been empirically evaluated for most drugs. Celecoxib may illustrate the utility of this type of data. The recommended and most frequently prescribed starting dose of celecoxib for acute pain is an initial single dose of 400 mg (e.g., given preoperatively for surgical patients) followed by another 200 mg on the day of surgery and twice daily doses on subsequent days (Recart, Issioui, White, et al., 2003). Single doses of 200 mg daily or 100 mg twice daily are recommended and most often prescribed for OA; doses of 100 mg to 200 mg twice daily are recommended for RA, and the most commonly prescribed daily dose is 400 mg (Schnitzer, Kong, Mitchell, et al., 2003). Generally, a starting dose of 200 mg daily is recommended for most patients with persistent pain (Laine, White, Rostom, et al., 2008). Higher doses may improve analgesia but can also result in more adverse effects (Bertagnolli, Eagle, Zauber, et al., 2006).

Celecoxib efficacy does not appear to be influenced by whether the drug is dosed once or twice daily, but as discussed in Chapter 6, a twice-daily dosing regimen may increase the incidence of CV adverse effects. Once-daily dosing may be preferable, particularly in patients at high risk for CV adverse events (Grosser, Fries, FitzGerald, 2006; Sowers, White, Pitt, et al., 2005; Vardeny, Solomon, 2008; Whelton, Fort, Puma, et al., 2001).

Acute Pain

NSAIDs vary in time to onset and duration of analgesia. Generally, NSAIDs with a longer half-life have a slower onset of analgesia. NSAIDs with shorter half-lives, which have a more rapid onset, are used most often for acute pain management (Helstrom, Rostom, 2006). Usually, higher doses result in a faster onset of analgesia, higher peak effect, and longer duration of analgesia. These kinetics would support the conclusion that the treatment of acute pain is most effectively managed by initiating treatment with the highest approved dose of a short half-life drug and then adjusting the dose downward. As noted, however, the increased safety of dose titration suggests that the alternative strategy—low initial dose combined with gradual exploration of the dose-response—is appropriate if therapy is started with the intent of long-term treatment, or if patients have important risk factors for adverse effects (see Chapter 8 for perioperative use of nonopioids).

Persistent (Chronic) Pain

NSAIDs with long half-lives should be considered for persistent pain because they require less frequent dosing and may enhance adherence as a result. Although some clinicians recommend a priming dose of a long half-life drug to increase blood levels and shorten onset of analgesia, others start with low doses to minimize adverse effects, especially in those patients at risk for adverse effects (also see discussion of celecoxib dosing regimen earlier in the chapter). Caution is recommended in administering long-acting NSAIDs in older adults (Simon, Lipman, Caudill-Slosberg, et al., 2002). Many clinicians recommend avoiding full doses of naproxen, piroxicam, and oxaprozin in older adults because of their long half-life and increased risk of GI toxicity (Fick, Cooper, Wade, et al., 2003; Hanlon, Backonja, Weiner, et al., 2009) (see Chapter 6).

Several weeks are necessary to evaluate the effectiveness of an NSAID when it is used to treat grossly inflammatory conditions such as rheumatoid arthritis (RA) (Burke, Smythe, FitzGerald, 2006). However, analgesia can occur with the first dose, and typically a week or less is sufficient to evaluate the global analgesic benefit of an NSAID regimen at a selected dose. The foregoing discussion of selection and dosing of nonopioids is summarized in Box 7-1.

Special Circumstances and Conditions

Osteoarthritis

OA is the most common form of arthritis in the United States (American College of Rheumatology (ACR). 2000). In 2000, the North American prevalence was 25 million; projections have this number doubling by 2020 (Hunter, Lo, 2008). OA is age-related, chronic, and often debilitating; pain is a major determinant of its impact on function and quality of life (AHRQ, 2006; Simon, Lipman, Caudill-Slosberg, et al., 2002).

The underlying disease process of OA is joint degeneration with loss of joint space, osteophyte formation, and subchondral sclerosis (Sun, Wu, Kalunian, 2007).

OA can be asymmetrical and affect just one or multiple joints. The associated pain usually is classified as nociceptive (see Section I), and nonopioid analgesics have a major role in its relief. The challenge, as with all types of pain, is to select nonopioid analgesics that will provide the greatest degree of pain relief with the fewest adverse effects (AHRQ, 2006).

Several professional organizations, including the ACR (Altman, Hochberg, Moskowitz, et al., 2000), APS (Simon, Lipman, Caudill-Slosberg, et al., 2002), and European League Against Rheumatism (EULAR) (Jordan, Arden, Doherty, et al., 2003; Zhang, Doherty, Arden, et al., 2005; Zhang, Doherty, Leeb, et al., 2007), have released evidence-based treatment recommendations for OA pain. More recently, a panel composed of 16 experts from around the world appointed by the Osteoarthritis Research Society International (OARSI) released recommendations (Zhang, Moskowitz, Nuki, et al., 2008). The OARSI panel appraised already published guidelines, systematically reviewed the research for treatment of knee and hip OA through January 2006, and issued guidelines that are considered by some to contain the most up-to-date recommendations (Hunter, Lo, 2008). The reader is referred to the OARSI document.

All of the guidelines agree that acetaminophen at doses up to 4 g/day is first line for the pharmacologic treatment of mild to moderate OA pain (Altman, Hochberg, Moskowitz, et al., 2000; NCC-CC, 2008; Roddy, Doherty, 2003; Simon, Lipman, Caudill-Slosberg, et al., 2002; Zhang, Moskowitz, Nuki, et al., 2008). The AGS also recommends acetaminophen as a first-choice analgesic for mild to moderate persistent musculoskeletal pain (AGS, 2009). Further, the OARSI promotes acetaminophen as a safe long-term analgesic if pain relief is satisfactory. However, some researchers question the appropriateness of acetaminophen as a first-line choice for OA and call for more studies that compare the drug to specific NSAIDs for pain treatment (Case, Baliunas, Block, 2003). Sun and colleagues (2007) recommend an NSAID as a primary drug in the treatment of patients with an inflammatory phenotype of OA.

NSAIDs are recommended as the next choice of analgesic if pain is uncontrolled by acetaminophen (Altman, Hochberg, Moskowitz, et al., 2000; American Academy of Orthopaedic Surgeons, 2008; NCC-CC, 2008; Roddy, Doherty, 2003; Simon, Lipman, Caudill-Slosberg, et al., 2002; Zhang, Moskowitz, Nuki, et al., 2008). Randomized controlled studies comparing acetaminophen and NSAIDs support this recommendation with findings of superior analgesia with NSAIDs for OA pain (Battisti, Katz, Weaver, et al., 2004; Case, Baliunas, Block, 2003; Pincus, Koch, Lei, et al., 2004; Pincus, Koch, Sokka, et al., 2001). A Cochrane Collaboration Review of 15 randomized controlled trials involving nearly 6000 patients concluded that NSAIDs were superior to acetaminophen in reduction of pain, global assessments, and improvements in functional status for both knee and hip OA pain (Towheed, Maxwell, Judd, et al., 2006). Safety and tolerability were essentially the same between the two types of analgesics, except that those taking an NSAID were more likely to experience a GI adverse effect (see Chapter 6 for NSAID-induced GI adverse effects). The AHRQ (2006) executive summary on the best evidence comparing the various common OA pain treatments also notes the benefits of NSAIDs (AHRQ, 2006).

Some of the literature comparing NSAIDs and acetaminophen has focused on the COX-2 selective drugs. A 6-week study randomized 288 patients with OA of the knee to receive acetaminophen, rofecoxib, or celecoxib and found that all treatments were safe and well tolerated; however, more patients receiving acetaminophen than the COX-2 selective NSAIDs discontinued treatment due to lack of efficacy (Geba, Weaver, Polis, et al., 2002). Rofecoxib (no longer available), followed closely by celecoxib, was associated with the most improvement in outcome indicators (e.g., pain relief, morning stiffness, physical function). Although acetaminophen is generally reserved for mild OA pain, it has been shown to produce an additive effect (Sun, Wu, Kalunian, 2007), and some clinicians advocate the continuation of acetaminophen therapy during NSAID treatment as part of a multimodal pain treatment plan (Simon, Lipman, Caudill-Slosberg, et al., 2002).

As discussed in Chapter 6, the risks and benefits of initiating NSAID therapy must be considered on an individual basis. If initiated, all guidelines stress the importance of administering the lowest NSAID dose for the shortest time necessary. This principle is particularly applicable in patients with OA, as treatment is likely to be long-term and the risk for adverse effects increases over time. Older adults are the most likely to be afflicted with OA and are at high risk for NSAID-induced GI adverse effects, and it is reasonable to consider those NSAIDs with relatively more favorable GI risk profiles as particularly preferable. Topical NSAIDs produce fewer GI adverse effects than oral drugs, and guidelines also recommend that they be considered another means of reducing risk. The United Kingdom's National Collaborating Centre for Chronic Conditions recommends that topical NSAIDs be the core treatment, along with acetaminophen, for knee and hand OA and should be tried before oral NSAIDs (NCC-CC, 2008).

For oral NSAID therapy, the OARSI recommends a COX-2 selective NSAID or a nonselective NSAID with a PPI or misoprostol, but cautions against long-term NSAID therapy because of the significant risk of GI adverse effects (Zhang, Moskowitz, Nuki, et al., 2008). Many older adults also have CV risk factors, and some have both GI and CV risk factors that must be considered. A placebo-controlled trial showed naproxen (440/660 mg/day), which is characterized as an NSAID with relatively low GI and CV adverse effect profiles, provided comparable satisfactory pain relief to ibuprofen (1200 mg/day) for mild to moderate OA knee pain (Schiff, Minic, 2004). Some researchers recommend avoiding full doses of NSAIDs with a long half-life, such as naproxen (Fick, Cooper, Wade, et al., 2003).

Several guidelines recommend the use of opioid analgesics for OA pain that is unrelieved by nonpharmacologic measures, acetaminophen, and NSAIDs (Altman, Hochberg, Moskowitz, et al., 2000; NCC-CC, 2008; Simon, Lipman, Caudill-Slosberg, et al., 2002; Zhang, Moskowitz, Nuki, et al., 2008). Tramadol is also suggested for more severe pain (Altman, Hochberg, Moskowitz, et al., 2000; Simon, Lipman, Caudill-Slosberg, et al., 2002). (See Section IV for more on the use of opioids and tramadol for OA pain.)

Rheumatoid Arthritis

RA is the second most common form of arthritis, with a prevalence of 1% to 2% of adults afflicted. It affects women more frequently than men and is diagnosed most often between the ages of 20 and 40 (Simon, Lipman, Caudill-Slosberg, et al., 2002). It is usually chronic, progressive, and can be extremely debilitating. Over 9 million physician visits and more than 250,000 hospitalizations annually are related to RA (Khanna, Arnold, Pencharz, et al., 2006).

RA is an autoimmune inflammatory disease with hallmark features of symmetrical erosive synovitis with an unknown etiology (Khanna, Arnold, Pencharz, et al., 2006). The disease begins in the synovial fluid but is systemic and can affect multiple organs and lead to premature death. Early and aggressive treatment is critical to prevent cartilage destruction (Simon, Lipman, Caudill-Slosberg, et al., 2002).

Pain, swelling, tenderness, and morning stiffness of various joints usually prompts individuals with RA to seek initial medical help. Urgent treatment with immunosuppressive agents, including a blocker of the cytokine tumor necrosis factor, typically is indicated. This treatment often is highly effective and may control pain to such a degree that further analgesic therapy is not needed. In some cases, other disease modifying therapies may be needed, among which is an NSAID at antiinflammatory doses. In other cases, synovitis appears to be stemmed by immunosuppressive therapy, but additional treatment for pain is necessary to allow optimal functioning.

A Cochrane Collaboration Review found only four studies comparing acetaminophen and NSAIDs for RA pain (Wienecke, Gotzsche, 2004). The poor quality of the studies made it impossible to draw conclusions about superiority; however, the patients in the trials preferred NSAIDs to acetaminophen far more often. Guidelines support the use of NSAIDs as first-line analgesics for RA pain; however, the choice of NSAID must be guided by thoughtful consideration of patient risk factors (Luqmani, Hennel, Estrach, et al., 2009; Simon, Lipman, Caudill-Slosberg, et al., 2002).

RA is associated with an increased risk for CV adverse events, such as myocardial infarction, and individuals with RA who have had a previous CV event or have other risk factors are of particular concern (Medscape Rheumatology, 2006) (see Table 6-4 and Chapter 6 for discussion of CV risk factors). Many individuals with RA take cardioprotective aspirin as a way of addressing the elevated CV risk. Aspirin therapy has the potential to produce an increase in GI adverse effects and also has implications for the choice of NSAID. Some clinicians favor the use of celecoxib given its pharmacologic profile (see discussion in Chapter 6), and a Cochrane Collaboration Review evaluating the use of celecoxib in patients with RA found that celecoxib produced pain relief similar to naproxen, diclofenac, and ibuprofen, and had fewer associated upper GI complications (Garner, Fidan, Frankish, et al., 2002). The latter benefit may or may not persist during long-term therapy, however, and presumably is attenuated or eliminated by aspirin co-therapy. Nonetheless, a recent study found a decline in NSAID-related GI adverse effects in patients with RA worldwide (Steen, Nurmohamed, Visman, et al., 2008), a change attributed to an increase in the use of COX-2 selective inhibitors, strict adherence to gastroprotective guidelines, and better general RA treatment regimens (see Chapter 6 for gastroprotective therapy and for selection of NSAID with consideration of CV and GI risk). Clearly, the selection of an NSAID for RA pain should favor those with relatively better risk profiles and the use of treatment strategies that minimize risk through careful dose selection and adverse effect management. Moreover, as with OA, the use of opioid analgesics should be considered when other analgesics do not produce adequate pain relief or are contraindicated by patient risk factors (Simon, Lipman, Caudill-Slosberg, et al., 2002). See Section IV for more on the use of opioid analgesics for RA.

Low Back Pain

At some point, most people will experience low back pain. It is reported that up to 90% of adults will have low back pain during their lifetime (Birbara, Puopolo, Munoz, et al., 2003). Next to upper respiratory infection, it is the most common reason for lost work. Although most acute low back pain is benign and resolves over time (Pepijn, Roelofs, Deyo, et al., 2008), it can persist and become disabling. The disability and costs associated with acute and persistent low back pain are in the range of 20 to 50 million dollars every year, with persistent pain accounting for up to 90% of this cost.

Nonopioid analgesics are commonly used to treat both acute and persistent low back pain, but the research supporting their efficacy for this type of pain is lacking. A Cochrane Collaboration Review of 65 trials (11,237 patients) found that acetaminophen and the various nonselective and COX-2 selective NSAIDs were more effective than placebo and equally effective to one another in reducing short-term acute low back pain and persistent low back pain without sciatica (Roelofs, Deyo, Koes, et al., 2008). In a joint clinical practice guideline, the American College of Physicians and the APS noted that acetaminophen is a less efficacious analgesic than NSAIDs but

recommended it for initial low back pain treatment because of its more favorable safety profile (Chou, Qaseem, Snow, et al., 2007). The guideline recommends NSAID therapy in the lowest effective dose after a careful assessment of CV and GI risk and opioids or tramadol for severe, disabling acute or persistent low back pain. European evidence-based guidelines for the management of persistent low back pain recommend short-term use (e.g., 3 months) of NSAIDs and opioid analgesics (Airaksinen, Brox, Cedraschi, et al., 2006). The guideline panel stated that more research, specifically of functional outcomes, is needed before recommendations for long-term use of acetaminophen and NSAIDs could be made.

At least two studies have been conducted to evaluate the effect of the COX-2 selective NSAID etoricoxib (Arcoxia) on persistent low back pain. The first study randomized 319 patients with persistent low back pain to receive 60 mg or 90 mg of etoricoxib or placebo daily for 12 weeks (Birbara, Puopolo, Munoz, et al., 2003). The patients who took either dose of etoricoxib demonstrated significantly more pain relief and improvement in multiple functional and quality of life indicators compared with placebo. Pain relief and reductions in disability were noticeable within 1 week, maximal at 4 weeks, and maintained over the 3-month study period. A multicenter (46 sites) study of very similar design also reported improvements in pain and physical functioning that were maintained over 3 months with etoricoxib (Pallay, Seger, Adler, et al., 2004).

Combination opioid-nonopioid formulations are frequently administered for acute and persistent low back pain, but more research is needed to support their use. A multicenter, randomized, controlled study of 147 individuals with moderate-to-severe acute low back pain found similar efficacy and tolerability with the combination of hydrocodone (7.5 mg) and ibuprofen (200 mg) and the combination of oxycodone (5 mg) and acetaminophen (325 mg) (Palangio, Morris, Doyle, et al., 2002). The analgesics were administered over a period of 8 days.

Renal Colic

Ureteral obstruction such as from urolithiasis (renal calculi) is usually accompanied by the acute severe flank or abdominal pain of renal colic (Serinken, Karcioglu, Turkcuer, et al., 2008). Prostaglandins mediate ureteral contractility and stretching, which potentiates the pain associated with the obstruction (Jerde, Calamon-Dixon, Bjorling, et al., 2005). This suggests that NSAIDs may be useful in this condition beyond their nonspecific analgesic effects.

A Cochrane Collaboration Review of 20 randomized controlled trials (1613 patients) concluded that both NSAIDs and opioids are effective for pain associated with renal colic (Holdgate, Pollock, 2005). Research comparing pain relief in 130 patients who were given ketorolac or morphine or a combination of the two showed that the combination of ketorolac and morphine produced superior pain relief and a need for less rescue analgesia compared with either drug alone (Safdar, Degutis, Landry, et al., 2006). Experimental research has shown that parenteral ketorolac significantly reduces ureteral contractility, which may account for the effectiveness of this drug on this type of pain (Wen, Coyle, Jerde, et al., 2008). Diclofenac also has been shown to be effective (Yencilek, Aktas, Goktas, et al., 2008), but one study failed to show any morphine-sparing effects with the drug when used for treatment of renal colic pain (Engeler, Ackermann, Osterwalder, et al., 2005). A randomized placebo-controlled trial compared IV acetaminophen (1 g) with IV morphine (0.1 mg/kg) in 146 patients presenting in the emergency department (ED) with renal colic and found that IV acetaminophen and IV morphine produced comparable pain relief with no adverse events in any patients (Bektas, Eken, Karadeniz, et al., 2009).

Biliary Colic

Obstruction to gallbladder drainage is the underlying mechanism for acute cholecystitis (Yusoff, Barkun, Barkun, 2003). Enhanced prostaglandin production is reported to mediate the associated inflammation, and NSAID-induced inhibition of prostaglandins has been shown to reduce this process and the pain that accompanies the condition (Yusoff, Barkun, Barkun, 2003). In the past, meperidine has been the drug of choice for treatment of biliary colic in the ED; however, the drug does not appear to offer any advantages over NSAIDs and may have disadvantages (see Chapter 13). One study showed that ketorolac (30 mg IV) and meperidine (50 mg IV) produced equivalent pain relief for treatment of acute biliary colic in the ED, but ketorolac was better tolerated; those receiving meperidine experienced more nausea and dizziness (Henderson, Swadron, Newton, 2002). Another small study (N = 30) showed similar effective analgesia when meperidine and ketorolac were compared; however, patients in the ketorolac group required less rescue medication (Dula, Anderson, Wood, 2001). A randomized, controlled trial comparing the agonist-antagonist opioid butorphanol (Stadol) and ketorolac reported excellent pain relief with both drugs and more dizziness and sedation with butorphanol and nausea with ketorolac (Olsen, McGrath, Schwarz, et al., 2008). Effective pain relief and a lack of sedation with ketorolac may be important in helping to achieve the goal of short length of stay in the ED.

Pregnancy

The use of nonopioid analgesics during pregnancy has increased and appears to be commonplace today (Alano, Ngougmna, Ostrea, et al., 2001; Freyer, 2008; Werler, Mitchell, Hernandez-Diaz, et al., 2005). A case-control study of 101 newborn infants revealed a high presence of NSAIDs (49.5%) in meconium, particularly aspirin (43.6%), ibuprofen (22.8%), and naproxen (18.8%) (Alano, Ngougmna, Ostrea, et al., 2001). Analysis of data on over 10,500 women from two case-control studies on birth defects revealed that acetaminophen and ibuprofen were among the most commonly used over-the-counter (OTC) medications during pregnancy in the United States, with 65% and 18% of the women saying they used acetaminophen and ibuprofen, respectively (Werler, Mitchell, Hernandez-Diaz, et al., 2005). An increase in the use of naproxen during pregnancy also has been noted (Werler, Mitchell, Hernandez-Diaz, et al., 2005). A Canadian study (N = 36,387) showed that the most common nonopioids used by pregnant women were naproxen (35%), ibuprofen (26%), rofecoxib (15%), diclofenac (9%), and celecoxib (9%) (Ofori, Oraichi, Blais, et al., 2006).

More research is needed to determine the short- and long-term effects of NSAIDs in pregnancy (Andrade, Gurwitz, Davis, et al., 2004; Larsen, Pedersen, 2006; Li, Lui, Odouli, 2003; Werler, Mitchell, Hernandez-Diaz, et al., 2005). At present, the U.S. FDA (2008) lists the nonselective NSAIDs in risk category B (no controlled studies showing adverse effect, or controlled studies in women fail to demonstrate risk) and the COX-2 selective NSAIDs in risk category C (no controlled studies in women) (Temprano, Bandlamudi, Moore, 2005). It should also be noted that the FDA lists misoprostol, a gastroprotective therapy sometimes coadministered with NSAIDs, as a Category X drug, which means research and clinical experience has shown a definite fetal risk that clearly outweighs any possible benefit (Andrade, Gurwitz, Davis, et al., 2004).

Although the lack of data is noteworthy, enough evidence exists to recommend against NSAID use during pregnancy (Temprano, Bandlamudi, Moore, 2005). Not all of the effects of NSAIDs in the fetus are known, but NSAIDs do cross the placental barrier and can have a long half-life in the fetus. Research has shown an association between NSAID use during the first trimester and interference with implantation and increased rates of miscarriage (Li, Liu, Odouli, 2003). Cardiac malformations (Larsen, Pedersen, 2006; Ofori, Oraichi, Blais, et al., 2006) and reduced renal function in the fetus have also been reported (Freyer, 2008). Through meconium analysis, the previously mentioned case-control study of 101 newborn infants confirmed an association between the maternal use of NSAIDs and the development of persistent pulmonary hypertension of the newborn (PPHN) (Alano, Ngougmna, Ostrea, et al., 2001). A case report described renal tubular dysgenesis, a rare and lethal autosomal recessive disorder, in a neonate exposed in utero to naproxen (Koklu, Gurgoze, Akgun, et al., 2006). A study evaluating neonatal morbidity associated with prolonged use of indomethacin during pregnancy in 124 women demonstrated that 6.5% of the neonates developed ductal constriction and 7.3% had oligohydraminos (Savage,

Anderson, Simhan, 2007). Composite neonatal morbidity was 29%. Ibuprofen also has been associated with premature ductal closure and oligohydraminos (Freyer, 2008). Aspirin has been associated with premature closure of the ductus arteriosis as well as fetal gastroschisis (James, Brancazio, Price, 2008).

Taken during the last trimester, NSAIDs, and particularly aspirin, even in low doses, can cause maternal and fetal bleeding and increase the risk of placental abruption (James, Brancazio, Price, 2008; Moore, 2008). Through prostaglandin inhibition, NSAIDs can relax uterine contractions and prolong gestation, which is the rationale for the use of indomethacin for premature labor (Temprano, Bandlamudi, Moore, 2005). If an NSAID must be taken for a disease process, such as severe RA, it should be stopped preferably by 32 weeks gestation and no later than 8 weeks prior to delivery (Temprano, Bandlamudi, Moore, 2005).

It has been noted that pregnant women may not realize the potential dangers of NSAIDs, and many do not even know they are taking a nonopioid because the drug is often hidden within a formulation of a medication they are taking for symptoms other than pain relief (e.g., common cold remedies) (Alano, Ngougmna, Ostrea, et al., 2001). This underscores the need for obstetrical care providers to take time during the initial prenatal visit, if not earlier, to discuss the common OTC medications and their ingredients and explain the risks associated with taking them during pregnancy.

Acetaminophen is widely recommended as a safe alternative to NSAIDs during pregnancy (Freyer, 2008; Li, Liu, Odouli, 2003; Rebordosa, Kogevinas, Horvath-Puho, et al., 2008). Analysis of a Danish study of over 88,000 delivered women revealed no association between acetaminophen intake during pregnancy and congenital abnormalities (Rebordosa, Kogevinas, Horvath-Puho, et al., 2008). However, research has shown that children who were exposed in utero to acetaminophen taken by their mothers during middle to late (but not early) pregnancy have an increased risk of wheezing (Persky, Piorkowski, Hernandez, et al., 2008; Shaheen, Newson, Henderson, et al., 2005).

Opioids are recommended as an alternative to nonopioids for moderate to severe pain in the pregnant woman (Freyer, 2008). A large retrospective study (N = 152,531) found that acetaminophen is frequently prescribed with an opioid for relief of moderate pain during pregnancy (Andrade, Gurwitz, Davis, et al., 2004).

Breast-Feeding

The pharmacodynamic characteristics of a drug determine whether and how much of it will be absorbed by an infant during breast-feeding (Wilbeck, Schorn, Dailey, 2008). In general, oral drugs have poor bioavailability because of GI metabolism ("first-pass effect"), which results in less drug reaching the mother's systemic circulation to be passed on to the infant via breast milk. On the other hand, parenteral administration results in rapid and 100% bioavailability (see Chapter 11 for more on first-pass effect and drug pharmacodynamics). Unlike other NSAIDs, ketorolac has 100% bioavailability by both the oral and parenteral routes of administration (Wilbeck, Schorn, Dailey, 2008). Topical analgesics are poorly absorbed into the plasma, making the dose transferred to the infant almost negligible.

Other factors that determine how much drug is transferred into breast milk include drug dose and dosing regimen, molecular weight, lipid solubility, and protein binding (Wilbeck, Schorn, Daley, 2008). As the dose of the drug increases, the serum concentration and diffusion into the milk compartment increases. For this reason, any drug administered during breast-feeding should be given at the lowest dose possible. Drugs with a long half-life produce a greater risk to the nursing infant of cumulative exposure, and drugs with a short half-life (e.g., acetaminophen, ibuprofen) are preferred. Medications that are not very fat soluble but are highly protein bound and have a high molecular weight (e.g., ibuprofen, ketorolac) also are less likely to transfer into breast milk.

Most NSAIDs are safe for use during lactation, although they have been known to displace bilirubin and increase the risk of jaundice and kernicterus in the newborn (Temprano, Bandlamudi, Moore, 2005). In its policy statement on the transfer of drugs and other chemicals into human milk, the American Academy of Pediatrics (AAP) approved the use of acetaminophen, ibuprofen, indomethacin, ketorolac, naproxen, and piroxicam and recommended caution in the use of aspirin (AAP, 2001). There are no nonopioids listed in the AAP policy statement as drugs that are of concern or that would require cessation of breast-feeding. General consensus is that an appropriate choice of nonopioid is one with a short half-life and inactive metabolites that are rapidly excreted, such as acetaminophen or ibuprofen (Wilbeck, Schorn, Daley, 2008).

In summary, a few basic principles can be applied to nonopioid use during breast-feeding. First, the safest drug should be selected such as acetaminophen or ibuprofen rather than aspirin. A good rule of thumb is that a drug that is safe to give to an infant is likely to be safe to give to a breast-feeding mother (Wilbeck, Schorn, Daley, 2008). Second, mothers can be advised to plan feedings around times when the drug concentration in the breast milk is lowest. Taking the medication immediately before (Wilbeck, Schorn, Daley, 2008) or immediately after (AAP, 2001) breast-feeding is recommended. Avoiding drugs with a long half-life is advised, but if this is not possible, the drug should be taken once daily and just prior to an infant's lengthy sleep period (Wilbeck, Schorn, Daley, 2008). Finally, as always, the lowest effective nonopioid dose should be taken for the shortest time needed.

NSAIDs and Prevention of Cancer

Epidemiologic research has suggested a possible connection between NSAID use and the prevention or a lower incidence of some types of cancer (National Cancer Institute, 2004; Harris, 2009; Harris, Beebe-Donk, Alshafie, 2007, 2008; Harris, Beebe-Donk, Doss, et al., 2005; Pereg, Lishner, 2005). COX-2 activates signaling pathways that promote cell production and inhibit cell death through its mediation of prostaglandin E_2 (PGE_2). Though further research is needed to more clearly identify the underlying mechanisms, the inhibition of COX-2, such as by NSAIDs, is thought to prevent activation of this pathway and thereby decrease cell proliferation, reduce formation of vasculature to cancer cells, and alter the immune response (National Cancer Institute, 2004; Pereg, Lishner, 2005). A review of the literature revealed that daily intake of nonselective NSAIDs reduced risk for cancers of the colon (63%), breast (39%), lung (36%), esophagus (73%), stomach (62%), ovary (47%), and prostate (39%) (Harris, Beebe-Donk, Doss, et al., 2005). A more recent comprehensive review of the epidemiologic literature reported that regular intake of OTC nonselective NSAIDs produced significant risk reductions of 43% for colon cancer, 25% for breast cancer, 28% for lung cancer, and 27% for prostate cancer (Harris, 2009). A case control study revealed an association between COX-2 selective NSAID use and risk reductions for cancers of the breast (71%), prostate (55%), colon (70%), and lung (79%) with an overall 68% risk reduction for all 4 cancers (Harris, Beebe-Donk, Alshafie, 2007).

COX-2 is reported to be overexpressed in breast cancer tissues, and the greater the expression, the poorer the prognosis. This led researchers to study the impact of celecoxib on moderately and highly invasive breast cancer cell lines (Basu, Pathangey, Tinder, et al., 2005). In both cell types, celecoxib arrested cell growth and vascular channel formation and reduced vascular endothelial growth factor. A case control study demonstrated a 71% risk reduction for breast cancer with celecoxib and rofecoxib, but no significant reductions with acetaminophen or low-dose aspirin (Harris, Beebe-Donk, Alshafie, 2006). COX-2 selective NSAIDs in combination with standard breast cancer chemotherapy has shown promising results as well, but further research is needed to more clearly identify the role of COX-2 selective NSAIDs in cancer treatment (Pereg, Lishner, 2005).

Retrospective research has shown an association between nonselective NSAID use and reductions in breast cancer, with aspirin (analgesic doses) being the most commonly used NSAID in the research (Pereg, Lishner, 2005). A meta-analysis of six cohort studies and eight case-control studies showed an association between regular use of NSAIDs and a consistently reduced relative risk of breast cancer in the majority of the studies in the analysis (Khuder, Mutgi, 2001). Another meta-analysis (10 observational studies) also concluded that aspirin may reduce breast cancer; more frequent use was associated with lower risk (Mangiapane, Blettner, Schlattmann, 2008).

Studies have shown similar results in patients with lung cancer. A case-control study showed that regular use of NSAIDs over a 2-year period was associated with a 68% reduction in relative risk of lung cancer in heavy smokers (Harris, Beebe-Donk, Schuller, 2002). A similar effect was noted in another case-control study of 1038 patients (Muscat, Chen, Richie, et al., 2003). One-year intake of NSAIDs 3 or more times weekly demonstrated an odds ratio of 0.68 for the development of lung cancer. In contrast, another case-control study (N = 1884) showed that regular use (4 days or more week) of aspirin or other nonselective NSAIDs had no effect on risk of lung cancer (Kelly, Coogan, Strom, et al., 2008).

Numerous observational studies suggested a reduction in the incidence of colorectal cancer and cancer-related deaths with the use of NSAIDs. These findings led to the initiation of case-control studies and randomized controlled trials investigating the association (Bertagnolli, Eagle, Zauber, et al., 2006). The previously discussed Adenoma Prevention with Celecoxib (APC) trial (see Chapter 6) randomized over 2000 patients to receive twice-daily doses of either 200 mg or 400 mg celecoxib or placebo (Bertagnolli, Eagle, Zauber, et al., 2006). The cumulative incidence of adenomas by year 3 was 60.7%, 43.2%, and 37.5% in those receiving placebo, celecoxib 200 mg twice daily, and celecoxib 400 mg twice daily, respectively. The researchers concluded that celecoxib is an effective agent for the prevention of colorectal adenomas but could not recommend its routine use in prevention due to dose-related serious CV events. The Prevention of Colorectal Sporadic Adenomatous Polyps (PreSAP) trial randomized patients (N = 1561) to receive either 400 mg of celecoxib once daily or placebo (Arber, Eagle, Spicak, et al., 2006). Colonoscopy analysis revealed the cumulative rate of adenomas detected through year 3 was 33.6% and 49.3% in those who received celecoxib and placebo, respectively, and the cumulative rate of advanced adenomas through year 3 was 5.3% and 10.4% in those who received celecoxib and placebo, respectively.

A Cochrane Collaboration Review of 9 trials (24,143 patients) concluded that aspirin significantly reduced the recurrence of colorectal adenoma after 1 to 3 years; short-term studies also supported the regression but not elimination or prevention of colorectal adenoma (Asano, McLeod, 2004). A more recent case-control study of 326 patients with colon cancer demonstrated that both nonselective and COX-2 selective NSAIDs produced significant reductions in the risk of colon cancer and a potential for colon cancer prevention; no reduction was noted with acetaminophen or low-dose aspirin (Harris, Beebe-Donk, Alshafie, 2008).

In summary, there is no consensus at this time about the use of NSAIDs to reduce the risk of neoplasm. Concerns about cumulative risk of GI and CV events have prevented the promotion of routine treatment of asymptomatic patients for the purpose of cancer risk reduction, even with the positive findings noted.

NSAIDs and Long-Term Cognitive Function

Ongoing research in older adults has focused on a possible relationship between NSAID consumption and long-term cognitive function (Fotuhi, Zandi, Hayden, et al., 2008; Grodstein, Sharupski, Bienias, et al., 2008; Hayden, Zandi, Khachaturian, et al., 2007; Soininen, West, Robbins, et al., 2007), including a possible reduced risk of Alzheimer's dementia (ADAPT Research Group, 2008). This relationship may be due in part to the role of COX in the metabolism of arachidonic acid in the brain (Hoozemans, Rozemuller, van Haastert, et al., 2008; Tassoni, Kaur, Weisinger, et al., 2008). Inflammation has also been proposed to have a key role in neurodegeneration and cognitive disorders (Peila, Launer, 2006; Rogers, 2008).

Findings vary, however, and more well-designed research is needed to draw any firm conclusions. For example, although epidemiologic surveys have shown that NSAIDs may protect against the development of Alzheimer's disease, treatment trials in individuals with existing Alzheimer's disease have shown little or no effect on slowing or stopping the disease (Hoozemans, Rozemuller, van Haastert, et al., 2008; Rogers, 2008). A large study of veterans aged 55 years and older with Alzheimer's disease (49,349 cases and 196,850 controls) found that long-term (more than 5 years) NSAID use had a protective effect against the development of Alzheimer's disease (Vlad, Miller, Kowall, et al., 2008). In contrast, a 12-year follow-up study of 1019 Catholic clergy found no relationship between NSAID use and Alzheimer's disease or change in cognition (Arvanitakis, Grodstein, Bienias, et al., 2008). Similarly, the ADAPT Research Group (2008) conducted a randomized, double-blind trial in 2117 older men and women with a family history of Alzheimer's disease to evaluate the effect of celecoxib (200 mg twice daily), naproxen (220 mg twice daily), or placebo on cognitive function. The researchers concluded that neither of the drugs improved cognitive function and that naproxen produced a weak detrimental effect on cognitive function. This led to their suggestion that naproxen and celecoxib not be used for the prevention of Alzheimer's disease. A Cochrane Collaboration Review concluded that ibuprofen could not be recommended for the treatment of Alzheimer's disease either (Tabet, Feldman, 2003). Another Cochrane Collaboration Review found no evidence that aspirin improves cognitive function or prognosis in individuals with vascular dementia and suggested that the risk of hemorrhage associated with aspirin intake could worsen patient outcome should it occur (Rands, Orrell, Spector, 2000).

Need for Minimal Antipyretic Effect: Masking Infection

Occasionally, the antipyretic effect of NSAIDs is an undesirable adverse effect because it might mask an infection. If an NSAID is needed, a rapid onset, short half-life nonselective or COX-2 selective drug, or acetaminophen, can be used (Burke, Smythe, FitzGerald, 2006), and a temperature reading may be obtained at the end of the drug's duration of action. Alternatively, diflunisal (Dolobid) may be a preferred NSAID because it has minimal antipyretic effects (Burke, Smythe, FitzGerald, 2006). NSAID treatment also may be permissible if an infection can be detected by means other than a fever (e.g., visual inspection, increased pain, and elevated white blood cell count). Aspirin should be avoided for treatment of viral-related fever in individuals less than 20 years old due to an association with Reye's syndrome (Burke, Smythe, FitzGerald, 2006). Two consecutive randomized controlled, open label trials in healthy infants advised against prophylactic administration of acetaminophen prior to vaccinations, stating that although febrile reactions significantly decreased, antibody responses to several vaccine antigens also were reduced (Prymula, Siegrist, Chilbek, et al., 2009).

Conclusion

A key principle of establishing an optimal pain treatment plan is to individualize the selection of analgesics. General considerations in determining the best nonopioid to initiate therapy include the patient's type of pain, pain intensity, analgesic history, response to current treatments, and adverse effect risk profile, as well as the costs associated with nonopioid analgesic treatment. Doses are titrated according to patient response, and if an initial nonopioid is ineffective, another may be tried. In addition to their usefulness as primary analgesics for a wide variety of acute and persistent pain states, research is ongoing to determine whether or not nonopioids play a role in the prevention of other conditions, such as cancer and cognitive function decline.

Chapter 8 Perioperative Nonopioid Use

ACETAMINOPHEN and nonsteroidal antiinflammatory drugs (NSAIDs) have a long history as effective first-line analgesics for postoperative pain. The use of acetaminophen and NSAIDs alone or in combination with other analgesics, such as opioids, anticonvulsants, and local anesthetics, has become more common. This strategy is termed *multimodal analgesia*. The role of nonopioids in perioperative multimodal pain treatment plans is the focus of this chapter. (See Patient Medication Information Forms III-1 through III-5 on pp. 250-259.)

Effectiveness

As with other types of pain, acetaminophen is appropriate alone for mild postoperative pain. A Cochrane Collaboration Review evaluating 47 trials (2561 patients) concluded that single doses of acetaminophen were effective and had few adverse effects for this type of pain, but provided effective analgesia for only one-half of the patients with moderate to severe pain (Toms, McQuay, Derry, et al., 2008). A study of patients following Cesarean section produced similar results, with acetaminophen producing inferior pain relief compared with diclofenac (Siddik, Aouad, Jalbout, et al., 2001). Diclofenac, but not acetaminophen, also produced opioid-dose sparing effects. These studies support the recommendation of acetaminophen for mild pain and NSAIDs alone or in combination with other analgesics, including acetaminophen, for more severe pain (Bradley, Ellis, Thomas, et al., 2007; Cepeda, Carr, Miranda, et al., 2005; Helstrom, Rosow, 2006; Hyllested, Jones, Pedersen, et al., 2002; Issioui, Klein, White, et al., 2002; White, 2002).

Parenteral ketorolac (Toradol) is adequate alone for some moderate-to-severe postoperative pain (Breda, Bui, Liao, et al., 2007; Helstrom, Rosow, 2006). IV ibuprofen (Caldolor) is approved for treatment of acute pain, but clinical experience with this new formulation was sparse at the time of publication (see discussion of IV ketorolac and IV ibuprofen later in the chapter). Cochrane Collaboration Reviews over the years have shown that single doses of the various oral nonselective NSAIDs also produce effective postoperative analgesia alone, with little difference between them (Barden, Edwards, Moore, et al., 2004; Collins, Moore, McQuay, et al., 2000; Forrest, Camu, Greer, et al., 2002; Mason, Edwards, Moore, et al., 2004). One exception is piroxicam. A Cochrane Collaboration Review concluded that there is insufficient evidence to conclude that single doses of this drug provide adequate postoperative analgesia (Moore, Rees, Loke, et al., 2000). Ibuprofen (800 mg) was found to be equianalgesic to acetaminophen (800 mg) plus codeine (60 mg) following ambulatory surgery (Raeder, Steine, Vatsgar, 2001).

Nonselective and COX-2 selective NSAIDs appear to be equally efficacious for postoperative pain (Derry, Barden, McQuay, et al., 2008; Lenz, Raeder, 2008; Rasmussen, Malmstrom, Bourne, et al., 2005; Roy, Derry, Moore, 2007; Schug, 2006; Schug, Manopas, 2007). Etoricoxib (Arcoxia) was found to be superior in overall efficacy compared with acetaminophen plus oxycodone (Chang, Desjardins, King, et al., 2004).

An extensive review of the literature addressing the impact of several different analgesic techniques on patient outcomes concluded that both acetaminophen and NSAIDs used alone reduce pain and opioid requirements (Liu, Wu, 2007a). However, the researchers pointed out that problems with the research design in some of the studies made it difficult to draw concrete conclusions about the impact of the nonopioid analgesic group on postoperative patient-reported outcomes such as quality of recovery and satisfaction.

Perioperative Multimodal Analgesia

The analgesic ceiling effect that characterizes all nonopioids limits the effectiveness of this drug category following major surgical procedures. However, they do provide effective pain relief for a wide variety of major surgical procedures as part of a multimodal regimen that combines drugs with different underlying mechanisms of action (Andersen, Poulsen, Krogh, et al., 2007; Ashburn, Caplan, Carr, et al., 2004; Basse, Billesbolle, Kehlet, 2002; Basse, Hjort Jakobsen, Billesbolle, et al., 2000; Cepeda, Carr, Miranda, et al., 2005; Coloma, White, Huber, et al., 2000; Elia, Lysakowski, Tramer, 2005; Jensen, Kehlet, Lund, 2007; Nemergut, Durieux, Missaghi, et al., 2007; Schug, 2006; Schug, Manopas, 2007). In the perioperative setting, the most common analgesics in a multimodal approach are nonopioids, opioids, local anesthetics, and anticonvulsants.

Combinations of analgesics have been shown to provide greater pain relief than can be achieved with any single analgesic (Busch, Shore, Bhandari, et al., 2006; Cassinelli, Dean, Garcia, et al., 2008; Huang, Wang, Wang, et al., 2008; Merry, Gibbs, Edwards, et al., 2009; Schug, 2006; Tang, Evans, Chaput, et al., 2009). Several studies have shown that the multimodal approach can also result in lower opioid doses and fewer opioid-induced adverse effects than traditional single-agent approaches, particularly when NSAIDs are added to the treatment plan (Chen, Ko, Wen, et al., 2009; Kim, Kim, Nam, et al., 2008; Marret, Kurdi, Zufferey, et al., 2005; White, 2005; Tang, Evans, Chaput, et al., 2009). Although a meta-analysis of seven randomized controlled trials found that acetaminophen combined with morphine patient-controlled analgesia (PCA) produced a significant opioid-sparing effect, this did not result in a lower incidence of opioid-induced adverse effects (Remy, Marret, Bonnet, 2005). Similarly, a larger meta-analysis (33 trials, nearly 3000 patients) that reviewed data to evaluate whether multimodal analgesia with nonopioids plus IV PCA morphine offers advantages over morphine alone found that the addition of acetaminophen reduced 24-hour morphine consumption by an average of 8.3 mg but did not significantly decrease opioid-induced adverse effects (Elia, Lysakowski, Tramer, 2005). This same analysis reported that single doses of nonselective NSAIDs reduced 24-hour morphine consumption by 10.3 mg, postoperative infusions of ketorolac or diclofenac by 18.3 mg, and multiple-dose NSAID regimens by 19.7 mg. Reductions in postoperative nausea and vomiting and sedation were also noted with these NSAIDs. Similar to nonselective NSAIDs, the addition of COX-2 selective NSAIDs allows lower opioid doses, but more research is needed to conclude that this equates to fewer adverse effects (Elia, Lysakowski, Tramer, 2005; Kehlet, 2005; Liu, Wu, 2007a, 2007b; Romsing, Moiniche, Mathiesen, et al., 2005; Staube, Derry, McQuay, et al., 2005). The risk of serious postoperative bleeding was 0% in patients who received placebo or COX-2 selective NSAIDs but increased slightly to 1.7% in patients who received nonselective NSAIDs (ketorolac, diclofenac, ketoprofen) in the previously mentioned meta-analysis (Elia, Lyskowski, Tramer, 2005).

Preemptive Analgesia

In the early 1980s, studies of the spinal cord changes occurring in the context of peripheral afferent input, termed *central sensitization* (Woolf, 1983), generated interest in the therapeutic potential of interventions that could be implemented before tissue injury to block nociception (pain transmission) (Dahl, Moiniche, 2004; Grape, Tramer, 2007) (see Section I for a discussion of nociception). A multimodal approach (that includes NSAIDs to reduce activation of nociceptors, local anesthetics to block sensory input, and opioids to act within the CNS to interrupt pain) initiated preoperatively and continued intraoperatively and throughout the postoperative course was suggested as ideal preemptive analgesic treatment (Woolf, Chong, 1993). Since then, numerous studies have investigated a wide variety of agents and techniques in an attempt to show a preemptive analgesic effect (Dahl, Moiniche, 2004; Moiniche, Kehlet, Dahl, 2002).

Testing the hypothesis of preemptive analgesia requires comparing the effectiveness of an intervention applied before the surgical incision (experimental group) with the effectiveness of the same or very similar intervention applied only after the surgical incision (control group). The notion that such a simple approach could reduce or possibly prevent postoperative pain stimulated an abundance of research on preemptive analgesia; however, many of the studies had flawed research designs which led to flawed conclusions (Bromley,

2006; Grape, Tramer, 2007; Moiniche, Kehlet, Dahl, 2002; Dahl, Moiniche, 2004). For example, some studies compared preoperative analgesic administration with placebo or no treatment and claimed a preemptive effect when treatment was associated with a subsequent reduction in pain. These and other inaccurate claims of positive results led to an overly optimistic perception of the effectiveness of preemptive analgesia (Grape, Tramer, 2007).

An extensive review of the literature on preemptive analgesia concluded that there was very little evidence that preemptive (preincisional) administration of NSAIDs produced any analgesic benefit when compared with their administration postincision (Moiniche, Kehlet, Dahl, 2002). Similar conclusions were made for IV opioids, ketamine, continuous epidural analgesia, and peripheral local anesthetics. However, an updated review in 2004 found more encouraging results, with 6 of 8 studies published after 2001 showing that NSAIDs produced a preemptive effect (i.e., lower postoperative pain scores or supplementary opioid requirements with preoperative NSAID administration) (Dahl, Moiniche, 2004). For example, a study of patients undergoing ankle fracture surgery (Norman, Daley, Lindsey, 2001) found that those who received IV ketorolac before tourniquet inflation (preemptive) had no increase in pain, and those who received IV ketorolac after tourniquet inflation had significant increases in pain. There were no differences in supplemental opioid consumption, and the preemptive effect was gone within 6 hours. A meta-analysis reviewed 12 randomized controlled trials that compared preincisional with postincisional systemic NSAIDs and concluded that preoperative NSAID administration improved analgesic consumption and time to first rescue dose but not postoperative pain ratings (Ong, Lirk, Seymour, et al., 2005). A more recent randomized, placebo-controlled study of celecoxib showed effective postoperative pain control and improved speed and quality of recovery after major plastic surgery but no advantage to preoperative versus postoperative administration (Sun, Sacan, White, et al., 2008).

The general consensus is that preemptive administration of analgesics does not offer major clinical benefits (i.e., consistent immediate postoperative pain relief or reduced need for supplemental analgesia) (Bromley, 2006; Dahl, Moiniche, 2004; Grape, Tramer, 2007; Kelly, Ahmad, Brull, 2001). However, the disappointing research related to preemptive analgesia does not mean postoperative benefits cannot be realized with aggressive perioperative analgesic interventions. It has been suggested that research and clinical practice should redirect the focus from "preemptive" (timing of a single [most often] conventional intervention) to "protective" analgesia, whereby aggressive, sustained multimodal interventions are initiated preoperatively and continued throughout the intraoperative and postoperative periods (Moiniche, Kehlet, Dahl, 2002; Dahl, Moiniche, 2004).

Consistent with this approach are the goals of immediate postoperative pain reduction and prevention of prolonged and pathologic pain (Kelly, Ahmad, Brull, 2001). The key underlying pain management principles are to intervene before the onset of pain, use a multimodal approach, and administer analgesics in the proper dose and manner, on time, and for an adequate duration of time (Kelly, Ahmad, Brull, 2001).

Accelerated Multimodal Postoperative Rehabilitation

Advances in the field of pain management have led to more aggressive use of analgesics, but it is unclear if this has resulted in significant improvements in patient outcomes such as the quality of postoperative recovery and long-term function (Liu, Wu, 2007a). An unacceptable number of surgical patients continue to experience delays in recovery, complications, and the need for extended hospital stays (Kehlet, Wilmore, 2008). An extensive review of research (18 meta-analyses, 10 systematic reviews, 8 randomized controlled trials, and 2 observational database articles) revealed that there is insufficient data to show that high-quality postoperative pain management, such as regional analgesia and IV PCA, impacts the incidence and severity of postoperative complications (Liu, Wu, 2007a). The researchers suggested that improvements will depend on the integration of pain control into a comprehensive postoperative rehabilitation program that includes fluid balance and early mobilization and nutrition.

Patient outcomes have historically been reported as morbidity and mortality data; however, a focus on patient-reported assessments as a subset of morbidity and mortality events may provide unique insight into specific areas that need more intense research and clinical focus (Liu, Wu, 2007a, 2007b). An exhaustive review of the literature evaluated the effect of postoperative analgesia on patient-assessed indicators that included a variety of aspects of analgesia, presence of adverse effects, health-related quality of life, quality of recovery, and patient satisfaction (Liu, Wu, 2007a). The researchers concluded a general lack of high-quality data. They called for the development of validated tools to measure patient-reported outcomes and well-designed research that examines these as the primary study end points.

Establishing the link between good pain management and improvements in patient outcomes will require changes in the way health care is administered (Kehlet, Wilmore, 2008; Liu, Wu, 2007a, 2007b). Traditional practices in perioperative care, such as prolonged bed rest, withholding oral nutrition for extensive periods, and routine use of tubes and drains, are being increasingly challenged and replaced with evidence-based decision making (Pasero, Belden, 2006). This and other factors have led to the evolution of fast track surgery and enhanced postoperative

Box 8-1 | Key Components to Accelerated Multimodal Postoperative Recovery

1. Preoperative patient education outlining plan of care and emphasizing expectations of an active patient role in recovery
2. Perioperative optimization (e.g., preoperatively ensure optimal nutritional and hydration status; maximize pulmonary function; control underlying persistent pain; and reduce alcohol, tobacco, and medications that can cause intraoperative adverse events)
3. Surgical stress reduction (attenuation of neurohormonal response to the surgical procedure)
   - Intraoperative actions: Avoid hypothermia, optimize stroke volume, and prevent hyper- and hypovolemia
   - Neural blockades to reduce protein loss and minimize postoperative ileus
   - Minimally invasive surgery to reduce wound size and undesirable inflammatory responses, pain, and pulmonary compromise (e.g., transverse rather than vertical abdominal incision)
   - Thromboprophylaxis
   - Pharmacologic interventions to improve recovery (e.g., prevention of nausea and insulin resistance)
4. Pain reduction: Multimodal perioperative analgesic approaches that reduce postoperative pain and other discomforts, control the stress response, and allow early and aggressive recovery activities
   - Focus on strategies that allow the lowest effective opioid dose or avoidance of opioids (e.g., combinations of NSAIDs, ketamine, gabapentin, local anesthetic techniques)
5. Prevent and control nausea and other discomforts and adverse effects that interfere with recovery (e.g., implement multimodal strategies to prevent and treat nausea)
6. Aggressive postoperative rehabilitation measures (e.g., goal-directed ambulation, early discharge planning)
7. Evidence-based decision making with regard to care practices (e.g., challenge traditional practices that increase infection and pain, impede ambulation, and produce other adverse effects that impede recovery)
   - Avoid routine use of catheters (urinary), tubes (e.g., nasogastric), and drains (cause pain and infection and impede mobilization) or discontinue necessary catheters, tubes, and drains as soon as possible
   - Avoid prolonged fasting (contributes to catabolism); institute early enteral feeding to facilitate gastric emptying and build tissue

From Pasero, C., & McCaffery, M. *Pain assessment and pharmacologic management*, p. 230, St. Louis, Mosby. Data from Gan, T. J., Kovac, A. L., Lubarsky, D. A., et al. (2006). PONV management: Tackling the practical issues. Available at http://www.edscape.com/viewprogram/4990. Accessed September 1, 2009; Kehlet, H., & Wilmore, D. W. (2008). Evidence-based surgical care and the evolution of fast-track surgery. *Ann Surg, 248*(2), 189-198; Pasero, C. (2007). Procedure-specific pain management: PROSPECT. *J PeriAnesth Nurs, 22*(5), 335-340; Pasero, C., & Belden, J. (2006). Evidence-based perioperative care: Accelerated postoperative recovery programs. *J PeriAnesth Nurs, 21*(3), 168-177; PROSPECT: Procedure Specific Postoperative Pain Management. Available at http://www.postoppain.org. Accessed September 1, 2009. © 2011, Pasero C, McCaffery M. May be duplicated for use in clinical practice.

recovery (Kehlet, Wilmore, 2008). In a review of the literature, Kehlet and Wilmore (2008) describe the evidence that supports key principles of implementing what is referred to as *accelerated multimodal postoperative rehabilitation*. These are outlined in Box 8-1. Continuous multimodal pain relief with nonopioids and other analgesics is integral to this concept.

Tools that can be used to increase evidence-based perioperative pain management practice patterns are emerging. For example, a novel web-based program called PROSPECT (**P**rocedure **Spe**cific Postoperative Pain Management) *(http://www.postoppain.org)*, established by an international team of surgeons and anesthesiologists, posts evidence-based recommendations and algorithms to guide the health care team in decision making with regard to pain management according to specific surgical procedures (Pasero, 2007).

Selected Nonopioids and Routes of Administration

Nonopioid analgesics are given most often by the oral route of administration; however, many surgical patients are restricted from oral intake or suffer postoperative nausea and vomiting. These factors make the IV route the primary route of administration in the perioperative setting. Rectal administration is another option. Other novel routes of administration for postoperative analgesia include local infiltration (Coloma, White, Huber, et al., 2000); intraarticular injection (Andersen, Poulsen, Krogh, et al., 2007; Andersen, Pfeiffer-Jensen, Haraldsted, et al., 2007; Toftdahl, Nikolajsen, Haraldsted, et al., 2007); intranasal (Brown, Moodie, Bisley, et al., 2009; Moodie, Brown, Bisley, et al., 2008); and ocular (topical).

At the time of publication, an injectable form of diclofenac (Dyloject) was in development for approval in the United States (Colucci, Wright, Mermelstein, et al., 2009). Topical NSAIDs are used for acute pain associated with soft-tissue injury (see Chapter 7), but no research could be found regarding their use for postoperative analgesia. Following is a discussion of selected nonopioids and routes of administration as they relate to their use in the perioperative setting.

Ketorolac

Ketorolac is the only parenteral nonopioid available in the United States. An abundance of research has shown it to be effective as a first-line analgesic alone for moderate postoperative pain and in combination with other analgesics for more severe pain (Basse, Billesbolle, Kehlet, 2002; Basse, Hjort Jakobsen, Billesbolle, et al., 2000; Ben-David, Swanson, Nelson, et al., 2007; Breda, Bui, Liao, et al., 2007; Chen, Ko, Wen, et al., 2009; Helstrom, Rosow, 2006; Lenz, Raeder, 2008; White, 2002, 2005).

A dose of 30 mg of ketorolac is considered to be roughly equianalgesic to 10 mg of parenteral morphine, which is the standard parenteral postoperative adult morphine dose (Smith, Carroll, Edwards, et al., 2000). However, a large randomized trial of over 1000 patients following a variety of surgical procedures calculated the number of patients who achieved at least 50% reduction in pain intensity 30 minutes after analgesic administration and found that just 50% of those who received an IV morphine infusion (0.1 mg/kg, or approximately 7 mg in a 150 lb patient) and 31% of those who received IV ketorolac (30 mg) met this threshold (Cepeda, Carr, Miranda, et al., 2005). Rescue doses of morphine were given for pain intensity 5 or greater (0 to 10 scale) after the infusions, and fewer rescue doses were required by those who had received the ketorolac infusion. This study reinforces the appropriateness and value of using ketorolac in combination with other analgesics as part of a multimodal pain treatment plan for more severe pain.

Adverse effects associated with ketorolac are dose-dependent. Though 30 mg every 6 hours (120 mg/day maximum) is generally recommended for adults and 15 mg every 6 hours (60 mg/day maximum) for older adults, many clinicians routinely use a lower dose (i.e., 7.5 to 15 mg) or administer the drug less frequently (i.e., every 8 hours) in an effort to minimize adverse effects.

Like opioids, ketorolac doses can be titrated to effect if necessary. An initial loading dose is not necessary and should be avoided. Older adults should be started and maintained on lower doses than those recommended for younger patients. Around-the-clock (ATC) rather than PRN administration of ketorolac is recommended to prevent gaps in analgesia, and the drug should not be used for more than 5 days.

A common misconception is that duration of analgesia will be extended if ketorolac is administered by the intramuscular (IM) rather than the IV route of administration. With the exception of a one-time dose (e.g., office or emergency department (ED) setting) when IV access is not available, there is no advantage or rationale for administering ketorolac by the IM route. Nor is there any advantage to administering one-half of the dose via the IM route and the other half by the IV route, which is another occasional practice. If IV access is available, the drug should be administered by the IV route.

Ketorolac injected into the surgical site was found to produce similar analgesia and a shorter time to discharge compared with IV ketorolac following minor anorectal surgery (Coloma, White, Huber, et al., 2000). Oral ketorolac is reported to be as effective as acetaminophen plus codeine (McCormack, Power, 2009) but is rarely used, likely because more effective options are available.

Intranasal ketorolac was in clinical development at the time of publication and shown to be convenient, effective, and well tolerated for the treatment of acute pain in ambulatory patients (Brown, Moodie, Bisley, et al., 2009; Moodie, Brown, Bisley, et al., 2008). The ketorolac solution is provided in a disposable, multi-dose, metered-spray device that permits patients to self-administer the pain medication. A placebo-controlled study randomized 127 patients to receive 10 mg or 31.5 mg of intranasal ketorolac or intranasal placebo every 8 hours for 40 hours following major surgery (Moodie, Brown, Bisley, et al., 2008). Morphine consumption via IV PCA was significantly less in those who received ketorolac 31.5 mg (37.8 mg) compared with those who received ketorolac 10 mg (54.3 mg) or placebo (56.5 mg). Pain ratings and incidences of pyrexia and tachycardia were also significantly lower in those who received 31.5 mg of ketorolac. Other adverse effects were similar among the groups. The effectiveness of a 30 mg intranasal ketorolac dose was also established in a Phase 3, randomized placebo-controlled trial in which patients were provided a single 30 mg dose of intranasal ketorolac (N = 199) or intranasal placebo (N = 101) prior to a variety of surgical procedures (Brown, Moodie, Bisley, et al., 2009). Those who received ketorolac experienced a significant reduction in pain scores during the first 6 postoperative hours (the study period). Time to first request for analgesia was 3 hours in the ketorolac group compared with 1.3 hours in the placebo group, and morphine consumption via IV PCA was significantly lower with ketorolac.

IV Ibuprofen

A parenteral formulation of ibuprofen (Caldolor) was approved in the United States in 2009 for the treatment of fever and acute pain (Medscape Medical News, 2009); however, clinical experience and research were lacking regarding the use of parenteral ibuprofen for pain treatment at the time of publication. The recommended dosing regimen for acute pain treatment is 400 to 800 mg over 30 minutes every 6 hours; fever is treated with a 400 mg dose followed by 400 mg every 4 to 6 hours or 100 to 200 mg every 4 hours as needed (Medscape Medical News, 2009). Adverse effects, contraindications, and precautions are expected to be similar to those of other NSAIDs.

IV Acetaminophen

A major advantage of acetaminophen is that it can be administered by multiple routes of administration including the IV route (Bannwarth, Pehourcq, 2003). IV propacetamol, a prodrug that is rapidly metabolized to acetaminophen, has been used for pain management in countries other than the United States for several years. A randomized study of patients undergoing orthodontic surgery compared oral acetaminophen and IV propacetamol and found the latter to have an onset of analgesia of 3 minutes following a bolus dose and 5 minutes following a 15-minute infusion compared with 11 minutes following oral acetaminophen (Moller, Sindet-Pedersen, Petersen, et al., 2005). A dose of 2000 mg of propacetamol was equivalent to 1000 mg of oral acetaminophen. A higher incidence of adverse effects occurred with propacetamol, particularly injection site pain with bolus administration, which was experienced by 90% of the patients. Other adverse effects were dizziness and nausea, again more common with propacetamol bolus than with infusion or oral acetaminophen.

Another study established that 2000 mg of IV propacetamol produced similar pain relief with a faster onset of analgesia than 15 to 30 mg of IV ketorolac post total hip or knee replacement (Zhou, Tang, White, 2001). Other studies have shown an opioid dose-sparing effect with propacetamol, but this did not always result in reduced opioid adverse effects (Aubrun, Kalfon, Mottet, et al., 2003; Hernandez-Palazon, Tortosa, Martinez-Lage, et al., 2001; Lahtinen, Kokki, Hendolin, et al., 2002).

As noted, a major drawback of propacetamol is a high incidence of significant pain at the IV injection site. This is related to acetaminophen's poor water solubility, instability in solution, and pH of 3.5 (plasma is 7.3 to 7.4). Reconstitution of the drug for clinical use also is associated with mixing errors and a risk of contact dermatitis (Moller, Juhl, Payen-Champenois, et al., 2005). A stable, ready-to-use IV acetaminophen (paracetamol) has been developed to address these disadvantages. At the time of publication, the drug (Acetavance) was undergoing the approval process (Phase III trials) in the United States *(http://www.cadencepharm.com/products/apap.html)*. A randomized controlled study of patients undergoing orthodontic surgery demonstrated infusions of paracetamol (1000 mg) and propacetamol (2000 mg) produced similar pain relief and onset of analgesia (6 to 8 minutes) (Moller, Juhl, Payen-Champenois, et al., 2005). The more significant finding of this study, however, was that none of the patients who received paracetamol infusion experienced injection site pain compared with 49% of

the patients who received propacetamol. A randomized study of 151 patients who underwent hip or knee replacement demonstrated significant opioid dose-sparing effects with both paracetamol and propacetamol (Sinatra, Jahr, Reynolds, et al., 2005). As in other studies, the most common adverse effect was local injection pain associated with propacetamol (50%).

IV Parecoxib

The need for nonopioid analgesics that are available in IV formulation and do not increase bleeding time for postoperative pain management served as the impetus for the development and approval in Europe and other countries of the first parenteral COX-2 selective NSAID, parecoxib (Dynastat), a prodrug that is rapidly metabolized to its active form valdecoxib (Malan, Marsh, Hakki, et al., 2003). Parecoxib is reported to produce dose-dependent increases in pain relief and duration of analgesia; 40 mg of parecoxib provided 3 to 4 more hours of pain relief compared with 30 mg of IV ketorolac (Barden, Edwards, McQuay, et al., 2003). In 2005, the manufacturer of IV acetaminophen received a nonapproval letter by the United States Food and Drug Administration (U.S. FDA) that cited concerns about the adverse effects of valdecoxib (see Chapter 6 for discussion of cardiovascular [CV] effects) (U.S. FDA, 2005). At the time of this publication, it was unclear whether or not the manufacturer planned to address the FDA's concerns.

Perioperative Rectal Administration of Nonopioids

Although analgesic drugs rarely are administered rectally in adults in the perioperative setting, it is an attractive alternative when oral or parenteral nonopioid analgesics are not an option (Pasero, 2010). Rectal nonopioid administration also may be less costly than parenteral administration (White, 2002). Drawbacks include unreliable drug absorption by the rectal route, and the dislike of this route by some patients and nurses (Schug, Manopas, 2007).

Acetaminophen, aspirin, and indomethacin are available commercially in rectal formulation, and oral nonopioid analgesics can be administered rectally, either by using the intact tablet or by placing the intact or crushed tablet in a gelatin capsule for insertion (Pasero, McCaffery, 1999). (Note that modified-release analgesics should not be crushed.) Because of reduced bioavailability by the rectal route compared with the oral route (80% to 90% of oral bioavailability), higher nonopioid rectal doses may be required (Beck, Schenk, Hagemann, et al., 2000). One study showed that 1000 mg of rectal acetaminophen 4 times daily was too low to produce serum concentrations associated with opioid dose-sparing effects following abdominal hysterectomy (Kvalsvik, Borchgrevink, Hagen, et al., 2003). Maximum plasma concentrations are reached 2 to 3 hours after rectal administration, which is an important consideration when determining optimal time for preoperative administration (i.e., little immediate postoperative value is attained if administered immediately before induction for a 1-hour procedure) (Romsing, Moiniche, Dahl, 2002). Using criteria that excluded patients with known renal dysfunction, asthma, coagulopathy, peptic ulcer disease, or hepatic failure, and those who were receiving long-term NSAIDs or corticosteroids, a randomized controlled trial administered rectal indomethacin 100 mg or placebo to 200 patients 2 hours prior to undergoing open cholecystectomy and found that those who received indomethacin had significantly lower pain scores (VAS) and consumed significantly less opioid than those who received placebo (Bahar, Jangjoo, Soltani, et al., 2010). There were no NSAID-related adverse effects or complications.

Several studies have shown improved pain relief and reductions in opioid consumption with rectal nonopioid analgesics alone (Achariyapota, Titapant, 2008; Bahar, Jangjoo, Soltani, et al., 2010; Ng, Parker, Toogood, et al., 2002; Siddik, Aouad, Jalbout, et al., 2001). A review of randomized controlled trials concluded that rectal acetaminophen combined with NSAIDs was superior to acetaminophen alone, but there was no evidence of superiority when this combination was compared with NSAIDs alone (Romsing, Moiniche, Dahl, 2002). However, methodologic concerns preclude definitive conclusions from this review. Other studies have demonstrated highly effective pain control with combinations of rectal acetaminophen and various NSAIDs or other analgesics (Bannwarth, Pehourcq, 2003; Carli, Mayo, Klubien, et al., 2002; Ng, Swami, Smith, et al., 2008; Romsing, Moiniche, Dahl, 2002).

The recommendation that nonopioid analgesics be routinely administered to surgical patients (Ashburn, Caplan, Carr, et al., 2004) coupled with the lack of availability of parenteral nonopioids in the United States underscores the potential value of the rectal route. However, its use will require a new paradigm of practice—care providers must become familiar with prescribing the rectal administration of analgesics, pharmacists must support the use of this route for analgesic delivery with the necessary drugs and supplies, nurses must become competent in rectal drug administration technique, and patients must be taught the rationale and value of using this route of administration so that it is less objectionable to them (see Section IV for rectal administration technique).

Topical Ocular NSAIDs

Four topical ocular NSAIDs are approved in the United States for treatment of inflammation and pain after cataract surgery: ketorolac 0.4% (Acular), bromfenac 0.09% (Xibrom), diclofenac 0.1% (Voltaren), and nepafenac 0.1% (Nevanac). All four have been shown to produce safe and effective analgesia after the procedure (Smith, 2005; Lane, Modi, Lehmann, et al., 2007; Walters,

Raizman, Ernest, et al., 2007). One study showed that nepafenac, a prodrug, has the greatest ocular bioavailability and the most favorable anti-inflammatory profile compared with the other four (Walters, Raizman, Ernest, et al., 2007). However, another study showed that ketorolac produced significantly better patient satisfaction, compliance, and postoperative pain control when compared with nepafenac (Duong, Westfield, Chalkley, 2007). Other research has supported these findings with ketorolac (Kim, Lo, Hubbard, et al., 2008). Superior control of inflammation was found with ketorolac compared with bromfenac (Bucci, Waterbury, 2008).

A Cochrane Collaboration Review found that two trials demonstrated a positive effect of topical ketorolac on cystoid macular edema (CME), a complication and the most common cause of poor visual outcome after ophthalmic surgery (Sivaprasad, Bunce, Patel, 2005). More recently a 4-week randomized, multicenter study of 278 patients showed 6 cases of CME in patients who received topical steroid alone but none in those who received a combination of topical ketorolac and steroid (Wittpenn, Silverstein, Heier, et al., 2008). Another study showed increased corneal haze and delayed healing with nepafenac compared with ketorolac (Trattler, McDonald, 2007). Further research is required to more clearly establish the role of topical NSAIDs in preventing CME (Kim, Stark, 2008).

Adverse Effects

Short-term use of nonopioid analgesics is rarely associated with serious adverse effects (Schug, Manopas, 2007). As with long-term use, the patient's risk factors must be considered when determining whether and which nonopioid analgesics to use in the perioperative setting. See Box 8-2 for prevention and reduction of selected nonopioid analgesic adverse effects in the perioperative setting (see Chapter 6 for an in depth discussion of adverse effects).

Gastrointestinal (GI) Effects

NSAID-induced GI toxicity usually is addressed in the literature as an adverse effect resulting from long-term NSAID use; however, GI ulceration can occur with short-term perioperative administration as well (Schug, Manopas, 2007). This is particularly true in individuals with elevated risk for GI toxicity, such as older adults and those with a previous GI complication. The use of the least ulcerogenic nonselective NSAID or a COX-2 selective NSAID if not contraindicated by CV risk is encouraged. The underlying mechanisms, risk factors, and recommendations discussed previously in this section apply to patients in the perioperative setting (see Chapter 6). NSAID-induced GI bleeding as it relates to perioperative NSAID use will be addressed in the following sections.

Box 8-2 Prevention and Reduction of Nonopioid Analgesic Adverse Effects in the Perioperative Setting

1. Select the right nonopioid for the patient (also see Chapter 7).
   - Ask the patient about previous nonopioid use. If not contraindicated, administer a nonopioid that has been safe and effective for the patient in the past.
   - Consider patient risk factors.
   - Administer the least ulcerogenic NSAID (see Chapter 6 and Table 6-3 on p. 195).
   - Consider the type of surgery and anticipated pain intensity.
   - Administer acetaminophen alone or in combination with an NSAID when postoperative pain is expected to be mild to moderate.
   - Administer both acetaminophen and an NSAID with other analgesics as indicated by type of surgical procedure when pain is expected to be more severe.
2. Avoid NSAIDs in patients with very high CV and GI risk (see Chapter 6 and Table 6-1 on p. 192 and Table 6-4 on p. 199).
3. Administer gastroprotective co-therapy for patients at risk for GI complications (see Chapter 6).
4. Insure adequate hydration before initiation and during nonopioid treatment.
5. Increase nonopioid dose if initial dose is ineffective, tolerated well, and below maximum recommended dose.
6. Maximize the effectiveness of the nonopioid treatment plan with the lowest effective nonopioid doses.
   - Administer the nonopioid before pain begins (e.g., preoperatively when possible) and in ATC doses for the first 24 to 48 hours postoperatively then PRN depending on type of surgical procedure and pain intensity.
7. Systematically monitor for adverse effects.
   - Increase monitoring frequency in patients with elevated risk for adverse effects (e.g., older patients and patients with comorbidities).
   - Decrease the nonopioid dose 25% to 50% if adverse effects occur.
   - Discontinue nonopioid in presence of significant adverse effects (e.g., GI bleeding, acute renal failure).
8. Administer the nonopioid for the shortest time needed.

Hematologic Effects

The possibility of increased bleeding time is of special concern when NSAIDs are used for postoperative pain. Aspirin has an irreversible effect on platelets and will increase bleeding time for up to 7 days after the last dose (i.e., until the damaged platelets are replaced by new ones). For that reason, aspirin therapy is usually discontinued at 1 week or longer before surgery, and aspirin is not recommended for perioperative use (Ashraf, Wong, Ronayne, et al., 2004) (see following section for exceptions). Other nonselective NSAIDs are also sometimes withheld during the perioperative period because of their tendency to prolong bleeding time. However, COX-2 selective NSAIDs (e.g., celecoxib) have no effect on bleeding time and should be considered if not contraindicated by CV risk (Visser, Goucke, 2008). Another option is a nonselective NSAID with minimal effect on bleeding time. These include nabumetone, meloxicam, choline magnesium trisalicylate, magnesium salicylate, and salsalate.

Acetaminophen is another option. As mentioned, it can be given alone or in combination with NSAIDs that have minimal effect on bleeding time. It has been combined with the COX-2 selective NSAID celecoxib as part of an effective multimodal analgesic plan begun preoperatively for total knee arthroplasty (Dorr, Raya, Long, et al., 2008). It is important to note that acetaminophen has been shown to increase INR when administered concomitantly with warfarin (see Chapter 6); however, researchers note that acetaminophen inhibition of thromboxane A_2 is less than that of most nonselective NSAIDs, and the likelihood of surgical bleeding as a result of perioperative acetaminophen intake is low (Ashraf, Wong, Ronayne, et al., 2004; Munsterhjelm, Munsterhjelm, Niemi, et al., 2005). Nevertheless, some clinicians call for close monitoring of patients receiving acetaminophen and anticoagulation therapy (Mahe, Bertrand Drouet, et al., 2005, 2006; Ornetti, Ciappuccini, Tavernier, et al., 2005; Parra, Beckey, Stevens, 2007).

Preoperative Discontinuation of Aspirin and Other NSAID Therapy

Cessation of aspirin prior to surgery is recommended (except in patients with a history of unstable angina in whom cardioprotective aspirin should be continued) (Ashraf, Wong, Ronayne, et al., 2004), but the ideal timing of cessation is unclear. A randomized, placebo-controlled study of 51 healthy volunteers demonstrated no hemostatic defect by or beyond the sixth day after aspirin was discontinued (Cahill, McGreal, Crowe, et al., 2005). This led the researchers to recommend discontinuation of aspirin therapy 5 days preoperatively. Ashraf and colleagues (2004) recommend cessation of aspirin therapy 7 to 9 days before surgery (Ashraf, Wong, Ronayne, et al., 2004).

Sun and colleagues reviewed the research that supports both the risks and benefits of discontinuing cardioprotective aspirin pre–coronary artery bypass surgery and stated that the noted increased risk of hemorrhage when aspirin is not discontinued is supported by research that used aspirin doses well in excess of those used for cardioprotection (i.e., 81 mg) (Sun, Crowther, Warkentin, et al., 2005). However, they caution that further research is required to draw concrete conclusions on the practice of not discontinuing aspirin. They also point out that there is clear evidence that if aspirin is discontinued preoperatively, it should be restarted within 48 hours of surgery to improve graft patency and patient survival.

Patients with peripheral vascular disease are at increased risk for perioperative thrombotic complications, which led researchers to conduct a decision analysis (outcome-focused literature review) of aspirin therapy cessation 2 weeks prior to infrainguinal revascularization surgery compared with continuation of aspirin therapy throughout the perioperative course (Neilipovitz, Bryson, Nichol, 2001). They concluded that preoperative continuation of aspirin therapy in this population decreases perioperative mortality and increases life expectancy and called for further randomized controlled trials to confirm these findings.

Other NSAIDs have reversible effects on platelets, and inhibition of platelet aggregation only lasts as long as it takes to eliminate a sufficient quantity of the drug from the system. Guidelines recommend that nonaspirin nonselective NSAIDs be discontinued 3 to 7 days preoperatively, depending on how long it takes platelet function to normalize (Ashraf, Wong, Ronayne, et al., 2004). Platelets have been found to normalize within 24 hours after cessation of ibuprofen in healthy individuals who stopped the drug after taking it for 7 days (Goldenberg, Jacobson, Manco-Johnson, 2005).

GI Bleeding and Operative Site Bleeding

The safety and effectiveness of preoperative administration of nonopioid analgesics with minimal or no effect on bleeding time (see above) alone or as part of a multimodal pain treatment plan that extends into the postoperative period is supported by an abundance of research (Basse, Billesbolle, Kehlet, 2002; Basse, Hjort Jakobsen, Dorthe, et al., 2000; Dorr, Raya, Long, et al., 2009; Huang, Wang, Wang, et al., 2008; Meunier, Lisander, Good, 2007; Recart, Issioui, White, et al., 2003; Schug, 2006; Straube, Derry, McQuay, et al., 2005; Sun, Sacan, White, et al., 2008). As a group, however, nonselective NSAIDs have been identified as a risk factor of severe postoperative bleeding after some surgical procedures, such as tonsillectomy (Marret, Bonnet, 2007; Marret, Flahault, Samama, et al., 2003). Other researchers and clinicians have challenged the strength of the data cited to support this conclusion and question the extent and clinical significance of this risk (Dsida, Cote, 2004; Lake, Khater, 2004). Several other factors, including surgeon

skill and operative technique, may be the underlying cause of increased bleeding (Lake, Khater, 2004). A review of the medical records of 1025 patients who underwent laparascopic gastric bypass concluded that preoperative administration of low molecular weight heparin and laparoscopic approach may increase the incidence of bleeding with this procedure (Bakhos, Alkhoury, Kyriakides, et al., 2009).

Attention tends to center on the perioperative use of ketorolac as a primary cause of postoperative GI and incisional bleeding. However, a classic study by Strom and colleagues (35 hospitals, 9900 patients) in which 10,272 courses of parenteral ketorolac were compared with 10,247 courses of a parenteral opioid showed relatively little difference in the risk of GI bleeding, operative site bleeding, and other adverse effects in postoperative patients receiving ketorolac (Strom, Berlin, Kinman, et al., 1996). Other more recent studies also have shown that administration of ketorolac was not associated with significant intraoperative or postoperative blood loss (Cassinelli, Dean, Garcia, et al., 2008; Chin, Sundram, Marcotte, 2007; Diblasio, Snyder, Kattan, et al., 2004; El-Tahan, Warda, Yasseen, et al., 2007). Nevertheless, ketorolac is not recommended as a prophylactic drug prior to major surgery.

The dose of ketorolac is an important factor when considering risk of GI and incisional bleeding. Again, Strom and colleague's classic study provides insight into this aspect of treatment (Strom, Berlin, Kinman, et al., 1996). The use of ketorolac in patients younger than 65 years at an average dose of 105 mg/day or lower for 5 or fewer days was not associated with a detectable increase in risks. Factors that increased the risk of bleeding in the ketorolac group were advanced age (65 years with significant increase at 75 years), higher doses (120 mg/day or more), and therapy lasting longer than 5 days. Because ketorolac has been shown to provide effective analgesia with parenteral doses as low as 10 mg, the authors recommended using the lowest dose needed to obtain the desired analgesic effect rather than following a specific regimen. A dose of 15 mg parenteral ketorolac given every 6 hours would fulfill the criteria of keeping the dose at less than 105 mg/24 h while providing potentially effective analgesia. As mentioned previously, some clinicians administer doses as low as 7.5 mg, and frequency of dosing can be decreased from every 6 hours to every 8 hours to reduce the total dose and further minimize risk of bleeding.

Cardiovascular (CV) Effects

Shortly after the release of the COX-2 selective NSAIDs, studies revealed an association between their perioperative use and an increase in adverse CV events in patients who had undergone high-risk cardiac surgery. A multicenter study randomized nearly 1700 patients undergoing post coronary artery bypass graft (CABG) to receive IV parecoxib for at least 3 days postoperatively followed by oral valdecoxib through day 10, or IV placebo followed by oral valdecoxib or placebo for 10 days (Nussmeier, Whelton, Brown, et al., 2005). There was a higher rate of myocardial infarction (MI), cardiac arrest, stroke, and pulmonary embolism in those who received parecoxib and valdecoxib. Another multicenter, placebo-controlled 14-day study randomized 462 CABG patients to receive IV parecoxib and oral valdecoxib or placebo after surgery (Ott, Nussmeier, Duke, et al., 2003). Although those receiving parecoxib and valdecoxib experienced very effective pain relief, there was a higher incidence of CV adverse events in these patients, including four deaths caused by MI, cerebral infarction, pulmonary thromboembolism, or sternal wound infection.

As discussed previously, the CV risk associated with use of celecoxib is less than with rofecoxib and valdecoxib (Dajani, Islam, 2008; Joshi, Gertler, Fricker, 2007) and more similar to that of the nonselective NSAIDs (Frampton, Keating, 2007). Nevertheless, these two postoperative studies and others that showed elevated CV risk with NSAIDs in general led to recommendations against the use of any NSAIDs following high-risk open heart surgery (U.S. FDA, 2007). (See Chapter 6 for an explanation of underlying mechanisms and in-depth discussion of CV risk factors and adverse effects.)

Renal Effects and Acute Renal Failure

Renal toxicity is rarely associated with short-term perioperative acetaminophen use (Shug, Manopas, 2007). A lack of effect on platelet aggregation and low incidence of GI adverse effects make acetaminophen the nonopioid analgesic of choice in individuals with renal insufficiency, advanced chronic kidney disease, and end-stage renal disease (Kurella, Bennett, Chertow, 2003; Launay-Vacher, Karie, Fau, et al., 2005; Leo, 2008). Dose adjustment is not necessary in the presence of these conditions, but caution is recommended when it is used in patients with coexisting liver disease.

Adverse renal effects are also relatively rare in otherwise healthy individuals who are given NSAIDs during the perioperative period. Endogenous renal prostaglandin synthesis does not play a significant role in maintaining optimal glomerular filtration rate (GFR) and renal blood flow in individuals with normal CV, hepatic, endocrine, and renal function who have adequate volume and sodium stores (Helstrom, Rosow, 2006). In these individuals, NSAID-induced renal effects are usually minor and transient (Forrest, Camu, Greer, et al., 2002; Helstrom, Rosow, 2006; Lee, Cooper, Craig, et al., 2007), and there appears to be no difference in these effects between nonselective and COX-2 selective NSAIDs (Helstrom, Rosow, 2006; Launay-Vacher, Karie, Fau, et al., 2005). A Cochrane Collaboration Review could find no cases

of renal failure or serious kidney problems in individuals with normal preoperative renal function who were given NSAIDs following surgery in any of the 23 trials (1459 patients) reviewed (Lee, Cooper, Craig, et al., 2007).

In contrast, individuals with acute or chronic volume depletion or hypotension depend on prostaglandin synthesis to maintain adequate renal blood flow ("prostaglandin dependence") (Helstrom, Rosow, 2006), and NSAID inhibition of prostaglandin synthesis in such patients can cause acute renal ischemia and acute renal failure (ARF) (Helstrom, Rosow, 2006). ARF as a result of hypovolemia is usually reversed when the NSAID is stopped and volume is replenished (Miyoshi, 2001), but it underscores the importance of adequate hydration and maintenance of acceptable blood pressure (BP) before and during NSAID administration.

Patients at increased risk for perioperative ARF and who might be more susceptible to NSAID-induced renal injury include those with cardiac failure, liver cirrhosis, ascites, diabetes, or pre-existing hypertension, and patients being treated with ACE inhibitors (Brater, 2002; Brune, 2003; Forrest, Camu, Greer, et al., 2002; Helstrom, Rosow, 2006; Launay-Vacher, Karie, Fau, et al., 2005). Other risk factors include preexisting renal impairment, advanced age, and left ventricular dysfunction (Helstrom, Rosow, 2006).

Although age alone is not a risk factor for NSAID-induced renal impairment (Brater, 2002), older adults and anyone with risk factors should be assessed frequently for adverse renal effects during perioperative NSAID therapy. ARF can develop with the first NSAID dose in patients with elevated risk, and higher doses carry greater risk (Launay-Vacher, Karie, Fau, et al., 2005).

It is generally recommended that NSAIDs be avoided in patients with chronic renal failure and in any patient with a creatinine clearance below 30 mL/min (Launay-Vacher, Karie, Fau, et al., 2005; Laine, White, Rostom, et al., 2008). Acetaminophen, opioids (e.g., fentanyl), or other analgesics are a better choice in these patients (see Sections IV and V). If NSAID treatment is essential, other risk factors should be eliminated prior to initiating therapy (e.g., correct volume depletion and discontinue potassium-sparing diuretics). NSAIDs with a long half-life can cause persistent decreases in GFR and should be avoided. NSAIDs with a short half-life (e.g., ibuprofen) are preferred because declines in GFR return to baseline levels at the end of the dosing interval (Launay-Vacher, Karie, Fau, et al., 2005).

Although ketorolac is sometimes cited as a cause of perioperative ARF, retrospective data comparing perioperative administration of ketorolac with that of opioids in patients without preexisting risk factors do not show an elevated risk of ARF (Helstrom, Rosow, 2006). One prospective study randomized 11,245 patients undergoing major surgical procedures to receive parenteral and oral doses of ketorolac, ketoprofen, or diclofenac (Forrest, Camu, Greer, et al., 2002). Serious adverse outcomes occurred in 155 patients, which included 10 cases of ARF. Of the 10 who experienced ARF, three received ketorolac, three received ketoprofen, and four received diclofenac. Interestingly, there was no significant increase risk of ARF in patients with preexisting renal insufficiency or congestive heart failure in this study. Adequate hydration is essential before administration of ketorolac to avoid ARF. (See Chapter 6 for renal adverse effects associated with long-term NSAID use.)

Bone Healing and Formation

The inflammatory process is initiated when bone is fractured, just as it is with any other tissue trauma. Prostaglandins, particularly PGE_2, have a central role as mediators in bone healing, providing a balance between bone formation and resorption (Gajraj, 2003; Helstrom, Rosow, 2006). NSAIDs have been used for decades to control pain associated with fracture and for the prevention of heterotropic ossification (see the following section) (Fransen, Neal, 2004; Gajraj, 2003; Helstrom, Rosow, 2006). However, red flags were raised when animal research in the 1980s and 1990s suggested fracture healing might be delayed by NSAID administration (Gajraj, 2003; Helstrom, Rosow, 2006; O'Connor, 2003). Research published in the early 2000s established that COX-2 was indeed essential for fracture healing in animals and that delayed fracture healing and bone ingrowth could occur in animals given NSAIDs (Goodman, Ma, Trindade, et al., 2002; Simon, Manigrasso, O'Connor, 2002; Zhang, Schwarz, Young, et al., 2002). All of this research helped to lay the foundation for the current ongoing controversy over the safety of NSAIDs in humans following fracture and some orthopedic surgical procedures (Einhorn, 2002a, 2002b, 2003a, 2003b; Hochberg, Melin, Reicin, 2003; O'Connor, 2003).

The release of COX-2 selective NSAIDs stimulated animal research comparing the effects of the new NSAIDs and nonselective NSAIDs on bone healing. One study found a higher rate of experimental fracture nonunion with 21 days of daily ketorolac administration (25%) compared with 21 days of daily high-dose parecoxib (8%) (Gerstenfeld, Thiede, Seibert, et al., 2003). A significant finding was that despite evidence of early nonunion, all fractures in both groups showed union by 35 days. A more recent study compared the effects of 7- and 21-day treatments with ketorolac and valdecoxib to evaluate the hypothesis that delays in fracture healing associated with NSAID administration are reversible (Gerstenfeld, Al-Ghawas, Alkhiary, et al., 2007). Seven days of treatment demonstrated a trend for a higher nonunion rate in both NSAID-treated animals compared with controls, but no differences were noted at 35 days. After 21 days of treatment, the valdecoxib-treated group had more nonunions than either the control or the ketorolac-treated group; however, these differences also disappeared by 35 days. The researchers concluded that COX-2 selective

NSAIDs inhibit fracture healing more than nonselective NSAIDs and the longer the treatment, the greater the effect; however, prostaglandin levels essential for fracture healing and strength are regained and similar to controls when NSAID treatment is discontinued after 21 days.

Concern has been expressed about the problems in extrapolating animal research to the clinical treatment of humans (Kharasch, 2004), and it has been pointed out that millions of patients have been treated with NSAIDs for fracture-related and other orthopedic pain over many years without an association between their use and impaired bone healing in the clinical setting (Einhorn, 2002a, 2002b). Criticism of the animal research includes the observation that the NSAIDs in experiments were administered for several weeks to months at doses greater than approved or used for acute pain management in humans. Still, researchers have urged practitioners to exercise caution in the use of NSAIDs after fracture until human clinical trials indicate otherwise (O'Connor, 2003; Einhorn, 2003a).

Unfortunately, there are very few well-designed studies that examine the impact of NSAIDs on bone healing in humans. The studies that have been done are retrospective in design and present conflicting findings (Einhorn, 2002b; Einhorn, 2003a; Gerstenfeld, Einhorn, 2004). Retrospective studies are confounded by numerous factors, including surgical technique, bone graft composition, type of fracture, and patient risk factors (Gajraj, 2005; Giannoudis, MacDonald, Matthews, et al., 2000). In addition, there are inherent problems in conducting randomized controlled trials, including the challenge of obtaining the sample size necessary to investigate risk rather than benefit of a treatment (Einhorn, 2003a).

Studies in humans began to focus on NSAID use post-spinal fusion following a retrospective study published in 1998 that found an association between postoperative ketorolac and spinal fusion nonunion (Glassman, Rose, Dimar, et al., 1998). This finding was not confirmed, however, by a more recent retrospective review of 405 patients who received ketorolac 30 mg IV every 6 hours for 48 hours or no ketorolac; ketorolac treatment had no significant effect on fusion rates at the 24-month follow-up period (Pradhan, Tatsumi, Gallina, et al., 2008).

There have been no adequate studies evaluating NSAIDs and spinal fusion. In an effort to offer a balanced appraisal of the existing, limited data, Einhorn (2003a) suggests that short-term use of an NSAID after skeletal surgery, for a period less than 2 weeks, probably is safe and might be considered an option unless a patient has a comorbid condition that could negatively impact fracture healing, such as smoking, glucocorticoid use, or metabolic bone disease. Others endorse this view (Helstrom, Rosow, 2006; Langford, Mehta, 2006).

Heterotrophic Bone Formation (Ossification)

Heterotrophic ossification is pathologic formation of bone in soft tissue. It may be a complication following surgery or trauma. If it occurs after hip surgery, with bone formation in the muscles around the hip, reduced joint mobility ensues (Fransen, Neal, 2004; Gajraj, 2003). Heterotrophic ossification is thought to result when surgery or trauma activates dormant osteoprogenitor stem cells (Helstrom, Rosow, 2006). Approximately one third of individuals who undergo hip replacement experience this complication (Fransen, Neal, 2006).

A Cochrane Collaboration Review of 16 randomized trials and two quasi-randomized trials (4763 patients) concluded that perioperative prophylactic use of an NSAID (other than low-dose aspirin) reduces the risk of heterotrophic bone formation by one-half to two-thirds (Fransen, Neal, 2004). The researchers called for large-scale randomized trials to determine the risks and benefits for all outcomes. A small randomized, placebo-controlled study (N = 23) appeared to confirm the utility of COX-2 selective NSAIDs for this purpose (Buvanendran, Kroin, Berger, 2007). Patients with osteoarthritis (OA) undergoing total hip arthroplasty who received rofecoxib 4 days preoperatively plus a single dose on the morning of surgery experienced a lower incidence of heterotrophic ossification at 6-month follow up than those who received placebo for 4 days preoperatively plus a single rofecoxib dose or placebo on the day of surgery. The authors concluded that preoperative treatment with COX-2 selective NSAIDs is preferable to long-term postoperative nonselective or COX-2 selective NSAIDs, or postoperative irradiation for prevention of heterotrophic ossification.

Surgical Wound Healing

The processes involved in soft-tissue healing are different from those of bone healing and consist of three distinct phases: Acute, proliferative, and remodeling (Busti, Hooper, Amaya, et al., 2005). The acute phase involves the inflammatory response, characterized by release of prostaglandins and leukotrienes to facilitate hemostasis. The patient experiences symptoms of warmth, swelling, redness, and pain during this phase. Prostaglandins also impact the proliferation phase by influencing the permeability of endothelial cells (Busti, Hooper, Amaya, et al., 2005).

The inhibition of prostaglandins by NSAIDs is the basis for concerns regarding their effect on wound healing. However, similar to the research on NSAIDs and bone healing, research on NSAIDs and soft-tissue healing has been performed entirely in animals, and the doses and duration of NSAID treatment used in the studies are not used to treat pain in patients in the clinical setting (Busti, Hooper, Amaya, et al., 2005). Large randomized controlled studies in humans are needed to confirm the lack of a relationship; however, clinicians should be reassured by the fact that NSAIDs have been used for decades in the perioperative setting as first-line analgesics for all types of postoperative pain without recognition of an increased risk of surgical wound healing complications.

Conclusion

Perioperative multimodal analgesia includes the administration of nonopioid analgesics preoperatively whenever possible and staying on top of pain with scheduled ATC postoperative doses to maximize pain relief with the lowest effective doses. Regular assessment of adverse effects is critical to reducing complications. The overriding principle of administering the lowest effective dose for the shortest time necessary applies in the perioperative setting.

Chapter 9 Nonprescription Nonopioids

JUDGING from the rows of nonprescription analgesics found in a well-stocked pharmacy, millions of Americans are self-medicating with nonopioids to treat their aches and pains. As a group, these analgesics are marketed to the public as "pain relievers."

Many nonprescription pain relievers are merely different doses of either acetaminophen or aspirin. Quite a few contain both aspirin and acetaminophen. The combination of acetaminophen and aspirin has raised concern about enhanced renal toxicity, and some find this combination questionable. Other common ingredients in nonprescription pain relievers are buffering agents, caffeine, and antihistamines. (See Patient Medication Information Forms III-4 and III-5 on pp. 256-259).

Buffered Aspirin

Buffered aspirin has been compared with nonbuffered aspirin, and endoscopic evaluation shows no difference in the amount of gastric damage produced by either one. Enteric-coated aspirin does not decrease the incidence of local irritation either (Bhatt, Scheiman, Abraham, et al., 2008; Laine, 2001). Nevertheless, some individuals report less dyspepsia and prefer these formulations.

Caffeine

Caffeine has been used to augment pain relief since research in the early 1980s showed that it produced a 40% acetaminophen dose-sparing effect (Zhang, 2001). Other research found that caffeine in combination with acetaminophen (but not alone) produced a significant enhanced and prolonged analgesic effect with onset of analgesia within 30 minutes and lasting for up to 3 hours (Renner, Clarke, Grattan, et al., 2007). Caffeine produces a synergistic effect with a variety of other analgesics as well, including opioids and NSAIDs (Diamond, Freitag, 2001; Mitchell, van Zanten, Inglis, et al., 2008). Consumption of caffeinated coffee has even been found to enhance the analgesic effect of nicotine (Nastase, Ioan, Braga, et al., 2007) (see Section V for more on nicotine analgesia). The underlying mechanisms of caffeine's action are unclear, but theories include that it blocks adenosine receptors, inhibits COX-2, or simply changes emotional state (Zhang, 2001).

Caffeine is often combined with nonopioids for the treatment of migraine and tension-type headaches. Combinations produce better pain relief than any of the analgesics alone for this type of pain (Diamond, Balm, Freitag, 2000; Diamond, Freitag, 2001). Research has not confirmed the optimal dose of caffeine for increasing the analgesia of nonopioids, but the minimal effective dose appears to be 65 mg (APS, 2003; Zhang, 2001). While nonopioid analgesia may be enhanced with this amount of caffeine, patients often also experience dizziness and nervousness (Zhang, 2001).

A randomized controlled study found that a single dose (2 tablets) of the combination of aspirin (250 mg), acetaminophen (250 mg), and caffeine (65 mg) produced significantly better and faster pain relief than a single dose of ibuprofen (200 mg) or placebo for acute migraine (Goldstein, Silberstein, Saper, et al., 2006). In contrast, a study of patients following outpatient general surgery found that acetaminophen plus ibuprofen produced fewer adverse effects and higher patient satisfaction than the combination of acetaminophen, codeine, and caffeine (Mitchell, van Zanten, Inglis, et al., 2008). However, the difference in findings in this study may have been due to codeine, which is associated with a relatively high incidence of adverse effects and wide variability in efficacy due to dependence on CYP2D6 metabolism; 10% of Caucasians are poor metabolizers and derive little or no analgesia from codeine (Stamer, Stuber, 2006) (see Chapter 13 for more on codeine). Other research supports the use of caffeine in the postoperative setting; randomized-controlled trials and an extensive meta-analysis of 30 trials concluded that caffeine significantly enhanced postoperative pain relief when combined with other analgesics (Fitzgerald, Buggy, 2006). Despite this evidence, caffeine is rarely prescribed as a component of a postoperative multimodal analgesic regimen.

IV caffeine has been researched in advanced cancer patients experiencing adverse psychomotor effects associated with high doses of opioids and found to have little effect (Mercandante, Serretta, Casuccio, 2001). Pain significantly decreased, but this was not statistically superior to placebo. Caffeine produced improvements in speed of finger tapping, but there was no improvement in cognitive outcomes as measured by testing of visual memory and number and digit recall. (See Section V for use of caffeine to counteract opioid-induced sedation.)

Because caffeine is a CNS stimulant, its effect on the cardiovascular (CV) system has been a concern. Some adults are very sensitive to caffeine and respond to even small doses with tremors, increased heart rate, and insomnia. Individuals with CV risks must exercise caution in the amount of caffeine they consume or avoid it altogether. For most people, moderate intake of caffeine (e.g., 200 to 300 mg, which is more than the amount required to augment nonopioid analgesia) is considered safe (Mayo Clinic.com, 2008). Heavy use (500 to 600 mg/day; 5 to 7 cups of coffee/day) is associated with a significant increase in adverse effects. Chronic repeated exposure to caffeine can increase the risks for development of analgesic-overuse headache, chronic daily headache, and physical dependency (Shapiro, 2008). Discontinuing caffeine after long-term use can lead to a withdrawal syndrome with headache as a dominant symptom.

An inexpensive way to reap the benefits of a caffeine/nonopioid combination is to avoid commercially compounded preparations and simply buy generic forms of the ingredients separately (e.g., aspirin and acetaminophen) and ordinary caffeine-containing beverages as a source of the dose of caffeine required for enhanced analgesia. Individuals often report resolution of pain, particularly headache pain, after drinking caffeinated beverages. Stimulant products also often contain a sufficient amount of caffeine (e.g., No-Doz has 200 mg caffeine).

A variety of food products contain caffeine. Chocolate lovers may be dismayed to learn that most chocolate contains very little caffeine (e.g., 9 mg). However, 1.45 ounces of dark, semisweet chocolate contains 31 mg, requiring at least 3 ounces to obtain the desired analgesic effect. The popularity of energy drinks, which contain large amounts of caffeine (e.g., 300 mg), has prompted calls for changes in labeling to include stronger warnings of the dangers of excessive caffeine intake (Johns Hopkins Medicine, 2008). See Table 9-1 for the caffeine content of common beverages, food, and over-the-counter (OTC) drugs.

Analgesic Nephropathy

For several years, concerns have been raised regarding the potential for caffeine, co-formulated with non-opioids, to initiate or sustain analgesic overuse causing kidney disease (Feinstein, Heinemann, Dalessio, et al., 2000; Fox, Seibers, 2003; van der Woude, Heinemann, Graf, et al., 2007). This is widely referred to as "analgesic nephropathy" (van der Woude, Heinemann, Graf, et al., 2007). Extensive reviews of the literature, case control studies, and expert panel opinions have concluded that there is insufficient evidence to support the claim that caffeine (in the absence of phenacetin) causes analgesic nephropathy or that such a phenomenon even exists since clear criteria for it have not been established (Feinstein, Heinemann, Dalessio, et al., 2000; Fox, Seibers, 2003; Michielsen, Heinemann, Mihatsch, et al., 2009; van der Woude, Heinemann, Graf, et al., 2007; Zhang, 2001).

The true culprit of the controversy appears to be a chemical substance called *phenacetin*, which was introduced in the late 1800s as an analgesic and antipyretic. In the 1970s and 1980s it was available in combination with other agents, such as aspirin and caffeine, for OTC analgesia. Phenacetin has psychotropic properties, which have been blamed for reports of abuse and overdosing of phenacetin-containing analgesics (Fox, Seibers, 2003). The chemical was withdrawn from the U.S. market in 1983 after research and clinical observations showed an association between phenacetin and renal pelvis and bladder cancer (DHHS, 2008). There have been no approved commercially-available products containing phenacetin since its withdrawal.

Antihistamines

As discussed early in Section I, histamines promote pain transmission (Raffa, 2001). Further research is needed to clarify the underlying mechanisms, but three histamine receptors appear to be primary sites of action. The antinociceptive properties of morphine were enhanced in H_1 and H_2 receptor knockout mice (H_1 and H_2 receptors are genetically "turned off") indicating a role (Mobarakeh, Takahashi, Sakurada, et al., 2006). The analgesic action of the centrally-acting nonopioid nefopam was modulated by H_3 receptors but not H_1 and H_2 receptors in other animal research (Girard, Pansart, Coppe, et al., 2004).

Despite histamine's role in nociception, antihistamines are poor pain relievers, and there is little evidence to support common claims of enhanced pain relief and dose-sparing effects when they are combined with other analgesics (APS, 2003; Fitzgerald, Buggy, 2006). For example, very little research could be found to support the use of antihistamines for analgesia in the postoperative setting; however, the phenothiazine-derived antihistamine

Table 9-1 | Content of Caffeine in Selected Beverages, Food, and OTC Drugs

Beverages/Food	Serving Size	Caffeine Content Range (mg)	Caffeine Content Average (mg)
Coffee (generic)	8 ounces	102-200	133
Coffee (instant)	8 ounces	27-173	93
Coffee (decaffeinated)	8 ounces	3-12	5
Espresso (generic)	1 ounce	30-90	40
Tea (generic)	8 ounces	40-120	53
Bottled tea (variety)	16 ounces	10-100	
Coca Cola Classic (diet and regular)	12 ounces	–	35
Pepsi (regular)	12 ounces	–	38
Pepsi (diet)	12 ounces	–	36
Dr. Pepper	12 ounces	–	42
Dr. Pepper (diet)	12 ounces	–	44
7-Up (regular and diet)	12 ounces		0
Energy drinks (variety)	8-16 ounces	48-300	
Specialty ice creams and frozen yogurt (variety)	8 fluid ounces	50-84	
Energy gum	1 stick		33
Dark chocolate bar	1.45 ounces		31
Milk chocolate bar	1.55 ounces		9
Hot cocoa	8 ounces	3-13	9
No-Doz (maximum strength)	1 tablet		200
Excedrin (extra strength)	2 tablets		200
Excedrin Migraine	2 tablets		130
Anacin (maximum strength)	2 tablets		64

OTC, Over the counter.
Note: The analgesia of a dose of nonopioid may be augmented by 65 to 200 mg of caffeine. The ideal caffeine dose has not been established.
From Pasero, C., & McCaffery, M. *Pain assessment and pharmacologic management,* p. 241, St. Louis, Mosby. Data from *Center for Science in the Public Interest.* Available at http://www.cspinet.org/new/cafchart.htm. Accessed December 24, 2008; *Energy fiend.* Available at http://www.energyfiend.com/the-caffeine-database. Accessed December 24, 2008. © 2011, Pasero C, McCaffery M. May be duplicated for use in clinical practice.

promethazine (Phenergan) is commonly used in the postoperative setting based on a misconception that it potentiates opioid analgesia (APS, 2003). One study of patients following abdominal hysterectomy showed that those who received preoperative promethazine (0.1 mg/kg) consumed less postoperative PCA morphine than those who received the same dose of the drug postoperatively (Chia, Lo, Liu, et al., 2004). However, another study found no differences in opioid-sparing effects among patients following abdominal hysterectomy who were randomized to receive different amounts of diphenhydramine (Benadryl) or placebo at induction plus morphine PCA postoperatively (Lin, Yeh, Yen, et al., 2005).

The use of antihistamines in the postoperative setting, where patients are given anesthesia and other sedating medications, may be dangerous because it can produce an additive sedative effect and increase the risk of respiratory depression (Anwari, Iqbal, 2003). Patients must be watched very closely and antihistamine administration discontinued if increasing sedation is detected (see Chapter 19).

Antihistamines, such as phenyltoloxamine and diphenhydramine, are commonly combined with nonopioids, such as acetaminophen, aspirin, and ibuprofen, and promoted as night-time pain relievers (Table 9-2). Occasionally, antihistamines are administered for bone

Table 9-2 | Selected Nonprescription Analgesics: Acetaminophen, Aspirin, and Combination Analgesics

ACETAMINOPHEN ONLY, ORAL AND RECTAL FORMULATIONS

Formulation[1-5]	Amount of Acetaminophen/Dose	Dose Form/Comments
Acetaminophen regular strength	325 mg	Tablet, caplet, capsule, gelcap, geltab; most commonly used strength of acetaminophen
Acetaminophen extra strength	500 mg	Tablet, caplet, capsule, gelcap, geltab; appropriate when higher single doses are required
Acetaminophen extra strength fast- or rapid-release[5]	500 mg	Gel, gelcap; speed of disintegration varies[4]
Acetaminophen extended-release	650 mg	Caplet, geltab; 8-hour modified-release formulation; sometimes referred to as *arthritis formula*
Panadol Back + Neck Long Lasting	665 mg	Caplet; 8-hour modified-release formulation
Acetaminophen chewable tablet	80, 160 mg	May be swallowed whole or chewed; available in a variety of flavors
Acetaminophen dissolving/disintegrating tablet ("disc")	80, 160 mg	Dissolving tablet described for children but may be used in adults who require low doses or are unable to take other oral formulations; dissolves on tongue; available in a variety of flavors
Acetaminophen oral suspension drops	80 mg/0.8 mL	Solution described for infants but may be used in adults who require low doses or are unable to take other oral formulations; available in variety of flavors
Acetaminophen oral solution/elixir	80 mg/2.5 mL	Solution described for children but may be used in adults who require low doses or are unable to take other oral formulations; available in a variety of flavors
Acetaminophen oral elixir	160 mg/5 mL	Low-dose solution available in variety of flavors
Acetaminophen oral solution/liquid	500 mg/5 mL or 15 mL	Available in variety of flavors
Acetaminophen oral solution	1000 mg/30 mL	Low-dose solution described for sore throat relief; available in variety of flavors
Acetaminophen effervescent tablets (Bromo Seltzer)	650 mg	Packet; dissolvable in water; granular effervescent contains the antacids sodium bicarbonate and citric acid
Acetaminophen, rectal	80, 120, 325, 650 mg	Rectal suppository

Continued

| Table 9-2 | Selected Nonprescription Analgesics: Acetaminophen, Aspirin, and Combination Analgesics—cont'd |

ASPIRIN ONLY, ORAL

Formulation[1-5]	Amount of Aspirin/Dose	Dose Form/Comments
Aspirin regular strength	325 mg	Caplet, tablet; most commonly used strength of aspirin; also available in enteric coated and delayed release
Aspirin extra strength	500 mg	Caplet, tablet, gelcap
Aspirin extra strength	650 mg	Tablet
Aspirin	800 mg	Tablet
Aspirin extended-release	800 mg	Tablet, modified-release formulation
Aspirin, buffered	325 mg	Calcium carbonate, magnesium oxide, magnesium carbonate (buffering agents)
Aspirin, buffered	500 mg	Calcium carbonate (buffering agent)
Aspirin effervescent tablets (Alka-Seltzer)	325, 500 mg	Tablet dissolvable in water; contains the antacids sodium bicarbonate and citric acid; available in lemon flavor
Aspergum	227 mg/stick	Gum; available in variety of flavors
Aspirin low-dose (Halfprin)	160 mg	Tablet
Aspirin low-dose	81 mg	Caplet, tablet; available sugar free
Aspirin low-dose chewable tablet	81 mg	Caplet, tablet; available in variety of flavors
Aspirin, rectal	300, 600 mg	Rectal suppository

COMBINATION ANALGESIC BRANDS

Brand Name[1-5]	Amount of Acetaminophen/Dose	Amount of Aspirin/Dose	Other Analgesic Ingredients and Amount/Dose[6-12]	Dose Form/Comments
Goody's Body Pain	325 mg	500 mg		Powder
Pamprin Maximum Strength	250 mg		Pamabrom 25 mg, magnesium salicylate 250 mg	Caplet; for menstrual pain
Tylenol Menstrual Relief; Midol Teen	500 mg		Pamabrom 25 mg	Caplet; for menstrual pain
Pamprin Multisystem; Premsyn PMS; Midol Maximum Strength PMS	500 mg		Pamabrom 25 mg, pyrilamine maleate 15 mg	Caplet, tablet; for menstrual pain and PMS, can sedate

Continued

Table 9-2 | Selected Nonprescription Analgesics: Acetaminophen, Aspirin, and Combination Analgesics—cont'd

COMBINATION ANALGESIC BRANDS—CONT'D

Brand Name[1-5]	Amount of Acetaminophen/Dose	Amount of Aspirin/Dose	Other Analgesic Ingredients and Amount/Dose[6-12]	Dose Form/Comments
Midol Complete	500 mg		Caffeine 60 mg, pyrilamine maleate 15 mg	Caplet, gelcap; for menstrual pain and PMS; can cause CNS stimulation
Arthriten	250 mg		Caffeine 32.5 mg, magnesium salicylate 250 mg	Tablet; can cause CNS stimulation
Cafgesic Forte, Durabac Forte, Combiflex ES	500 mg		Caffeine 50 mg, magnesium salicylate 500 mg, phenyltoloxamine 20 mg	Tablet; contains both a CNS stimulant and an antihistamine that can sedate
Excedrin Tension Headache; Panadol Extra	500 mg		Caffeine 65 mg	Caplet; can cause CNS stimulation
Anacin Fast Pain Relief		400 mg	Caffeine 32 mg	Caplet, tablet; can cause CNS stimulation
Anacin Maximum Strength; Bayer Extra Strength Back and Body		500 mg	Caffeine 32 mg	Caplet, tablet; can cause CNS stimulation
Stanback, Original Formula		650 mg	Caffeine 32 mg, salicylamide, 200 mg	Powder; can cause CNS stimulation
BC Fast Pain Relief		650 mg	Caffeine 33.3 mg	Powder; dissolvable in water; can cause CNS stimulation
BC Arthritis Strength		742 mg	Caffeine 38 mg	Powder; dissolvable in water; can cause CNS stimulation
Alka Seltzer Wake-up Call		600 mg	Caffeine 65 mg, sodium 415 mg, phenylalanine 9 mg	Effervescent tablet dissolves in water; can cause CNS stimulation
Anacin Headache Formula; Excedrin Extra Strength or Express Gels; Excedrin Migraine	250 mg	250 mg	Caffeine 65 mg	Caplet, tablet, gelcap, gels; can cause CNS stimulation
Goody's Extra Strength	260 mg	520 mg	Caffeine 32.5 mg	Powder; ingredients also available in strengths of 130 mg/260 mg/16.25 mg per tablet; can cause CNS stimulation

Continued

Table 9-2 | Selected Nonprescription Analgesics: Acetaminophen, Aspirin, and Combination Analgesics—cont'd

COMBINATION ANALGESIC BRANDS—CONT'D

Brand Name[1-5]	Amount of Acetaminophen/Dose	Amount of Aspirin/Dose	Other Analgesic Ingredients and Amount/Dose[6-12]	Dose Form/Comments
Goody's Extra Strength	325 mg	500 mg	Caffeine 65 mg	Powder, orange flavored; can cause CNS stimulation
Percogesic Original Aspirin Free	325 mg		Phenyltoloxamine 30 mg	Caplet; can sedate
Percogesic Extra Strength	500 mg		Diphenhydramine 12.5 mg	Caplet; can sedate
Panadol Night; Tylenol PM	500 mg		Diphenhydramine 25 mg	Caplet, geltab; can sedate
Excedrin PM	500 mg		Diphenhydramine 38 mg	Caplet; can sedate
Tylenol PM Liquid	1000 mg/3 mL		Diphenhydramine 50 mg	Vanilla-flavored liquid; can sedate
Goody's PM	1000 mg		Diphenhydramine 76 mg	Powder dissolvable in water; can sedate
Bayer PM		500 mg	Diphenhydramine 38 mg	Caplet; can sedate
Alka Seltzer PM		325 mg	Diphenhydramine 38 mg, sodium 504 mg, phenylalanine 4 mg	Effervescent tablet dissolvable in water; can sedate
Bayer Women's Low-Dose Aspirin Plus Calcium		81 mg	Calcium 300 mg	Caplet; for cardioprotection

[1]The nonopioids listed in this table are available under a variety of brand names and manufactured by a variety of pharmaceutical companies. Active and inactive ingredients vary, and some oral solutions contain alcohol and dyes. Product availability changes frequently; this is not intended to be a comprehensive list. Reading specific product labeling is recommended.
[2]Tablets are round or oblong/elliptical-shaped; caplets are oblong/elliptical-shaped; capsules, geltabs, and gelcaps are usually oblong/elliptical-shaped and usually contain gelatin in coating.
[3]Many manufacturers offer caplets and tablets with delayed-release or enteric coating promoted as gastro-protective (see text for more about enteric coating and gastro-protection).
[4]Products vary in the time it takes to dissolve and release the active drug. This can range from less than 1 minute for non-enteric coated aspirin to more than 35 minutes for liqui-gels (see http://cruftbox.com/cruft/docs/dissolve.html).
[5]Some formulations are described as fast- or rapid-release. Formulations vary; some contain the active ingredient within liquid and some have holes in the coating or an exposed gelcap center which facilitates faster disintegration and release of the drug.
[6]Pamabrom is a diuretic.

[7]Pyrilamine maleate, diphenhydramine, and phenyltoloxamine are antihistamines.
[8]Caffeine is a central nervous system stimulant.
[9]Magnesium salicylate is an NSAID.
[10]Salicylamide has analgesic and antipyretic properties.
[11]Sodium is a buffering agent in this formulation.
[12]Phenylalanine is an amino acid.
From Pasero, C., & McCaffery, M. *Pain assessment and pharmacologic management*, pp. 242-245, St. Louis, Mosby. Data from Berardi, R. R., Kroon, L. A., McDermott, J. H., et al. (2006). *Handbook of non-prescription drugs: An interactive approach to self-care*, ed 15, Washington, DC, American Pharmacists Association; Brunton, L. L., Lazo, J. S., & Parker, K. L. (Eds.). (2006). *Goodman & Gilman's the pharmacological basis of therapeutics*, ed 11, New York, McGraw-Hill; Clinical Pharmacology Online. Gold Standard, Inc. Available at http://clinicalpharmacology.com. Accessed January 4, 2009; Lacy, C. F., Armstrong, L. L., & Goldman, M. P., et al. (Eds.). (2010). *Drug information handbook 2009-2010*, ed 8, Hudson, OH, American Pharmacists Association and Lexi-Comp; *United States Food and Drug Administration (FDA) orange book*. Available at www.fda.gov/cder/orange/. Accessed January 8, 2009. © 2011, Pasero C, McCaffery M. May be duplicated for use in clinical practice.

pain associated with chemotherapy-induced neutropenia when other strategies are ineffective; however, research is lacking on this approach (Pangilinan, 2008).

Conclusion

Analgesics available without a prescription (OTC) include many formulations and brands of aspirin and acetaminophen as well as ibuprofen, naproxen, and ketoprofen (see Tables 9-2 and 9-3) (see also Patient Medication Information Forms III-4 and III-5 on pp. 256-259). More NSAIDs are likely to become available as OTC analgesics. Clinicians need to be familiar with doses and ingredients of those used by the individual patient. Clinicians also should know that sometimes a nonprescription NSAID (e.g., ibuprofen) will be less expensive than the same dose by prescription.

Table 9-3 | Selected Nonprescription NSAIDs Other Than Acetaminophen and Aspirin

Brand Name[1-7]	Ingredient	Dose	Dose Form/Comments
Advil, Motrin, Midol	Ibuprofen	200 mg	Caplet, tablet, gelcap, liquid gels; most commonly used strength of ibuprofen
Advil, Motrin Junior	Ibuprofen	100 mg	Tablet; described for children but may be used in adults who require lower dose
Advil, Motrin Junior or Children's Chewables	Ibuprofen	50 mg, 100 mg	Tablet may be swallowed whole or chewed; available in a variety of flavors; described for children but may be used in adults who cannot take other oral formulations
Advil, Motrin Infants' Suspension	Ibuprofen	40 mg/mL, 50 mg/1.25 mL	Liquid; available in a variety of flavors; described for infants but may be used in adults who require a low dose and cannot take other oral formulations
Advil, Motrin Children's Suspension	Ibuprofen	100 mg/5 mL	Liquid; available in a variety of flavors
Aleve	Naproxen sodium	220 mg	Caplet, tablet, liquid gels
Midol Extended Relief	Naproxen sodium	220 mg	Modified-release tablet
Arthropan	Choline salicylate	870 mg/5 mL	Liquid
Momentum Maximum Strength	Magnesium salicylate	580 mg	Caplet
Doan's Extra Strength	Magnesium salicylate tetrahydrate	580 mg	Caplet
MST	Magnesium salicylate tetrahydrate	600 mg	Tablet
Masalate, Novasal	Magnesium salicylate	600 mg	Tablet

[1]Product availability changes frequently; this is not intended to be a comprehensive list.

[2]Many of the active ingredients in this table are available by prescription in other strengths and formulations (e.g., modified-release, suspensions).

[3]Active and inactive ingredients vary, and some oral solutions contain alcohol and dyes. Reading specific product labeling is recommended.

[4]Tablets are round or oblong/elliptical-shaped; caplets are oblong/elliptical-shaped; capsules, geltabs, and gelcaps are usually oblong/elliptical-shaped and usually contain gelatin in coating

[5]Many manufacturers offer caplets and tablets with delayed-release or enteric coating promoted as gastro-protective (see text for more about enteric coating and gastro-protection).

[6]Products vary in the time it takes to dissolve and release the active drug. This can range from less than 1 minute for non-enteric coated aspirin to more than 35 minutes for liqui-gels (see http://cruftbox.com/cruft/docs/dissolve.html).

[7]Some formulations are described as fast or rapid-release. Formulations vary; some contain the active ingredient within liquid and some have holes in the coating or an exposed gelcap center, which facilitates faster disintegration and release of the drug. From Pasero, C., & McCaffery, M. *Pain assessment and pharmacologic management*, p. 246, St. Louis, Mosby. Data from Berardi, R. R., Kroon, L. A., McDermott, J. H., et al. (2006). *Handbook of non-prescription drugs: An interactive approach to self-care*, ed 15, Washington, DC, American Pharmacists Association; Brunton, L. L., Lazo, J. S., & Parker, K. L. (Eds.). (2006). *Goodman & Gilman's the pharmacological basis of therapeutics*, ed 11, New York, McGraw-Hill; Clinical Pharmacology Online. Gold Standard, Inc. Available at *http://clinicalpharmacology.com*. Accessed January 4, 2009; Lacy, C. F., Armstrong, L. L., & Goldman, M. P., et al. (Eds.). (2010). *Drug information handbook 2009-2010*, ed 8, Hudson, OH, American Pharmacists Association and Lexi-Comp; *United States Food and Drug Administration (FDA) orange book*. Available at www.fda.gov/cder/orange/. Accessed January 8, 2009. © 2011, Pasero C, McCaffery M. May be duplicated for use in clinical practice.

Chapter 10 Acute Overdose

ASPIRIN and acetaminophen are widely used as self-medication for pain relief, and many products marketed for other conditions such as cold and flu (e.g., Advil Cold & Sinus) contain one or more of these nonopioids. Patient and family teaching about these products should warn about the maximum recommended doses and the signs of overdose and alert them to sources of "hidden" aspirin and acetaminophen (see Patient Medication Information Forms III-4 and III-5 on pp. 256-259).

Acetaminophen

Chronic acetaminophen overdose can occur with regular daily consumption of higher than recommended doses and is discussed earlier in this section (see Chapter 6). Acute acetaminophen toxicity is generally the result of taking a single dose that is significantly higher than the recommended dose and is considered a medical emergency because untreated acute acetaminophen toxicity can cause fatal hepatic necrosis. Hepatotoxicity can also occur with a single dose of the recommended amount of acetaminophen (e.g., 1000 to 1500 mg in adults) under certain conditions, such as malnutrition, fasting, or heavy alcohol consumption (Burke, Smyth, FitzGerald, 2006).

Prompt diagnosis and treatment of acute acetaminophen overdose will optimize outcome. Approximately 10% of individuals who overdose and do not receive treatment develop severe liver damage. Damage occurs when plasma concentrations are 300 mcg/mL or more at 4 hours or 45 mcg/mL at 15 hours after ingestion of acetaminophen (Burke, Smyth, FitzGerald, 2006). If the dose is not fatal, liver damage can be reversible over a period of weeks or months (Burke, Smyth, FitzGerald, 2006).

Early symptoms of acute acetaminophen overdose occur within 2 days of ingestion and include nausea, vomiting, drowsiness, confusion, and abdominal pain. Plasma transaminase levels become elevated within 12 hours. Clinical signs of hepatic damage are evident within 4 days of overdose by increasing jaundice, right subcostal pain, tender hepatomegaly, and coagulopathy (prolonged prothrombin time) (Burke, Smyth, FitzGerald, 2006). Toxicity may be accompanied by renal impairment. Poor prognosis is associated with hepatic encephalopathy or worsening coagulopathy.

A Cochrane Collaboration Review concluded that the evidence for support of any one method of acetaminophen overdose treatment is weak; activated charcoal, gastric lavage, and ipecac administration within 2 hours of acetaminophen ingestion reduce absorption, but the clinical implications are not clear (Brok, Buckley, Gluud, 2006). Others recommend initial administration of activated charcoal but do not recommend gastric lavage (Burke, Smyth, FitzGerald, 2006). N-acetylcysteine (NAC) (Mucomyst, Mucosol) should be given orally to individuals at risk of hepatic injury (Brok, Buckley, Gluud, 2006; Burke, Smyth, FitzGerald, 2006). The underlying mechanism of hepatic damage as a result of acetaminophen overdose is conversion of acetaminophen to the toxic metabolite N-acetyl-p-benzo-quinone imine (NAPQI), and NAC detoxifies NAPQI. Administration of NAC should not be delayed or avoided if activated charcoal has already been given; interaction between the two is not a concern (Burke, Smyth, FitzGerald, 2006).

Aspirin and Other Salicylates

Toxicity related to aspirin and other salicylates is also generally a result of taking higher than recommended doses. Symptoms of toxicity from chronic use (referred to as *chronic salicylism*) include headache, dizziness, ringing in the ears, difficulty hearing, dim vision, confusion, drowsiness, and sweating (Burke, Smyth, FitzGerald, 2006). Toxicity may go undetected because some of these symptoms mimic the disease being treated. All are reversible by lowering the dose.

Acute salicylate overdose, on the other hand, is considered a medical emergency, and prognosis depends on prompt diagnosis and treatment. The American Association of Poison Control Centers recommends that any suspected or confirmed salicylate overdose in the outpatient setting be immediately referred to an emergency department for treatment (Chyka, Erdman, Christianson, et al., 2007). Fatal doses vary significantly and depend on the aspirin formulation; however, death has been reported with doses of 10 to 30 gm in adults (Burke, Smyth, FitzGerald, 2006).

Symptoms of acute toxicity include lethargy, ringing in the ears, nausea and vomiting, and convulsions. Gastric irritation may not be evident. Hyperventilation and tachycardia are sometimes mistaken for anxiety (O'Malley, 2007). However, co-ingestion of CNS-depressant drugs, such as opioids, can blunt respiratory symptoms. Serum aspirin levels may be normal or modestly elevated, and blood gas analysis will likely demonstrate respiratory alkalosis. Patients in the late stages of salicylate toxicity are often misdiagnosed as having sepsis, myocardial infarction (MI), or a psychiatric disturbance (O'Malley, 2007). Postmortem examination has shown myocardial necrosis, pulmonary congestion, hemorrhagic gastritis and ulceration, cerebral edema, and muscle rigidity.

There is no specific antidote for salicylate overdose. Emesis should not be induced (Chyka, Erdman, Christianson, et al., 2007). A combination of gastric irritation, nausea, and lethargy places the patient at high risk for vomiting, which can result in aspiration; therefore, the benefits and risks of gastric decontamination must be weighed. The most commonly used method for gastric decontamination consists of administering multidose activated charcoal (25 mg without sorbitol every 3 hours) to prevent further absorption of the drug from the GI tract (O'Malley, 2007). Doses are repeated if bowel sounds are absent when the next dose is due. Administration of activated charcoal is particularly important if enteric-coated aspirin, which has delayed absorption, has been ingested (Burke, Smyth, FitzGerald, 2006). Alkanized IV fluids (sodium bicarbonate + potassium chloride) are infused rapidly to counteract acidity and prevent hypokalemia (O'Malley, 2007). Maintaining high urine alkalinity (i.e., pH greater than 8) will facilitate salicylate excretion. Supplemental glucose should be administered to patients with altered mental status as this may indicate decreased CNS glucose despite normal plasma glucose levels. Hemodialysis is required if these simpler methods are ineffective (Burke, Smyth, FitzGerald, 2006; O'Malley, 2007).

Other NSAIDs

An overdose of a proprionic acid derivative, such as ibuprofen, ketoprofen, or naproxen, usually produces minimal symptoms of toxicity and is rarely fatal. However, there are case reports of multisystem organ failure and death after consumption of massive amounts of ibuprofen (e.g., 105-gm sustained-release ibuprofen) (Holubek, Stolbach, Nurok et al., 2007; Wood, Monaghan, Streete, et al., 2006). Management of suspected ibuprofen overdose accounts for 5% of the calls to poison control centers in the United Kingdom, and the fatalities associated with ibuprofen overdose are often complicated by comorbidities and co-ingestion of other drugs (Volans, Monaghan, Colbridge, 2003). There have been single reports of acute pancreatitis induced by an overdose of ibuprofen (Magill, Ridgway, Conlon et al., 2006) and naproxen (Aygencel, Akbuga, Keles, 2006).

Common symptoms of mild NSAID (e.g., ibuprofen, naproxen) overdose include nausea, vomiting, and abdominal pain. However, many patients are completely asymptomatic (Volans, Monaghan, Colbridge, 2003). Acute massive overdose produces severe metabolic acidosis, hypotension, hypothermia, and reduced level of consciousness, or the patient may be unresponsive. Treatment of acute toxicity includes gastric decontamination with activated charcoal, vasopressors, correction of metabolic acidosis, and dialysis (Wood, Monaghan, Streete, et al., 2006). Overdose of other NSAIDs appears to be similar to that seen with the proprionic acid derivatives.

Conclusion

Chronic nonopioid overdose can occur with regular daily intake of higher than recommended doses. Acute toxicity usually occurs when a single dose that is significantly higher than the recommended dose is consumed. Prognosis depends on prompt and appropriate treatment dependent on the type of nonopioid involved.

Section III | Conclusion

USE of acetaminophen and NSAIDs for pain relief is usually on an outpatient basis. Patients are often discharged from the hospital with nonopioids, and they are frequently prescribed or recommended to patients during an office or clinic visit. Because many are available without a prescription, the patient may decide independently to use them.

A review of the literature revealed numerous reasons why patients do not adhere to a variety of medications prescribed for pain (Monsivais, McNeil, 2007). In addition to an introductory review of the literature, these authors examined 42 abstracts and 17 full-text articles. Some of the concerns revealed are pertinent to nonopioid analgesics and may be diminished by providing the patient with written information about their medications. (See patient education forms for selected medications on pp. 250-255.) A common reason for nonadherence was a high level of concern about the medication, such as adverse effects, "dependency," and questions about the real need for the medication. Patients also had misconceptions about how long it should take for the drug to be effective, and they would stop taking it if no benefits occurred by the expected time. Patients also feared tolerance, that is, that the medication might cease to work if taken on a regular basis.

Nonopioids can cause serious adverse effects underscoring the need to provide accurate and complete information to patients and their families regarding safe use.

The usual teaching about drug, name, dose, timing, and adverse effects is important. Written information may be particularly helpful because it reminds the patient of what was said. It can be shared with interested family members and any health care providers the patient may see. Forms III-1 to III-3 are teaching tools specific to ibuprofen, naproxen, and celecoxib. Forms III-4 and III-5 (pp. 256-259) are teaching tools for prescription and nonprescription products containing acetaminophen and NSAIDs, respectively.

The information in the Patient Medication Information forms that follow is based on content from this chapter and the following five references:

- Clinical Pharmacology Online. Gold Standard, Inc. Available at *http://clinicalpharmacology.com.*
- Drug inserts, available online for each medication.
- Fox Chase Cancer Center/Pain Management. Patient Education Forms, celecoxib (2007), ibuprofen (2007), prescription and nonprescription products containing acetaminophen (2008), prescription and nonprescription products containing NSAIDs (2007), Philadelphia, PA.
- Clinical Pharmacology Online. Gold Standard, Inc. Available at *http://clinicalpharmacology.com.*
- Lacy, C. F., Armstrong, L. L., Goldman, M. P., et al. (Eds.) (2009-2010). *Drug information handbook*, ed 18, American Pharmacists Association, Lexi-Comp.

PATIENT MEDICATION INFORMATION

Celecoxib (generic name)

BRAND NAME: Celebrex®

TYPE OF PAIN MEDICINE: COX-2 selective nonsteroidal antiinflammatory (NSAID), nonopioid (not a narcotic)

DESCRIPTION: Celebrex comes in two strengths: 100 mg and 200 mg capsules

USES:
- Relieves mild to moderate pain such as muscle and bone injuries, after surgery, and arthritis.
- Decreases inflammation.
- Reduces fevers.

DOSE AND ADMINISTRATION:
- Take only as directed.
- May be taken alone or with other types of pain medicines, such as opioids, but do not take with other nonsteroidal medicines (NSAIDs).
- Take with a full glass of water.
- May be taken with or without food.
- Take with food if the medicine upsets your stomach or if you take 400 mg at once.
- Try not to lie down for at least 10 minutes after you take the medicine.
- If you miss a dose, take the missed dose as soon as possible. Skip the missed dose if it is almost time for the next dose.
- Do not take two doses at the same time.
- Before taking Celebrex tell your pharmacist, nurse, or doctor if you are taking:
  - Aspirin
  - Steroids such as Decadron® or Prednisone®
  - Antiinflammatory medicines such as ibuprofen (Motrin®, Advil®), fluriprofen (Ansaid®), nambuetone (Relafen®), naproxen (Naprosyn®, Anaprox®, Aleve®), or others
  - Blood pressure medicines called ACE inhibitors such as captopril, enalapril, lisinopril, and others
  - Other medicines, such as furosemide (Lasix®), rifampin (Rifadin®), methotrexate, warfarin (Coumadin®), lithium, phenytoin, fluconazole, or ketoconazole
- Tell your pharmacist, nurse, or doctor if you have any of the following conditions:
  - allergy to aspirin or other antiinflammatory drugs (NSAIDs)
  - asthma
  - stomach ulcers
  - kidney, heart, or liver disease
  - pregnant, trying to get pregnant, or breast-feeding

Continued

Form III-1 | Patient medication information: Celecoxib.

PATIENT MEDICATION INFORMATION—cont'd

Celecoxib (generic name)

POSSIBLE SIDE EFFECTS:
- Stomach irritation such as heartburn
- Nausea and vomiting
- Swelling in the ankles or feet
- <u>Report the following side effects to your nurse or doctor as soon as possible:</u> allergic reactions such as rash and swelling of the face, lips, or tongue

PRECAUTIONS:
- Do not take Celebrex if:
  - you are allergic to aspirin or other antiinflammatory drugs.
  - you are allergic to sulfa drugs or salicylates or have asthma.
  - you are pregnant or breast-feeding.
  - you had recent heart surgery.
- Drinking alcohol or smoking tobacco while taking Celebrex may increase the risk of bleeding stomach ulcers.

STOPPING MEDICATION: Do not suddenly stop taking your medicine. Call your pharmacist, nurse, or doctor before you stop taking your medicine.

REMEMBER!
- Keep count of your medicine.
- Do not run out of medicine.
- Do not mix medicines in the same container.
- Get a **new** prescription filled a few days before you will run out of medicine.
- **Call** your nurse or doctor if side effects occur or if pain changes or does not go away. Your medicine may need to be changed.
- Take unused, unneeded, or expired medicines out of their original containers and flush them down the toilet. Do not put them in the trash.

COMMENTS:

WARNING: Keep this and all medicines out of reach of children!

Form III-1 | Cont'd.

PATIENT MEDICATION INFORMATION

Ibuprofen (generic name)

BRAND NAMES: Some of the brand names are Advil®, Motrin®, Nuprin®, Rufen®, Ibu-Tab®, and Ibupren®.

TYPE OF PAIN MEDICINE: Nonsteroidal antiinflammatory (NSAID), nonopioid (not a narcotic)

DESCRIPTION: Ibuprofen comes in regular tablets, gelcaps, coated tablets, and liquids.

Non-prescription strength—200 mg tablets, 100 mg per teaspoon (5 mL) liquid
Prescription strength—300 mg, 400 mg, 600 mg, 800 mg

USES:
• Relieves mild to moderate pain such as muscle and bone injuries, after surgery, arthritis, and bone pain.
• Decreases inflammation.
• Reduces fevers.

DOSE AND ADMINISTRATION:
• <u>Take only as directed.</u>
• May be taken alone or with other types of pain medicines, such as opioids, but do not take with other nonsteroidal antiinflammatory medicines (NSAIDs).
• Take with a full glass of water.
• May be taken with or without food.
• If the medicine upsets your stomach, try taking it with food.
• Try not to lie down for at least 10 minutes after you take ibuprofen.
• If you miss a dose, take the missed dose as soon as possible. Skip the missed dose if it is almost time for the next dose.
• Do not take two doses at the same time.
• Before taking ibuprofen tell your pharmacist, nurse, or doctor if you are taking:
  - Aspirin. If you take low-dose (81 mg per day) aspirin to protect your heart or prevent stroke and it is not coated, take ibuprofen 30 minutes after or 8 hours before you take your aspirin. If you don't take ibuprofen on a regular basis, it probably will not interfere with effects of low dose aspirin.
  - Steroids such as Decadron® or Prednisone®
  - Antiinflammatory medicines such as fluriprofen (Ansaid®) nambuetone (Relafen®), naproxen (Naprosyn®, Anaprox®, Aleve®), or others
  - Blood pressure medicines called ACE inhibitors such as captopril, enalapril, lisinopril, and others
  - Other medicines, such as furosemide (Lasix®), rifampin (Rifadin®), methotrexate, warfarin (Coumadin®), lithium, phenytoin, fluconazole, or ketoconazole

Continued

Form III-2 | Patient medication information: Ibuprofen.

PATIENT MEDICATION INFORMATION—cont'd

Ibuprofen (generic name)

- Tell your pharmacist, nurse, or doctor if you have any of the following conditions:
  - allergy to aspirin or other antiinflammatory drugs (NSAIDs)
  - asthma
  - stomach ulcers
  - kidney, heart, or liver disease
  - pregnant, trying to get pregnant, or breast-feeding

POSSIBLE SIDE EFFECTS:
- Stomach irritation: can usually be prevented by taking it with food, milk, or antacids
- Nausea and vomiting: can be controlled with medicines
- Change in color of bowel movement
- Swelling in the ankles or feet
- Ringing in the ears
- Report the following side effects to your nurse or doctor as soon as possible:
  black or bloody stools; blood in the urine or in vomit; allergic reactions like skin rash, hives, swelling of face; breathing problems

PRECAUTIONS:
- Avoid alcohol while taking ibuprofen. Alcohol may increase risk of liver damage or stomach irritation.
- This medicine can increase your risk of bleeding. Avoid ibuprofen 7 days before surgery.

STOPPING MEDICATIONS: Do not suddenly stop taking your medicine. Call your pharmacist, nurse, or doctor before you stop taking your medicine.

REMEMBER!
- Keep count of your medicine.
- Do not run out of medicine.
- Do not mix medicines in the same container.
- Get a **new** prescription filled a few days before you will run out of medicine.
- **Call** your nurse or doctor if side effects occur or if pain changes or does not go away. Your medicine may need to be changed.
- Take unused, unneeded, or expired medicines out of their original containers and flush them down the toilet. Do not put them in the trash.

COMMENTS:

WARNING: Keep this and all medicines out of reach of children!

PATIENT MEDICATION INFORMATION

Naproxen (generic name)

BRAND NAMES: Some of the brand names are Aleve® (non-prescription), Anaprox® (prescription), Naprosyn® (prescription), EC-Naproxen® (prescription), and Naprolan® (prescription)

TYPE OF PAIN MEDICINE: Nonsteroidal antiinflammatory (NSAID), nonopioid (not a narcotic)

DESCRIPTION: Naproxen comes in regular tablets, long-acting tablets, and liquid. Some products contain naproxen alone and others contain naproxen and sodium.

Nonprescription strength—naproxen sodium 220 mg tablet (contains naproxen 200 mg plus 20 mg of sodium)
Prescription strength—tablet strengths: 250 mg, 375 mg, 500 mg
delayed release tablets: 375 mg, 500 mg
oral suspension: 25 mg per teaspoon (5 mL)

USES:
- Relieves mild to moderate pain such as muscle and bone injuries, after surgery, and arthritis.
- Decreases inflammation.
- Reduces fevers.

DOSE AND ADMINISTRATION:
- Take only as directed.
- May be taken alone or with other types of pain medicines, such as opioids, but do not take with other nonsteroidal antiinflammatory medicines (NSAIDs).
- Take with a full glass of water.
- May be taken with or without food
- If the medicine upsets your stomach, try taking it with food.
- Try not to lie down for at least 10 minutes after you take naproxen.
- If you miss a dose, take the missed dose as soon as possible. Skip the missed dose if it is almost time for the next dose.
- Do not take two doses at the same time.
- Before taking naproxen tell your pharmacist, nurse, or doctor if you are taking:
  - Aspirin. If you take low-dose (81 mg per day) aspirin to protect your heart or prevent stroke, take naproxen 30 minutes after or 8 hours before you take your aspirin. If you don't take naproxen on a regular basis, it probably will not interfere with effects of low-dose aspirin.
  - Steroids, such as Decadron® or Prednisone®
  - Antiinflammatory medicines such as fluriprofen (Ansaid®), nambuetone (Relafen®), and ibuprofen such as Advil®, Motrin®, Nuprin®, or others
  - Blood pressure medicines called ACE inhibitors such as captopril, enalapril, lisinopril, and others
  - Other medicines, such as furosemide (Lasix®), rifampin (Rifadin®), methotrexate, warfarin (Coumadin®), lithium, phenytoin, fluconazole, or ketoconazole

Continued

Form III-3 | Patient medication information: Naproxen.

From Pasero, C., & McCaffery, M. *Pain assessment and pharmacologic management*, pp. 254-255, St. Louis, Mosby. © 2011, McCaffery M, Pasero C. May be duplicated for use in clinical practice.

PATIENT MEDICATION INFORMATION—cont'd

Naproxen (generic name)

- Tell your pharmacist, nurse, or doctor if you have any of the following conditions:
  - allergy to aspirin or other antiinflammatory drugs (NSAIDs)
  - asthma
  - stomach ulcers
  - kidney, heart, or liver disease
  - pregnant, trying to get pregnant, or breast-feeding

POSSIBLE SIDE EFFECTS:
- Stomach irritation: can usually be prevented by taking it with food, milk, or antacids
- Nausea and vomiting: can be controlled with medicines
- Change in color of bowel movement
- Swelling in the ankles or feet
- Ringing in the ears
- <u>Report the following side effects to your nurse or doctor as soon as possible:</u>
  black or bloody stools; blood in the urine or in vomit; allergic reactions like skin rash,
  hives, swelling of face; breathing problems

PRECAUTIONS:
- Avoid alcohol while taking naproxen. Alcohol may increase the risk of
  liver damage or stomach irritation.
- This medicine can increase your risk of bleeding. Avoid naproxen 7 days before surgery.

STOPPING MEDICATIONS: Do not suddenly stop taking your medicine. Call your
pharmacist, nurse, or doctor before you stop taking your medicine.

REMEMBER!
- Keep count of your medicine
- Do not run out of medicine.
- Do not mix medicines in the same container.
- Get a **new** prescription filled a few days before you will run out of medicine.
- **Call** your nurse or doctor if side effects occur or if pain changes or does not go
  away. Your medicine may need to be changed.
- Take unused, unneeded, or expired medicines out of their original containers
  and flush them down the toilet. Do not put them in the trash.

COMMENTS:

WARNING: Keep this and all medicines out of reach of children!

Form III-3 | Cont'd.

PATIENT MEDICATION INFORMATION

Products with Acetaminophen (such as Tylenol®)

Please refer to this sheet if:

- you are taking a product with acetaminophen.
- your doctor tells you not to take acetaminophen and products with acetaminophen.

<u>You should not take more than 4000 milligrams (mg) of acetaminophen a day.</u> You need to read the label to check the milligrams. Too much acetaminophen can be harmful to your liver.

Prescription Products with Acetaminophen

- Acetaminophen and codeine
- Anexsia® tablets
- APAP, acetaminophen uniserts/suppositories
- Axocet® capsules
- Butalbital, acetaminophen and caffeine
- Capital® and codeine oral suspension
- Darvocet-N® 100 tablets
- Endocet tablets
- Esgic® capsules and tablets and Esgic-Plus™ tablets
- Fioricet® tablets
- Hycomine® compound
- Hydrocet® capsules
- Hydrocodone bitartrate and acetaminophen tablets, capsules, elixir
- Lorcet® tablets, capsules, HD, plus
- Lortab® tablets and elixir
- Midrin® capsules
- Norco® tablets
- Norel plus® capsules
- Oxycodone and acetaminophen tablets and capsules
- Pentazocine HCl & acetaminophen tablets
- Percocet® tablets
- Phenaphen® with codeine capsules
- Phrenilin® tablets, Forte capsules
- Propoxyphene HCl and acetaminophen tablets
- Propoxyphene napsylate and acetaminophen tablets
- Roxicet™ tablets, caplets, oral solution
- Talacen® caplets
- Tylenol® with codeine tablets and elixir
- Tylox® capsules
- Ultracet™ tablets
- Vicodin®, Vicodin ES®, Vicodin HP® tablets
- Wygesic® tablets
- Zebutal® capsules
- Zydone® tablets

Non-Prescription Products with Acetaminophen (such as Tylenol®)

- Actifed®: Cold & Allergy Sinus
- Alka-Seltzer Plus®: all products
- Anacin®: Aspirin-Free Formula
- Benadryl®: Allergy Sinus Headache, Severe Allergy & Sinus Headache
- Comtrex®: all products
- Contact®: Severe Cold and Flu Maximum Strength Caplets, Non-Drowsy Caplets, Day & Night Cold & Flu
- Coricidin® D Cold, Flu & Sinus tablets; HBP Cold & Flu tablets
- Dimetapp®: Non-Drowsy Flu syrup
- Dristin®: Cold Multi-Symptom Formula
- Drixoral®: Allergy Sinus, Cold & Flu
- Excedrin®: all products
- Feverall®: suppositories
- Goody's® Powders: all products

Continued

Form III-4 | Patient medication education: Products with acetaminophen.

PATIENT MEDICATION INFORMATION—cont'd

Non-Prescription Products with Acetaminophen (such as Tylenol®)

- Midol®: Maximum Strength Menstrual Formula, Maximum Strength PMS Formula
- NyQuil®/DayQuil®: Cold/Flu Relief Liquid and LiquiCaps
- Pamprin®: all products
- Percogesic®: all products
- Robitussin: Cold, Multi-Symptom Cold & Flu, Multi-Symptom Honey Flu Liquid, Nighttime Honey Flu Liquid
- Singlet® tablets
- Sinutab® Sinus: Sinus Allergy Medication Maximum Strength Formula
- Sudafed®: Cold & Cough Liquid Caps, Cold & Sinus Liquid Caps, Severe Cold Caplets and Tablets, Sinus caplets and tablets

- Tavist®: Sinus Non-Drowsy coated caplets
- TheraFlu®: all regular and maximum strength caplets and hot liquid
- Triaminic®: Cold, Cough & Fever Liquid; Cough & Sore Throat Liquid, Cough & Sore Throat Softchews
- Tylenol®: Allergy Sinus Formula, Severe Allergy; Arthritis Pain Extended Relief; Cold Formula, Cold & Flu; Extra Strength Pain Reliever; Flu Formula; Maximum Strength Sore Throat Adult Liquid; PM Pain Reliever/Sleep Aid; Regular Strength; Sinus; Women's Tylenol
- Vanquish®: caplets
- Vicks®: Vicks 44M Cough, Cold & Flu Relief Liquid and Liquicaps

Form III-4 | Cont'd.

PATIENT MEDICATION INFORMATION

Products with NSAIDs (nonsteroidal antiinflammatory drugs)

Please refer to this sheet if:

- you are taking NSAIDs.
- your doctor tells you not to take NSAIDs.

Too much NSAID can be harmful to your kidneys and cause stomach ulcers and bleeding.

Prescription Products with NSAIDs

- Alor® 5/500 tablets
- Anaprox® tablets, DS tablets
- Ansaid® tablets
- Arthrotec®
- ASA w/codeine
- Butalbital, aspirin, caffeine, and codeine phosphate capsules
- Carisoprodol and aspirin tablets
- Cataflam® tablets
- Celebrex® capsules
- Choline Magnesium Trisalicylate tablets, liquid
- Clinoril® tablets
- Darvon® Compound-65, pulvules®
- Daypro® caplets
- Diclofenac Potassium tablets
- Diclofenac sodium, XR tablets
- Disalcid™ capsules and tablets
- Dolobid® tablets
- Easprin® tablets
- EC-Naprosyn® delayed-release tablets
- Endodan tablets
- Equagesic® tablets
- Fedene capsules
- Fiorinal and fiorinal w/codeine capsules
- Flurbiprofen tablets
- Ibuprofen tablets 400/600/800 mg
- Indocin® capsules, IV oral suspension, suppositories
- Indomethacin, SR capsules, suspension
- Ketoprofen tablets
- Lodine® capsules, tablets, XL extended-release tablets
- Lortab® ASA tablets
- Methocarbamol and aspirin tablets
- Mobic® tablets
- Motrin® tablets 400/600/800 mg
- Nalfon® capsules
- Naprelan® tablets
- Naprosyn® suspension, tablets
- Naproxen sodium tablets
- Norgesic™ and Norgesic™ Forte tablets
- Orphenadrine citrate, aspirin and caffeine tablets
- Orudis® capsules
- Oruvail® extended-release capsules
- Oxycodone and aspirin tablets
- Pentazocine HCl and ASA
- Percodan® tablets
- Piroxicam capsules
- Ponstel® capsules
- Propoxyphene hydrochloride, aspirin and caffeine capsules
- Relafen® tablets
- Robaxisal® tablets
- Soma® compound and Soma® compound with codeine tablets
- Sulindac® tablets
- Synalgos®-DC capsules
- Talwin® compound caplets
- Tolectin® 200 and 600 tablets, DS capsules
- Tolmetin sodium tablets, capsules
- Toradol® IM, IV injection and tablets
- Trilisate® liquid and tablets
- Vicoprofen® tablets
- Voltaren® and Voltaren®-XR tablets

Continued

Form III-5 | Patient medication education: Products with NSAIDs.

As appears in Pasero, C., & McCaffery, M. *Pain assessment and pharmacologic management*, pp. 258-259, St. Louis, Mosby. Modified from Fox Chase Cancer Center/Pain Management, 2007, Philadelphia. © 2011, Pasero C, McCaffery M. May be duplicated for use in clinical practice.

PATIENT MEDICATION INFORMATION—cont'd

Non-Prescription Products with NSAIDs

- **Advil®:** Cold and Sinus caplets and tablets; Ibuprofen tablets, caplets, and gel caplets; Flu and Body Ache caplets; migraine liquidgels
- **Aleve®:** tablets, caplets, and gelcaps; Cold and Sinus caplets
- **Alka-Seltzer®:** Original, Extra Strength, Cherry and Lemon/Lime Effervescent Antacid and Pain Reliever; Alka-Seltzer PM
- **Anacin®:** Regular Strength, Extra Strength tablets
- **Bayer®:** Genuine Aspirin tablets and caplets, Extra Strength Plus Aspirin caplets, Extra Strength PM Aspirin Plus Sleep Aid, Extra Strength Arthritis Pain Regimen Formula, Extra Strength Aspirin caplets and tablets, Vanquish caplets

- **BC®:** Arthritis Strength Powder, Allergy Sinus Cold Powder, BC Powder, Sinus Cold Powder
- **Bufferin®:** all products
- **Dristan®:** Sinus Pain Formula
- **Ecotrin®:** Enteric Coated Aspirin Regular Strength, Enteric Coated Aspirin Maximum Strength
- **Excedrin®:** Extra Strength caplets, geltabs, tablets; migraine tablets
- **Goody's®:** Body Pain Formula powder, Extra Strength Headache powder, Extra Strength Pain Relief tablets
- **Halfprin®:** tablets
- **Midol®:** Maximum Strength Cramp Formula tablets
- **Motrin®:** IB caplets, tablets, and gelcaps; IB Pain Reliever/Fever Reducer tablets, caplets, and gelcaps; Migraine Pain caplets; Sinus/Headache caplets

Form III-5 | Cont'd.

References

Achariyapota, V., & Titapant, V. (2008). Relieving perineal pain after perineorrhaphy by diclofenac rectal suppositories: A randomized double-blinded placebo-controlled trial. *Journal of the Medical Association of Thailand*, 91(6), 799–804.

Agency for Healthcare Research and Quality (AHRQ). (2006). *Comparative effectiveness and safety of analgesics for osteoarthritis: Executive summary from AHRQ*. Available at http://www.medscape.com/viewarticle/547970. Accessed October 26, 2008.

Agency for Healthcare Research and Quality (AHRQ). (2007). Choosing non-opioid analgesics for osteoarthritis. *Clinician's Guide*. Available at http://effectivehealthcare.ahrq.gov/healthInfo.cfm?infotype=sg&DocID=5&ProcessID=2. Accessed July 24, 2008.

Agrawal, N. M., Campbell, D. R., Safdi, M. A., et al. (2000). Superiority of lansoprazole vs ranitidine in healing nonsteroidal anti-inflammatory drug-associated gastric ulcers: Results of a double-blind, randomized, multicenter study. *Archives of Internal Medicine*, 160(10), 1455–1461.

Airaksinen, O., Brox, J. I., Cedraschi, C., et al. (2006). European guidelines for the management of chronic nonspecific low back pain. *European Spine Journal*, 15(Suppl. 2), S192–S300.

Alano, M. A., Ngougmna, E., Ostrea, E. M., et al. (2001). Analysis of nonsteroidal antiinflammatory drugs in meconium and its relation to persistent pulmonary hypertension in the newborn. *Pediatrics*, 107(3), 519–523.

Altman, R. D. (2004). A rationale for combining acetaminophen and NSAIDs for mild-to-moderate pain. *Clinical and Experimental Rheumatology*, 22(1), 110–117.

Altman, R. D., Dreiser, R. L., Fisher, C. L., et al. (2009). Diclofenac sodium gel in patients with primary hand osteoarthritis: A randomized, double-blind, placebo-controlled trial. *The Journal of Rheumatology*, 36(9), 1991–1999.

Altman, R. D., Hochberg, M. C., Moskowitz, R. W., et al. (2000). Recommendations for the medical management of osteoarthritis of the hip and knee. *Arthritis and Rheumatism*, 43(9), 1905–1915.

Alzheimer's Disease Anti-inflammatory Prevention Trial Research Group. (2008). Cognitive function over time in the Alzheimer's Disease Anti-inflammatory Prevention Trial (ADAPT): Results of a randomized, controlled trial of naproxen and celecoxib. *Archives of Neurology*, 65(7), 896–905.

Ambler, J. J. S., Zideman, D. A., & Deakin, C. D. (2005). The effect of topical non-steroidal anti-inflammatory cream on the incidence and severity of cutaneous burns following external DC cardioversion. *Resuscitation*, 65(2), 173–178.

American Academy of Orthopaedic Surgeons (AAOS). (2008). *Treatment of osteoarthritis of the knee (non-arthroplasty)*. Available at http://www.aaos.org/Research/guidelines/GuidelineOAKnee.asp. Accessed March 9, 2009.

American Academy of Pediatrics (AAP). (2001). The transfer of drugs and other chemicals into human milk. *Pediatrics*, 108(3), 776–789. Available at http://aappolicy.aappublications.org/cgi/content/full/pediatrics%3b108/3/776. Accessed November 21, 2008.

American College of Rheumatology (ACR) Subcommittee on Osteoarthritis Guidelines. (2000). Recommendations for the medical management of osteoarthritis of the hip and knee:

2000 update. *Arthritis and Rheumatism*, 43(9), 1905–1915. Available at http://www.rheumatology.org/publications/guidelines/oa-mgmt/oa-mgmt.asp?aud=mem. Accessed July 23, 2008.

American Geriatrics Society (AGS). (2002). The management of persistent pain in older persons. *Journal of the American Geriatrics Society*, 50(1), 1–20.

American Geriatrics Society (AGS) Panel on Pharmacological Management of Persistent Pain in the Older Persons. (2009). The pharmacological management of persistent pain in older persons. *Journal of the American Geriatrics Society*, 57(8), 1331–1346.

American Pain Society (APS). (2003). *Principles of analgesic use in the treatment of acute pain and cancer pain.* (ed 5), Glenview, IL: APS.

Andersen, K. V., Pfeiffer-Jensen, M., Haraldsted, V., et al. (2007). Reduced hospital stay and narcotic consumption, and improved mobilization with local and intraarticular infiltration after hip arthroplasty: A randomized clinical trial of an intraarticular technique versus epidural infusion in 80 patients. *Acta Orthopaedica*, 78(2), 180–186.

Andersen, L. J., Poulsen, T., Krogh, B., et al. (2007). Postoperative analgesia in total hip arthroplasty: A randomized, double-blinded, placebo-controlled study on preoperative and postoperative ropivacaine, ketorolac, and adrenaline wound infiltration. *Acta Orthopaedica*, 78(2), 159–161.

Andersohn, F., Suissa, S., & Garbe, E. (2006). Use of first- and second-generation cyclooxygenase-2-selective nonsteroidal antiinflammatory drugs and risk of acute myocardial infarction. *Circulation*, 113(16), 1950–1957.

Anderson, J. L., Adams, C. D., Antman, E. M., et al. (2007). ACC/AHA 2007 guidelines for the management of patients with unstable angina/non-ST-elevation myocardial infarction: Executive summary. *Circulation*, 116(7), 803–877.

Andrade, R. J., Lucena, I., Fernandez, C. M., et al. (2005). Drug-induced liver injury: An analysis of 461 incidences submitted to the Spanish registry over a 10-year period. *Gastroenterology*, 129(2), 512–521.

Andrade, S. E., Gurwitz, J. H., Davis, R. L., et al. (2004). Prescription use in pregnancy. *American Journal of Obstetrics and Gynecology*, 191(2), 398–407.

Andri, L., & Falagiani, P. (2007). Safety of celecoxib in patients with cutaneous reactions due to ASA-NSAIDs intolerance. *Allergol Immunopathol (Madrid)*, 35(4), 126–129.

Antman, E. M., Bennett, J. S., Daugherty, A., et al. (2007). Use of nonsteroidal antiinflammatory drugs: An update for clinicians: A scientific statement from the American Heart Association. *Circulation*, 115(12), 1634–1642.

Antman, E. M., DeMets, D., & Loscalzo, J. (2005). Cyclooxygenase inhibition and cardiovascular risk. *Circulation*, 112(5), 759–770.

Anwari, J. S., & Iqbal, S. (2003). Antihistamines and potentiation of opioid induced sedation and respiratory depression. *Anaesthesia*, 58(5), 494–495.

Arber, N., Eagle, C. J., Spicak, J., et al. (2006). Celecoxib for the prevention of colorectal adenomatous polyps. *The New England Journal of Medicine*, 355(9), 885–895.

Arvanitakis, Z., Grodstein, F., Bienias, J. L., et al. (2008). Relation of NSAIDs to incident AD, change in cognitive function and AD pathology. *Neurology*, 70(23), 2219–2225.

Asano, T. K., & McLeod, R. S. (2004). Non steroidal anti-inflammatory drugs (NSAID) and aspirin for preventing colorectal adenomas and carcinomas. *Cochrane Database of Systematic Reviews*, (2) CD004079.

Ashburn, M. A., Caplan, R. A., Carr, D. B., et al. (2004). Practice guidelines for acute pain management in the perioperative setting. An updated report by the American Society of Anesthesiologists task force on acute pain management. *Anesthesiology*, 100(6), 1573–1581.

Ashraf, W., Wong, D. T., Ronayne, M., et al. (2004). Guidelines for preoperative administration of patients' home medications. *Journal of Perianesthesia Nursing*, 19(4), 228–233.

Atzori, L., Pinna, A. L., Pau, M., et al. (2006). Adverse cutaneous reactions to selective cyclooxygenase 2 inhibitors: Experience of an Italian drug-surveillance center. *Journal of Cutaneous Medicine and Surgery*, 10(1), 31–35.

Aubrun, F., Kalfon, F., Mottet, P., et al. (2003). Adjunctive analgesia with intravenous propacetamol does not reduce morphine-related adverse effects. *British Journal of Anaesthesia*, 90(3), 314–319.

Aygencel, G., Akbuga, B., & Keles, A. (2006). Acute pancreatitis following naproxen intake. *European Journal of Emergency Medicine*, 13(6), 372.

Babu, K. S., & Salvi, S. S. (2000). Aspirin and asthma. *Chest*, 118(5), 1470–1476.

Baer, P. A., Thomas, L. M., & Shainhouse, Z. (2005). Treatment of osteoarthritis of the knee with a topical diclofenac solution: A randomized controlled, 6-week trial. *BMC Musculoskeletal Disord*, 6, 44.

Bahar, M. M., Jangjoo, A., Soltani, E., et al. (2010). Effect of preoperative rectal indomethacin on postoperative pain reduction after open cholecystectomy. *Journal of Perianesthesia Nursing*, 25(1), 4–8.

Baker, J., Cotter, J. D., Gerrard, D. F., et al. (2005). Effects of indomethacin and celecoxib on renal function in athletes. *Medicine and Science in Sports and Exercise*, 37(5), 712–717.

Bakhos, C., Alkhoury, F., Kyriakides, T., et al. (2009). Early postoperative hemorrhage after open and laparascopic roux-en-y gastric bypass. *Obesity Surgery*, 19(2), 153–157.

Banning, M. (2008). Topical diclofenac: Clinical effectiveness and current uses in osteoarthritis of the knee and soft tissue injuries. *Expert Opinion on Pharmacotherapy*, 9(16), 2921–2929.

Bannwarth, B. (2006). Acetaminophen or NSAIDs for the treatment of osteoarthritis. *Clinical Rheumatology*, 20(1), 117–129.

Bannwarth, B. (2008). Safety of the nonselective NSAID nabumetone: Focus on gastrointestinal tolerability. *Drug Safety*, 31(6), 485–503.

Bannwarth, B., & Pehourcq, F. (2003). Pharmacologic basis for using paracetamol: Pharmacokinetics and pharmacodynamic issues. *Drugs*, 63(2), 5–13.

Barden, J., Edwards, J., McQuay, et al. (2003). Oral valdecoxib and injected parecoxib for acute postoperative pain: A quantitative systematic review. *BMC Anesthesiol*, 3(1), 1.

Barden, J., Edwards, J., Moore, R. A., et al. (2004). Single dose oral diclofenac for postoperative pain. *Cochrane Database of Systematic Reviews*, (2) CD004768.

Barkin, R. L., & Buvanendran, A. (2004). Focus on the COX-1 and COX-2 agents: Renal events of nonsteroidal and anti-inflammatory drugs—NSAIDs. *American Journal of Therapeutics*, 11(2), 124–129.

Basse, L., Billesbolle, P., & Kehlet, H. (2002). Early recovery after abdominal rectopexy with multimodal rehabilitation. *Diseases of the Colon and Rectum*, 45(2), 195–199.

Basse, L., Hjort Jakobsen, D., Billesbolle, P., et al. (2000). A clinical pathway to accelerate recovery after colonic resection. *Annals of Surgery*, 232(1), 51–57.

Basu, G. D., Pathangey, L. B., Tinder, T. L., et al. (2005). Mechanisms underlying the growth inhibitory effects of the cyclooxygenase-2 inhibitor celecoxib in human breast cancer cells. *Breast Cancer Research*, 7(4), R422–R435.

Bataller, R. M. (2007). Evidence for practice: Education about the dangers of acetaminophen. *Journal of Emergency Nursing*, 33(4), 327–330.

Battisti, W. P., Katz, N. P., Weaver, A. L., et al. (2004). Pain management in osteoarthritis: A focus on onset of efficacy— a comparison of rofecoxib, celecoxib, acetaminophen, and nabumetone across four clinical trials. *The Journal of Pain*, 5(9), 511–520.

Beck, D. H., Schenk, M. R., Hagemann, K., et al. (2000). The pharmacokinetics and analgesic efficacy of larger dose rectal acetaminophen (40 mg/kg) in adults: A double-blinded, randomized study. *Anesthesia and Analgesia*, 90(2), 431–436.

Bektas, F., Eken, C., Karadeniz, O., et al. (2009). Intravenous paracetamol or morphine for the treatment of renal colic: A randomized, placebo-controlled trial. *Annals of Emergency Medicine*, 54(4), 568–574.

Ben-David, B., Swanson, J., Nelson, J. B., et al. (2007). Multimodal analgesia for radical prostatectomy provides better analgesia and shortens hospital stay. *Journal of Clinical Anesthesia*, 19(4), 264–268.

Bennett, J. S., Daugherty, A., Herrington, D., et al. (2005). The use of nonsteroidal anti-inflammatory drugs (NSAIDs). A science advisory from the American Heart Association. *Circulation*, 111(13), 1713–1716.

Bertagnolli, M. M., Eagle, C. J., Zauber, A. G., et al. (2006). Celecoxib for the prevention of sporadic colorectal adenomas. *The New England Journal of Medicine*, 355(9), 873–884.

Bhatt, D. L., Scheiman, J., Abraham, N. S., et al. (2008). ACCF/ACG/AHA 2008 expert consensus document on reducing the gastrointestinal risks of antiplatelet therapy and NSAID use. *The American Journal of Gastroenterology*, 103(18), 2890–2907.

Birbara, C. A., Puopolo, A. D., Munoz, D. R., et al. (2003). Treatment of chronic low back pain with etoricoxib, a new cyclo-oxygenase selective inhibitor: Improvement in pain and disability—a randomized, placebo-controlled, 3-month trial. *The Journal of Pain*, 4(6), 307–315.

Bjornsson, E., & Olsson, R. (2005). Outcome and prognostic markers in severe drug-induced liver disease. *Hepatology (Baltimore, Md.)*, 42(2), 481–489.

Bolesta, S., & Haber, S. L. (2002). Hepatotoxicity associated with chronic acetaminophen administration in patients without risk factors. *The Annals of Pharmacotherapy*, 36(2), 331–333.

Bombardier, C., Laine, L., Reicin, A., et al. (2000). Comparison of upper gastrointestinal toxicity of rofecoxib and naproxen in patients with rheumatoid arthritis. *The New England Journal of Medicine*, 343(21), 1520–1528.

Bookman, A. A. M., Williams, K. S. A., & Shainhouse, J. Z. (2004). Effect of a topical solution for relieving symptoms of primary osteoarthritis of the knee: A randomized controlled trial. *Canadian Medical Association Journal*, 171(14), 333–338.

Botting, R. (2003). COX-2 and COX-3 inhibitors. *Thrombosis Research*, 110(5–6), 269–272.

Bradley, R. L., Ellis, P. E., Thomas, P., et al. (2007). A randomized clinical trial comparing the efficacy of ibuprofen and paracetamol in the control of orthodontic pain. *American Journal of Orthodontics and Dentofacial Orthopedics, 132*(4), 511–517.

Bradshaw, H. (2010). CB1-induced side effects of specific COX-2 inhibitors: A feature, not a bug. (Commentary). *Pain, 148*(1), 5.

Brater, D. C. (2002). Renal effects of cyclooxygenase-2-selective inhibitors. *Journal of Pain and Symptom Management, 23*(4 Suppl. 1), S15–S20.

Breda, A., Bui, M. H., Liao, J. C., et al. (2007). Association of bowel rest and ketorolac analgesia with short hospital stay after laparascopic donor nephrectomy. *Urology, 69*(5), 828–831.

Bresalier, R. S., Sandler, R. S., Quan, H., et al. (2005). Cardiovascular events associated with rofecoxib in a colorectal adenoma chemoprevention trial. *The New England Journal of Medicine, 352*(11), 1092–1102.

Brok, J., Buckley, N., & Gluud, C. (2006). Interventions for paracetamol (acetaminophen) overdose. *Cochrane Database of Systematic Reviews,* (2) CD003328.

Bromley, L. (2006). Pre-emptive analgesia and protective premedication. (2006). What is the difference? *Biomedicine & Pharmacotherapy, 60*(7), 336–340.

Brophy, J. M., Levesque, L. E., & Zhang, B. (2007). The coronary risk of cyclooxygenase-2 inhibitors in patients with a previous myocardial infarction. *Heart (British Cardiac Society), 93*(2), 189–194.

Brown, C., Moodie, J., Bisley, E., et al. (2009). Intranasal ketorolac for postoperative pain: A phase 3, double-blind, randomized study. *Pain Medicine (Malden, Mass.), 10*(6), 1106–1114.

Brown, T. J., Hooper, L., Elliott, R. A., et al. (2006). A comparison of the cost-effectiveness of five strategies for the prevention of non-steroidal anti-inflammatory drug-induced gastrointestinal toxicity: A systematic review with economic modeling. *Health Technology Assessment (Winchester, England), 10*(38), 1–202.

Brune, K. (2003). COX-2 inhibitors and the kidney: A word of caution. *IASP Pain Clinical Updates, 11*(4), 1–2.

Bucci, F. A., & Waterbury, L. D. (2008). Comparison of ketorolac 0.4% and bromfenac 0.09% at trough dosing: Aqueous drug absorption and prostaglandin E2 levels. *Journal of Cataract and Refractive Surgery, 34*(9), 1509–1512.

Burke, A., Smyth, E., & FitzGerald, G. A. (2006). Analgesic-antipyretic agents: Pharmacotherapy of gout. In L. L. Brunton, J. S. Lazo, & K. L. Parker (Eds.), *Goodman & Gilman's the pharmacological basis of therapeutics.* (11th ed.). New York, NY: McGraw-Hill.

Busch, C. A., Shore, B. J., Bhandari, R., et al. (2006). Efficacy of periarticular multimodal drug injection in total knee Arthroplasty. *Journal of Bone and Joint Surgery, 88a*(5), 959–963.

Busti, A. J., Hooper, J. S., Amaya, C. J., et al. (2005). Effects of perioperative antiinflammatory and immunomodulating therapy on surgical wound healing. *Pharmacotherapy, 25*(11), 1566–1591.

Buvanendran, A., Kroin, J. S., & Berger, R. A. (2007). Preoperative cyclooxygenase-2 inhibitor treatment reduces the incidence of heterotropic ossification after hip arthroplasty: Six-month follow-up. (Correspondence). *Anesthesiology, 107*(2), 358–359.

Cahill, R. A., McGreal, G. T., Crowe, B. H., et al. (2005). Duration of increased bleeding tendency after cessation of aspirin therapy. *Journal of the American College of Surgeons, 200*(4), 564–573.

Cairns, B. E., Mann, M. K., Mok, E., et al. (2008). Diclofenac exerts local anesthetic-like actions on rat masseter muscle afferent fibers. *Brain Research, 1194*(4), 56–64.

Cannon, C. P., Curtis, S. P. O., FitzGerald, G. A., et al. (2006). Cardiovascular outcomes with etoricoxib and diclofenac in patients with osteoarthritis and rheumatoid arthritis in the multinational etoricoxib and diclofenac arthritis long-term (MEDAL) programme: A randomized comparison. *Lancet, 368*(9549), 1771–1781.

Capone, M. L., Sciulli, M. G., Tacconelli, S., et al. (2005). Pharmacodynamic interaction of naproxen with low-dose aspirin in healthy subjects. *Journal of the American College of Cardiology, 45*(8), 1295–1301.

Carli, F., Mayo, N., Klubien, K., et al. (2002). Epidural analgesia enhances functional exercise capacity and health-related quality of life after colonic surgery. *Anesthesiology, 97*(3), 540–549.

Case, J. P., Baliunas, A. J., & Block, J. A. (2003). Lack of efficacy of acetaminophen in treating symptomatic knee osteoarthritis. *Archives of Internal Medicine, 163*(2), 169–178.

Cassinelli, E. H., Dean, C. L., Garcia, R. M., et al. (2008). Ketorolac use for postoperative pain management following lumbar decompression surgery: A prospective, randomized, double-blinded, placebo-controlled trial. *Spine, 33*(12), 1313–1317.

Catella-Lawson, F., Reilly, M. P., Kapoor, S. C., et al. (2001). Cyclooxygenase inhibitors and the antiplatelet effects of aspirin. *The New England Journal of Medicine, 345*(25), 1809–1817.

Celiker, R., Arslan, S., & Inanici, F. (2002). Corticosteroid injection vs. nonsteroidal antiinflammatory drug and splinting in carpal tunnel syndrome. *American Journal of Physical Medicine & Rehabilitation, 81*(3), 182–186.

Cepeda, M. S., Carr, D. B., Miranda, N., et al. (2005). Comparison of morphine, ketorolac, and their combination for postoperative pain. *Anesthesiology, 103*(6), 1225–1232.

Chan, A. T., Manson, J. E., Albert, C. M., et al. (2006). Nonsteroidal antiinflammatory drugs, acetaminophen, and risk of cardiovascular events. *Circulation, 113*(12), 1578–1587.

Chan, F. K., Abraham, N. S., Scheiman, J. M., et al. (2008). Management of patients on nonsteroidal anti-inflammatory drugs: A clinical practice recommendation from the first international working party on gastrointestinal and cardiovascular effects of nonsteroidal anti-inflammatory drugs and anti-platelet agents. *The American Journal of Gastroenterology, 103*(11), 2908–2918.

Chan, F. K. L., & Graham, D. Y. (2004). Prevention of nonsteroidal anti-inflammatory drug gastrointestinal complications—Review and recommendations based on risk assessment. *Alimentary Pharmacology & Therapeutics, 19*(10), 1051–1061.

Chan, F. K. L., Hung, L. C. T., Suen, B. Y., et al. (2004). Celecoxib versus diclofenac plus omeprazole in high-risk arthritis patients: Results of a randomized double-blind trial. *Gastroenterology, 127*(4), 1038–1043.

Chan, F. K. L., To, K. F., Wu, J. C. Y., et al. (2002). Eradication of helicobacter pylori and risk of peptic ulcers in patients starting long-term treatment with non-steroidal anti-inflammatory drugs: A randomised trial. *Lancet, 359*(9300), 9–13.

Chan, F. K. L., Wong, V. W., Suen, B. Y., et al. (2007). Combination of a cyclo-oxygenase-2 inhibitor and a proton-pump inhibitor for prevention of recurrent ulcer bleeding in patients at very high risk: A double-blind, randomised trial. *Lancet, 369*(9573), 1621–1626.

Chang, D. J., Desjardins, P. J., King, T. R., et al. (2004). The analgesic efficacy of etoricoxib compared with oxycodone/acetaminophen in an acute postoperative pain model: A randomized, double-blind clinical trial. *Anesthesia and Analgesia, 99*(3), 807–815.

Chantler, I., Mitchell, D., & Fuller, A. (2009). Diclofenac potassium attenuates dysmenorrhea and restores exercise performance in women with primary dysmenorrhea. *The Journal of Pain, 10*(2), 191–200.

Chen, J. Y., Ko, T. L., Wen, Y. R., et al. (2009). Opioid-sparing effects of ketorolac and its correlation with the recovery of postoperative bowel function in colorectal surgery patients. A prospective randomized double-blinded study. *The Clinical Journal of Pain, 25*(6), 485–489.

Chia, Y. Y., Lo, Y., Liu, K., et al. (2004). The effect of promethazine on postoperative pain: A comparison of preoperative, postoperative, and placebo administration in patients following total abdominal hysterectomy. *Acta Anaesthesiologica Scandinavica, 48*(5), 625–630.

Chibnall, J. T., Tait, R. C., Harman, B., et al. (2005). Effect of acetaminophen on behavior, well-being, and psychotropic medication use in nursing home residents with moderate-to-severe dementia. *Journal of the American Geriatrics Society, 53*(11), 1921–1929.

Chin, K. R., Sundram, H., & Marcotte, P. (2007). Bleeding risk with ketorolac after lumbar microdiscectomy. *Journal of Spinal Disorders & Techniques, 20*(2), 123–126.

Chou, R., Qaseem, A., Snow, V., et al. (2007). Diagnosis and treatment of low back pain: A joint clinical practice guideline from the American College of Physicians and the American Pain Society. *Annals of Internal Medicine, 147*(7), 478–491.

Chyka, P. A., Erdman, A. R., Christianson, G., et al. (2007). Salicylate poisoning: An evidence-based consensus guideline for out-of-hospital management. *Clinical Toxicology (Phila), 45*(2), 95–131.

Colditz, G. A. (1995). The Nurses' Health Study: A cohort of U.S. women followed since 1976. *Journal of the American Medical Women's Association, 50*(2), 40–44.

Collins, S., Moore, R. A., McQuay, H. J., et al. (2000). Single dose oral ibuprofen and diclofenac for postoperative pain. *Cochrane Database of Systematic Reviews,* (2) CD001548.

Coloma, M., White, P. F., Huber, P. J., et al. (2000). The effect of ketorolac on recovery after anorectal surgery: Intravenous versus local administration. *Anesthesia and Analgesia, 90*(5), 1107–1110.

Colucci, R. D., Wright, C., Mermelstein, F. H., et al. (2009). Dyloject, a novel injectable diclofenac solubilised with cyclodextrin: Reduced incidence of thrombophlebitis compared to injectable diclofenac solubilised with polyethylene glycol and benzyl alcohol. *Acute Pain, 11*(1), 15–21.

Coyne, P. J., Hansen, A. L., Watson, A. C. (2003). Compounded drugs. *The American Journal of Nursing, 103*(5), 78–79 81, 84–85.

Critchley, J. A. J. H., Critchley, L. A. H., Anderson, P. J., et al. (2005). Differences in the single-oral-dose pharmacokinetics and urinary excretion of paracetamol and its conjugates between Hong Kong Chinese and Caucasian subjects. *Journal of Clinical Pharmacy and Therapeutics, 30*(2), 179.

Crofford, L. J., Oates, J. C., McCune, W. J., et al. (2000). Thrombosis in patients with connective tissue diseases treated with specific cyclooxygenase 2 inhibitors: A report of four cases. *Arthritis and Rheumatism, 43*(8), 1891–1896.

Cryer, B. (2004). COX-2-specific inhibitor or proton pump inhibitor plus traditional NSAID: Is either approach sufficient for patients at highest risk of NSAID-induced ulcers? *Gastroenterology, 127*(4), 1256–1262.

Cryer, B., Berlin, R. G., Cooper, S. A., et al. (2005). Double-blind, randomized, parallel, placebo-controlled study of ibuprofen effects on thromboxane b2 concentrations in aspirin-treated healthy adult volunteers. *Clinical Therapeutics, 27*(2), 185–191.

Curhan, G. C., Knight, E. L., Rosner, B., et al. (2004). Lifetime nonnarcotic analgesic use and decline in renal function in women. *Archives of Internal Medicine, 164*(14), 1519–1524.

Curhan, G. C., Willett, W. C., Rosner, B., et al. (2002). Frequency of analgesic use and risk of hypertension in younger women. *Archives of Internal Medicine, 162*(19), 2204.

Curtis, S. P., Bockow, B., Fisher, C., et al. (2005). Etoricoxib in the treatment of osteoarthritis over 52-weeks: A double-blind, active-comparator controlled trial. *BMC Musculoskeletal Disorders, 6,* 58.

D'Cruz, D. P. (2006). Systemic lupus erythematosus. *BMJ (Clinical Research Ed.), 332*(7546), 890–894.

Dahl, J. B., & Moiniche, S. (2004). Pre-emptive analgesia. *British Medical Bulletin, 71*(1), 13–27.

Dahl, V., Dybvik, T., Steen, T., et al. (2004). Ibuprofen vs. acetaminophen vs. Ibuprofen and acetaminophen after arthroscopically assisted anterior cruciate ligament reconstruction. *European Journal of Anaesthesiology, 21*(6), 471–475.

Dahlen, B., Szczeklik, A., Murray, J. J. (2001). Celecoxib in patients with aspirin-induced asthma (letter). *The New England Journal of Medicine, 344*(2), 142.

Dajani, E. Z., & Islam, K. (2008). Cardiovascular and gastrointestinal toxicity of selective cyclo-oxygenase-2 inhibitors in man. *Journal of Physiology and Pharmacology, 59*(Suppl. 1), 117–133.

Daly, F. F., O'Malley, G. F., Heard, K., et al. (2004). Prospective evaluation of repeated supratherapeutic acetaminophen (paracetamol) ingestion. *Annals of Emergency Medicine, 44*(4), 399–400.

Dawson, W. (2010). *Diclofenac sodium topical gel (Voltaren)—Stronger hepatic toxicity warning.* http://updates.pain-topics.org/2010/01/jan2010-pain-product-announcements.html. Accessed January 4, 2010.

de Carvalho, J. F., Bonfa, E., & Borba, F. F. (2008). Systemic lupus erythematosus and "lupus dyslipoproteinemia". *Autoimmunity Reviews, 7*(3), 246–250.

Dedier, J., Stampfer, M. J., Hankinson, S. E., et al. (2002). Nonnarcotic analgesic use and the risk of hypertension in US women. *Hypertension, 40*(5), 604–608.

DeMaria, A. N., & Weir, M. R. (2003). Coxibs—beyond the GI tract: Renal and cardiovascular issues. *Journal of Pain and Symptom Management, 25*(2S), S41–S45.

Department of Health and Human Services (DHHS). (2008). *Phenacetin and analgesic mixtures containing phenacetin. Report on carcinogens.* (11th ed.). Available at http://ntp.niehs.nih.gov/ntp/roc/eleventh/profiles/s143phen.pdf. Accessed December 24, 2008.

Derry, S., Barden, J., McQuay, H. J., et al. (2008). Single dose oral celecoxib for acute postoperative pain in adults. *Cochrane Database of Systematic Reviews*, (4) CD004233.

Diamond, S., Balm, T. K., & Freitag, F. G. (2000). Ibuprofen plus caffeine in the treatment of tension-type headache. *Clinical Pharmacology and Therapeutics*, 68(3), 312–319.

Diamond, S., & Freitag, F. G. (2001). The use of ibuprofen plus caffeine to treat tension-type headache. *Current Pain and Headache Reports*, 5(5), 472–478.

Diblasio, C. J., Snyder, M. E., Kattan, M. W., et al. (2004). Ketorolac: Safe and effective analgesia for the management of renal cortical tumors with partial nephrectomy. *The Journal of Urology*, 17(3), 1062–1065.

Dong, X. D., Svensson, P., & Cairns, B. E. (2009). The analgesic action of topical diclofenac may be mediated through peripheral NMDA receptor antagonism. *Pain*, 147(1–3), 36–45.

Dorr, L. D., Raya, J., Long, W. T., et al. (2008). Multimodal analgesia without parenteral narcotics for total knee arthroplasty. *The Journal of Arthroplasty*, 23(4), 502–508.

Drago, F., Brusati, C., Desirello, G., et al. (2004). Cutaneous vasculitis induced by cyclo-oxygenase-2 selective inhibitors. *Journal of the American Academy of Dematology*, 51(6), 1029–1030.

Drug facts and comparisons. (2006). St. Louis, MO: Wolters Kluwer Health.

Dsida, R., & Cote, C. J. (2004). Nonsteroidal antiinflammatory drugs and hemorrhage following tonsillectomy: Do we have the data? *Anesthesiology*, 100(3), 749–751.

Dula, D. J., Anderson, R., & Wood, G. C. (2001). A prospective study comparing IM ketorolac with IM meperidine in the treatment of acute biliary colic. *The Journal of Emergency Medicine*, 20(2), 121–124.

Duong, H. V. Q., Westfield, K. C., & Chalkley, T. H. F. (2007). Ketorolac tromethamine LS 0.4% versus nepafenac 0.1% in patients having cataract surgery: Prospective randomized double-masked clinical trial. *Journal of Cataract and Refractive Surgery*, 33(11), 1925–1929.

Dworkin, R. H., O'Connor, A. B., Backonja, M., et al. (2007). Pharmacologic management of neuropathic pain: Evidence-based recommendations. *Pain*, 132(3), 237–251.

Edwards, J. E., Loke, Y. K., Moore, R. A., et al. (2000). Single dose oral piroxicam for acute postoperative pain. *Cochrane Database of Systematic Reviews*, (4) CD002762.

Edwards, J. E., Oldman, A., Smith, L., et al. (2000). Single dose oral aspirin for acute pain. *Cochrane Database of Systematic Reviews*, (2) CD002067.

Einhorn, T. A. (2002a). Use of COX-2 inhibitors in patients with fractures. Is there a trade off between pain relief and healing? *Am Acad Orthop Surg Bull*, 50(5).

Einhorn, T. A. (2002b). Do inhibitors of cyclooxygenase-2 impair bone healing? *Journal of Bone and Mineral Research*, 17(6), 977–978.

Einhorn, T. A. (2003a). Cox-2 inhibitors and fracture healing: Arguments for such an effect and a suggestion about caution in use. *Journal of Bone and Mineral Research*, 18(3), 584.

Einhorn, T. A. (2003b). Cox-2. Where are we in 2003? The role of cyclooxygenase-2 in bone repair. *Arthritis Research*, 5(1), 5–7.

Elia, N., Lysakowski, C., & Tramer, M. R. (2005). Does multimodal analgesia with acetaminophen, nonsteroidal antiinflammatory drugs, or selective cyclooxygenase-2-inhibitors and patient-controlled analgesia morphine offer advantages over morphine alone? Meta-analyses of randomized trials. *Anesthesiology*, 103(6), 1295–1304.

El Miedany, Y., Youssef, S., Ahmed, I., et al. (2006). Safety of etoricoxib, a specific cyclooxygenase-2 inhibitor, in asthmatic patients with aspirin-exacerbated respiratory disease. *Annals of Allergy, Asthma & Immunology*, 97(1), 105–109.

El-Tahan, M. R., Warda, O. M., Yasseen, A. M., et al. (2007). A randomized study of the effects of preoperative ketorolac on general anaesthesia for Caesarean section. *International Journal of Obstetric Anesthesia*, 16(3), 214–220.

Emery, P., Zeidler, H., Kvien, K. D., et al. (1999). Celecoxib versus diclofenac in long-term management of rheumatoid arthritis: Randomised double-blind comparison. *Lancet*, 354(9196), 2106–2111.

Engeler, D. S., Ackermann, D. K., Osterwalder, J. J., et al. (2005). A double-blind, placebo controlled comparison of the morphine sparing effect of oral rofecoxib and diclofenac for acute renal colic. *The Journal of Urology*, 174(3), 933–936.

Esparza, F., Cobian, C., Jimenez, J. F., et al. (2007). Topical ketoprofen TDS patch versus diclofenac gel: Efficacy and tolerability in benign sport related soft-tissue injuries. *British Journal of Sports Medicine*, 41(3), 134–139.

Farkouh, M. E., Kirshner, H., Harrington, R. A., et al. (2004). Comparison of lumiracoxib with naproxen and ibuprofen in the therapeutic arthritis research and gastrointestinal event trial (TARGET), cardiovascular outcomes: Randomised controlled trial. *Lancet*, 364(9435), 675–684.

Feinstein, A. R., Heinemann, A. L., Dalessio, D., et al. (2000). Do caffeine-containing analgesics promote dependence? A review and evaluation. *Clinical Pharmacology and Therapeutics*, 68(5), 457–467.

Fick, D. M., Cooper, J. W., Wade, W. E., et al. (2003). Updating the Beers criteria for potentially inappropriate medication use in older adults. *Archives of Internal Medicine*, 163(22), 2716–2724.

FitzGerald, G. A. (2004). Coxibs and cardiovascular disease. *The New England Journal of Medicine*, 351(17), 1709–1711.

FitzGerald, G. A., & Patrono, C. (2001). The coxibs, selective inhibitors of cyclooxygenase-2. *The New England Journal of Medicine*, 345(6), 433–442.

Fitzgerald, K., & Buggy, D. (2006). Nonconventional and adjunctive analgesia. In G. Shorten, D. B. Carr, & D. Harmon, et al. (Eds.), *Postoperative pain management: An evidence-based guide to practice*. Philadelphia: Saunders.

Fontana, R. J. (2008). Acute liver failure due to drugs. *Seminars in Liver Disease*, 28(2), 175–187.

Fored, C. M., Ejerblad, E., Lindblad, P., et al. (2001). Acetaminophen, aspirin, and chronic renal failure. *The New England Journal of Medicine*, 345(25), 1801–1808.

Forman, J. P., Rimm, E. B., & Curhan, G. C. (2007). Frequency of analgesic use and risk of hypertension among men. *Archives of Internal Medicine*, 167(4), 394–399.

Forman, J. P., Stampfer, M. J., & Curhan, G. C. (2005). Non-narcotic analgesic dose and risk of incident hypertension in US women. *Hypertension*, 46(3), 500–507.

Forrest, J. B., Camu, F., Greer, I. A., et al. (2002). Ketorolac, diclofenac, and ketoprofen are equally safe for pain relief after major surgery. *British Journal of Anaesthesia*, 88(2), 227–233.

Forster, U., & Olze, H. (2008). Analgesic intolerance. Key position of ENT physicians for early detection of this condition (translated from German). *HNO*, 56(4), 443–450.

Fotuhi, M., Zandi, P. P., Hayden, K. M., et al. (2008). Better cognitive performance in elderly taking antioxidant vitamins

E and C supplements in combination with nonsteroidal anti-inflammatory drugs: The Cache County Study. *Alzheimers Dement*, 4(3), 223–227.

Fox, C. S., Coady, S., Sorlie, P. D., et al. (2007). Increasing cardiovascular disease burden due to diabetes mellitus. The Framingham heart study. *Circulation*, 115(12), 1544–1550.

Fox, J. M., & Siebers, U. (2003). Caffeine as a promoter of analgesic-associated nephropathy—where is the evidence? *Fundamental & Clinical Pharmacology*, 17(3), 377–392.

Frampton, J. E., & Keating, G. M. (2007). Celecoxib: A review of its use in the management of arthritis and acute pain. *Drugs*, 67(16), 2433–2472.

Fransen, M., & Neal, B. (2004). Non-steroidal anti-inflammatory drugs for preventing heterotopic bone formation after hip arthroplasty. *Cochrane Database of Systematic Reviews*, (3) CD001160.

Freyer, A. M. (2008). Drug-prescribing challenges during pregnancy. *Obstetrics and Gynecology*, 18(7), 180–186.

Gabriel, S. E., Jaakkimainen, L., & Bombardier, C. (1991). Risk for serious gastrointestinal complications related to use of nonsteroidal anti-inflammatory drugs. A meta-analysis. *Annals of Internal Medicine*, 115(10), 787–796.

Gajraj, N. M. (2003). The effect of cyclooxygenase-2 inhibitors on bone healing. *Regional Anesthesia and Pain Medicine*, 28(5), 456–465.

Galer, B. S., Rowbotham, M., Perander, J., et al. (2000). Topical diclofenac patch relieves minor sports injury pain: Results of a multicenter controlled clinical trial. *Journal of Pain and Symptom Management*, 19(4), 287–294.

Garner, S. E., Fidan, D. D., Frankish, R. R., et al. (2002). Celecoxib for rheumatoid arthritis. *Cochrane Database of Systematic Reviews*, (4) CD003831.

Geba, G. P., Weaver, A. L., Polis, A. B., et al. (2002). Efficacy of rofecoxib, celecoxib, and acetaminophen in osteoarthritis of the knee. A randomized trial. *JAMA: The Journal of the American Medical Association*, 286(24), 64–71.

Gebauer, M. G., Nyfort-Hansen, K., Henschke, P. J., et al. (2003). Warfarin and acetaminophen interaction. *Pharmacotherapy*, 23(1), 109–112.

Gerstenfeld, L. C., Al-Ghawas, M., Alkhiary, Y. M., et al. (2007). Selective and nonselective cyclooxygenase-2 inhibitors and experimental fracture healing. Reversibility of effects after short-term treatment. *The Journal of Bone and Joint Surgery. American Volume*, 89(1), 114–125.

Gerstenfeld, L. C., & Einhorn, T. A. (2004). COX inhibitors and their effects on bone healing. *Expert Opinion on Drug Safety*, 3(2), 131–136.

Gerstenfeld, L. C., Thiede, M., Seibert, K., et al. (2003). Differential inhibition of fracture healing by non-selective and cyclooxygenase-2 selective non-steroidal anti-inflammatory drugs. *Journal of Orthopaedic Research*, 21(4), 670–675.

Gianni, W., Madaio, R. A., Di Cioccio, L., et al. (2009). Prevalence of pain in elderly hospitalized patients. *Archives of Gerontology and Geriatrics*, doi: 10.1016/jarchger.2009.11.016.

Giannoudis, P. V., MacDonald, D. A., Matthews, S. J., et al. (2000). Nonunion of femoral diaphysis. *The Journal of Bone and Joint Surgery*, 82B(5), 655–658.

Girard, P., Pansart, Y., Coppe, M. C., et al. (2004). Role of the histamine system in nefopam-induced antinociception in mice. *European Journal of Pharmacology*, 503(1), 63–69.

Gislason, G. H., Jacobsen, S., Rasmussen, J. N., et al. (2006). Risk of death or reinfarction associated with the use of selective cyclooxygenase-2 inhibitors and nonselective nonsteroidal antiinflammatory drugs after acute myocardial infarction. *Circulation*, 113(25), 2906–2913.

Glasser, D. L., & Burroughs, S. H. (2003). Valdecoxib-induced toxic epidermal necrolysis in a patient allergic to sulfa drugs. *Pharmacotherapy*, 23(4), 551–553.

Glassman, S. D., Rose, S. M., Dimar, J. R., et al. (1998). The effect of postoperative antiinflammatory drug administration on spinal fusion. *Spine*, 23(7), 834–838.

Goldenberg, N. A., Jacobson, L., & Manco-Johnson, M. J. (2005). Platelet function after taking ibuprofen for 1 week. *Annals of Internal Medicine*, 142(7), 506–509.

Goldstein, J., Silberstein, S. D., Saper, J. R., et al. (2006). Acetaminophen, aspirin, and caffeine in combination versus ibuprofen for acute migraine: Results from a multicenter, double-blind, randomized, parallel-group, single-dose, placebo-controlled study. *Headache*, 46(3), 444–453.

Goldstein, J. L., Eisen, G. M., Burke, T. A., et al. (2002). Dyspepsia tolerability from the patients' perspective: A comparison of celecoxib with diclofenac. *Alimentary Pharmacology & Therapeutics*, 16(4), 819–827.

Goldstein, J. L., Eisen, G. M., Lewis, B., et al. (2005). Video capsule endoscopy to prospectively assess small bowel injury with celecoxib, naproxen plus omeprazole, and placebo. *Clinical Gastroenterology and Hepatology*, 3(2), 133–141.

Goldstein, J. L., Eisen, G. M., Lewis, B., et al. (2007). Small bowel mucosal injury is reduced in healthy subjects treated with celecoxib compared with ibuprofen plus omeprazole, as assessed by video capsule endoscopy. *Alimentary Pharmacology & Therapeutics*, 25(10), 1211–1222.

Goldstein, L. B., Adams, R., Alberts, M. J., et al. (2006). Primary prevention of ischemic stroke. A guideline from the American Heart Association/American Stroke Association Stroke Council: Cosponsored by the Atherosclerotic Peripheral Nursing Council; Clinical Cardiology Council; Nutrition, Physical Activity, and Metabolism Council; and the Quality of Care and Outcomes Research Interdisciplinary Working Group. *Circulation*, 113(24), e873–e923.

Goodman, S., Ma, T., Trindade, M., et al. (2002). COX-2 selective NSAID decreases bone ingrowth in vivo. *Journal of Orthopaedic Research*, 20(6), 1164–1169.

Graham, D. J. (2006). COX-2 inhibitors, other NSAIDs, and cardiovascular risk. The seduction of common sense. (Editorial). *JAMA: The Journal of the American Medical Association*, 296(13), 1653–1656.

Graham, D. J., Agrawal, N. M., Campbell, D. R., et al. (2002). Ulcer prevention in long-term users of nonsteroidal anti-inflammatory drugs. *Archives of Internal Medicine*, 162(2), 169–175.

Graham, D. J., Campen, D., Hui, R., et al. (2005). Risk of acute myocardial infarction and sudden cardiac death in patients treated with cyclo-oxygenase 2 selective and non-selective non-steroidal anti-inflammatory drugs: Nested case-control study. *Lancet*, 365(9458), 475–481.

Graham, G. G., Scott, K. F., & Day, R. O. (2005). Tolerability of paracetamol. *Drug Safety*, 28(3), 227–240.

Grape, S., & Tramer, M. R. (2007). Do we need preemptive analgesia for the treatment of postoperative pain? *Best Practice & Research. Clinical Anaesthesiology*, 21(1), 51–63.

Grodstein, F., Sharupski, K. A., Bienias, J. L., et al. (2008). Anti-inflammatory agents and cognitive decline in a bi-racial population. *Neuroepidemiology*, 30(1), 45–50.

Grosser, T., Fries, S., & FitzGerald, G. A. (2006). Biologic basis for cardiovascular consequences of COX-2 inhibition: Therapeutic challenges and opportunities. *The Journal of Clinical Investigation*, 116(1), 4–15.

Hanlon, J. T., Backonja, M., Weiner, D., et al. (2009). Evolving pharmacological management of persistent pain in older persons. *Pain Medicine (Malden, Mass.)*, 10(6), 959–961.

Hardt, J., Jacobsen, C., Goldberg, J., et al. (2008). Prevalence of chronic pain in a representative sample in the United States. *Pain Medicine (Malden, Mass.)*, 9(7), 803–812.

Harris, R. E. (2009). Cyclooxygenase-2 (COX-2) blockade in the chemoprevention of cancers of the colon, breast, prostate, and lung. *Inflammopharmacology*, 17(2), 55-67.

Harris, R. E., Beebe-Donk, J., & Alshafie, G. A. (2006). Reduction in the risk of human breast cancer by selective cyclooxygenase-2 (COX-2) inhibitors. *BMC Cancer*, 6, 27.

Harris, R. E., Beebe-Donk, J., & Alshafie, G. A. (2007). Cancer chemoprevention by cyclooxygenase 2 (COX-2) blockade: Results of case control studies. *Sub-cellular Biochemistry*, 42, 193–212.

Harris, R. E., Beebe-Donk, J., & Alshafie, G. A. (2008). Similar reductions in the risk of human colon cancer by selective and nonselective cyclooxygenase-2 (COX-2) inhibitors. *BMC Cancer*, 8, 237.

Harris, R. E., Beebe-Donk, J., Doss, H., et al. (2005). Aspirin, ibuprofen, and other non-steroidal anti-inflammatory drugs in cancer prevention: A critical review of non-selective COX-2 blockade. *Oncology Reports*, 13(4), 559–583.

Harris, R. E., Beebe-Donk, J., & Schuller, H. M. (2002). Chemoprevention of lung cancer by non-steroidal anti-inflammatory drugs among cigarette smokers. *Oncology Reports*, 9(4), 693–695.

Hassani, A., Ponvert, C., Karila, C., et al. (2008). Hypersensitivity to cyclooxygenase inhibitory drugs in children. A study of 164 cases. *European Journal of Dermatology*, 18(5), 561–565.

Hawkcy, C. J., Ell, C., Simon, B., et al. (2008). Less small-bowel injury with lumiracoxib compared with naproxen plus omeprazole. *Clinical Gastroenterology and Hepatology*, 6(5), 536–544.

Hawkey, C. J., Karrasch, J. A., Szczepanski, L., et al. (1998). Omeprazole compared with misoprostol for ulcers associated with nonsteroidal antiinflammatory drugs. *The New England Journal of Medicine*, 338(11), 727–734.

Hayashi, Y., Yamamoto, H., Kita, H., et al. (2005). Non-steroidal anti-inflammatory drug-induced small bowel injuries identified by double-balloon endoscopy. *World Journal of Gastroenterolology*, 11(2), 4861–4864.

Hayden, K. M., Zandi, P. P., Khachaturian, A. S., et al. (2007). Does NSAID use modify cognitive trajectories in the elderly? The Cache County Study. *Neurology*, 69(3), 275–282.

Hedner, T., Samulesson, O., Wahrborg, P., et al. (2004). Nabumetone: Therapeutic use and safety profile in the management of osteoarthritis and rheumatoid arthritis. *Drugs*, 64(20), 2315–2343.

Helstrom, J., & Rosow, C. E. (2006). Nonsteroidal anti-inflammatory drugs in postoperative pain. In G. Shorten, D. B. Carr, & D. Harmon, et al. (Eds.), *Postoperative pain management: An evidence-based guide to practice*. Philadelphia: Saunders.

Henderson, S. O., Swadron, S., & Newton, E. (2002). Comparison of intravenous ketorolac and meperidine in the treatment of biliary colic. *The Journal of Emergency Medicine*, 23(3), 237–241.

Hermann, M., Krum, H., & Ruschitzka, F. (2005). To the heart of the matter. Coxibs, smoking, and cardiovascular risk. *Circulation*, 112(7), 941–945.

Hernandez-Diaz, S., Varas-Lorenzo, C., & Rodriguez, L. A. (2006). Non-steroidal antiinflammatory drugs and the risk of acute myocardial infarction. *Basic & Clinical Pharmacology & Toxicology*, 98(3), 266–274.

Hernandez-Palazon, J., Tortosa, J. A., Martinez-Lage, J. F., et al. (2001). Intravenous administration of propacetamol reduces morphine consumption after spinal fusion surgery. *Anesthesia and Analgesia*, 92(6), 1473–1476.

Heyneman, C. A., Lawless-Liday, C., & Wall, G. C. (2000). Oral versus topical NSAIDs in rheumatic diseases: A comparison. *Drugs*, 60(3), 555–574.

Hochberg, M. C., Melin, J. M., & Reicin, A. (2003). Cox-2 inhibitors and fracture healing: An argument against such an effect. (Letter to Editor). *Journal of Bone and Mineral Research*, 18(3), 583.

Holdgate, A., & Pollock, T. (2005). Nonsteroidal anti-inflammatory drugs (NSAIDS) versus opioids for acute renal colic. *Cochrane Database of Systematic Reviews*, 18(2) CD004137.

Holubek, W., Stolbach, A., Nurok, S., et al. (2007). A report of two deaths from massive ibuprofen ingestion. *Journal of Medical Toxicology*, 3(2), 52–55.

Hong, Y., Gengo, F. M., Rainka, M. M., et al. (2008). Population pharmacodynamic modeling of aspirin- and ibuprofen-induced inhibition of platelet aggregation in healthy subjects. *Clinical Pharmacokinetics*, 47(2), 129–137.

Hoozemans, J. J., Rozemuller, J. M., van Haastert, E. S., et al. (2008). Cyclooxygenase-1 and -2 in the different stages of Alzheimer's disease pathology. *Current Pharmaceutical Design*, 14(14), 1419–1427.

Hsieh, L. F., Hong, C. Z., Chern, S. H., et al. (2010). Efficacy and side effects of diclofenac patch in treatment of patients with myofascial pain syndrome of the upper trapezius. *Journal of Pain and Symptom Management*, 39(1), 116–125.

Huang, J. Q., Sridhar, S., & Hunt, R. H. (2002). Role of helicobacter pylori infection and nonsteroidal anti-inflammatory drugs in peptic ulcer disease: A meta-analysis. *Lancet*, 359(9300), 14–22.

Huang, Y. M., Wang, C. M., Wang, C. T., et al. (2008). Perioperative celebrex administration for pain management after total knee arthroplasty—A randomized, controlled study. *BMC Musculoskeletal Disorders*, 9, 77.

Hudson, M., Rahme, E., Richard, H., et al. (2007). Risk of congestive heart failure with nonsteroidal antiinflammatory drugs and selective COX 2 inhibitors: A class effect? *Arthritis and Rheumatism*, 15(57), 516–523.

Hughes, S. (2006). MEDAL: Etoricoxib shows same thrombotic cardiovascular risk as diclofenac. *Heartwire*. Available at http://www.medscape.com/viewarticle/547814. Accessed August 15, 2008.

Hughes, S. (2007). COX-2 inhibitors with low-dose aspirin for patients at risk of CV events? *Heartwire*. Available at http://www.medscape.com/viewarticle/567951. Accessed August 16, 2008.

Hunter, D. J., & Lo, G. H. (2008). The management of osteoarthritis: An overview and call to appropriate conservative treatment. *Rheumatic Diseases Clinics of North America,* *34*(3), 689–712.

Hyllested, M., Jones, S., Pedersen, J. L., et al. (2002). Comparative effect of paracetamol, NSAIDs or their combination in postoperative pain management: A qualitative review. *British Journal of Anaesthesia,* *88*(2), 199–214.

Issioui, T., Klein, K. W., White, P. F., et al. (2002). The efficacy of celecoxib and acetaminophen in preventing pain after otolaryngologic surgery. *Anesthesia and Analgesia,* *94*(5), 1188–1193.

Jacobsen, R. B., & Phillips, B. B. (2004). Reducing clinically significant gastrointestinal toxicity associated with nonsteroidal antiinflammatory drugs. *The Annals of Pharmacotherapy,* *38*(9), 1469–1481.

James, A. H., Brancazio, L. R., & Price, T. (2008). Aspirin and reproductive outcomes. *Obstetrical & Gynecological Survey,* *63*(1), 49–57.

James, T. N. (2000). Homage to James B. Herrick: A contemporary look at myocardial infarction and at sickle-cell heart disease. *Circulation,* *101*(15), 1874–1887.

Jensen, K., Kehlet, H., & Lund, C. M. (2007). Post-operative recovery profile after laparoscopic cholecystectomy: A prospective, observational study of a multimodal anaesthetic regime. *Acta Anaesthesiologica Scandinavica,* *51*(4), 464–471.

Jerde, T. J., Calamon-Dixon, J. L., Bjorling, D. E., et al. (2005). Celecoxib inhibits ureteral contractility and prostanoids release. *Urology,* *65*(1), 185–190.

Johns Hopkins Medicine. (2008). *Caffeine experts at Johns Hopkins call for warning labels on energy drinks.* (Press Release). Available at http://www.hopkinsmedicine.org/Press_releases/2008/09_24_08.html. Accessed December 24, 2008.

Jordan, K. M., Arden, N. K., Doherty, M., et al. (2003). EULAR Recommendations 2003: an evidence based approach to the management of knee osteoarthritis: Report of a Task Force of the Standing Committee for International Clinical Studies Including Therapeutic Trials (ESCISIT). *Annals of the Rheumatic Diseases,* *62*(12), 1145–1155.

Jorgensen, B., Gottrup, F., Karlsmark, T., et al. (2008). Combined use of an ibuprofen-releasing foam dressing and silver dressing on infected leg ulcers. *Journal of Wound Care,* *17*(5), 210–214.

Joshi, G. P., Gertler, R., & Fricker, R. (2007). Cardiovascular thromboembolic adverse effects associated with cyclooxygenase-2 selective inhibitors and nonselective antiinflammatory drugs. *Anesthesia and Analgesia,* *105*(6), 1793–1804.

Jousilahti, P., Vartiainen, E., Tuomilehto, J., et al. (1999). Sex, age, cardiovascular risk factors, and coronary heart disease. *Circulation,* *99*(9), 1165–1172.

Kauser, F., & Davis, M. P. (2006). Ketorolac in neuropathic pain. *Journal of Pain and Symptom Management,* *32*(3), 202–204.

Kearney, P. M., Baigent, C., Godwin, J., et al. (2006). Do selective cyclo-oxygenase-2 inhibitors and traditional non-steroidal anti-inflammatory drugs increase the risk of atherothrombosis? Meta-analysis of randomised trials. *BMJ (Clinical Research Ed.),* *332*(7553), 1302–1308.

Kehlet, H. (2005). Postoperative opioid sparing to hasten recovery (Editorial). *Anesthesiology,* *102*(6), 1083–1085.

Kehlet, H., & Wilmore, D. W. (2008). Evidence-based surgical care and the evolution of fast-track surgery. *Annals of Surgery,* *248*(2), 189–198.

Kelly, D. J., Ahmad, M., & Brull, S. J. (2001). Preemptive analgesia II: Recent advances and current trends. *Canadian Journal of Anaesthesia,* *48*(11), 1091–1101.

Kelly, J. P., Coogan, P., Strom, B. L., et al. (2008). Lung cancer and regular use of aspirin and nonaspirin nonsteroidal anti-inflammatory drugs. *Pharmacoepidemiology and Drug Safety,* *17*(4), 322–327.

Khanna, D., Arnold, E. L., Pencharz, J. N., et al. (2006). Measuring process of arthritis care: The Arthritis Foundation's quality indicator set for rheumatoid arthritis. *Seminars in Arthritis and Rheumatism,* *35*(4), 211–237.

Kharasch, E. D. (2004). Perioperative COX-2 inhibitors: Knowledge and challenges. *Anesthesia and Analgesia,* *98*(1), 1–3.

Khuder, S. A., & Mutgi, A. B. (2001). Breast cancer and NSAID use: A meta-analysis. *British Journal of Cancer,* *84*(9), 1186–1192.

Kim, A., & Stark, W. J. (2008). Are topical NSAIDs needed for routine cataract surgery? *Am J Opthalmol,* *146*(4), 483–485.

Kim, S. J., Lo, W. R., Hubbard, G. B., et al. (2008). Topical ketorolac in vitreoretinal surgery: A prospective, randomized, placebo-controlled, double-masked trial. *Arch Opthalmol,* *126*(9), 1203–1208.

Kim, S. Y., Kim, E. M., Nam, K. H., et al. (2008). Postoperative intravenous patient-controlled analgesia in thyroid surgery: Comparison of fentanyl and ondansetron regimens with and without the nonsteroidal anti-inflammatory drug ketorolac. *Thyroid,* *18*(12), 1285–1290.

Knowles, S. R., Drucker, A. M., Weber, E. A., et al. (2007). Management options for patients with aspirin and nonsteroidal antiinflammatory drug sensitivity. *The Annals of Pharmacotherapy,* *41*(7), 1191–1200.

Knowles, S. R., Phillips, E. J., Wong, G., et al. (2004). Serious dermatologic reaction associated with valdecoxib: Report of two cases. *Journal of the American Academy of Dermatology,* *51*(6), 1028–1029.

Koklu, E., Gurgoze, M., Akgun, H., et al. (2006). Renal tubular dysgenesis with atypical histology and in-utero exposure to naproxen sodium. *Annals of Tropical Paediatrics,* *26*(3), 241–245.

Kovac, S. H., Mikuls, T. R., Mudano, A., et al. (2006). Health-related quality of life among self-reported arthritis sufferers: Effects of race/ethnicity and residence. *Quality of Life Research,* *15*(3), 451–460.

Kuffner, E. K., & Dart, R. C. (2001). Acetaminophen use in patients who drink alcohol: Current study evidence. *Pharmacy Times,* 4–8.

Kurella, M., Bennett, W. M., & Chertow, G. M. (2003). Analgesia in patients with ESRD: A review of available evidence. *American Journal of Kidney Diseases,* *42*(2), 217–228.

Kurth, T., Glynn, R. J., Walker, A. M., et al. (2003). Inhibition of clinical benefits of aspirin on first myocardial infarction by nonsteroidal antiinflammatory drugs. *Circulation,* *108*(10), 1191–1195.

Kurth, T., Hennekens, C. H., Sturmer, T., et al. (2005). Analgesic use and subsequent risk of hypertension in apparently healthy men. *Archives of Internal Medicine,* *165*(16), 1903–1909.

Kvalsvik, O., Borchgrevink, P. C., Hagen, L., et al. (2003). Randomized, double-blind, placebo-controlled study of the effect of rectal paracetamol on morphine consumption after abdominal hysterectomy. *Acta Anaesthesiologica Scandinavica,* *47*(4), 451–456.

Lahtinen, P., Kokki, H., Hendolin, H., et al. (2002). Propacetamol as adjunctive treatment for postoperative pain after cardiac surgery. *Anesthesia and Analgesia,* *95*(4), 813–819.

Laine, L. (2001). Approaches to nonsteroidal anti-inflammatory drug use in the high-risk patient. *Gastroenterology*, 120(3), 594–606.

Laine, L., Curtis, S. P., Cryer, B., et al. (2007). Assessment of upper gastrointestinal safety of etoricoxib and diclofenac in patients with osteoarthritis and rheumatoid arthritis in the multinational etoricoxib and diclofenac arthritis long-term (MEDAL) programme: A randomised comparison. *Lancet*, 369(9560), 465–473.

Laine, L., Curtis, S. P., Langman, M., et al. (2008). Lower gastrointestinal events in a double-blind trial of the cyclo-oxygenase-2 selective inhibitor etoricoxib and the traditional nonsteroidal anti-inflammatory drug diclofenac. *Gastroenterology*, 135(5), 1517–1525.

Laine, L., White, W. B., Rostom, A., et al. (2008). COX-2 selective inhibitors in the treatment of osteoarthritis. *Seminars in Arthritis and Rheumatism*, 38(3), 165–187.

Lake, A. P. J., & Khater, M. (2004). Effects of postoperative nonsteroidal antiinflammatory drugs on bleeding risk after tonsillectomy (Letter to the Editor). *Anesthesiology*, 100(3), 748–749.

Lanas, A., Bajador, E., Serrano, P., et al. (2000). Nitrovasodilators, low-dose aspirin, other nonsteroidal antiinflammatory drugs, and the risk of upper gastrointestinal bleeding. *The New England Journal of Medicine*, 343(12), 834–839.

Lane, S. S., Modi, S. S., Lehmann, R. P., et al. (2007). Nepafenac opthalmic 0.1% for the prevention and treatment of ocular inflammation associated with cataract surgery. *Journal of Cataract and Refractive Surgery*, 33(1), 53–58.

Langford, R. M., & Mehta, V. (2006). Selective cyclooxygenase inhibition: Its role in pain and anaesthesia. *Biomedicine & Pharmacotherapy*, 60(7), 323–328.

Larsen, J. B., & Pedersen, S. T. (2006). Non-steroidal anti-inflammatory agents—potential risks of use during pregnancy. *Ugeskrift for Laeger*, 168(43), 3709–3711.

Larson, A. M., Polson, J., Fontana, R. J., et al. (2005). Acetaminophen-induced acute liver failure: Results of a United States multicenter, prospective study. *Hepatology (Baltimore, Md.)*, 42(6), 1364–1372.

Launay-Vacher, V., Karie, S., Fau, J. B., et al. (2005). Treatment of pain in patients with renal insufficiency: The World Health Organization three-step ladder adapted. *The Journal of Pain*, 6(3), 137–148.

Layton, D., Marshall, V., Boshier, A., et al. (2006). Serious skin reactions and selective COX-2 inhibitors: A case series from prescription-event monitoring in England. *Drug Safety*, 29(8), 687–696.

Lee, A., Cooper, M. G., Craig, J. C., et al. (2007). Effects of nonsteroidal anti-inflammatory drugs on postoperative renal function in adults with normal renal function. *Cochrane Database of Systematic Reviews*, 18(2) CD002765.

Leimgruber, A. (2008). Allergic reactions to nonsteroidal anti-inflammatory drugs (translated from French). *Revue Medicale Suisse*, 4(140), 100–103.

Lenz, H., & Raeder, J. (2008). Comparison of etoricoxib vs. ketorolac in postoperative pain relief. *Acta Anaesthesiologica Scandinavica*, 52(9), 1278–1284.

Leo, R. J. (2008). Safe analgesic use in patients with renal dysfunction. *Pract Pain Manage*, 12(22), 27.

Li, D. K., Liu, L., & Odouli, R. (2003). Exposure to non-steroidal anti-inflammatory drugs during pregnancy and risk of miscarriage: Population based cohort study. *BMJ (Clinical Research Ed.)*, 327(7411), 368–372.

Liccardi, G., Cazzola, M., De Giglio, C., et al. (2005). Safety of celecoxib in patients with adverse skin reactions to acetaminophen (paracetamol) and other non-steroidal anti-inflammatory drugs. *Journal of Investigational Allergology & Clinical Immunology*, 15(4), 249–253.

Lin, J., Zhang, W., Jones, A., et al. (2004). Efficacy of topical non-steroidal anti-inflammatory drugs in the treatment of osteoarthritis: Meta-analysis of randomized controlled trials. *BMJ (Clinical Research Ed.)*, 329(7461), 324–327.

Lin, T. F., Yeh, Y. C., Yen, Y. H., et al. (2005). Antiemetic and analgesic-sparing effects of diphenhydramine added to morphine intravenous patient-controlled analgesia. *British Journal of Anaesthesia*, 94(6), 835–839.

Linton, M. F., & Fazio, S. (2002). Cyclooxygenase-2 and atherosclerosis. *Current Opinion in Lipidology*, 13(5), 497–504.

Liu, S. S., & Wu, C. L. (2007a). The effect of analgesic technique on postoperative patient-reported outcomes including analgesia: A systematic review. *Anesthesia and Analgesia*, 105(3), 789–808.

Liu, S. S., & Wu, C. L. (2007b). Effect of postoperative analgesia on major postoperative complications: A systematic update of the evidence. *Anesthesia and Analgesia*, 104(3), 689–702.

Luqmani, R., Hennell, S., Estrach, C., et al. (2009). British Society for Rheumatology and British Health Professionals in Rheumatology guideline for the management of rheumatoid arthritis (after the first 2 years). *Rheumatology*, 48(4), 436–439.

Magill, P., Ridgway, P. F., Conlon, K. C., et al. (2006). A case of probable ibuprofen-induced acute pancreatitis. *JOP: Journal of the Pancreas*, 7(3), 311–314.

Mahe, I., Bertrand, N., Drouet, L., et al. (2005). Paracetamol: An haemorrhagic risk factor in patients on warfarin. *British Journal of Clinical Pharmacology*, 59(3), 371–374.

Mahe, I., Bertrand, N., Drouet, L., et al. (2006). Interaction between paracetamol and warfarin in patients: A double-blind, placebo controlled, randomized study. *Haematologica*, 91(12), 1621–1627.

Malan, T. P., Marsh, G., Hakki, S. I., et al. (2003). Parecoxib sodium, a parenteral cyclooxygenase-2 selective inhibitor, improves morphine analgesia and is opioid-sparing following total hip arthroplasty. *Anesthesiology*, 98(4), 950–956.

Manek, N. J., & MacGregor, A. J. (2005). Epidemiology of back disorders: Prevalence, risk factors, and prognosis. *Current Opinion in Rheumatology*, 17(2), 134–140.

Mangiapane, S., Blettner, M., & Schlattmann, P. (2008). Aspirin use and breast cancer risk: A meta-analysis and meta-regression of observational studies from 2001 to 2005. *Pharmacoepidemiology and Drug Safety*, 17(2), 115–124.

Marchand, S. (2008). The physiology of pain mechanisms: From the periphery to the brain. *Rheumatic Diseases Clinics of North America*, 34(2), 285–309.

Marjoribanks, J., Proctor, M. L., & Farquhar, C. (2003). Nonsteroidal anti-inflammatory drugs for primary dysmenorrhoea. *Cochrane Database of Systematic Reviews*, (2) CD003855.

Marks, F., Harrell, K., & Fischer, R. (2001). Successful use of cyclooxygenase-2 inhibitor in a patient with aspirin-induced asthma. *Southern Medical Journal*, 94(2), 256–257.

Marret, E., & Bonnet, F. (2007). Perioperative anti-inflammatory drug use: Which evidences for their utility and safety? *Annales Francaises d'anesthesie et de Reanimation*, 26(6), 535–539.

Marret, E., Flahault, A., Samama, C. M., et al. (2003). Effects of postoperative, nonsteroidal, antiinflammatory drugs on bleeding risk after tonsillectomy. *Anesthesiology, 98*(6), 1497–1502.

Marret, E., Kurdi, O., Zufferey, P., et al. (2005). Effects of nonsteroidal antiinflammatory drugs on patient-controlled analgesia morphine side effects. *Anesthesiology, 102*(6), 1249–1260.

Mason, L., Edwards, J. E., Moore, R. A., et al. (2004a). Single dose oral naproxen and naproxen sodium for acute postoperative pain. *Cochrane Database of Systematic Reviews, 18*(4) CD004234.

Mason, L., Moore, R. A., Edwards, J. E., et al. (2004b). Systematic review of efficacy of topical rubefacients containing salicylates for the treatment of acute and chronic pain. *BMJ (Clinical Research Ed.), 328*(7446), 991–994.

Mason, L., Moore, R. A., Edwards, J. E., et al. (2004c). Topical NSAIDs for acute pain: A meta-analysis. *BMC Family Practice, 5*, 10.

Mason, L., Moore, R. A., Edwards, J. E., et al. (2004). Topical NSAIDs for chronic musculoskeletal pain: Systematic review and meta-analysis. *BMC Musculoskeletal Disorders, 5*, 28.

Mayo Clinic.com. (2008). *Caffeine: How much is too much?* Available at http://www.mayoclinic.com/health/caffeine/NU00600. Accessed December 24, 2008.

Mazieres, B. (2005). Topical ketoprofen patch. *Drugs in R&D, 6*(6), 337–344.

Mazieres, B., Rouanet, S., Guillon, Y., et al. (2005). Topical ketoprofen patch in the treatment of tendinitis: A randomized, double blind, placebo controlled study. *The Journal of Rheumatology, 32*(8), 1563–1570.

McAdam, B. F., Byrne, D., Morrow, J. D., et al. (2005). Contribution of cyclooxygenase-2 to elevated biosynthesis of thromboxane A2 and prostacyclin in cigarette smokers. *Circulation, 112*(7), 1024–1029.

McAdam, B. F., Catella-Lawson, F., Mardini, I. A., et al. (1999). Systemic biosynthesis of prostacylin by cyclooxygenase (COX)-2: The human pharmacology of a selective inhibitor of COX-2. *Proceedings of the National Academy of Sciences of the United States of America, 96*(1), 272–277.

McAleer, S. D., Majid, O., Venables, E., et al. (2007). Pharmacokinetics and safety of ketorolac following single intranasally and intramuscular administration in healthy volunteers. *Journal of Clinical Pharmacology, 47*(1), 13–18.

McCleane, G. (2008). Topical analgesic agents. *Clinics in Geriatric Medicine, 24*(2), 299–312.

McCormack, J., & Power, I. (2009). Nonsteroidal antiinflammatory drugs and acetaminophen: Pharmacology for the future. In R. S. Sinatra, O. A. de Leon-Casasola, Ginsberg, et al. (Eds.), *Acute pain management.* New York, NY: Cambridge University Press.

McDermott, M. M., Fried, L., Simonsick, E., et al. (2000). Asymptomatic peripheral artery disease is independently associated with lower extremity functioning. The women's health and aging study. *Circulation, 101*(9), 1007–1012.

McGettigan, P., & Henry, D. (2006). Cardiovascular risk and inhibition of cyclooxygenase: A systematic review of the observational studies of selective and nonselective inhibitors of cyclooxygenase 2. *JAMA: The Journal of the American Medical Association, 296*(13), 1633–1644.

McNicol, E. D., Strassels, S., Goudas, L., et al. (2005). NSAIDS or paracetamol, alone or combined with opioids, for cancer pain. *Cochrane Database of Systematic Reviews, 25*(1) CD005180.

McQuay, H. J., & Moore, A. (2004). Non-opioid analgesics. In D. Doyle, G. Hanks, & I. Cherny, et al. (Eds.), *Oxford textbook of palliative medicine.* (3rd ed.)New York, NY: Oxford Press.

McQuay, H. J., & Moore, R. A. (2006). Dose-response in direct comparisons of different doses of aspirin, ibuprofen, and paracetamol (acetaminophen) in analgesic studies. *British Journal of Clinical Pharmacology, 63*(3), 271–278.

Medscape Medical News. (2005). *FDA brief shows CV risk with etoricoxib and uncertainty over lumiracoxib.* Available at http://www.medscape.com/viewarticle/53811. Accessed August 13, 2008.

Medscape Medical News. (June 12, 2009). *FDA approves ibuprofen injection to treat pain and fever.* Available at http://www.medscape.com/viewarticle704331. Accessed June 25, 2009.

Medscape Rheumatology. (2006). *Update on pain management with COX-2 inhibitors: An expert interview with Michael E. Farkouh, MD, MSc, FAAC.* Available at http://www.medscape/com/viewarticle/548669. Accessed December 13, 2006.

Mellemkjaer, L., Biot, W., & Sorensen, H. (2002). Upper gastrointestinal bleeding among users of NSAIDs: A population based cohort study in Denmark. *British Journal of Clinical Pharmacology, 53*(2), 173–181.

Mercadante, S., Serretta, R., & Casuccio, A. (2001). Effects of caffeine as an adjunct to morphine in advanced cancer patients: A randomized, double-blind, placebo-controlled, crossover study. *Journal of Pain and Symptom Management, 21*(5), 369–372.

Merry, A. F., Gibbs, R. D., Edwards, J., et al. (2009). Combined acetaminophen and ibuprofen for pain relief after oral surgery in adults: A randomized controlled trial. *British Journal of Anaesthesia, 104*(1), 80–88.

Meunier, A., Lisander, B., & Good, L. (2007). Effects of celecoxib on blood loss, pain, and recovery of function after total knee replacement: A randomized placebo-controlled trial. *Acta Orthopaedica, 78*(5), 661–667.

Miaskowski, C., Cleary, J., Burney, R., et al. (2005). *Guideline for the management of cancer pain in adults and children.* Glenview, IL: American Pain Society.

Michielsen, P., Heinemann, L., Mihatsch, M., et al. (2009). Non-phenacetin analgesics and analgesic nephropathy: Clinical assessment of high users from a case-control study. *Nephrology, Dialysis, Transplantation, 24*(4), 1253–1259.

Miranda, H. F., Puig, M. M., Prieto, J. C., et al. (2006). Synergism between paracetamol and non steroidal anti-inflammatory drugs in experimental acute pain. *Pain, 121*(1–2), 22–28.

Mitchell, A., van Zanten, S. V., Inglis, K., et al. (2008). A randomized controlled trial comparing acetaminophen plus ibuprofen versus acetaminophen plus codeine plus caffeine after outpatient general surgery. *Journal of the American College of Surgeons, 206*(3), 472–479.

Miyoshi, H. R. (2001). Systemic nonopioid analgesics. In J. D. Loeser, S. H. Butler, & R. Chapman, et al. (Eds.), *Bonica's management of pain.* (3rd ed.). Philadelphia: Lippincott Williams & Wilkins.

Mobarakeh, J. I., Takahashi, K., Sakurada, S., et al. (2006). Enhanced antinociceptive effects of morphine in histamine H2 receptor gene knockout mice. *Neuropharmacology, 51*(3), 612–622.

Moiniche, S., Kehlet, H., & Dahl, J. B. (2002). A qualitative and quantitative systematic review of preemptive analgesia for postoperative pain relief. *Anesthesiology, 96*(3), 725–741.

Moller, P. L., Juhl, G. I., Payen-Champenois, C., et al. (2005). Intravenous acetaminophen (paracetamol): Comparable analgesic efficacy, but better local safety than its prodrug, propacetamol, for postoperative pain after third molar surgery. *Anesthesia and Analgesia, 101*(1), 90–96.

Moller, P. L., Sindet-Pedersen, S., Petersen, C. T., et al. (2005). Onset of acetaminophen analgesia: Comparison of oral and intravenous routes after third molar surgery. *British Journal of Anaesthesia, 94*(5), 642–648.

Monsivais, D., & McNeill, J. (2007). Multicultural influences on pain medication attitudes and beliefs in patients with nonmalignant chronic pain syndromes. *Pain Management Nursing, 8*(2), 64–71.

Moodie, J. E., Brown, C. R., Bisley, E. J., et al. (2008). The safety and analgesic efficacy of intranasal ketorolac in patients with postoperative pain. *Anesthesia and Analgesia, 107*(6), 2025–2031 See Erratum in *Anesthesia and Analgesia, 108*(3), 991 (corrected dose from 30 mg to 31.5 mg).

Moore, L. E. (2008). Recurrent risk of adverse pregnancy outcome. *Obstetrics and Gynecology Clinics of North America, 35*(3), 458–471.

Moore, R. A., Derry, S., & McQuay, H. J. (2008). Topical agents in the treatment of rheumatic pain. *Rheumatic Diseases Clinics of North America, 34*(2), 415–432.

Moore, R. A., Derry, S., Phillips, C. J., et al. (2006). Nonsteroidal anti-inflammatory drugs (NSAIDs), cyclooxygenase-2-selective inhibitors (coxibs) and gastrointestinal harm: Review of clinical trials and clinical practice. *BMC Musculoskeletal Disorders, 7*, 79.

Moore, R. A., Rees, J., Loke, Y., et al. (2010). Single dose oral piroxicam for acute postoperative pain. *Cochrane Database of Systematic Reviews* 2000, Issue 2. Art. No.: CD002762. DOI: 10.10002/14651858.CD002762.

Motov, S. M., & Ast, T. D. (2008). Is there a limit to the analgesic effect of pain medications. *Medscape Emergency Medicine,* . Available at http://www.medscape.com/viewarticle/574279. Accessed June 30, 2008.

Moulin, D. E., Clark, A. J., Gilron, I., et al. (2007). Pharmacological management of chronic neuropathic pain—Consensus statement and guidelines from the Canadian Pain Society. *Pain Research & Management, 12*(1), 13–21.

Munsterhjelm, E., Munsterhjelm, N. M., Niemi, T. T., et al. (2005). Dose-dependent inhibition of platelet function by acetaminophen in healthy volunteers. *Anesthesiology, 103*(4), 712–717.

Munsterhjelm, E., Niemi, T. T., Syrjala, M. T., et al. (2003). Propacetamol augments inhibition of platelet function by diclofenac in volunteers. *British Journal of Anaesthesia, 91*(3), 357–362.

Muscat, J. E., Chen, S. Q., Richie, J. P., et al. (2003). Risk of lung carcinoma among users of nonsteroidal antiinflammatory drugs. *Cancer, 97*(7), 1732–1736.

Muth-Selbach, U. S., Tegeder, I., Brune, K., et al. (1999). Acetaminophen inhibits spinal prostaglandin E2 release after peripheral noxious stimulation. *Anesthesiology, 91*(1), 231–239.

Myers, R. P., Shaheen, M., Li, B., et al. (2008). Impact of liver disease, alcohol abuse, and unintentional ingestions on the outcomes of acetaminophen overdose. *Clinical Gastroenterology and Hepatology, 6*(8), 918–925.

Nastase, A., Ioan, S., Braga, R. I., et al. (2007). Coffee drinking enhances the analgesic effect of cigarette smoking. *Neuroreport, 18*(9), 921–924.

National Cancer Institute. (2004). *COX-2 inhibitors and cancer: Questions and answers.* Available at http://www.cancer.gov/cancertopics/factsheet/APCtrialCOX2QandA. Accessed October 26, 2008.

National Collaborating Centre for Chronic Conditions (NCC-CC). (2008). *Osteoarthritis: National clinical guideline for care and management in adults.* London: Royal College of Physicians. Available at http://www.nice.org.uk/nicemedia/pdf/CG059FullGuideline.pdf. Accessed November 29, 2008.

National Institutes of Health (NIH). (2004). *Use of nonsteroidal antiinflammatory drugs suspended in large Alzheimer's disease prevention trial.* Available at http://www.nih.gov/news/pr/dec2004/od-20.htm. Accessed August 17, 2008.

Neilipovitz, D. T., Bryson, G. L., & Nichol, G. (2001). The effect of perioperative aspirin therapy in peripheral vascular surgery: A decision analysis. *Anesthesia and Analgesia, 93*(3), 573–580.

Nemergut, E. C., Durieux, M. E., Missaghi, N. B., et al. (2007). Pain management after craniotomy. *Best Practice & Research. Clinical Anaesthesiology, 21*(4), 557–573.

Ng, A., Parker, J., Toogood, L., et al. (2002). Does the opioid-sparing effect of rectal diclofenac following total abdominal hysterectomy benefit the patient? *British Journal of Anaesthesia, 88*(5), 714–716.

Ng, A., Swami, A., Smith, G., et al. (2008). Early analgesic effects of intravenous parecoxib and rectal diclofenac following laparoscopic sterilization: A double-blind, double-dummy randomized controlled trial. *Journal of Opioid Management, 4*(1), 49–53.

Niethard, F. U., Gold, M. S., Solomon, G. S., et al. (2005). Efficacy of topical diclofenac diethylamine gel in osteoarthritis of the knee. *Journal of Rheumatology, 32*(12), 2384–2392.

Norman, P. H., Daley, M. D., & Lindsey, R. W. (2001). Preemptive analgesic effects of ketorolac in ankle fracture surgery. *Anesthesiology, 94*(4), 599–603.

Nussmeier, N. A., Whelton, A. A., Brown, M. T., et al. (2005). Complications of the COX-2 inhibitors parecoxib and valdecoxib after cardiac surgery. *The New England Journal of Medicine, 352*(11), 1081–1091.

O'Connor, J. P. (2003). Cox-2 inhibitors and fracture healing: Arguments for such an effect and a suggestion about caution in use (Reply). *Journal of Bone and Mineral Research, 18*(3), 585–586.

Ofori, B., Oraichi, D., Blais, L., et al. (2006). Risk of congenital anomalies in pregnant users of non-steroidal anti-inflammatory drugs: A nested case-control study. *Birth Defects Research. Part B, Development and Reproductive Toxicology, 77*(4), 268–279.

Olsen, J. C., McGrath, N. A., Schwarz, D. G., et al. (2008). A double-blind randomized clinical trial evaluating the analgesic efficacy of ketorolac versus butorphanol for patients with suspected biliary colic in the emergency department. *Academic Emergency Medicine, 15*(8), 718–722.

O'Malley, G. F. (2007). Emergency department management of the salicylate-poisoned patient. *Emergency Medicine Clinics of North America, 25*(2), 333–346.

Ong, C. K. S., Lirk, P., Seymour, R. A., et al. (2005). The efficacy of preemptive analgesia for acute postoperative pain management: A meta-analysis. *Anesthesia and Analgesia*, *100*(3), 757–773.

Ornetti, P., Ciappuccini, R., Tavernier, C., et al. (2005). Interaction between paracetamol and oral anticoagulants. *Rheumatology (Oxford)*, *44*(12), 1584–1585.

Ott, E., Nussmeier, N. A., Duke, P. C., et al. (2003). Efficacy and safety of the cyclooxygenase 2 inhibitors parecoxib and valdecoxib in patients undergoing coronary artery bypass surgery. *The Journal of Thoracic and Cardiovascular Surgery*, *125*(6), 1481–1492.

Palangio, M., Morris, E., Doyle, R. T., et al. (2002). Combination hydrocodone and ibuprofen versus combination oxycodone and acetaminophen in the treatment of severe acute low back pain. *Clinical Therapeutics*, *24*(1), 87–99.

Palao, I., Domenech, R., Romanelli, M., et al. (2008). Effect of an ibuprofen-releasing foam dressing on wound pain: A real-life RCT. *Journal of Wound Care*, *17*(8), 342, 344–348.

Pallay, R. M., Seger, W., Adler, J. L., et al. (2004). Etoricoxib reduced pain and disability and improved quality of life in patients with chronic low back pain: A 3 month, randomized, controlled trial. *Scandinavian Journal of Rheumatology*, *33*(4), 257–266.

Pangilinan, J. M. (2008). Do antihistamines relieve drug-induced bone pain? *Medscape Pharmacists*. Available at http://www/medscape.com/viewarticle/566300. Accessed January 23, 2008.

Parra, D., Beckey, N. P., & Stevens, G. R. (2007). The effect of acetaminophen on the international normalized ratio in patients on warfarin therapy. *Pharmacotheraphy*, *27*(5), 675–683.

Pasero, C. (2007). Procedure-specific pain management: PROSPECT. *Journal of Perianesthesia Nursing*, *22*(5), 335–340.

Pasero, C. (2010). Perioperative rectal administration of analgesics. *Journal of Perianesthesia Nursing*, *25*(1), 1–3.

Pasero, C., & Belden, J. (2006). Evidence-based perioperative care: Accelerated postoperative recovery programs. *Journal of Perianesthesia Nursing*, *21*(3), 168–177.

Pasero, C., & McCaffery, M. (1999). Opioids by the rectal route. *The American Journal of Nursing*, *99*(11), 20.

Pasero, C., & McCaffery, M. (2007). Orthopaedic postoperative pain management. *Journal of Perianesthesia Nursing*, *22*(3), 160–173.

Patrono, C., Patrignani, P., & Rodriguez, L. A. (2001). Cyclooxygenase-selective inhibition of prostanoid formation: Transducing biochemical selectivity into clinical readouts. *The Journal of Clinical Investigation*, *108*(1), 7–13.

Paulson, S. K., Hribar, J. D., Liu, N. W., et al. (2000). Metabolism and excretion of [(14)C] celecoxib in healthy male volunteers. *Drug Metabolism and Disposition*, *28*(3), 308–314.

Pearson, T. A., Blair, S. N., Daniels, S. R., et al. (2002). AHA guidelines for primary prevention of cardiovascular disease and stroke: 2002 update. Consensus panel guide to comprehensive risk reduction for adult patients without coronary or other atherosclerotic vascular diseases. *Circulation*, *106*(4), 388–391.

Peila, R., & Launer, L. J. (2006). Inflammation and dementia: Epidemiologic evidence. *Acta Neurologica Scandinavica. Supplementum*, *185*(S185), 102–106.

Pereg, D., & Lishner, M. (2005). Nonsteroidal anti-inflammatory drugs for the prevention and treatment of cancer. *Journal of Internal Medicine*, *258*(2), 115–123.

Persky, V., Piorkowski, J., Hernandez, E., et al. (2008). Prenatal exposure to acetaminophen and respiratory symptoms in the first year of life. *Ann Allergy Asthma Immunol*, *101*(3), 271–278.

Pickering, G. (2005). Age differences in clinical pain states. In S. J. Gibson, & D. K. Weiner (Eds.), *Pain in older persons*. Seattle: International Association for the Study of Pain (IASP) Press.

Pickering, G., Loriot, M., Libert, F., et al. (2006). Analgesic effect of acetaminophen in humans: First evidence of a central serotonergic mechanism. *Clinical Pharmacology and Therapeutics*, *79*(4), 371–378.

Pincus, T., Koch, G. G., Lei, H., et al. (2004). Patient preference for placebo, acetaminophen, or celecoxib efficacy studies (PACES): Two randomized, double blind, placebo controlled, crossover clinical trials in patients with knee or hip osteoarthritis. *Annals of the Rheumatic Diseases*, *63*(8), 931–939.

Pincus, T., Koch, G. G., Sokka, T., et al. (2001). A randomized, double-blind, crossover clinical trial of diclofenac plus misoprostol versus acetaminophen in patients with osteoarthritis of the hip or knee. *Arthritis and Rheumatism*, *44*(7), 1587–1598.

Porter, V. (2005). NSAIDs still under surveillance—Celecoxib, valdecoxib, and naproxen have been added to the list of suspects. *Medscape Cardiology*, *9*(1). Available at http://www.medscape.com/viewarticle/496951. Accessed August 1, 2008.

Pradhan, B. B., Tatsumi, R. L., Gallina, J., et al. (2008). Ketorolac and spinal fusion: Does the perioperative use of ketorolac really inhibit spinal fusion? *Spine*, *33*(19), 2079–2082.

Pratico, D., & Dogne, J.-M. (2005). Selective cyclooxygenase inhibitors development in cardiovascular medicine. *Circulation*, *112*(7), 1073–1079.

Predel, H. G., Koll, R., Pabst, H., et al. (2004). Diclofenac patch for topical treatment of acute impact injuries: A randomised, double blind placebo controlled, multicentre study. *British Journal of Sports Medicine*, *38*(3), 318–323.

Prymula, R., Siegrist, C. A., Chilbek, R., et al. (2009). Effect of prophylactic paracetamol administration at time of vaccination on febrile reactions and antibody responses in children: Two open-label, randomised controlled trials. *Lancet*, *374*, 1339–1350.

Psaty, B. M., & Furberg, C. D. (2005). COX-2 inhibitors—lessons in drug safety. *The New England Journal of Medicine*, *352*(11), 1133–1135.

Raeder, J. C., Steine, S., & Vatsgar, T. T. (2001). Oral ibuprofen versus paracetamol plus codeine for analgesia after ambulatory surgery. *Anesthesia and Analgesia*, *92*(6), 1470–1472.

Raffa, R. B. (2001). Antihistamines as analgesics. *Journal of Clinical Pharmacy and Therapeutics*, *26*(2), 81–85.

Rahme, E., Bardou, M., Dasgupta, K., et al. (2007). Hospitalization for gastrointestinal bleeding associated with non-steroidal anti-inflammatory drugs among elderly patients using low-dose aspirin: A retrospective cohort study. *Rheumatology (Oxford)*, *46*(2), 265–272.

Rahme, E., Pettitt, D., & LeLorier, J. (2002). Determinants and sequelae associated with utilization of acetaminophen versus traditional nonsteroidal antiinflammatory drugs in an elderly population. *Arthritis and Rheumatism*, *46*(11), 3046–3054.

Rainsford, K. D., Kean, W. F., & Ehrlich, G. E. (2008). Review of the pharmaceutical properties and clinical effects of the topical NSAID formulation diclofenac epolamine. *Current Medical Research and Opinion*, 24(10), 2967–2992.

Ramanuja, S., Breall, J. A., & Kalaria, V. G. (2004). Approach to "aspirin allergy" in cardiovascular patients. *Circulation*, 110(1), e1–e4.

Ramsoekh, D., Van Leerdam, M. E., Rauws, E. A., et al. (2005). Outcome of peptic ulcer bleeding, nonsteroidal anti-inflammatory drug use, and helicobacter pylori infection. *Clinical Gastroenterology and Hepatology*, 3(9), 859–864.

Rands, G., Orrell, M., & Spector, A. E. (2000). Aspirin for vascular dementia. *Cochrane Database of Systematic Reviews*, (4) CD001296.

Rao, S. G., & Bennett, R. M. (2003). Pharmacological therapies in fibromyalgia. *Best Practice & Research. Clinical Rheumatology*, 17(4), 611–627.

Rasmussen, G. L., Malmstrom, K., Bourne, M. H., et al. (2005). Etoricoxib provides analgesic efficacy to patients after knee or hip replacement surgery: A randomized, double-blind, placebo-controlled study. *Anesthesia and Analgesia*, 101(4), 1104–1111.

Rauscher, M. (2007). *OTC naproxen doesn't interfere with aspirin's cardioprotection.* (Report on poster presentation by Schiff M at ACR meeting.) Available at http://www.medscape.com/viewarticle/565518. Accessed August 17, 2008.

Ray, W. A., Stein, C. M., Hall, K., et al. (2002). Non-steroidal anti-inflammatory drugs and risk of serious coronary heart disease: An observational cohort study. *Lancet*, 359(9301), 118–132.

Rebordosa, C., Kogevinas, M., Horvath-Puho, E., et al. (2008). Acetaminophen use during pregnancy: Effects on risk for congenital abnormalities. *American Journal of Obstetrics and Gynecology*, 198(2), 178–180.

Recart, A., Issioui, T., White, P. F., et al. (2003). The efficacy of celecoxib premedication on postoperative pain and recovery times after ambulatory surgery: A dose-ranging study. *Anesthesia and Analgesia*, 96(6), 1631–1635.

Reginster, J. Y., Malmstrom, K., Mehta, A., et al. (2007). Evaluation of the efficacy and safety of etoricoxib compared with naproxen in two, 138-week randomised studies of patients with osteoarthritis. *Annals of the Rheumatic Diseases*, 66(7), 945–951.

Remy, C., Marret, F., & Bonnet, F. (2005). Effects of acetaminophen on morphine side-effects and consumption after major surgery: Meta-analysis of randomized controlled trials. *British Journal of Anaesthesia*, 94(4), 505–513.

Renner, B., Clarke, G., Grattan, T., et al. (2007). Caffeine accelerates absorption and enhances the analgesic effect of acetaminophen. *Journal of Clinical Pharmacology*, 47(6), 715–726.

Rexrode, K. M., Buring, J. E., Glynn, R. J., et al. (2001). Analgesic use and renal function in men. *JAMA: The Journal of the American Medical Association*, 286(3), 315–321.

Roberts, L. J., & Morrow, J. D. (2001). Analgesic-antipyretic and antiinflammatory agents and drugs employed in the treatment of gout. In J. L. Hardman, & L. E. Limbird (Eds.), *Goodman & Gilman's the pharmacological basis of therapeutics.* (10th ed.). New York, NY: McGraw-Hill.

Roddy, E., & Doherty, M. (2003). Guidelines for the management of osteoarthritis published by the American College of Rheumatology and the European League Against Rheumatism: Why are they so different? *Rheumatic Diseases Clinics of North America*, 29(4), 717–731.

Rodriguez, L. A. (2001). The effect of NSAIDs on the risk of coronary heart disease: Fusion of clinical pharmacology and pharmacoepidemiologic data. *Clinical and Experimental Rheumatology*, 19(S25), S41–S44.

Rodriguez, L. A., & Patrignani, P. (2006). The ever growing story of cyclo-oxygenase inhibition. *Lancet*, 368(9549), 1745–1747.

Roelofs, P. D. D. M., Deyo, R. A., Koes, B. W., et al. (2008). Non-steroidal anti-inflammatory drugs for low back pain. *Cochrane Database of Systematic Reviews*, 23(1) CD000396.

Rogers, J. (2008). The inflammatory response in Alzheimer's disease. *Journal of Periodontology*, 78(Suppl. 8), 1535–1543.

Romsing, J., Moiniche, S., & Dahl, J. B. (2002). Rectal and parenteral paracetamol, and paracetamol in combination with NSAIDs, for postoperative analgesia. *British Journal of Anaesthesia*, 88(2), 215–226.

Romsing, J., Moiniche, S., Mathiesen, O., et al. (2005). Reduction of opioid-related adverse events using opioid-sparing analgesia with COX-2 inhibitors lacks documentation: A systematic review. *Acta Anaesthesiologica Scandinavica*, 49(2), 133–142.

Rostom, A., Dube, C., Wells, G., et al. (2002). Prevention of NSAID-induced gastroduodenal ulcers. *Cochrane Database of Systematic Reviews*, (4) CD002296.

Rostom, A., Goldkind, L., & Laine, L. (2005). Nonsteroidal anti-inflammatory drugs and hepatic toxicity: A systematic review of randomized controlled trials in arthritis patients. *Clinical Gastroenterology and Hepatology*, 3(5), 489–498.

Roth, S. H., & Shainhouse, J. Z. (2004). Efficacy and safety of a topical diclofenac solution (Pennsaid) in the treatment of primary osteoarthritis of the knee: A randomized, double-blind vehicle-controlled clinical trial. *Archives of Internal Medicine*, 164(18), 2017–2023.

Rovensky, J., Micekova D., Gubzova, Z., et al. (2001). Treatment of knee osteoarthritis with a topical non-steroidal antiinflammatory drug: Results of a randomized, double-blind, placebo-controlled study on the efficacy and safety of a 5% ibuprofen cream. *Drugs under Experimental and Clinical Research*, 27(5–6), 209–221.

Roy, Y. M., Derry, S., & Moore, R. A. (2007). Single dose oral lumiracoxib for postoperative pain. *Cochrane Database of Systematic Reviews*, (4) CD006865.

Rozsasi, A., Polzehl, D., Deutschle, T., et al. (2008). Long-term treatment with aspirin desensitization: A prospective clinical trial comparing 100 mg and 300 mg aspirin daily. *Allergy*, 63(9), 1228–1234.

Rubenstein, J. H., & Laine, L. (2004). Systematic review: The hepatotoxicity of non-steroidal anti-inflammatory drugs. *Alimentary Pharmacology & Therapeutics*, 20(4), 373–380.

Rumack, B. H. (2002). Acetaminophen hepatotoxicity: The first 35 years. *Journal of Clinical Toxicology*, 40(1), 3–20.

Russo, M. W., Galanko, J. A., Shrestha, R., et al. (2004). Liver transplantation for acute liver failure from drug-induced liver injury in the United States. *Liver Transplantation*, 10(8), 1018–1023.

Safdar, B., Degutis, L. C., Landry, K., et al. (2006). Intravenous morphine plus ketorolac is superior to either drug alone for treatment of acute renal colic. *Annals of Emergency Medicine*, 48(2), 173–181.

Salpeter, S. R., Gregor, P., Ormiston, T. M., et al. (2006). Meta-analysis: Cardiovascular events associated with nonsteroidal anti-inflammatory drugs. *The American Journal of Medicine, 119*(7), 552–559.

Savage, A. H., Anderson, B. L., & Simhan, H. N. (2007). The safety of prolonged indomethacin therapy. *American Journal of Perinatology, 24*(4), 207–213.

Sawynok, J. (2003). Topically and peripherally acting analgesics. *Pharmacological Reviews, 55*(1), 1–20.

Scharbert, G., Gebhardt, K., Sow, Z., et al. (2007). Point-of-care platelet function tests: Detection of platelet inhibition induced by nonopioid analgesic drugs. *Blood Coagulation & Fibrinolysis, 18*(8), 775–780.

Scheiman, J. M. (2006). *Cardiovascular risks associated with cyclooxygenase-2 selective inhibitors and traditional nonsteroidal antiinflammatory drugs.* Available at http://www.medscape.com/viewarticle/543804_1. Accessed August 10, 2008.

Scheiman, J. M., & Fendrick, A. M. (2005). Practical approaches to minimizing gastrointestinal and cardiovascular safety concerns with COX-2 inhibitors and NSAIDs. *Arthritis Research & Therapy, 7*(Suppl. 4), 23–29.

Schiff, M., & Minic, M. (2004). Comparison of analgesic efficacy and safety of nonprescription doses of naproxen sodium and ibuprofen in the treatment of osteoarthritis of the knee. *The Journal of Rheumatology, 31*(7), 1373–1383.

Schneider, F., Meziani, F., Chartier, C., et al. (2002). Fatal allergic vasculitis associated with celecoxib. *Lancet, 359*(9305), 852–853.

Schneider, V., Levesque, L. E., Zhang, B., et al. (2006). Association of selective and conventional nonsteroidal antiinflammatory drugs with acute renal failure: A population-based, nested case-control analysis. *Am J Epidiol, 164*(9), 881–889.

Schnitzer, T. J., Burmester, G. R., Mysler, E., et al. (2004). Comparison of lumiracoxib with naproxen and ibuprofen in therapeutic arthritis research and gastrointestinal event trial (TARGET), reduction in ulcer complications: Randomised controlled trial. *Lancet, 364*(9435), 665–674.

Schnitzer, T. J., Kong, S. X., Mitchell, J. H., et al. (2003). An observational, retrospective, cohort study of dosing patterns for rofecoxib and celecoxib in the treatment of arthritis. *Clinical Therapeutics, 25*(12), 3162–3172.

Schoken, D. D., Benjamin, E. J., Fonarow, G. C., et al. (2008). Prevention of heart failure. A scientific statement from the American Heart Association Councils on Epidemiology and Prevention, Clinical Cardiology, Cardiovascular Nursing, and High Blood Pressure Research; Quality of Care and Outcomes Research Interdisciplinary Working Group; and Functional Genomics and Translational Biology Interdisciplinary Working Group. *Circulation, 117*(19), 2544–2565.

Schug, S. A. (2006). The role of COX-2 inhibitors in the treatment of postoperative pain. *Journal of Cardiovascular Pharmacology, 47*(Suppl. 1), S82–S86.

Schug, S. A., & Manopas, A. (2007). Update on the role of non-opioids for postoperative pain treatment. *Best Prac Res Clin Anesth, 21*(1), 15–30.

Schwartz, J. I., Vandormael, K., Malice, M. P., et al. (2002). Comparison of rofecoxib, celecoxib, and naproxen on renal function in elderly subjects receiving a normal-salt diet. *Clinical Pharmacology and Therapeutics, 72*(1), 50–71.

Segev, G., & Katz, R. (2004). Selective COX-2 inhibitors and risk of cardiovascular events. *Hospital Physician, 40*(2), 39–46.

Serinken, M., Karcioglu, O., Turkcuer, I., et al. (2008). Analysis of clinical and demographic characteristics of patients presenting with renal colic in the emergency department. *BMC Res Notes, 16*(1), 79.

Shaheen, S. O., Newson, R. B., Henderson, A. J., et al. (2005). Prenatal paracetamol exposure and risk of asthma and elevated immunoglobulin E in childhood. *Clinical and Experimental Allergy, 325*(6), 700–702.

Shapiro, L. E., Knowles, S. R., Weber, E., et al. (2003). Safety of celecoxib in individuals allergic to sulfonamide: A pilot study. *Drug Safety, 26*(3), 187–195.

Shapiro, R. E. (2008). Caffeine and headaches. *Current Pain and Headache Reports, 12*(4), 311–315.

Shen, H., Sprott, H., Aeschlimann, A., et al. (2006). Analgesic action of acetaminophen in symptomatic osteoarthritis of the knee. *Rheumatology, 45*(6), 765–770.

Shi, Q., Langer, G., Cohen, J., et al. (2007). People in pain: How do they seek relief? *The Journal of Pain, 8*(8), 624–636.

Siddik, S. M., Aouad, M. T., Jalbout, M. I., et al. (2001). Diclofenac and/or propacetamol for postoperative pain management after Cesarean delivery in patients receiving patient controlled analgesia morphine. *Regional Anesthesia and Pain Medicine, 26*(4), 310–315.

Silverstein, F. E., Faich, G., Goldstein, J. L., et al. (2000). Gastrointestinal toxicity with celecoxib vs nonsteroidal anti-inflammatory drugs for osteoarthritis and rheumatoid arthritis. The CLASS study: A randomized controlled trial. *JAMA: The Journal of the American Medical Association, 284*(10), 1247–1255.

Simon, A. M., Manigrasso, M. B., & O'Connor, J. P. (2002). Cyclo-oxygenase 2 function is essential for bone fracture healing. *J Bone Res, 17*(6), 963–976.

Simon, L. S. (2007). *Risks and benefits of COX-2 selective inhibitors.* Available at http://www.medscape.com/viewprogram/6872/. Accessed August 5, 2007.

Simon, L. S. (2008). Do topical NSAIDs work? *Nature Clinical Practice Rheumatology, 4*(9), 458–459.

Simon, L. S., & Fox, R. I. (2005). What are the options available for anti-inflammatory drugs in the aftermath of rofecoxib's withdrawal? *Medscape Rheumatology, 6*(1). Available at http://www.medscape.com/viewarticle/500056. Accessed August 16, 2005.

Simon, L. S., Lipman, A. G., Caudill-Slosberg, M., et al. (2002). *Guideline for the management of pain in osteoarthritis, rheumatoid arthritis, and juvenile chronic arthritis.* Glenview, IL: American Pain Society.

Simon, L. S., Weaver, A. L., Graham, D. Y., et al. (1999). Anti-inflammatory and upper gastrointestinal effects of celecoxib in rheumatoid arthritis. A randomized controlled trial. *JAMA: The Journal of the American Medical Association, 282*(20), 1921–1928.

Sinatra, R. S., Jahr, J. S., Reynolds, L. W., et al. (2005). Efficacy and safety of single and repeated administration of 1 gram intravenous acetaminophen injection (paracetamol) for pain management after major orthopedic surgery. *Anesthesiology, 102*(4), 822–831.

Singh, G., Fort, J. G., Goldstein, J. L., et al. (2006). Celecoxib versus naproxen and diclofenac in osteoarthritis patients: SUCCESS-I study. *The American Journal of Medicine, 119*(3), 255–266.

Sivaprasad, S., Bunce, C., & Patel, N. (2005). Non-steroidal anti-inflammatory agents for treating cystoid macular oedema following cataract surgery. *Cochrane Database of Systematic Reviews*, (1) CD004239.

Smith, A. L., Carroll, J. E., Edwards, J. E., et al. (2000). Single-dose ketorolac and pethidine in acute postoperative pain: Systematic review with meta-analysis. *British Journal of Anaesthesia*, *84*(1), 48–58.

Smith, H. S., & Baird, W. (2003). Meloxicam and selective COX-2 inhibitors in the management of pain in the palliative care population. *The American Journal of Hospice & Palliative Care*, *20*(4), 297–306.

Smith, S. E. (2005). Ocular NSAIDs. *Cataract Refrac Surg Today*, 124–127.

Soininen, H., West, C., Robbins, J., et al. (2007). Long-term efficacy and safety of celecoxib in Alzheimer's disease. *Dementia and Geriatric Cognitive Disorders*, *23*(1), 8–21.

Solomon, D. H., Glynn, R. J., Rothman, K. J., et al. (2008). Subgroup analyses to determine cardiovascular risk associated with nonsteroidal antiinflammatory drugs and coxibs in specific patient groups. *Arthritis and Rheumatism*, *59*(8), 1097–1104.

Solomon, D. H., Karlson, E. W., Rimm, E. B., et al. (2003). Cardiovascular morbidity and mortality in women diagnosed with rheumatoid arthritis. *Circulation*, *107*(9), 1303–1307.

Solomon, D. H., Schneeweiss, S., Levin, R., et al. (2004). Relationship between COX-2 specific inhibitors and hypertension. *Hypertension*, *44*(2), 140–145.

Solomon, S. D., McMurray, J. J. V., Pfeffer, M. A., et al. (2005). Cardiovascular risk associated with celecoxib in a clinical trial for colorectal adenoma prevention. *The New England Journal of Medicine*, *352*(11), 1071–1080.

Solomon, S. D., Pfeffer, M. A., McMurray, J. J. V., et al. (2006). Effect of celecoxib on cardiovascular events and blood pressure in two trials for the prevention of colorectal adenomas. *Circulation*, *114*(10), 1028–1035.

Solomon, S. D., Schneeweiss, S., Glynn, R. J., et al. (2004). Relationship between selective cyclooxygenase-2 inhibitors and acute myocardial infarction in older adults. *Circulation*, *109*(17), 2068–2073.

Solomon, S. D., Wittes, J., Finn, P. V., et al. (2008). Cardiovascular risk of celecoxib in 6 randomized placebo-controlled trials. The cross trial safety analysis. *Circulation*, *117*(16), 2104–2113.

Sowers, J. R., White, W. B., Pitt, B., et al. (2005). The effects of cyclooxygenase-2 inhibitors and nonsteroidal anti-inflammatory therapy on 24-hour blood pressure in patients with hypertension, osteoarthritis, and type 2 diabetes mellitus. *Archives of Internal Medicine*, *165*(2), 161–168.

Soylu, A., Dolapcioglu, C., Dolay, K., et al. (2008). Endoscopic and histopathic evaluation of acute gastric injury in high-dose acetaminophen and nonsteroidal anti-inflammatory drug ingestion with suicidal intent. *World Journal of Gastroenterology: WJG*, *14*(43), 6704–6710.

Stamer, U. M., & Stuber, F. (2006). Postoperative pain—genetics and genomics. In G. Shorten, D. B. Carr, & D. Harmon, et al. (Eds.), *Postoperative pain management: An evidence-based guide to practice*. Philadelphia: Saunders.

Stanos, S. P. (2007). Topical agents for the management of musculoskeletal pain. *Journal of Pain and Symptom Management*, *33*(3), 342–355.

Steen, K. S. S., Nurmohamed, M. T., Visman, I., et al. (2008). Decreasing incidence of symptomatic gastrointestinal ulcers and ulcer complications in patients with rheumatoid arthritis. *Annals of the Rheumatic Diseases*, *67*(2), 256–259.

Steinbach, B., Lynch, P. M., Phillips, R. K., et al. (2000). The effect of celecoxib, a cyclooxygenase-2 inhibitor, in familial adenomatous polyposis. *The New England Journal of Medicine*, *342*(26), 1946–1952.

Strand, V. (2007). Are COX-2 inhibitors preferable to non-selective non-steroidal anti-inflammatory drugs in patients with risk of cardiovascular events taking low-dose aspirin? *Lancet*, *370*(9605), 2138–2151.

Straube, S., Derry, S., McQuay, H. J., et al. (2005). Effect of preoperative COX-II-selective NSAIDs (coxibs) on postoperative outcomes: A systematic review of randomized studies. *Acta Anaesthesiologica Scandinavica*, *49*(5), 601–613.

Strom, B. L., Berlin, J. A., Kinman, J. L., et al. (1996). Parenteral ketorolac and risk of gastrointestinal and operative site bleeding. *JAMA: The Journal of the American Medical Association*, *275*(5), 376–382.

Sun, B. H., Wu, C. W., & Kalunian, K. C. (2007). New developments in osteoarthritis. *Rheumatic Diseases Clinics of North America*, *33*(1), 135–148.

Sun, J. C. J., Crowther, M. A., Warkentin, T. E., et al. (2005). Should aspirin be discontinued before coronary artery bypass surgery? *Circulation*, *112*(7), e85–e90.

Sun, T., Sacan, O., White, P. F., et al. (2008). Perioperative versus postoperative celecoxib on patient outcomes after major plastic surgery procedures. *Anesthesia and Analgesia*, *106*(3), 950–958.

Svenungsson, E., Jensen-Urstad, K., Heimburger, M., et al. (2001). Risk factors for cardiovascular disease in systemic lupus erthematosus. *Circulation*, *104*(16), 1887–1893.

Szczeklik, A., Nizankowska, E., Bochenek, G., et al. (2001). Safety of a specific COX-2 inhibitor in aspirin-induced asthma. *Clinical and Experimental Allergy*, *31*(2), 219–225.

Tabet, N., & Feldman, H. (2003). Ibuprofen for Alzheimer's disease. *Cochrane Database of Systematic Reviews*, (2) CD004031.

Tang, R., Evans, H., Chaput, A., et al. (2009). Multimodal analgesia for hip arthroplasty. *The Orthopedic Clinics of North America*, *40*(3), 377–387.

Tannenbaum, H., Bombardier, C., Davis, P., et al. (2006). An evidence-based approach to prescribing nonsteroidal antiinflammatory drugs. Third Canadian Consensus Conference. *The Journal of Rheumatology*, *33*(1), 140–157.

Tassoni, D., Kaur, G., Weisinger, R. S., et al. (2008). The role of eicosanoids in the brain. *Asia Pacific Journal of Clinical Nutrition*, *17*(Suppl. 1), 220–228.

Telleria-Diaz, A., Schmidt, M., Kreusch, S., et al. (2010). Spinal antinociceptive effects of cyclooxygenase inhibition during inflammation: Involvement of prostaglandins and endocannabinoids. *Pain*, *148*(1), 26–35.

Temprano, K. K., Bandlamudi, R., & Moore, T. L. (2005). Antirheumatic drugs in pregnancy and lactation. *Seminars in Arthritis and Rheumatism*, *35*(2), 112–121.

Thiagarajan, P. (2001). Atherosclerosis, autoimmunity, and systemic lupus erythematosus. *Circulation*, *104*(16), 1876–1877.

Thijssen, H. H., Soute, B. A., Vervoort, L. M., et al. (2004). Paracetamol (acetaminophen) warfarin interaction: NAPQI, the toxic metabolite of paracetamol, is an inhibitor of enzymes in the vitamin K cycle. *Thrombosis and Haemostasis*, *92*(4), 797–802.

Toftdahl, K., Nikolajsen, L., Haraldsted, V., et al. (2007). Comparison of peri- and intraarticular analgesia with femoral nerve block after total knee arthroplasty: A randomized clinical trial. *Acta Orthopaedica, 78*(2), 159–161.

Toms, L., McQuay, H. J., Derry, S., et al. (2008). Single dose oral paracetamol (acetaminophen) for postoperative pain in adults. *Cochrane Database of Systematic Reviews,* (4) CD004602.

Topol, E. J., & Falk, G. W. (2004). A coxib a day won't keep the doctor away. *Lancet, 364*(9435), 639–640.

Towheed, T. E., Maxwell, L., Judd, M. G., et al. (2006). Acetaminophen for osteoarthritis. *Cochrane Database of Systematic Reviews,* (1) CD004257.

Trattler, W., & McDonald, M. (2007). Double-masked comparison of ketorolac tromethamine 0.4% versus nepfanac sodium 0.1% for postoperative healing rates and pain control in eyes undergoing surface ablation. *Cornea, 26*(6), 665–669.

Trnavsky, K., Fischer, M., Vogtle-Junkert, U., et al. (2004). Efficacy and safety of 5% ibuprofen cream treatment in knee osteoarthritis: Results of a randomized, double-blind, placebo-controlled study. *The Journal of Rheumatology, 31*(3), 565–572.

Underwood, M., Ashby, D., Cross, P., et al. (2008). Advice to use topical or oral ibuprofen for chronic knee pain in older people: Randomised controlled trial and patient preference study. *BMJ (Clinical Research Ed.), 336*(7636), 138–142.

United States Food and Drug Administration (FDA) Website. (2005). *Alert for healthcare professionals: Valdecoxib (marketed as Bextra).* Available at http://www.fda.gov/Cder/drug/InfoSheets/HCP/valdecoxibHCP.pdf. Accessed August 21, 2008.

United States Food and Drug Administration (FDA) Website. (2006). *Concomitant use of ibuprofen and aspirin: Potential for the attenuation of anti-platelet effect of aspirin.* Available at http://www.fda.gov/cder/drug/infopage/ibuprofen/science:paper.htm. Accessed August 16, 2007.

United States Food and Drug Administration (FDA) Website. (2007). *Medication guide for non-steroidal anti-inflammatory drugs (NSAIDs).* Available at http://www.fda.gov/cder/drug/infopage/COX2/NSAIDmedguide.htm. Accessed August 10, 2008.

United States Food and Drug Administration (FDA) Website. (2008). *Pregnancy and lactation labeling.* Available at http://www.fda.gov/cder/regulatory/pregnancy_labeling/default.htm. Accessed December 1, 2008.

United States Food and Drug Administration (FDA) Website. (2009). *Organ specific warnings: Internal analgesic, antipyretic, and antirheumatic drug products for over-the-counter human use.* Final monograph. Available at http://edocket.access.gpo.gov/2009/pdf/E9-9684.pdf. Accessed September 8, 2009.

van der Woude, F. J., Heinemann, A. L., Graf, H., et al. (2007). Analgesic use and ESRD in younger age: A case-control study. *BMC Nephrology, 8,* 15.

van Haselen, R. A., & Fisher, P. A. G. (2000). A randomized controlled trial comparing topical piroxicam gel with a homeopathic gel in osteoarthritis of the knee. *Rhematology, 39*(7), 714–719.

Vane, J. R., & Warner, T. D. (2000). Nomenclature for COX-2 inhibitors. (Commentary). *Lancet, 356*(9239), 1373–1374.

Vardeny, O., & Solomon, S. D. (2008). Cyclooxygenase-2-inhibitors, nonsteroidal anti-inflammatory drugs, and cardiovascular risk. *Cardiology Clinics, 26*(4), 589–601.

Vasan, R. S., Sullivan, L. M., Roubenoff, R., et al. (2003). Inflammatory markers and risk of heart failure in elderly subjects without prior myocardial infarction: The Framingham Heart Study. *Circulation, 107*(11), 1486–1491.

Verhamme, K. M. C., Dieleman, J. P., Van Wijk, M. A. M., et al. (2005). Nonsteroidal anti-inflammatory drugs and increased risk of acute urinary retention. *Archives of Internal Medicine, 165*(13), 1547–1551.

Visser, E. J., & Goucke, C. R. (2008). Acute pain and medical disorders. In P. E. Macintyre, S. M. Walker, & D. J. Rowbotham (Eds.), *Clinical pain management: Acute pain.* (2nd ed.). London: Hodder Arnold.

Vlad, S. C., Miller, D. R., Kowall, N. W., et al. (2008). Protective effects of NSAIDs on the development of Alzheimer disease. *Neurology, 70*(19), 1672–1677.

Volans, G., Monaghan, J., & Colbridge, M. (2003). Ibuprofen overdose. *International Journal of Clinical Practice Suppl, 135*(Apr), 54–60.

Walters, T., Raizman, M., Ernest, P., et al. (2007). In vivo pharmacokinetics and in vitro pharmacodynamics of nepafenac, amfenac, ketorolac, and bromfenac. *Journal of Cataract and Refractive Surgery, 33*(9), 1539–1545.

Warner, T. D., & Mitchell, J. A. (2004). Cyclooxygenases: New forms, new inhibitors, and lessons from the clinic. *The FASEB Journal, 18*(7), 790–804.

Warner, T. D., & Mitchell, J. A. (2008). COX-2 selectivity alone does not define the cardiovascular risks associated with nonsteroidal anti-inflammatory drugs. (Viewpoint). *Lancet, 371*(9608), 270–273.

Watkins, P. B., Kaplowitz, N., Slattery, J. T., et al. (2006). Aminotransferase elevations in healthy adults receiving 4 grams of acetaminophen daily. *JAMA: The Journal of the American Medical Association, 296*(1), 87–93.

Wen, C. C., Coyle, T. L., Jerde, T. J., et al. (2008). Ketorolac effectively inhibits ureteral contractility in vitro. *Journal of Endourology/Endourological Society, 22*(4), 739–742.

Werler, M. M., Mitchell, A. A., Hernandez-Diaz, S., et al. (2005). Use of over-the-counter medications during pregnancy. *American Journal of Obstetrics and Gynecology, 193*(Part 1), 771–777.

Whelton, A., Fort, J. C., Puma, J. A., et al. (2001). Cyclooxygenase-2-specific inhibitors and cardiorenal function: A randomized, controlled trial of celecoxib and rofecoxib in older hypertensive osteoarthritis patients. *American Journal of Therapeutics, 8*(2), 85–96.

Whelton, A., Lefkowith, J. L., West, C. R., et al. (2006). Cardiorenal effects of celecoxib as compared with the nonsteroidal anti-inflammatory drugs diclofenac and ibuprofen. *Kidney International, 70*(8), 1495–1502.

Whelton, A., White, W. B., Bello, A. E., et al. (2002). Effects of celecoxib and rofecoxib on blood pressure and edema in patients ≥65 years of age with systemic hypertension and osteoarthritis. *The American Journal of Cardiology, 90*(9), 959–963.

White, P. F. (2002). The role of nonopioid analgesic techniques in the management of pain after ambulatory surgery. *Anesthesia and Analgesia, 94*(3), 577–585.

White, P. F. (2005). The changing role of non-opioid analgesic techniques in the management of postoperative pain. *Anesthesia and Analgesia, 105*(Suppl. 5), S5–S22.

White, W. B., Kent, J., Taylor, A., et al. (2002). Effects of celecoxib on ambulatory blood pressure in hypertensive patients on ACE inhibitors. *Hypertension, 39*(4), 929–934.

White, W. B., West, C. R., Borer, J. S., et al. (2007). Risk of cardiovascular events in patients receiving celecoxib: A meta-analysis of randomized clinical trials. *The American Journal of Cardiology, 99*(1), 91–98.

Whitefield, M., O'Kane, C. J. A., & Anderson, S. (2002). Comparative efficacy of a proprietary topical ibuprofen gel and oral ibuprofen in acute soft tissue injuries: A randomized, double-blind study. *Journal of Clinical Pharmacy and Therapeutics, 27*(6), 409–417.

Wienecke, T., & Gøtzsche, P. C. (2004). Paracetamol versus nonsteroidal anti-inflammatory drugs for rheumatoid arthritis. *Cochrane Database of Systematic Reviews,* (1) CD003789.

Wilbeck, J., Schorn, M. N., & Daley, L. (2008). Pharmacologic management of acute pain in breastfeeding women. *Journal of Emergency Nursing, 34*(4), 340–344.

Wilcox, C. M., Allison, J., Benzuly, K., et al. (2006). Consensus development conference on the use of nonsteroidal anti-inflammatory agents, including cyclooxygenase-2 enzyme inhibitors and aspirin. *Clinical Gastroenterology and Hepatology, 4*(9), 1082–1089.

Wilner, K. D., Rushing, M., Walden, C., et al. (2002). Celecoxib does not affect the antiplatelet activity of aspirin in healthy volunteers. *Journal of Clinical Pharmacology, 42*(9), 1027–1030.

Wittpenn, J. R., Silverstein, S., Heier, J., et al. (2008). A randomized, masked comparison of topical ketorolac 0.4% plus steroid vs steroid alone in low-risk cataract surgery patients. *Am J Opthalmol, 146*(4), 554–560.

Woo, W. W. K., Man, S. Y., Lam, P. K. W., et al. (2005). Randomized double-blind trial comparing oral paracetamol and oral nonsteroidal antiinflammatory drugs for treating pain after musculoskeletal injury. *Annals of Emergency Medicine, 46*(4), 352–361.

Wood, D. M., Monaghan, J., Streete, P., et al. (2006). Fatality after deliberate ingestion of sustained-release ibuprofen: A case report. *Critical Care (London, England), 10*(2), R44.

Wood, S. (2007). FDA advisory panel votes "no" to etoricoxib. *Medscape Heartwire.* Available at http://www.medscape.com/viewarticle/555141. Accessed August 13, 2008.

Woolf, C. J. (1983). Evidence for a central component of post-injury pain hypersensitivity. *Nature, 306*(5944), 686–688.

Woolf, C. J., & Chong, M. S. (1993). Preemptive analgesia: Treating postoperative pain by preventing the establishment of central sensitization. *Anesthesia and Analgesia, 77*(2), 362–379.

Yencilek, F., Aktas, C., Goktas, C., et al. (2008). Role of papaverine hydrochloride administration in patients with intractable renal colic: Randomized prospective trial. *Urology, 72*(5), 987–990.

Yeomans, N. D., Tulassay, Z., Juhasz, L., et al. (1998). A comparison of omeprazole with ranitidine for ulcers associated with nonsteroidal antiinflammatory drugs. *The New England Journal of Medicine, 338*(11), 719–726.

Yusoff, I. F., Barkun, J. S., & Barkun, A. N. (2003). Diagnosis and management of cholecystitis and cholangitis. *Gastroenterology Clinics of North America, 32*(4), 1145–1168.

Zacher, J., Altman, R., Bellamy, N., et al. (2008). Topical diclofenac and its role in pain and inflammation: An evidence-based review. *Current Medical Research and Opinion, 24*(4), 925–950.

Zembowicz, A., Mastalerz, L., Setkowicz, M., et al. (2003). Safety of cyclooxygenase 2 inhibitors and increased leukotriene synthesis in chronic idiopathic urticaria with sensitivity to nonsteroidal anti-inflammatory drugs. *Archives of Dermatology, 139*(12), 1577–1582.

Zhang, J., Ding, E. L., & Song, Y. (2006). Adverse effects of cyclooxygenase-2 inhibitors on renal and arrhythmia events: Meta-analysis of randomized trials. *JAMA: The Journal of the American Medical Association, 296*(13), 1619–1632.

Zhang, W., Doherty, M., Arden, N., et al. (2005). EULAR evidence based recommendations for the management of hip osteoarthritis: Report of a task force of the EULAR Standing Committee for International Clinical Studies Including Therapeutics (ESCISIT). *Annals of the Rheumatic Diseases, 64*(5), 669–681.

Zhang, W., Doherty, M., Leeb, B. F., et al. (2007). EULAR evidence based recommendations for the management of hand osteoarthritis: Report of a Task Force of the EULAR Standing Committee for International Clinical Studies Including Therapeutics (ESCISIT). *Annals of the Rheumatic Diseases, 66*(3), 377–388.

Zhang, W., Moskowitz, R. W., Nuki, G., et al. (2008). OARSI recommendations for the management of hip and knee osteoarthritis, Part II: OARSI evidence-based, expert consensus guidelines. *Osteoarthritis and Cartilage, 16*(2), 137–162.

Zhang, W. Y. (2001). A benefit-risk assessment of caffeine as an analgesic adjuvant. *Drug Safety, 24*(15), 1127–1142.

Zhang, X., Schwarz, E. M., Young, D. A., et al. (2002). Cyclooxygenase-2 regulates mesenchymal cell differentiation into the osteoblast lineage and is critically involved in bone repair. *The Journal of Clinical Investigation, 109*(911), 1405–1415.

Zhao, S. Z., Reynolds, M. W., Lejkowith, J., et al. (2001). A comparison of renal-related adverse drug reactions between rofecoxib and celecoxib, based on the World Health Organization/Uppsala Monitoring Centre safety database. *Clinical Therapeutics, 23*(9), 1478–1491.

Zhou, T. J., Tang, J., & White, P. F. (2001). Propacetamol versus ketorolac for treatment of acute postoperative pain after total hip or knee replacement. *Anesthesia and Analgesia, 92*(6), 1569–1575.

Ziemer, M., Wiesend, C. L., Vetter, R., et al. (2007). Cutaneous adverse reactions to valdecoxib distinct from Stevens-Johnson syndrome and toxic epidermal necrolysis. *Archives of Dermatology, 143*(6), 711–716.

Opioid Analgesics

Chris Pasero, Thomas E. Quinn,
Russell K. Portenoy, Margo McCaffery,
and Albert Rizos

Terminology

Acetaminophen Other generic names include *paracetamol* and *acetylparaaminophenol* (APAP). Also referred to as "aspirin-free."

Addiction A chronic neurologic and biologic disease. As defined by pain specialists, it is characterized by behaviors that include one or more of the following: impaired control over drug use, compulsive use, continued use despite harm, and craving. Continued craving for an opioid and the need to use the opioid for effects other than pain relief. Physical dependence and tolerance are not the same as addiction.

Adjuvant analgesic A drug that has a primary indication other than pain (e.g., anticonvulsant, antidepressant, sodium channel blocker, and muscle relaxant) but is analgesic for some painful conditions.

Agonist-antagonist A type of opioid (e.g., nalbuphine and butorphanol) that binds to the kappa opioid receptor site acting as an agonist (capable of producing analgesia) and simultaneously to the mu opioid receptor site acting as an antagonist (reversing mu agonist effects).

Allodynia Pain due to a stimulus that does not normally provoke pain such as touch. Typically experienced in the skin around areas affected by nerve injury, commonly seen with many neuropathic pain syndromes.

Analgesic ceiling A dose beyond which further increases in dose do not provide additional analgesia.

Antagonist Drug that competes with agonists for opioid receptor binding sites; can displace agonists, thereby inhibiting their action. Examples include naloxone, naltrexone, and nalmefene.

Bioavailability The extent to which a dose of a drug reaches its site of action.

Blood-brain barrier A barrier that exists between circulating blood and brain, preventing damaging substances from reaching brain tissue and cerebrospinal fluid.

Breakthrough dose (BTD) Also referred to as *supplemental dose* or *rescue dose;* the dose of analgesic taken to treat breakthrough pain.

Breakthrough pain (BTP) A transitory increase in pain that occurs on a background of otherwise controlled persistent pain.

Ceiling effect A dose above which further dose increments produce no change in effect.

Comfort-function goal The pain rating identified by the individual patient above which the patient experiences interference with function and quality of life, that is, activities that the patient needs or wishes to perform.

Controlled release See **modified release.**

Crescendo pain A period of rapid pain escalation often associated with increasing distress and functional impairment.

Distribution half-life The time it takes a drug to move from the blood and plasma to other tissues. Distribution half-life differs from half-life (terminal) (see **half-life**).

Dysesthesia An unpleasant abnormal sensation (spontaneous or evoked) that is usually associated with neuropathic pain. It is usually described as "pins and needles" (e.g., a limb "falling asleep," burning, electric shock–like, tingling) and may be intermittent or continuous and experienced in an area of sensory loss. A dysesthesia should always be unpleasant; whereas, a paresthesia should not be unpleasant. It may be difficult to differentiate dysesthesias from paresthesias.

Efficacy The extent to which a drug or another treatment "works" and can produce the effect in question— analgesia in this context. To determine whether this is the case, the treatment must be compared to another, typically a placebo, but sometimes an active comparator. Maximal efficacy refers to the maximum effect that can be produced by a drug, and comparative efficacy refers to the relative effects of two or more treatments compared at comparable treatment intensities.

Extended release See **modified release**.

Half-life The time it takes for the plasma concentration (amount of drug in the body) to be reduced by 50%. After starting a drug or increasing its dose, four to five half-lives are required to approach a steady-state level in the blood, irrespective of the dose, dosing interval, or route of administration; after four to five half-lives, a drug that has been discontinued generally is considered to be mostly eliminated from the body.

Hand-off Communication The process by which nurses share pertinent information about their patients when care is transferred from one nurse to another.

Hydrophilic Readily absorbed in aqueous solution.

Hyperalgesia Increased pain response to noxious stimuli.

Immediate release See **short acting**.

Incomplete cross-tolerance Because similar drugs (like the mu agonists), have different intrinsic efficacies (how they produce effects after binding to a receptor) at the same receptors, and because each also interacts with a different group of receptor subtypes, a switch from one drug to another similar drug (e.g., from one mu agonist to another) is associated with a variable degree of tolerance to different effects; for example, in an animal model, tolerance to morphine's analgesic effect can be produced and be made very profound, but analgesia will reappear on switching to another mu agonist like hydromorphone.

Independent double check process An individual, e.g., nurse or pharmacist, checks the analgesic, solution, concentration, dose, and/or programming of analgesic device against the written prescription without prompting from the person administering the analgesic or anyone else. This safety measure is done at specified (by institutional policy) intervals to ensure accuracy of drug delivery, e.g., prior to initiation of IV PCA.

Intractable In reference to pain that is unresponsive to all other recommended therapeutic options (e.g., first-line and second-line analgesics).

Intraspinal "Within the spine"; term referring to the spaces or potential spaces surrounding the spinal cord into which medications can be administered. Most often, the term is used when referring to the epidural and intrathecal routes of administration. Sometimes used interchangeably with the term **neuraxial**.

Lipophilic Readily absorbed in fatty tissues.

Medically ill patients Patients with existing debilitating pathologic condition/illness that may be progressive or stable, as opposed to those who have only the symptom of pain and are otherwise healthy.

Metabolite The product of biochemical reactions during drug metabolism.

Modified release Oral opioid analgesics that are formulated to release over a prolonged period of time; often used interchangeably with the terms **extended release**, **sustained release**, and **controlled release**. The term **modified release** will be used in this book to describe these drugs.

Mu agonist Any opioid that binds to the mu opioid receptor subtype and produces effects. Includes morphine and other opioids that relieve pain by binding to the mu receptor sites in the nervous system. Used interchangeably with the terms **full agonist, pure agonist,** and **morphine-like drug**.

Narcotic See **Opioid**. Obsolete term for **opioid**, in part because the government and media use the term loosely to refer to a variety of substances of potential abuse. Legally, controlled substances classified as narcotics include opioids, cocaine, and various other substances.

Neuralgia Pain in the distribution of a nerve (e.g., sciatica, trigeminal neuralgia). Often felt as an electrical shock–like pain.

Neuropathic pain Pain sustained by injury or dysfunction of the peripheral or central nervous systems.

NMDA N-methyl-D-aspartate. In this book, the term is used in conjunction with drugs that are NMDA receptor antagonists or blockers, such as ketamine or dextromethorphan.

Nociceptive pain Pain that is sustained by ongoing activation of the sensory system that subserves the perception of noxious stimuli; implies the existence of damage to somatic or visceral tissues sufficient to activate the nociceptive system.

Nociceptor A primary afferent nerve that has the ability to respond to a noxious stimulus or to a stimulus that would be noxious if prolonged.

Nonopioid Used instead of **nonnarcotic**. Refers to acetaminophen and nonsteroidal antiinflammatory drugs (NSAIDs).

Normal release See **short acting**.

NSAID An acronym for nonsteroidal antiinflammatory drug. (Pronounced "in said.") Also referred to as "aspirin like" drugs.

Opioid This term is preferred to **narcotic**. Opioid refers to codeine, morphine, and other natural, semisynthetic, and synthetic drugs that relieve pain by binding to multiple types of opioid receptors.

Opioid dose-sparing effect The dose of opioid may be lowered when another analgesic, such as a nonopioid, is added.

Opioid-induced hyperalgesia (OIH) A phenomenon clearly demonstrated in experimental models, but of uncertain significance in humans, by which exposure to the opioid induces increased sensitivity, or a lowered threshold, to the neural activity subserving pain perception; it is the "flip side" of analgesic tolerance, which is defined by the loss of analgesic activity due to exposure to the drug.

Opioid-naïve An opioid-naïve person has not recently taken enough opioid on a regular enough basis to become tolerant to the effects of an opioid.

Opioid-tolerant An opioid-tolerant person has taken opioids long enough at doses high enough to develop tolerance to many of the effects of the opioid, including analgesia and sedation, but there is no timeframe for developing tolerance.

Paresthesia An abnormal sensation, whether spontaneous or evoked, manifested by sensations of numbness, prickling, tingling, and heightened sensitivity that is typically not unpleasant.

Paroxysmal Sudden periodic attack or recurrence.

Physical dependence Potential for withdrawal symptoms if the opioid is abruptly stopped or an antagonist is administered; not the same as **addiction**.

Potency The dose required to produce a specified effect; relative potency is the ratio of the doses of two or more analgesics required to produce the same analgesic effect.

Preemptive analgesia Preinjury pain treatments (e.g., preoperative epidural analgesia and preincision local anesthetic infiltration) to prevent the establishment of peripheral and central sensitization of pain.

Primary afferent neuron See definition of **nociceptor**.

Prodrug An inactive precursor of a drug, converted into its active form in the body by normal metabolic processes.

Protective analgesia An aggressive, sustained multimodal intervention administered perioperatively (e.g., local anesthetic block, acetaminophen, NSAID, and anticonvulsant initiated preoperatively and continued throughout the intraoperative and postoperative periods) and directed toward prevention of pathologic pain (e.g., persistent neuropathic postsurgical pain syndromes).

Pseudoaddiction A mistaken diagnosis of addiction in which patients exhibit behaviors often seen in addictive disease, such as escalating demands for larger doses of opioids, but actually reflect undertreated pain; may co-exist with the disease of addiction and drive relapse behaviors.

Refractory Nonresponsive or resistant to therapeutic interventions such as first- and second-line analgesics.

Rescue dose Also referred to as *supplemental dose* or *breakthrough dose*. Administered on a PRN basis (as needed) in combination with the regularly scheduled analgesic to relieve pain that exceeds, or breaks through, the ongoing pain.

Short acting Oral opioid analgesics with a relatively fast onset of action (e.g., 30 minutes) and short duration (3 to 4 hours) and often referred to a "normal release" and inaccurately as "immediate release." The term *immediate release* is particularly problematic because none of the oral opioid analgesics have an immediate onset of action. The term *short acting* will be used in this book.

Supraspinal Involving the brainstem or cerebrum.

Sustained release See modified release.

Systemic drug treatment; systemic administration Administration of a drug by a given route that allows absorption into the systemic circulation. Routes include oral, parenteral (IV, IM, SC), rectal, vaginal, topical application, transdermal, intranasal, and transmucosal. By contrast, the spinal route of administration deposits the drug directly into the central nervous system, minimizing the amount of drug that reaches the systemic circulation.

Titration Adjusting the amount (e.g., adjusting the dose of opioid).

Tolerance A process characterized by decreasing effects of a drug at its previous dose, or the need for a higher dose of drug to maintain an effect; not the same as **addiction**.

Upregulation An increase in a cellular component, e.g., increase in the number of receptors making the cells more sensitive to a particular drug or other agent.

Terminology Related to Research

Anecdotal evidence Evidence derived from clinical observations, clinical experience, or published case reports.

Case reports Published reports of one or more patient cases describing patient experiences, circumstances, or situations that infer specific outcomes that are not based on any scientific method of study.

Case-control study A retrospective observational study used most often to evaluate risk factors that may help explain the appearance or presentation of a disease or condition. Subjects with a known disease or condition are matched with similar individuals who do not possess it. Various potential risk factors, such as age or sex, or lifestyle factors, are then statistically evaluated to determine their levels of association with the disease or condition.

Cohort study A retrospective or prospective study in which a group of subjects who have a specific condition or receive a particular treatment are evaluated over time for a defined period. Data may be compared with another group of subjects who do not have the same condition or receive the same treatment, or subgroups within the cohort may be compared.

Controlled studies/trials Research studies that exert some or total control over the various treatment effects by using a comparison group (placebo group or comparator treatment group) and may use a single- or double-blind design, or random assignment of subjects.

Double-blind study Neither the investigator nor the subject know the critical aspects of the study (e.g., in a placebo-controlled trial, neither the person administering the intervention nor the subject receiving the intervention know if the intervention is experimental or placebo); used to reduce investigator and subject bias.

Meta-analysis Data analysis in which the results of several studies that address related research are combined and analyzed to arrive at one overall measurement of treatment effect.

Number needed to treat (NNT) A parameter that is often used in reporting the results of epidemiologic studies, clinical trials, systematic reviews, and meta-analyses. It is an estimate of how many people would need to receive an intervention to prevent one undesirable outcome or how many people need to receive a treatment in order that one derives a well-defined benefit (e.g., a 50% reduction in pain). NNT is calculated by using a formula that involves a known risk reduction or benefit analysis. Investigators typically determine and define the outcome that is used to compute the NNT for their study.

Open-label Both the investigators and the subjects know what treatment subjects are receiving. An investigator studies the response to an analgesic in a sample of patients and follows them through the treatment phase, observing and recording the effects. A disadvantage of this study design is potential bias for patient selection, observations, and conclusions.

Placebo-controlled trial A study that compares a treatment to a placebo, which is a treatment with no known therapeutic value. The placebo typically resembles the active intervention and is used as the control to determine the active intervention's efficacy.

Randomized controlled trial (RCT) A study in which subjects are randomly assigned (by chance alone) to receive the various interventions in a study. Randomization increases the likelihood that factors that could influence the effects produced by a treatment are distributed evenly across treatment groups, thereby limiting the risk of bias.

Relative risk (RR) A measure of the risk of a certain event happening in one group compared with the risk of the same event happening in another group. For example, in cancer research, relative risk is used in prospective (forward looking) studies, such as cohort studies and clinical trials. A relative risk of 1 means there is no difference between groups in terms of their risk of cancer, based on whether or not they were exposed to a certain substance or factor, or how they responded to two treatments being compared. A relative risk of greater than 1 or less than 1 means that being exposed to a certain substance or factor either increases (relative risk greater than 1) or decreases (relative risk less than 1) the risk of cancer, or that the treatments being compared do not have the same effects (e.g., a relative risk of 2 would mean that those exposed to a certain substance or factor have twice the risk of cancer compared with those who are not exposed to a certain substance or factor). Relative risk is also often called *relative ratio*.

Sequential trials One drug is tried and if the results are unfavorable, it is discontinued and another drug is tried. A trial-and-error approach in which one drug after another is tried until the desired effects occur.

Single-blind study The investigators know what treatment conditions to which subjects are assigned, but subjects are "blinded" (not aware) of what they are receiving.

Some of the most persistent barriers to the effective treatment of pain come from clinician and patient fears and misconceptions surrounding the use of opioid analgesics. Abundant research shows that physicians and others underprescribe opioid analgesics, nurses give inadequate doses (often less than prescribed), and patients take too little to control their pain (Ardery, Herr, Hannon, et al., 2003; Dix, Sandhar, Murdoch, et al., 2004; Jacobsen, Sjogren, Moldrup, et al., 2007; Roth, Burgess, 2008; Schumacher, West, Dodd, et al., 2002). (See Section II for more on the undertreatment of pain.)

A key to effective pain management is that opioid doses must be individualized to meet each patient's unique analgesic needs. To accomplish this, a collaborative approach to managing pain is recommended (Pasero, Portenoy, McCaffery, 1999). As discussed in Section II, high-quality pain control requires patients with pain and the health care team members who care for them to share common goals, a common knowledge base, and a common language with regard to the use of opioid drugs in managing pain.

This section of the book is based on the assumption that nurses have an active and pivotal role in the daily, ongoing use of opioid analgesics. For the nurse to fulfill this role, it is essential that institutional policies, analgesic orders, and regulatory agencies support the nurses' role in teaching patients about pain and in assessing and managing it. This is especially critical with regard to titrating opioid doses and treating adverse effects (Pasero, 2009b; Pasero, Eksterowicz, Primeau, et al., 2007; Pasero, Manworren, McCaffery, 2007).

This section presents the underlying mechanisms of opioid analgesics and their adverse effects (see Section I for more detail on this). Relevant pharmacologic concepts are explained. The indications for opioid analgesic use and guidelines and strategies for administering them are discussed, including how to determine the right opioid drug, dose, interval, and route for patients. The differences in using opioid analgesics for acute pain, cancer pain, and persistent noncancer pain are delineated throughout the section. Important points to include in patient and family teaching are presented, including guidelines for discussing addiction. The controversies and conclusions regarding withholding opioid analgesic treatment are discussed. Misconceptions related to the use of opioid analgesics are presented and corrected in the following table. Selected terms and definitions are listed at the beginning of this section to facilitate an understanding of the section content.

Misconceptions about Opioid Analgesics

Misconception	Correction
Taking opioids for pain relief leads to addiction.	Addiction occurring as a result of taking opioids for pain relief is rare (<1%).
How much analgesia opioids can produce is limited.	The dose and the analgesic effect of mu agonist opioids have no ceiling, but dose may be limited by adverse effects.
Not all pain responds to opioids.	All pain responds to opioids, but some types of pain are more responsive than others. Opioids are particularly effective in relieving visceral and somatic pain and less effective in relieving neuropathic pain. Although a number of factors can affect opioid responsiveness, no evidence exists that any characteristic of the pain or the patient causes uniform opioid resistance.
Opioid treatment should be withheld in the early stages of a progressive disease to prevent the development of tolerance and lack of analgesia in the later stages.	Tolerance to opioid analgesia may or may not be evident during opioid treatment; dose usually stabilizes if pain is stable. In addition, tolerance is treatable, usually by increasing the opioid dose; no ceiling to the analgesia of opioids exists, and patients develop tolerance to respiratory depression. Clinicians should not withhold opioid treatment from patients with long life expectancies or delay initiating opioid therapy for fear of encountering unmanageable tolerance.
The more potent opioids are the more therapeutically superior opioids.	Potency does not determine efficacy. Potency can be viewed as the ratio of the dose of two analgesics required to produce the same analgesic effect. All mu agonist opioids are capable of producing the same degree of analgesia when given at equianalgesic doses. Increased potency alone does not provide any advantage because the more potent drugs also exhibit a parallel increase in their ability to produce undesirable effects.
When pain is no longer relieved by a given opioid dose, the opioid should be discontinued to allow the receptors to "reset" and become more sensitive to opioids.	Continued stimulation of opioid receptors does not result in desensitization. Stopping the opioid will not make the receptors more sensitive to opioids. When a given dose is safe but ineffective, the dose should be increased by appropriate percentages, keeping in mind that no ceiling to the analgesia of mu agonist opioids exists.
Long-term opioid therapy places the patient at high risk for developing opioid-induced hyperalgesia (OIH) and is a reason for avoiding long-term use of opioids.	The actual incidence of OIH is unknown, but it appears to be a rare outcome of long-term opioid therapy and at this time cannot be predicted.
When OIH occurs, all opioids must be stopped.	Treatment of OIH does involve reduction in the dose of the original opioid, but resumption of satisfactory pain relief may be achieved in some patients by rotation to another opioid, especially methadone.
Opioids frequently cause clinically significant respiratory depression.	Opioid-induced respiratory depression is rare if opioid doses are titrated slowly and decreased when increased sedation is detected. Clinically significant opioid-induced respiratory depression can be avoided in opioid-naïve patients by careful nurse monitoring of sedation levels. Tolerance to the respiratory depressant effect of opioids develops within 72 hours of regular daily doses. Therefore in patients who have been taking opioids on a long-term basis, a wider margin of safety exists. The fear of causing death from respiratory depression by administering opioids to the terminally ill also is exaggerated. Opioids given to relieve pain during the withholding and withdrawal of life support in terminally ill patients do not hasten death.

Continued

Misconceptions about Opioid Analgesics—cont'd

Misconception	Correction
Agonist-antagonist opioid analgesics are safer than other opioids because they do not produce respiratory depression and will prevent addiction and discourage drug-seeking behavior.	At equianalgesic doses all opioids cause equal respiratory depression. The agonist-antagonist opioid drugs have a ceiling for the amount of analgesia and respiratory depression they cause (i.e., beyond a certain dose, no further analgesia or respiratory depression is produced), but this is usually above recommended doses. Furthermore, respiratory depression from buprenorphine is not readily reversed by naloxone. Agonist-antagonist opioids can produce significant sedation and extremely unpleasant dysphoria. Addiction is no less likely with agonist-antagonist drugs than with other opioids. Finally, the practice of administering agonist-antagonist opioid analgesics to known drug abusers to discourage drug-seeking behavior is not appropriate because it may precipitate withdrawal. Because agonist-antagonist drugs antagonize at the mu opioid receptor site, they should be avoided in patients who are physically dependent on opioid drugs.
Endorphins and enkephalins are effective analgesics.	Endorphins and enkephalins bind to opioid receptor sites and prevent the release of the neurotransmitters, thereby inhibiting the transmission of pain impulses. Unfortunately, endogenous opioids degrade too quickly to be considered useful analgesics. Although administering morphine and other opioids probably temporarily decreases production of endogenous opioids, belief that use of opioids, such as morphine, should be avoided for this reason is unfounded.

Chapter 11 Physiology and Pharmacology of Opioid Analgesics

THIS chapter expands on the underlying mechanisms of the opioid analgesics presented in Section I of this book. Several pharmacokinetic and pharmacodynamic concepts are explained. Terms such as *opioid naïve* and *opioid tolerant* are distinguished, and *addiction, pseudo-addiction, physical dependence, tolerance,* and *cross tolerance* are defined. The research and recommended diagnostic and treatment approaches for *opioid-induced hyperalgesia* are presented.

Groups of Opioids

The opioid agonist drugs can be divided into two major groups. The largest group is the morphine-like agonists. The terms *morphine-like drugs, mu agonists, pure agonists,* and *full agonists* are used interchangeably. Throughout this book, the term *mu agonist* will be used when referring to opioid drugs in this group. The other group of opioids is the agonist-antagonist group and is further divided into the mixed agonist-antagonists and the partial agonists. Opioid agonist drugs can be distinguished from opioid compounds more generally. Opioid compounds include both drugs and endogenous chemicals (generically called the *endorphins*); they also refer to

both agonists, which produce effects at opioid receptors, and antagonists, which block or reverse effects produced by the agonists.

Underlying Mechanisms of Opioid Analgesia and Adverse Effects

To understand the appropriate use of opioids in the treatment of pain, it is valuable to review the mechanisms that are described by the term *nociception*. Nociception refers to the normal functioning of physiologic systems that lead to the perception of noxious stimuli as painful. In short, it means "normal" pain transmission. Nociception is described in Section I of this book. Review of Section I is advised so that the following discussion of the underlying mechanisms of the analgesia and adverse effects of opioids is clear.

Endogenous Opioid System

As explained in the discussion of nociception in Section I, the modulation (inhibition) of pain involves the release of dozens of neurochemicals by peripheral and central systems. Endogenous opioids (internal naturally-occurring), for example, are found throughout the periphery and central nervous system (CNS), including in the cardiovascular (CV) and gastrointestinal (GI) systems, pituitary gland, and in immune cells (Machelska, 2007; Mousa, 2003; Murphy, 2006; Rittner, Brack, 2007). It is thought that opioids given therapeutically activate endogenous pain-modulating systems and produce analgesia and other effects by binding to opioid receptor sites and mimicking the action of endogenous opioid compounds. Endogenous opioids are composed of three distinct families of peptides (naturally occurring compounds of two or more amino acids), all pharmacologically related to morphine: enkephalins, dynorphins, and β-endorphins (Gutstein, Akil, 2006; Inturrisi, 2002). Other endogenous peptides that have been more recently discovered—the endomorphins and orphanin-FQ—also appear to be important in pain processing, but their roles are yet poorly understood; the endomorphins bind selectively to the mu receptor, and orphanin-FQ is a ligand for another receptor, which is known as *opioid receptor–like 1* (ORL1).

Although discovered in the 1970s (Gutstein, Akil, 2006), not everything is known about the physiologic role of endogenous opioids (Fine, Portenoy, 2007). They may serve as neurotransmitters, neuromodulators, and neurohormones (Inturrisi, 2002). Research is ongoing to identify more endogenous opioid compounds and add to the understanding of this role and the potential for new analgesics (Noble, Roques, 2007; Wisner, Dufour, Messaoudi, et al., 2006). Among other important activities, they are involved in hemostasis and the stress response.

Opioid Receptors

Drugs exert their effects on the body by interacting with specialized macromolecular components in cells called *drug receptors*. Drug receptors usually are cellular proteins, but can be enzymes, carbohydrate residues, and lipids. The binding of drug molecules to their specific receptor molecules often is described as similar to a key fitting a lock (Figure 11-1). Binding affinity refers to the strength of attachment of a drug to the receptor site, and

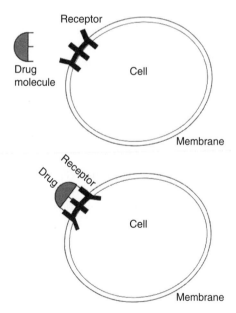

Figure 11-1 | Drug and receptor interaction. The binding of drug molecules to their specific receptor molecules, often described as similar to a key fitting a lock, is shown. The electromagnetic forces produced by the bond between a drug and receptor distort the configuration of the receptor molecule, changing its biochemical properties and functions. The body's responses to the drug are a result of these changes.

From Spencer, R. T. Pharmacodynamics and pharmacokinetics. In *Clinical pharmacology and nursing management*, ed 4, Philadelphia, 1993, Lippincott Williams & Wilkins.) As appears in Pasero, C., & McCaffery, M. *Pain assessment and pharmacologic management*, p. 284, St. Louis, Mosby. May be duplicated for use in clinical practice.

drugs bind with varying strength. The electromagnetic forces produced by the bond between a drug and receptor distort the configuration of the receptor molecule, changing its biochemical properties and functions. The body's responses to the drug are a result of these changes (Bateman, Eddleston, 2007).

Researchers think that receptors evolved for the purpose of interacting with endogenous compounds. The endogenous opioid system is an excellent example of this interaction. Opioid receptors are particularly abundant in the periacqueductal gray (PAG) and dorsal horn of the spinal cord. They are also located in the brainstem, thalamus, and cortex. Their presence in the midbrain PAG, nucleus raphe magnus, and the rostral ventral medulla help to inhibit pain via the descending modulatory system (Inturrisi, 2002). (See Section I and Figure I-2, *D* on pp. 4-5.)

Nociceptors—the primary afferent neurons that carry information about noxious stimuli from the periphery—terminate in the dorsal horn of the spinal cord. These cells release neurotransmitters, such as adenosine triphosphate, glutamate, and substance P, to further pain transmission. This is one of the sites at which endogenous and exogenous opioids play an important role in pain control by binding with opioid receptors, reducing the influx of calcium at the cellular level, and, among other functions, blocking the release of presynaptic neurotransmitters, principally substance P (Inturrisi, 2002). They also increase potassium influx, resulting in a decrease in synaptic transmission.

Opioids also reduce pain transmission by activating inhibitory pathways that originate segmentally (in the spinal cord) and supraspinally (Inturrisi, 2002). For example, the gamma aminobutyric acid (GABA) pathway is one of the major inhibitory neurotransmitter systems (see Section I), and opioids can activate the GABA system, leading to inhibition of pain transmission (Bridges, Thompson, Rice, 2001).

For many years, opioid analgesics were thought to produce analgesia only through the CNS. However, more recently, opioid receptors have been found also on peripheral terminals of sensory nerves and cells of the immune system (Fine, Portenoy, 2007; Inturrisi, 2002; Machelska, 2007; Mousa, 2003; Rittner, Brack, 2007). Their location in peripheral tissues has led to research suggesting that opioids also can produce analgesia following local administration by binding to the peripheral opioid receptors (Inturrisi, 2002; Zajaczkowska, Wlodzimierz, Wordliczek, et al., 2004). This may account for the antiinflammatory actions of opioid drugs on peripheral tissues (Nunez, Lee, Zhang, et al., 2007).

Classes of Opioid Receptor Sites

Three major classes or types of opioid receptor sites are involved in analgesia: mu, delta, and kappa. The pharmacologic differences in the various opioids are the result of their interaction with these three opioid receptor types

(Inturrisi, 2002). A fourth receptor, structurally similar to the opioid receptor and designated as ORL-1 (opioid receptor–like 1), has been identified (Fine, Portenoy, 2007). The ligand for ORL-1, orphanin FQ or OFQ, induces spinal analgesia and appears to be involved in the modulation of pain but is not associated with respiratory depression. Research is needed to develop drugs that take advantage of this receptor site (Murphy, 2006). Subtypes of each of the main opioid receptor types have also been identified and may account for the wide variability in patient response to the various opioid analgesics (Fine, Portenoy, 2007; Pasternak, 2005).

When an opioid binds to the mu, delta, or kappa opioid receptor sites as an agonist, it produces analgesia as well as unwanted effects, such as nausea, constipation, and respiratory depression. Antagonists are drugs that also bind to opioid receptors but produce no analgesia. If an antagonist is present, it competes with opioid molecules for binding sites on the receptors. When a drug binds to any of the opioid receptor sites as an antagonist, analgesia and other effects are blocked. For example, naloxone, an opioid antagonist, can bind to the mu site and reverse analgesia and other opioid adverse effects, such as respiratory depression and sedation (Gutstein, Akil, 2006). See Table 11-1 for a summary of actions at opioid receptor type.

Opioid drugs that produce analgesia all have agonist effects at one or more of the opioid receptor site types and are classified based on the receptors to which they bind and act (Pasternak, 2005). Most of the clinically useful opioid analgesics bind primarily to mu opioid receptor sites (Gutstein, Akil, 2006). These are the mu agonist opioid analgesics, which are considered the mainstay of analgesia for acute pain and cancer pain. Examples of mu agonist opioid analgesics are morphine, hydromorphone (Dilaudid), fentanyl, oxycodone, hydrocodone, codeine, methadone (Dolophine), and meperidine (Demerol). Mu agonists can be administered by numerous routes, and onset of analgesia is within minutes by some routes. They can be combined with almost any of the nonopioid and adjuvant analgesics.

The mixed agonist-antagonist opioid analgesics are designated as mixed because they bind to more than one opioid receptor site. They bind as agonists, producing analgesia at the kappa opioid receptor sites, and as weak antagonists at the mu opioid receptor sites (Gutstein, Akil, 2006). Mixed agonist-antagonists opioid analgesics include butorphanol (Stadol), nalbuphine (Nubain), pentazocine (Talwin), and dezocine (Dalgan). Their clinical usefulness is limited because of undesirable adverse effects (Gutstein, Akil, 2006). Some of the mixed agonist-antagonists produce more dysphoria

Table 11-1 | Summary of Actions at Opioid Receptor Type

Opioid Receptor Site	Activity	Opioids with Agonist Action	Opioids with Antagonist Action
Mu (μ)	Spinal and supraspinal analgesia, respiratory depression, CV effects, physical dependence, tolerance, decreased GI motility, urinary retention, pruritus, euphoria	Pure: e.g., morphine, methadone, codeine, fentanyl, sufentanil, alfentanil, oxycodone, levorphanol, oxymorphone, hydromorphone (Dilaudid), meperidine (Demerol)	Pure: naloxone (Narcan), naltrexone (Trexan), nalmefene (Revex), methylnaltrexone (Relistor), alvimopan (Entereg), butorphanol (Stadol), nalbuphine (Nubain), pentazocine (Talwin), dezocine (Dalgan) Partial: buprenorphine, (Buprenex)
Kappa (κ)	Spinal and supraspinal analgesia, miosis, psychotomimetic effects (dysphoria, agitation), and sedation without pronounced respiratory depression, euphoria, or gastrointestinal effects	Butorphanol, nalbuphine, pentazocine, buprenorphine, oxycodone, sufentanil (weak affinity), methadone (weak affinity)	Pure: naloxone, naltrexone, nalmefene
Delta (δ)	Spinal and supraspinal analgesia without respiratory compromise. (Effects are under investigation.)	Levorphanol, dezocine, sufentanil (weak affinity), morphine (weak affinity) methadone (weak affinity), oxymorphone (weak affinity)	Naloxone, naltrexone, nalmefene, pentazocine

CV, Cardiovascular; *GI*, gastrointestinal.
The effects (activity) a drug produces depends on the type(s) of opioid receptor(s) to which the drug binds and whether the drug acts as an agonist or an antagonist at that opioid receptor type. When a drug binds to any of these receptor sites as an agonist, it produces analgesia and other effects. When a drug binds to any of the opioid receptor sites as an antagonist, analgesia and other effects are blocked. Table 11-1 summarizes the activity of drugs when they bind to any of three opioid receptor types that are involved in analgesia.

From Pasero, C., & McCaffery, M. *Pain assessment and pharmacologic management*, p. 285, St. Louis, Mosby. Data from Fine, P., & Portenoy, R. K. (2007). *A clinical guide to opioid analgesia*. New York, Vendome Group, LLC; Gutstein, H. B., & Akil, H. (2006). Opioid analgesics. In L. L. Brunton, J. S. Lazo, & K. L. Parker (Eds.), *Goodman & Gilman's the pharmacological basis of therapeutics*, ed 11, New York, McGraw-Hill; Hanks, G., Cherny, N. I., & Fallon, M. Opioid analgesic therapy. In D. Doyle, G. Hanks, N. I. Cherny, et al. (Eds.), *Oxford textbook of palliative medicine*, ed 3, New York, Oxford Press. © 2011, Pasero C, McCaffery M. May be duplicated for use in clinical practice.

and psychotomimetic effects than the pure mu agonists, and all appear to have a ceiling effect to the respiratory depression effects.

Although buprenorphine (Buprenex) has some kappa agonist activity, it is known primarily as a partial mu agonist drug. It is referred to as *partial* because it binds as an agonist at the mu opioid receptors but has limited intrinsic efficacy (Gutstein, Akil, 2006). In the clinical setting, this means that analgesia plateaus as the dose is increased. Buprenorphine also has very high affinity for the mu receptor. It is not readily reversed by opioid antagonists, such as naloxone, which suggests the drug dissociates very slowly from the mu opioid receptor sites (Gutstein, Akil, 2006). The drug is used most often as a maintenance drug for the treatment of addictive disease (Suboxone, Subutex) (see Chapter 13).

Opioid Receptors and Adverse Effects

The type of opioid receptor site and its location determine the effects an opioid drug produces. As mentioned, in addition to producing analgesia, opioid drugs produce a number of other effects, including constipation, nausea and vomiting, sedation, respiratory depression, and urinary retention (Gutstein, Akil, 2006) (see Table 11-1).

The main GI effect of opioid drugs is inhibition of GI peristalsis and diminished GI, biliary, and pancreatic secretions, which can lead to constipation and predispose to ileus and other adverse effects as a result of opioid binding to receptors located in the GI tract and CNS (Gutstein, Akil, 2006; Kraft, 2007; Thomas, 2008). Opioid bowel syndrome is described as a "constellation" of undesirable outcomes, including but not limited to constipation (McNicol, Boyce, Schumann, et al., 2008). Nausea and vomiting are the result of opioid binding to receptors located in the fourth ventricle of the brain and direct stimulation of the chemoreceptor trigger zone in the area postrema of the medulla (Freye, 2008). Urinary retention may occur when opioid binding leads to inhibition of the release of acetylcholine (Freye, 2008). Respiratory depression may follow binding in the pontine and ventral medulla of the brainstem (Freye, 2008), and sedation occurs from binding to receptors in the brain (Gutstein, Akil, 2006) (see Chapter 19 for discussion of opioid adverse effects).

Pharmacologic Concepts

After systemic (oral or parenteral) administration, an opioid drug is absorbed into the vascular system. For the drug to produce a pharmacologic effect, it must leave the plasma, diffuse into tissue, reach opioid receptors, and activate them (Gutstein, Akil, 2006). Topical administration may rely on both peripheral and systemic absorption (LeBon, Zeppetella, Higginson, et al., 2009; Ribeiro, Joel, Zeppetella, 2004; Sawynok, 2003). When administered by intraspinal routes of administration, opioids are carried

via the cerebrospinal fluid (CSF) to opioid receptor sites in the spinal cord and brain (Freye, 2008). Appropriate use of opioid analgesics requires an understanding of these processes and some important pharmacologic concepts. The following is a discussion of pharmacokinetics (the movement of the drug through the body) and pharmacodynamics (what effects are produced). Tolerance, cross-tolerance, opioid-induced hyperalgesia, physical dependence, addiction, pseudoaddiction, and equianalgesia also are discussed.

Pharmacokinetics

Pharmacokinetics is the science of what the body does to a drug after its administration. Pharmacokinetic processes include absorption, distribution, metabolism, and elimination and are discussed in the following sections along with other related key concepts.

Absorption, Bioavailability, First Pass Effect, and Solubility

Absorption is the rate and extent to which a drug leaves its site of administration and moves to plasma or other tissues. A more clinically important concept than absorption is bioavailability, which is the extent to which a dose of a drug reaches its site of action (Buxton, 2006), or how much drug is available for therapeutic effect. Opioid drugs are 100% bioavailable when administered intravenously because they are introduced directly into the systemic circulation. After oral administration, opioids are absorbed from the GI tract and transported by the portal vein to the liver, the primary site of drug metabolism, before they reach systemic circulation. This process reduces the bioavailability of an opioid when administered orally (Buxton, 2006). Oral bioavailability depends on how much of the drug is absorbed in the GI tract and inactivated as it passes through the liver. This is called first pass effect. First pass effect is why the dose of an opioid drug by the oral route must be much larger than by the parenteral route to produce equal analgesia (Buxton, 2006). For example, the bioavailability of morphine when given orally usually is between 20% and 30% because of first pass losses (De Pinto, Dunbar, Edwards, 2006; Gutstein, Akil, 2006; Stevens, Ghazi, 2000) (Figure 11-2).

Many factors influence a drug's absorption and bioavailability besides route of administration. The site of absorption, including its surface area and vascularity, is important. Drugs are absorbed rapidly from large surface areas, such as the intestinal mucosa, and when there is increased blood flow at the site (Buxton, 2006). A high concentration of drug in a small volume leads to faster absorption compared with a low concentration in a large volume. The presence of a pathologic condition also affects bioavailability. For example, bioavailability is increased in hepatic dysfunction because the liver cannot metabolize and excrete the drug efficiently (Johnson, 2007).

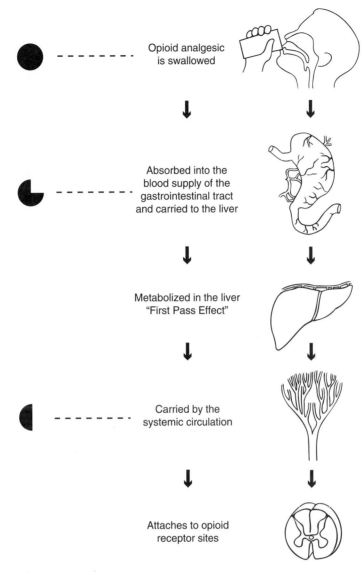

Opioid analgesic
is swallowed

Absorbed into the
blood supply of the
gastrointestinal tract
and carried to the liver

Metabolized in the liver
"First Pass Effect"

Carried by the
systemic circulation

Attaches to opioid
receptor sites

Figure 11-2 | Drug absorption and metabolism by the oral route. The solid sphere represents an opioid analgesic pill. The decreasing size of the pill represents loss through absorption to the gastrointestinal tract and metabolism in the liver. The half sphere represents the dose of opioid available for analgesia at the opioid receptor sites (bioavailability) after it has been diminished by absorption and metabolism.

From Pasero, C., & McCaffery, M. *Pain assessment and pharmacologic management*, p. 287, St. Louis, Mosby. © 2011, Pasero C, McCaffery M. May be duplicated for use in clinical practice.

Characteristics of the drug itself also help to determine its bioavailability (Buxton, 2006). A drug's bioavailability will be decreased if it is a drug for which the liver has a great capacity to metabolize and excrete, such as hydromorphone. When given intravenously, hydromorphone is 100% bioavailable and the recommended starting adult dose for severe pain is 1.5 mg given over a 4-hour period; when given orally, which subjects the drug to a significant first-pass effect, the equianalgesic dose is approximately five times greater at 7.5 mg (see later in this chapter for more on equianalgesia).

A drug's solubility also influences its bioavailability. The more lipid soluble (also referred to as *lipophilic*, meaning readily dissolved into fatty tissues) the drug, the more readily it moves through membranes, which may increase bioavailability. Lipid solubility also is related to other pharmacokinetic parameters, which may be more important in practice (Buxton, 2006). For example, when highly lipid soluble opioids, such as fentanyl and sufentanil, are administered to opioid-naïve patients, the analgesic and other effects have a rapid onset and a short duration; in contrast, comparable doses of drugs that are less lipid soluble, like morphine and hydromorphone, lead to effects that have a slower onset of action and longer duration; meperidine is intermediate between these drugs. Lipophilicity and all the other factors discussed in this section can affect the efficacy and toxicity of a drug and therefore must be considered when establishing an opioid analgesic regimen.

Protein Binding

Many drugs are bound to plasma proteins, primarily albumin (Buxton, 2006). Plasma protein binding can be viewed as a transport mechanism that delivers drugs to their sites of metabolism. Plasma protein binding limits a drug's concentration in tissues and at its site of action because only unbound drug is in equilibrium across membranes and can move freely. Bound drug is devoid of pharmacologic activity; drug responses, whether efficacious or toxic, are a function of unbound concentrations (Buxton, 2006).

Metabolism, Metabolites, and Prodrugs

When a drug passes through the liver, and often through other tissues, it is subjected to multiple biochemical processes and reactions (metabolism) that change part of the drug into different compounds. Enzymes mediate most of these processes and reactions. The resulting products are called *metabolites*. Many opioid analgesics have metabolites, including morphine (morphine-6-glucuronide [M6G] and morphine-3-glucuronide [M3G]), meperidine (normeperidine), and propoxyphene (norpropoxyphene). Metabolites are referred to as being active (having pharmacologic action) or inactive (having no pharmacologic action) (Buxton, 2006).

Metabolites often have properties and characteristics different from their parent drug. Sometimes their pharmacologic actions are indistinguishable from the parent drug, but their biologic activity may be increased, decreased, or eliminated. For example, the major metabolite of morphine, M6G, is analgesic like its parent but is significantly more potent (Buxton, 2006) (see Chapter 13).

Prodrugs are pharmacologically inactive compounds (sometimes called *inactive precursors*) that are converted quickly to active metabolites following administration (Buxton, 2006). Prodrugs are sometimes used to maximize the amount of the active drug that reaches the site of action. Codeine is an example of a prodrug. To produce analgesia, it must be catalyzed by the cytochrome (CY) P450 enzyme CYP2D6 to morphine.

Cytochrome P450 Enzyme System. Two major hepatic enzyme systems are responsible for metabolism of opioids: CYP450 and, to a lesser extent, the UDP-glucuronosyltransferases (UGTs) (Holmquist, 2009). The UGTs are involved in the formation of glucuronides and the metabolism of hydromorphone, morphine, and oxymorphone. The CYP450 enzyme system is important to the metabolism of codeine, fentanyl, methadone, oxycodone,

and oxymorphone (Holmquist, 2009). CYP450 enzymes also are located in other tissues of the body and are the primary enzymes involved in drug metabolism and the production of cholesterol, steroids, prostacylins, and other essential substances (Holmquist, 2009).

Drugs interact with the CYP450 enzyme system by acting as a substrate (metabolized by one or more of the CYP450 enzymes); an inhibitor (slowing the activity of CYP450 enzyme metabolism); or an inducer (boosting the activity of CYP450 metabolism) (Holmquist, 2009). There are more than 50 different CYP450 enzymes, but not all are involved in drug metabolism. The CYP2D6 and CYP3A4 are the most important to opioid metabolism (Fine, Portenoy, 2007). Patients may lack normal levels of these enzymes as a result of genetics, hepatic disease, or competition with other medications that are metabolized by the same enzymes (Fine, Portenoy, 2007).

There are four major CYP2D6 phenotypes, which render patients poor, intermediate, extensive, or ultra-rapid metabolizers (Holmquist, 2009). There are interethnic variations in phenotypes (Palmer, Giesecke, Body, et al., 2005); it is estimated that 7% to 10% of Caucasians and 1% of Asians are poor metabolizers (Holmquist, 2009; Paice, 2008). Patients who are poor metabolizers have altered pharmacokinetics of 2D6-metabolized drugs, which may cause clinically important effects in some. For example, whereas hydromorphone, morphine, and oxymorphone are not metabolized by the CYP450 enzymes to a great extent (UGT is their primary metabolic pathway) and genetic polymorphisms of the CYP450 enzymes have little effect, the prodrug codeine relies on 2D6 to become the active compound morphine, and slow metabolizers may not respond well to codeine as a result (Fine, Portenoy, 2007; Palmer, Giesecke, Body, et al., 2005). Ultra-rapid metabolizers at 2D6 may have an exaggerated (i.e., toxic) response to codeine (Voronov, Przybylo, Jagannathan, et al., 2007; United States Food and Drug Administration [U.S. FDA], 2007a; Palmer, Giesecke, Body, et al., 2005).

Some drugs compete with opioids for metabolism by specific enzymes, which may result in drug-drug interactions. Table 11-2 lists potential drug interactions for the CYP2D6 and CYP3A4 enzymes. Box 11-1 provides websites where information can be found regarding drugs that are metabolized by the cytochrome P450 enzyme system and their potential drug-drug interactions.

Half-Life, Clearance, Steady State, and Accumulation

Drugs are eliminated from the body either unchanged or as metabolites. The kidney is the primary organ for elimination of drugs and metabolites. Drugs are also excreted in the feces, breast milk, sweat, saliva, tears, hair, and skin. The pulmonary route of excretion is important mainly for anesthetic gases and vapors (Buxton, 2006).

Terminal half-life provides an estimate of how fast a drug leaves the body. By definition, half-life is the time it takes for the amount of drug in the body to be reduced by

Table 11-2 | Potential Drug Interactions for Major Cytochrome P-450 Enzymes CYP3A4 and CYP2D6

Enzyme	Substrates	Inhibitors	Inducers
CYP3A4	Alprazolam, amitriptyline, bupropion, dexamethasone, dextromethorphan, diazepam, fentanyl, fluoxetine, ketamine, lidocaine, meperidine, methadone, prednisone, sertraline, venlafaxine	Fluoxetine, paroxetine, propoxyphene, venlafaxine	Carbamazepine, dexamethasone, phenytoin, rifampin
CYP2D6	Amitriptyline, bupropion, codeine, desipramine, dextromethorphan, doxepin, fluoxetine, haloperidol, hydrocodone, methadone, morphine, nortriptyline, oxycodone, paroxetine, sertraline, tramadol, venlafazine	Celecoxib, bupropion, desipramine, haloperidol, metoclopramide, paroxetine, venlafaxine	Carbamazepine, dexamethasone, phenytoin, rifampin

From Pasero, C., & McCaffery, M. *Pain assessment and pharmacologic management*, p. 289, St. Louis, Mosby. Data from Clinical Pharmacology Online. Gold Standard, Inc. Available at http://clinicalpharmacology.com; Cytochrome P450 Interactions ©GlobalRPh Inc. Available at http://www.globalrph.com/cytochrome. htm; Cytochrome P450 and Drug Interactions (Drugs that Induce or Inhibit Various Cytochrome P-450 Systems). Available at http://www.edhayes.com/CYP450-3.html. © 2011, Pasero C, McCaffery M. May be duplicated for use in clinical practice.

Box 11-1 | Cytochrome P450 Enzyme System: Information Websites

- CYP450 Interactions: Flockhart, D. A. Drug Interactions: Cytochrome P450 Drug Interaction Table. Indiana University School of Medicine (2007). http://medicine.iupui.edu/flockhart/table.htm
- Cytochrome P450 and Drug Interactions (Drugs that Induce or Inhibit Various Cytochrome P-450 Systems): http://www.edhayes.com/CYP450-3.html
- P450 Enzyme Drug Interactions By Erowid: http://www.erowid.org/psychoactives/pharmacology/pharmacology_enzymes1.shtml#4
- An excellent resource for information about drug interactions and that contains a list of online sites that offer specific information about drug interactions can be found in Leavitt SB. (2005). *Methadone-drug interaction*, ed 3. Addiction Treatment Forum. http://www.atforum.com/SiteRoot/pages/addiction_resources/Drug_Interactions.pdf

The following are interactive websites and require the user to enter the drug the patient is taking (or the drug that is being considered). The application returns a list of potential interactions.

- Cytochrome P450 Interactions ©GlobalRPh Inc.: http://www.globalrph.com/cytochrome.htm
- DrugDigest Drug Interaction Checker: http://www.drugdigest.org/wps/portal/ddigest (click on Check Interactions)
- Medscape Drug Interaction Checker: http://www.medscape.com/druginfo/druginterchecker
- Drugs.com Drug Interaction Checker: http://www.drugs.com/drug_interactions.php

From Pasero, C., & McCaffery, M. *Pain assessment and pharmacologic management*, p. 289, St. Louis, Mosby. © 2011, Pasero C, McCaffery M. May be duplicated for use in clinical practice.

50% (Buxton, 2006). Half-life varies significantly from one drug to another. For example, the half-life of morphine is 2 to 4 hours, whereas the half-life of methadone ranges from 4.2 hours to 130 hours in some individuals (Lynch, 2005). Terminal half-life is different from, but sometimes confused with, distribution half-life, which reflects the time necessary for a drug to move from the blood and plasma to other tissues.

Clearance is also a measure of the body's ability to eliminate a drug from the body. The clearance of a drug depends on the organs of elimination coming in contact with the blood or plasma containing the drug (Buxton, 2006). Because the kidney is the major organ of elimination, renal insufficiency can alter drug clearance. Creatinine clearance analysis is a measure of kidney function and a tool to determine the body's ability to handle drugs that are primarily eliminated by the kidney. A high creatinine level may be an indication of reduced kidney function and, therefore, a reduced ability to eliminate a drug. Normally, men tend to have higher creatinine levels than women. Aging is associated with decreased body mass and total body water and an increased proportion of body fat which can alter the rates of clearance and elimination (American Geriatrics Society [AGS], 2009; Cook, Rooke, 2003). Box 11-2 provides serum creatinine and creatinine clearance values for all age groups and the formula for calculating creatinine clearance.

A drug's half-life changes according to the body's ability to clear the drug; therefore, both half-life and clearance are important to consider when developing a regimen for long-term opioid analgesic administration. Both are influenced by age, gender, disease, and body composition. For example, because clearance decreases with age, half-life can be expected to increase (AGS, 2009).

A concept closely related to half-life is steady state. A steady state is approached when the rate of excretion of a drug equals the rate at which the drug enters the system. Long-term opioid analgesic treatment is intended to maintain a steady state of opioid within the therapeutic range.

Half-life determines how long it will take for a given opioid drug to reach steady state. For example, the full effects of a change in dose of an opioid drug will not be seen until the time equal to four to five times the half-life of the opioid drug has passed (Bateman, Eddleston, 2007; Buxton, 2006).

Accumulation (or cumulation) of drug occurs when doses are administered but steady state has not yet been approached; less drug is excreted than is absorbed. When this happens, serum drug levels rise. The phenomenon of accumulation occurs whenever dosing is initiated or the dose is increased during the course of therapy; it also can occur if drug metabolism or excretion changes and clearance declines as a result. Because four to five half-lives are required to approach steady state, opioids that have a relatively long half-life can require a prolonged period of time to stabilize in the blood. During this period, the drug concentration is slowly rising and patients must be carefully monitored. If the dose is increased in an effort to produce analgesia, but the blood level continues to rise for a while after the dose is stable (until four to five half-lives pass), it is possible that unanticipated toxic effects can occur. This scenario can occur with long half-life opioids, like methadone. Problems also can occur if a drug has an active metabolite with a half-life longer than the parent compound. For example, meperidine's metabolite, normeperidine, has a long half-life (15 to 20 hours) compared with the half-life of its parent, meperidine (2 to 3 hours). If meperidine is administered for a few days, accumulation of the normeperidine may lead to adverse effects, which include irritability, tremors, and seizures (see Chapter 13).

Pharmacodynamics

Pharmacodynamics refers to the effects of drugs on the body after their administration. Pharmacodynamic phenomena include potency, efficacy, tolerance, cross tolerance, and physical dependence and are discussed in the following sections along with other conditions, such as opioid-induced hyperalgesia and addiction.

Opioid Responsiveness: Potency and Efficacy

Terms that are sometimes confused when discussing opioid analgesics and their patients' responses to opioid analgesic treatment include efficacy, potency, responsiveness, and resistance. The meaning of efficacy varies, depending on the context in which it is used. Intrinsic efficacy is a pharmacology term defined as the proportion of opioid receptors that must be occupied by a drug to produce a given effect. The receptor occupancy required for an agonist to produce a response is inversely proportional to its intrinsic efficacy.

In the clinical setting, efficacy refers to the extent to which a drug or another treatment "works" and can produce the effect in question—analgesia in this context. To determine whether this is the case, the treatment must be compared with another, typically a placebo, but sometimes an active comparator. *Maximal efficacy* refers to the maximum effect that can be produced by a drug, and *comparative efficacy* refers to the relative effects of two or more treatments compared at comparable treatment intensities.

The term *efficacy* often is contrasted and confused with the term *potency,* which refers to the dose of a drug required to produce a specified effect (Fine, Portenoy, 2007). Relative potency is the ratio of doses required to produce the same analgesic effect (Freye, 2008). For example, parenteral hydromorphone is more potent than parenteral morphine because the dose of hydromorphone required to achieve the same analgesia as morphine is about one sixth that of the morphine dose. On the basis of single-dose studies, the relative potency of parenteral hydromorphone and parenteral morphine is 1.5:10 (see later in this chapter for a discussion on equianalgesia).

A common misconception is that the more potent a drug is, the more therapeutically superior it is. In reality, all opioid analgesics are theoretically capable of producing the same degree of analgesia if doses are appropriately adjusted. Increased potency alone does not provide any advantage because the more potent drugs also exhibit a parallel increase in their ability to produce undesirable effects (Bateman, Eddleston, 2007).

The clinical relevance of efficacy and potency and why potency is less important than efficacy in the clinical setting is better understood by comparing the differences between butorphanol, a mixed agonist-antagonist opioid analgesic, and morphine, a mu agonist opioid analgesic. Although butorphanol is five times more potent than morphine (2 mg of butorphanol produces analgesia comparable to 10 mg of morphine), it has a maximal efficacy far lower than that of morphine. That is, butorphanol's analgesic effect plateaus as the dose is increased, and further dose increases for unrelieved pain will produce no increase in analgesia (analgesic ceiling). On the other hand, morphine, like other mu agonist opioid analgesics, has no analgesic ceiling, and the only limiting factor in increasing its dose is the incidence and severity of adverse effects (Fine, Portenoy, 2007).

The term *efficacy* often is used when clinicians discuss the patient's response to opioid analgesic treatment. A better term to describe clinical response is opioid responsiveness. Opioid responsiveness refers to the probability that adequate analgesia (an overall favorable balance between satisfactory pain relief and adverse effects that are considered tolerable and manageable) can be achieved during dose titration. This is influenced by patient characteristics and the particular type of pain or pain syndrome being treated.

It is a common misconception that certain patient characteristics, such as advancing age (AGS, 2009), or types of pain, such as neuropathic (Finnerup, Otto, McQuay, et al., 2005; Rowbotham, Twilling, Davies, et al., 2003), render a group of patients "opioid-resistant." No evi-

dence exists that this phenomenon of opioid-resistance occurs, and clinicians should not withhold a trial of an opioid on the basis of a priori certainty that an opioid drug will be inefficacious. It is more accurate to proceed on the assumption that all individuals and types of pain are potentially opioid responsive, but they vary in the degree to which they respond, i.e., in the probability that a favorable balance between analgesia and adverse effects will occur if an effort is made to individualize the dose. In short, it is best to view opioid responsiveness on a continuum rather than as an all-or-none phenomenon.

Opioid analgesics should be considered for the treatment of all types of pain. Presumed responsiveness should be one consideration among many in making a decision to proceed with a treatment trial (see the paragraphs that follow). For example, nociceptive somatic pains, such as cancer pain, usually are highly responsive to opioid analgesics, and this observation combined with a worldwide consensus that pain associated with active cancer should be treated with an opioid supports the view that opioid therapy is first-line in this context (Miaskowski, Cleary, Burney, et al., 2005). In contrast, although opioids clearly work in neuropathic pain, guidelines consider them as second-line approaches in most settings (Dworkin, O'Connor, Backonja, et al., 2007). This has many reasons, but one relates to the view that neuropathic pain may be relatively less responsive to opioid therapy than other types of pain and that the opioid doses needed to control neuropathic pain may be more likely to cause intolerable adverse effects (Rowbotham, Twilling, Davies, et al., 2007).

Opioid responsiveness is affected by both the inherent response of the pain to the therapy and also to the predisposition to opioid-related adverse effects. Any factor that increases the risk of dose-limiting toxicity, such as advanced age or major organ dysfunction, will reduce responsiveness.

Significant variation exists in patients' responsiveness to opioid analgesics (interindividual differences). With the same opioid, one patient may achieve excellent analgesia with few adverse effects, whereas another patient experiences intolerable adverse effects with minimal or no analgesia. Patients can vary also in their individual responsiveness to different opioid analgesics (intraindividual differences). For example, a patient may experience unacceptable nausea and poor analgesia with one opioid analgesic and no nausea but unacceptable somnolence and lesser, equal, or better analgesia with another.

Tolerance

In a consensus statement developed by the American Academy of Pain Medicine (AAPM), the American Pain Society (APS), and the American Society of Addiction Medicine (ASAM), tolerance is defined as "a state of adaptation in which exposure to a drug induces changes that result in a diminution of one or more of the drug's effects over time" (ASAM, 2001). In other words, tolerance is a state of adaptation characterized by decreasing effects of the drug at a constant dose or, conversely, the need for a higher dose of drug to maintain an effect (Fine, Portenoy, 2007). The development of acute tolerance, such as may occur when remifentanil is used in surgical patients, has recently been recognized, but the implications of this phenomenon remain uncertain (Fukuda, 2005). In humans, it is likely that tolerance to a variety of opioid effects, including analgesia, can begin to develop after the first dose of opioid, but this is seldom clinically significant (Webster, Dove, 2007). The focus in the clinical setting is on tolerance that develops following continued exposure to opioids, i.e. continued exposure to the drug is the primary cause.

Clinicians often incorrectly conclude that patients with chronic disease who experience diminished analgesia after a period of stable dosing have developed tolerance. A diagnosis of tolerance cannot be made until other causes of decreased pain relief, such as new pathology, disease progression, or lack of adherence to the medication treatment plan, can be ruled out (Fine, Portenoy, 2007). A differential diagnosis is required.

The underlying mechanism of tolerance is not well understood. Several theories involving changes in opioid receptors have been proposed (DuPen, Shen, Ersek, 2007). For example, one theory proposes that opioid receptors become desensitized. However, no agreement has been reached, and the issue remains complex (Angst, Chu, Tingle, et al., 2009; Simonnet, 2009).

Tolerance should not be confused with addiction or physical dependence (described in the following paragraphs), and it is not a predictor of abuse (Fine, Portenoy, 2007). Further, opioid-induced hyperalgesia (discussed in the following paragraphs) and tolerance are two distinct, albeit related, phenomena (Chu, Angst, Clark, 2008).

Although many clinicians suggest that opioid tolerance should be expected with long-term opioid treatment (Miaskowski, Cleary, Burney, et al., 2005), tolerance to the analgesic effects of an opioid may or may not be evident during long-term therapy. Patients who do not have progressive painful disease often achieve a stable dose after titration and require no increase in opioid doses, unless other reasons occur, as mentioned earlier in the chapter (Portenoy, Foley, 1986; Portenoy, Maldonado, Fitzmartin, et al., 1989). There is no specific timeframe for the development of tolerance (Wu, 2005), and, although there may be patient characteristics associated with an increased likelihood of analgesic tolerance (e.g., tolerance may develop more quickly in younger individuals than in older individuals [Buntin-Mushock, Phillip, Moriyana, et al., 2005]), there is great variation among individuals (Webster, Dove, 2007), and clinicians cannot predict those patients who will or will not develop a pattern of opioid response consistent with this phenomenon.

Tolerance develops to both the desirable and undesirable effects of opioids. Tolerance to the various effects of

opioids differs, and the rate at which tolerance develops varies (Webster, Dove, 2007). Tolerance to the nonanalgesic effects of an opioid drug (i.e., adverse effects) occurs and can be beneficial in achieving a balance between analgesia and adverse effects. Tolerance usually develops quickly to respiratory depression (ASAM, 2001), and tolerance to respiratory depression may precede or be more profound than tolerance to sedation; as a result, observations of sedation level are a good way to monitor for impending opioid-induced respiratory depression (see Chapter 19).

Although tolerance to respiratory depression is never complete, it allows patients to escalate doses to a level required for analgesia. Studies have shown that patients with cancer pain may require and safely receive daily doses ranging from 30 to 7000 mg of morphine (or equivalent) (Foley, 1995). In a study of 435 home-care hospice patients, 7 required doses equal to or exceeding 600 mg of oral morphine a day (Bercovitch, Adunsky, 2004). In a study of patients on very high doses of IV methadone, one patient received 1920 mg per day (Vadalouca, Moka, Argyra, et al., 2008). Obviously, these high doses are not common, but they demonstrate the degree of tolerance to respiratory depression that some patients develop. Although there appears to be no limit to the degree of tolerance to respiratory depression that may develop, there is always a lethal dose for the individual.

In contrast to the tolerance to respiratory depression, somnolence and mental clouding, and nausea, all of which usually occur within days or weeks (Foley, 1995; Portenoy, 1996), tolerance to constipation more typically occurs far more slowly, or not at all. It is generally accepted that patients, especially those who are otherwise predisposed to constipation, e.g., older adults, should be routinely treated with a preventative bowel regimen if long-term opioid analgesic therapy is undertaken (Coyle, Cherny, Portenoy, 1995) (see Chapter 19).

Tolerance to analgesia may be evident after a few days of treatment. The first indication of tolerance is most commonly a decrease in the duration of analgesia for a given opioid dose (Miaskowski, Cleary, Burney, et al., 2005) followed by a decrease in analgesic effect. This can be treated easily, usually by increasing the opioid dose or decreasing the interval between doses.

After the opioid is titrated to an acceptable dose, the dose stabilizes if the pain is stable. Further dose escalation in patients with stable pain syndromes is unusual. Thus, stable pain leads to stable doses (Foley, 1993; Levy, 1989; Miaskowski, Cleary, Burney, et al., 2005). If analgesia does decline, it is handled easily, usually by increasing the dose. "There is no arbitrary ceiling beyond which a dose of opioids is unsafe." (p. 23, Webster, Dove, 2007). Further, as stated by ASAM (2001), "Tolerance to the analgesic effects of opioids is variable in occurrence but is never absolute; thus no upper limit to dosage of pure opioid agonists can be established." For these reasons, clinicians should not withhold opioid analgesia from patients with long life expectancies or delay initiating opioid analgesic treatment for fear of producing tolerance or reaching a dose beyond which no further analgesia can be obtained (see Chapter 20).

It is important to reinforce information about tolerance and lack of a ceiling effect to patients and families. They are frequently reluctant to begin opioid analgesic treatment because they are concerned that the effectiveness of opioid analgesics will diminish over time and that the patient will be subjected to severe pain in later stages of disease if the opioid is started in the early stages (Portenoy, 1996). The patient and family should be reassured that as pain increases, the opioid dose probably can be increased and other analgesics, such as nonopioids and adjuvants, can be added.

Pain itself may diminish the adverse effects of opioids. Evidence exists that patients thought to be tolerant to the adverse effects of an opioid drug can experience a return of adverse effects if the pain is lessened or eliminated. Consider a patient who is tolerant to opioid-induced sedation and nausea associated with high doses of morphine taken for pain related to a malignant lesion. The patient may once again experience all of the adverse effects of morphine, including respiratory depression, if an intervention such as cordotomy suddenly eliminates the pain. Under these circumstances, patients may develop signs and symptoms of overdose if the opioid dose is not reduced promptly after the intervention (Portenoy, 1996).

The treatment of acute pain in those receiving long-term opioid therapy for persistent (chronic) pain may be a challenge. It is impossible to predict the degree of tolerance to analgesia and to other effects such as respiratory depression. In opioid-tolerant patients with acute pain, such as postoperative pain, high pain ratings are common (Patanwala, Jarzyna, Miller, et al., 2008). The clinician needs to treat pain based on these pain ratings but also on the observation of safety factors such as sedation levels and respiratory status. Ideally a treatment plan is created preoperatively that assures continuation of the patient's baseline opioid requirements and also considers the use of additional drugs, such as nonopioids and local anesthetics (Patanwala, Jarzyna, Miller, et al., 2008; Wu, 2005). This is discussed in more detail later in the section (see Chapters 16 and 20).

Incomplete Cross-Tolerance

Drugs that act at the same receptor can produce different levels of tolerance, in part because similar drugs (such as the mu agonists) have different intrinsic efficacies. Additionally, each opioid drug interacts with a different group of receptor subtypes (de Leon-Casasola, 2008; Pasternak, 2001, 2005). For these reasons, a switch from one opioid to another similar drug (e.g., from one mu agonist to another) is associated with a variable degree of tolerance to different effects. For example, an animal can be made tolerant to morphine's analgesic effect, but

partial analgesia will reappear on switching to another mu agonist such as hydromorphone.

Clinicians have wondered why analgesics that act at the same mu opioid peptide receptor can result in such a range of responses in individuals, such as differences in adverse effects, and why switching from one mu agonist to another results in incomplete cross-tolerance. One reason is related to the presence of multiple mu opioid peptide receptor subtypes that may be genetically different (de Leon-Casasola, 2008; Pasternak, 2001, 2005). Thus, incomplete-cross-tolerance among mu opioids may be explained in part by their different selectivities for the receptor subtypes.

In opioid rotation, or switching from one mu agonist to another, the principle of incomplete cross-tolerance is said to be the keystone to success. Patients with persistent pain who have been on high-dose opioid therapy are likely to be significantly sensitive to a new opioid (Knotkova, Fine, Portenoy, 2009; Vadalouca, Moka, Argyra, et al., 2008). Therefore, when switching to another opioid, it is vital for clinicians to assume that cross-tolerance exists but will be incomplete (Foley, 1995). This means that the starting dose of the new opioid must be reduced by at least 25% to 50% of the calculated equianalgesic dose to prevent overdosing; otherwise the full calculated equianalgesic dose of the new opioid could lead to effects such as sedation that would be greater than expected (Fine, Portenoy, Ad Hoc Expert Panel on Evidence Review and Guidelines for Opioid Rotation, 2009; Knotkova, Fine, Portenoy, 2009; Indelicato, Portenoy, 2002; Vadalouca, Moka, Argyra, et al., 2008). A methadone dose may need to be reduced by as much as 90% (Fine, Portenoy, Ad Hoc Expert Panel on Evidence Review and Guidelines for Opioid Rotation, 2009) (see Chapter 13 for conversion to methadone). Then the dose is gradually increased as needed to the point of pain relief and tolerable, manageable adverse effects (Coyle, Cherny, Portenoy, 1995; Levy, 1993; Indelicato, Portenoy, 2002).

An example of a clinical implication of incomplete cross-tolerance is that a patient receiving morphine may have developed tolerance to nausea, but when switched to the new opioid drug may experience severe nausea. Thus surveillance of all of the opioid's effects is warranted when switching to an alternative opioid (see Chapter 18).

Opioid-Tolerant versus Opioid-Naïve

The terms *opioid-tolerant* and *opioid-naïve* are used to distinguish between patients who have, or have not, respectively, been taking opioid drugs regularly. Whereas an opioid-naïve individual has not recently taken enough opioid on a regular basis to become opioid-tolerant (i.e., tolerant to the effects of an opioid), an opioid-tolerant individual has taken opioids long enough at doses high enough to develop tolerance to many of the effects of the opioid, including analgesia and sedation. Unfortunately, as mentioned earlier in the chapter, there is no set time for the development of tolerance (Wu, 2005), and there is great variation among individuals, with some not developing tolerance (Webster, Dove, 2007). Therefore, it is difficult to determine if and when an individual on regular doses of opioids has become tolerant. Consequently, there is no widely accepted definition for classifying a patient as opioid-tolerant (Patanwala, Jarzyna, Miller, et al., 2008).

Clinicians appear to agree that if a patient has been on long-term opioid therapy, opioid tolerance should be expected (Miaskowski, Cleary, Burney, et al., 2005). By convention, many clinicians will consider a patient who has used opioids regularly for approximately seven days or more to be opioid-tolerant. For example, in a study of patients undergoing total knee arthroplasty, patients were considered opioid-tolerant if they had taken 30 mg or more of oral morphine a day, or its equivalent, for one week prior to surgery (Patanwala, Jarzyna, Miller, et al., 2008). Patients who took 10 mg or less of oral morphine a day, or its equivalent, for the week preceding surgery were considered opioid-naïve. Grades of opioid tolerance are seldom discussed, but a few clinicians have suggested that patients requiring the equivalent of 1 mg or more of intravenous (IV) morphine or 3 mg or more of oral morphine per hour for longer than 1 month may be considered to have a high grade of opioid tolerance (Mitra, Sinatra, 2004).

Failing to appreciate the differences between opioid-tolerant and opioid-naïve individuals can lead to overdosing opioid-naïve patients and underdosing opioid-tolerant patients (Pantanwala, Jarzyna, Miller, et al., 2008). This is especially evident with the use of IV patient-controlled analgesia (PCA). A continuous infusion postoperatively is recommended for opioid-tolerant patients (Rozen, DeGaetano, 2006). In the use of opioids to manage persistent cancer pain, patients often receive the major portion of their opioid requirement as a continuous infusion without experiencing adverse effects such as sedation (APS, 2003). Many clinicians have discovered that the doses of opioid analgesics tolerated well by postoperative opioid-tolerant patients can produce significant adverse effects in opioid-naïve postoperative patients (Parker, Holtmann, White, 1991). For example, compared with opioid-tolerant patients, some studies have shown that opioid-naïve postoperative patients may be more likely to experience opioid-induced sedation with a continuous opioid infusion (APS, 2003). However, others have found that the addition of a low continuous infusion to IV PCA can be done safely in many opioid-naïve patients (Pasero, McCaffery, 2004) (see Chapter 17).

Clinicians unfamiliar with caring for opioid-tolerant patients are likely to be fearful of the high doses often required, and as a result, the patient may be underdosed. However, the opioid-tolerant patient has developed tolerance to most of the opioid adverse effects. Tolerance to the adverse effects of opioids develops more rapidly than to analgesia, meaning that opioids may be safely titrated to high doses to provide adequate analgesia (Mehta, Langford, 2006). Most importantly, the occurrence of respiratory depression is rare in opioid-tolerant individuals whose doses are carefully titrated. The fear of producing respiratory depression in these individuals usually is overstated. This fear should not interfere with adequate opioid dosing. In addition, compared with opioid-naïve individuals, opioid-tolerant individuals are generally able to tolerate faster escalation of larger doses of opioid drugs without experiencing life-threatening adverse effects (Foley, 1995).

Unfortunately, there are no evidence-based guidelines for predicting postoperative opioid requirements on the basis of the opioid dose consumed before surgery. A small prospective observational study (N = 29) classified patients as opioid tolerant or opioid naïve based on their preoperative daily opioid requirements; those taking 10 mg or less of oral morphine equivalent were designated opioid naïve, and those taking at least 30 mg of oral morphine equivalent were designated opioid tolerant (Pantanwala, Jarzyna, Miller, et al., 2008). Significantly higher pain scores and postoperative opioid consumption were noted in the opioid tolerant patients compared with the opioid naïve patients; median IV morphine equivalents were 56 mg, 108 mg, and 152.3 mg for the opioid tolerant patients and 8.2 mg, 20.5 mg, and 25 mg in opioid naïve in the PACU, during the first 24 hours after discharge from the PACU, and 24 to 48 hours after discharge from the PACU, respectively. One suggestion is to expect opioid requirements postoperatively in the opioid-tolerant patient to be two to four times the dose required in an opioid-naïve individual (Carroll, Angst, Clark, 2004). Clearly, more research is needed on opioid dose requirements in opioid tolerant patients in the postoperative setting and those who require high postoperative opioid doses in addition to their usual preoperative dose must be watched closely for sedation and respiratory depression (see Chapter 19).

Doses of opioid required by the opioid-tolerant patient with cancer pain also are sometimes extremely high. In one study, the maximum doses required for acceptable analgesia were 80 mg/h of morphine, 50 mg/h of meperidine (use of this drug is not recommended; see Chapter 13), and 60 mg/h of hydromorphone. Adverse effects and safety profiles were acceptable (Kerr, Sone, DeAngelis, et al., 1988). Some cancer patients have required as much as 40,000 mg of IV morphine per 24 hours to achieve adequate analgesia (Weinstein, 1994). These findings reinforce that in many patients no ceiling on analgesia exists when mu agonist opioid analgesics are used, and "high" doses are safe and appropriate in many opioid-tolerant individuals. It is prudent to note, however, that new information about the phenomenon of opioid-induced hyperalgesia obligates the clinician to be particularly careful when doses need to be escalated to relatively high levels.

Opioid-Induced Hyperalgesia (OIH)

Hyperalgesia means increased sensitivity to pain. Opioid-induced hyperalgesia (OIH) is a paradoxical situation in which increasing doses of opioid result in increasing sensitivity to pain (Compton, 2008). OIH has only recently been identified as a clinical reality (Mitra, 2008). The incidence of clinically significant OIH has not been determined, but it appears to be a rare but serious consequence of opioid administration (Angst, Clark, 2006; Chu, Angst, Clark, 2008). Compton (2008) has hypothesized that the incidence of OIH may be much greater, since the large number of patients with persistent noncancer pain who fail to get relief from opioids or discontinue opioid therapy may actually have undiagnosed OIH. As yet, it is not possible to predict who will develop OIH as a result of opioid exposure.

Some experts characterize OIH and analgesic tolerance as "opposite sides of the coin." In tolerance, increasing doses of opioid are needed to provide the same level of pain relief because opioid exposure induces neurophysiologic changes that reverse analgesia; in OIH, opioid exposure induces neurophysiologic changes that produce pain or increase sensitivity to noxious input (Angst, Clark, 2006). In other words, tolerance may be inferred clinically when opioid treatment leads to decreased sensitivity to opioid analgesia over time (in the absence of another process that would explain this), whereas OIH may be inferred clinically when opioid treatment leads to increased pain or sensitivity to pain over time (DuPen, Shen, Ersek, 2007).

Individuals with OIH may not have increased sensitivity to all types of pain. One study showed that individuals with OIH had increased sensitivity to cold but not heat (Chu, Clark, Angst, 2006). Another study of methadone-maintained patients found more pronounced hyperalgesia to cold than electrical pain (Doverty, White, Somogyi, et al., 2001).

The mechanisms underlying OIH remain largely unknown. In general, OIH is thought to be the result of changes in the central and peripheral nervous systems that upregulate pain-processing mechanisms, which results in increased transmission of nociceptive signals (Compton, 2008). The mechanism presumably involves neuroexcitatory and possibly pronociceptive (pain facilitation) effects of specific molecules in the brain and spinal cord (Compton, 2008; Mitra, 2008). The best studied OIH mechanism involves the upregulation of excitatory N-methyl-D-aspartate (NMDA) receptors in dorsal horn neurons (Compton, 2008). Another mechanism involves neuroplastic changes that result in part from the activation of descending pain facilitation mechanisms arising in the brain (Mitra, 2008).

A small prospective study of opioid-naïve patients with moderate to severe persistent low back pain suggested that OIH could occur within 4 weeks after exposure to moderate doses (median dose 75 mg/day) of oral morphine (Chu, Clark, Angst, 2006). A few studies have examined the occurrence of OIH after acute perioperative opioid exposure, but the results have been mixed (Chu, Angst, Clark, 2008).

Although the majority of case reports of OIH concern systemic or intrathecal administration of morphine, raising the possibility that morphine metabolites may be involved in OIH (Chu, Angst, Clark, 2008), hyperalgesia has also been demonstrated in patients with opioid addiction receiving methadone maintenance therapy (Chu, Angst, Clark, 2008), and it has been observed anecdotally during treatment with other opioids. Development of OIH may vary between different opioid medications, but which opioids are most likely to contribute to OIH is as yet unknown (Compton, 2008). Some evidence suggests that not all opioids produce OIH, and efforts are being made to identify these (Yaksh, Harty, 1988).

OIH is suspected when increasing doses (usually high, rapidly escalating doses) of opioid fail to relieve pain and actually make pain worse at the original site of pain or at other sites (Chu, Angst, Clark, 2008; Mitra, 2008). OIH may involve unexplained pain, diffuse pain (even the whole body), and diffuse allodynia (Compton, 2008; Chu, Angst, Clark, 2008; Mitra, 2008). Allodynia may be so severe that gentle touch or movement causes generalized tenderness of the skin and soft tissue (Angst, Clark, 2006). OIH may be accompanied by generalized neuroexcitation such as agitation, multifocal myoclonus, seizures, and even delirium (Mitra, 2008).

Similar to the suspicion of tolerance, the possibility that OIH is occurring demands a careful re-evaluation to determine whether other reasons for failure of the opioid to relieve pain exist. These include increase in pain pathology, opioid or other types of withdrawal, opioid addiction or pseudoaddiction, and other phenomena (Compton, 2008). Table 11-3 gives a brief description of these conditions compared with OIH and suggests some distinguishing characteristics. More detail is presented in the paragraphs that follow. Each of these conditions merits a different response or treatment. In all of these conditions, except OIH, pain will improve with increasing opioid doses.

When an opioid analgesic appears to lose its effectiveness, one obvious reason is that the *pain pathology has worsened*. This situation requires a careful evaluation of possible causes of an increase in existing pain or new sites of pain. In a patient with persistent cancer-related pain, this may involve increased tumor growth or a new tumor site. This simple example illustrates how important it is to the treatment of this patient to determine if OIH exists or if pain pathology underlies the appearance of decreasing effectiveness of current opioid treatment. In this patient example, appropriate responses may include adding or adjusting adjuvant analgesics, radiologic treatment, surgical excision, or increase in opioid dose.

Although the phenomena may be intricately related mechanistically, OIH should be distinguished from *opioid tolerance*. Initially it may seem that a patient with OIH has developed tolerance to analgesia, and that the best course of action is to increase the opioid dose. Careful evaluation is needed to exclude the possibility that the increases in opioid dose are actually worsening pain. If adverse effects of the original opioid are absent, manageable, or

GUIDELINES

Table 11-3 | Differential Assessment of Opioid-Induced Hyperalgesia vs. Other Conditions

Condition	Nature of Pain	Presentation of Onset of Pain	Response to Opioid Administration
Worsening pain pathology*	Localized to site of pre-existing pain or new site of pathology.	Variable, depending on source of pain	Pain improves.
Opioid tolerance*	Localized to site of pre-existing pain.	Gradual onset	Pain improves.
Opioid withdrawal*	Increased sensitivity to pain; diffuse pain extending beyond distribution of pre-existing pain.	Abrupt with short-acting opioids or antagonist administration; gradual with long-acting opioids	Pain improves.
Opioid addictive disease*	Increased sensitivity to pain; diffuse, may extend beyond the distribution of pre-existing pain.	Gradual onset	Pain may improve, but function may worsen.
Pseudoaddiction*	Localized to site of pre-existing pain.	Variable, depending on source of pain	Pain improves.
Opioid-induced hyperalgesia	Increased sensitivity to pain; diffuse pain, extending beyond the distribution of pre-existing pain; possibly allodynia.	Abrupt onset with rapid opioid escalation or high-dose opioid administration	Pain worsens.

*If careful evaluation reveals that none of the above conditions is causing increased pain sensitivity and the following characteristics are largely descriptive of the current presentation, then it is reasonable to suspect the existence of OIH.
As appears in Pasero, C., & McCaffery, M. *Pain assessment and pharmacologic management*, p. 296, St. Louis, Mosby. Modified from Compton, P. (2008). The OIH paradox:

Can opioids make pain worse? *Pain Treatment Topics.* Available at: http://pain-topics.org/pdf/Compton-OIH-Paradox.pdf. Accessed February 16, 2009. © 2011, Pasero C, McCaffery M. May be duplicated for use in clinical practice.

tolerable, a practical approach to making the differential diagnosis is to continue to increase the dose of the same opioid until pain is finally controlled with higher or more frequent doses of opioid, signifying tolerance that can be overcome by dose escalation, or until it is obvious that increased doses result in increased pain, indicating OIH. Opioid tolerance may be treated by increasing the dose or frequency of opioid, by opioid rotation, or by combining opioids (Compton, 2008; Mitra, 2008). Opioid rotation or combining opioids is also used in the treatment of OIH but must be accompanied by a decrease in the dose of the original opioid (Mitra, 2008).

Withdrawal symptoms that occur when the opioid dose is decreased or when an opioid antagonist is given result in increased pain in patients with physical dependence. This pain is similar to that of OIH in that increased sensitivity to pain may be diffuse and may extend beyond the pre-existing pain. This increase in pain needs to be differentiated from OIH. Pain associated with opioid withdrawal may be abrupt if the opioid is short acting or an antagonist is given, or it may be gradual if the opioid is long acting. Obviously, when the opioid dose is increased, pain improves, and this observation distinguishes it from OIH (Compton, 2008).

Opioid addictive disease must also be distinguished from OIH. As with pain associated with opioid withdrawal and OIH, increased sensitivity to pain in individuals with opioid addictive disease may be diffuse and extend beyond the distribution of pre-existing pain. This pain may have a

gradual onset (Compton, 2008). Patients may request an increased dose, more frequent doses, or a specific opioid. This behavior is usually attributed to the addictive disease, and clinicians are reluctant to provide what the patient requests. However, a trial of increased opioid doses may result in pain relief. Unfortunately in some patients, function may worsen, and, despite their admissions of satisfactory pain relief, they may demonstrate behaviors typical of addiction such as inability to control opioid use, requests for opioids from multiple prescribers, or repeated unauthorized escalations in dose despite discussions with the patients about these behaviors.

OIH must also be differentiated from *pseudoaddiction,* defined as a mistaken diagnosis of addictive disease in patients with undertreated pain who manifest behaviors very similar to those typical of addictive disease, described in the previous paragraph (Weissman, Haddox, 1989). Pseudoaddiction can be distinguished from true addictive disease in that the behaviors resolve when pain is effectively treated.

If the above conditions have been ruled out and OIH is suspected, several strategies may be considered to manage it. These strategies overlap those used to address poor opioid responsiveness and include opioid rotation and efforts to reduce the opioid dose by concurrent administration of a nonopioid analgesic (Mitra, 2008), an adjuvant analgesic, or a nonpharmacologic treatment. OIH is not reversed by administration of an opioid antagonist (Angst, Clark, 2006).

Opioid rotation is one possible strategy for treating OIH. The original opioid dose is reduced, and another opioid is introduced. Incomplete cross-tolerance between opioids often allows comparable analgesia with another opioid at a lower equianalgesic opioid dose, in effect lowering the amount of opioid required for satisfactory analgesia (Compton, 2008).

In case reports of patients receiving large doses of morphine for intractable pain who had developed opioid-induced allodynia, reduction or elimination of the allodynia was achieved by reducing the morphine dose or substituting another opioid (fentanyl, sufentanil, methadone) (Angst, Clark, 2006). However, in this overview of case reports, it was not clear whether opioid-induced allodynia was always associated with OIH. The authors discussed the two as potentially separate entities.

Methadone may be particularly useful for opioid rotation because its NMDA antagonist activity reduces neuronal excitability (Compton, 2008). Many clinicians choose methadone for opioid rotation, and several case reports have shown that this is an effective way to reduce OIH (Chu, Angst, Clark, 2008). However, methadone is not a panacea and has actually worsened the patient's condition in some situations. Note that switching from one opioid to methadone is a complex process (Fine, Portenoy, Ad Hoc Expert Panel on Evidence Review and Guidelines for Opioid Rotation, 2009; Knotkova, Fine, Portenoy, 2009), which is discussed in Chapter 13. Several conversions involving ratios depending upon the dose of the first opioid have been developed, but research has not established which is the most reliable.

Studies of the use of the NMDA antagonist dextromethorphan in OIH have shown conflicting results (Compton, 2008). A trial of this drug may be helpful for some patients, but it is not a first-line choice. In a study using ketamine, another NMDA antagonist, OIH was completely reversed, but the potential for unpleasant adverse effects with ketamine may make it a less attractive alternative (Mitra, 2008) (see Chapter 23). Although there is some evidence that perioperative use of ketamine modulates OIH or opioid tolerance and that it reduces postoperative wound hyperalgesia, some researchers think that the clinical significance of ketamine's benefits requires larger prospective studies (Chu, Angst, Clark, 2008).

Research has begun to identify potential approaches to preventing OIH. These include proper timing of COX-2 selective NSAIDs in postoperative patients, NMDA antagonists, opioid dose-sparing medications such as certain adjuvant analgesics, and avoidance of rapid opioid dose escalation when possible. Studies have shown that COX-2 selective NSAIDs may partially reduce OIH and that proper timing of the administration is critical in producing this effect (Mitra, 2008); in postoperative pain, 40 mg of parenteral parecoxib (a COX-2 selective drug not available in the United States) 30 minutes prior to the opioid, may be helpful in preventing OIH (Troster, Sittl, Singler,

et al., 2006) (see Section III). Continued use of COX-2 selective NSAIDs, as in persistent pain, is not only opioid dose-sparing but also may help prevent OIH because these medications reduce the spinal release of excitatory neurotransmitters (Mitra, 2008). Additional opioid dose-sparing approaches include gabapentin for both acute pain and neuropathic pain. Other useful adjuvants for neuropathic pain may involve other anticonvulsants and antidepressants (see Section V).

Rapid escalations in opioid plasma levels have been associated with the development of OIH. For that reason, the use of long-acting opioids seems preferable to short-acting opioids for persistent pain. The more gradual onset and offset of long-acting opioids helps avoid rapid escalations in opioid plasma levels and may minimize the development of OIH (Compton, 2008). On the other hand, one study comparing around-the-clock (ATC) opioid dosing with PRN ("as needed") dosing in patients with persistent pain found that scheduled opioid dosing resulted in 12.4 times more opioid than the PRN dosing group (Miaskowski, Mack, Dodd, et al., 2002). No differences in pain relief were found between the two groups. Since higher doses are associated with OIH, PRN versus scheduled dosing needs to be evaluated as a strategy to prevent OIH (Chu, Angst, Clark, 2008).

It has been proposed that use of very low doses of an opioid antagonist in combination with opioid agonists may counteract the development of OIH. This approach is in the investigational stages (Compton, 2008; Sloan, Harmann, 2006). Some evidence suggests that clonidine preoperatively reduces development of opioid tolerance, but no evidence has substantiated its usefulness in OIH (Mitra, 2008).

In summary, the knowledge that long-term opioid therapy (especially if doses escalate rapidly) may actually worsen pain for selected patients adds to the list of reasons to be cautious about the use of opioids and particularly vigilant if a patient appears to require relatively high doses. Prescribers need to be aware of ways to prevent or minimize OIH and implement these when possible. They should also be alert to symptoms of OIH and know how to make a differential diagnosis. Fortunately, if correctly diagnosed, OIH can be treated and satisfactory pain relief restored in most patients.

Physical Dependence

Physical dependence is defined in a consensus statement published by the ASAM (2001) as "a state of adaptation that is manifested by a drug class specific withdrawal syndrome that can be produced by abrupt cessation, rapid dose reduction, decreasing blood level of the drug, and/or administration of an antagonist." (p. 2). The focus here is on opioids, but other drugs that patients may become physically dependent on include all of the sedative-hypnotics (including alcohol and benzodiazepines), beta blockers, corticosteroids, and antidepressants.

Physical dependence is one of the most frequently misunderstood terms and is often confused with addiction or "dependence" (Webster, Dove, 2007). The term *dependence* should be avoided since it is used by specialists in addiction medicine as a synonym for addiction and creates confusion between physical dependence and the type of psychological dependence that is associated with addictive disease (Fine, Portenoy, 2007). Because of this confusion, patients should not be referred to as dependent.

One source of confusion over the term *dependence* is related to definitions in the *Diagnostic and Statistical Manual of Mental Disorders,* Fourth Edition, Text Revised (DSM-IV-TR) (American Psychiatric Association [APA], 2000). The manual lists withdrawal symptoms and tolerance as "defining features" of addiction, thus failing to distinguish addictive disease from the normal physiologic responses of physical dependence and tolerance. Tolerance and physical dependence are likely to be present in an individual addicted to opioids, but neither tolerance nor physical dependence is required for addiction to be present, and either phenomenon may occur independently of addictive disease. In short, physical dependence and addiction are distinct; the term *physical dependence* should only be applied to the overt or potential capacity to have withdrawal, the term *addiction* should never be used when the term *physical dependence* is appropriate, and the term *dependence* should not be used at all.

To reduce the fear that may prevent patients and families from seeking appropriate pain management, it is important that caregivers understand and reinforce to patients and families the differences between addiction and physical dependence. Patients on long-term opioid therapy are appropriately told not to stop taking their opioid medication. This offers an opportunity to discuss the reason for not stopping their medication and assure the patient and family that it does not indicate possible addiction. The patient needs to understand that the potential for withdrawal symptoms is not a problem when opioid doses are tapered as opposed to suddenly stopped (APS, 2003).

Physical dependence is an expected result of opioid use. However, how long it takes to develop physical dependence and the dose of drug required is unknown (Fine, Portenoy, 2007). Certainly in long-term therapy with opioids, physical dependence should be expected (Miaskowski, Cleary, Burney, et al., 2005). It may also occur after opioids have been administered for only a few days (Fine, Portenoy, 2007).

The presence of physical dependence is not evident until some event such as abrupt cessation of the opioid occurs that causes the withdrawal, or abstinence, syndrome. Thus, physical dependence is not problematic as long as measures are taken to avoid abrupt cessation or administration of an opioid antagonist (Fine, Portenoy, 2007).

Symptoms of acute withdrawal include anxiety, irritability, salivation, rhinorrhea, insomnia, chills alternating with hot flashes, joint and muscle pain, tearing of the eyes, sweating, nausea, vomiting, diarrhea, and abdominal cramps (APS, 2003; Miaskowski, Cleary, Burney, et al., 2005). Acute withdrawal has been likened to having the "flu" and may be mild or severe and may manifest with any combination of the precipitated phenomena (e.g., abrupt cessation of the opioid or administration of an antagonist) or with all of them. Although as a rule, higher opioid doses and longer duration of opioid treatment are associated with a more severe syndrome, there also is substantial individual variation, with some patients experiencing only mild withdrawal symptoms, even if the opioid dose is relatively high, and some experiencing such a degree of physical dependence that they have withdrawal between doses of opioid and find it difficult to stop a low-dose PRN regimen.

The onset of withdrawal symptoms after abrupt cessation of an opioid depends upon the half-life of the opioid being used. For example, codeine, hydrocodone, morphine, and hydromorphone have short half-lives, and symptoms may begin within 6 to 12 hours and peak at 24 to 72 hours. With a long half-life opioid, such as methadone or levorphanol, the onset of withdrawal symptoms may not occur for 24 hours or longer, and the symptoms are usually less severe (APS, 2003; Miaskowski, Cleary, Burney, et al., 2005).

When opioids become unnecessary because pain has been resolved, the withdrawal syndrome can be avoided by slowly tapering the dose, i.e., weaning the patient off the regimen. This process should not be referred to as *detoxification* because of the use of the latter term in relation to the treatment of addiction (Webster, Dove, 2007).

Several guidelines for tapering the opioid dose are available, but most offer similar plans for gradual decreases in opioid doses. The longer the patient has been taking the opioid, the longer it takes to complete the weaning process. One suggested approach to tapering the opioid in an adult is to start with one-half the previous total daily dose, and administer this for 2 days. Then decrease the dose by 25% every two days until the patient reaches a total daily dose of 30 mg a day of oral morphine or its equivalent. After 2 days at this minimum dose, the opioid may be discontinued (Miaskowski, Cleary, Burney, et al., 2005).

If anxiety, sweating, or other withdrawal symptoms are problematic, the tapering can be slowed, medications can be added to treat the symptoms (e.g., a drug for nausea or diarrhea), the patient can be "rotated" to another opioid and tapering recommenced, or clonidine (a specific treatment for opioid withdrawal) can be added, starting at a dose of 0.1 mg to 0.2 mg per day (APS, 2003).

Addiction and Pseudoaddiction

No universally accepted definition of opioid addiction exists. A consensus statement published by ASAM (2001), defines addiction as "a primary chronic, neurobiologic disease, with genetic, psychosocial, and environment factors influencing its development and manifestations. It is characterized by behaviors that include one or more of the following: impaired control over drug use, compulsive use, continued use despite harm, and craving." (p. 2) An important message in this definition is that taking opioids for pain relief is not addiction, no matter how long an individual takes opioids or at what doses. Individuals taking opioid drugs for relief of pain are using them therapeutically. Addiction is discussed at length in Section II. A brief summary of important points is presented here.

How likely is it that addiction will occur as a result of using opioids for pain relief? This is a difficult question to frame and to answer. The specifics of the question must be clarified. Is the phenomenon being considered a diagnosis of "substance dependence disorder" as described by the APA's *Diagnostic and Statistical Manual of Mental Disorders* (DSM)? This diagnosis, which requires compulsive use of a substance, is usually said to be synonymous with addiction and is distinguished from substance abuse disorder. In non-DSM language, the lack of an international consensus on the definition of addiction obviously complicates questions related to the incidence of addiction during medical treatment of pain.

During long-term therapy, the clinical concern relates not only to the occurrence of addiction per se, but also to the development of drug abuse, or even nonadherence behaviors that are too "mild" to be labeled abuse, but still raise a "red flag" for clinicians. The more clinically relevant question, therefore, is not limited to the incidence of addiction but rather to the broader occurrence of nonadherence and the extent to which this can be related to the abuse liability of these drugs.

The question is further complicated by the heterogeneity of the population. Is the issue the de novo appearance of an addictive pattern of medication use among the population of patients who have no prior history of addiction? If so, the question revolves around the incidence of iatrogenic addiction rather than relapse, and the data used to answer this must include a careful screening for prior drug abuse. Should a patient with a prior history of drug abuse, but not addiction, be in the denominator of patients treated for pain who are evaluated for the incidence of addiction?

Finally, the question is complicated by treatment issues. The incidence of addiction after short-term treatment of pain following surgery is very unlikely to be relevant to the incidence during the long-term treatment of persistent pain.

Given the uncertainties surrounding the nature of the question, the data extant to evaluate the incidence of addiction are very limited and difficult to interpret (see Section II). In an evidence-based review of all available studies on the development of drug abuse behaviors, addiction, *and* aberrant drug-related behavior in patients with persistent noncancer pain being treated with opi-

oids, only four studies preselected patients for no past or present history of abuse/addiction (Fishbain, Cole, Lewis, et al., 2008). In these studies, the percentage of abuse/addiction following opioid therapy was calculated at 0.19%. These data are reassuring, suggesting that patients with no past or present history of abuse/addiction usually remain responsible medication users over time.

A recent registry study of oxycodone (OxyContin)-treated patients who were followed for up to 3 years after participating in a clinical trial also showed a very low occurrence of problematic drug-related behavior (of 227 cases, just 6 cases of misuse and none of addiction) (Portenoy, Farrar, Backonja, et al., 2007). Because this registry included only those patients who had previously been in trials that had excluded patients with significant drug abuse, the data can only be used to evaluate the incidence of addiction among those with no (or very limited) history of abuse. Again, this number is very reassuring in terms of the rate of iatrogenic addiction among those with no history of abuse, but is not relevant to the general population of patients.

Pseudoaddiction, as the name implies, is a mistaken diagnosis of addictive disease. The term was first used and the behaviors described in a case report by Weissman and Haddox (1989). When a patient's pain is not well controlled, the patient may begin to manifest symptoms suggestive of addictive disease. In an effort to obtain adequate pain relief, the patient may respond with demanding behavior, escalating demands for more or different medications, repeated requests for opioids before the prescribed interval between doses has elapsed, and frequent visits to the emergency department. (See Table 2-2, p. 36, for other behaviors that may be mistaken as addictive disease but actually reflect undertreated pain.)

As an example, patients who receive opioid doses that are too low or at intervals greater than the opioid's duration of action may understandably try to manipulate the staff into giving them more analgesic. Pain relief typically eliminates these behaviors and is often accomplished by increasing opioid doses, decreasing intervals between doses, or providing an extra prescription in case it is needed.

Although pseudoaddiction can be distinguished from true addictive disease in that the behaviors resolve when pain is effectively treated, the challenge in the clinical setting typically relates to patients who may be manifesting both pseudoaddiction and drug abuse (unrelieved pain may be driving a relapse of addiction, or increased abuse among those with a history of drug abuse, and it may be exceedingly difficult to know whether an effort to relieve pain by adding medication will both lessen pain and lessen newly established abuse behaviors). Another challenge exists in the decision to call more severe behaviors pseudoaddiction, rather than addiction. Although it is probable that the patient with a history of addiction may be more likely to buy heroin if pain is unrelieved, it is obviously difficult to address this behavior as a case of pseudoaddiction. These challenges indicate that a careful assessment must be done before consideration is given to labeling a patient's behavior as pseudoaddiction, that there must be a willingness to diagnosis both pseudoaddiction and addiction (and to treat accordingly), and that an effort should always be made to determine whether the unrelieved pain can be addressed using a treatment other than an opioid.

Equianalgesia

The term *equianalgesia* means approximately "equal analgesia." Equianalgesic doses refer to the doses of various opioid analgesics that provide approximately the same pain relief. An equianalgesic chart (see Table 16-1, pp. 444-446) provides a list of analgesic doses, both oral and parenteral, that are approximately equal to each other in ability to provide pain relief. These doses are also referred to as *equianalgesic dose units*. Most of the doses in equianalgesic charts are based on single-dose studies, often conducted with opioid-naïve surgical patients, using morphine, 10 mg IM, for comparison (Knotkova, Fine, Portenoy, 2009). The parenteral doses listed are typical of IM doses given approximately every 3 to 4 hours. Equianalgesic dose calculation provides a basis for selecting the appropriate starting dose when changing from one opioid drug or route of administration to another. However, these calculations are just estimates and vary with repeated dosing and opioid rotation (Knotkova, Fine, Portenoy, 2009; Shaheen, Walsh, Lasheen, et al., 2009). The optimal dose for the patient is determined always by titration (Fine, Portenoy, 2007).

Conversion Charts. Conversion charts for opioid analgesics are provided by drug manufacturers to assist clinicians in converting from various other opioids to the opioid being marketed. They usually provide a conservative estimate of the dose of the new opioid that will be required. The charts often assume that the switch to the new opioid is likely to be taking place in an opioid-tolerant patient. The reasoning behind using conversion charts is that cross tolerance is not complete and patients respond differently to different opioids as discussed earlier in this chapter. Adverse effects and overdosing can be more readily avoided by using conservative estimates of the dose of the new drug. Thus conversion charts are not the same as equianalgesic charts. Rather they take into consideration equianalgesic doses and reduce that estimate.

Because conversion charts are conservative in their estimate of what the initial dose of the new drug should be, many patients require titration upward to achieve satisfactory analgesia. For example, one manufacturer of transdermal fentanyl cautions that when using the estimates from its conversion chart, 50% of the patients switched from other opioids by other routes to transdermal fentanyl will require an increase in dose after the initial dose of transdermal fentanyl (Janssen, 2008). The manufacturer of OxyContin provides a table with multiplication factors to determine the starting dose when converting from a variety of opioids to OxyContin; however, it appropriately cautions that no fixed conversion ratio will fit all patients, and the doses are a starting point and should be titrated as needed (Purdue Pharma, 2007). It is also important to note that the doses recommended in conversion tables do not yield equianalgesic doses (see Chapter 16 for more on equianalgesia).

Conclusion

This chapter lays the foundation for the content presented in the rest of the chapters in this section. An understanding of the underlying mechanisms of opioids as well as the key concepts related to pharmacokinetics and pharmacodynamics of drugs as presented here is essential to initiating and maintaining a sound pain treatment plan.

Chapter 12 Key Concepts in Analgesic Therapy

THIS chapter presents the key concepts of opioid analgesic administration. Included is a discussion of the recommended approach to managing all types of pain: multimodal analgesia. The research related to preemptive analgesia, accelerated multimodal postoperative rehabilitation, and prevention of persistent postsurgical pain is reviewed. The pros and cons of the various methods for opioid analgesic dosing are described, and an introduction to the concept of patient-controlled analgesia (PCA) and alternative uses of analgesic devices is provided.

Multimodal Analgesia

As discussed in Section III, a multimodal regimen combines drugs with different underlying mechanisms, such as nonopioids, opioids, local anesthetics, and anticonvulsants. This approach allows lower doses of each of the drugs in the treatment plan, which lowers the potential for each to produce adverse effects (Ashburn, Caplan, Carr, et al., 2004; Kim, Kim, Nam, et al., 2008; Marret, Kurdi, Zufferey, et al., 2005; Schug, 2006; Schug, Manopas, 2007; White, 2005). Further, multimodal analgesia can result in comparable or greater pain relief than can be achieved with any single analgesic (Busch, Shore, Bhandari, et al., 2006; Cassinelli, Dean, Garcia, et al., 2008; Huang, Wang, Wang, et al., 2008).

Multimodal analgesia is discussed most often in the context of acute pain treatment; however, pain has multiple underlying mechanisms and is a multifaceted phenomenon, underscoring the importance of using a multimodal approach to manage all types of pain; this should be the rule, rather than the exception (Argoff, Albrecht, Irving, et al., 2009; Kehlet, Wilmore, 2008; Kehlet, Jensen, Woolf, 2006) (see Section I). A sound treatment plan relies on the selection of appropriate analgesics from the opioid, nonopioid, and adjuvant analgesic groups.

WHO Analgesic Ladder for Cancer Pain Relief

Probably the most well-known example of combining analgesics from the nonopioid, opioid, and adjuvant analgesic groups is the World Health Organization (WHO) analgesic ladder (Figure 12-1), which was proposed in the early 1980s as a guide to the management of persistent cancer pain (WHO, 1986; Meldrum, 2005). Still today, it is the clinical model for pain therapy (Ripamonti, Bandieri, 2009). The analgesic ladder focuses on selecting analgesics on the basis of the intensity of the pain using analgesics from each of the analgesic groups and, to some extent, building on previously effective analgesics.

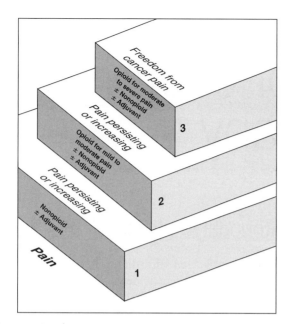

Figure 12-1 | WHO three-step analgesic ladder.

From World Health Organization (1996). *Cancer pain relief,* ed 2, Geneva, World Health Organization.

Steps 1, 2, and 3

The three steps of the WHO analgesic ladder address different intensities of pain. However, patients do not always have mild pain at the bottom of the ladder and do not necessarily progress through each of the three levels of pain intensity. Some patients with cancer pain will have moderate to severe pain initially, whereas others may progress directly from mild pain to severe pain. Therefore, treatment of cancer pain does not necessarily begin with step 1, progress to step 2, and follow with step 3 (Eisenberg, Marinangeli, Birkhahn, et al., 2005). If the patient initially has severe pain, step 3 treatment considerations are appropriate (Marinangeli, Ciccozzi, Leonardis, et al., 2004).

Step 1 of the analgesic ladder addresses mild pain by suggesting a nonopioid analgesic, such as acetaminophen or an NSAID, and the possibility of an adjuvant analgesic, particularly if the patient has neuropathic pain. It should be noted, however, that the term *adjuvant,* when used in this ladder, refers to both the adjuvant analgesics and the adjuvant drugs that are added to analgesics to reduce adverse effects (e.g., laxatives for opioid-induced constipation; see Chapter 19).

If pain is mild to moderate and not relieved by a nonopioid (with or without an adjuvant), step 2 recommends adding an opioid. In other words, the next level of analgesia builds on the previous analgesics. If a nonopioid relieves some but not enough pain, it is continued and an opioid is added. This action, of course, must be predicated on an assessment that indicates the favorable risk:benefit ratio for the continued treatment with

the nonopioid drug. Although, in the past, the decision to stop the nonopioid and start an opioid rather than add an opioid to the nonopioid often was considered merely a common mistake, new information about the gastrointestinal (GI) and the cardiovascular (CV) risk of NSAID therapy alters this view. Rather, the decision to use or continue an NSAID cannot be mostly determined by the pain intensity, or the analgesic ladder guideline, but rather, must be decided based on an evaluation of cumulative risk over the remaining time (see Chapter 6).

The clinical usefulness of step 2 is frequently debated (Ripamonti, Bandieri, 2009). An early meta-analysis demonstrated no differences between the safety and efficacy of NSAIDs (step 1 analgesics) and so-called "weak" opioids (step 2 analgesics) (Eisenberg, Berkey, Carr, et al., 1994). Pharmacologically, no difference exists between most of the drugs used on step 2 and those used on step 3. Because the same three groups of analgesics are considered at both steps, the ladder could be reduced to only 2 steps.

In clinical practice, the reason for having step 2 is to assist the clinician in selecting an opioid that may be conventionally preferred for the treatment of moderate to severe pain in the patient who is opioid-naïve, or nearly so. For example, mild to moderate pain is often treated with oral analgesics in a fixed combination of opioid and nonopioid, usually acetaminophen or sometimes aspirin (see Chapter 5). Although the problem with fixed combinations is that the dose of acetaminophen (or other nonopioid) limits the escalation of the opioid dose, the benefit is that it helps the clinician to select a formulation that is generally safe for the patient with very limited opioid exposure (and also allows a potentially more convenient way of combining the nonopioid and opioid). Common examples of opioid/nonopioid fixed combinations are as follows:

- Lortab 5/500 (hydrocodone 5 mg, and acetaminophen 500 mg)
- Percocet (oxycodone 5 mg, and acetaminophen 325 mg)
- Tylenol No. 3 (codeine 30 mg, and acetaminophen 300 mg)
- Tylox (oxycodone 5 mg, and acetaminophen 500 mg)
- Vicodin (hydrocodone 5 mg, and acetaminophen 500 mg)

To avoid exceeding the recommended maximum daily dose of 4 g of acetaminophen, the patient cannot take more than 8 tablets per day of those containing 500 mg of acetaminophen or 12 tablets per day of those containing 325 mg of acetaminophen. Recent discussions by the United States Food and Drug Administration (U.S. FDA) encourage clinicians to consider the maximum daily dose of acetaminophen to be 2.6 g, or 8 tablets per day of those formulations containing 325 mg of acetaminophen (U.S. FDA, 2009b; Harris, 2008). This provides more of a safety margin if the patient unintentionally takes other acetaminophen-containing (usually over-the-counter) drugs.

Oxycodone is commonly used in these fixed combinations and is also considered a step 3 drug, a useful opioid for escalating pain. Therefore if a fixed combination of acetaminophen and oxycodone is used at step 2, plain (single-entity) oxycodone may be continued at step 3. Plain acetaminophen can also be continued at appropriate doses.

To avoid step 2 and the need to change opioids or formulations as pain increases, mild to moderate pain may be treated with low doses of plain oxycodone, morphine, or hydromorphone. These mu agonists may be continued throughout the course of therapy because doses of these may be escalated for the relief of increasingly severe pain. Studies have demonstrated the effectiveness of this approach. In 110 opioid-naïve patients with moderate to severe cancer pain, oral morphine at a starting dose of 15 mg/day (10 mg in older adults) followed by titration was found to be well tolerated and effective (Mercadante, Porzio, Ferrera, et al., 2006). A randomized controlled study showed that first-line use of so-called "strong" opioids (e.g., morphine, fentanyl, or methadone) in terminally ill cancer patients resulted in significantly better pain relief and patient satisfaction and necessitated fewer changes in the pain treatment plan than when patients followed the 3-step WHO ladder approach (Marinangeli, Ciccozzi, Leonardis, et al., 2004). Similarly, another study of patients with moderate cancer pain compared the 3-step WHO ladder approach with a modified version that moved patients directly from step 1 to step 3 as pain increased (Maltoni, Scarpi, Modonesi, et al., 2005). Direct progression from step 1 to step 3 resulted in a lower percentage of days with worst pain but were associated with a higher incidence of anorexia and constipation despite laxative treatment. The researchers promoted this approach but underscored the importance of attention to careful management of adverse effects.

Opioid analgesics recommended at step 3 should be available orally and by a variety of other routes of administration so that the opioid need not be changed if the route of administration must change. For example, if a patient taking oral morphine has a temporary episode of nausea and vomiting, morphine may be continued by administering it by other routes, such as rectally or subcutaneously. Many opioids, such as morphine, hydromorphone, and fentanyl, are available by a variety of routes of administration (see Chapter 14).

In much of the world, opioids used at step 3 are either available in a modified-release formulation, or they are long half-life drugs. After dose titration (which in the case of the modified-release drugs often can be accomplished using short-acting formulations),

these drugs can be administered with relatively long dosing intervals, which may be more convenient and support adherence to the therapy. For example, morphine and oxycodone have fairly short half-lives—2 to 4 hours (Gutstein, Akil, 2006)—and are available in modified-release formulations that allow dosing every 12 hours.

The existence of active metabolites should be considered when selecting an opioid for long-term therapy. Morphine has active metabolites: morphine-6-glucuronide [M6G] and morphine-3-glucuronide [M3G]. These metabolites accumulate in patients with renal dysfunction and may be associated with toxicity (Johnson, 2007). Hydromorphone (Dilaudid) is a common alternative to morphine, and a modified-release formulation is available in some countries and most recently in the United States. Hydromorphone's metabolite (hydromorphone-3-glucouronide) can also accumulate in patients with renal dysfunction (Johnson, 2007), but the clinical consequences appear to be limited (Kurella, Bennett, Chertow, 2003). Nonetheless, it has been noted that opioid toxicity can recur when morphine is replaced with hydromorphone in patients with renal dysfunction, and dose should be reduced in such patients (Launay-Vacher, Karie, Fau, et al., 2005). Cautious use of fentanyl in patients with renal dysfunction has been suggested as an alternative when metabolite accumulation is a concern (Dean, 2004; Launay-Vacher, Karie, Fau, et al., 2005) (see Chapter 13 for more on morphine, hydromorphone, and fentanyl).

Other important recommendations that accompany the WHO analgesic ladder are to administer analgesics orally whenever possible and to administer them "by the clock" or around the clock (ATC) to prevent the return of pain.

Patient Example: WHO Ladder

A 59-year-old man has arm, shoulder, and chest pain as a result of invasion of the chest wall and brachial plexus by an apical lung cancer. He has not responded to radiation therapy and chemotherapy. History is remarkable for a major gastrointestinal hemorrhage from a gastric ulcer 2 years earlier. Analgesic use is limited to an occasional acetaminophen for headaches. He is married and has two adult children.

PATIENT ENCOUNTER 1

Pain severity and descriptors: Mild, aching (1 to 2/10) in arm, shoulder, and chest.
Inferred pain pathophysiology: Somatic and neuropathic.

Analgesic selection: Acetaminophen, 650 mg orally (PO), every 4 hours.

Step on analgesic ladder: 1.

Rationale: Step 1 of the "analgesic ladder" indicated because patient had mild pain. Analgesic history indicated that he had done well with acetaminophen in the past. NSAIDs relatively contraindicated because of history of ulcer. (NOTE: if patient's pain was moderate to severe on the first encounter, it would have been appropriate to start the patient on Step 2 or Step 3 of the "analgesic ladder.")

Potential adverse effects: None.

Outcome: Good pain relief for 3 to 4 weeks.

PATIENT ENCOUNTER 2

Pain severity and descriptors: The patient returns to the clinic with reports of escalating chest wall pain. The pain was described as aching and constant, moderate in severity (5 to 6/10).

Inferred pain pathophysiology: Somatic.

Analgesic selection: Oxycodone begun in addition to acetaminophen and given in combination form (oxycodone, 5 mg, + acetaminophen, 325 mg [Percocet]); to take 1 to 2 tablets PO, every 4 hours.

Step on analgesic ladder: 2.

Rationale: Step 2 chosen because pain was moderate to severe.

Potential adverse effects: Constipation, sedation, nausea.

Outcome: Pain progressed over the next 2 to 3 days and its quality changed. Percocet intake was 12 tablets per day. No adverse effects were reported.

PATIENT ENCOUNTER 3

Pain severity and descriptors: Aching, burning, constant, radiating from chest and shoulder into arm, moderate to severe (7 to 8/10). Disturbed sleep and ability to concentrate.

Inferred pain pathophysiology: Neuropathic and somatic.

Analgesic selection: Percocet was changed to morphine sulfate, 15 mg, + acetaminophen, 650 mg PO, every 4 hours, ATC, with morphine sulfate, 15 mg, breakthrough doses (BTDs) every 1 to 2 hours as needed (PRN). An adjuvant, desipramine 25 mg was added at night.

Step on analgesic ladder: 3.

Rationale: Step 3 of the analgesic ladder was selected because the patient's pain was severe. An adjuvant drug was added because of the neuropathic component of the pain. The opioid dose was determined as follows: 10 mg of morphine PO is considered to be equianalgesic to 7 to 10 mg of oxycodone PO (= 2 Percocet). Because the pain was not controlled, the equianalgesic dose was increased by 50%. The BTD of morphine

sulfate of 15 mg PO every 1 to 2 hours PRN was selected on the basis of a 5% to 15% ratio of his 24-hour baseline morphine dose. The dose, 15 mg, is in fact 17% of the 24-hour dose but was chosen because of the available tablet size.

Possible adverse effects: Constipation, sedation, nausea, dry mouth.

Outcome: Thirty-six hours later, the patient called to say that his pain control had markedly improved but only in the setting of frequent BTDs. Overall, with BTDs, pain was 75% better. He had required nine BTDs in the previous 24 hours (15 mg × 9 = an additional 135 mg of morphine). Consequently, his baseline morphine dose was increased by approximately the equivalent amount, to 30 mg PO every 4 hours. The dose chosen was a slightly lower dose than the total of the baseline plus BTDs but reflected the available tablet size and was considered likely to provide adequate analgesia. Rescue medication continued to be available. His BTD was adjusted to reflect 5% to 15% of the new 24-hour baseline dose of 180 mg, at 30 mg every 2 hours PRN. Again, this dose, 30 mg, is in fact 17% of the 24-hour dose but was chosen because of the available tablet size. Adjustment was undertaken because the 15 mg dose was not providing effective analgesia.

Good pain control was reached with BTDs used only once or twice a day in relation to a specific activity. Once stable pain relief was established, he was switched to a modified-release oral morphine preparation, allowing for 12-hour dosing. The equivalent dose he received was 90 mg q12h; the BTD dose was left unchanged. The desipramine was increased every 3 to 4 days until the analgesia it provided seemed maximal and he was sleeping well; the dose reached was 100 mg q hs. Mild nausea and mental clouding resolved after a few days. Constipation was treated with a bowel regimen (refer to Chapter 19).

He did relatively well for several months; however, his disease was progressing, and intermittent upward titration of his baseline dose was undertaken on the basis of his BTD requirement. Four months later he was taking modified-release morphine, 180 mg every 12 hours, and the BTD remained at 30 mg short-acting morphine every 1 to 2 hours PRN (within 5% to 15% of baseline and providing effective analgesia).

PATIENT ENCOUNTER 4

A fall at home resulted in a fractured femur. The patient elected to have surgery as a means of allowing prompt mobilization that could facilitate an improved quality of life. Preoperatively his leg pain was severe, and analgesic therapy needed to be adjusted.

Pain severity and descriptors: Sharp, 9 to 10/10 on movement.

Inferred pain pathophysiology: Somatic. Acute pain superimposed on persistent chest wall and arm pain.

Analgesic selection: Morphine was continued, but the route of administration was changed from an oral to an IV infusion. His infusion rate was started at 7.5 mg/h with 4 mg BTDs available every 30 minutes PRN.

Step on analgesic ladder: 3.

Rationale: Because of the severity of the pain, the equianalgesic dose was increased by 50% when switching from the oral to the IV route. Using a 3:1 oral/IV ratio, his infusion rate was started at 7.5 mg/h (360 mg + 180 mg = 540 mg oral morphine/24 h = 180 mg IV morphine/24 h = 7.5 mg/h), with 4 mg BTDs available every 30 minutes PRN. (The total hourly BTD was approximately 5% of the total daily dose, and the first dose given provided effective analgesia. If it had not, the rescue dose would have been escalated by 30% to 50%.) Although several BTDs were required in the first few hours, the need for these subsided. Surgical recovery was uneventful. Five days after surgery, he was able to take PO medications and was using very occasional BTDs. He was, however, anxious about the planned switch to oral pain medication and requested that it be done gradually. The IV infusion was initially decreased to approximately half (3.5 mg/h), and he was given the equivalent oral dose, 130 mg every 12 hours, in a modified-release oral morphine preparation. He continued to have IV BTDs available to him as before. Forty-eight hours later, his IV infusion had been discontinued, and he was taking the equivalent modified-release morphine dose of 260 mg every 12 hours by mouth. BTDs of oral short-acting morphine sulfate, 60 mg (5% to 15% of 24-hour opioid dose) were available to him every 1 to 2 hours PRN. Desipramine was restarted at 25 mg q hs and gradually titrated up to its previous level of 100 mg.

Outcome: The patient's pain remained well controlled at home on oral analgesics until his death 4 weeks after discharge. Ongoing assessment and reassessment by the nurse in liaison with the patient's primary physician were critical components in managing the analgesic approach to this man's pain. The assessment included the effectiveness of relief, the duration of relief, the effectiveness of BTDs, and the presence and management of adverse effects.

Adapted from Coyle, N., & Portenoy, R. K. (1996). Pharmacologic management of cancer pain. In R. McCorkle, M. Grant, M. Frank-Stromborg M, et al. (Eds.), *Cancer nursing: A comprehensive textbook*, Philadelphia, Saunders.

Effectiveness of the WHO Analgesic Ladder

The use of the WHO ladder in combination with appropriate dosing guidelines is capable of providing adequate pain relief in 70% to 90% of individuals with persistent cancer pain (Hanks, Cherny, Fallon, 2004). This was demonstrated in a 10-year study of 2118 patients, which further

indicated that clinically significant pain reduction usually occurred within the first week of treatment (Zech, Grond, Lynch, et al., 1995). Good to satisfactory pain relief was maintained in 88% of the patients over the entire treatment period, and only 12% required invasive procedures for pain relief, such as nerve blocks. Of note is the fact that both opioids and nonopioids were prescribed in 73% of the patients. Also, oral opioid doses reported in this study suggest that the clinicians understood that no ceiling exists on the analgesia of mu agonists because some patients received up to 2400 mg/day of oral morphine. A more recent retrospective study of 3238 patients with advanced cancer reported good pain relief (VAS scores less than 30) in 89% of those following the principles of the WHO analgesic ladder (Bhatnagar, Mishra, Srikanti, et al., 2008). The WHO ladder approach has also been adapted to effectively treat phantom limb pain (Mishra, Bhatnagar, Gupta, et al., 2008) and pain in patients with end-stage renal disease (Salisbury, Game, Al-Shakarchi, et al., 2009).

Preemptive Analgesia for Postoperative Pain Management

In the early 1980s, studies of the spinal cord changes occurring in the context of peripheral afferent input—changes that were termed *central sensitization* (Woolf, 1983)—generated interest in the therapeutic potential of interventions that could be implemented before tissue injury occurred, in the hope of blocking or reducing this phenomenon (Dahl, Moiniche, 2004; Grape, Tramer, 2007) (see Section I for more on central sensitization). A multimodal approach that includes local anesthetics to block sensory input and NSAIDs and opioids, which act in the periphery and in the CNS, initiated preoperatively and continued intraoperatively and throughout the postoperative course, was suggested as ideal preemptive analgesic treatment (Woolf, Chong, 1993). Since then, numerous studies have investigated a wide variety of agents and techniques in an attempt to show a preemptive analgesic effect (Dahl, Moiniche, 2004; Moiniche, Kehlet, Dahl, 2002). Unfortunately, these studies showed that this approach alone did not result in major benefits postoperatively.

Testing the hypothesis of preemptive analgesia requires comparing the effectiveness of an intervention applied before the surgical incision (experimental group) with the effectiveness of the same or very similar intervention applied only after the surgical incision (control group). The notion that such a simple approach could reduce or possibly prevent postoperative pain stimulated an abundance of research on preemptive analgesia; however, many of the studies had flawed research designs and led to flawed conclusions (Bromley, 2006; Grape, Tramer, 2007; Moiniche, Kehlet, Dahl, 2002; Dahl, Moiniche, 2004). For example, some studies compared preoperative analgesic administration with placebo or no treatment and claimed a preemptive effect when treatment was associated with a subsequent reduction in pain. These and other inaccurate claims of positive results led to an overly optimistic perception of the effectiveness of preemptive analgesia (Grape, Tramer, 2007).

An extensive review of the literature on preemptive analgesia concluded that preoperative (preemptive) administration of systemic opioids did not improve postoperative analgesia (Moiniche, Kehlet, Dahl, 2002). None of the studies reviewed demonstrated a reduction in pain intensity scores in the groups of patients who received preemptive (preincision) analgesia; analysis of the weighted mean differences in pain scores favored the groups who received postoperative (postincision) analgesia. An updated review in 2004 reported the same results (Dahl, Moiniche, 2004).

The general consensus is that preemptive administration of analgesics does not offer major clinical benefits (i.e., consistent immediate postoperative pain relief or reduced need for supplemental analgesia) (Bromley, 2006; Dahl, Moiniche, 2004; Grape, Tramer, 2007; Kelly, Ahmad, Brull, 2001; Moiniche, Kehlet, Dahl, 2002). However, the disappointing research related to preemptive analgesia does not mean that postoperative benefits cannot be realized with aggressive perioperative analgesic interventions. It has been suggested that research and clinical practice should redirect the focus from "preemptive" (timing of a single [most often] conventional intervention) to "protective" analgesia whereby aggressive, sustained multimodal interventions are initiated preoperatively and continued throughout the intraoperative and postoperative periods (Moiniche, Kehlet, Dahl, 2002; Dahl, Moiniche, 2004). Consistent with this approach are the goals of immediate postoperative pain reduction and prevention of prolonged and pathologic pain (Kelly, Ahmad, Brull, 2001). The key underlying pain management principles are to intervene before the onset of pain, use a multimodal approach, and administer analgesics in the proper dose and manner, on time, and for an adequate duration of time (Kelly, Ahmad, Brull, 2001).

Accelerated Multimodal Postoperative Rehabilitation

Advances in the field of pain management have led to more aggressive use of analgesics, but it is unclear if this has resulted in significant improvements in patient outcomes such as the quality of postoperative recovery and long-term function (Liu, Wu, 2007a). An unacceptable number of surgical patients continue to experience delays in recovery, complications, and the need for extended hospital stays (Kehlet, Wilmore, 2008). An extensive review of research (18 meta-analyses, 10 systematic reviews, 8 randomized controlled trials, and 2 observa-

tional database articles) revealed that there are insufficient data to show that high-quality postoperative pain management, such as regional analgesia and IV PCA, impacts the incidence and severity of postoperative complications (Liu, Wu, 2007b). The researchers suggested that improvements will depend on the integration of pain control into a comprehensive postoperative rehabilitation program that includes fluid balance and early mobilization and nutrition. For example, a variety of positive outcomes, such as early return of GI function and shortened length of hospital stay, have been observed in patients undergoing major surgery when epidural analgesia is combined in a multimodal postoperative rehabilitation plan (Basse, Billesbolle, Kehlet, 2002; Basse, Hjort Jakobsen, Billesbolle et al., 2000; Brodner, Van Aken, Hertle, et al., 2001; Kehlet, Wilmore, 2004). The use of multimodal strategies that attack the specific physiologic insults of surgery should be considered when developing postoperative treatment plans, particularly for patients who undergo major surgical procedures. For example, the IV administration of hypocaloric dextrose (glucose) 10% in addition to continuous epidural analgesia has been shown to inhibit the catabolic effects of surgery as demonstrated by postoperative suppression of whole-body protein breakdown (Lattermann, Wykes, Eberhart, et al., 2007; Schricker, Meterissian, Wykes et al., 2004).

Patient outcomes have historically been reported as morbidity and mortality data; however, a focus on patient-reported assessments as a subset of morbidity and mortality events may provide unique insight into specific areas that need more intense research and clinical focus (Liu, Wu, 2007a, 2007b). An exhaustive review of the literature evaluated the effect of postoperative analgesia on patient-assessed indicators, which included a variety of aspects of analgesia, presence of adverse effects, health-related quality of life, quality of recovery, and patient satisfaction (Liu, Wu, 2007b). The researchers identified a lack of high-quality data and called for the development of validated tools to measure patient-reported outcomes and well-designed research that examines these as the primary study end points.

Establishing the link between good pain management and improvements in patient outcomes will require changes in the way health care is administered (Kehlet, Wilmore, 2008; Liu, Wu, 2007a, 2007b). Traditional practices in perioperative care, such as prolonged bed rest, withholding oral nutrition for extensive periods, and routine use of tubes and drains, are being increasingly challenged and replaced with evidence-based decision making (Pasero, Belden, 2006). This and other factors have led to the evolution of fast track surgery and enhanced postoperative recovery (Kehlet, Wilmore, 2008). In a review of the literature, Kehlet and Wilmore (2008) describe the evidence that supports key principles of implementing what is referred to as *accelerated multimodal postoperative rehabilitation*. These are outlined in Box 12-1. Continuous multimodal pain relief is integral to this concept.

Box 12-1 | Key Components to Accelerated Multimodal Postoperative Recovery

1. Preoperative patient education outlining the plan of care and emphasizing expectations of an active patient role in recovery
2. Perioperative optimization (e.g., preoperatively ensure optimal nutritional and hydration status; maximize pulmonary function; control underlying persistent pain; and reduce alcohol, tobacco, and medications that can cause intraoperative adverse events)
3. Surgical stress reduction (attenuation of neurohormonal response to the surgical procedure)
   - Intraoperative actions: Avoid hypothermia, optimize stroke volume, and prevent hyper- and hypovolemia
   - Neural blockades to reduce protein loss and minimize postoperative ileus
   - Minimally invasive surgery to reduce wound size and undesirable inflammatory responses, pain, and pulmonary compromise (e.g., transverse rather than vertical abdominal incision)
   - Thromboprophylaxis
   - Pharmacologic interventions to improve recovery (e.g., prevention of nausea and insulin resistance)
4. Pain reduction: Multimodal perioperative analgesic approaches that reduce postoperative pain and other discomforts, control the stress response, and allow early and aggressive recovery activities
   - Focus on strategies that allow the lowest effective opioid dose or avoidance of opioids (e.g., combinations of NSAIDs, ketamine, gabapentin, local anesthetic techniques)
5. Prevent and control nausea and other discomforts and adverse effects that interfere with recovery

(e.g., implement multimodal strategies to prevent and treat nausea)
6. Aggressive postoperative rehabilitation measures (e.g., goal-directed ambulation, early discharge planning)
7. Evidence-based decision making with regard to care practices (e.g., challenge traditional practices that increase infection and pain, impede ambulation, and produce other adverse effects that impede recovery)
   - Avoid routine use of catheters (urinary), tubes (e.g., nasogastric), and drains (cause pain and infection and impede mobilization) or discontinue necessary catheters, tubes, and drains as soon as possible
   - Avoid prolonged fasting (contributes to catabolism); institute early enteral feeding to facilitate gastric emptying and build tissue

From Pasero, C., & McCaffery, M. *Pain assessment and pharmacologic management*, p. 308, St. Louis, Mosby. Data from Gan, T. J., et al. (2006). *PONV management*. http://www.medscape.com/viewprogram/4990. Accessed December 8, 2009; Jensen, K., Kehlet, H., & Lund, C. M. (2007). Post-operative recovery profile after laparoscopic cholecystectomy: A prospective, observational study of a multimodal anaesthetic regime. *Acta Anaesthesiol Scand, 51*(4), 464-471; Kehlet, H., & Wilmore, D. W. (2002). Multimodal strategies to improve surgical outcome. *Am J Surg, 183*(6), 630-641; Kehlet, H., & Wilmore, D. W. (2008). Evidence-based surgical care and the evolution of fast-track surgery. *Ann Surg, 248*(2), 189-198; Pasero, C. (2007). Procedure-specific pain management: PROSPECT. *J PeriAnesth Nurs, 22*(5), 335-340; Pasero, C., & Belden, J. (2006). Evidence-based perioperative care: Accelerated postoperative recovery programs. *J PeriAnesth Nurs, 21*(3), 168-177; PROSPECT: Procedure Specific Postoperative Pain Management. http://www.postoppain.org. Accessed December 8, 2009. © 2011, Pasero C, McCaffery M. May be duplicated for use in clinical practice.

Tools that can be used to increase evidence-based perioperative pain management practice patterns are emerging. For example, a novel web-based program called PROSPECT (**Pro**cedure **Spec**ific Postoperative Pain Management) *(http://www.postoppain.org)*, established by an international team of surgeons and anesthesiologists, posts evidence-based recommendations and algorithms to guide the health care team in decision making with regard to pain management according to specific surgical procedures (Pasero, 2007).

Persistent Postsurgical Pain

As many as 50% of patients undergoing surgical procedures, such as inguinal hernia repair; breast, cardiac, or thoracic surgery; leg amputation; and coronary artery bypass, experience persistent pain; in 2% to 10% of these individuals, the intensity of persistent postsurgical pain is severe (Kehlet, Jensen, Woolf, 2006). A study of 90 women who underwent abdominal hysterectomy pain for noncancer conditions found that 16.7% experienced persistent postoperative pain (Brandsborg, Dueholm, Nikolajsen, et al., 2009). The incidence of persistent post-mastectomy pain is reported to be as high as 65% (Smith, Bourne, Squair, et al., 1999).

Pain following traumatic injury is common as well. A multicenter study conducted in 69 hospitals in 14 states in the United States found that 62.7% of patients (N = 3047) reported injury-related pain at 12 months after a traumatic injury (Rivara, MacKenzie, Jurkovich, et al., 2008). A quarter of patients in an earlier study (N = 397) described pain that interfered with daily activity 7 years following limb-threatening lower extremity trauma; 40% reported high pain intensities (Castillo, MacKenzie, Wegener, et al., 2006).

Further research is needed, but multiple factors are thought to contribute to the likelihood of postsurgical pain, including surgical nerve injury, preexisting pain, and genetic susceptibility. For example, severe pre-amputation pain has long been associated with a higher incidence of phantom limb pain (Bach, Noreng, Tjellden, 1988; Katz, 1997; Nikolajsen, Ilkjaer, Kroner, et al., 1997). A 2-year study of 57 patients who underwent lower extremity amputation revealed that high levels of both pre-amputation pain and acute pain after amputation predicted persistent post-amputation pain (Hanley, Jensen, Smith, et al., 2007). Greater analgesic requirements during the immediate postoperative period following coronary artery bypass surgery predicted persistent pain (multiple anatomic sites) in a study of 736 patients (Taillefer, Carrier, Belisle, et al., 2006). Older patients tend to have a lower risk of developing persistent postsurgical pain than younger patients (Poobalan, Bruce, Smith, et al., 2003; Smith, Bourne, Squair, et al., 1999). For example, one study showed that patients under the age of 40 years old were at increased risk for persistent post-inguinal hernia repair pain (Poobalan, Bruce, King, et al., 2001). Another found that the prevalence of persistent chest and leg pain following cardiac surgery was 55% in patients who were less than 60 years of age and 34% in those over 70 years old (Bruce, Drury, Poobalan, et al., 2003). The reader is referred to an excellent review by Perkins and Kehlet (2000) that includes predictive factors, etiology, and progression of postsurgical pain conditions.

The presence of pain at 3 months after injury was a predictive factor for both the presence and the high severity of persistent pain following major trauma (Rivara, MacKenzie, Jurkovich, et al., 2008). Although the presence of persistent pain varied with age, it was more common in women and in those who had untreated depression before the traumatic injury in this study. Another study found that multiple factors influenced the likelihood of persistent pain 7 years after major lower extremity trauma (Castillo, MacKenzie, Wegener, et al., 2006). These included having less than a high school education, having less than a college education, low self-efficacy for return to usual major activities, a high level of alcohol consumption in the month prior to injury, and high pain intensity, high levels of sleep and rest dysfunction, and elevated levels of depression and anxiety at three months after hospital discharge. Interestingly, those who were treated with opioid analgesics during the first three months after discharge in this study had lower levels of persistent pain at 7 years, underscoring the importance of early initiation of aggressive pain management approaches.

The clinical presentation of persistent postsurgical or post-trauma pain is primarily the patient's report of the features characteristic of neuropathic pain, such as continuous burning pain and pain beyond the expected time of pain resolution (see Section II for assessment of neuropathic pain). Strategies for preventing these persistent pain states are being investigated, but sustained multimodal pharmacologic approaches that target the underlying mechanisms of neuropathic pain described earlier in this section are recommended (Kehlet, Jensen, Woolf, 2006). See Section I for the underlying mechanisms of the pathology of pain and more on persistent postsurgical pain, and Sections III, IV, and V for discussion of the role of the various analgesics and techniques in the prevention of persistent postsurgical and posttrauma pain.

Around-the-Clock (ATC) Dosing

Two basic principles of providing effective pain management are preventing pain and maintaining a pain rating that allows the patient to accomplish functional or quality of life goals with relative ease (see Section II for goal setting). These may require that the mainstay analgesic be administered on a scheduled ATC basis, rather than PRN ("as needed"), to maintain stable analgesic blood levels. ATC dosing regimens are designed to control baseline pain, defined as the pain the patient reports as being the average pain intensity experienced for 12 hours or more during a 24-hour period (Foley, 2004). In other words, ATC dosing should be considered when pain itself is ATC (continuous) or present for 12 or more hours each day. The use of continuous analgesia prevents the undertreatment of pain in patients who are hesitant to request pain medication and eliminates delays patients encounter waiting for caregivers to prepare and administer pain medication. Another benefit is that patients have been shown to be more adherent with their analgesic regimen when analgesics are prescribed ATC. A 5-week study of oncology outpatients with pain who kept a daily diary to record level of pain and analgesic intake showed that overall adherence rates for those who took their analgesics ATC ranged from 84.5% to 90.8%, compared with 22.2% to 26.6% in those who took them PRN (Miaskowski, Dodd, West, et al., 2001). The researchers pointed out that one might speculate that the reason for lower adherence rates for the PRN regimen was because those patients were experiencing less pain and, therefore, needed less analgesics; however, no significant differences were found in the percentage of patients who reported severe pain (NRS 7 or higher) in the ATC compared with the PRN group.

ATC dosing for continuous pain may be accompanied by provision of additional analgesic doses (called *breakthrough doses, supplemental doses,* or *rescue doses*) as needed to relieve pain that exceeds, or breaks through, the ongoing pain (discussed in the following paragraphs). For example, when analgesia is provided orally, ATC dosing often is accomplished with a combination of modified-release opioid given at scheduled times with breakthrough doses of short-acting opioid given if pain breaks through (Cousins, 2007). When invasive routes are used to manage pain, a continuous infusion with PCA boluses or clinician-administered supplemental doses accomplishes the same objectives as this oral approach (see Chapter 17 for more on PCA). Supplemental dosing for breakthrough pain is conventional practice during the management of pain associated with active cancer or other advanced medical illness. It is not considered to be the standard of care in the management of patients with persistent non-cancer pain, and in this large and diverse population, the use of this approach requires a separate, careful assessment of potential benefits and burdens (Devulder, Jacobs, Richarz, et al., 2009; Fine, Portenoy, 2007).

Surprisingly, little research has been conducted on the use of ATC dosing. An early cross-over study showed that scheduled ATC dosing of analgesics improved pain relief and mood level compared with on-demand PRN dosing in patients with persistent noncancer pain (Berntzen, Gotestam, 1987). A more recent parallel-design study of medical inpatients with pain from a variety of origins compared ATC scheduled opioid doses with PRN opioid doses and found that those who received ATC doses experienced lower pain intensity ratings (Paice, Noskin, Vanagunas, et al., 2005). As might be expected, a significantly greater percentage of the prescribed opioid was administered when it was given ATC (70.8%) compared with PRN (38%). There were no differences in adverse effects between the two groups. A randomized controlled trial (N = 227) showed that early oral analgesia (first postoperative day) with scheduled 20 mg doses of short-acting morphine every 4 hours and an additional 10 mg dose every 2 hours PRN was safe and effective, producing similar analgesia as IV PCA with a basal rate after intra-abdominal surgery (Pearl, McCauley, Thompson, et al., 2002). An observational, prospective study administered ATC oral short-acting morphine to patients (N = 95) following orthopedic surgery and reported average pain scores were 2.4 at rest and 4.0 during movement in bed (Zaslansky, Eisenberg, Peskin, et al., 2006). Nausea and vomiting, the most common adverse effects, were reported by 22%, and no one required naloxone.

Other research has shown conflicting results. A study of outpatients with pain from bone metastases found no significant differences in average, least, or worst pain intensity in patients taking ATC or PRN opioids, but significantly higher opioid prescriptions and intake (12.4 times more) were reported in patients who took ATC opioids (Miaskowski, Mack, Dodd, et al., 2002). The researchers noted that their findings challenge the accepted principle of treating continuous pain with ATC analgesics but offered a number of possible explanations. These included that the opioid analgesic regimens may not have been effective for the type of pain the patients had (bone pain), analgesic doses were not titrated to optimal effect, and the possibility that comparisons were difficult because the two groups were not receiving the same analgesics (PRN received short-acting opioids and ATC received long-acting opioids). Another study randomized children to receive ATC or PRN acetaminophen plus codeine following tonsillectomy and found no differences in pain intensity ratings or pain relief scores

(Sutters, Miaskowski, Holdridge-Zeuner, et al., 2004, 2005). Both groups experienced moderate to severe pain, and similar to the previous study, more analgesic (two times more) was consumed by those in the ATC group. There were no differences in adverse effects, such as nausea and vomiting, sedation, and dizziness, which were described as moderate to severe. An interesting finding was that the parents of children receiving PRN analgesia decreased the dose of analgesic they gave to their children over time despite high pain intensity and poor pain relief.

These studies suggest the need for more research evaluating the best method for analgesic dose administration in a variety of populations and for a variety of types of pain. Until research proves otherwise, prevention of the recurrence of pain with scheduled ATC dosing is recommended for continuous types of pain.

Awakening Patients for Analgesic Administration

Nurses often wonder if patients taking ATC short-acting opioids should be awakened and given pain medication and if they should teach patients in the home setting to wake themselves up during their normal sleep time to take their pain medications to keep pain under control. There is very little research guiding this practice, and none could be found in opioid-naïve patients with acute pain. The consensus expert opinion of the European Association for Palliative Care (EAPC) regarding palliative care patients with moderate to severe pain is to give a double dose of short-acting opioid at bedtime rather than a single dose and awaken the patient for a second dose 4 hours later (Hanks, De Conno, Cherny, et al., 2001). This is based on the assumption that doubling the dose will prolong the duration of analgesia long enough to prevent awakening with pain.

Some research on the efficacy of double dosing vs. usual dosing has been done in patients with cancer pain. A double-blind, randomized, cross-over study that compared the two methods found that average pain, strongest night pain, and sleep quality were slightly better in those who took a double dose compared with those who took a single dose, but the difference was not clinically significant (Dale, Piribauer, Kaasa, et al., 2009). The researchers suggested that the slight difference may have been due to initial higher exposure to morphine's metabolite M6G (see Chapter 13). An earlier prospective study of palliative care patients found that all pain scores were worse in patients who took a double dose of opioid compared with those who took a single dose at bedtime followed by another dose 4 hours later (Todd, Rees, Gwilliam, et al., 2002). Further, those in the double-dose group required more breakthrough analgesia and experienced more adverse effects.

Double doses of opioids should not be given to opioid-naïve patients, but patients who are opioid tolerant can be told to try double dosing and usual dosing as described above and see which works best to keep their pain under control. Alternatively, the patient who has access to long-acting, modified-release formulations can be switched to one of these in an effort to improve sleep at night. Occasional patients in the ambulatory setting prefer to have a short-acting drug during the day and a dose of a long-acting drug at night; this unconventional practice can be explored on a case-by-case basis. Both opioid-naïve and opioid-tolerant patients with persistent pain in the hospital setting should be awakened to take their pain medication (see Chapter 19 for assessment of sedation and respiratory status before opioid administration). Awakening postoperative patients with moderate-to-severe pain to take their pain medication is especially important during the first 24 to 48 hours of therapy to keep pain under control. Patients should be told that this helps to avoid waking up with severe pain and that if their pain is well controlled, they are more likely to go back to sleep quickly. The patient can transition gradually to PRN dosing and sleeping during the night as pain resolves.

Breakthrough Pain

Breakthrough pain (sometimes called *pain flare, episodic pain,* or *transient pain*) is defined as a transitory exacerbation of pain in a patient who has relatively stable and adequately controlled baseline pain (Portenoy, Forbes, Lussier, et al., 2004). The intensity of pain is sometimes included in the definition of breakthrough pain, i.e., a transient increase in pain to greater than moderate intensity occurring on a baseline pain of moderate intensity or less (Foley, 2004). Breakthrough pain is not routinely recognized, evaluated, and treated, and research has revealed a need for standardized methods for diagnosing it (Caraceni, Martini, Zecca, et al., 2004; Mercadante, 2006a, 2006b; Mercadante, Radbruch, Caraceni, et al., 2002) (see Section II for assessment tools).

Like its definition, there is variation in the description of breakthrough pain. Some describe it as occurring spontaneously (not related to activity), rapidly increasing to a high intensity level, and having a short duration (30 to 45 minutes) (de Leon-Casasola, 2008). Others describe subtypes of breakthrough pain, noting that it can have a sudden or gradual onset and can be brief or prolonged; some episodes are spontaneous, and others are associated with an identifiable precipitant (Bennett, Burton, Fishman, et al., 2005a; Payne, 2007). When breakthrough pain is brief and precipitated by a voluntary action, such as movement, it is referred to as *incident pain*. One study of patients with persistent noncancer pain showed this to be the most common type of breakthrough pain with an identifiable precipitant in 69% of the episodes, and 92% of these were activity-related (Portenoy, Bennett, Rauck, et al., 2006). Incident pain can also be unpredictable and associated with involuntary activity, such as sneezing or coughing. This type of breakthrough pain is also common,

with no predictable onset in 45% and sometimes a predictable onset in 31% of the episodes (Portenoy, Bennett, Rauck, et al., 2006). Another subtype, idiopathic pain, is not associated with a known cause and often has a longer duration than incident pain. End-of-dose failure, the last of the subtypes, is characterized by a return of pain before the next analgesic dose is due. The occurrence of increased pain at the end of the scheduled dosing period suggests a need to maintain a higher plasma drug concentration throughout the dosing interval (Portenoy, Forbes, Lussier, et al., 2004). In these cases, the dose of the scheduled analgesic should be increased, or, in some patients, the interval between doses should be shortened, which results ultimately in an increased dose.

The incidence of breakthrough pain in cancer patients is reported to be between 50% and 90% (Portenoy, Bennett, Rauck, et al., 2005). A prospective international survey of patients with cancer pain (N = 1095) in 24 countries reported breakthrough pain in 64.8% of those surveyed (Caraceni, Martini, Zecca, et al., 2004). Most of these studies were performed in inpatient environments or in populations with advanced illness; the prevalence of breakthrough cancer pain in the population of patients undergoing treatment in the community is largely unknown. A longitudinal study (N = 101) of breakthrough pain in advanced cancer patients at home found that on admission to the study, 49% reported breakthrough pain, and 78% reported that the breakthrough pain strongly limited their activity; most had no prescription for breakthrough analgesia (Mercadante, Costanzo, Fusco, et al., 2009). The researchers described breakthrough pain as a dynamic entity dependent on several factors, including analgesic treatment and the course of disease.

Individuals with persistent noncancer pain also may experience a high incidence of breakthrough pain. A telephone questionnaire administered to patients with well-controlled baseline persistent noncancer pain revealed that 74% experienced breakthrough pain (Portenoy, Bennett, Rauck, et al., 2006). The median number of episodes was two per day, and the median time to maximum intensity was 10 minutes with a median duration of 60 minutes. The type of breakthrough pain was somatic (38%), neuropathic (18%), visceral (4%), or mixed (40%). These patients were undergoing treatment at pain clinics, and this prevalence may overstate the rate that exists in the general population.

Although much about the epidemiology of breakthrough pain remains to be elucidated, some early data strongly suggest that, if not addressed adequately, breakthrough pain can have significant negative effects on function and quality of life (Fine, Portenoy, 2007; Mercadante, Villari, Ferrera, et al., 2004; Taylor, Webster, Chun, et al., 2007; Zeppetella, Ribeiro, 2006). One study also indicated that the presence of breakthrough pain in U.S. cancer patients increases the economic burden for patients and the health care system (Portenoy, Bennett, Rauck, et al., 2006).

Treatment of Breakthrough Pain

The routine treatment of breakthrough pain generally is considered to be conventional practice in populations for which opioid therapy is the mainstay for the long-term management of moderate to severe pain—specifically those with active cancer or other types of advanced medical illness. The treatment of breakthrough pain in other populations has yet garnered no consensus, and the prudent approach is to consider this strategy as a separate intervention requiring its own assessment of benefit and burden (Devulder, Jacobs, Richarz, et al., 2009; Fine, Portenoy, 2007).

Addressing the cause of breakthrough pain can eliminate the need for analgesic therapy in some patients (Portenoy, Forbes, Lussier, et al., 2004). For example, surgery, chemotherapy, or radiation therapy in some cancer patients may eliminate the cause. Adjusting the scheduled analgesic regimen, such as by increasing the dose, is another approach that targets cause. Even breakthrough pain that does not appear to be associated with end-of-dose failure (e.g., pain occurring in patients receiving continuous infusions) may be amenable to a dose increase. As a trial, the scheduled analgesic dose should be increased until either acceptable pain relief or intolerable and unmanageable adverse effects supervene (Portenoy, Forbes, Lussier, et al., 2004). If the frequency or intensity of breakthrough pain episodes decline, this change can be continued.

If the decision is made to treat the breakthrough pain specifically, a variety of analgesic interventions may be considered (Portenoy, Forbes, Lussier, et al., 2004). NSAIDs can be used, again based on an analysis of benefit and burden. More often, a short-acting mu agonist opioid is selected and provided on a PRN basis (Mercadante, 2004; Portenoy, Forbes, Lussier et al., 2004). Comparative studies sufficient to guide drug selection and dosing for breakthrough pain are lacking, and guidelines are empirical. Often, a short-acting formulation of the same drug given as a modified-release formulation is selected. For example, short-acting oral morphine is prescribed for breakthrough pain in patients taking modified-release morphine. Although cases have been published that suggest the safety and efficacy of methadone for the treatment of breakthrough pain (Fisher, Stiles, Hagen, 2004), concern about accumulation of this drug with repeated doses suggests that an alternative short half-life opioid drug be selected instead (see Chapter 13). Similarly, a short-acting oral or transmucosal drug usually is prescribed when baseline pain is treated with transdermal fentanyl. (See Chapter 16 for calculation of breakthrough doses and Chapter 18 for patient examples that demonstrate the clinical management of breakthrough pain.)

There is a mismatch between the time-action relationship of oral opioids and the temporal profile of most breakthrough pains. Oral drugs typically have an analgesic onset of at least 20 minutes. Most breakthrough pains reach a maximum intensity in just a few minutes and disappear within an hour. A prospective survey of hospice patients identified this mismatch as a potential barrier to effective management (Zeppetella, 2008). Most patients in this study described their breakthrough pain as sudden and unpredictable, lasting an average of 35 minutes. By the time the oral analgesic was deemed effective, the pain may already have spontaneously resolved. This phenomenon was noted in another study that showed patients often failed to take breakthrough doses when they had breakthrough pain episodes (Davies, Vriens, Kennett, et al., 2008). The mean duration of the breakthrough episodes was 30 minutes. The patients reported that the pain improved before the drug could take effect; most were prescribed an opioid with an onset of 20 to 30 minutes. A perplexing finding was that the most commonly cited explanation for not taking a breakthrough dose in this study was a lack of sufficient pain intensity for breakthrough pain medication even though the breakthrough episodes were described as usually moderate to severe in intensity. The researchers underscored the need for appropriate prescriptions for breakthrough pain and focused education about breakthrough pain for both health care professionals and patients and their caregivers.

Lipophilic transmucosal formulations are undergoing development with the intent of addressing the temporal mismatch by providing a more rapid onset of effect. Oral transmucosal fentanyl (OTFC, Actiq) and buccal fentanyl tablet (Fentora) are both commercially available in many countries, a sublingual fentanyl tablet and a fentanyl nasal spray are available in some countries, and a buccal patch of fentanyl (Onsolis) was recently approved in the United States. Similar formulations of other lipophilic drugs, such as sufentanil, are undergoing development (see Chapter 14 for intranasal and oral transmucosal formulations).

The rapid-onset transmucosal fentanyl formulations have a faster onset of analgesia than the oral formulations; peak effect is substantially earlier, and duration of action is relatively short (Fine, Portenoy, 2007). Patients have reported improvement in breakthrough pain within 15 minutes with OTFC (Mystakidou, Katsouda, Parpa, et al., 2005) and buccal fentanyl (Portenoy, Taylor, Messina, et al., 2006). Oral transmucosal and intranasal sufentanil formulations presumably will have similarly rapid onset (Gardner-Nix, 2001a; Jackson, Ashby, Keech, 2002). A Cochrane Collaboration Review of opioids used for breakthrough cancer pain identified only four randomized controlled trials for analysis, and all four examined the use of OTFC and showed it to be safe and effective (Zeppetella, Ribeiro, 2006). This review underscored the need for more research to evaluate the effectiveness of the opioids used to manage breakthrough pain.

Much is not known about the rapid-onset transmucosal formulations for breakthrough pain. Direct comparisons with oral formulations are very limited, and the extent to which the more rapid onset yields clinically meaningful benefit is uncertain. Presumably, there is a subpopulation that could benefit greatly, but empirical definition of this group has not yet been done. The various formulations (e.g., buccal vs. sublingual vs. intranasal) appear to vary in onset such that the proportion of patients who report meaningful benefit at 5 minutes, 10 minutes, or later points varies by drug; as yet, it is unknown whether these differences will translate into clinical preferences for any formulation or group of formulations. As implied previously, all these formulations have been approved by the regulatory authorities for cancer-related breakthrough pain; there is very little evidence of efficacy in populations with noncancer pain, and the appropriate positioning of these drugs remains a matter of clinical judgment only. Finally, there is concern about the abuse liability of the rapid-onset formulations, but the extent to which these drugs may drive aberrant behavior, relapse into addiction, or diversion now is unknown.

In short, the rapid-onset transmucosal formulations appear to be a therapeutic advance given their likely ability to improve the management of breakthrough pain, at least those with rapid onset. At present, their role relative to conventional oral rescue medication is uncertain and is evolving as studies appear and experience accumulates.

The IV route has also been used to rapidly treat breakthrough pain and optimize the control of baseline pain. In an open-label study, patients (N = 25) with poorly controlled baseline metastatic (bone) cancer pain and movement-related breakthrough pain received rapid IV opioid titration to obtain pain relief (Mercadante, Villari, Ferrera, et al., 2004). The dose was then increased further to challenge the therapeutic ceiling, which was determined by the development of adverse effects rather than pain relief at rest. The daily IV dose was converted to a daily oral dose and administered in modified-release formulation every 8 to 12 hours (mean oral morphine equivalents were 102 mg). This titration approach resulted in significant improvements in movement-related pain. A minority of patients experienced adverse effects that required treatment or decreases in opioid dose. A later open-label study showed similar results in patients with advanced cancer who were administered IV morphine in doses proportional to their ATC regimen (Mercadante, Intravaia, Villari, et al., 2008). The mean IV morphine dose was 12 mg (range of 9 mg to 14 mg), and more than 60% of the patients in this study experienced a > 33% reduction in pain intensity (see Section II for more on meaningful pain relief). There were no adverse events with this approach.

Alternative methods may be necessary when systemic (oral, IV) opioids fail to relieve breakthrough pain. A report of 12 patients with advanced cancer receiving intrathecal analgesia described treatment of breakthrough pain unresponsive to high doses of IV morphine (Mercadante, Arcuri, Ferrera, et al., 2005). The patients were titrated with intrathecal boluses of local anesthetics (levobupivacaine 0.25%, mean, 1.5 mg) or with doses of

sublingual ketamine (25 mg), depending on patient preference. Breakthrough pain was achieved for all episodes within 10 minutes by either method. Treatment was well tolerated, but the researchers suggested reserving these alternative methods for select patients and administering them in a setting that can support frequent monitoring and skilled nursing. (See Chapter 15 for more on intraspinal analgesia and Chapter 23 for more on ketamine.)

PRN Dosing

PRN ("as needed") dosing requires patients to request analgesia. Effective PRN dosing relies on the patient's active participation. Patient teaching must include reminding patients to "stay on top of pain" and request analgesia before pain is severe and out of control. Obviously crucial to the effective use of PRN dosing is a rapid response to reports of pain and to requests for an analgesic.

In addition to its use for breakthrough pain, PRN dosing of opioid analgesics may be appropriate for other types of pain, such as intermittent pain. It also is useful when initiating opioid analgesic therapy in opioid-naïve patients with moderate to severe persistent pain, especially when pain is escalating rapidly. In these cases, PRN dosing allows for a rapid response to the patient's need for pain relief while minimizing the chance of overdose. PRN dosing is also helpful when pain is decreasing rapidly (Coyle, Cherny, Portenoy, 1995). When patients with acute pain recover and pain resolves, ATC dosing may be replaced with PRN dosing (Pasero, Portenoy, McCaffery, 1999).

Although PRN dosing may be effective in these scenarios, there is abundant clinical experience suggesting the potential for negative outcomes. A study of outpatient oncology patients with pain who kept a daily diary to record level of pain and analgesic intake showed overall adherence rates for those who took their analgesics ATC ranged from 84.5% to 90.8% compared with 22.2% to 26.6% in those who took them PRN, respectively (Miaskowski, Dodd, West, et al., 2001). When PRN dosing is used in the inpatient setting, patients may be reluctant to ask for pain medication for a variety of reasons (Salmon, Hall, 2001) and request it when pain is severe and out of control despite instructions to stay on top of the pain. After the patient's request, the nurse must check the record to ensure that enough time has elapsed since the last dose the patient received; then the nurse must obtain and prepare the analgesic, and, if it is an opioid, account for removal of the drug from the drug security system. These activities are time-consuming and result in further loss of pain control.

Research shows that the most vulnerable of patients are at high risk for undertreatment of pain when the PRN approach is used for continuous pain. A study of older adults hospitalized for hip fracture found that most of the analgesics were prescribed for PRN administration and the nurses were unaware that ATC administration of PRN-prescribed analgesics would be preferable for this type of pain; only 22.3% of the patients received ATC analgesic administration of the PRN analgesics, and less than 25% of the *minimum* morphine equivalents of the opioids prescribed were administered (Titler, Herr, Schilling, et al., 2003). Patients with dementia received significantly less pain medication than those without dementia, and 8 patients with dementia in this study received no opioid at all during the first 72 hours after admission (Ardery, Herr, Hannon, et al., 2003). It is important for nurses to recognize that PRN-prescribed analgesics may be administered ATC within the parameters of the PRN prescription and that this is the preferred dosing method for patients with continuous pain. Because there are so many disadvantages to PRN dosing, the appropriateness of its use should be carefully evaluated in all cases.

Patient-Controlled Analgesia (PCA)

PCA is an interactive method of pain management that permits patients to treat their pain by self-administering doses of analgesics. It has been used to manage all types of pain, most commonly acute pain and less often cancer pain because most cancer pain can be managed with oral opioid analgesics. Procedural sedation has also been delivered via PCA (Lehmann, 2005). Although patients with pain often self-administer their oral analgesics (see Inpatient Oral PCA, later in this chapter), the term *PCA* is applied usually when dosing opioids by IV, subcutaneous (SC), perineural (i.e., patient-controlled regional analgesia, PCRA), epidural (PCEA), and intranasal routes of administration. Typically, a special infusion pump is used to deliver PCA by most of these routes of administration. In this context, PCA refers to the bolus dose the patient controls when pressing a button on or attached to the pump. PCA can be delivered by two modes: PCA bolus doses with a continuous infusion (basal rate) or PCA bolus doses alone.

The PCA approach recognizes that only the patient can feel the pain and only the patient knows how much analgesic will relieve it (Pasero, McCaffery, 1993; Pasero, Portenoy, McCaffery, 1999). By allowing patients to determine dosing, PCA addresses the significant variations in analgesic requirements between individuals (Grass, 2005; Lehmann, 2005).

PCA is similar to responsive PRN dosing in that it requires patients to recognize that they are experiencing pain and request analgesia (e.g., by pressing a button on a pump to deliver a PCA bolus). The difference between PRN and PCA dosing is that with PCA the patient rather than a caregiver administers the analgesic, so the delay in waiting for a caregiver's response to the request for analgesia is eliminated. Just as with effective PRN dosing, patients are reminded to "stay on top of the pain" to maintain a steady analgesic level and administer doses before pain is severe and out of control.

Mu agonist opioid analgesics, specifically morphine, hydromorphone, and fentanyl, are the most common analgesics administered by PCA. Frequently, local anesthetics and sometimes the alpha$_2$-adrenergic drug clonidine are added to an opioid for PCEA (see Chapter 15), and local anesthetics are used for PCRA (see Chapter 26).

PCA has been studied extensively, particularly IV PCA in postoperative patients (Gilron, 2008). A meta-analysis of 32 trials comparing opioids via IV PCA with opioids via conventional (intramuscular [IM], IV, SC) methods for postoperative pain management found that IV PCA was associated with improved analgesia, decreased pulmonary complications, and higher patient preference for the method of pain control (Walder, Schafer, Henzi, et al., 2001). A later Cochrane Collaboration Review of 55 randomized controlled studies concluded that IV PCA resulted in better pain control, increased patient satisfaction, and a higher incidence of pruritus compared with conventional methods of pain control (Hudcova, McNicol, Quah, et al., 2006). There were no differences in other adverse effects or length of hospital stay. Patients who used PCA consumed higher opioid doses suggesting that the less effective analgesia from conventional methods may have been related to inadequate dosing. A meta-analysis concluded that IV PCA was associated with higher cumulative morphine consumption at 24 and 48 hours and improved VAS scores compared with nurse-administered analgesia in patients following cardiac surgery (Bainbridge, Martin, Cheng, 2006). One study randomized patients (N = 122) following gynecologic surgery to receive IV hydromorphone by PCA or IV or SC hydromorphone by scheduled nurse-administered doses and reported no differences in pain scores and patient satisfaction (Bell, Shaffer, Schrickel-Feller, 2007). PCA was associated with higher opioid doses, but unlike the previous analysis, this did not result in better pain control. Another randomized controlled trial (N = 93) showed that oral oxycodone plus acetaminophen provided superior pain control with fewer adverse effects compared with IV PCA morphine following cesarean section (Davis, Esposito, Meyer, 2006).

A Cochrane Collaboration Review compared IV PCA with continuous epidural analgesia and found the latter produced superior postoperative pain relief and a higher incidence of pruritus following intra-abdominal surgery, but comparisons of other outcomes were not possible because of a lack of research (Werawatganon, Charuluxananan, 2005). A study (N = 92) comparing continuous peripheral nerve block vs. IV PCA showed a 74% and 35% reduction in postoperative opioid requirement, respectively (Chelly, Greger, Gebhard, et al., 2001). Continuous peripheral nerve block also produced less blood loss, better functional outcomes, fewer complications, and a shorter length of hospital stay than IV PCA (see Chapter 26 for more on continuous peripheral nerve block).

Some have suggested that PCA provides an opportunity for nurses to "distance" themselves from the responsibilities of assessing and managing their patients' pain

(Salmon, Hall, 2001); however, PCA does not absolve nurses from their role as the patient's primary pain manager. Successful PCA therapy depends on the nurse's systematic assessment of the patient's pain, adverse effects, and use of the technology followed by adjustments in the prescription if necessary to optimize pain control (see Chapter 17 for the clinical use of PCA).

Appropriateness of PCA

A number of factors need to be considered in determining whether a patient is a candidate for PCA (Box 12-2). Great care must be taken to ensure that PCA is appropriate, especially the additional cost of a PCA pump and the risks (e.g., infection, programming errors) associated with its use (Macario, 2005).

Clinicians often hesitate to prescribe PCA for children believing that they are too young to understand the concept of PCA and how to use the pump appropriately. However, PCA has been used effectively and safely in developmentally normal children as young as 4 years old (Wellington, Chia, 2009). Although IV PCA has been shown for many years to be safe in older patients (Egbert, Parks, Short, et al., 1990; Gagliese, Gauthier, Macpherson, et al., 2008; Gagliese, Jackson, Ritvo, et al., 2000; Mann, Pouzeratte, Boccara, et al., 2000), clinicians often do not prescribe it for fear of producing confusion in these patients. Although the opioid (by whatever approach it is delivered) can contribute to confusion, the factors that may be responsible are numerous (Bagri, Rico, Ruiz, 2008; Redelmeier, 2007; Sharma, Sieber, Zakriya, et al., 2005; Zakriya, Christmas, Wenz, et al., 2002), and the development of confusion should not be assumed to be related to either the drug or the delivery approach. For example, a study of 333 older (mean age 74) postoperative patients revealed that the presence of postoperative pain and increased intensity of postoperative pain were independent predictors of postoperative delirium (Vaurio, Sands, Wang, et al., 2006). There was also an ordered relationship between the severity of preoperative persistent pain and the risk of postoperative delirium in this study; those with severe preoperative pain were at greater risk than those with moderate preoperative pain. It is important to also note that naloxone administration does not improve postoperative delirium, further suggesting that opioids often are not a primary underlying cause (Redelmeier, 2007) (see Chapter 19 for cognitive effects).

To be considered a candidate for PCA, patients must be able to understand the relationships between pain, pushing the PCA button, and pain relief (Pasero, Portenoy, McCaffery, 1999). In cases when PCA is warranted, patients should not be denied access to this modality simply because of their age. Instead, they should be carefully screened for their cognitive and physical ability to manage their pain by PCA.

It is important that clinicians regularly assess an individual's ability to self-administer analgesia after PCA is initiated. Patients who are deemed appropriate candidates for the therapy may prove unable to maintain adequate analgesia with this method. Although patient independence in controlling pain has been described as a benefit of PCA, research and clinical experience has shown that not all patients want this responsibility (Salmon, Hall, 2001). Further, it has been noted that a number of factors influence the variation seen in patients' ability to use PCA successfully (Katz, Buis, Cohen, 2008; Salmon, Hall, 2001). For example, some patients may fear adverse effects or mistrust the technology. Some populations warrant particularly close attention to dosing patterns to help ensure adequate pain relief with PCA. For example, research has shown that older patients tend to self-administer less opioid via PCA than younger patients (Gagliese, Gauthier, Macpherson, et al., 2008; Gagliese, Jackson, Ritvo, et al., 2000). There were no age-related differences in pain intensity in this study. PCA should be discontinued, and alternative methods for managing pain, such as nurse-administered scheduled ATC doses, should be promptly initiated if patients are unable or unwilling to use PCA.

PCA by Proxy

PCA by proxy is the *unauthorized* administration of a PCA dose by another person. This has the potential to produce significant patient harm because it circumvents an important safeguard of PCA, i.e., the excessively sedated patient will drop the PCA button, thereby preventing further opioid administration and subsequent respiratory depression (Pasero, McCaffery, 2005a). Over the years, there have been reports of the dangers of PCA by proxy. One early report evaluated 3785 patients who received IV PCA and reported 14 critical events, 3 of which involved unauthorized family members pressing the PCA button (Ashburn, Love, Pace, 1994). A review of nearly 6000 patients who had received IV PCA with no basal rate identified unauthorized PCA delivery to sleeping patients by relatives as the cause of 2 of 14 cases of respiratory depression (Sidebotham, Dijkhuizen, Schug, 1997).

These types of reports prompted The Joint Commission (TJC), an independent accrediting body of health care facilities in the United States, to issue a "sentinel event alert" on unauthorized PCA administration. This alert identified 460 PCA-related adverse events over a 5-year period; 15 of these events were the result of unauthorized family or staff members pressing the PCA button (TJC, 2004). Others have echoed concerns regarding this phenomenon (Institute for Safe Medication Practices, 2003a, 2003b).

Given the risks associated with PCA by proxy, TJC now expects to see proof that institutions take steps to minimize the potential for this outcome. These include patient education about the use of PCA prior to initiation of therapy and the use of verbal and written instruction warning against individuals other than the patient

Box 12-2 | Use of Intravenous (IV) Patient-Controlled Analgesia (PCA)

PATIENT SELECTION

- For patients with cancer and noncancer pain, oral and other noninvasive routes produce unmanageable and intolerable adverse effects.
- For patients with acute pain (e.g., surgery, trauma), the oral and other noninvasive routes have been considered and are not an option because they would produce unmanageable and intolerable adverse effects at the anticipated doses required for adequate analgesia, or the oral route is not an option because the patient is fasting (NPO).
- In the patient with persistent cancer or noncancer pain or who is terminally ill, the patient's need for parenteral administration of an opioid analgesic is expected to be longer than 1 or 2 days.
- Patient is able to understand the relationships between pain, pushing the PCA button, and pain relief; is motivated to manage his or her pain; and is cognitively and physically able to self-administer a PCA dose using the available equipment.

OTHER CONSIDERATIONS

- Pumps are available.
- Cost is not prohibitive.
- Staff (or family) is trained to explain, assess, manage, and document IV PCA analgesia, adverse effects, and complications.

SURGICAL PROCEDURES FOR WHICH IV PCA IS PRESCRIBED

- Cesarean section when epidural anesthesia/analgesia is not used
- Abdominal, vaginal hysterectomy
- Anterior and posterior repair
- Bladder surgery
- Ureteral reimplantation
- Penile implant
- Radical prostatectomy
- Mastectomy
- Gastroplasty
- Abdominoplasty
- Inpatient rectal surgeries
- Major plastic surgeries and skin grafts
- Major hand, ankle, or foot repair
- Joint replacement
- Long bone surgery
- Laminectomy
- Shoulder repair
- Radical neck surgery

MEDICAL CONDITIONS FOR WHICH IV PCA IS PRESCRIBED

- Cancer pain
- Sickle cell pain
- Burn pain
- HIV pain
- Fractures
- Pancreatitis
- Nephrolithiasis

HIV, Human immunodeficiency virus; *IV*, intravenous; *PCA*, patient-controlled analgesia.
From Pasero, C., & McCaffery, M. *Pain assessment and pharmacologic management*, p. 315, St. Louis, Mosby. Data from Cashman, J. N. (2006). Patient-controlled analgesia. In G. Shorten, D. B. Carr, D. Harmon, et al. (Eds.), *Postoperative pain management: An evidence-based guide to practice*, Philadelphia, Saunders; Grass, J. A. (2005). Patient-controlled analgesia. *Anesth Analg, 101*(Suppl 1), S44-S61; Lehmann, K. A. (2005). Recent developments in patient-controlled analgesia. *J Pain Symptom Manage, 29*(Suppl 5), S72-S89; Macintyre, P. E., & Coldrey, J. (2008). Patient-controlled analgesia. In R. S. Sinatra, O. A. de Leon-Casasola, B. Ginsberg, et al. (Eds.), *Acute pain management*, Cambridge, New York, Cambridge University Press; Macintyre, P. E., & Coldrey, J. (2008). Patient-controlled analgesia. In P. E. Macintyre, S. M. Walker, & D. J. Rowbotham. (Eds.), *Clinical pain management: Acute pain*, ed 2, London, Hodder Arnold; Sherman, B., Enu, I., & Sinatra, R. S. (2009). Patient-controlled analgesia devices and analgesic infusion pumps. In R. S. Sinatra, O. A. de Leon-Casasola, Ginsberg, B., et al. (Eds.), *Acute pain management*, Cambridge, New York, Cambridge University Press. © 2011, Pasero C, McCaffery M. May be duplicated for use in clinical practice.

---

pressing the PCA button (Box 12-3). The observation that most PCA by proxy is initiated by well-intentioned family members who want to ensure that their loved one is comfortable underscores the importance of frequent assessment of patients during PCA therapy to identify those who are unable to manage their own pain effectively as well as telling family members to contact staff if they have concerns about the patient's pain.

Authorized Agent-Controlled Analgesia: Unconventional Use of the PCA Pump

When patients are unable or unwilling to self-administer analgesics, another individual may be authorized to manage the patient's pain using the PCA technology. For example, family-controlled analgesia (FCA) or caregiver-controlled analgesia (CCA) designates *one* person to be the patient's primary pain manager with the responsibility

| **Box 12-3** | Safe Use of Patient-Controlled Analgesia (PCA) Pumps |

1. Develop criteria for selecting appropriate patients to receive:
   - Patient-controlled analgesia (PCA) (see Box 12-2)
   - Authorized agent-controlled analgesia (AACA) (see Box 12-4)
     - Family-controlled analgesia (FCA) or caregiver-controlled analgesia (CCA) (one designated person)
     - Nurse-activated dosing (NAD) (primary nurse)
2. Teach patients, family members, and visitors about the proper use of PCA and the dangers of anyone other than the patient or an authorized person pressing the button. Instruct them to tell staff if a patient appears to have unrelieved pain.
3. Alert all health care professionals and other staff members to the dangers of pressing the PCA button unless they are authorized to do so.
4. PCA
   - Provide patient and family members with written instructions that stipulate the patient-only aspect of PCA (see pp. 544-545 at the end of Section IV).
   - Place warning signs in the room or tags on PCA buttons that state, "Only the patient should press the PCA button."
5. AACA[1] (see Box 12-4)
   - Authorize one person at a time (primary pain manager) to manage the pain.
   - Assign a secondary pain manager to provide respite for the primary pain manager.
   - Teach pain manager to assess pain and look for adverse effects before bolus dose administration
   - Provide written instructions
6. Monitor patient's level of sedation and respiratory status q 1 h × 12 h, q 2 h × 12 h, then q 4 h if stable.[2] If patient is excessively sedated (see POSS, Box 19-4, p. 510):
   - Treat life-threatening respiratory depression if present (see Box 19-6, p. 521).

- Decrease opioid dose; stop basal infusion if in use.
- Increase monitoring until sedation level is 2 or lower; consider capnography
- Evaluate patient's (PCA) or pain manager's (FCA, CCA) ability to manage pain safely and effectively.
  - Promptly switch to an alternative pain management approach if increased sedation is thought to be related to the patient's or family member's or caregiver's inability to manage pain safely.

ATC, Around the clock; *h,* hour; *POSS,* Pasero Opioid-induced Sedation Scale; *q,* every

[1]Prior to the use of AACA, institutional policies and procedures should be approved and staff (and patients and families when indicated) trained to assess and manage the therapies. Note that AACA is not PCA; policies and procedures, orders, and teaching materials should be entitled with the correct name of the therapy (e.g., family-controlled analgesia; caregiver-controlled analgesia, nurse-activated dosing).

[2]This guideline should be adjusted as appropriate for patient condition. For example, the suggested level of monitoring and actions for treatment of sedation may need to be adjusted for terminally ill patients.

From Pasero, C., & McCaffery, M. *Pain assessment and pharmacologic management,* p. 316, St. Louis, Mosby. Data from Joint Commission (JC). (2004). *Sentinel event alert: Patient-controlled analgesia by proxy.* http://www.jointcommission.org/SentinelEvents/SentinelEventAlert/sea_33.htm. Accessed January 9, 2005; Pasero, C., & McCaffery, M. (1993). Unconventional PCA: Making it work for your patient. *Am J Nurs, 93*(9), 38-41; Pasero, C., & McCaffery, M. (2002). Monitoring opioid-induced sedation. *Am J Nurs, 102*(2), 67-68; Pasero, C., & McCaffery, M. (2005). Authorized and unauthorized use of PCA pumps. *Am J Nurs, 105*(7), 30-33; Pasero, C., Portenoy, R. K., & McCaffery, M. (1999). Opioid analgesics. In M. McCaffery, & C. Pasero: *Pain: Clinical manual,* ed 2, St. Louis, Mosby; Wuhrman, E., Cooney, M. F., Dunwoody, C. J., et al. (2007). Authorized and unauthorized ("PCA by proxy") dosing of analgesic infusion pumps: Position statement with clinical practice recommendations. *Pain Manage Nurs, 8*(1), 4-11. © 2011, Pasero C, McCaffery M. May be duplicated for use in clinical practice.

---

of pressing the PCA button (on the face of the pump or pendant attached to the pump) (Pasero, McCaffery, 1993; Pasero, Portenoy, McCaffery, 1999). With nurse-activated dosing (NAD) (also called *nurse-controlled analgesia*), the patient's primary nurse has that responsibility. These methods have collectively been called "authorized agent-controlled analgesia" (AACA) (Wuhrman, Cooney, Dunwoody, et al., 2007) and have been safely and effectively used for many years in patients of all ages. AACA is supported by a position paper with clinical practice recommendations developed by the American Society for Pain

Management Nursing (Wuhrman, Cooney, Dunwoody, et al., 2007) and endorsed by other nursing specialty organizations such as the Oncology Nursing Society and the Hospice and Palliative Care Nurses Association (see Boxes 12-3 and 12-4 for guidelines for the use of PCA and AACA).

Although FCA and CCA have long been used in adults (Cohen, Smetzer, 2005; Pasero, McCaffery, 1993; Pasero, Portenoy, McCaffery, 1999), clinical experience and research is most abundant in the use of parent-controlled analgesia, another form of AACA, in pediatric patients (Anghelescu, Burgoyne, Oakes, et al., 2005; Czarnecki, Ferrise, Jastrowski Mano, et al., 2008; Lehr, BeVier, 2003; Monitto, Greenberg, Kost-Byerly, et al., 2000; Voepel-Lewis, Marinkovic, Kostrzewa, et al., 2008). When any of these methods are used, it is particularly important to designate a secondary pain manager to provide respite for the primary pain manager. Alternately, in the hospital setting, NAD may be used during the primary pain manager's rest periods. However, essential to safe use of these methods is to ensure that only one person is managing the patient's pain at a time (Pasero, McCaffery, 2005a).

NAD may be used in patients who have no family member or significant other who can manage their pain (Pasero, McCaffery, 2005a). It is ideally suited for critically ill patients who experience significant, continuous pain from surgery or underlying pathology and undergo numerous repetitive, painful procedures. Rarely do these patients meet the cognitive or physical criteria for managing PCA, but the PCA pump can be used to administer a continuous infusion and the nurse can press the PCA button to administer supplemental doses for breakthrough pain and prior to painful procedures (Pasero, McCaffery, 2001; 2005a). This is not only effective and convenient but saves nursing time that would be spent preparing and administering analgesia by conventional methods. In all cases of AACA, the control of analgesia is returned to patients (i.e., PCA) if and as soon as they are able to assume it.

Criteria for determining which patients are candidates for AACA and for selecting a pain manager, policies and procedures, teaching strategies for pain managers and staff, and monitoring guidelines should be developed prior to the use of AACA (see Box 12-4). It is important to note that these methods are not patient controlled, and it is inaccurate and confusing to refer to them as patient controlled (e.g., "PCA by caregiver" or "PCA by nurse"). Attention should be given to insuring that policies and procedures, orders, and patient education material are entitled with the correct name of the therapy (e.g., "caregiver-controlled analgesia" or "nurse-activated dosing").

Some institutions have adapted PCA equipment for patients who are cognitively able to use PCA but are physically unable to press the PCA button, such as patients with rheumatoid arthritis (Pasero, Portenoy, McCaffery, 1999). One publication described the development of a pneumatic trigger for an 8-year-old child and an 11-year-old child who were unable to activate PCA otherwise because of major burn injuries of both hands and arms (Lehr, BeVier, 2003). The device was activated by pressing the heel of the foot against the trigger. The legal implications of altering infusion devices must be carefully considered before implementing these novel approaches.

Inpatient Oral PCA

A major advantage of using PCA is the elimination of the delay period between the patient's request for analgesia and the nurse administering it. As mentioned, the use of PCA in the hospital is administered most often by the IV, SC, or epidural routes. Although patients commonly self-administer oral pain medications in the home setting, oral PCA in the hospital setting is a relatively new concept (Kastanias, Snaith, Robinson, 2006; Pasero, Portenoy, McCaffery, 1999). However, it has been used safely and effectively in this setting for the treatment of all types of pain.

Perhaps the first description of inpatient oral PCA was a study of 48 adult patients admitted for orthopedic surgery; 26 patients were allowed to self-administer 5 mg oxycodone + 500 mg acetaminophen (Tylox) from a bedside supply of 25 tablets, and 22 were given the same drug on a PRN basis by the nursing staff (Jones, 1987). There were no significant differences in amount of analgesic the patients took, but older patients took less. Although pain was not formally assessed (common practice in the 1980s), 100% of the patients taking oral PCA stated they would request the same method of analgesic administration in the future. The majority of nurses expressed satisfaction with the method citing benefits such as greater patient independence, improved nurse-patient relationship, and time saved related to the tasks required for conventional opioid drug administration. There were no cases of drug loss or diversion.

Other creative approaches for using oral PCA have been described. One hospital provided selected patients with a Velcro wrist pouch in which one or two doses of opioid analgesic could be stored for PRN self administration (Pasero, Portenoy, McCaffery, 1999). The hospital reported that not one incident of patient noncompliance or loss or diversion of analgesics occurred with the program. Further, the hospital saw a 10% increase in patient satisfaction with oral analgesics with the use of oral PCA. A study of general surgical patients was undertaken to compare this same oral PCA approach (N = 19) with nurse-administered oral analgesia (NAOA) (N = 17) (Riordan, Beam, Okabe-Yamamura, 2004). Despite taking more doses (acetaminophen + hydrocodone), only 65% of the patients in the NAOA group achieved their pain rating goal within 1 hour compared with 93% in the oral PCA group. There were no adverse effects or episodes of missing or diverted analgesics.

A randomized controlled study compared oral PCA and IV PCA in 60 patients following orthopedic surgery (Striebel, Scheitza, Philippi, et al., 1998). After titration to comfort, patients were randomly assigned to self-administer IV doses of morphine via a portable IV PCA device or doses of oral morphine solution via a modified version of the same PCA device. Patients reported comparable pain relief and satisfaction and had a similar low incidence of adverse effects and no respiratory depression. The researchers described oral PCA as "an attractive, simple, inexpensive, and patient-convenient mode of opioid administration for patients who are permitted to drink oral fluids after surgery" (p. 1053).

Box 12-4 Authorized Agent-Controlled Analgesia (AACA): Unconventional Use of the PCA Pump[1-4]

PATIENT SELECTION (ANY ONE OF THE FOLLOWING)

- Patient is unable to understand the relationships between pain, pushing the PCA button, and pain relief.
- Patient is not cognitively or physically able to self-administer a PCA dose using the available equipment.
- Patient is not motivated to manage his or her own pain.

NURSE-ACTIVATED DOSING (NAD)

1. The patient's primary nurse is designated to be the patient's primary pain manager (the primary nurse is the only person who presses the PCA button during that nurse's shift).
2. The nurse is competent in the use of the equipment used to deliver NAD.
3. This method may be used:
   - In addition to a basal rate. Patients are assessed every 30 to 60 minutes for the need for a bolus dose for breakthrough pain.
   - Without a basal rate as a means of maintaining analgesia with ATC bolus doses
   - To administer PRN bolus doses prior to painful procedures.

FAMILY-CONTROLLED ANALGESIA (FCA) OR CAREGIVER-CONTROLLED ANALGESIA (CCA)

- *One* family member or significant other is designated to be the patient's primary pain manager and has the responsibility of pressing the PCA button.

- Guidelines for selecting a primary pain manager for FCA:
  1. Spends a significant amount of time with the patient.
  2. Is willing to assume responsibility of being primary pain manager.
  3. Is willing to accept and respect patient's reports of pain (if able to provide) as the best indicator of how much pain the patient is experiencing.
  4. Demonstrates understanding of the educational content below.

EDUCATION OF THE PAIN MANAGER (FCA, CCA)

- Select and teach the pain manager the appropriate method for assessment of the patient's pain (see Section II for appropriate tools).
  - If the patient is able to report, teach the pain manager to use a 0-to-10 numerical or faces pain rating scale or another self-report tool appropriate to the patient's ability.
  - If the patient is unable to report, a behavioral assessment tool may be used.
- Discuss the purpose and goals of the patient's pain management plan.
- Explain the concept of maintaining a steady analgesic blood level.
- Teach the pain manager to look for adverse effects, such as nausea, sedation, and respiratory depression, before administering a bolus dose. Explain when it is safe and unsafe to administer a PCA bolus dose and to promptly notify the staff if any adverse effects are detected.

Continued

A Canadian hospital reported success with an oral PCA program for patients after laminectomy or spinal fusion (Kastanias, Snaith, Robinson, 2006). Patients were allowed to keep a single dose of an oral short-acting opioid analgesic at the bedside in a child-resistant container. Patients were told to take the analgesic as needed as often as every 2 hours, record their pain ratings before and after taking a dose, and notify the nurse as soon as a dose was taken so the nurse could replace it with another. There were no reports of diversion or medication loss. A majority (92%) of the patients were satisfied or very satisfied with this method of pain control. Those who were not satisfied cited difficulty completing the flow sheet as the reason.

A mechanical device called the "MOD" (Medication on Demand) may be a solution to system barriers to the use of oral PCA. The MOD is the first device that allows patients access at the bedside to secured oral analgesics when needed for pain (Figure 12-2, *A*). The device is loaded with a cartridge containing eight doses of the selected analgesic and programmed according to prescribed parameters (dosing frequency [lockout, delay interval]). A green light on the device indicates to the patient that a dose may be accessed. The patient must enter the current pain intensity rating on a large 0 to 10 numerical rating scale and swipe a radio frequency identification wristband over a reader, both located on the face of the device, to request a dose of analgesic

- Explain that sedation precedes opioid-induced respiratory depression and that the patient's sedation level should be assessed using a sedation scale that includes appropriate interventions at each level of sedation such as the one shown below.[3] Provide the pain manager with a copy of the sedation scale with interventions as a reference during therapy.

PASERO OPIOID-INDUCED SEDATION SCALE (POSS) (MODIFIED FOR AACA)

S = Sleep, easy to arouse
   Action: Awaken patient to determine arousability (1 to 4 below) before administering a PCA bolus dose

1 = Awake and alert
   Action: Acceptable; may administer PCA bolus dose

2 = Slightly drowsy, easily aroused
   Action: Acceptable; may administer a PCA bolus dose

3 = Frequently drowsy, arousable, drifts off during conversation
   Action: Unacceptable; notify nurse immediately.

4 = Somnolent, minimal or no response to physical stimulation
   Action: Unacceptable; notify nurse immediately.

TREATMENT OF EXCESSIVELY SEDATED PATIENT[3-4]

- Treat life-threatening significant respiratory depression if present (see Box 19-6, pp. 521).
- Decrease opioid dose; stop basal infusion if in use.
- Increase monitoring until sedation level is 2 or lower; consider capnography.
- Evaluate pain manager's (FCA, CCA) ability to manage pain safely and effectively.

- Promptly switch to an alternative pain management approach if increased sedation is thought to be related to the family member's or caregiver's inability to manage pain safely.

ATC, Around the clock

[1]Prior to the use of AACA, institutional policies and procedures should be approved and staff (and patients and families when indicated) trained to assess and manage the therapies. Note that AACA is not PCA; policies and procedures, orders, and teaching materials should be entitled with the correct name of the therapy (e.g., family-controlled analgesia; caregiver-controlled analgesia, nurse-activated dosing)

[2]In all cases of AACA, the control of analgesia is returned to patients (i.e., PCA) if and as soon as they are able to assume it.

[3]This guideline should be adjusted as appropriate for patient condition. For example, the suggested level of monitoring and actions for treatment of sedation may need to be adjusted for terminally ill patients.

[4]See Chapter 19 for discussion of opioid-induced sedation and respiratory depression including patient examples using the POSS.

From Pasero, C., & McCaffery, M. *Pain assessment and pharmacologic management*, pp. 318-319, St. Louis, Mosby. Data from Nisbet, A. T., & Mooney-Cotter, F. (2009). Selected scales for reporting opioid-induced sedation. *Pain Manage Nurs, 10*(3), 154-164; Pasero, C., & McCaffery, M. (1993). Unconventional PCA: Making it work for your patient. *Am J Nurs, 93*(9), 38-41; Pasero, C., & McCaffery, M. (2005). Authorized and unauthorized use of PCA pumps. *Am J Nurs, 105*(7), 30-33; Pasero, C., Portenoy, R. K., & McCaffery, M. (1999). Opioid analgesics. In M. McCaffery, & C. Pasero. *Pain: Clinical manual*, ed 2, St. Louis, Mosby; Wuhrman, E., Cooney, M. F., Dunwoody, C. J., et al. (2007). Authorized and unauthorized ("PCA by proxy") dosing of analgesic infusion pumps: Position statement with clinical practice recommendations. *Pain Manage Nurs, 8*(1), 4-11. © 2011, Pasero C, McCaffery M. May be duplicated for use in clinical practice.

(see Figure 12-2, *B*). If enough time has elapsed since the last dose, the device will allow the patient to take another dose (Figure 12-2, *C*). The nurse can query the device to obtain and print the patient's pain ratings and dosing history.

The MOD was evaluated in 20 oncology patients who were anticipated to require PRN analgesics for at least 48 hours (Rosati, Gallagher, Shook, et al., 2007). Eligibility criteria included age 21 years or older, no history of drug abuse, ability to understand and use the oral PCA device, and agreement to maintain security of the device. Physicians prescribed one from a choice of oral opioid analgesics (i.e., hydrocodone/acetaminophen, hydromorphone, morphine, oxycodone, or propoxyphene) and the frequency of PRN

administration. The device was loaded with a pharmacy-prepared cartridge containing eight analgesic doses and programmed with the prescribed lockout interval. The device also allowed nurses to override the lockout time to make an immediate dose available if needed. All of the patients (100%) in the study preferred using the device to calling a nurse for each PRN dose and said they would choose to use the device again if rehospitalization was necessary. There were no reports of diversion. Nurses were also surveyed, and 90% stated the device was reliable and easy to query, 88% said it was easy to program, and 98% thought the patient's pain was better controlled than with the traditional nurse-administered method. Although the pharmacy staff found loading of the device simple, most did not think it saved pharmacy

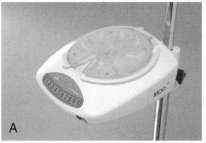 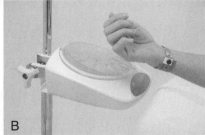 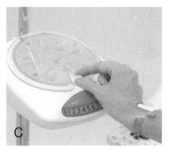

Figure 12-2 | **A,** The MOD (medication on demand) oral PCA device. **B,** Patient activation of the MOD. **C,** Patient taking tablet from the MOD.

Courtesy Avancen MOD Corporation.

GUIDELINES

Box 12-5 | Inpatient Oral PCA

PATIENT SELECTION

1. Patient has no contraindications to using the oral route of administration.
2. Patient appears to be cognitively able to self-administer oral analgesia: Understands the relationships between pain, taking a dose of pain medication, and pain relief.
3. Can cognitively understand how and physically use the necessary supplies (e.g., access the PCA device or open the wrist pouch and document appropriately in the pain relief diary).
4. Acknowledges understanding that because of substance control regulations, noncompliance with oral PCA policy and procedure (e.g., loss of controlled substance) will necessitate discontinuing oral PCA, and staff will administer analgesics.

OTHER CONSIDERATIONS

1. Supplies, equipment, and analgesics are available.
2. Staff is trained to explain to patient, and assess, manage, and document oral PCA.

PATIENT TEACHING

1. Review prescription including analgesic and PRN dosing frequency.
2. Explain procedure:
   • If oral PCA device is used: Demonstrate and have the patient return demonstrate the use of the device.
   • If wrist pouch is used: Explain that one dose at a time will be given to store in pouch, and any doses left over when oral PCA is discontinued must be returned to nurse.
3. If pain diary is used, show patients how and what to document:
   • Time and amount of dose taken
   • Pain rating
   • Adverse effects
4. Remind patients to "stay on top of pain" by taking dose before pain becomes severe.
5. Tell patients why, when, and what information needs to be reported to nurse:
   • If wrist pouch is used, notify nurse after taking a dose so that nurse can provide the next dose to keep in pouch

• Inadequate pain relief so that nurse can perform assessment and take appropriate action
   • Adverse effects so that nurse can perform assessment and take appropriate action
   • Inability to perform recovery activities at expected level of function
   • Loss of medication
6. Explain to patient that because of substance control regulations, noncompliance with oral PCA policy and procedure (e.g., loss of controlled substance) will necessitate discontinuing oral PCA, and staff will administer analgesics.
7. Provide written prescription and instructions.

NURSING RESPONSIBILITIES RELATED TO ASSESSMENT, DOCUMENTATION, SUBSTANCE CONTROL

• Respond promptly to patient needs (i.e., replace used doses/cartridges, assess inadequate pain relief, adverse effects and reactions).
   • Report to prescriber and document adverse effects, lack of pain relief, patient noncompliance, inability to perform responsibilities, and if oral PCA is discontinued for any reason other than patient discharge.
   • Document assessments, interventions, discontinuation of oral PCA, and dispensation of controlled substances according to hospital policy.
   • Count and document amount remaining in patient's oral PCA device or wrist pouch at end of shift.
   • Count, waste, and document unused medication according to hospital policy.
   • Report to pharmacy unaccounted-for doses.

PCA, Patient-controlled analgesia.
Although patients commonly self-administer oral pain medications in the home setting, oral PCA in the hospital setting is a relatively new concept.

From Pasero, C., & McCaffery, M. *Pain assessment and pharmacologic management,* p. 320, St. Louis, Mosby. © 2011, Pasero C, McCaffery M. May be duplicated for use in clinical practice.

PATIENT PAIN RELIEF DIARY

PATIENT INFORMATION

Take 1 or 2 _____ Every _____ Hour(s)
if Needed for Pain

COMMENTS
_____
_____
_____
_____
_____

My goals include:

☐ A pain rating of _____

☐ Take _____ deep breaths and cough every hour

☐ Walk _____ times per day

☐ _____

DATE	TIME	HOW MANY PILLS I TOOK?	RATE YOUR PAIN 1 HOUR AFTER TAKING YOUR PAIN PILLS — PAIN RATING — None Mod. Severe	ARE YOU MEETING YOUR RECOVERY GOALS?	REVIEWED & ACTION TAKEN, IF ANY	DATE TIME	NURSE SIGNATURE
			0 1 2 3 4 5 6 7 8 9 10	YES NO			
			0 1 2 3 4 5 6 7 8 9 10	YES NO			
			0 1 2 3 4 5 6 7 8 9 10	YES NO			
			0 1 2 3 4 5 6 7 8 9 10	YES NO			
			0 1 2 3 4 5 6 7 8 9 10	YES NO			
			0 1 2 3 4 5 6 7 8 9 10	YES NO			
			0 1 2 3 4 5 6 7 8 9 10	YES NO			
			0 1 2 3 4 5 6 7 8 9 10	YES NO			
			0 1 2 3 4 5 6 7 8 9 10	YES NO			
			0 1 2 3 4 5 6 7 8 9 10	YES NO			
			0 1 2 3 4 5 6 7 8 9 10	YES NO			
			0 1 2 3 4 5 6 7 8 9 10	YES NO			
			0 1 2 3 4 5 6 7 8 9 10	YES NO			

I understand and agree to follow the instructions as written on the back of this form

Patient Signature _____ Date _____

Pills not recorded as taken by the patient in the hospital must be returned.

_____ # of pills returned

nurse initials   date/time

Form 12-1 | Patient pain relief diary.

As appears in Pasero, C., & McCaffery, M. *Pain assessment and pharmacologic management*, p. 321, St. Louis, Mosby. Courtesy Wellmont Health System, Holston Valley Medical Center, Kingsport, TN, 1998. May be duplicated for use in clinical practice.

time compared with traditional delivery of medications. The use of commercially-available dose cartridges and refinement of dispensing procedures may help to ease the workload for the pharmacy staff.

Prior to the use of oral PCA, hospitals must establish guidelines for safe use. Box 12-5 provides a framework for the development of an inpatient oral PCA policy and procedure. Form 12-1 provides an example of a pain diary that patients can complete if paper documentation is required.

Conclusion

This chapter has presented some of the basic concepts and principles of pain management and provided suggestions for the appropriate use of PRN and ATC dosing, PCA, and AACA. A working knowledge of the many strategies available for managing pain allows clinicians to individualize the pain treatment plan to meet the patient's unique needs and capabilities.

Chapter 13 Guidelines for Opioid Drug Selection

SAFE and effective use of opioid analgesics requires the development of an individualized treatment plan. This begins with a comprehensive pain assessment, which includes clarifying the goals of treatment and discussing options with the patient and family. The need for periodic reevaluation of the goals is common and should be expected as disease progresses or, in the case of acute pain, as pain resolves (Portenoy, 1996).

Goals are stated as simply as possible and shared among the patient, family, and caregivers. Goals ordinarily include the patient's desired pain rating and the activities that accompany this pain level. For example, a postoperative patient may identify a comfort-function goal of 3/10 to enable regular use of the incentive spirometer and may state that the mild sedation accompanying this level of analgesia is acceptable. A patient with persistent pain may identify a comfort-function goal of 2/10 as necessary for engaging in employment and may state that sedation is not compatible with this goal (see Section II).

Many factors are considered when determining the appropriate opioid analgesic for the patient with pain (Box 13-1). These include the unique characteristics of the various opioids and patient characteristics, such as pain intensity, patient age, coexisting disease, current drug regimen and potential drug interactions, prior treatment outcomes, and patient preference.

Because pain has multiple underlying mechanisms and is a multifaceted phenomenon, the use of a multimodal approach to managing all types of pain should be the rule, rather than the exception (Argoff, Albrecht, Irving, et al., 2009; Kehlet, Jensen, Woolf, 2006; Kehlet, Wilmore, 2008) (see Section I and Chapter 12). A sound treatment plan relies on the selection of appropriate analgesics from the opioid, nonopioid, and adjuvant analgesic groups.

Box 13-1 | Use of Opioids

- Perform a comprehensive assessment that addresses pain, all co-morbidities, and functional status.
- Develop an individualized treatment plan that includes specific goals related to pain intensity, activities (function), and adverse effects (e.g., pain rating of 3/10 to ambulate or walk the dog accompanied by minimal or no sedation, and other adverse effects are tolerable and manageable).
- Use multimodal analgesia (i.e., this should be the rule more than the exception for treatment of most types of pain).
- Assess for presence preoperatively of underlying persistent pain in surgical patients, and optimize its treatment.
- Consider the potential for development of persistent postsurgical pain associated with type of surgery in surgical patients and provide preemptive analgesia (see Chapter 12).
- Consider preemptive analgesics before surgery for all patients (e.g., provide nonopioid analgesics preemptively, intraoperatively, or as soon as a patient is admitted to the PACU).
- Provide analgesics prior to painful procedures.
- Drug selection
  - Consider diagnosis, condition, or surgical procedure, current or expected pain intensity, age, whether major organ failure is present (especially renal, hepatic, or respiratory), and presence of coexisting disease.
  - Consider pharmacologic issues (e.g., accumulation of metabolites and effects of concurrent drugs, including over-the-counter drugs, and possible interactions).

- Consider individual differences (note prior treatment outcomes) and patient preference.
  - Be aware of available routes of administration (e.g., oral, transdermal, rectal, IV, SC, perineural, intraspinal) and formulation (e.g., short-acting or modified-release).
  - Be aware of cost differences.
- Route selection
  - Use least invasive route possible.
  - Consider convenience and patient's ability to adhere to the regimen (ease of use).
  - Consider staff's (or family's, patient's) ability to monitor and provide care required (e.g., parenteral and intraspinal routes in the home setting).
- Dosing and dose titration
  - Consider previous dosing requirement and relative analgesic potencies when initiating therapy.
  - Use pain intensity and equianalgesic chart to determine starting dose with consideration of patient's current status (e.g., sedation and respiratory status) and co-morbidities (e.g., medical frailty), and then titrate until adequate analgesia is achieved or dose-limiting adverse effects are encountered (see Chapter 16).
  - Use appropriate dosing schedule (e.g., ATC or PRN).
  - When a dose is safe but additional analgesia is desired, titrate upward by 25% for slight increase, 50% for moderate increase, and 100% for considerable increase in analgesia.
  - Provide supplemental doses for breakthrough pain.
  - Consider PCA (see Box 12-2, p. 315).

Continued

Characteristics of Selected Mu Agonist Opioids

As discussed previously, the mu agonist opioid analgesics are capable of managing all pain intensities and are effective for many different painful conditions. They are the most common analgesics used to manage moderate to severe nociceptive pain, but they have also been shown to be effective for some neuropathic pain (Dworkin, Barbano, Tyring, et al., 2009; Dworkin, O'Connor, Backonja, et al., 2007; Eisenberg, McNicol, Carr, 2006; Gimbel, Richards, Portenoy, 2003; Maier, Hildebrandt, Klinger, et al., 2002; Watson, Moulin, Watt-Watson, et al., 2003). Mu

agonists are also recommended for the management of breakthrough pain. See Table 13-1 for a summary of information on selected mu opioid analgesics. For more detail about the characteristics of the various opioid analgesics as they relate to route of administration, see Chapter 14. The equianalgesic chart in Table 16-1 on pp. 444-446 contains dosing and pharmacokinetic information on the various opioid analgesics.

The previously used classification of opioid analgesics as "weak" or "strong" is outdated. Instead, opioid analgesics are conventionally labeled as being appropriate for the treatment of mild, moderate, or severe pain. In reality, however, all the various full mu agonists are capable of producing comparable analgesia if the dose is adjusted appropriately.

- Recognize that for persistent cancer or noncancer pain, tolerance is rarely the "driving force" for dose escalation; consider disease progression when increasing dose requirements occur.
- Trials of alternative opioids
  - Trial of another opioid should be done only after the first opioid has been titrated upward to determine whether adequate analgesia can be obtained without intolerable adverse effects.
  - Be aware of incomplete cross-tolerance, and start the new opioid at about 50% of the estimated equianalgesic dose (see later in this chapter and Box 13-3 for switching to methadone).
- Treatment of adverse effects (see Chapter 19)
  - Be aware of the prevalence and impact of opioid adverse effects.
  - Remember that most opioid adverse effects are dose dependent; always consider decreasing the opioid dose as a method of treating or eliminating an adverse effect; adding nonopioid analgesics for additive analgesia facilitates this approach.
  - Use a preventive approach in the management of constipation, including for patients receiving short-term opioid treatment (e.g., postoperative patients).
  - Use a preventive, multimodal antimetic approach for patients with moderate to high risk for postoperative nausea and vomiting.
  - Prevent respiratory depression by monitoring sedation levels in opioid-naïve patients and decreasing the opioid dose as soon as increased sedation is detected.

- Advise patient/family which adverse effects are likely to subside with long-term opioid treatment (e.g., nausea, cognitive effects).
- Consider changing the opioid if adverse effects overshadow efficacy.
- Monitoring
  - Continually and consistently evaluate the treatment plan on the basis of the specific goals identified at the outset and assess pain intensity, adverse effects, and activity levels. Focus on functional improvement and clinically meaningful pain relief (see Section II).
  - Make necessary modifications to treatment plan.
- Tapering and cessation of treatment
  - If a decrease in dose or cessation of treatment is appropriate, do so in accordance with decreased pain ratings and after evaluation of functional outcomes.
  - Be aware of potential for withdrawal syndrome and need for tapering schedule in patients who have been receiving opioid therapy for more than a few days.
  - Use equianalgesic dosing to determine appropriate decreases in doses (see Chapter 16).

ATC, Around-the-clock; *IV,* intravenous; *PACU,* post anesthesia care unit; *PCA,* patient-controlled analgesia; *SC,* subcutaneous.

From Pasero, C., & McCaffery, M. *Pain assessment and pharmacologic management,* pp. 324-325, St. Louis, Mosby. Data from Argoff, C. E., Abrecht, P., Irving, G., et al. (2009). Multimodal analgesia for chronic pain: Rationale and future directions. *Pain Med, 10*(Suppl 2), S53-S66; Coyle, N., Cherny, N., & Portenoy, R. K. (1995). Pharmacologic management of cancer pain. In D. McGuire, C. H. Yarbro, & B. R. Ferrell (Eds.), *Cancer pain management,* ed 2, Boston, Jones and Bartlett; Fine, P. G., Mahajan, G., & McPherson, M. L. (2009). Long-acting opioids and short-acting opioids: Appropriate use in chronic pain management. *Pain Med, 10*(Suppl 2), S79-S88. © 2011, Pasero C, McCaffery M. May be duplicated for use in clinical practice.

The terms *short acting, immediate release,* and *normal release* have been used interchangeably to describe oral opioids that have an onset of action of approximately 30 minutes and a relatively short duration of 3 to 4 hours. The term *short acting* will be used in this book to describe oral opioids with these characteristics. It should be noted that the term *immediate release* is misleading because none of the oral opioid analgesics have an immediate onset of analgesia. The term *rapid onset* may accurately be applied to drugs such as oral transmucosal fentanyl (OTFC) or buccal fentanyl because of their significantly faster onset of action compared with other short-acting opioids. The terms *modified release,* *extended release, sustained release,* and *controlled release* are used to describe opioids that are formulated to release over a prolonged period of time. Most often, the terms are applied to oral formulations or to transdermal formulations. The term *modified release* will be used in this book to describe these drugs.

Some of the generic and brand name opioid formulations have sound-alike/look-alike name similarities (e.g., hydromorphone and morphine, hydromorphone and hydrocodone, OxyContin and MSContin; Roxanol and Roxicodone), which have been blamed as a cause of medication errors (Institute for Safe Medication Practices, 2009). Some ways to avoid confusion when prescribing opioids are

Table 13-1 | Characteristics of Selected Mu Opioid Agonist Drugs[1]

Mu Opioid Agonist Drug	Routes Administered	Comments
Morphine	PO (short-acting and modified-release), SL, R, IV, IM, SC, E, I, IA	Standard for comparison. Multiple routes of administration. Several modified-release formulations available, but they are not therapeutically equivalent. Begin with lower doses in older adults. Active metabolite M6G can accumulate with repeated dosing in renal failure. 20% to 30% oral bioavailability.
Codeine	PO, IM, SC	Limited usefulness. Usually compounded with nonopioid (e.g., Tylenol No. 3). Used orally for mild to moderate pain, but analgesia is inferior to that of ibuprofen. IM has unpredictable absorption and high adverse effect profile; IV route not recommended, SC rarely used, and IM administration of any opioid is discouraged.
Fentanyl	OT, B, IV, IM, TD, E, I, IN	Fast-acting; short half-life (except TD). At steady state, slow elimination from tissues can lead to a prolonged half-life (up to 12 h). On the basis of clinical experience, fentanyl 1 mcg/h transdermally is roughly equivalent to morphine 2 mg/24 h orally[2]; fentanyl, 100 mcg/h parenterally and transdermally is roughly equivalent to 4 mg/h morphine parenterally.[2] Opioid-naïve patients should be started on no more than 25 mcg/h transdermally. Transdermal fentanyl is not appropriate for acute pain management. OTFC and buccal fentanyl are approved for management of breakthrough pain in opioid tolerant individuals.
Hydrocodone	PO	Used for mild to moderate pain; available in nonopioid combination only (e.g., Vicodin, Lortab) (see Table 13-3).
Hydromorphone (Dilaudid)	PO, R, IV, IM, SC, E, I	Useful alternative to morphine. Metabolite may accumulate with long-term, high dose administration. Available in high-potency parenteral formulation (10 mg/mL) useful for SC infusion; 3 mg R roughly equivalent to 650 mg aspirin; oral modified-release formulation available.
Levorphanol (Levo-Dromoran)	PO, IV, IM, SC	Long half-life can lead to accumulation within 2 to 3 days of repetitive dosing.
Meperidine (Demerol)	PO, IV, IM, SC, E, I	No longer recommended for the management of any type of pain because of potential toxicity from accumulation of metabolite, normeperidine. Half-life of normeperidine is approximately 15 to 20 h; NR in older adults or patients with impaired renal function; continuous IV infusion NR. The most appropriate candidates for meperidine use are patients with acute pain who are otherwise healthy with no risk factors and are allergic to or intolerant of other opioids, such as morphine, fentanyl, and hydromorphone, or have demonstrated a more favorable outcome with meperidine than other opioid drugs.
Methadone (Dolophine)	PO, SL, R, IV, SC, IM, E, I	Long half-life can lead to delayed toxicity from accumulation. See text for information on methadone.
Oxycodone (OxyIR, OxyContin)	PO (short-acting and modified-release), IV, IM, R	Used for mild to moderate pain when combined with a nonopioid (e.g., Percocet, Tylox) (see Table 13-9). As single entity, can be used like oral morphine for severe pain. Rectal and parenteral formulation not available in the United States. Oral formulation can be administered rectally.

Continued

Table 13-1 | Characteristics of Selected Mu Opioid Agonist Drugs—cont'd.

Mu Opioid Agonist Drug	Routes Administered	Comments
Oxymorphone (Opana, Opana ER [oral], Numorphan [parenteral, rectal])	PO (short-acting and modified-release) IV, IM, SC, R	Used for moderate to severe pain. Available in 5 mg rectal suppositories.
Propoxyphene (Darvocet, Darvon)	PO	Used in combination with acetaminophen (Darvocet) and aspirin (Darvon Compound). Long half-life. Accumulation of toxic metabolite norpropoxyphene with repetitive dosing. Inappropriate for use in older adults (see Table 13-4).

B, Buccal; *E*, epidural analgesia; *h*, hour; *IM*, intramuscular; *I*, intrathecal analgesia; *IA*, intraarticular; *IN*, intranasal; *IV*, intravenous; *mcg*, microgram; *mg*, milligram, *mL*, milliliter; *M6G*, morphine-6-glucuronide; *NR*, not recommended; *OTFC*, oral transmucosal fentanyl citrate; *PO*, oral; *q*, every; *R*, rectal; *SC*, subcutaneous; *SL*, sublingual; *TD*, transdermal; *UK*, unknown.

¹See Table 16-1 on pp. 444-446, for dosing and pharmacokinetic information.
²These are the ratios used in clinical practice.
From Pasero, C., & McCaffery, M. *Pain assessment and pharmacologic management*, pp. 326-327, St. Louis, Mosby. Data from American Society of Health System Pharmacists. Available at http://www.ashp.org/import/news/HealthSystemPharmacyNews/newsarticle.aspx?id=3037. Accessed December 9, 2009. Barkin, R. L., Barkin, S. J., & Barkin, D. S. (2006). Propoxyphene (dextropropoxyphene), A critical review of a weak opioid analgesic that should remain in antiquity. *Am J Ther, 13*(6), 534-542; Burnham, R., McNeil, S., Hegedus, C., et al. (2006). Fibrous myopathy as a complication of repeated intramuscular injection for chronic headache. *Pain Res Manage, 11*(4), 249-252; Chamberlin, K. W., Cottle, M., Neville, R., et al. (2007). Oral oxymorphone for pain management. *Ann Pharmacother, 41*(7), 1144-1152; Coda, B. A. (2006). Opioids. In P. G. Barash, B. F. Cullen, & R. K. Stoelting (Eds.), *Clinical anesthesia*, ed 5, Philadelphia, Lippincott, Williams & Wilkins; Dale, O., Hjortkjær, R., & Kharasch, E. D. (2002). Nasal administration of opioids for pain management in adults. *Acta Anaesthesiol Scand, 46*(7), 759-770; Davis, M. P., Varga, J., Dickerson, D., et al. (2003). Normal-release and controlled-release oxycodone: pharmacokinetics, pharmacodynamics, and controversy. *Support Care Cancer, 11*(2), 84-92; De Pinto, M., Dunbar, P. J., & Edwards, W.T. (2006). Pain management. *Anesthesiology Clin N Am, 24*(1), 19-37; Du Pen, S., Du Pen, A., & Hillyer, J. (2006). Intrathecal hydromorphone for intractable nonmalignant pain: a retrospective study. *Pain Med, 7*(1), 10-15; Fick, D. M., Cooper, J. W., Wade, W. E., et al. (2003). Updating the Beers criteria for potentially inappropriate use in older adults: Results of a US consensus panel of experts. *Arch Intern Med, 163*(22), 2716-2724; Fong, H. K., Sands, L. P., & Leung, J. M. (2006). The role of postoperative analgesia in delirium and cognitive decline in elderly patients: A systematic review. *Anesth Analg, 102*(4), 1255-1266; Fukuda, K. (2005). Intravenous opioid anesthetics. (2005). In R. D. Miller (Ed.), *Miller's anesthesia*, ed 6, St. Louis, Churchill Livingstone; Furlan, A. D., Sandoval, J. A., Mailis-Gagnon, A., et al. (2006). Opioids for chronic noncancer Pain a meta-analysis of effectiveness and side effects. *Can Med Assoc J, 174*(11), 1589-1594; Gupta, S., & Sathyan, G. (2007). Providing constant analgesia with OROS hydromorphone. *J Pain Symptom Manage, 33*(2S), S19-S24; Gutstein, H., & Akil, H. (2006). Opioid analgesics. In L. L. Brunton (Ed.), *Goodman & Gilman's the pharmacological basis of therapeutics*, ed 11, New York, McGraw-Hill; Hagen, N. A., & Babul, N. (1997). Comparative clinical efficacy and safety of a novel controlled-release oxycodone formulation and controlled-release hydromorphone in the treatment of cancer pain. *Cancer, 79*, 1428-1437; Hale, M. E., Ahdieh, H., Ma, T., et al. (2007). Efficacy and safety of OPANA ER (oxymorphone extended release) for relief of moderate to severe chronic low back pain in opioid-experienced patients: A 12-week, randomized, double-blind, placebo-controlled study. *J Pain, 8*(2), 175-184; Hanks, G., Cherny, N. I., & Fallon, M. (2004). Opioid analgesics. In D. Doyle, G. Hanks, N. I. Cherny (Eds.), *Oxford textbook of palliative medicine*, ed 3, New York, Oxford University Press; Kalso, E. (2005). Oxycodone. *J Pain Symptom Manage, 29*(Suppl 5), S47-S56; Kumar, M. G., & Lin, S. (2007). Hydromorphone in the management of cancer-related pain: An update on routes of administration and dosage forms. *J Pharm Sci, 10*(4), 504-518; Latta, K. S., Ginsberg, B., & Barkin, R. L. (2002). Meperidine: A critical review. *Am J Ther, 9*(1), 53-68; Lugo, R. A., & Kern, S. E. (2004). The pharmacokinetics of oxycodone. *J Pain Palliat Care Pharmacother, 18*(4), 17-30; McIlwain, H., & Ahdieh, H. (2005). Safety, tolerability, and effectiveness of oxymorphone extended release for moderate to severe osteoarthritis pain. A one year study. *Am J Therap, 12*(2), 105-112; Miller, M. G., McCarthy, N., O'Boyle, C. A., et al. (1999). Continuous subcutaneous infusion of morphine vs. hydromorphone: A controlled trial. *J Pain Symptom Manage, 18*(1), 9-16; Mitchell, A., van Zanten, S. V., Inglis, K., et al. (2008). A randomized controlled trial comparing acetaminophen plus ibuprofen versus acetaminophen plus codeine plus caffeine after outpatient general surgery. *J Am Coll Surg, 206*(3), 472-479; Murray, A., & Hagen, N. A. Hydromorphone. (2005). *J Pain Symptom Manage, 29*(Suppl 5), S57-66; Prommer, E. (2006). Oxymorphone: A review. *Support Care Cancer, 14*(2), 109-115; Prommer, E. (2007). Levorphanol: The forgotten opioid. *Support Care Cancer, 15*, 259-264; Prommer, E. E. (2007). Levorphanol revisited. *J Palliat Med, 10*(6), 1228-1230; Quigley, C. (2002). Hydromorphone for acute and chronic pain. *Cochrane Database of Systematic Reviews*, issue 1. Art. No.: CD003447. DOI: 10.1002/14651858.CD003447; Quigley, C., & Wiffen, P. (2003). A systematic review of hydromorphone in acute and chronic pain. *J Pain Symptom Manage, 5*(2), 169-178; Riley, J., Eisenberg, E., Müller-Schwefe, G., et al. (2008). Oxycodone: A review of its use in the management of pain. *Curr Med Res Opin, 24*(1), 175-192; Sarhill, N., Walsh, D., & Nelson, K. A. (2001). Hydromorphone: Pharmacology and clinical applications in cancer patients. *Support Care Cancer, 9*(2), 84-96; Susce, M. T., Murray-Carmichael, E., & de Leon, J. (2006). Response to hydrocodone, codeine and oxycodone in a CYP2D6 poor metabolizer. *Prog Neuropsychopharmacol Biol Psychiatry, 30*(7), 1356-1358; United States Food and Drug Administration. Available at http://www.fda.gov/downloads/AdvisoryCommittees/CommitteesMeetingMaterials/Drugs/AnestheticAndLifeSupportDrugsAdvisoryCommittee/UCM120095.pdf. Accessed December 10, 2009. Wright, A. W., Mather, L. E., & Smith, M. T. (2001). Hydromorphone-3-glucuronide: A more potent neuro-excitant than its structural analogue, morphine-3-glucuronide. *Life Sci, 69*(4), 409-420. © 2011, Pasero C, McCaffery M. May be duplicated for use in clinical practice.

to use tall-man lettering (e.g., HYDROmophone, oxyCONTIN, oxyCODONE), never express doses of liquid opioids in mL alone (include mg amount), and write out opioid name modifiers (e.g., "extended release" rather than "ER" or "immediate release" rather than "IR") (Institute for Safe Medication Practices, 2009).

The characteristics of opioid analgesics vary widely. There have been few randomized controlled trials comparing the different opioids head to head (Fine, Portenoy, 2007; Hanks, De Conno, Cherny, et al., 2001). There are also well-known, wide variations in patient response to all opioids. Therefore, no opioid can be said to be clinically superior to all others in providing analgesia across settings, indications, and populations. Understanding the unique characteristics of each helps to determine the optimal opioid analgesic for the individual patient. This chapter of the book presents a general overview of selected mu agonists that are commonly used for pain management beginning with morphine and followed by the other opioid analgesics presented in alphabetical order.

Morphine

Morphine is the prototype mu agonist opioid (Fine, Portenoy, 2007) and is the standard against which all other opioid drugs are compared (Hanks, De Conno, Cherny, et al., 2001; Inturrisi, 2002; Knotkova, Fine, Portenoy, 2009). It is the most widely used opioid throughout the world (Andersen, Christrup, Sjøgren, 2003), particularly for cancer pain (Flemming, 2010). Its role is supported by extensive research, clinical experience with its use, the availability of formulations for multiple routes of administration, and early development of modified-release formulations. In 1984, the World Health Organization designated morphine as the preferred drug for cancer pain management (WHO, 1996), and still today it is referred to as the "gold standard" for opioid analgesics (Quigley, Wiffen, 2003). This characterization can be viewed as educational; as noted previously, it is not based on comparative effectiveness or safety data. Although some guidelines continue to advocate for morphine as the preferred first-choice "strong" opioid (Hanks, De Conno, Cherny, et al., 2001; Donnelly, Davis, Walsh, et al., 2002), others recognize the lack of evidence to support a preferred status and are less definitive, instead preferring to recommend mu agonist opioids as a class (American Pain Society [APS], 2003; National Comprehensive Cancer Network, 2008). A Cochrane Collaboration Review of 54 studies of oral morphine for cancer pain concluded that well-controlled research with large numbers of patients is lacking, but that existing studies generally confirm that morphine is effective, with the most common adverse effects being constipation, nausea, and vomiting (Wiffen, McQuay, 2007).

In addition to the large role that it plays in the worldwide treatment of cancer pain (Donnelly, Davis, Walsh, et al., 2002; Hanks, Cherny, Fallon, 2004), morphine has a long history as a primary drug for acute postoperative pain management (McCartney, Niazi, 2006) and has been used to treat a wide range of other painful conditions including severe angina pectoris (Mouallem, Schwartz, Farfel, 2000), AIDS-related pain (Kaplan, Slywka, Slagle, et al., 2000), and prehospital admission trauma and medical conditions (Ricard-Hibon, Belpomme, Chollet, et al., 2008). As part of a standard anesthetic regimen, IV morphine, but not IV fentanyl, suppressed several components of the inflammatory response to cardiopulmonary bypass in patients undergoing coronary artery bypass graft surgery (Murphy, Szokol, Marymont, et al., 2007).

Although opioids are not first-line analgesics for neuropathic pain, morphine has been shown to effectively treat this type of pain, particularly in combination with first-line adjuvant analgesics for neuropathic pain, such as the gabapentinoids (i.e., gabapentin and pregabalin) and the analgesic antidepressants (Dworkin, O'Connor, Backonja, et al., 2007; Gilron, Bailey, Tu, et al., 2005; Maier, Hildebrandt, Klinger, et al., 2002). One randomized, placebo-controlled, double-blind, cross-over study (N = 76) found that opioids (morphine or methadone) and tricyclic antidepressants (despiramine or nortriptyline) were effective in treating postherpetic neuralgia with a nonsignificant trend toward greater reduction in pain with opioids (Raja, Haythornthwaite, Pappagallo, et al., 2002).

Even with a higher incidence of adverse effects such as nausea and constipation, patients preferred opioid treatment. Cognitive decline during opioid administration was not observed.

Morphine has been administered by several routes of administration: oral, intranasal, intrapulmonary, rectal, IV, SC, IM, intraspinal (epidural and intrathecal), intraarticular, vaginal, sublingual/buccal, and topical (Christensen, Cohen, Mermelstein, et al., 2008; Donnelly, Davis, Walsh, et al., 2002; Hanks, Cherny, Fallon, 2004; Lavelle, Lavelle, Lavelle, 2007; Stoker, Reber, Waltzman, et al., 2008). Poor lipid solubility precludes transdermal absorption and also complicates reliable delivery through mucous membranes, such as the sublingual/buccal route (Donnelly, Davis, Walsh, et al., 2002; Reisfield, Wilson, 2007). The evidence for vaginal administration of morphine is limited to case reports (Ostrop, Lamb, Reid, 1998). Topical application of morphine is reported for painful wounds, in which case it is presumed to have a primary local action; there is a dearth of systematic research on this use, and it should not be considered an approach for systemic analgesic therapy (Paice, Von Roenn, Hudgins, et al., 2008; Zeppetella, Porzio, Aielli, 2007). Nebulized morphine has been used for dyspnea; case reports suggest a favorable local action exists, but the data overall are mixed, and there are no research reports describing this route as a means to provide systemic analgesia (see Chapters 14 and 20).

Morphine's effectiveness as an analgesic, therefore, is established for specific systemic routes of administration—oral and parenteral—and intraspinal routes. Of the parenteral routes, IM administration is not recommended for morphine or for any other drug because of the painful injection and unreliable absorption (APS, 2003) (see Chapter 14). Short-term and long-term parenteral use can be easily accomplished with the IV or SC routes. The oral formulations of morphine are available in liquids, tablets, and capsules and in both short-acting and modified-release preparations. (See Chapter 14 for a detailed discussion of oral morphine formulations.)

Morphine is metabolized primarily in the liver. It has two main metabolites, morphine-3-glucuronide (M3G) and morphine-6-glucuronide (M6G) (Gutstein, Akil, 2006). M3G is the primary metabolite of morphine, but it is not active at the opioid receptor and does not produce analgesia (South, Smith, 2001; Andersen, Christrup, Sjogren, 2003); M6G is active at the opioid receptor and produces analgesia (Dahan, van Dorp, Smith, et al., 2008; Smith, Binning, Dahan, 2009; Vaughn, Connor, 2003). Both metabolites have been implicated in morphine toxicity in animals and in patients with advanced disease (Morita, Tei, Tsunoda, et al., 2002), but the studies in humans have not established a clear association (Andersen, Christrup, Sjøgren, 2003). The mechanism by which toxicity, which is evidenced most often by delirium or myoclonus, occurs has not been fully described, and it has been noted that these symptoms are also seen with other opioids (Harris,

2008; Okon, George, 2008) (see Chapter 19 for treatment). Renal insufficiency presumably increases the risk of morphine toxicity because both the parent compound and its major metabolites are renally excreted (Dean, 2004) and there is a direct correlation between creatinine clearance and morphine, M6G, and M3G serum levels.

Administration of M3G directly into the CNS has been shown to produce neuroexcitability and anti-analgesic effects in animals (Sharke, Geisslinger, Lotsch, 2005). This metabolite has been implicated as the cause of the neuroexcitability noted in some patients who receive large doses of morphine on a long-term basis (Inturrisi, 2002). Some have suggested that opioid-induced hyperalgesia (see Chapter 11) may be due in part to M3G activity (Hemstapat, Monteith, Smith, et al., 2003; South, Smith, 2001); however, further research in humans is needed to draw firm conclusions (Andersen, Christrup, Sjogren, 2003; Sharke, Geisslinger, Lotsch, 2005).

M6G is thought to produce at least some (e.g., 10%) of the analgesic effect of a dose of morphine, but potency and effectiveness studies in humans have produced mixed results (Andersen, Christup, Sjogren, 2003; Smith, South, 2001; Wittwer, Kern, 2006). M6G is absorbed and eliminated from the CNS more slowly than morphine, which may account for the observed increase in potency with long-term morphine administration (Donnelly, Davis, Walsh, et al., 2002; Smith, South, 2001). It may be that the adverse effect profile of M6G is better than that of morphine (Donnelly, Davis, Walsh, et al., 2002). Specific adverse effects that have been investigated include respiratory depression, sedation, nausea and vomiting, hyperalgesia, and myoclonus. A randomized study of 170 patients with moderate to severe postoperative pain demonstrated that M6G produced long-lasting, dose-related analgesia with minimal cardiorespiratory or opioid-like adverse effects (Smith, Binning, Dahan, 2009). In another study (N = 100), M6G was compared with morphine and was found to produce less sedation and respiratory depression, and to have a slower initial onset of effect, with no significant difference in mean pain intensity between groups at 24 hours, but higher pain intensities at 30 minutes and 1 hour after M6G administration (Hanna, Elliott, Fung, 2005). The various factors that influence blood levels of morphine, M6G, and M3G are listed in Table 13-2.

Morphine is hydrophilic (soluble in aqueous solution), which contributes to its slow onset and long duration of action compared with the more lipophilic (soluble in fatty tissue) opioid drugs, such as fentanyl and sufentanil. This is not relevant after steady state is reached during continuous dosing but may be important when intermittent boluses are used systemically or intraspinally (see Chapters 15 through 17). The longer time that it takes morphine to reach its analgesic site of action must be considered when determining how quickly to administer doses during titration (IV); adequate time must be allowed to assess response to one dose before administration of another (Lotsch, Dudziak, Freynhagen, et al., 2006). Morphine

Table 13-2 | Factors That Influence Blood Levels of Morphine, M6G, and M3G

Factor	Morphine	M6G	M3G
Oral route		↑	
Age older than 70 years		↑	↑
Male sex	↓	↓	
Concurrent use of rifampin	↓	↓	↓
Concurrent use of tricyclic antidepressants			↓
Concurrent use of ranitidine	↓		
Renal failure		↑	

↑, Increased blood level; ↓, decreased blood level; *M3G*, morphine-3-glucuronide; *M6G*, morphine-6-glucuronide.

Morphine has two main metabolites, morphine-3-glucuronide (M3G) and morphine-6-glucuronide (M6G). M3G is the primary metabolite of morphine, but it is not active at the opioid receptor, M6G is active at the opioid receptor. With long-term oral morphine dosing, blood levels of M6G typically exceed those of morphine; the concentration ratios of M3G to morphine are inconsistent and variable. Unanticipated opioid toxicity and adverse effects are attributed to accumulation and high blood concentrations of M6G (see text regarding M3G).

From Pasero, C., & McCaffery, M. *Pain assessment and pharmacologic management*, p. 329, St. Louis, Mosby. Data from Buxton, I. L. O. (2006). Pharmacokinetics and pharmacodynamics. The dynamics of drug absorption, distribution, action, and elimination. In L. L. Brunton, J. S. Lazo, & K. L. Parker (Eds.), *Goodman & Gilman's the pharmacological basis of therapeutics*, ed 11, New York, McGraw-Hill; Gutstein, H., & Akil, H. (2006). Opioid analgesics. In L. L. Brunton (Ed.), *Goodman & Gilman's the pharmacological basis of therapeutics*, ed 11, New York, McGraw-Hill; Portenoy, R. K., & Kanner, R. M. (Eds.). (1996). *Pain management: Theory and practice*, Philadelphia, FA Davis; Sharke, C., Geisslinger, G., & Lotsch, J. (2005). Is morphine-3-glucuronide of therapeutic relevance? *Pain*, 116(3), 177-180. © 2011, Pasero C, McCaffery M. May be duplicated for use in clinical practice.

has a short half-life of 2 to 4 hours; the half-life of M6G is somewhat longer (Andersen, Christup, Sjøgren, 2003). It is estimated that approximately 20% to 30% of the given dose of oral morphine is available for therapeutic effect because of first-pass effect (De Pinto, Dunbar, Edwards, 2006; Gutstein, Akil, 2006) (see Chapter 11). This is why the recommended dose of morphine by the oral route is higher than that by the parenteral route (APS, 2003) (see Table 16-1 on pp. 444-446).

IV morphine has been observed to have an increased analgesic efficacy and longer duration of action in older patients than in younger patients for reasons that are thought to be multifactorial; slow, steady titration is recommended (Villesen, Banning, Petersen, et al., 2007). A general practice is to reduce the starting dose of morphine (and other opioids) in older patients because of physiologic changes associated with aging, such as diminished first pass effect, enhanced bioavailability, and 20% to 40% decrease in clearance (Aubrun, Marmion, 2007).

Codeine

Codeine is the prototypical "weak" opioid used primarily for short-term acute pain. It is usually prescribed as an oral combination product that also contains aspirin or acetaminophen. Codeine combination products may also include caffeine or a muscle relaxant.

Combination preparations that include codeine are not appropriate for moderate to severe or escalating pain because of the dosing limitations inherent in the nonopioid constituent. The ceiling on the maximum safe daily doses of acetaminophen (4000 mg) and aspirin (4000 mg) limits dose increases for inadequate pain control (see Section III). In addition, aspirin is contraindicated for patients with a number of underlying conditions, such as those with a bleeding disorder or history of asthma. See Patient Education Form VI-2 (pp. 547-548) on codeine with acetaminophen at the end of Section IV.

Although a single-entity codeine formulation could theoretically undergo dose escalation sufficient to manage severe persistent pain, this is not pursued in practice. At the customary doses used, codeine provides analgesia for mild to moderate pain. A common oral dose of 60 mg produces analgesia equal to 600 mg of aspirin (less than two 325 mg tablets) (Gutstein, Akil, 2006). A systematic literature search concluded that acetaminophen/codeine (e.g., 300 mg/30 mg) was less efficacious and associated with more adverse effects than NSAIDs (e.g., ibuprofen, naproxen) for postpartum and postlaparotomy analgesia (Nauta, Landsmeer, Koren, 2009). One double-blind study randomized patients to receive codeine (30 mg) plus acetaminophen (300 mg) and caffeine (15 mg) per dose or ibuprofen (400 mg) plus acetaminophen (325 mg) per dose four times daily for 7 days or until pain free following outpatient hernia repair or laparascopic cholecystectomy (Mitchell, van Zanten, Inglis, et al., 2008). Those who received ibuprofen plus acetaminophen had lower pain ratings and fewer adverse effects throughout the treatment period and were more satisfied and less likely to discontinue treatment due to adverse effects or ineffectiveness compared with those who received codeine. A Cochrane Collaboration Review concluded that single doses of dihydrocodeine, a synthetic opioid with structure and pharmacokinetics very similar to codeine, is not sufficient for postoperative pain relief and that 400 mg of ibuprofen was superior to 30 or 60 mg of dihydrocodeine (Edwards, McQuay, Moore, 2004).

There also is evidence that higher doses of codeine would be relatively less effective than other opioids. Doses above 65 mg have been described as providing diminishing incremental analgesia but continued increase in adverse effects (Miaskowski, Cleary, Burney, et al., 2005).

The IM route has been used to administer codeine, but absorption is unreliable and is associated with a five-fold variation in peak blood level; the peak occurs approximately 30 to 60 minutes after IM administration.

Nine-fold differences in minimum effective analgesic concentration have been found by this route, and late respiratory depression can occur. These properties make the IM route unfavorable for use in postoperative pain management (Cousins, Umedaly, 1996). It has also long been regarded as inappropriate for IV administration, with low doses of IV morphine recommended instead (Semple, Macintyre, Hooper, 1993) (see Table 13-1). The dose ratio for total analgesic effect between IM and oral codeine is 0.6:1, and a comparison between parenteral codeine and oxycodone found an equianalgesic dose ratio of 10:1; however, its relative potency varies with the extent to which it is converted to its active metabolite (Knotkova, Fine, Portenoy, 2009).

Codeine is a prodrug and is approximately 60% bioavailable orally (as compared, for example, with morphine, which has oral bioavailability of 20% to 30%). This is because codeine, like levorphanol, oxycodone, and methadone, undergoes less first-pass metabolism than morphine (Gutstein, Akil, 2006) (see Chapter 11). Once absorbed, 10% of codeine is metabolized in the liver to morphine, its active form (Somogyi, Barratt, Coller, 2007), which probably provides the bulk of its analgesic effect. However, as with other opioids, extremely wide variations exist between individuals in terms of absorption and analgesic requirements of codeine.

The metabolism of codeine to morphine depends on the presence of the enzyme cytochrome P450 2D6 (Fine, Portenoy, 2007) (see Chapter 11 for a detailed discussion of this enzyme system). There is population variation in phenotype of cytochrome P450 2D6, distinguishing patients intermediate, extensive (or rapid), ultra-rapid metabolizers, or poor metabolizers. Extensive metabolizers are the norm and are able to perform catalyzed biotransformation of codeine (and other drugs). Approximately 10% of Caucasians and varying frequencies in other ethnic groups are poor metabolizers. These individuals have a very limited ability to convert codeine to morphine, and as a consequence, are relatively less responsive to codeine's analgesic effect (Palmer, Giesecke, Body, et al., 2005). In contrast, ultra-rapid metabolizers, who biotransform codeine more rapidly or more completely and most of the population, may have an exaggerated (i.e., toxic) response to codeine (Voronov, Przybylo, Jagannathan, 2007; United States Food and Drug Administration [U.S. FDA], 2007a; Palmer, Giesecke, Body, et al., 2005).

The impact of the biotransformation via P450 2D6 can vary according to circumstances. Although biotransformation at this isoenzyme occurs at the same rate in neonates and adults, neonates can develop toxicity from codeine because the clearance of morphine is relatively reduced and it can accumulate in the blood. In 2007, the U.S. FDA issued a warning that nursing mothers who are ultra-rapid metabolizers of codeine can transfer sufficient morphine to their breast-feeding infants to cause life-threatening or fatal adverse effects (U.S. FDA, 2007a) (see Chapter 20 for more on opioid use during breast-feeding). In adults, the efficiency of the enzyme can be affected by certain drugs, leading to changes in the production of morphine from codeine. Drugs such as paroxetine (Paxil) and fluoxetine (Prozac), for example, may inhibit cytochrome P450 2D6, and therefore, could potentially interfere with the metabolism of codeine. Case reports suggest that hydrocodone may be effective in CPY2D6 poor metabolizers for whom codeine was ineffective (Susce, Murray-Carmichael, de Leon, 2006).

Codeine Post-Craniotomy

The incidence of moderate-to-severe postoperative pain after craniotomy is common, and the surgical procedure is associated with the development of persistent postsurgical pain (Gottschalk, 2009). Pain management is complicated by concerns about opioid-related adverse effects, such as sedation, miosis, nausea, and vomiting, in this patient population. Codeine has been used for the treatment of postcraniotomy and other types of neurosurgical pain for decades, but its unpredictable absorption, variability in demethylation, and high incidence of nausea and sedation at effective doses make it a particularly poor choice in this population (Roberts, 2004). A review of randomized controlled trials revealed two studies that showed more consistent pain control with morphine compared with codeine and no differences in respiratory depression, sedation, pupillary size, and cardiovascular (CV) effects in patients following craniotomy (Nemergut, Durieux, Missaghi, et al., 2007). A study comparing IV morphine PCA, IV tramadol PCA, and IM codeine in postcraniotomy patients found that morphine produced significantly better analgesia with less vomiting than the other two drugs (Sudheer, Logan, Terblanche, et al., 2007). Roberts (2004) points out that patients are admitted to the intensive care setting where close monitoring is standard following craniotomy. This and thoughtful titration to minimize adverse effects help to ensure the safety of morphine in this population (see also discussion of remifentanil later in this chapter and Chapter 26 for discussion of gabapentin as a component of a multimodal analgesic regimen for craniotomy pain).

Fentanyl

Fentanyl is the prototype in a subset of mu agonists which includes sufentanil, alfentanil, and remifentanil (see separate discussions for the latter three). All of these drugs are characterized by high potency and high lipophilicity (fat solubility). When administered parenterally to the opioid-naïve patient, the effects are characterized by rapid onset and short duration of action. The injectable formulations of these drugs are administered via the IV, epidural, and intrathecal routes and typically are used for acute pain in the perioperative and procedural

settings, often in conjunction with anesthetic or sedating agents; they are the most commonly used opioids in anesthesia (Coda, 2006). They also may be administered transmucosally, e.g., by the buccal, sublingual, or intranasal routes (see Chapter 14).

As a class, fentanyl and comparable drugs are versatile, although none are commercially available in an oral or rectal formulation. There are pharmacologic and cost differences that are considered in drug selection for each therapeutic application. With rapid IV administration of high doses, these drugs can produce chest wall rigidity and subsequent difficult ventilation (Lalley, 2005; Fukuda, 2005); this is a concern when fentanyl is used for intraoperative anesthesia (see Chapter 16 for more on speed of injection). Likely related is cough, which has been reported as a complication of both fentanyl and sufentanil (Agarwal, Gautam, Nath, et al., 2007); this effect has been successfully suppressed with IV lidocaine 0.5 mg/kg (Pandey, Raza, Ranjan, et al., 2005).

Fentanyl differs in many ways from morphine. Its lipophilicity means that there is wide and rapid distribution after IV administration, as well as ready passage through the blood-brain barrier. When given as a single IV bolus, fentanyl's onset (within 1 to 5 minutes) is faster and its duration (sometimes less than 1 hour) is shorter than morphine as the drug moves from blood to lungs, muscle, and fat (Taylor, 2005). It also is approximately 100 times more potent than morphine, so that a single IV bolus of 100 mcg produces roughly the same analgesia as morphine 10 mg; however, caution is recommended when converting to and from fentanyl as studies demonstrate considerable variability in conversion ratios (see Knotkova, Fine, Portenoy, 2009 for a discussion of this research).

The lipophilicity and potency of fentanyl makes it an excellent candidate for transdermal and oral transmucosal formulation. The fentanyl transdermal patch is commonly used in long-term pain treatment (see Chapter 14). Oral transmucosal fentanyl formulations are used in the treatment of breakthrough pain: oral transmucosal fentanyl and buccal fentanyl; a buccal patch was recently approved in the United States, and a sublingual formulation and an intranasal formulation are available in some other countries (see Chapter 14 for oral transmucosal formulations).

After repetitive dosing or continuous infusion of fentanyl, a steady state is approached. Although some clinicians believe that fentanyl has a very short half-life, this is a misconception. When fentanyl or some other very lipophilic drug is administered to the patient who is not receiving regular dosing, the blood levels decline quickly as the drug redistributes into fatty tissue. This redistribution, or "alpha" phase, is associated with a short half-life and a brief duration of clinical effects. With fentanyl, it is typically only minutes long. In contrast, regular dosing of fentanyl or any other lipophilic drug eventually leads to a steady state in which there is equilibrium between the blood and fatty tissues. A bolus injection in this setting still has a redistribution phase, but most of the elimination time, the "beta" phase, results from metabolism and redistribution of drug from fat back into blood. As a result, the half-life, and the duration of effect after the bolus, is much longer. The so-called *terminal elimination half-life* is the half-life that is obtained after the redistribution has taken place.

Given these kinetics, the half-life of fentanyl varies in the literature depending on whether the study that yielded the value measured the decline in concentration in a steady-state situation or not. Although it has been reported that fentanyl has a terminal half-life of approximately 3 to 4 hours, it is much longer—four to five times longer—after steady state has been approached (Dershwitz, Landow, Joshi-Ryzewicz, 2003; Liu, Gropper, 2003). After steady state is achieved using transdermal fentanyl, half-life also is affected by continued absorption from the skin depot under the patch; the half-life is therefore even longer, typically over 24 hours (see Table 13-1).

Fentanyl's lipophilicity and storage in fatty tissue has significant implications for obese patients in the perioperative setting. If perioperative dosing is based on body weight alone, obese patients are likely to receive too high a dose. Dosing based on a calculated "pharmacokinetic mass" (i.e., for patients weighing 140 to 200 kg, dosing weights of 100 to 108 kg are projected) has been shown in two clinical studies to provide safe and effective intraoperative and postoperative analgesia at lower doses than would be predicted by actual weight (Shibutani, Inchiosa, Sawada, et al., 2004, 2005). This is a result of a nonlinear relationship between total body weight and fentanyl clearance.

Fentanyl is metabolized in the liver, has no active metabolites, and produces minimal hemodynamic effects (Fukuda, 2005). These characteristics have made fentanyl a favorite in the critically ill, including older critically ill adults, and especially patients who are hemodynamically unstable or have renal failure (Graf, Puntillo, 2003; Jacobi, Fraser, Coursin, et al., 2002). It is recommended for patients with end-stage renal disease who need opioid analgesia (Dean, 2004; Johnson, 2007; Murtagh, Chai, Donohoe, et al., 2007). Though more research is needed, fentanyl appears safe in patients with hepatic dysfunction as well (Johnson, 2007).

When used for pain, fentanyl typically is given either parenterally (by the IV route usually) or intraspinally (see Chapter 15). Its rapid onset and short duration in the non–steady state situation make fentanyl the most commonly used opioid in combination with benzodiazepines for procedural analgesia and sedation. Along with morphine and hydromorphone, fentanyl has become a first-line choice for postoperative pain management via IV PCA in many institutions (Pasero, 2005) (see Chapter 17 for PCA dosing). There have been no randomized controlled trials comparing these drugs. A retrospective analysis of medical records compared adverse effects associated with morphine (N = 93), hydromorphone (N = 89), and fentanyl

(N = 72) via postoperative IV PCA and found lower mean rates of nausea, pruritus, urinary retention, and sedation with fentanyl; there were no differences among the opioids in incidence of respiratory depression, headache, agitation, confusion, and hallucinations (Hutchison, Chon, Tucker, et al., 2006). However, well-controlled research is needed to draw conclusions regarding differences.

Parenteral fentanyl can be administered by SC infusion (Anderson, Shreve, 2004). A small study comparing continuous SC infusions of morphine followed by fentanyl (N = 13) and fentanyl followed by morphine (N = 10) in hospice cancer patients revealed that fentanyl is as efficacious as morphine with no differences in adverse effects except less constipation in patients receiving fentanyl (Hunt, Fazekas, Thorne, et al., 1999). The researchers recommended a conversion ratio of morphine 10 mg to fentanyl 150 mcg as appropriate but emphasized that further research is needed in this area.

Although fentanyl's properties of high lipophilicity, rapid onset, and short duration in the non–steady state situation make it an attractive option for pain management in a variety of settings, populations, and conditions, these properties also necessitate careful patient selection, appropriate monitoring, and adherence to the safety warnings that accompany fentanyl products, especially the patches and oral transmucosal products. A number of fatalities have occurred due to improper prescribing and use. See Chapter 14 for specific information on indications, patient selection, administration, monitoring, and precautions for the various fentanyl products.

Hydrocodone

Hydrocodone is available in several proprietary products (e.g., Lortab, Vicodin, Lorcet, Hydrocet, and Norco) and generic preparations, and in several different fixed-dose combinations with acetaminophen, aspirin, and ibuprofen. Most are available in tablet form, while others are available in capsule or liquid form (Table 13-3). Combination drugs containing hydrocodone and a nonopioid drug can provide more effective relief than either drug alone. Ibuprofen combined with a variety of hydrocodone doses was shown to increase the effectiveness of hydrocodone seven-fold in animal research (Kolesnikov, Wilson, Pasternak 2003). See Patient Education Form IV-6 on hydrocodone with acetaminophen on pp. 556-557 at the end of Section IV.

Hydrocodone is not available in single-entity form. The dose is limited by the ceiling on safety and efficacy inherent in the nonopioid constituent. The dose limitation, in turn, typically means that the drug is useful for the management of mild to moderate pain in the opioid-naïve patient. Use in persistent pain (except for breakthrough dosing) should be carefully evaluated. Long-acting analgesics without a fixed dose co-analgesic are preferred for moderate to severe persistent cancer or noncancer pain.

Table 13-3 | Commercially Available Combinations of Hydrocodone and Nonopioids

Brand	Hydrocodone (mg)	Acetaminophen (mg)	Aspirin (mg)	Ibuprofen (mg)	Dose Form
Anexia 5/325; Norco; Generic	5	325			Tablet
Co-Gesic 5/500; Lortab 5/500; Generic	5	500			Tablet
Hycet; Norco; Generic	7.5	325			Oral solution (per 15 mL)
Lorcet 10/650	10	650			Tablet
Lorcet Plus; Generic	7.5	650			Tablet
Damason-P; Lortab ASA; Panasal; Generic	5		500		Tablet
Lortab 7.5/500; Generic	7.5	500			Elixir (per 15 mL)
Lortab 10/500; Generic	10	500			Tablet
Margesic H	5	500			Capsule
Maxidone; Generic	10	750			Tablet
Norco; Generic	10	325			Tablet
Reprexain	5			200	Tablet
Stagesic	5	500			Capsule
Vicodin	5	500			Tablet
Vicodin ES; Generic	7.5	750			Tablet
Vicodin HP; Generic	10	660			Tablet
Vicoprofen; Generic	7.5			200	Tablet
Xodol 5/300	5	300			Tablet
Xodol 7/300	7	300			Tablet
Xodol 10/300	10	300			Tablet
Zydone	5	400			Tablet
Zydone	7.5	400			Tablet
Zydone	10	400			Tablet
Generic	2.5	500			Tablet
Generic	10	650			Tablet

From Pasero, C., & McCaffery, M. *Pain assessment and pharmacologic management*, p. 333, St. Louis, Mosby. © 2011, Pasero C, McCaffery M. May be duplicated for use in clinical practice.

A modified-release (12-hour) oral formulation of hydrocodone 15 mg plus acetaminophen 500 mg has been studied in clinical trials but has not been approved in the United States (Coddings, Levinsky, Hale, et al., 2008; Golf, Robson, Pollak, et al., 2008).

Hydrocodone with acetaminophen is not only the most commonly prescribed analgesic in the United States, it is by far the most commonly prescribed medication in all classes (Lamb, 2008). In 2008, hydrocodone plus acetaminophen was first in the list of the 200 most commonly prescribed drugs (Drug Topics, 2008). It is critical to avoid prescribing or administering amounts that would exceed the daily maximum dose for acetaminophen (4000 mg), aspirin (4000 mg), or ibuprofen (3200 mg) and teach the patient the dangers of exceeding these amounts (see Section III).

Hydrocodone has an onset of action of approximately 20 minutes, reaches peak effectiveness by 60 minutes, and has a half-life of 3.8 hours (Gutstein, Akil, 2006). It is metabolized by the cytochrome P450 2D6 (CYP2D6) enzyme. Case reports suggest that hydrocodone may be effective in CPY 2D6 poor metabolizers for whom codeine was ineffective (Susce, Murray-Carmichael, de Leon, 2006). (See Chapter 11 for more on the cytochrome P450 enzyme system and drug-drug interactions.)

The adverse effects of hydrocodone are comparable to that of other opioids. It has been shown to have similar efficacy (when titrated to effect) and a lower incidence of adverse effects compared with tramadol and codeine (Rodriguez, Bravo, Castro, et al., 2007; Rodriguez, Castillo, Del Pilar Castillo, et al., 2007). Several cases of an unusual adverse effect (hearing loss) have been reported in patients taking hydrocodone and in hydrocodone abusers (Ho, Vrabec, Burton, 2007). No causative mechanism, if it exists, has been identified for this association.

To ensure safety, it should be specifically noted that the name *hydrocodone* is similar in appearance and sound to oxycodone, oxymorphone, and hydromorphone. An increased level of alertness is required to prevent medication errors with these opioids.

Hydromorphone

Hydromorphone is often considered an alternative to morphine, especially for acute pain (Chang, Bijur, Meyer, et al., 2006; Rapp, Egan, Ross, et al., 1996). Although there are few head-to-head studies, morphine and hydromorphone appear to provide equivalent analgesic effects and very similar adverse effect profiles (Ripamonti, Bandieri, 2009; Quigley, Wiffen, 2003); there is some evidence that hydromorphone may be associated with less nausea and pruritus (Chang, Bijur, Meyer, et al., 2006).

IV hydromorphone is a first- or second-choice opioid (after morphine) for postoperative pain management via PCA (Quigley, 2002). When given IV as a bolus, its onset of action is 5 minutes, its peak effect occurs in 8 to 20 minutes, and its duration is approximately 4 hours (Sarhill, Walsh, Nelson, 2001).

Oral short-acting hydromorphone is available in 2, 4, and 8 mg tablets and in a 1 mg/mL oral solution. It is approximately 60% bioavailable with an onset of action of 30 minutes via the oral route (Kumar, Lin, 2007) and a duration of approximately 3 to 4 hours; maximum plasma concentrations are reached within 1 hour of dosing (Gupta, Sathyan, 2007). Modified-release formulations of oral hydromorphone are available in Canada and Europe and most recently on the U.S. market (Gupta, Sathyan, 2007) (see Chapter 14 for modified-release hydromorphone). See Patient Education Form IV-3 on short-acting hydromorphone at the end of Section IV.

Hydromorphone also has been administered via a variety of other routes. Its greater potency compared with morphine, as well as its availability in concentrated parenteral form (10 mg/mL), has made it attractive for SC administration, especially when high doses are needed. It was found to be comparable to morphine by SC continuous infusion for persistent cancer pain in terminally

ill patients (Miller, McCarthy, O'Boyle, et al., 1999). Absorption via the IM route is erratic and not recommended (Golembiewski, 2003). The epidural and intrathecal routes have been utilized for acute and persistent cancer and noncancer pain (DuPen, DuPen, Hillyer, 2006). Hydromorphone given rectally (3 mg suppository) is as effective as by the oral route; it is not, however, absorbed well by the oral mucosa (Kumar, Lin, 2007; Sarhill, Walsh, Nelson, 2001) (see Table 13-1).

Hydromorphone is metabolized in the liver and eliminated via the kidneys (Sarhill, Walsh, Nelson, 2001). It has a neuroexcitatory metabolite, hydromorphone-3-glucuronide (H3G), and it may be speculated that neurotoxicity at high doses is related to this molecule (Thwaites, McCann, Broderick, 2004; Wright, Mather, Smith, 2001; Smith, 2000). Although neurotoxic symptoms can occur in advanced disease and decreased renal clearance, hydromorphone appears to be a safer choice than morphine under these conditions (Dean, 2004). Hydromorphone is often recommended as the first alternative for opioid rotation when these symptoms occur during morphine administration (Hanks, Reid, 2005). Some clinicians will use hydromorphone in older adults as a first-line opioid instead of morphine because of the theoretically improved tolerance in the presence of decreased renal function; however, this practice has not been studied and has not been recommended by published guidelines. A prospective, randomized study (N = 50) comparing morphine and hydromorphone via postoperative IV PCA found no difference in efficacy, adverse effects, or patient satisfaction (Hong, Flood, Diaz, 2008). A retrospective analysis of medical records found the mean rates of nausea, pruritus, urinary retention, and sedation with postoperative IV PCA hydromorphone to be similar to that of IV PCA morphine and more common than with IV PCA fentanyl; there were no differences among the three opioids in incidence of respiratory depression, headache, agitation, confusion, and hallucinations (Hutchison, Chon, Tucker, et al., 2006). Well-controlled research is needed to draw conclusions regarding differences among the various opioids.

The equianalgesic dose conversion between morphine and hydromorphone is unclear and likely varies with the length of time a patient has been on one drug or the other (Berdine, Nesbit, 2006; Knotkova, Fine, Portenoy, 2009). Published equianalgesic tables typically show oral hydromorphone to be 5 times more potent than oral morphine. This is the most common ratio used when preparing equianalgesic solutions for PCA administration (e.g., 0.2 mg hydromorphone per 1 mL solution is considered approximately equal to 1 mg morphine per 1 mL solution) (Golembiewski, 2003). However, these data are generally derived from acute pain treatment in opioid-naïve patients or healthy volunteers (APS, 2003). An early study of morphine-hydromorphone equivalence showed that after a week of PCA treatment, the ratio was 3:1 (morphine 10 mg to hydromorphone 3.3 mg) (Dunbar, Chapman, Buckley, et al., 1996). Subsequent research found that when switching from long-term dosing of either oral or parenteral morphine to hydromorphone, the ratio was approximately 5.5:1 (morphine 10 mg to hydromorphone 2 mg) (Lawlor, Turner, Hanson, et al., 1997). However, when switching from hydromorphone to morphine, the ratio was 3.7:1 (morphine 10 mg to hydromorphone 2.7 mg). Still others suggest that an equianalgesic dose conversion of parenteral morphine to hydromorphone for long-term dosing is probably 4:1 (morphine 10 mg to hydromorphone 2.5 mg) (Hanks, Cherny, Fallon, 2004). A systematic review of hydromorphone for various types of pain concluded that there is insufficient evidence to recommend specific ratios of hydromorphone (Quigley, Wiffen, 2003) (see also Knotkova, Fine, Portenoy, 2009). (See Table 16-1).

When using equianalgesic dosing to switch a patient from another opioid to hydromorphone, the general condition of the patient and the severity of pain must be considered when choosing a starting dose (Fine, Portenoy, the Ad Hoc Expert Panel on Evidence Review and Guidelines for Opioid Rotation, 2009). In general, it is safest to use a conservative conversion ratio then titrate to effect. No matter what ratio or method for conversion is used, it is vital to take into account that hydromorphone is significantly more potent than morphine, there is great interindividual variability (Murray, Hagen, 2005), and individualization and monitoring are essential elements of prescribing and administering these agents. Deaths have occurred because of confusion between the two agents and a failure to take their inherent differences into account (Institute for Safe Medication Practices, 2004a).

It also should be noted that the name *hydromorphone* is similar in appearance and sound to oxycodone, oxymorphone, and hydrocodone. An increased level of alertness is required to prevent medication errors with these opioids.

Levorphanol

Like methadone, levorphanol (Levo-Dromoran) is considered a second-line drug for cancer pain (Hanks, Cherny, Fallon, 2004). It has not been widely used clinically since the modified-release formulations of morphine and oxycodone became available in the 1990s (McNulty, 2007). Most clinicians are unfamiliar with its pharmacology, which is somewhat different than the more commonly used opioids (McNulty, 2007; Prommer, 2007a; Prommer, 2007b). It is an agonist at both the mu and kappa opioid receptor sites and, like methadone, it also is an N-methyl-D-aspartate (NMDA) antagonist. In addition, it is an inhibitor of serotonin and norepinephrine reuptake (see Section I).

Levorphanol is available for oral (2 mg/tablet) and parenteral administration (2 mg/mL) and has a parenteral-to-oral ratio of 1:2 (Prommer, 2007a).

Its metabolism is similar to morphine's. It undergoes glucuronidation in the liver and is not affected by the CYP 450 system. For this reason, it has fewer potential drug-drug interactions than methadone but is subject to the effects of inducers and inhibitors of glucuronidation (Prommer, 2007a).

Levorphanol's duration of analgesia is reported to range from a low of 3 hours to a high of 15 hours (Fine, Portenoy, 2007; Hanks, Cherny, Fallon, 2004; Prommer, 2007a) with both IV and oral dosing. Importantly, levorphanol has a longer half-life (15 hours) than morphine (2 to 4 hours), and it is likely that at least some patients can attain sustained analgesia with a relatively long dosing interval. Like methadone, the discrepancy between analgesic duration and half-life can predispose levorphanol to accumulation. Although outliers with half-lives that can extend to as much as 30 hours (Prommer, 2007a) are likely to pose substantial risk, accumulation overall appears to be less of a problem than it can be with methadone (Hanks, Cherny, Fallon, 2004). Excretion is by the kidneys.

A study using levorphanol at two dose levels established that neuropathic pain is responsive to opioid treatment (Rowbotham, Twilling, Davies, et al., 2003). In fact, all types of neuropathic pain responded to levorphanol except central poststroke pain in the study. In the higher-dose arm (mean was approximately 9 mg/day) apparent CNS toxicity occurred (irritability, mood changes, confusion, weakness). The reasons and risk factors for these changes were unknown. Close monitoring as well as dose and interval changes are indicated for older adults and those with impaired renal function.

Levorphanol is available in the United States orally only in 2 mg tablets, which can make titration difficult. It is no longer available in the United Kingdom or Canada (Hanks, Cherny, Fallon, 2004). (See Table 16-1 on pp. 444-446.)

Meperidine

Meperidine (Demerol) was once the most widely used opioid analgesic. In recent years, it has been either removed from or severely restricted on hospital formularies, the result of concerted efforts to improve patient safety during opioid use (Gordon, Jones, Goshman, et al., 2000; Raymo, Camejo, Fudin, 2007) (see the paragraphs that follow). The Beers Criteria of inappropriate medication use in older individuals, originally developed in 1991 (Beers, Ouslander, Rollingher, et al., 1991), described meperidine as having many disadvantages and continues to advise against the use of the drug in older adults (Beers, 1997; Fick, Cooper, Wade, et al., 2003) (Table 13-4). A refinement of the 1996 Medical Expenditure Panel Survey designated the drug as one to "always avoid" in older adults (Zhan, Sangl, Bierman, et al., 2001). Meperidine has some positive attributes, but it

Table 13-4 | Beers Criteria for Inappropriate Medication Use in Older Adults: Selected Analgesics

Drug	Concerns	Severity Rating
Propoxyphene (Darvon, Darvocet, Darvon Compound)	Offers no advantages over other opioids; toxic metabolite; high adverse effect profile.	Low
Meperidine (Demerol)	Offers few if any advantages over other opioids; toxic metabolite that can cause CNS disturbances.	High
Pentazocine (Talwin)	Low analgesic efficacy; high incidence of CNS adverse effects (e.g., hallucinations, delirium).	High
Short-acting benzodiazepines (e.g., Ativan, Restoril, Serax, Xanax)	Increased sensitivity in older adults; dose-related adverse CNS effects.	High
Long-acting benzodiazepines (e.g., Librium, Valium)	Increased sensitivity in older adults; long half-life; dose-related adverse CNS effects; associated with falls and fractures. Short-acting is preferred if a benzodiazepine is needed.	High
Flurazepam (Dalmane)	Very long half-life in older adults (often days); prolonged.	High
Anticholinergics and antihistamines (e.g., Benadryl, Atarax, Vistaril)	Most antihistamines have potent anticholinergic effects. Noncholinergic antihistamines are preferred. Hydroxyzine (Vistaril, Atarax) and diphenhydramine (Benadryl) can cause confusion and sedation. If antihistamine is necessary, use low dose.	High
Amitriptyline (Elavil)	High incidence of anticholinergic and sedative adverse effects; rarely appropriate in older adults.	High
Daily fluoxetine (Prozac)	Long half-life; can produce CNS stimulation, sleep disturbances, and agitation.	High
Clonidine (Catapres)	Can cause orthostatic hypotension and CNS adverse effects.	Low
Orphenadrine (Norflex)	Can cause significant sedation and anticholinergic effects.	High
Muscle relaxants (e.g., Soma, Flexeril, Skelaxin)	Most have anticholinergic effects and are poorly tolerated by older adults. Can cause sedation and muscle weakness, which may contribute to falls.	High
Long-term use of full-dose, longer half-life, nonselective NSAIDs (e.g., Naprosyn, Aleve, Feldene)	Potential GI, renal, CV adverse effects.	High
Ketorolac (Toradol)	High incidence of GI adverse effects in older adults.	High
Indomethacin (Indocin)	High incidence of CNS adverse effects.	High

CNS, Central nervous system; *CV*, cardiovascular; *GI*, gastrointestinal,
From Pasero, C., & McCaffery, M. *Pain assessment and pharmacologic management*, p. 336, St. Louis, Mosby. Data from Beers, M. H. (1997). Explicit criteria for determining potentially inappropriate medication use by the elderly. An update. *Arch Intern Med, 157*(14), 1531-1536; Beers, M. H., Ouslander, J. G., Rollingher, I, et al. (1991). Explicit criteria for determining inappropriate medication use in nursing home residents. UCLA Division of Geriatric Medicine. *Arch Intern Med,* 151(9), 1825-1832; Fick, D. M., Cooper, J. W., Wade, W. E., et al. (2003). Updating the Beers criteria for potentially inappropriate medication use in older adults: Results of a US consensus panel of experts. *Arch Intern Med, 163*(22), 2716-2724; Zhan, C., Sangl, J., Bierman, A. S., et al. (2001). Potentially inappropriate medication use in the community-dwelling elderly: Findings from the 1996 Medical Expenditure Panel Survey. *JAMA, 286*(22), 2823-2829. © 2011, Pasero C, McCaffery M. May be duplicated for use in clinical practice.

continues to be overused (Kornitzer, Manace, Fischberg, 2006) and misused (Hubbard, Wolfe, 2003) because of lack of knowledge about its pharmacology. Numerous misconceptions about meperidine persist (Table 13-5).

Meperidine has a rapid onset and short duration of action, which would seem to make it an attractive option for limited use, such as IV analgesia for short procedures. Indeed, this is now its most commonly approved use in some institutions, although other opioids, such as fentanyl, hydromorphone, or morphine are usually favored for procedural pain. In low doses (12.5 to 25 mg IV), meperidine also has a role in alleviating the shivering associated with general anesthesia and drugs, such as amphoteracin and some biologic agents; other

Table 13-5 | Misconceptions: Meperidine

Misconception	Correction
Meperidine causes less respiratory depression than morphine.	At equianalgesic doses, opioid analgesics produce equal respiratory depression.
Meperidine is less likely than morphine to cause addiction.	The abuse liability for meperidine is at least as high as that for morphine. In other words, people addicted to opioids find morphine and meperidine equally attractive. Several early reports suggested meperidine may be the more addictive of the two.
Meperidine causes less constriction of the sphincter of Oddi and the biliary tract than does morphine.	Both meperidine and morphine cause constriction of the sphincter of Oddi and the biliary tract. Laboratory studies show that morphine may cause more constriction in animals, but this has never been shown to be clinically relevant in humans. In humans, morphine and meperidine caused a rise in bile duct pressure of 52.7% and 61.3%, respectively.
Meperidine is less constipating than morphine.	Meperidine may be less constipating but only when used on a long-term basis, and long-term use is not recommended.
Long-term clinical experience with meperidine proves it is safe and effective.	Meperidine prescribing has declined, but the drug continues to be used despite ample evidence that it has no advantages over other opioids and has toxicities that make it undesirable for almost any use. Historically, therapeutic doses (e.g., 100 mg IM for adults) were seldom used, and studies show that during decades of use, many patients were undertreated for pain. Furthermore, problems may have gone unnoticed because the existence of the metabolite normeperidine was not known and patients were not assessed for signs of neurotoxicity. Meperidine cannot be used safely if pain is treated aggressively.
Meperidine is the only drug effective for treatment of perioperative and postdelivery shivering.	Although low-dose meperidine is widely used to treat perioperative and post-delivery shivering, other drugs are also effective. These include clonidine, ondansetron, and tramadol.

IM, Intramuscular; *mg*, milligram.

Meperidine (Demerol) continues to be used despite sufficient evidence that it is not appropriate as a first-line opioid analgesic for the management of any type of pain.

From Pasero, C., & McCaffery, M. *Pain assessment and pharmacologic management*, p. 337, St. Louis, Mosby. Data from Austin, K. L., Stapleton, J. V., & Mather, L. E. (1980). Relationship between blood meperidine concentrations and analgesic response: A preliminary report. *Anesthesiology, 53*(6), 460-466; Beaulé, P. E., Smith, M. I., & Nguyen, V. N. (2004). Meperidine-induced seizure after revision hip arthroplasty. *J Arthroplasty, 19*(4), 516-519; Burnham, R., McNeil, S., Hegedus, C., et al. (2006). Fibrous myopathy as a complication of repeated intramuscular injection for chronic headache. *Pain Res Manage, 11*(4), 249-252; Coelho, J. C., Senninger, N., Runkel, N., et al. (1986). Effect of analgesic drugs on electromyographic activity of the gastrointestinal tract and sphincter of Oddi and on biliary pressure. *Ann Surg, 204*(1), 53-58; Fong, H. K., Sands, L. P., & Leung, J. M. (2006). The role of postoperative analgesia in delirium and cognitive decline in elderly patients: A systematic review. *Anesth Analg 102*(4), 1255-1266; Hubbard, G. P., & Wolfe, K. R. (2003). Meperidine misuse in a patient with sphincter of Oddi dysfunction. *Ann Pharmacother, 37*(4), 534-537; Kornitzer, B. S., Manace, L. C., Fischberg, D. J., et al. (2006). Prevalence of meperidine use in older surgical patients. *Arch Surg, 141*(8), 76-81; Latta, K. S., Ginsberg, B., & Barkin, R. L. (2002). Meperidine: A critical review. *Am J Ther, 9*(1), 53-68; Lee, F., & Cundiff, D. (1998). Meperidine vs morphine in pancreatitis and cholecystitis. *Arch Intern Med, 158*(21), 2399; Mohta, M., Kumari, N., Tyagi, A., et al. (2009). Tramadol for prevention of postanaesthetic shivering: A randomised double-blind comparison with pethidine. *Anaesthesia, 64*(2), 141-146; Kranke, P., Eberhart, L. H., Roewer, N., et al. (2004). Single-dose parenteral pharmacological interventions for prevention of postoperative shivering: A quantitative systematic review of randomized controlled trials. *Anesth Analg, 99*(3), 718-727; Radnay, P. A., Brodman, E., Mankikar, D., et al. (1980). The effect of equianalgesic doses of fentanyl, morphine, meperidine, and pentazocine on common bile duct pressure. *Anaesthetist 29*, 26-29; Schwarzkopf, K. R. G., Hoff, H., Hartmann, M., et al. (2001). A comparison between meperidine, clonidine and urapidil in the treatment of postanesthetic shivering. *Anesth Analg, 92*(1), 257-260. © 2011, Pasero C, McCaffery M. May be duplicated for use in clinical practice.

agents, including clonidine, ondansetron, and tramadol, among others, are also effective for treatment of shivering (Kranke, Eberhart, Roewer, et al., 2004; Mohta, Kumari, Tyagi, et al., 2009; Schwarzkopf, Hoff, Hartmann, et al., 2001).

Meperidine is one fourth as potent orally as parenterally (APS, 2003). By the SC and IM routes, it has an onset of action of 10 minutes, a peak effect of 30 minutes, and a duration of up to 4 hours. When given orally, the analgesic effects of meperidine are felt within 30 minutes. Its peak effect is within 1 to 2 hours, and its duration of action is approximately 3 hours (Latta, Ginsberg, Barkin, 2002). Regardless of route, it has a half-life of 2 to 3 hours. Although absorbed by all routes of administration, the rate of absorption is erratic after IM injec-

tion, with a wide range of peak plasma concentrations (Gutstein, Akil, 2006; Latta, Ginsberg, Barkin, 2002). In addition, repeated IM injection is associated with fibrous myopathy (Burnham, McNeil, Hegedus, et al., 2006; Latta, Ginsberg, Barkin, 2002) (see Tables 13-1 and 13-5; also see Table 16-1 on pp. 444-446).

A major drawback to the use of meperidine is its active metabolite, normeperidine (Latta, Ginsberg, Barkin, 2002). Normeperidine is a CNS stimulant and can cause delirium, irritability, tremors, myoclonus, muscle twitches, shaky feelings, and generalized seizures (Simopoulos, Smith, Peeters-Asdourian, et al., 2002). Because normeperidine is eliminated by the kidneys, meperidine should not be used in patients with decreased renal function (APS, 2003; Latta, Ginsberg,

Barkin, 2002; Simopoulos, Smith, Peeters-Asdourian, et al., 2002). It is a particularly poor choice in older patients and individuals with sickle cell disease because most have some degree of renal insufficiency. Because normeperidine has a half-life that is usually more than four times longer than meperidine itself, repeated dosing leads to an initial accumulation of normeperidine. This accumulation increases the risk of normeperidine toxicity during the early period (first several days) of repetitive dosing with meperidine. The effects of normeperidine have been observed even in young, otherwise healthy patients given sufficiently high doses of meperidine postoperatively (Simopoulos, Smith, Peeters-Asdourian, et al., 2002). The risk of toxicity overall, particularly risk that increases in the setting of progressive renal insufficiency, has led to the recommendation that meperidine should not be prescribed for patients requiring long-term opioid treatment, such as those with persistent cancer or noncancer pain (Hanks, Cherny, Fallon, 2004; Miaskowski, Cleary, Burney, et al., 2005).

Research shows that meperidine is more likely than other opioid drugs to cause delirium in postoperative patients of all ages (Fong, Sands, Leung, 2006). In a case-control study (N = 91 with 1 to 2 controls) meperidine more than doubled the risk of delirium when given either epidurally or IV (Marcantonio, Juarez, Goldman, et al., 1994). It has also been suggested to have a relatively severe negative impact on mood (Latta, Ginsberg, Barkin, 2002), which is sometimes the first sign of neurotoxicity. A prospective, randomized controlled study found that IV meperidine produced more nausea and vomiting than IV morphine in 200 women following gynecologic surgery (Ezri, Lurie, Stein, et al., 2002).

The most appropriate candidates for meperidine use are patients with acute pain who are otherwise healthy and do not tolerate other opioids, such as morphine and hydromorphone (Simopoulos, Smith, Peeters-Asdourian, et al., 2002), or those with normal renal function who already have demonstrated a favorable outcome with meperidine. If meperidine is used in these patients, frequent high doses should be avoided, the course of treatment should be restricted to no more than 2 days if possible, and the total daily dose should be limited to 600 mg (APS, 2003). A similar guideline, based on a retrospective chart review, is proposed when meperidine is given via PCA to patients unable to take morphine or hydromorphone: 10 mg/kg/day for no more than 3 days in patients with normal renal function (Simopoulos, Smith, Peeters-Asdourian, et al., 2002).

Patients who are taking meperidine should be evaluated frequently, probably every 8 to 12 hours, for signs of CNS irritability, specifically restlessness, shakiness, tremors, twitching, and jerking. Tremors are assessed by asking patients to stretch out their arms in front and noting a postural tremor in the hands. Patients should also be questioned about being awakened at night by twitching or jerking. If symptoms are present and have occurred after the initiation of meperidine doses, they may be due to normeperidine toxicity. The patient should be switched to another opioid analgesic, such as morphine or hydromorphone. Further accumulation of normeperidine may result in seizures (Beaule, Smith, Nguyen, 2004).

Because the half-life of the normeperidine is much longer than that of the meperidine, and the depressant effects of the latter drug may be partially suppressing the effects of the former, symptoms of toxicity may paradoxically worsen as the dose of meperidine is initially decreased. Naloxone should be avoided because it does not reverse the action of normeperidine and may even exacerbate the CNS hyperexcitability by decreasing the level of the depressant meperidine (Gordon, Jones, Goshman, et al., 2000). If meperidine has been used repeatedly and there are signs of toxicity, careful monitoring is necessary if the dose is suddenly lowered or if, in rare circumstances, naloxone is needed; if increased agitation or tremulousness appears, consideration should be given to administration of a sedative-hypnotic or an anticonvulsant.

Meperidine is frequently dosed inadequately, which may be one of the reasons it has been considered a safe drug despite ample evidence to the contrary (Latta, Ginsberg, Barkin, 2002). The habitual under-dosing is somewhat surprising since meperidine has relatively low potency and a very short duration of action (Latta, Ginsberg, Barkin, 2002). In one study, a 75 mg parenteral dose was found to be effective for only 30 minutes (Fairlie, Marshall, Walker, et al., 1999). In another study, a 50 mg parenteral dose was found to be no more effective than placebo (Austin, Stapleton, Mather, 1980a). The initial optimal dose of meperidine recommended for adults with moderate to severe pain is 75 to 100 mg, with some adults requiring 150 mg. The effective interval between doses ranges from 2 to 4 hours, with 3 hours as the average. These doses would quickly exceed the 600 mg/24 h maximum recommended by the APS and produce numerous adverse effects.

As mentioned, meperidine can be administered by the oral route, but just as with the parenteral route, it is rarely dosed appropriately. Oral meperidine is less than one fourth as potent as parenteral meperidine. This means that if a patient is receiving 75 mg of meperidine by the IV or IM route over a 3- to 4-hour period, 300 mg orally would be required to produce equianalgesia (see Table 16-1 on pp. 444-446). Even if the patient's pain had decreased by 50% at the time the switch was made from parenteral to oral, 150 mg would be required orally. Obviously, doses required for analgesia by the oral route produce a significant risk of accumulation of normeperidine (Latta, Ginsberg, Barkin, 2002), making oral meperidine inappropriate for any type of pain management.

Meperidine is contraindicated in children, older adults, patients with impaired renal function, and those who have taken MAOIs in the past 14 days (APS, 2003; Gutstein,

Akil, 2006). It is also contraindicated in patients with untreated hypothyroidism, Addison's disease, benign prostatic hypertrophy, or urethral stricture. It should be used with extreme caution in patients with preexisting convulsive disorders and in patients with atrial flutter or other supraventricular tachycardias (Antonopolous, Bollinger, Goshman, 1996).

Meperidine continues to be commonly used for procedural analgesia, particularly for GI procedures, based on the misconception that it produces less biliary spasm than other opioids (Lee, Cundiff, 1998) (see Table 13-5). It is important to note that all opioids are capable of causing constriction of the sphincter of Oddi and the biliary tract, and there is no clinical advantage to using meperidine from this perspective (see Chapter 19 for a detailed discussion).

In summary, meperidine has no advantages over any other opioid (Latta, Ginsberg, Barkin, 2002) and it has no place in the treatment of persistent pain or in delivery systems such as PCA. Oral meperidine undergoes extensive first-pass metabolism, leaving the patient with poor analgesia but even more rapid normeperidine accumulation than the IV preparation (Latta, Ginsberg, Barkin, 2002). In healthy adults, meperidine should not be used for more than 48 hours or at doses exceeding 600 mg/24 h (APS, 2003). Given the multiple alternative opioids available, there is little rationale to continue using meperidine as an analgesic except in extraordinary cases.

Meperidine Use in Sickle Cell Patients

Although meperidine has been used for many years to treat pain in patients with sickle cell disease, it is a particularly poor choice in this population because the toxic metabolite is renally excreted and most individuals with sickle cell disease have renal insufficiency. Current guidelines recommend morphine as the opioid of choice for treatment of sickle cell pain (Platt, Eckman, Beasley, et al., 2002; Rees, Olujohungbe, Parker, et al., 2003). The Georgia Comprehensive Sickle Cell Center, well known for its research and clinical treatment of sickle cell disease, provides a protocol for rapid management of pain that includes IV morphine 3 to 5 mg every 10 minutes until pain is controlled plus IV ketorolac, followed by IV PCA morphine (with basal rate as needed) or ATC oral morphine dosing (Platt, Eckman, Beasley, et al., 2002). A common and recommended practice is to store a specified number of PCA pumps, drug reservoirs, and infusion tubings (number is dependent on the size of the institution) in the emergency department so that the therapy can be initiated without delay in sickle cell patients as well as other patients who are admitted for treatment of severe pain crises.

The British Committee for Standards in Haematology General Haematology Task Force by the Sickle Cell Working Party guideline calls for rapid assessment and treatment of painful episodes, a designated nursing staff who are trained and experienced with the management of patients with sickle cell disease, and multidisciplinary consultation as needed (Rees, Olujohungbe, Parker, et al., 2003). The guideline recommends treatment of acute pain based on pain intensity (see Chapter 12 for the WHO Ladder) and a multimodal approach that includes IV morphine titration (0.1 mg/kg every 20 minutes until pain is controlled) plus acetaminophen and NSAIDs, such as IV ketorolac. Ongoing analgesia is also based on pain intensity and may include nonopioids for mild to moderate pain and long-acting opioids with short-acting opioid breakthrough doses for more severe pain. Anticonvulsants are considered if neuropathic pain is present.

Patients who have received meperidine in the past may be resistant to changing from meperidine to safer analgesics, such as morphine. Understandably, patients will request what has been effective in relieving their pain in the past. It is important for clinicians to have patience and realize that change can be frightening especially when it occurs during a painful episode. Providing pain relief by the method preferred by the patient and then discussing changes in the treatment plan after pain is controlled is apt to be met with more patient acceptance (see Section II).

Methadone

Methadone (Dolophine; Methadose) is a unique opioid analgesic that may have advantages over other opioids in carefully selected and closely monitored patients (Table 13-6). In all countries except Germany, methadone is sold as a racemic mixture containing two mirror-image molecules—the l-isomer and the d-isomer. The l-isomer of methadone is a mu receptor agonist that has properties similar to other mu agonists but also has a long and variable half-life. The d-isomer of methadone is not an opioid compound, but instead, is an antagonist at the N-methyl-D-aspartate (NMDA) receptor. Based on extensive preclinical science, it is believed that NMDA receptor antagonism has the potential to produce analgesic effects independent of the opioid effect, at least in some neuropathic pain states; it also has been shown in animal models to reduce opioid tolerance. The combined effects of the l-isomer and d-isomer lead to effects from methadone that may be different than other opioids and potentially may make it a useful choice as a second- or third-line opioid for syndromes that have been poorly responsive to other opioids, including neuropathic pain syndromes (Dworkin, O'Connor, Backonja, et al., 2007). In other words, these effects may make methadone a favorable drug to consider when planning opioid rotation (switching) to an alternative opioid in the setting of poor opioid responsiveness due to inadequate analgesia (Mannino, Coyne, Swainey, et al., 2006) or when unacceptable adverse effects occur (Manfredi, Houde, 2003) (see Chapter 18).

Given the observation that up to 80% of cancer patients will require rotation to another opioid during the course of pain treatment and that 44% may need

Table 13-6 | Methadone Advantages and Disadvantages

Advantages	Disadvantages
Multiple mechanisms of action • Agonist at mu, delta, and kappa opioid receptors • NMDA receptor antagonist • Serotonin and norepinephrine reuptake inhibitor	Very wide interindividual pharmacokinetic and pharmacodynamic variability
Recommended for neuropathic as well as nociceptive pain	Long half-life and wide distribution may cause accumulation and potential toxicity with improper prescribing and/or inadequate monitoring
Onset of action comparable to morphine (30 to 60 minutes)	Large number of drug-drug interactions due to metabolism by multiple CYP450 pathways
Prolonged analgesia (usually 8 to 12 hours but for some patients only 6 hours) once steady state is reached	Variable dose ratio when converting from other opioids
Increased effectiveness with long-term dosing	No consensus on best procedure for switching from another opioid; requires specific expertise or consultation with expert
Excellent option when rotating from other opioids due to ineffectiveness or adverse effects	Not appropriate for use in pain emergency
Oral bioavailability of 85%	Requires patient/family who can remain adherent to prescribed regimen
No neurotoxic metabolites	Requires close monitoring, especially during titration phase
May be used in most patients with renal insufficiency	Tablets are available only in 5 and 10 mg strengths*
May be used in most patients with hepatic insufficiency	Potential for QTc prolongation and torsade de pointes
Relative potency of methadone increases with rising dose of other opioid (dose ratio decreases as prior opioid dose increases)	Reluctance to prescribe and use due to perceived stigma of a drug used to treat addiction
Relatively inexpensive	
Multiple routes of administration*	
May be alternative when patient is allergic to other opioids (is structurally unrelated to other opioids)	
May be less constipating than morphine and hydromorphone	
Available in tablet, parenteral, and liquid formulations; may be compounded for rectal administration*	

*Available dose forms/strengths may vary in different countries.
From Pasero, C., & McCaffery, M. (2011). *Pain assessment and pharmacologic management*, p. 340, St. Louis, Mosby. Data from Daeninck, P. J., & Bruera, E. (1999). Reduction in constipation and laxative requirements following opioid rotation to methadone: A report of four cases. *J Pain Symptom Manage, 18*(4), 303-309; Davis, M. P., & Walsh, D. (2001). Methadone for relief of cancer pain: A review of pharmacokinetics, pharmacodynamics, drug interactions and protocols of administration. *Support Care Cancer, 9*(2), 73-83; Krantz, M. J., Martin, J., Stimmel, B., et al. (2009). QTc interval screening in methadone treatment. *Ann Intern Med, 150*(6), 387-395; Lynch, M. E. (2005). A review of the use of methadone for the treatment of chronic noncancer pain. *Pain Res Manag, 10*(3), 133-144; Mannino, R., Coyne, P., Swainey, C., et al. (2006). Methadone for cancer-related neuropathic pain: A review of the literature. *J Opioid Manage, 2*(5), 269-276; Weschules, D. J., & Bain, K. T. (2008). A systematic review of opioid conversion ratios used with methadone for the treatment of pain. *Pain Med, 9*(5), 595-612. © 2011, Pasero C, McCaffery M, Quinn TE. May be duplicated for use in clinical practice.

more than one switch (Foley, Houde, 1998), methadone could potentially assume an important role in long-term opioid therapy. In a prospective controlled trial, 25% of patients were considered nonresponders to morphine, but after one, two, or three switches to alternative opioids, 96% of patients were able to achieve adequate analgesia with tolerable adverse effects (Riley, Ross, Rutter, et al., 2006). A 10-year review of opioid switching showed a dozen studies in which the range of success in switching from another opioid to methadone was 75% to 100% (Mercadante, Bruera, 2006).

Methadone is most often used by the oral route for persistent cancer and noncancer-related pain. Although usually considered a second- or third-line treatment (Mannino, Coyne, Swainey, et al., 2006; Fredheim, Moksnes, Borchgrevink, et al., 2008), some experts suggest that methadone can be used as a first-line opioid for cancer pain (Bruera, Palmer, Bosnjak, et al., 2004; Mercadante, Porzio, Ferrera, et al., 2008) and some types of neuropathic pain (Dworkin, O'Connor, Backonja, et al., 2007; Mannino, Coyne, Swainey, et al., 2006; Raja, Haythornthwaite, Pappagallo, et al., 2002).

For many people, the more familiar use of methadone is as maintenance therapy to reduce craving and prevent withdrawal in patients with addiction. Despite significantly increased use of methadone as an analgesic, some patients are reluctant to take it because of the perceived stigma of taking a medication that is used by opioid addicts (Davis, Walsh, 2001; Fredheim, Moksnes, Borchgrevink, et al., 2008). It is important to elicit patient and family concerns and provide clarification. The indication ("For Pain") should be written on the prescription to avoid misunderstanding at the pharmacy.

It is extremely important that acute pain episodes, such as following trauma or surgery, be treated adequately in individuals who are taking methadone, including those who are receiving it for treatment of addictive disease. Individuals with addiction have been observed to have exaggerated pain responses (Savage, Schofferman, 1995), which may necessitate frequent dose adjustments if pain is treated with an opioid (Peng, Tumber, Gourlay, 2005; Savage, Schofferman, 1995). (See further discussion of pain in individuals with addictive disease in Chapter 20.)

After an oral dose, methadone has an onset of analgesia comparable to morphine (30 to 60 minutes). Plasma concentrations peak at approximately 2 hours after oral administration (Davis, Walsh, 2001). Methadone is extensively metabolized in the liver via the cytochrome P450 enzyme system, which has important implications for drug-drug interactions (see the paragraphs that follow and Box 11-1). Its oral bioavailability is 80% to 85%, which is significantly higher than that of morphine. This is reflected in a lower parenteral/oral potency ratio of 1:2 compared with 1:6 for morphine for initial dosing in an opioid-naïve patient. The elimination half-life of methadone is long and highly variable (5 to 130 hours; mean 20 to 35) (Lugo, Satterfield, Kern, 2005).

Methadone does not have neurotoxic metabolites, unlike morphine and hydromorphone. It may be less likely to cause severe constipation than other opioids, but this has not been confirmed (Daeninck, Bruera, 1999; Leppert, 2009). Methadone is synthetic and structurally unrelated to other opioids, and for this reason, it may be an alternative for the rare patient with a true allergy to another opioid.

Although methadone usually is administered orally (tablets and liquid are available), it can be given intravenously, intramuscularly, subcutaneously, sublingually, rectally, and topically. A guideline for the use of parenteral methadone in pain and palliative care has been published (Shaiova, Berger, Blinderman, et al., 2008). Most published reports on continuous SC administration indicate that local irritation is a significant management problem (Makin, 2000; Mathew, Storey, 1999; Centeno, Vara, 2005); flushing of the access site with normal saline has been reported to minimize irritation so that sites can be maintained for prolonged periods without the need for dose limitation or medications added to prevent irritation (Hum, Fainsinger, Bielech, 2007) (see Chapter 14 for the SC route). Although a commercial product is not available, rectal administration of methadone is very effective. The rectal to oral dose ratio is 1:1, with rapid absorption (Davis, Walsh, 2001). Methadone has been investigated for breakthrough pain via both oral and sublingual routes. In a pilot study, all patients reported that oral methadone was at least as effective as their usual breakthrough opioid, and remarkably, some reported onset of analgesia in as short as 10 minutes. The authors acknowledged

that an explanation for such rapid relief is uncertain (Fisher, Stiles, Hagen, 2004). A pilot study of liquid sublingual methadone for breakthrough pain demonstrated a median time to meaningful pain reduction of 5 minutes (Hagen, Fisher, Stiles, 2007).

As described previously, the racemic mixture of methadone, which is available in the United States and most other countries, has multiple mechanisms of action. The opioid constituent, which is primarily an agonist at the mu opioid receptor, also has agonist effects at the delta and kappa receptors, which may contribute to analgesia (Davis, Walsh, 2001). In morphine-insensitive mice, methadone provided analgesia via the mu receptor, indicating that methadone and morphine occupy the mu receptor differently (Chang, Emmel, Rossi, et al., 1998). It also suggests a partial explanation for the observed incomplete cross-tolerance between methadone and morphine (and other opioids) (Pasternak, 2001). Clinically this means that when switching from another opioid to methadone, the effective methadone dose will be lower than predicted by equianalgesic calculations (Davis, Walsh, 2001).

Methadone's analgesia also may be related to its antagonism of the NMDA receptor (Manfredi, Houde, 2003; Trafton, Ramani, 2009). This mechanism, which may involve both a direct analgesic effect and a partial reversal of opioid tolerance, is likely to be another factor that produces analgesia at lower than expected doses. The proposed mechanisms for reduced development of tolerance by methadone compared with other opioids is suggested by animal studies but have not yet been conclusively demonstrated in humans (Trafton, Ramani, 2009; Leppert, 2009).

Finally, the analgesic effects of methadone could be related to its inhibition of the reuptake of serotonin and norepinephrine at central synapses. Serotonin/norepinephrine reuptake inhibitors have been found to be effective in alleviating neuropathic pain, similar to NMDA receptor antagonism (Manfredi, Houde, 2003) (see Section I and Chapter 22). Although there is no evidence that methadone is more effective for neuropathic pain than other opioid drugs, it has been speculated that these unique mechanisms on other receptors may yield such an effect. More research is needed to determine whether there are drug-selective differences in opioid efficacy for neuropathic pain.

Another important methadone characteristic is its lipophilicity. Methadone readily crosses the blood-brain barrier, is widely distributed throughout the body, and is highly protein-bound (Lynch, 2005). Lipophilicity makes methadone a potential candidate for sublingual (Hagen, Fisher, Stiles, 2007) and topical (Gallagher, Arndt, Hunt, 2005) administration.

The duration of analgesia after an oral dose of methadone usually is just 3 to 6 hours, particularly in those who have not been receiving regular doses (Davis, Walsh, 2001; Lugo, Satterfield, Kern, 2005; Bruera, Palmer, Bosnjak, et al., 2004); it may extend to 8 to 12 hours (or longer) with continued dosing. The half-life, as noted previously, typically is about 24 hours and has an upper limit more than 6 times this duration. These characteristics impact clinical management, especially during the initial titration phase. After dosing begins, or is increased, accumulation may occur for many days, or even weeks, before a steady state is approached. Clearance can increase with long-term dosing (Davis, Walsh, 2001). Even after accumulation, some patients may continue to need dosing four times a day (Peng, Tumber, Stafford, et al., 2008). These characteristics are manageable, but require close attention, as described in the following paragraphs and in Box 13-2. Some authors suggest that a few "priming" (Mercadante, Casuccio, Fulfaro, et al., 2001) or "loading" (Ayonrinde, Bridge, 2000; Blackburn, Somerville, Squire, 2002) doses on the first day or two of treatment will decrease the amount of time it takes to distribute the drug and reach steady state.

Elimination of methadone is primarily via feces. Unlike morphine and hydromorphone, there are no methadone toxic metabolites to accumulate in renal failure, and dose adjustment in the presence of renal insufficiency is generally not necessary (Davis, Walsh, 2001). However, as with other opioids, initial doses for older adults should be lower and dosing intervals longer than for healthy younger adults (Lugo, Satterfield, Kern, 2005); the half-life in older adults is likely to be relatively longer than in younger patients (Leppert W, 2009). Some methadone metabolism occurs in the intestine rather than the liver. Therefore, methadone doses may not need to be adjusted in cirrhosis and stable chronic liver disease (Lugo, Satterfield, Kern, 2005).

Drug-Drug Interactions

One of the major safety and clinical management limitations of methadone is the large number of medications with which it interacts. However, these drug interactions are still poorly understood in that many of the reports are theoretical and not clinically supported with case reports or clinical trials (Weschules, Bain, Richeimer, 2008; Gourevitch, Friedland, 2000). It is important to remember as well that these pharmacokinetic interactions may be compounded by pharmacodynamic interactions, or effects that are overlapping but have nothing to do with changes in blood levels. For example, methadone and benzodiazepines both cause sedation and should be used together with caution (Webster, Choi, Desai et al., 2008).

Box 13-2 | Summary of Clinically Important Methadone Characteristics

- Highly lipophilic
  - Oral bioavailability 85%
  - Wide distribution
  - Readily crosses blood-brain barrier
- Highly protein bound
- Wide distribution due to lipophilicity and protein binding
  - Slow elimination
  - Long but highly variable half-life (5 to 100+ hours; average 20 hours)
  - Accumulation and potential resultant toxicity
- Short duration of action (4 to 6 hours) with initial dosing; longer duration (8 to 12 hours) with accumulation
- When switching from another opioid (e.g., morphine), the morphine-methadone dose ratio varies with the morphine dose; methadone potency increases significantly as the morphine dose increases; published dose ratios vary from 4:1 (less than 90 mg morphine/day) to 20:1 (more than 1000 mg morphine/day)
- Multiple analgesic mechanisms of action
  - Active at mu, kappa, and delta opioid receptors
  - NMDA receptor antagonist
    Effective in neuropathic pain states
    Potential decreased level of physiologic tolerance
  - Serotonin and norepinephrine reuptake inhibitor
- Elimination mostly via nonrenal routes; dose adjustment not normally necessary for renal insufficiency

- Urine pH affects excretion: Urine pH less than 6 increases urinary excretion of methadone
- Metabolism in intestines as well as liver; dose adjustment not normally required in hepatic failure
- Wide interindividual variability in pharmacokinetics and response
- Large number of drug-drug interactions mediated by cytochrome (CY) P450 system (primarily via C4A, but also 2D6 and 1A2; other CYP450 enzymes may have a smaller role in metabolism)
- Potential for cardiac arrhythmia, especially at methadone doses more than 100 mg/day (extended QTc interval with potential to induce torsades de pointes)
- No active metabolites

From Pasero, C., & McCaffery, M. (2011). *Pain assessment and pharmacologic management*, p. 342, St. Louis, Mosby. Data from Davis, M. P., & Walsh, D. (2001). Methadone for relief of cancer pain: A review of pharmacokinetics, pharmacodynamics, drug interactions and protocols of administration. *Support Care Cancer, 9*(2), 73-83; Fredheim, O. M., Moksnes, K., Borchgrevink, P. C., et al. (2008). Clinical pharmacology of methadone for pain. *Acta Anaesthesiol Scand, 52*(7), 879-889; Krantz, M. J., Martin, J., Stimmel, B., et al. (2009). QTc interval screening in methadone treatment. *Ann Intern Med, 150*(6), 387-395; Lynch, M. E. (2005). A review of the use of methadone for the treatment of chronic noncancer pain. *Pain Res Manag, 10*(3), 133-144; Mannino, R., Coyne, P., Swainey, C., et al. (2006). Methadone for cancer-related neuropathic pain: A review of the literature. *J Opioid Manage, 2*(5), 269-276; Mercadante, S., & Bruera, E. (2006). Opioid switching: A systematic and critical review. *Cancer Treat Rev, 32*(4), 304-315; Weschules, D. J., & Bain, K. T. (2008). A systematic review of opioid conversion ratios used with methadone for the treatment of pain. *Pain Med, 9*(5), 595-612. © 2011, Quinn TE, Pasero C, McCaffery M. May be duplicated for use in clinical practice.

The monoamine oxidase inhibitors (MAOIs) should be avoided in patients receiving methadone because of the risk of inducing serotonin syndrome (Weschules, Bain, Richeimer, 2008; Leavitt, 2005, 2006) (see Chapter 22). Methadone is partially metabolized in the liver via multiple cytochrome P450 (CYP450) pathways, primarily CYP3A4, but also CYP1A2 and CYP2D6. Most methadone drug-drug interactions are related to CYP3A4 (Davis, Walsh, 2001). Methadone has the potential to induce or inhibit the metabolism of other drugs that use the same pathways. In turn, methadone metabolism can be induced or inhibited by drugs that use these enzyme pathways (see Chapter 11). Inducing metabolism has the effect of lowering serum concentration and decreasing the intended effect. Inhibiting metabolism has the effect of increasing serum concentration and increasing the intended effect or causing toxicity (Armstrong, Cozza, Sandson, 2003; Weschules, Bain, Richeimer, 2008). In the case of methadone, decreasing serum concentration may cause an increase in pain or even cause withdrawal syndrome. Increasing methadone serum concentration can cause adverse effects such as sedation and respiratory depression. The potential for either toxicity or undermedication and withdrawal from the previous opioid may be substantial in some instances (Lugo, Satterfield, Kern, 2005). A known food interaction (grapefruit juice inhibits gut-wall

CYP3A4) and herb interaction (St. John's wort induces CYP3A4 metabolism) further underscores the complexity of methadone and reinforces the need for thorough history taking and patient teaching (Armstrong, Wynn, Sandson, 2009; Zhou, Chan, Pan, et al., 2004). A drug interaction should be suspected whenever a new drug or remedy is introduced and there is a sudden increase in pain or increase in sedation when the methadone dose is stable.

Sharing a metabolic pathway is not an absolute contraindication for two drugs being taken concurrently, but close observation is necessary and dose adjustment of one medication may be required. Alternative medications with the same intended effect and which are metabolized differently should also be considered (Weschules, Bain, Richeimer, 2008) (Table 13-7). A particularly complex population is patients with HIV/AIDS. Research has shown that interactions are common between methadone and antiretroviral therapies and certain other medications commonly used in this population (Gourevitch, Friedland, 2000; Bruce, Altice, Gourevitch et al., 2006).

Renal excretion of methadone is affected by urine pH. Methadone renal clearance is increased three-fold in a low pH environment (Davis, Walsh, 2001). Medications that lower urine pH such as furosemide, and drugs that increase urine pH such as sodium bicarbonate and acetazolamide (Diamox) must therefore be used with caution.

Table 13-7 | Methadone: Drug-Drug Interactions[1]

Medication Class	Selected Medications with Known or Theoretical Interaction with Methadone	Potential Alternatives (Low or No Pharmacokinetic Interaction Potential)
Anticonvulsants	Phenytoin, phenobarbital, carbamazepine	Valproic acid, gabapentin, lamotrigine, levetiracetam
Antidepressants	Fluvoxamine, fluoxetine, paroxetine, desipramine, amitriptyline, imipramine	Sertraline, citalopram, escitalopram, venlafaxine, mirtazapine
Neuroleptics	Risperidone	Olanzapine
Anxiolytics	Alprazolam, diazepam	Buspirone, lorazepam, oxazepam, triazolam
H$_2$ receptor blockers	Cimetidine	Famotidine, ranitidine
Antituberculosis antibiotics	Rifamycins (e.g., rifampin)	Rifabutin
Antifungals	Ketoconazole, fluconazole, itraconazole	Terbinafine, caspofungin
Macrolide antibiotics	Erythromycin, clarithromycin	Azithromycin
Quinolone antibiotics	Ciprofloxacin	Levofloxacin
Antiretrovirals	Most	See Bruce et al. and Gourevitch et al. below for extensive discussion of management

[1]This table contains selected drugs and their potential for interaction with methadone. It is not a comprehensive list and is meant to be a quick reference for clinicians treating multiple diagnoses.
From Pasero, C., & McCaffery, M. (2011). *Pain assessment and pharmacologic management*, p. 343, St. Louis, Mosby. Data from Bruce, R. D., Altice, F. L., Gourevitch, M. N., et al. (2006). Pharmacokinetic drug interactions between opioid agonist therapy and antiretroviral medications: implications and management for clinical practice. *J Acquir Immune Defic Syndr, 41*(5), 563-572; Gourevitch, M. N., & Friedland, G. H. (2000).

Interactions between methadone and medications used to treat HIV infection: A review. *Mt Sinai J Med, 67*(5-6), 429-436; Leavitt, S. B. (2005). *Methadone-drug interactions*, ed 3. Addiction Treatment Forum. Available at http://www.atforum.com/SiteRoot/pages/addiction_resources/Drug_Interactions.pdf. Accessed December 20, 2009; Leppert, W. (2009). The role of methadone in cancer pain treatment—A review. *Int J Clin Pract, 63*(7), 1095-1109; Weschules, D. J., Bain, K.T., & Richeimer, S. (2008). Actual and potential drug interactions associated with methadone. *Pain Med, 9*(3), 315-344. © 2011, Quinn TE, Pasero C, McCaffery M. May be duplicated for use in clinical practice.

An additional potential concern with methadone and drug-drug interaction that is only partially related to its metabolic pathway is an association with cardiac arrhythmia, specifically, prolongation of the QTc interval seen on electrocardiogram (ECG). A critically prolonged QTc interval—one greater than 500 ms—can lead to the potentially fatal cardiac arrhythmic disorder torsades de pointes (Krantz, Martin, Stimmel, et al., 2009). Many drugs, including methadone, can prolong the interval and potentially increase this risk (University of Arizona, 2009).

The U.S. FDA issued an *FDA Alert* in 2006 to warn health professionals about the potential for cardiac arrhythmias with methadone use (United States Food and Drug Administration, 2006). The risk of QTc prolongation is presumably dose-dependent and related to other factors, including co-morbid heart disease, the use of other drugs with effects on cardiac conduction, and genetic factors. The degree of risk must be balanced with severity of pain and goals of care (Moryl, Coyle, Foley, 2008; Sekine, Obens, Coyle, et al., 2007).

There is no consensus on routine screening with ECG prior to starting methadone (Schmittner, Krantz, 2006; Cruciani, 2008). It is prudent to obtain an ECG if the patient has a history of significant heart disease or if the patient is older. Routine serial ECG is recommended by one recent guideline (Krantz, Martin, Stimmel, et al., 2009), but is considered controversial (Gourevitch, 2009). Periodic ECG monitoring of patients on doses of methadone greater than 100 mg/day also has been recommended (Krantz, Martin, Stimmel, et al., 2009).

Rotating to Methadone

Safely switching a patient from another opioid to methadone is a clinical challenge (Fine, Portenoy, Ad Hoc Expert Panel on Evidence Review and Guidelines for Opioid Rotation, 2009) (Box 13-3; also see Patient Examples). The most common reason for making the switch is adverse effects from the previous opioid. Another reason is ineffectiveness of another opioid despite appropriate titration. Because of its long half-life, the titration of methadone takes at least several days, during which strict adherence to the dose and schedule are required and close monitoring of the patient is essential. A short-acting opioid may be used for breakthrough pain (Lugo, Satterfield, Kern, 2005). Careful patient selection and clear instructions are required.

Determining the starting morphine to methadone dose ratio and using a systematic method of patient selection and monitoring are related but distinct elements of the conversion process. Factors to consider in planning the switch:

- Onset of action is comparable to other oral opioids, about 30 to 60 minutes.
- Duration of analgesia with acute dosing (e.g., the beginning of the titration period) is 4 to 6 hours.

- Duration of analgesia with long-term dosing may be 8 to 12 hours or longer.
- Peak effect is at about 2.5 hours.
- Steady state will not be reached for several days, and in occasional patients with longer half-lives, as long as several weeks.
- Drug accumulation occurs during initial titration when the concentration in the blood continues to increase above the effective analgesic level and into the toxic range as a result of the relatively prolonged period required to approach steady state. Toxic accumulation is more likely if a relatively high dose or short dosing interval is used in an effort to quickly identify an analgesic dose; accumulation-related adverse effects can include excessive sedation and respiratory depression.
- Clinical experience indicates that the greatest incidence of serious adverse effects occurs on days 3 to 5. There is great interindividual pharmacokinetic variability.
- There is no fixed equianalgesic ratio between methadone and other opioids, contrary to the experience with most other opioids.

It is now widely agreed among pain specialists that published equianalgesic dose tables that include methadone do not reflect the pharmacology of methadone and the clinical reality of patient management (Knotkova, Fine, Portenoy, 2009; Pereira, Lawlor, Vigano, et al., 2001). Several attempts have been made in the past decade to determine the equianalgesic dose ratio of other opioids, principally morphine, to methadone (Mercadante, Bruera, 2006; Benítez-Rosario, Salinas-Martín, Aguirre-Jaime, et al., 2009). It is clear that the new dose of methadone is dependent on the prior dose of morphine, but not in a fixed ratio. As the dose of morphine increases, the equianalgesic dose of methadone decreases (see the discussion of tolerance in Chapter 11 for possible explanations of this phenomenon). This has been described as a "dynamic inverse potency relationship between methadone and other opioids" (Weschules, Bain, 2008). For example, with a daily morphine dose of 80 mg, the morphine to methadone ratio was found to be 4:1 (Ripamonti, Groff, Brunelli, et al., 1998). As the daily morphine dose rises, the morphine to methadone ratio increases to as much as 14:1 or higher (Pereira, Lawlor, Vigano, et al., 2001; Soares, 2005; Ayonrinde, Bridge, 2000). Clinical research-derived tables that match morphine dose ranges to morphine-methadone ratios are in close, but not complete, agreement (see examples in Table 13-8). Use of these tables is intended to find a safe starting dose, but does not predict the final effective methadone dose, which varies widely across patients (Benítez-Rosario, Salinas-Martín, Aguirre-Jaime, et al., 2009).

Attempts have been made to simplify the process of determining the morphine to methadone dose ratio that is necessary to calculate the starting dose of methadone for

GUIDELINES

Box 13-3 Switching from Another Opioid to Oral Methadone

Note: Consult with an expert in pain management with methadone. Familiarity with methadone and individualization of care are essential to safe management. As shown in Table 13-8, other methods of switching have been published.

PATIENT SELECTION FOR OUTPATIENT INITIATION OF METHADONE FOR PAIN

1. Patients who live alone are generally not good candidates. If the patient lives alone, strong consideration to how monitoring and reporting will occur is necessary.
2. Is the patient reliable? Able to follow instructions? Willing to have daily monitoring by phone?
3. Does the patient have a reliable family member who can monitor and communicate with you? Make sure you have current contact information.
4. Is there a personal or family cardiac history? Consider baseline ECG.
5. Review all current medications for potential drug-drug interactions.
6. Give written instructions (see patient education Form IV-4) as well as a written schedule of doses and times, your contact information during office hours, and when your practice is closed.
7. Confirm the patient's phone number(s), which may be different than what you already have in your records. Make sure you have contact information for at least one family member.

DETERMINE STARTING DOSE

1. Convert current opioid(s) to oral morphine equivalent using standard equianalgesic table.
2. Determine total opioid dose in previous 24 hours (Note: if there has been rapid dose escalation in past few days, consider using the 24-hour dose from the most recent stable day).
3. Match the 24-hour morphine dose to a morphine-methadone dose ratio table to approximate the equianalgesic dose of methadone.

Morphine Dose Range (24 h)	Morphine-Methadone Ratio
Less than or equal to 100 mg	3:1
101-300 mg	5:1
301-600 mg	10:1
601-800 mg	12:1
801-1000 mg	15:1
more than 1000 mg	20:1

From Ayonrinde, O. T., & Bridge, D. T. (2000). The rediscovery of methadone for cancer pain management. *Med J Aust, 173*(10), 536-540.

IMPLEMENT SWITCH

1. Stop the previous scheduled opioid.
2. At the time that the prior opioid dose would have been due, administer the calculated methadone dose (rounded to nearest 2.5 to 5 mg[1]); continue dosing at fixed intervals of 6 hours for the first 24 hours.
3. Extend the interval for subsequent doses to 8 hours.[2]
4. Do not increase the methadone dose for at least 3 days (significant toxicity from accumulation becomes evident on days 3 to 5); may decrease the dose by 50% for excess sedation (consider also skipping a dose; consider increasing the interval to 12 hours).
5. Use a short-acting opioid for breakthrough pain.
6. Monitor patient daily by phone. Assess for pain level, use of breakthrough analgesic, sedation, and any other symptoms.
7. Continue to monitor closely until pain and methadone dose are stable for 3 to 5 days after the last dose or increment adjustment.

---

[1]Methadone is available in 5 and 10 mg tablets.
[2]Experience of 5 or more days with a particular patient may indicate that returning to a 6-hour interval is needed. Most studies report success with 8- to 12-hour dosing.

From Pasero, C., & McCaffery, M. (2011). *Pain assessment and pharmacologic management*, p. 345, St. Louis, Mosby. Data from Ayonrinde, O. T., & Bridge, D. T. (2000). The rediscovery of methadone for cancer pain management. *Med J Aust, 173*(10), 536-540; Davis, M. P., & Walsh, D. (2001). Methadone for relief of cancer pain: A review of pharmacokinetics, pharmacodynamics, drug interactions and protocols of administration. *Support Care Cancer, 9*(2), 73-83; Weschules, D. J., & Bain, K. T. (2008). A systematic review of opioid conversion ratios used with methadone for the treatment of pain. *Pain Med, 9*(5), 595-612; Zimmermann, C., Seccareccia, D., Booth, C. M., et al. (2005). Rotation to methadone after opioid dose escalation: How should individualization of dosing occur? *J Pain Palliat Care Pharmacother, 19*(2), 25-31. *Med J Aust, 173*(10), 536-540; Weschules, D. J., & Bain, K. T. (2008). A systematic review of opioid conversion ratios used with methadone for the treatment of pain. *Pain Med, 9*(5), 595-612; Zimmermann, C., Seccareccia, D., Booth, C. M., et al. (2005). Rotation to methadone after opioid dose escalation: How should individualization of dosing occur? *J Pain Palliat Care Pharmacother, 19*(2), 25-31. © 2011, Quinn TE, Pasero C, McCaffery M. May be duplicated for use in clinical practice.

Table 13-8 | Comparison of Selected Methods of Converting Morphine to Methadone

	Bruera & Sweeney, 2002	Morley & Makin, 1998	Mercadante, et al., 2001	Ayonrinde & Bridge, 2000	Ripamonte et al., 1998	Blackburn et al., 2002	Indelicato & Portenoy, 2002
Conversion ratio (MS*:methadone) (All doses in mg) *MS =morphine sulphate	1:1 (MS dose <100) 10:1 (MS dose >500)	10:1	4:1 (MS dose <90) 8:1 (MS dose 90-300) 12:1 (MS dose >300)	3:1 (MS dose <100) 5:1 (MS dose 101-300) 10:1 (MS dose 301-600) 12:1 (MS dose 601-800) 15:1 (MS dose 801-1000) 20:1 (MS dose >1001)	4:1 (MS dose <90) 8:1 (MS dose 90-300) 12:1 (MS dose >300)	10:1	1.5:1 (oral) 1:1 (parenteral)
Starting dose	10% of daily oral MS dose × 0.33 or 0.5	10% of daily oral MS dose	As above + additional 20%-30% as "priming dose" on day 1-2	As above + additional 25%-50% as "loading dose" × 2 days	10% of daily oral MS dose × 0.33	Loading dose of 1/10 of the total morphine equivalent dose of previous 24 hours; additional loading dose may be given at 12 hours for severe pain. Subsequent doses are ½ of loading dose	Reduce calculated dose by 75%-90%
Starting dose limit	None	30 mg/dose	None	None	None	30 mg/dose	None
Dosing interval	8 hours	q3h PRN × 6 days; then q12h fixed dose based on previous 48 hour total dose	8 hours	6 hours increasing to 8-12 hours over several days	8 hours	12 hours	
Breakthrough interval		As above	Up to 3 doses per day			"Ideally" 3 hours, but may be decreased if necessary or incorporated in the 12-h dose	
Breakthrough drug	Use short-acting drug initially, then 10% of daily methadone	Methadone	Methadone: 1/6 of daily dose	Short-acting opioid	Use short-acting opioid initially, then 10% of daily methadone	Methadone: 1/8 of loading dose	

Gradual substitution vs acute conversion	⅓ – ½ reduction in MS each day for 2-3 days; only increase methadone dose on day 2 or 3 if pain is moderate to severe	Stop previous opioid	Regular doses of previous opioid stopped, but short-acting opioids (morphine or oxycodone) used for breakthrough pain	⅓ reduction in MS each day for 3 days; only increase methadone dose on day 2 or 3 if pain is moderate to severe	Stop previous opioid	
Additional reduction after conversion calculation					Reduce calculated dose by 75%-90%	
Planned conversion period	3 days	6 days	4 days	"Several days"	5+ days; regular 12-h doses should not be increased for 5 days, but may be decreased for toxicity	
Route	Oral or rectal	Oral	Oral			
Study method	Review	Prospective N = 146	Prospective N = 50	Prospective N = 14	Prospective N = 49	Prospective N = 9	Review

N, Number.
From Pasero, C., & McCaffery, M. (2011). *Pain assessment and pharmacologic management*, pp. 346-347. St. Louis, Mosby. Data from Ayonrinde, O. T., & Bridge, D. T. (2000). The rediscovery of methadone for cancer pain management. *Med J Aust*, 173(10), 536-540; Blackburn, D., Somerville, E., & Squire, J. (2002). Methadone: An alternative conversion regime. *Eur J Palliat Care*, 9(3), 92-96; Bruera, E., & Sweeney, C. (2002). Methadone use in cancer patients with pain: A review. *J Palliat Med*, 5(1), 127-138; Indelicato, R. A., & Portenoy, R. K. (2002). Opioid rotation in the management of refractory cancer pain. *J Clin Oncol*, 20(1), 348-352; Mercadante, S., Casuccio, A., Fulfaro, F., et al. (2001). Switching from morphine to methadone to improve analgesia and tolerability in cancer patients: A prospective study. *J Clin Oncol*, 19(11), 2898-2904; Morley, J. S., & Makin, M. K. (1997). Comments on Ripamonti et al. *Pain*, 73(1), 114; Ripamonti, C., Groff, L., Brunelli, C., et al. (1998). Switching from morphine to oral methadone in treating cancer pain: What is the equianalgesic dose ratio? *J Clin Oncol*, 16(10), 3216-3221. © 2011, Quinn TE, Pasero C, McCaffery M. May be duplicated for use in clinical practice.

a particular patient. Nomograms (Toombs, 2008; New Hampshire Hospice and Palliative Care Organization at *http://www.nhhpco.org/opioid.htm*) and formulas (Plonk, 2005) have been derived using values from published research. These methods yield more precise values than matching ratios to a table of dose ranges, but it is not known whether such precision has clinical relevance. In their extensive review, Weschules and Bain (2008) conclude that the actual dose ratio used to determine the starting dose of methadone is probably less important than careful patient selection and close systematic monitoring of the patient during the titration period.

An additional safety consideration is found in the setting of rapid dose escalation of the previous opioid. If the previous opioid dose is relatively stable, any of the morphine-methadone ratio tables described above could be used. However, if the previous opioid has recently been escalated, it may be prudent to use the dose prior to escalation as the starting point for calculating the starting methadone dose in order to avoid methadone adverse effects (Zimmermann, Seccareccia, Booth, et al., 2005).

The dose ratio between methadone and other opioids is not bidirectional. In other words, the ratio used to switch a patient *to* methadone cannot be used to switch a patient *from* methadone to another opioid (Bhimji, 2005; Prommer, 2006a; Walker, Palla, Pei, et al., 2008). Clearly, this area of practice requires clinical expertise, individualization of care, and close monitoring.

There are widely differing approaches to systematically switch a patient to methadone from another opioid (see Table 13-8). There is no evidence of superiority of one conversion method over another (Weschules, Bain, 2008). In general, these regimens can be divided into two groups: a gradual substitution of methadone for the other opioid over 3 days (Bruera, Sweeney, 2002; Ripamonti, Groff, Brunelli, et al., 1998) and completely stopping the previous opioid while initiating titration of methadone ("stop and go" method) (Morley, Makin, 1997; Ayonrinde, Bridge, 2000; Mercadante, Casuccio, Calderone, 1999; Mercadante, Casuccio, Fulfaro, et al., 2001). The latter approach is particularly appropriate if the reason for switching is opioid toxicity and the previous opioid must be stopped quickly.

A consensus guideline (Fine, Portenoy, the Ad Hoc Expert Panel on Evidence Review and Guidelines for Opioid Rotation, 2009) concludes that a two-step approach guided by a careful clinical assessment is a safe strategy when switching from any pure mu agonist opioid to methadone. The first step involves calculation of the equianalgesic dose using a generally accepted equianalgesic table, followed by reduction in this calculated dose by 75% to 90% (with high dose therapy and some other factors suggesting the use of the upper bound of the calculated reduction). After this first step, a possible second step is undertaken, which involves another dose adjustment of 15% to 30%, either decrease or increase, depending on whether the assessment reveals any of a set of clinical characteristics (e.g., presence of severe pain

would suggest adding to the calculation, whereas presence of medical comorbidities would suggest subtracting further). Studies are needed to provide an empirical basis to this and other conversion strategies. Pending these studies, however, the most important consideration must be safety, which requires significant reduction in the calculated equianalgesic dose, followed by dose titration.

Some experts have concluded that the risk associated with a switch to methadone is sufficient to institute additional requirements for safety. These include limiting any single dose to 30 mg during the initial titration, even if the calculated dose is higher (Morley, Makin, 1997) and switching gradually over 3 days (Lawlor, Turner, Hanson, et al., 1998).

Generally, an opioid other than methadone, specifically one with a short half-life, is desirable for the treatment of severe, escalating pain, when rapid titration is needed. The risk of accumulation of drug levels into the toxic range is greater with an opioid drug with a long half-life, such as methadone. Deaths have been reported among patients in the community experiencing too-rapid dose increases without adequate follow up (Institute for Safe Medication Practices, 2008).

A variety of additional dosing schemes have been suggested in an effort to provide analgesic doses while avoiding toxic accumulation (Mercadante, Bruera, 2006). These include using a higher "loading" or "priming" dose (so that steady state can be reached sooner) (Mercadante, Casuccio, Calderone, 1999; Ayonrinde, Bridge, 2000; Blackburn, Somerville, Squire, 2002); the use of a PRN methadone regimen to start, which is then converted to fixed dosing after titration; and the use of an initial fixed dosing interval of 3 or 6 hours, which is lengthened to 8 to 12 hours after analgesia is obtained (Ayonrinde, Bridge, 2000; Morley, Makin, 1997; Lugo, Satterfield, Kern, 2005). Additionally, a second, short-acting drug, such as morphine, oxycodone, or hydromorphone, also can be provided for rescue doses (Lugo, Satterfield, Kern, 2005). The rescue dose may require titration in terms of size or frequency during the initial period of methadone titration.

The factors outlined above strongly support the use of a systematic procedure and the assistance of a clinician experienced in the use of methadone when switching from another opioid (Leppert, 2009). In addition, the patient and family must be willing and able to follow the regimen, and a process for regular monitoring must be incorporated in the procedure.

Methadone is a complex analgesic. To be used optimally and safely, a clinician well versed in its characteristics should be involved in care planning and implementation. Patient selection and close monitoring during the titration phase are critical elements in pain management with this drug. The reader is referred to an excellent website for information on methadone safety, Pain Treatment Topics, *http://pain-topics.org/opioid_rx/methadone.php*. See Patient Education Form IV-8 on methadone on pp. 560-561 at the end of Section IV.

Following are two patient examples to illustrate how patients may be switched from other opioids to methadone using morphine-methadone dose ratios and other pointers from Box 13-3 and Table 13-8.

Patient Example: Methadone

Mr. A. is a 48-year-old man with cancer metastatic to liver and bone in several locations. In addition, he has severe chemotherapy-induced peripheral neuropathy. His analgesics include gabapentin and short-acting oxycodone. He takes oxycodone 30 to 60 mg approximately every 3 to 4 hours for pain. His sleep is interrupted by pain, and he takes at least one dose of oxycodone during the night. His pain is continuous, but his insurance does not cover any modified-release opioids. In addition, the insurance limits the number of tablets that can be dispensed at any one time, requiring frequent prescriptions. A decision is made to convert his oxycodone to methadone. Because his current medication pattern is to take oxycodone PRN, there is no need to stop the current opioid; Mr. A. will continue to use oxycodone for breakthrough pain.

Mr. A. had a significant problem with sedation from both gabapentin and oxycodone when those medications were being titrated to effect. It is therefore decided that a very conservative approach to a starting methadone dose will be used. Mr. A's pain diary indicates that he averaged 200 mg of oxycodone a day for the previous 3 days.

Using a standard equianalgesic table (see Table 16-1), 20 mg oral oxycodone equals 30 mg oral morphine, so the 200 mg of oxycodone is changed to oral morphine equivalents (300 mg/day).

Using a dose-range table (see Box 13-3 or Table 13-8), 300 mg morphine per day yields a morphine to methadone dose ratio of 5:1.

In this case, however, we are being intentionally conservative. We will use the next increment, 10:1. This yields a daily methadone starting dose of 30 mg.

Methadone comes in 5 and 10 mg tablets. It would be convenient to use a schedule of 10 mg every 8 hours. We could consider a loading dose or shorter interval, but in this case rapid conversion is not a goal.

The nurse calls Mr. A. daily at about the same time. After the first 4 doses, Mr. A. reports reduction in pain and less use of oxycodone; however, he also reports falling asleep watching television, which is unusual for him. At the patient's request, the dose is reduced to 5 mg every 8 hours.

On day 4, the patient continues to report improved pain but also sleepiness and requests another decrease in dose, to 2.5 mg every 8 hours.

Over the next few days, the adverse effect of sleepiness varies but does not go away, contrary to the experience of most patients. Several more days of experimenting with extending dose intervals to 12 and even 18 hours prove ineffective at alleviating the symptom of sleepiness. After 3 weeks, Mr. A. elects to resume PRN oxycodone as his only opioid analgesic.

Patient Example

Ms B. is a 60 year-old obese cancer survivor with persistent back pain due to ruptured disks. She has severe chemotherapy-induced peripheral neuropathy. Because of pulmonary disease unrelated to the cancer, she is not a surgical candidate for the back. Her pain has been reasonably well-controlled with pregabalin, tramadol, modified-release oxycodone, and short-acting oxycodone. She was referred to the pain management nurse during a shortage of oxycodone when her short-acting analgesic was changed to hydromorphone. She was unhappy with the "funny feeling in my head" attributed to the hydromorphone. Multiple attempts to increase the dose of modified-release oxycodone in order to reduce the amount of short-acting opioid resulted in unacceptable sedation. It was decided that methadone would be a reasonable option that would also take advantage of its effectiveness in treating neuropathic pain.

Current regimen: Modified-release oxycodone 120 mg every 8 hours (360 mg/day); hydromorphone 40 to 48 mg approximately 2 to 4 times per day; tramadol 50 mg every 8 hours. **Plan:** Discontinue tramadol and modified-release oxycodone, substitute methadone on a conservative regimen that will be titrated to need, continue hydromorphone for the present.

Using a standard equianalgesic table (see Table 16-1 on pp. 444-456), 20 mg oral oxycodone equals 30 mg oral morphine, so the oxycodone 360 mg is changed to oral morphine equivalents (540 mg/day).

Using a dose-range table (see Box 13-3 or Table 13-8), 540 mg morphine/day yields a morphine to methadone dose ratio of 10:1, with a calculated methadone dose of 54 mg/day (540 divided by 10 = 54).

Taking age and multiple co-morbidities into account, the calculated dose is reduced by 50%, for a starting dose of 27 mg/day. Since methadone comes in 5 and 10 mg tablets, a loading dose of 10 mg every 6 hours for 6 doses will be used, then 5 mg every 8 hours for 3 days. (See Table 13-8 for examples of how to calculate a loading dose.) Hydromorphone will be used liberally for breakthrough pain.

The nurse calls Ms. B. daily at about the same time. For the first 3 days Ms. B. reports that pain is the same or worse than before the switch, with more frequent use of hydromorphone. On day 4, the methadone dose is increased to 10 mg every 8 hours. On this regimen Ms. B. reports that her pain is improved, but she still needs to take about half the amount of hydromorphone as before the switch. On day 6, the methadone dose is increased to 15 mg every 8 hours. There is continued improvement, but Ms. B. notes that she doesn't get a full 8 hours of relief following the methadone doses. On day 8, the dose increment is reduced to every 6 hours with the dose remaining at 15 mg.

On day 10, Ms. B. is very happy to report that she had not taken any breakthrough doses in the prior 24 hours. After several weeks at 15 mg methadone every 6 hours, breakthrough dosing is rare and Ms. B. has resumed care of her young grandchildren 3 afternoons a week.

Oxycodone

Oxycodone is used to treat acute cancer and noncancer-related persistent pain. It is commercially available in single entity oral formulations and a variety of fixed combinations with acetaminophen, aspirin, and ibuprofen (Table 13-9). When taken in fixed combination with a nonopioid, it is critical to patient safety and treatment efficacy to establish exactly what dose of the nonopioid the patient is taking. Care should be taken to avoid prescribing or administering amounts that would exceed the daily maximum dose for acetaminophen (4000 mg), aspirin (4000 mg), or ibuprofen (3200 mg). Patients should also be told not to take additional nonopioid that could result in excess dosing (see Section III).

As a single agent, oxycodone is available as a tablet, capsule, and elixir, and also in a modified-release (every 12-hour) formulation (OxyContin) (see Chapter 14 for a detailed discussion of specific oral oxycodone formulations). A once-daily oxycodone was in development at the time of publication. Oxycodone is not available in the United States in suppository form for rectal administration; however, oral preparations are commonly administered rectally. It is given via the IV route outside of the United States and has been shown to be effective for postoperative pain by this route (Lenz, Sandvik, Qvigstad, et al., 2009).

Oxycodone is metabolized in the liver primarily by the CYP450 2D6 enzyme and excreted by the kidneys. The starting dose should be reduced and the dosing interval may need to be increased for patients with hepatic or renal insufficiency (Riley, Eisenberg, Müller-Schwefe, et al., 2008). One of the metabolic products of oxycodone is oxymorphone, but it does not account for a significant proportion of oxycodone's analgesic effect (Kalso, 2007; Lalovic, Kharasch, Hoffer, et al., 2006). Although it is known that there is significant

genetic polymorphism at P450 2D6—leading to intermediate, extensive (or rapid), ultra-rapid metabolizers, or poor metabolizers (Palmer, Giesecke, Body, et al., 2005)—CYP450 polymorphism probably is not responsible when pain in an individual seems not to be oxycodone-responsive. Unchanged oxycodone and multiple metabolites produced by other pathways appear to produce oxycodone's pharmacodynamic effects, although the role of the several metabolites has not been well described (Lalovic, Kharasch, Hoffer, et al., 2006). Nonetheless, interactions at this enzyme potentially could be responsible for adverse effects and interactions with other drugs affected by the same metabolic pathway (Foster, Mobley, Wang, 2007). For example, rifampin was shown to greatly reduce the plasma concentrations of both IV and oral oxycodone (Nieminen, Hagelberg, Saari, et al., 2009). Drug-drug interaction lists (see Table 11-2 and Box 11-1 on p. 289) should be consulted when oxycodone is initiated or other medications, especially selective serotonin reuptake inhibitor (SSRI) antidepressants, are started in a patient taking oxycodone (Davis, Varga, Dickerson, et al., 2003) (see Chapter 11 for more on the cytochrome P450 enzyme system and drug-drug interactions).

Compared with morphine, oxycodone is more potent (Boström, Hammarlund-Udenaes, Simonsson, 2008; Davis, Varga, Dickerson, et al., 2003; Kalso 2007), has greater oral bioavailability (~60%) (Kalso 2007), comparable onset of action (30 to 60 minutes) and half-life (3 to 4 hours), and a similar adverse effect profile (see Table 16-1 on pp. 444-446). Older equianalgesic tables used a 1:1 ratio for morphine to oxycodone, but more typically a 1.5:1 ratio is now used (APS, 2003). However, similar to hydromorphone, the ratio between oxycodone and morphine may be influenced by the direction of the change in opioid. Some research suggests that when converting from morphine to oxycodone, a ratio of 2:1 might be used, but when converting from oxycodone to morphine, a ratio of 1:1 might be better (Knotkova, Fine, Portenoy, 2009).

Absorption and peak blood levels by the rectal route appear to be comparable to that of the oral route, but maximum blood concentration is prolonged. Bioavailability by the rectal route is estimated to be 45% to 60% (Lugo, Kern, 2004). Although further research is needed, morphine may cause more nausea and oxycodone more constipation (Riley, Eisenberg, Müller-Schwefe, et al., 2008; Davis, Varga, Dickerson, et al., 2003). Women may have a greater analgesic response to oxycodone than men (Davis, Varga, Dickerson, et al., 2003). A study comparing the adverse effects of short-acting oxycodone found no gender- or age-related differences between the adverse effects experienced by healthy older and middle-aged adults without pain, which led the researchers to reinforce to clinicians that they should not avoid prescribing oral opioids to older adults based on the belief that older adults are at higher risk of adverse effects than younger adults (Cherrier, Amory, Ersek, et al., 2009).

Table 13-9 | Commercially Available Fixed Combination Doses of Oxycodone and Nonopioids

Brand	Oxycodone (mg)	Acetaminophen (mg)	Aspirin (mg)	Ibuprofen (mg)	Dose Form
Combunox 5/400	5			400	Tablet
Endocet 5/325; Percocet 5/325; Generic	5	325			Tablet
Endocet 7.5/325; Percocet 7.5/325; Generic	7.5	325			Tablet
Endocet 7.5/500; Percocet 7.5/500; Generic	7.5	500			Tablet
Endocet 10/650; Percocet 10/650; Generic	10	650			Tablet
Endodan; Percodan	4.8		325		Tablet
Magnacet 2.5/400	2.5	400			Tablet
Magnacet 5/400	5	400			Tablet
Magnacet 7.5/400	7.5	400			Tablet
Magnacet 10/400	10	400			Tablet
Percocet 2.5/325	2.5	325			Tablet
Percocet 10/325; Generic	10	325			Tablet
Roxicet	5	325			Oral solution (per 5 mL)
Roxicet	5	325			Tablet
Roxicet 5/500	5	500			Caplet
Tylox	5	500			Capsule

From Pasero, C., & McCaffery, M. (2011). *Pain assessment and pharmacologic management*, p. 351, St. Louis, Mosby. © 2011, Pasero C, McCaffery M. May be duplicated for use in clinical practice.

In contrast to morphine, oxycodone binds to the kappa receptor as well as the mu receptor (Lauretti, Oliveira, Pereira, 2003). This kappa affinity is relatively weak, compared to its mu affinity, but the dual action and interaction between receptor types theoretically may provide clinical advantages in some pain states. For example, it may be speculated that the kappa activity could render oxycodone relatively more effective than morphine for visceral pain and some types of neuropathic pain (Riley, Eisenberg, Muller-Schwefe, et al., 2008; Nielsen, Ross, Lotfipour, et al., 2007). Further research will be needed to determine whether these differences exist and are clinically meaningful.

There is also evidence of synergy between morphine and oxycodone (Ross, Wallis, Smith, 2000). A combined morphine-oxycodone tablet is currently in clinical trials. A small study of patients with cancer pain (N = 22) compared modified-release formulations of oxycodone and morphine (Lauretti, Oliveira, Pereira, 2003). Those who took oxycodone consumed 38% less short-acting morphine for breakthrough pain to achieve the primary outcome of achieving and maintaining a VAS of 4 or less and reported less nausea and vomiting compared with those who took morphine only. The researchers concluded that a combination of opioids with different receptor action sites (i.e., morphine and oxycodone) may produce better analgesia than the use of an opioid that has one action site.

There is a lack of head-to-head studies comparing oxycodone with other analgesics (Ripamonti, Bandieri, 2009). A large (N = 456) randomized, placebo-controlled, single-dose study of women with moderate to severe pain after abdominal or pelvic surgery found that the combination of oxycodone (5 mg) plus ibuprofen (400 mg) provided significantly better pain relief than either agent taken alone (Singla, Pong, Newman, et al., 2005). A meta-analysis identified just four randomized controlled trials that compared oral oxycodone with either oral morphine (N = 3) or oral hydromorphone (N = 1) and concluded that there were no significant differences in efficacy and tolerability between the opioids (Reid, Martin, Sterne, et al., 2006). A more recent Cochrane Collaboration Review concluded that single oxycodone doses higher than 5 mg are effective for postoperative pain and two to three times stronger than codeine (Gaskell, Derry, Moore, et al., 2009). Efficacy was increased when oxycodone was combined with acetaminophen. Oxycodone 10 mg plus acetaminophen (650 mg) provided good analgesia to half of those treated, comparable to NSAIDs but with a longer duration of action.

It should be noted that the name *oxycodone* is similar in appearance and sound to oxymorphone, hydrocodone, and hydromorphone. An increased level of alertness is required to prevent medication errors with these opioids.

Oxymorphone

Oxymorphone is a semi-synthetic opioid indicated for moderate to severe cancer and noncancer pain (Smith, 2009). It is an agonist at both the mu and delta opioid receptors (Prommer, 2006b). Although the clinical implications of these interactions with different types of opioid receptors are unclear, it is possible that delta receptor agonism may potentiate mu receptor analgesic effects (Chamberlin, Cottle, Neville, et al., 2007; Fishbain, 2009; Smith, 2009).

Oxymorphone is available in parenteral and rectal forms (Numorphan) (Smith, 2009). In 2006, it was released in short-acting (Opana) and modified-release (Opana ER) oral formulations (see Chapter 14 for discussion of these formulations of oral oxymorphone).

Parenterally, oxymorphone is 10 times more potent than IV morphine (Fukuda, 2005). When given IV, it has a quick onset (5 to 10 minutes). Its peak time is 15 minutes, and its duration is 3 to 6 hours. It sometimes is used as a preoperative medication and a supplement for balanced anesthesia but is less popular for this purpose than the faster-acting opioids such as fentanyl and sufentanil (White, Freire, 2005). Oymorphone has been shown to provide effective pain relief via IV PCA (Farragher, Laffey, 2006), and it is well absorbed subcutaneously and intramuscularly, although IM administration of any opioid is discouraged (see Chapter 14).

The safety, efficacy, and adverse effect profiles of oral oxymorphone are similar to that of other mu agonist opioids (Chamberlin, Cottle, Neville, et al., 2007). When converting from morphine or oxycodone, the suggested oral conversion ratios are 3:1 and 2:1, respectively (Smith, 2009). Oxymorphone is more lipophilic than morphine, which may account for its slightly faster onset of action (30 to 45 minutes for oral short-acting) (Smith, 2009). A mean time to peak effect of 30 minutes has been associated with all doses of short-acting oxymorphone (Smith, 2009). Its half-life (7 to 11 hours) is longer than morphine's (2 to 4 hours) (Chamberlin, Cottle, Neville, 2007) and significantly longer than parenteral oxymorphone's (2 hours) (Smith, 2009). The oral bioavailability of oxymorphone is 10% (Prommer, 2006b); therefore, parenteral oxymorphone is 10 times more potent than oral oxymorphone.

Food, particularly food with a high fat content, can increase the plasma concentration of oral oxymorphone by as much as 50%, so the drug should be taken on an empty stomach (1 hour before or 2 hours after a meal). Alcohol ingestion at the time of dosing can accelerate the drug delivery from the modified-release formulation and lead to increased serum levels (Smith, 2009). These are important considerations when selecting an opioid; oral oxymorphone would not be a good choice in those who

are unable to follow these restrictions concerning the timing of food consumption or alcohol intake. Given an upper bound of half-life measurements that approaches 11 hours, time to steady state with both short-acting and modified-release oxymorphone could be as long as almost 3 days (Smith, 2009) (see Chapter 14 for pharmacokinetic information on modified-release oxymorphone).

Besides morphine and hydromorphone, oxymorphone is the only other opioid analgesic commercially available in the United States as a rectal suppository (Numorphan). By the rectal route, its onset of action is 15 to 30 minutes, with a peak time of 120 minutes. In one study, rectal oxymorphone was found to be one-tenth as potent as IM oxymorphone but one twentieth as potent in terms of peak effect (Beaver, Frise, 1977).

Oxymorphone is extensively metabolized in the liver and produces clinically inert metabolites (Smith, 2009). A major metabolite, noroxymorphone, is a potent mu opioid receptor agonist when administered intrathecally but lacks systemic efficacy most likely because of its inability to penetrate the blood-brain barrier (Lemberg, Siiskonen, Kontinen, et al., 2008). Though further research is needed, dose adjustments are likely necessary in patients with renal and hepatic disease (Smith, 2009); Guay (2007) recommends avoiding oxymorphone entirely in patients with moderate-to-severe hepatic impairment. The drug was shown in one study to be removed by hemodialysis (Smith, 2009). There appears to be a low risk for interaction with concurrent medications that are metabolized by the CYP450 enzyme system, which may be a significant benefit in patients who are poor metabolizers or those who take multiple medications that rely on this enzyme system for metabolism, such as some antidepressants, beta blockers, antipsychotics, chemotherapeutic agents, and some other opioids (Adams, Pieniaszek, Gammaitoni, et al., 2005; Chamberlin, Cottle, Neville, 2007; McIlwain, Ahdieh, 2005) (see Chapter 11 for more on cytochrome P450 enzymes and drug-drug interactions).

It should be noted that the name *oxymorphone* is similar in appearance and sound to oxycodone, hydrocodone, and hydromorphone. An increased level of alertness is required to prevent medication errors with these opioids.

Propoxyphene

Propoxyphene (Darvon) is prescribed for mild to moderate pain but has fallen out of favor over the years (Barkin, Barkin, Barkin, 2006) (discussed later in this section). It is often used in combination with acetaminophen (Darvocet) or aspirin (Darvon Compound). Propoxyphene is one half to one third as potent as codeine. Its recommended dose of 100 mg is equal in analgesic effect to 60 mg of codeine, which is known to be equal to 600 mg of aspirin (less than two 325 mg tablets). A systematic review of 26 randomized trials showed that adding propoxyphene to acetaminophen improved analgesia by an average of only 7.3% compared with acetaminophen alone (Li Wan Po, Zhang, 1997). Despite having antagonist effects at the NMDA receptor, it is no better for neuropathic pain than any comparable drug (Scott, 2005; Patt, 1998). In a meta-analysis of opioids for all types of noncancer pain, the so-called "weak" opioids, including propoxyphene, were found to be better than placebo but less effective than acetaminophen, NSAIDs, and strong opioids (Furlan, Sandoval, Mailis-Gagnon, et al., 2006).

At equianalgesic doses, propoxyphene has the same incidence of adverse effects as codeine and a longer half-life (6 to 12 hours) (see Table 13-1; also see Table 16-1 on pp. 444-446). It also is metabolized in the liver by the CYP2D6 enzyme system, and therefore, has the potential for interaction with many other drugs. Serious interactions are also possible with several other drugs that may have additive adverse effects (Barkin, Barkin, Barkin, 2006). (See Chapter 11 for more on the CYP2D6 enzyme system and drug-drug interactions.)

Propoxyphene has an active metabolite, norpropoxyphene, which has a half-life of 30 to 36 hours and can accumulate with repeated dosing, particularly in patients with renal insufficiency (Strassels, McNicol, Suleman 2008). Norpropoxyphene can produce pulmonary edema and cardiotoxicity, including arrhythmias (Strassels, McNicol, Suleman 2008). Apnea, cardiac arrest, and death have been reported. Seizures and other CNS toxicities have occurred (Barkin, Barkin, Barkin, 2006). These effects are not reversed by naloxone (Barkin, Barkin, Barkin, 2006), and even dialysis may not help (Bailie, Johnson, 2002).

Because of the toxicity related to norpropoxyphene, propoxyphene is no longer favored for the routine treatment of pain. It is an especially poor choice for use in older individuals because most have some degree of renal insufficiency. It has caused adverse events in residents in nursing homes (Perri, Menon, Deshpande, et al., 2005) and community-dwelling older adults (Gallagher, Barry, Ryan, et al., 2008; Kamal-Bahl, Stuart, Beers, 2006) and has been associated with hip fractures, possibly because of the CNS adverse effects of dizziness and sedation (Kamal-Bahl, Stuart, Beers, 2006). Since 1991, it has been listed in the Beers Criteria as an inappropriate medication for older adults (Beers, 1997; Beers, Ouslander, Rollinger, et al., 1991; Fick, Cooper, Wade, et al., 2003) (see Table 13-4). Others have similarly designated the drug as "rarely appropriate" in older adults (Zhan, Sangl, Bierman, et al., 2001). In Europe, propoxyphene was associated with accidental deaths and suicide and was withdrawn in the United Kingdom (Committee on the Safety of Medicines of the UK, 2006). A review of prescribing data in England and Wales reported that changes in prescribing after the withdrawal of co-proxamol (propoxyphene plus acetaminophen) resulted in a reduction in mortality involving the drug and little evidence of substitution of suicide method related to increased prescribing of other analgesics (Hawton, Bergen, Simkin, et al., 2009).

Unfortunately, despite its inappropriateness and published guidelines recommending against its use in older adults (APS, 2003; American Geriatrics Society [AGS], 2002; Fick, Cooper, Wade, et al., 2003; Zhan, Sangl, Bierman, et al., 2001), propoxyphene continues to be commonly prescribed for this population group (Singh, Sleeper, Seifert, 2007; Kamal-Bahl, Stuart, Beers, 2006; Liu, Christensen, 2002). Most recently, the U.S. FDA decided to require manufacturers to strengthen their warning to emphasize the risk of overdose with propoxyphene but allowed continued marketing of the drug despite agreement among a majority of FDA advisers that propoxyphene-containing products offer little benefit and should be removed from the market (Traynor, 2009).

In summary, despite a history of widespread use and occasional anecdotal reports in its favor (Scott 2005; Patt, 1998), the overwhelming evidence strongly suggests that this drug should not be a first-line analgesic and should be avoided in older adults, those with renal insufficiency, and those likely to need multiple medications for comorbidities. Oxycodone (Mercadante, Arcuri, 2007) and tramadol (Mullins, Wild, 2003) have been suggested as safer alternatives for older adults. See Patient Education Form IV-5 on propoxyphene at the end of Section IV.

Other Mu Opioid Analgesics

Some mu opioid analgesics are seldom used for pain but may offer options for selected patients. They include alfentanil, remifentanil, and sufentanil.

Alfentanil

Alfentanil is rarely used for pain management today (Gutstein, Akil, 2006). It is the least potent of the fentanils: one-fortieth as potent as fentanyl (Mildh, Scheinin, Kirvelä, 2001). It is lipophilic and has a faster onset but a shorter duration of action (30 minutes) than fentanyl (Duncan, 2002; Murphy, 2006; Upton, 2007). It is used primarily in the intraoperative and procedural settings via the IV route (Fukuda, 2005). Patients who received a mixture of alfentanil and morphine in the PACU achieved equal but faster comfort with no increase in opioid-induced adverse effects, compared with those who received morphine alone (Alkhazrajy, Macintyre, Upton, et al., 2007).

Given its wide distribution in the body, alfentanil is like fentanyl in having a short duration of effect when administered in a non–steady state situation when the decline in blood level after the dose is largely determined by redistribution into fat, rather than by metabolism. In this setting, given rapid clearance from its site of analgesic action in the brain (Upton, 2007) and its resultant short duration of action, it is considered a poor choice for postoperative analgesia. SC alfentanil infusions in palliative care settings have been reported (Urch, Carr, Minton, 2004), and there are anecdotal reports of its use for breakthrough pain in palliative care via intranasal and buccal administration, although there are no commercial preparations available for this use (Dale, Hjortkjær, Kharasch, 2002; Duncan, 2002). The drug is metabolized in the liver, has no clinically significant metabolites (Murphy, 2006), and is one of the few drugs (along with fentanyl and methadone) to have been recommended for patients with end-stage renal disease who need opioid analgesia (Murtagh, Chai, Donohoe, et al., 2007).

Remifentanil

Remifentanil is in the same mu agonist subclass as fentanyl, sufentanil, and alfentanil but has unique pharmacokinetic properties. It is available for IV use only. Current formulations of the drug contain glycine and are not approved for intrathecal or epidural use (Fukuda, 2005).

Remifentanil is unique in that its structure includes an ester linkage, which is broken down in the blood. As a result, it is rapidly cleared from the blood after a dose. It is not metabolized in the liver and is minimally affected by renal and hepatic function; accumulation does not occur (Beers, Camporesi, 2004; Pitsiu, Wilmer, Bodenham, et al., 2004). Its principle metabolite, remifentanil acid, has low potency and is excreted by the kidneys. Although remifentanil acid clearance is markedly reduced in patients with renal failure, increasing the half-life of the metabolite from 2 hours to 26 hours, this has not been shown to produce adverse effects (Hoke, Shlugman, Dershwitz, et al., 1997). For example, clearance of remifentanil acid was reduced in critically ill patients (N = 40) with moderate to severe renal impairment to about 25% that of patients with no to mild renal impairment; however, prolonged opioid effects were not noted (Pitsiu, Wilmer, Bodenham, et al., 2004). With these pharmacokinetics, the elimination half-life of remifentanil is only 3.2 minutes (25% longer in older adults), and this short half-life exists even after a long-duration (more than 8 hours) infusion (Beers, Camporesi, 2004).

Remifentanil is slightly more potent than fentanyl (Servin, Billard, 2008), quickly crosses the blood-brain barrier (Beers, Camporesi, 2004), and has an ultra rapid onset of action (1.5 minutes in young adults, increasing with age). The pharmacokinetic profile appears to be unaltered by obesity (Beers, Camporesi 2004). A study comparing remifentanil pharmacokinetics in 12 obese and 12 lean patients undergoing surgery demonstrated no significant differences between the 2 groups (Egan, Huizinga, Gupta, et al., 1998). The researchers recommended dosing regimens based on ideal body weight, or lean body mass, rather than total body weight.

Remifentanil's characteristics allow easy titration for intraoperative sedation and analgesia; it has been given via patient-controlled sedation (Fong, Kwan, 2005) and target-controlled infusions (titrated

according to respiratory rate) (Beers, Camporesi 2004). The drug is capable of providing extremely rapid and intense analgesia with minimal effect on cognition, making it suitable for procedures during which patient response to instruction is required, such as fiberoptic intubation (Beers, Camporesi 2004; Johnson, Swenson, Egan, et al., 2002). Several studies have found remifentanil to be safe and effective for analgesia and sedation during extracorporeal shockwave lithotripsy (ESWL) (Beloeil, Corsia, Coriat, et al., 2002; Cortinez, Munoz, De al Fuente, et al., 2005; Medina, Galvin, Dirckx, et al., 2005) and a variety of other painful procedures. A comparison of infusion doses led one group of researchers to recommend a regimen of 0.05 mcg/kg/minute with 10 mcg PCA doses for ESWL (Medina, Galvin, Dirckx, et al., 2005). It has been used successfully for sedation and analgesia in critically ill patients after organ transplantation as well (Evans, Park, 1997).

Similar to fentanyl and sufentanil, remifentanil allows rapid extubation in critically ill medical and surgical patients (Cheng, Newman, Duke, et al., 2001; Dahaba, Grabner, Rehak, et al., 2004; Engoren, Luther, Fenn-Buderer, 2001). In these populations, it has been shown to be superior to morphine in terms of ease of titration, hours of optimal sedation, amount of supplemental sedation required, and time to extubation with comparable adverse effects (Muellejans, Lopez, Cross, et al., 2004). Remifentanil has been shown to allow more rapid awakening and shorter time to neurologic testing after cessation of infusion compared with other short-acting opioids (Soltesz, Biedler, Silomon, et al., 2001; Wilhelm, Schlaich, Harrer, et al., 2001). This has led researchers to suggest it as an option for intermittent, rapid neurologic assessment in those with intracranial disease (Soletz, Biedler, Silomon, et al., 2001). By continuous infusion, the drug was not found to be effective in blocking cough response to endotracheal suctioning, resulting in increased intracranial pressure in mechanically-ventilated head-injured patients (Leone, Albanese, Viviand, et al., 2004).

The short duration of action of remifentanil after a dose, or after discontinuation of an infusion, is a major disadvantage when the need for analgesia is anticipated following painful medical or surgical procedures. Patients consistently report severe pain shortly after cessation of remifentanil administration (Litman, 2000; Soltesz, Biedler, Silomon, et al., 2001). In such cases, a proactive, preventive approach that includes administration of local or regional anesthesia, nonopioids, or the use of a longer-acting opioid is essential (Beers, Camporesi, 2004).

Like other mu opioids, remifentanil produces dose-related analgesia and adverse effects; nausea and pruritus are common. Of more concern is the high incidence of adverse respiratory events (Joo, Perks, Kataoka, et al., 2001; Litman, 2000). Incidence of respiratory depression has been reported to be as high as 29% in the postoperative setting

(Bowdle, Camporesi, Maysick, et al., 1996), and apnea with oxygen desaturation is common (Bowdle, Camporesi, Maysick, et al., 1996; Joo, Perks, Kataoka, et al., 2001; Litman, 2000). Like the other fentanils, muscle rigidity, in particular chest wall rigidity requiring resuscitation, can occur with rapid bolus administration (Beers, Camporesi, 2004). A randomized, double-blind study of 64 healthy volunteers (16 over 60 years old) led researchers to conclude that bolus doses of remifentanil (up to 200 mcg) can be highly effective for clinical situations requiring intense analgesia; however, older adults experienced more respiratory depression than younger subjects, and 4 older subjects experienced significant but short-lived and easily managed respiratory depression at 75 mcg (Egan, Kern, Muir, et al., 2004). The researchers reinforced the need for careful monitoring of respiratory function when this drug is used. In addition, remifentanil bolus dosing was associated with severe hemodynamic instability and 1 case of myocardial infarction (MI) in a group of patients scheduled for coronary artery bypass graft (CABG) surgery, leading the researchers to terminate the study after 8 patients and recommend remifentanil administration only by slow infusion in this population (Elliott, O'Hare, Bill, et al., 2000). (See the following on PCA use after CABG.)

For severe postoperative pain treatment, a continuous infusion of 0.1 mcg/kg/min of remifentanil (N = 15) resulted in the need for less rescue medication than 0.05 mcg/kg/min (N = 15) (Calderon, Pernia, De Antonio, et al., 2001). The 2 infusion rates yielded 1 case of nausea and vomiting each and no cases of respiratory depression. Despite low dosing recommendations, several have advised against the use of remifentanil for postoperative pain management outside of a monitored setting, such as the intensive care unit (ICU), citing the absence of around-the-clock, readily available anesthesia providers and a potential for life-threatening dose errors or equipment malfunction as barriers to safe use (Beers, Camporesi, 2004).

A randomized controlled trial compared IV PCA remifentanil (0.05 mcg/kg/min basal rate, 0.25 mcg/kg PCA bolus, lockout 5 minutes) with IV PCA morphine (0.3 mg/h, 1 mg PCA bolus, lockout 5 minutes) in 60 patients after CABG and found better analgesia with cough and movement in those receiving remifentanil and concluded that remifentanil is a safe alternative to morphine in this patient population (Baltali, Turkoz, Bozdogan, et al., 2009). Although remifentanil has been found to produce effective pain relief via PCA during labor and delivery (Blair, Hill, Fee 2001; Douma, Verwey, Kam-Endtz, et al., 2010; Evron, Glezerman, Sadan, et al., 2005), wide variation in analgesic requirements and adverse effects, such as maternal oxygen desaturation and nausea, and the need for very close monitoring (Saunders, Glass 2002; Volmanen, Akural, Raudaskoski, et al., 2002) would seem to limit its use in this setting. However, an observational study of 205 women in active labor who received remifentanil via a titrated continuous IV infusion (0.025 mcg/kg/minute

increased in a stepwise approach to a maximum dose of 0.15 mcg/kg/minute) reported reductions in mean visual analog scores from 9.4 to 5.1 after 5 minutes and to 3.6 after 30 minutes of infusion (D'Onofrio, Novelli, Mecacci, et al., 2009). This was accomplished with minimal maternal opioid-related adverse effects (e.g., 3 patients reported nausea), no hemodynamic instability, and no fetal or neonatal adverse effects. The researchers recommended this stepwise titration regimen and suggested that fixed-dose regimens of remifentanil in this setting may have led to the underdosing and inadequate analgesia or overdosing and maternal desaturation reported in other studies.

Remifentanil has provided some observations intended to elucidate the controversial clinical effect of opioid-induced hyperalgesia. For many years, animal and healthy human volunteer studies have documented secondary hyperalgesia after acute and long-term opioid exposure (Angst, Koppert, Pahl, et al., 2003; Joly, Richebe, Guignard, et al., 2005) (see Chapter 11 for a detailed discussion of opioid-induced hyperalgesia). Postoperative secondary hyperalgesia has also been reported in the clinical setting, as evidenced by increased pain and morphine consumption in patients who received high intraoperative doses of remifentanil compared with those who did not (Guignard, Bossard, Coste, et al., 2000; Joly, Richebe, Guignard, et al., 2005). Other studies have not confirmed this (Lahtinen, Kokki, Hynynen 2008). The underlying mechanisms of opioid-induced hyperalgesia may involve a pain facilitator system mediated by the NMDA receptor (Angst, Koppert, Pahl, et al., 2003; Joly, Richebe, Guignard, et al., 2005) (see Section I). Indeed, co-administration of the NMDA receptor antagonist ketamine with remifentanil has been shown to abolish hyperalgesia (Angst, Koppert, Pahl, et al., 2003; Joly, Richebe, Guignard, et al., 2005).

Sufentanil

Sufentanil is a very potent, lipophilic mu agonist opioid analgesic usually used in perioperative or procedural settings as an IV, epidural, or intrathecal infusion. It is the most lipid-soluble opioid (twice that of fentanyl) and, being approximately 1000 times more potent than morphine (Gutstein, Akil, 2006), is the most potent of the fentanyl analogs (White, Hardy, Boyd, et al., 2008) (see Knotkova, Fine, Portenoy, 2009 for research on potency ratios). It has no active metabolites and, like other highly lipophilic drugs, is fast acting (IV peak analgesic effect is ~5 minutes) and has a short duration of action (approximately 1 hour), because it moves rapidly from plasma to opioid receptor action sites (Fukuda, 2005; Gutstein, Akil, 2006; Murphy, 2006). These qualities have attracted investigators and clinicians to consider it for alternative routes that require high potency and low volume, such as intranasal administration for acute postoperative pain (Mathieu, Cnudde, Engelman, et al., 2006; Dale, Hjortkjaer, Kharasch, 2002) and SC infusion in palliative care settings (Urch, Carr, Minton, 2004; White, Hardy, Boyd, et al., 2008). These characteristics also make the drug suitable for breakthrough pain. Indeed, sufentanil has been given via the oral transmucosal route (Gardner-Nix, 2001a) and the intranasal route (Jackson, Ashby, Keech, 2002) to provide rapid and effective analgesia for breakthrough cancer pain. Intraarticular administration of a single bolus of sufentanil at the end of arthroscopic knee surgery produced effective pain relief for up to 24 hours; the addition of methylprednisolone (e.g., Solu-Medrol, Depo-Medrol) further prolonged analgesia (Kizilkaya, Yildirim, Dogan, et al., 2004). A transdermal sufentanil patch for long-term pain treatment was in development at the time of publication (Freye, 2008).

Sufentanil is sometimes combined with a local anesthetic when administered epidurally (Bauer, Hentz, Ducrocq, et al., 2007). In the postoperative setting, sufentanil is reported to be more potent via the intrathecal route than the IV route of administration. A randomized, double-blind study of 40 patients older than 75 years undergoing total hip replacement showed that those who received intrathecal sufentanil had significantly faster pain relief and required less rescue medication than those who received IV sufentanil (Fournier, Weber, Gamulin, 2005). Whereas oxygen desaturation was common with IV sufentanil, pruritus was common with intrathecal sufentanil. In another study (N = 20) comparing epidural and IV sufentanil, approximately 50% more sufentanil was required epidurally than intravenously to produce comparable pain relief (Menigaux, Guignard, Fletcher, et al., 2001). The researchers suggested that the bioavailability of epidural sufentanil is reduced and much of the lipophilic drug may be absorbed into the epidural fat (see Chapter 15 for more on intraspinal sufentanil). The effects of sufentanil's lipophilicity could also be seen in a small study comparing 8 obese and 8 control patients in which IV sufentanil's half-life was 208 minutes and 135 minutes, respectively (Schwartz, Matteo, Ornstein, et al., 1991).

As with fentanyl, there is a wide volume of distribution, but clearance is much faster. When given by continuous IV infusion as part of a sedation/analgesia protocol, distribution and clearance were extended compared with bolus or short infusion in the perioperative setting (Ethuin, Boudaoud, Leblanc, et al., 2003). Sufentanil has been shown to be sufficiently hypnotic to be used as a long-term (12 days) sedative agent in critically ill mechanically-ventilated patients without renal or hepatic disease (Ethuin, Boudaoud, Leblanc, et al., 2003). In critically ill trauma patients, analgesia was easier to maintain following discontinuation of sufentanil/propofol (N = 10) infusion compared with remifentanil/propofol (N = 10) infusion, although awakening was more rapid with the latter (Soltesz, Biedler, Silomon, et al., 2001). Sufentanil does not interfere with hemodynamic stability (Fukuda, 2005); however, adverse effects, such as respiratory depression and nausea and vomiting, were more common compared with remifentanil when sufentanil was used for procedural pain management (Beloeil, Corsia, Coriat, et al., 2002).

Characteristics of Selected Agonist-Antagonist Opioids

Historically, agonist-antagonist opioids have been discouraged as first-line drugs for any type of pain (APS, 2003) and contraindicated in patients receiving a mu agonist opioid, because of their ability to antagonize at the mu opioid receptor and reverse analgesia and precipitate withdrawal (Miaskowski, Cleary, Burney, et al., 2005). This perspective continues to be held with regard to the mixed agonist-antagonist opioids, such as pentazocine (Butorphanol), but has been evolving with the advent of new formulations of the partial mu agonist buprenorphine. Some clinicians use agonist-antagonist opioid analgesics believing that they cause no respiratory depression or less than the mu agonist opioids (see the misconceptions table in the Introduction to Section IV). Rather, they have a ceiling on the respiratory depression; they can produce respiratory depression comparable to morphine at a relatively low dose (e.g., 10 mg of parenteral morphine), and patients who would be at risk from morphine at this dose presumably also would be at risk from an agonist-antagonist opioid. The agonist-antagonists also have a ceiling on their analgesic effects (see discussion in the following buprenorphine section) (APS, 2003), which is why they are especially inappropriate for severe, escalating pain.

All agonist-antagonist opioids are available parenterally. Pentazocine is the only agonist-antagonist available in oral formulation, and this is in combination with naloxone (Talwin NX). Buprenorphine is formulated for sublingual administration as a single-entity drug (Subutex) and in combination with naloxone (Suboxone); these drugs are indicated for the office-based treatment of opioid addiction. Buprenorphine also is available in some countries as a transdermal patch. Butorphanol (Stadol) is available by nasal spray.

The division of the agonist-antagonists into partial agonists (buprenorphine) and mixed agonist-antagonists (butorphanol, nalbuphine [Nubain], and pentazocine) is clinically important. This is apparent in reviewing the pharmacology of the individual drugs.

Buprenorphine

Buprenorphine is the only partial mu agonist with high affinity for the mu opioid receptor. As such, it binds tightly to the mu opioid receptor but does not "turn on" that receptor as completely as a full mu agonist opioid, such as morphine (Heit, Gourlay, 2008; Johnson, Strain, Amass, 2003; Johnson, Fudala, Payne, 2005). It has a complex pharmacology and probably also has antagonist effects at other opioid receptors, such as the kappa receptor. In opioid-naïve individuals, low-dose buprenorphine acts like a potent mu agonist opioid. As the dose is increased, the drug has a ceiling effect (Johnson, Strain, Amass, 2003). As mentioned, this is believed to limit its usefulness for the treatment of severe, escalating pain. If it is administered to a patient who already has physical dependence to another mu agonist drug, it has the potential to produce acute withdrawal.

Buprenorphine can be given parenterally (Buprenex) and, being highly lipophilic, is absorbed well by the oral mucosa (Subutex, Suboxone) (Center for Drug Evaluation and Research, 2002) and can be administered transdermally. The transdermal buprenorphine patch currently is available in several European and other countries and is used for the treatment of persistent pain. Research and clinical experience is lacking on transdermal buprenorphine, but a large multicenter (110 centers) study of cancer patients (N = 1801) demonstrated that the formulation was well tolerated and produced analgesia similar to mu opioid agonists (Apolone, Corli, Negri, et al., 2009). A clinical trial that compared pain relief and adverse effects in 82 adults ages 65 years and older with equal numbers of adults between the ages of 51 and 64 and 50 years or younger found that transdermal buprenorphine was equally effective, tolerable, and safe in all age groups for moderate to severe noncancer pain (Likar, Vadlau, Breschan, et al., 2008). Buprenorphine is not offered in an oral formulation because of low oral bioavailability from significant first-pass metabolism (Johnson, Fudala, Payne, 2005) (see Chapter 11).

Sublingual absorption of a liquid buprenorphine formulation, which is not available in the United States, occurs within 5 minutes. In contrast, sublingual tablets, approved for treatment of opioid addiction (discussed in the next section), require at least 20 minutes, with peak plasma concentrations measured over a wide range of 60 to 360 minutes. Bioavailability is 51% to 55% with the sublingual formulations, but with wide interpatient variability (Johnson, Fudala, Payne, 2005).

IV buprenorphine has a slow onset of action with a peak effect that can be as long as 3 hours and a terminal half-life of 5 to 6 hours (Johnson, Fudala, Payne, 2005). The duration of buprenorphine varies significantly depending on route of administration. Acceptable postoperative pain was attained via every-3-hour dosing with sublingual buprenorphine, while patients receiving IM buprenorphine reported analgesia lasting for approximately 12 hours (Johnson, Fudala, Payne, 2005).

Buprenorphine's principle metabolite norbuprenorphine has not been studied extensively in humans but has been found to be a potent partial agonist in animals (Huang, Kehner, Cowan, et al., 2001), though less potent

and with a lower affinity for the mu opioid receptor than buprenorphine (Fukuda, 2005). Norbuprenorphine's analgesic effect is one-fiftieth that of buprenorphine via IV administration, and it has a slower elimination than buprenorphine (Johnson, Strain, Amass, 2003).

Buprenorphine has been used for postoperative pain, administered by IM and IV injection and by IV PCA (Wu, 2005). It also has been given epidurally (Johnson, Fudala, Payne, 2005) and intrathecally (Vadivelu, Hines, 2007). It has some local anesthetic effects and has been added to local anesthetic blocks to prolong the effect (Candido, Franco, Khan, et al., 2001; Candido, Winnie, Ghaleb, et al., 2002). Neuropathic pain and cancer-related pain have been successfully treated with buprenorphine by all routes of administration (Johnson, Fudala, Payne, 2005; Davis, 2005; Hans, 2007). Concern about the ability to reverse this high affinity drug with typical doses of naloxone has led to the recommendation that it not be used in laboring patients (APS, 2003).

Sedation, nausea, vomiting, dizziness, sweating, and headache are the most common adverse effects of parenteral buprenorphine. It may be less constipating and less likely to alter the levels of sex hormones than other opioids (Davis, 2005). Like other opioids, it may produce dysphoric and psychomimetic effects (Johnson, Fudala, Payne, 2005). In contrast to butorphanol and pentazocine, buprenorphine does not produce adverse cardiac effects (Fukuda, 2005). It also has a lower incidence of prolonged QT interval than methadone (Wedam, Bigelow, Johnson, et al., 2007). Safety in renal failure and in older adults has not been studied. Neither buprenorphine nor its active metabolites are excreted by the kidneys, so some speculate that dose reductions may not be necessary in those with renal insufficiency (Davis, 2005).

Parenteral buprenorphine is about 30 times more potent than morphine, but at usual doses is less likely to cause respiratory depression (Johnson, Fudala, Payne, 2005). A ceiling on respiratory depression after 0.15 to 1.2 mg IV in adults is reported (Fukuda, 2005). Dahan and colleagues (2005) found a respiratory ceiling effect at IV doses equal to or greater than 2.9 $mcg\,kg^{-1}$; the administration of IV doses as high as 7 mg without respiratory depression have also been described (Johnson, Fudala, Payne, 2005). Peak respiratory depression has been found to occur between 150 to 180 minutes after IV infusion (Dahan, Yassen, Romberg, et al., 2006). Respiratory depression plateaus have also been noted between 0.4 and 0.8 mg sublingually (Dahan, Yassen, Bijl, et al., 2005). High doses of buprenorphine may stimulate respiration via its antagonist characteristic (Fukuda, 2005).

Some studies provide empirical support for the conclusion that the ceiling dose for respiratory depressant effects is relevant in the context of acute pain management (Dahan, Yassan, Bijl, et al., 2005; Dahan, Yassen, Romberg, et al., 2006). Researchers administered 0.2 mg and 0.4 mg IV doses to 20 healthy male volunteers (age 22 to 35 years, weight 62 to 92 kg) for the purpose of examining buprenorphine's respiratory and analgesic effects during experimental pain induced by electrical current via surface electrodes (Dahan, Yassen, Romberg, et al., 2006). Doubling the buprenorphine dose (from 0.2 mg to 0.4 mg) increased its peak analgesic effect by a factor of 3.5, but did not change the respiratory effects. These findings suggest that the doses that are effective for pain are in a range that yields a plateau on respiratory depression. Further research in patients in the clinical setting is warranted.

Though clinically significant respiratory depression is rare with buprenorphine and associated most often with the use of other sedating drugs, such as benzodiazepines (Dahan, Yassen, Bijl, et al., 2005), the unusual times that it happens may pose a significant challenge in management because buprenorphine is not readily reversed by naloxone. In fact, very high doses (10 to 35 mg) of naloxone may be required to reverse respiratory depression due to buprenorphine's strong affinity for the mu opioid receptor (Johnson, Fudala, Payne, 2005).

Buprenorphine for Treatment of Opioid Addiction

There are two sublingual buprenorphine formulations (Subutex and Suboxone). They are the only agents approved for treatment of opioid addictive disease by the Drug Addiction Treatment Act of 2000 (DATA) (methadone maintenance programs are approved and licensed under a different law). Suboxone contains buprenorphine and the opioid antagonist naloxone, a combination intended as an abuse deterrent. Suboxone is available in two tablet strengths: 2 mg buprenorphine plus 0.5 mg naloxone and 8 mg buprenorphine plus 2 mg naloxone. Subutex contains buprenorphine alone in 2 and 8 mg strength tablets. Sublingual buprenorphine tablets are placed under the tongue until dissolved, for about 2 to 10 minutes (Center for Drug Evaluation and Research, 2002) (see Chapter 14). Because buprenorphine is approved as a treatment for addiction and clinicians who prescribe it for this purpose must indicate on the prescription that they have been certified to do so, it is best that the words "For Pain" be written on the prescription if the drug is to be used as an analgesic (Heit, Gourlay, 2008). This is frequent practice when using methadone for pain as well.

It is extremely important that acute pain episodes, such as following trauma or surgery, be treated adequately in individuals who are taking buprenorphine for addictive disease. There is very little experience in the use of morphine or some other pure mu agonist drug to augment the effects of buprenorphine. Theoretically, relatively high doses of a pure mu opioid would be needed because buprenorphine binds so tightly to the opioid receptor that fewer receptors will be available for activation. In addition, there is concern that patients with the disease of addiction may be predisposed to experience relatively more pain after injury as a result of pain facilitation through mechanisms linked to withdrawal (Savage, Schofferman, 1995). Whatever the reason, patients who are receiving buprenorphine, or methadone, and require opioid administration for the management of acute severe pain, may need a relatively aggressive treatment protocol, with quick dose escalation based on observed response to the therapy. (See Chapter 20 for more discussion of treatment of pain in individuals with addictive disease.)

Butorphanol

Butorphanol is a mixed agonist-antagonist opioid with an affinity for mu, delta, and kappa receptors. It is an agonist at the kappa receptor and either an antagonist or partial agonist at the mu opioid receptor (Fukuda, 2005). As discussed, the antagonistic characteristic can lead to withdrawal symptoms if butorphanol is administered to an individual who is physically dependent on a mu opioid.

Butorphanol is available for IV (Stadol) and intranasal (Stadol NS) administration. Though there is no clear advantage of butorphanol over the first-line mu agonist opioids, it has been used in perioperative (Wu, 2005) and labor settings (Birnbach, Browne, 2005) and as a treatment for migraine (Davis, Rudy, Archer, et al., 2005; Rapoport, Bigal, Tepper, et al., 2004). There are experimental data suggesting that women may achieve better analgesia than men with butorphanol (Miller, Ernst, 2004).

The onset, peak, and duration of analgesic action of IV butorphanol are similar to that of IV morphine, and it has a plasma half-life of approximately 3 hours (Gutstein, Akil, 2006). It has been shown to be effective for IV PCA following abdominal hysterectomy (Thakore, D'Mello, Saksena, et al., 2009). Dose adjustment is not needed in renal or hepatic insufficiency or in the older patient, but extending the dosing interval may be advisable (Asenjo, Brecht, 2005; Vachharajani, Shyu, Garnett, et al., 1996).

Intranasal butorphanol is absorbed rapidly, detectable in serum in 5 minutes or less, but onset of analgesia may be as much as 15 minutes (Asenjo, Brecht, 2005). It is approximately 60% to 70% bioavailable (Cashman, 2008). Adverse effects are typical of opioids, with the addition of an unpleasant taste (Davis, Rudy, Archer, et al., 2005). In opioid-naïve patients who are taking occasional mu agonist opioids, such as codeine or oxycodone, the addition of butorphanol nasal spray may provide additive analgesia. However, in opioid-tolerant patients, such as those receiving ATC morphine, the addition of butorphanol nasal spray should be avoided because it may reverse analgesia and precipitate withdrawal.

Adverse effects of butorphanol include headache, vertigo, lethargy, and lightheadedness. Psychomimetic effects are possible and include a feeling of floating, confusion, hallucinations, unusual dreams, and depersonalization (Dawn, Yosipovitch, 2006). Parenteral butorphanol is associated with a high degree of sedation (Coda, 2006). Therapeutic doses of butorphanol can produce levels of respiratory depression equal to mu opioid agonist drugs until a ceiling for respiratory depression is reached, typically at doses of 30 to 60 mcg/kg (Fukuda, 2005). Butorphanol by any route is not recommended for use in the treatment of MI or patients with hypertension because it produces multiple adverse effects on cardiac function, including increased pulmonary arterial pressure and cardiac workload (Fukuda, 2005; Gutstein, Akil, 2006).

Butorphanol and other agonist-antagonist opioids are sometimes used at low doses for treatment of opioid-induced adverse effects, particularly pruritus. However, studies on the effectiveness of butorphanol on opioid-induced pruritus have been mixed. Two small uncontrolled trials suggest that intranasal butorphanol may be effective against pruritus related to opioid agonists and to skin conditions (Dawn, Yosipovitch, 2006; Dunteman, Karanikolas, Filos, 1996). Others have reported that IV butorphanol reduced analgesia but not itching (Sakai, Fukano, Sumikawa, 2001). The risk of adding adverse effects, and inadvertently reversing analgesia and inducing withdrawal, must be weighed against the benefit of a small reduction in the severity of a minor adverse effect that quite often can be treated effectively with opioid dose reduction or other methods (see Chapter 19 for more on management of pruritus).

Dezocine

Approved in 1989, dezocine (Dalgan) has not been widely used for the treatment of pain, and there is very little clinical research on the drug. It was discontinued in the United States in 1999 (APS, 2003). Although it is classified as an agonist-antagonist opioid, some researchers question the existence of antagonist properties. Experimental research using human embryonic kidney cells concluded that it is an antagonist at the kappa opioid receptor, rather than an agonist like butorphanol (Gharagozlou, Hashemi, DeLorey, et al., 2006), and earlier studies in animals showed that large doses of naloxone failed to antagonize the drug (Picker, 1997). It has been administered with mu opioid agonists and other agonist-antagonists without precipitating withdrawal symptoms (Barkin Lubenow, Bruehl, et al., 1996; Wilson, Cohen, Kezer, et al., 1995). These are confusing data, and most experts continue to classify dezocine as a mixed agonist-antagonist, with properties similar to other drugs of this type.

Dezocine undergoes extensive first-pass hepatic metabolism and is without active metabolites. An early review of dezocine described the drug as having extensive distribution, high clearance, and short half-life (3 hours) over a range of IV doses and being well absorbed by all parenteral routes (Locniskar, Greenblatt, Zinny, 1986). Peak effect was 0.6 hours, and bioavailability was 97% following IM injection. Doses should be reduced if used in patients with hepatic or renal dysfunction. No evidence exists of changes in pressure within the common bile duct or ampulla of Vater in patients after biliary surgery. Mental status changes and delirium have been reported with use of dezocine in older adults (Barkin, Lubenow, Bruehl, et al., 1996).

Nalbuphine

Nalbuphine (Nubain) is a mixed agonist-antagonist opioid and like butorphanol is a kappa receptor agonist and a mu receptor antagonist (Fukuda, 2005). Similar to the other drugs in this subclass, nalbuphine can reverse analgesia or precipitate withdrawal if administered to an individual who is physically dependent on a mu opioid, and it has a ceiling dose for both analgesia and respiratory depressant effects (Gunion, Marchionne, Anderson, 2004). It is available for administration only by the parenteral route (IM, SC, IV).

Although there is no advantage over the first-line mu agonist opioids, nalbuphine is occasionally used for postoperative pain (Coda, 2006; Gunion, Marchionne, Anderson, 2004; Wu, 2005). It also has been administered for labor pain (Birnbach, Browne, 2005), but a warning was issued by the manufacturer in 2005 noting a risk of serious fetal and neonatal adverse effects (including fetal bradycardia, respiratory depression at birth, apnea, cyanosis, and hypotonia) associated with its use during labor and delivery. As a result, the drug should not be used during labor and delivery unless clearly indicated and only if the benefits outweigh the risks *(http://www.fda.gov/medwatch/safety/2005/aug_PI/Nubain_PI.pdf)*. (See Chapter 20 for opioid use during pregnancy and breast-feeding.)

Nalbuphine has an IV onset of 2 to 3 minutes, a duration of 4 to 6 hours (Birnbach, Browne, 2005), and a half-life of 2 to 3 hours (Guinon, Marchionne, Anderson, 2004). It has no clinically significant metabolites (Guinon, Marchionne, Anderson, 2004). In contrast to butorphanol and pentazocine, nalbuphine does not produce adverse cardiac effects, so it is acceptable for use when MI is suspected (Fukuda, 2005; Gutstein, Akil, 2006).

Nalbuphine may cause less nausea and vomiting than other opioids (Birnbach, Browne, 2005); however, compared with fentanyl for outpatient anesthesia, nalbuphine produced more unpleasant dreams during surgery and more postoperative nausea, anxiety, and sedation (White, Freire, 2005). At equianalgesic doses, nalbuphine and morphine produce a similar degree of respiratory depression. The ceiling for respiratory depression is reached at doses of more than 30 mg of nalbuphine; however, no increase in analgesia beyond 30 mg occurs (Gutstein, Akil, 2006). Like other agonist-antagonists, this property means that there is no safeguard against respiratory depression if this adverse effect occurs at a dose below the ceiling dose.

Single low dose (2.5 to 5 mg) and continuous infusions of parenteral nalbuphine sometimes are used to prevent or treat opioid-induced adverse effects, primarily pruritus, associated with mu agonist opioid epidural analgesia; however, reversal of analgesia can occur (Coda, 2006). Although nalbuphine has been reported to reverse morphine-induced respiratory depression while maintaining analgesia (Coda, 2006), others report that nalbuphine does not reverse and may actually increase respiratory depression after morphine (Fukuda, 2005). Even more report severe pain, hypertension, and tachycardia requiring pharmacologic intervention following administration of nalbuphine for treatment of opioid-induced adverse effects (Fukuda, 2005). In an attempt to reduce adverse effects, a nalbuphine and naloxone mixture was administered by slow IV push upon awakening from gynecologic surgery in a study of 12 patients (Gordon, Levine, Dubois, et al., 2007); all but two of the patients required rescue analgesia within 50 minutes of receiving the mixture. The risk of adding adverse effects and inadvertently reversing analgesia must be weighed against the benefit of a small reduction in the severity of a minor adverse effect (see Chapter 19 for more on management of pruritus and other adverse effects).

Pentazocine

Pentazocine is the only agonist-antagonist opioid to have an oral formulation. Although originally intended as an opioid with low abuse potential, abuse occurred after the drug was marketed, and this was addressed by reformulating it into a combination product containing pentazocine (50 mg) and naloxone (0.5 mg) (Talwin Nx). This markedly reduced crushing and IV injection of the oral formulation (Gutstein, Akil, 2006). A generic pentazocine combined with acetaminophen is also available.

Pentazocine has one-fourth the potency of morphine and a duration of action of 3 hours. As with other agonist-antagonist opioids, it has a ceiling effect on analgesia and respiratory depression; this probably occurs in the 30 to 70 mg range (Fukuda, 2005). When given to patients with respiratory depression from morphine, respiratory depression is not reversed, but patients who are dependent on other opioids may experience withdrawal symptoms (Gutstein, Akil, 2006). Pentazocine is associated with a relatively high incidence of psychotomimetic effects, and doses above 60 mg are associated with dysphoria (Gutstein, Akil, 2006), especially in older adults (Fukuda, 2005). The dysphoric effects are reversible with naloxone. Pentazocine also can produce negative CV effects, and it should not be used for analgesia in patients with MI (Fukuda, 2005). It has been used most often in labor and delivery and perioperative settings in the past, but it is very rarely used today.

Dual Mechanism Analgesics

Analgesics with a dual mechanism of action are relatively new to pain management. They bind weakly to the mu opioid receptor site and, similar to antidepressants, inhibit serotonin and/or norepinephrine. The two commercially available at the time of publication, tramadol and tapentadol, are discussed here.

Tramadol

Tramadol is a synthetic atypical opioid analgesic, indicated for moderate to some moderately severe pain. As mentioned, it has a dual mechanism of action: binding weakly to the mu opioid receptor site and inhibiting serotonin and norepinephrine reuptake, which in turn activates the descending inhibitory spinal pathway (Leppert, Luczak, 2005; Scott, Perry, 2000) (see Section I).

Tramadol has 68% oral bioavailability, is subject to first-pass effect, and is metabolized via the CYP2D6 pathway. Both tramadol and its active metabolite, M1, are excreted by the kidneys. M1 has 200 times stronger affinity for the mu receptor, is 2 to 4 times more potent, and has a longer half-life than tramadol (Sinatra, 2009). The onset of action of the short-acting formulation is as long as 60 minutes, which is slower than morphine (Sarbu, Radulescu, Robertson, et al., 2007), and its duration is longer (6 hours).

Tramadol is equipotent with codeine and five times less potent than morphine (Leppert, Luczak, 2005). A study comparing tramadol/acetaminophen to hydrocodone/acetaminophen and placebo in adults with partial ankle ligament tear showed 1 to 2 capsules of 37.5 mg tramadol/325 mg acetaminophen provided equivalent analgesia and comparable adverse effects to 7.5 mg hydrocodone/650 mg acetaminophen (Hewitt, Todd, Xiang, et al., 2007).

Tramadol is one of the most widely used analgesics throughout the world (Raffa, Stone, 2008). Despite reports of abuse, it is not a controlled substance under the Controlled Substances Act in the United States (Drug Enforcement Administration, 2008). In the United States, tramadol is available in short-acting (Ultram) and modified-release tablets (Ultram ER, Ryzolt) and in a combination tablet with acetaminophen (Ultracet). Acetaminophen combined with tramadol appears to enhance effectiveness beyond the degree expected, demonstrating a "supra-additive effect" (Filitz, Ihmsen, Gunther, et al., 2007; McClellan, Scott, 2003). There are conflicting findings regarding synergism with other opioids (Marinangeli, Ciccozzi, Aloisio, et al., 2007; Marcou, Marque, Mazoit, et al., 2005; Webb, Leong, 2005). In Europe and Australia, in addition to the oral formulations, tramadol is used intravenously and epidurally for perioperative pain, for postoperative pain via IV PCA, and to relieve postoperative shivering (Kaya, Sariyildiz, Karakus, et al., 2003). It is also available in

Europe for rectal administration (Mercadante, Arcuri, Fusco, et al., 2005).

Short-acting tramadol is available in 50 mg tablets. Modified-release tramadol (100, 200, and 300 mg) is effective for 24 hours. The maximum recommended dose of tramadol is 400 mg/day (Dworkin, O'Connor, Backonja, et al., 2007). A maximum dose limit of 300 mg/day for older adults over age 75 (AGS, 2002; Dworkin, O'Connor, Backonja, et al., 2007) and in the acute pain setting (Sinatra, 2009) is recommended.

Tramadol has been found to be effective in a variety of pain states, including postoperative pain (McCartney, Niazi, 2006; Scott, Perry, 2000), minor musculoskeletal trauma (Hewitt, Todd, Xiang, et al., 2007), migraine/headache (Alemdar, Pekdemir, Selekler 2007), cancer-related pain (Prommer, 2005; Leppert, Luczak, 2005), and pain from rheumatoid arthritis (Lee, Lee, Park, et al., 2006) and osteoarthritis (OA) (Vorsanger, Xiang, Jordan, et al., 2007). It is regarded as a first- or second-line analgesic in guidelines for neuropathic pain (Argoff, Backonja, Belgrade, et al., 2006; Dworkin, O'Connor, Backonja, et al., 2007; Finnerup, Otto, McQuay, et al., 2005; Moulin, Clark, Gilron, et al., 2007), although it is acknowledged that it may not be effective against severe neuropathic pain (Dworkin, O'Connor, Backonja, et al., 2007). It is not considered appropriate for severe pain associated with major surgical procedures either (Sinatra, 2009). Tramadol has been used for treatment of mild to moderate acute pain associated with sickle cell disease (Varadarajan, Weisman, 2009) and is listed as an option for persistent pain in older adults (AGS, 2002, 2009). The drug is widely prescribed to older adults with moderate to severe pain. In the only study to stratify patients by age (younger than 65, 65, younger than 75, 75 or older), the drug was well tolerated and effective for moderate to severe cancer and noncancer pain, and there were no significant differences in tolerability and effectiveness across age groups (Likar, Wittels, Molnar, et al., 2006). A Cochrane Collaboration Review and a later systematic review and meta-analysis by the same researchers concluded that the analgesic and functional outcome benefits are small and adverse events are reversible and not life-threatening but are often a cause of treatment cessation for OA (Cepeda, Camargo, Zea, et al., 2006, 2007).

The most common adverse effects of tramadol are nausea and vomiting, dizziness, drowsiness, and dry mouth. The risk of respiratory depression is lower than with pure mu agonist opioids (Scott, Perry, 2000). Because tramadol is largely dependent on the CYP2D6 metabolic pathway for analgesic activation, drug interactions must be taken into consideration. The selective serotonin reuptake inhibitors (SSRIs) (e.g., fluoxetine, paroxetine) may inhibit tramadol metabolism (see Chapter 11 for more on the CYP2D6 enzyme system and drug-drug interactions). During prolonged therapy at high doses, combined tramadol and SSRIs has led to life-threaten-ing serotonin syndrome, evidenced by shivering, nausea, low-grade fever, sweating, mental confusion, and delirium. It should not be administered with MAOIs, as this has been associated with the development of psychosis (Sinatra, 2009). As with other opioids, additive toxicity is seen with concurrent use of CNS depressants (Hersh, Pinto, Moore, 2007). Starting with a low dose (12.5 mg to 25 mg) and titrating to effect may limit the development of adverse effects.

Early reports of a significant risk of tramadol-induced seizures have been questioned (Raffa, Stone, 2008; Marquardt, Alsop, Albertson, 2005; Gasse, Derby, Vasilakis-Scaramozza, et al., 2000). There may not be a greater risk than that associated with other opioids (Gasse, Derby, Vasilakis-Scaramozza, et al., 2000), and attempts to induce seizures with tramadol in mice were unsuccessful (Raffa, Stone, 2008). However, tramadol should be taken within the recommended dose range and used with caution in patients with a history of seizure and when concurrently taking SSRIs and other drugs that can lower the seizure threshold (AGS, 2009). There have been anecdotal reports of the need to gradually taper doses to prevent withdrawal if the drug is to be discontinued.

Tapentadol

Tapentadol (Nucynta) is another centrally-acting analgesic with a dual mechanism of action, binding as an agonist to the mu opioid receptor site and also blocking the reuptake of norepinephrine. Tapentadol is a Schedule II drug indicated for moderate to severe pain and available in short-acting formulation in 50, 75, and 100 mg tablets. Dosing is recommended every 4 to 6 hours, and doses higher than 600 mg are not recommended because they have not been studied. A modified-release formulation of tapentadol was in development at time of publication. One phase III study showed that when compared with placebo and modified-release oxycodone (20 to 50 mg), significantly more patients taking modified-release tapentadol (100 to 250 mg) experienced 30% or greater and 50% or greater pain relief and a lower incidence of adverse effects and discontinuations due to adverse effects (Etropolski Rauschkolb-Loffler, Shapiro, et al., 2009).

The pharmacokinetics of a single 100 mg dose of tapentadol were studied in 4 healthy males (Terlinden, Ossig, Fliegert, et al., 2007). Absorption of the drug was described as rapid (time to peak plasma concentration was 1.25 to 1.5 hours), and elimination was almost exclusively by the renal system; it was excreted in the urine in the form of unconjugated metabolites (no clinically relevant metabolites). Other research revealed an oral bioavailability of 32% and a time to steady state of 25 to 30 hours with 4-hour dosing (Tzschentke, De Vry, Terlinden, et al., 2006). Although the manufacturer warns of possible interactions with drugs that are metabolized by the cytochrome P450 enzyme system (Pricara, 2008), research that evaluated tapentadol for protein binding and induction and inhibition of cytochrome P450 enzymes concluded that no clinically relevant drug-drug interactions are likely to occur through these mechanisms (Kneip, Terlinden, Beier, et al., 2008). Tapentadol has not been evaluated for use in patients with renal or hepatic impairment; the manufacturer advises not to use the drug in patients with these conditions.

Because this is a relatively new drug, clinical experience is lacking and there were only a few clinical trials at the time of publication. A single-dose (25, 50, 75, 100, or 200 mg) study of 400 patients with moderate to severe pain following dental surgery demonstrated that 75 mg or more of the drug produced effective dose-related analgesia and was well tolerated (Kleinert, Lange, Steup, et al., 2008). Tapentadol 200 mg produced higher total pain relief scores and a faster onset of action than 60 mg of oral morphine. Nausea and vomiting were also less common with all doses of tapentadol than with morphine. Another large trial randomized 901 patients to receive tapentadol 50 or 75 mg, oxycodone 10 mg, or placebo every 4 to 6 hours for 72 hours following bunionectomy (Daniels, Casson, Stegmann, et al., 2009). Acetaminophen was allowed during the study. Both doses of tapentadol and oxycodone were superior to placebo, and both doses of tapentadol produced similar pain relief as oxycodone. Nausea and vomiting were statistically significantly lower with tapentadol 50 mg and numerically lower (not statistically significant) with tapentadol 75 mg compared with oxycodone.

The drug has also been studied in patients with persistent pain. A 10-day, phase III, randomized, placebo-controlled study found tapentadol 50 and 75 mg produced similar analgesia as oxycodone 10 mg in patients awaiting joint replacement for uncontrolled arthritis pain (Hartrick, Van Hove, Stegmann, et al., 2009). As in other studies, GI adverse effects, such as nausea, vomiting, and constipation, were less frequent with both doses of tapentadol than with oxycodone. Another phase III study randomized 849 patients with lower back pain or hip or knee OA to receive tapentadol or oxycodone using a flexible dosing regimen for 90 days (Hale, Upmalis, Okamoto, et al., 2009). Pain relief was similar among the groups. CNS symptoms such as dizziness and somnolence were similar, but, again, GI adverse effects were less likely with tapentadol than with oxycodone. The researchers noted that dose tapering after treatment with tapentadol for 90 days did not appear to be necessary.

Tapentadol differs from tramadol in that it does not directly block the reuptake of serotonin; however, elevated norepinephrine levels can result in elevated levels of serotonin, which can lead to the development of serotonin syndrome evidenced by shivering, nausea, low-grade fever, sweating, mental confusion, and delirium. The same precautions for tramadol apply to tapentadol (i.e., avoid combining tapentadol with other drugs that increase serotonin level, such as tramadol and SSRIs). Tapentadol should also not be administered with MAOIs. As with other opioids, additive toxicity may occur with concurrent use of CNS depressants.

Effects of Patient Characteristics on Opioid Drug Selection

Other important factors to consider when selecting the optimum opioid analgesic are intrinsic to the patient. These factors include pain intensity, patient age, coexisting disease, current drug regimen and potential drug interactions, prior treatment outcomes, patient preference and convenience, and cost.

Pain Intensity

Evaluation of the patient's report of pain intensity is critical to the development of an individualized opioid analgesic treatment plan. A variety of pain rating scales exist for the purpose of assessing pain intensity (see Section II). For some types of mild to moderate pain, the options to consider typically include the dual-mechanism drugs tramadol or tapentadol, or one of the pure mu agonists. There also is extensive experience with the agonist-antagonist drugs in some types of pain, such as the use of the agonist-antagonist butorphanol (Stadol nasal spray) for migraine headache pain (Rapoport, Bigal, Tepper, et al., 2004). For moderate to severe persistent pain that already has been treated with an opioid, the preferred drug is a pure mu agonist; the preferred route is oral or transdermal. Severe acute pain is treated with pure mu agonist opioids.

Guidelines usually underscore the conclusion that most patients with mild pain do not require an opioid. A nonopioid such as ibuprofen or celecoxib may be sufficient (see Section III). If an opioid is appropriate, mild pain theoretically could be treated with any of the opioids, even morphine, if the dose is kept low; however, it is far more customary to use an opioid-nonopioid combination, such as oxycodone or hydrocodone compounded with a nonopioid such as acetaminophen (see Tables 13-3 and 13-9), or one of the dual-mechanism drugs.

Some pain of moderate intensity may also be satisfactorily relieved with a nonopioid (e.g., IV ketorolac). If an opioid is required, an opioid-nonopioid combination may be selected; however, as mentioned previously, the dose of the opioid will be restricted by the dose of the nonopioid with which it is compounded. In patients with moderate pain associated with progressive illness and in whom it may be predicted that pain will worsen over time, it is reasonable to select a single-entity opioid because it will allow the opioid dose to be titrated upward without concern about exceeding the recommended total daily dose of a nonopioid.

In addition to providing valuable information needed to select the correct analgesic for a patient, evaluating the severity of pain may suggest the underlying mechanism and pain syndrome. For example, the pain associated with radiation-induced nerve injury usually is not severe. The occurrence of severe pain in a previously irradiated area suggests recurrent or new pathology in the patient with cancer (Coyle, Cherny, Portenoy, 1995; Portenoy, 1996).

In the case of postoperative pain management, research and clinical experience determine the expected or usual pain intensity associated with surgical procedures and are used as guides for opioid selection and determining appropriate starting doses for pain relief. For example, pain associated with a thoracotomy is expected to be severe. Preplanning for severe postthoracotomy pain may include the placement of an epidural catheter for intraoperative and postoperative pain management using a mu agonist opioid analgesic and a local anesthetic. (See Chapter 16 for determining an appropriate starting dose.)

Patient Age

For the younger adult with no major organ failure, any of the available mu agonist opioids can be selected. For the older adult and those with major organ failure, changes in metabolism and elimination of drugs must be considered. Opioids with a short half-life are recommended, such as morphine, hydromorphone, and oxycodone. These drugs will achieve stable plasma concentrations within 24 hours (4 to 5 half-lives) and are, therefore, simpler to titrate and monitor (Coyle, Cherny, Portenoy, 1995). Mu agonists with a long half-life, such as methadone and levorphanol, are more challenging to dose and monitor in older patients and may be avoided on this basis. Drugs with active metabolites, such as meperidine and propoxyphene, are also avoided in older adults (see Table 13-4) and in all patients with renal dysfunction.

Coexisting Disease

Major organ failure, particularly cardiac, hepatic, and renal failure, influences the distribution, clearance, and excretion of opioids (Wellington, Chia, 2009) (see Chapter 11). Opioids, in turn, have adverse effects that may interact with dysfunctional organ systems. For example, opioids decrease the cough reflex, dry secretions, and release histamine (leading rarely to bronchial constriction) (Gutstein, Akil, 2006)—effects that increase the need for caution in patients with compromised respiratory function, including those with obstructive sleep apnea syndrome (American Society of Anesthesiologists, 2006) (also see Chapter 19).

When an opioid is prescribed to a patient with major organ failure, it is appropriate to start with less than the usual recommended dose and titrate the dose gradually. Extended dosing intervals are also advisable in some patients, particularly when multiple daily doses are required (Johnson, 2007).

All opioid drugs are metabolized to some extent by the liver. In patients with liver disease, clearance is decreased and bioavailability and half-life of opioids are increased (Wellington, Chia, 2009). This can lead to adverse effects from higher than expected plasma concentrations of these drugs. Higher plasma concentrations can also occur following liver surgery (Rudin, Lundberg, Hammarlund-Udenaes, et al., 2007). Administration of reduced doses (e.g., 50% less) or increased interval (e.g., twice the usual time period) and close monitoring of sedation and respiratory status is advised in the setting of liver dysfunction (Johnson, 2007). Propoxyphene, codeine, and meperidine should be avoided in patients with hepatic disease (Johnson, 2007). Johnson (2007) recommends also avoiding methadone in patients with hepatic disease, but others suggest that methadone may be used and doses may not need to be adjusted in cirrhosis and stable chronic liver disease because some methadone metabolism occurs in the intestine rather than the liver (Lugo, Satterfield, Kern, 2005).

Fentanyl is considered relatively safer in patients with hepatic dysfunction, and dose adjustment is not usually needed (Johnson, 2007). Remifentanil has also been suggested as an option for those with hepatic impairment (Wellington, Chia, 2009), but further research and clinical experience with this drug in patients with this condition is warranted.

Patients with renal disease may accumulate the active metabolites of drugs. For example, patients with renal insufficiency can develop relatively high concentrations of normeperidine during meperidine treatment, norpropoxyphene during propoxyphene treatment, and the glucuronidated metabolites during morphine treatment. Metabolite accumulation happens with all routes of administration, but the concentrations of the metabolites are greatest during oral administration. Metabolite accumulation is most problematic with meperidine (Marcantonio, Juarez, Goldman, et al., 1994). The accumulation of M6G and M3G can produce clinical effects (Dean, 2004), and a trial of an alternative opioid (e.g., hydromorphone or fentanyl) often is recommended if morphine toxicity occurs in a patient with renal disease (Portenoy, 1996). Morphine should be avoided in patients with end-stage renal disease (Dean, 2004). See Table 13-10 for recommendations regarding the use of selected mu opioids in patients with renal failure or undergoing dialysis.

When indicated by the type and severity of pain, the use of alternative routes may be a solution for some patients with major organ failure. Opioids can be given in lower doses by the epidural and intrathecal routes compared with the doses needed when given by the

Table 13-10 | Opioid Use During Renal Failure and Dialysis

Opioid	Comments about Use During Renal Failure	Comments about Use During Dialysis
Morphine	Do not use. Metabolites can accumulate, and adverse effects can be prolonged.	Choose another opioid, e.g., see fentanyl and methadone. Parent drug and metabolites are removed by dialysis, but "rebound" accumulation can occur between dialysis sessions as drug and metabolites re-equilibrate between CNS and plasma.
Codeine	Do not use. Metabolites can accumulate and cause serious adverse effects.	Do not use. Parent drug and metabolites can accumulate and cause serious adverse effects.
Fentanyl[1,2]	Appears safe, particularly for short-term use. Metabolites are inactive, but accumulation of parent drug may occur. Cautious use and careful monitoring of adverse effects is advised with long-term use and continuous IV or intraspinal infusion.	Not removed by dialysis. Appears safe, particularly for short-term use. Metabolites are inactive, and no adverse effects have been reported during dialysis. In most cases, no dose adjustments are necessary, but use caution during and after titration. Fentanyl may absorb onto one type of filter in which changing the filter is recommended. If this is not possible, switch to methadone.
Hydrocodone	Use cautiously, monitor adverse effects closely, and adjust dose as needed. Metabolite can accumulate causing neuroexcitation.	Parent drug can be removed, but metabolite can accumulate and may pose risk.
Hydromorphone	Use cautiously, carefully monitor for adverse effects, and adjust dose as needed. Metabolite can accumulate causing neuroexcitation, but the drug has been used safely in patients with renal failure. May be an option in patients with ESRD who are unable to tolerate other opioids.	Parent drug can be removed, but metabolite can accumulate and may pose a risk. Use cautiously and monitor patient closely during dialysis.
Meperidine	Do not use. Metabolite accumulation increases adverse effects.	Do not use. No data on drug or metabolites during dialysis, but risk of adverse effects is plausible.
Methadone[1]	Appears to be safe. Eliminated primarily by hepatic metabolism, but more research regarding its excretion is needed. Parent drug and metabolites are excreted into the gut, and renal excretion varies widely.	Metabolites are inactive, but use with caution as parent drug is not removed by dialysis.
Oxycodone	Further research is needed to make conclusive recommendations. Parent drug and metabolite (oxymorphone) can accumulate. If used, administer with great caution and carefully monitor adverse effects.	Avoid until research provides conclusive evidence of safety.
Propoxyphene	Do not use. Potential for significant toxicities from both the parent drug and its metabolite. Associated with hypoglycemia, cardiac conduction problems, and CNS and respiratory depression.	Do not use. Propoxyphene and its metabolite are not removed by dialysis. Potential for significant toxicities from both the parent drug and its metabolite. Associated with hypoglycemia, cardiac conduction problems, and CNS and respiratory depression.

CNS, Central nervous system; ESRD, end-stage renal disease.
[1]Not dialyzed; considered "safe", but cautious titration and close monitoring for a protracted period are recommended in patients with renal failure or undergoing dialysis (Dean, 2004).
[2]The other fentanils (i.e., remifentanil, sufentanil, and alfentanil) have been designated as safe for use in patients with renal impairment (Wellington and Chia, 2009), but further research and clinical experience with their use in these patients is warranted.
From Pasero, C., & McCaffery, M. (2011). *Pain assessment and pharmacologic management*, p. 364, St. Louis, Mosby. Data from Dean, M. (2004). Opioids in renal failure and dialysis patients. *J Pain Symptom Manage, 28*(5), 497-504; Johnson, S. J. (June, 2007). Opioid safety in patients with renal or hepatic dysfunction. Pain Treatment Topics. www.pain-topics.org. Accessed February 2, 2009; Kurella, M., Bennett, W. M., & Chertow, G. M. (2003). Analgesia in patients with ESRD: A review of available evidence. *Am J Kidney Dis, 42*(2), 217-228; Wellington, J., & Chia Y. Y. (2009). Patient variables influencing acute pain management. In R. S. Sinatra, O.A. de Leon-Casasola, B. Ginsberg, et al (Eds.), *Acute pain management*, Cambridge, New York, Cambridge University Press. © 2011, Pasero C, McCaffery M. May be duplicated for use in clinical practice.

oral and parenteral routes. Because of this, patients with major organ failure sometimes are able to tolerate opioids by an intraspinal route that they were unable to tolerate by the oral or parenteral routes. Lipophilic drugs, such as fentanyl and sufentanil, can accumulate, particularly when administered on a long-term basis or by continuous infusion (Kurella, Bennett, Chertow, 2003); morphine and hydromorphone may be better choices by the epidural route in patients with hepatic dysfunction and CNS depression. Continuous peripheral nerve block may be an alternative for postoperative patients in whom opioids must be avoided entirely (see Chapter 26).

Current Drug Regimen and Potential Drug Interactions

Many patients with pain, especially those with co-existing disease and continuous cancer or persistent noncancer pain, take several medications. Co-administration of two or more drugs often can result in a change in the metabolism, clearance, or both of the drugs (Pasero, Portenoy, McCaffery, 1999). It is extremely important when developing an opioid treatment plan to know all the medications the patient is taking and how they will interact with the opioid, and to monitor on an ongoing basis for drug interactions.

As discussed in Chapter 11, many opioid drugs are metabolized by the liver's cytochrome P450 (CYP) system, and the most important enzymes responsible for opioid metabolism are CYP2D6 and CYP3A4. Concomitant administration of a drug that induces one of these enzymes can lead to decreased levels of the opioid, and treatment with a drug that inhibits one of these enzymes can lead to increased levels (Fine, Portenoy, 2007) (see Tables 11-2 and 11-3, pp. 289 and 296).

The tricyclic antidepressants, including clomipramine (Anafranil) and amitriptyline (Elavil), may increase the bioavailability and half-life of morphine. This would cause a rise in plasma morphine levels (Coyle, Cherny, Portenoy, 1995). Phenytoin and the antitubercular drug, rifampin, increase the metabolism of methadone, and phenobarbital and phenytoin increase the metabolism of meperidine. This can result in decreased plasma levels of these opioids. Treatment with rifampin can result in complete loss of the analgesic effects of morphine (Fromm, Eckhardt, Li, et al., 1997). In the presence of MAOIs, meperidine can precipitate excitation, hyperpyrexia, convulsions, and death (Coyle, Cherny, Portenoy, 1995).

When drugs with anticholinergic effects, such as some antihistamines, phenothiazines, tricyclic antidepressants, and antiparkinsonian drugs, are administered with opioids, adverse effects, including dry mouth and constipation, may increase. It is important to emphasize the need for a bowel management regimen in patients taking any of these drugs with opioids (Coyle, Cherny, Portenoy, 1995) (see Chapter 19).

Seizures have been identified as a risk associated with the use of tramadol. Although the severity of this risk is uncertain, it is presumably enhanced when patients are taking tricyclic antidepressants, MAOIs, neuroleptics, and other drugs that reduce the seizure threshold. Serotonin syndrome can also occur when drugs that increase the serotonin level, such as tramadol, tapentadol, and SSRIs, are taken concomitantly.

Additive effects when opioid drugs are combined with other drugs also must be considered when implementing a pain treatment plan. Close monitoring of sedation is indicated when opioids are combined with antidepressants, phenothiazines, benzodiazepines, or neuroleptics. Because of their sedative and respiratory depressive effects, the amount of opioid that can be safely administered may be limited (APS, 2003; Anwari, Iqbal, 2003; Coyle, Cherny, Portenoy, 1995; Webster, Choi, Desai, et al., 2008).

Combining drugs can also have a positive effect on analgesia and adverse effects (APS, 2003; Inturrisi, 2002). For example, a review of the literature between 1996 and 2002 concluded that methylphenidate (Ritaline) attenuated opioid-induced somnolence, augmented opioid analgesia, treated depression, and improved cognitive function in cancer patients and recommended its use in palliative care (Rozans, Dreisbach, Lertora, et al., 2002). Co-administration of amphetamine has been reported to enhance the analgesic effects while counteracting the sedative effects of both morphine and meperidine (APS, 2003). (See Chapter 19 for treatment of opioid-induced sedation and Section V for more on the effects of adjuvant drugs.) NSAIDs combined with opioids can improve pain relief, and if this allows reduction in the opioid dose, the combination can reduce opioid-induced adverse effects (Ashburn, Caplan, Carr, et al., 2004; Kim, Kim, Nam, et al., 2008; Marret, Kurdi, Zufferey, et al., 2005; Schug, 2006; Schug, Manopas, 2007; White, 2005) (see Section III).

Prior Treatment Outcomes

In some cases, the prior experiences with opioids can be used to predict the response to future therapy. If a patient reports having previously experienced unmanageable adverse effects with an opioid, explore with the patient the occurrence, severity, and management of the adverse effects. An attempt should be made to determine whether the adverse effects were really unmanageable (e.g., nausea unresponsive to antiemetics) or simply unmanaged (e.g., no attempt made to relieve nausea). A drug that has been associated with intensely negative effects in the past usually is not preferred during later therapy. This is comparable to the decision to switch to another opioid if intolerable and unmanageable adverse effects occur during therapy, the strategy known as *opioid rotation* (Hanks, Cherny, Fallon, 2004) (see Chapter 18).

A true allergy to an opioid is extremely rare (Amabile, Bowman, 2006; Hanks, Cherny, Fallon, 2004; Woodall, Chiu, Weissman, 2008). Generalized erythema and bronchospasm within 4 hours of application of transdermal fentanyl were reported in an allergic patient (Dewachter, Lefebvre, Kalaboka, et al., 2009). Often, patients erroneously report being "allergic" to an opioid after experiencing adverse effects from it in the past. For example, patients commonly mistake nausea and vomiting after an opioid bolus dose as an allergy to the opioid. Patients also frequently assume that flushing, itching, or hives after initiation of opioid therapy reflects allergy. In most cases, this effect is believed to be related to a direct histamine-releasing effect of these drugs, an effect distinct from true hypersensitivity. In the absence of evidence of allergy, patients should be educated about the outcomes they experience and reassured that an adverse effect such as nausea or itching is an adverse effect and not an allergy.

Patient Preferences and Convenience

Often, patients have preferences when it comes to the choice of opioid, route of administration, and scheduling of doses. Unfortunately, a patient's request for a specific opioid is sometimes misinterpreted as a sign of addiction (see Section II). Respecting patients' preferences whenever feasible and making the opioid treatment regimen as convenient as possible may help the patient adhere better to the plan. Occasionally preferences are based on myths and misconceptions that can be corrected by providing factual information. During the initial interview with the patient, time can be taken to determine whether this is the case and ensure that the patient has an accurate understanding of pain management.

The oral and transdermal routes are the preferred routes of administration for continuous cancer and noncancer pain management. Occasionally, an alternative is needed. Although the rectal route is safe and effective, some patients with family caregivers are uncomfortable with the thought of a family member administering rectal medications to them. Occasionally patients who can self-administer their medications object to doing so by the rectal route. In these cases, alternative opioid delivery systems, such as continuous subcutaneous infusion, may provide a solution (see Chapter 14 for these alternative routes of administration).

Complying with the established opioid treatment regimen can become a problem for some patients, especially if the regimen requires the patient to take several pills several times a day. Older patients in particular may forget to take their pills at the prescribed intervals or object to taking so many pills. For these patients, a modified-release preparation of the opioid may be ideal. This will allow the patient to take pills once or twice daily instead of several times a day required by short-acting preparations. Scheduling doses along with

other medications the patient is already accustomed to taking also is recommended. For example, individuals can take their morning opioid dose with their daily vitamin. Nonopioids and opioids may be given at the same time (staggered dosing is not necessary). The fentanyl transdermal patch, which is changed only every 3 days in most individuals (see Chapter 14), can be considered also for patients who are unreliable in taking oral medications.

Cost

The cost of an opioid is an important consideration in selecting the optimal opioid for the pain treatment plan, especially for long-term opioid therapy. The cost of medications can vary greatly. Several years ago, an analysis of equianalgesic doses of opioids revealed a 19-fold price difference among opioid prescriptions (Ferrell, Griffith, 1994). A later cost comparison of routes of administration showed the cost for one day of opioid treatment; oral or rectal MS Contin 120 mg twice daily was $18.16; IV morphine at 3.3 mg/h was $17.08; SC hydromorphone at 0.9 mg/h was $24.33; and transdermal fentanyl at 50 mcg/h was $8.16 (Stevens, Ghazi, 2000). The authors pointed out that IV and SC infusions also incur the expense of supplies and equipment (e.g., tubings and pumps).

A number of factors influence the cost of drugs, including packaging of the drug, wholesale prices, and pharmacy dispensing fees. The cost of prescription opioids varies from one pharmacy to another, but the newer opioids without generic equivalents tend to be more expensive (Chamberlin, Cottle, Neville, et al., 2007). There are numerous websites, such as PharmacyChecker.com (http://www.pharmacychecker.com/), that compare drug costs worldwide. Some pain guidelines include tables displaying the costs of analgesics at the time of publication. Although listed prices in guidelines are likely to be different from current prices, they provide an idea of relative cost.

As a rule, morphine and especially methadone are significantly less expensive than other opioids, bulk containers of drugs are less expensive than prefilled syringes and unit dose or blister packs, and large hospitals or urban chain pharmacies that can purchase drugs in large quantities are likely to charge less than small independent pharmacies (Kunz, 1994). The use of multiple prescriptions (polypharmacy) to manage pain is more costly than single prescriptions. Although combined modalities are recommended, single opioids in sufficient doses may provide adequate pain control and certainly should be tried before adding adjuvant analgesics (Ferrell, Griffith, 1994).

Today, most individuals assume all or at least part of the cost of their medications. The insured patient's ability to pay depends on the amount of their co-payment. Great care should be taken to ensure cost savings for patients with end-stage disease so that appropriate pain management is not prohibitive and does not overburden patients and families with excessive costs. Many pharmaceutical companies have financial assistance programs that allow reduced purchase prices for patients who qualify. Prescribers can find information about this in the *Physician's Desk Reference* and at most pharmaceutical company websites. If drug costs are a significant issue, prices should be checked with the pharmacy.

Conclusion

There are many opioid analgesics to choose from when developing a pain treatment plan. The first-line opioids are mu agonist opioids; in most cases, there is no advantage to using an agonist-antagonist opioid for pain management. Selection of the optimal opioid analgesic is influenced by a number of patient factors, including age, coexisting disease, potential for drug-drug interaction, and previous experience with opioids. Cost of the drug is also a major consideration.

Chapter 14 Guidelines for Selection of Routes of Opioid Administration

before other routes because it is relatively safe, convenient, and inexpensive (Coyle, Cherny, Portenoy, 1995; Hanks, Cherny, Fallon, 2004; Stevens, Ghazi, 2000). The transdermal route is an accepted alternative for long-term therapy. If pain is severe and a rapid onset of analgesia is desired, the IV route can be used for rapid titration with close monitoring; the patient can be transitioned to the oral route when pain is under control.

Over time, it is often necessary to switch routes of administration (Hanks, Cherny, Fallon, 2004). For example, in a postoperative patient, the process of transitioning from IV or epidural to oral may require the use of both the old and the new routes to ensure continuous analgesia. For example, the patient may be started on the oral formulation while receiving PRN boluses by the IV route. When the oral route is established and at the approximate required dose, the IV route is discontinued.

In a survey of patients with cancer pain, more than half required more than one route of administration to maintain pain control during the last 4 weeks of life. This occurred usually when patients were unable to swallow. The routes used included rectal, SC, IV, and epidural. Sometimes patients required more than one route at a time (Coyle, Adelhardt, Foley, et al., 1990). Table 14-1 summarizes the advantages and disadvantages to some of the routes of opioid administration. This chapter presents most of the routes by which opioids are administered. The intraspinal routes are discussed separately in Chapter 15.

Oral

The oral route is the most commonly employed for patients with continuous cancer or noncancer pain, or mild to moderate acute pain (Fine, Portenoy, 2007; Hanks, Cherny, Fallon, 2004; Menefee, Katz, Zacharoff, 2007). The many oral formulations available provide convenience and flexibility (American Pain Society [APS], 2003). Given the potential to titrate the oral dose to whatever level is necessary, the most common reason for failure to achieve analgesia by

REGARDLESS of the type of pain being treated, opioids should be administered by the least invasive and safest route capable of producing satisfactory analgesia. The oral route is the most common and generally is selected

Table 14-1 | Routes of Opioid Administration

Route	Comments
Oral	Inexpensive, simple, noninvasive; should be considered before all other routes. Preferred in cancer and persistent noncancer pain management. Opioids are subject to extensive hepatic metabolism; slow onset but just as effective as other routes if doses are high enough and given ATC.
Oral transmucosal	Lipophilic drugs absorbed well by this route. Oral transmucosal fentanyl citrate (OTFC) has been shown to be effective and convenient in managing breakthrough pain in opioid-tolerant patients with cancer and noncancer pain. Opioid bypasses significant hepatic metabolism.
Buccal	Buccal fentanyl (BF) has been shown to be effective and convenient in managing breakthrough pain in opioid-tolerant patients with cancer and noncancer pain. A lack of other opioids in suitable preparations limits the usefulness of this route.
Sublingual	Buprenorphine, fentanyl, and methadone absorbed well; currently only buprenorphine is available in the United States. Morphine is commonly used by the sublingual route, but absorption of hydrophilic drugs is poor.
Rectal	Currently morphine, oxymorphone, and hydromorphone are commercially available in the United States. Alternative route for patients unable or unwilling to take analgesics orally. Considerable variation in dose required to produce effect and time to reach effect. Starting dose usually is same dose as oral dose. Any opioid may be compounded by pharmacy for rectal administration or given in an aqueous solution, unmodified tablet, or crushed and placed in gelatin capsule for rectal insertion; modified-release formulations should not be crushed or dissolved.
Vaginal	No commercially available formulations; research lacking, but absorption does occur by this route.
Transdermal	Available in fentanyl citrate drug delivery system incorporated within an adhesive patch. Can provide analgesia for 48 to 72 hours by continuous drug release via the skin to systemic circulation. Slow onset when patch is initially applied, gradual decline after patch is removed. Difficult to titrate; must use short-acting opioid until analgesia is achieved. Alternative for patients unable or unwilling to take analgesics orally. Not suitable for acute pain or severe escalating pain. Heat should not be applied to patch as this increases absorption and has resulted in life-threatening respiratory depression and death.
Intranasal	Butorphanol is available in the United States but not recommended for cancer or persistent noncancer pain. Sufentanil has been administered intranasally for breakthrough pain. Major drawback, especially in children, is burning and stinging on instillation. Bypasses significant hepatic metabolism.
Nebulized	Nebulization is not recommended as a primary route for analgesia, primarily because current administration techniques result in very small amounts of analgesic being absorbed; however, case reports suggest some analgesic efficacy, and nebulized morphine is used for management of dyspnea in end-stage terminal illness (e.g., chronic lung disease, heart failure).
Subcutaneous • Single or repetitive bolus • CI with or without PCA	Morphine and hydromorphone most common opioids administered subcutaneously, although fentanyl has also been administered by this route. Alternative when patient is unable to take opioid orally or parenteral route is indicated but venous access is limited. Easy to access, but technique and care require more skill and expertise than oral or rectal administration. Infusion pumps add expense, but are more convenient and allow for CI and PCA capability.
Intravenous • Single or repetitive bolus • CI with or without PCA	Indicated when rapid titration is required. Provides steady blood levels. Opioids with short half-life recommended. Boluses or PCA commonly used for postoperative pain management. Duration is dose dependent. When steady state is reached by continuous infusion, the various opioids differ little in terms of duration. For long-term CI, permanent venous access is recommended; indicated for cancer and persistent noncancer pain when patient has dose-limiting adverse effects from other systemic routes.

Continued

Table 14-1 | Routes of Opioid Administration—cont'd

Route	Comments
Epidural • Single or repetitive bolus • PCEA with or without CI • Chronic: Implanted for CI with side port for bolus injection	Indicated for major abdominal, thoracic, and joint surgeries when severe acute pain is anticipated; rarely indicated for cancer and persistent noncancer pain management (e.g., may be alternative for patients with dose-limiting adverse effects from systemic opioid analgesics). Infusion pumps add expense, but are more convenient and allow for continuous infusion and PCA capability. Duration is dose dependent. When steady state is reached by continuous infusion, the various opioids differ little in terms of duration. May be cost-effective for patients with cancer or persistent noncancer pain and long life expectancy; may be administered by external catheter and pump or by implanted infusion pump. Local anesthetics frequently added to opioids by this route.
Intrathecal • Acute: Single bolus • Chronic: Implanted for CI with side port for bolus injections	Indicated for some acute pain (single bolus most commonly used because temporary indwelling catheters are difficult to maintain); rarely indicated for cancer and persistent noncancer pain management (e.g., may be alternative for patients with dose-limiting adverse effects from systemic opioid analgesics). May be cost-effective for patients with cancer or persistent noncancer pain and long life expectancy; usually administered by implanted infusion pump.
Intraarticular (joint)	Shown to produce adequate analgesia for joint surgeries, but further studies are needed to establish best opioids and local anesthetics to use by this route.

ATC, Around-the-clock; *CI,* continuous infusion; *FDA,* Food and Drug Administration; *PCA,* patient-controlled analgesia.

Opioid analgesics can be administered by a wide variety of routes. This table summarizes the advantages and disadvantages to some of these. See text for detailed discussion.

From Pasero, C., & McCaffery, M. (2011). *Pain assessment and pharmacologic management,* pp. 369-370, St. Louis, Mosby. Data from Buxton, I. L. O. (2006). Pharmacokinetics and pharmacodynamics. The dynamics of drug absorption, distribution, action, and elimination. In L. L. Brunton, J. S. Lazo, & K. L. Parker KL (Eds.), *Goodman & Gilman's the pharmacological basis of therapeutics,* ed 11, New York, McGraw-Hill; Darwish, M., Kirby, M., Jiang, J. G., et al. (2008). Bioequivalence following buccal and sublingual placement of fentanyl buccal tablet 400 microg in healthy subjects. *Clin Drug Investig, 28*(1), 1-7.; Darwish, M., Kirby, M., Robertson, P. Jr, et al. (2007). Absolute and relative bioavailability of fentanyl buccal tablet and oral transmucosal fentanyl citrate. *J Clin Pharmacol, 47*(3), 343-350; Dale, O., Hjortkjær, R., & Kharasch, E. D. (2002). Nasal administration of opioids for pain management in adults. *Acta Anaesthesiol Scand, 46*(7), 759-770; Gordon, D. B. (2008). New opioid formulations and delivery systems. *Pain Manage Nurs, 8*(3, Suppl 1), S6-S13; Gutstein, H. B., & Akil, H. (2006). Opioid analgesics. In L. L. Brunton, J. S. Lazo, & K. L. Parker (Eds.), *Goodman & Gilman's the pharmacological basis of therapeutics,* ed 11, New York, McGraw-Hill; Hanks, G., Cherny, N. I., & Fallon, M. (2004). Opioid analgesic therapy. In D. Doyle, G. Hanks, N. I. Cherny, et al. (Eds.), *Oxford textbook of palliative medicine,* ed 3, New York, Oxford Press; Holmquist, G. (2009). Opioid metabolism and effects of cytochrome P450. *Pain Med, 10*(Suppl 1), S20-S29; Shelley, K., & Paech, M. J. (2008). The clinical applications of intranasal opioids. *Curr Drug Deliv, 5*(1), 55-58; Smith, H. S. (2003). *Drugs for pain.* Philadelphia, Hanley & Belfus; Stevens, R. A., & Ghazi, S. M. (2000). Routes of opioid analgesic therapy in the management of cancer pain. www.medscape.com/viewarticle/408974. Accessed January 9, 2009; Swarm, R. A., Karanikolas, M., & Cousins, M. J. (2004). In D. Doyle, G. Hanks, N. I. Cherny, et al. (Eds.), *Oxford textbook of palliative medicine,* ed 3, New York, Oxford Press; Vascello, L., & McQuillan, R. J. (2006). Opioid analgesics and routes of administration. In O. A. de Leon-Casasola (Ed.), *Cancer pain. Pharmacological, interventional and palliative care approaches,* Philadelphia, Saunders. © 2011, Pasero C, McCaffery M. May be duplicated for use in clinical practice.

this route is insufficient dose administration. There is wide interindividual variation in response to opioids, however, and if attempts to escalate the oral dose of opioid do not achieve the desired response or result in unacceptable adverse effects, switching to a different oral opioid should be considered, as unresponsiveness to one opioid does not predict response to others (Fine, Portenoy, 2007).

Most first-line mu agonists and dual-mechanism drugs are available in oral form; fentanyl is not. Of the agonist-antagonist opioids, only pentazocine is available orally. Oral opioids in tablet form can be taken by most patients. Capsules and liquids are available for some opioids. Liquids should be carefully measured using an oral medication syringe or graduated liquid measuring spoon. Both of these measuring devices are available free from most pharmacies. When prescribing, dispensing, and administering opioids, care should be taken to ensure that the correct concentration and milligram amount are specified. Liquids should be ordered by milligram amount, not just volume, to avoid serious dosing errors (Institute for Safe Medication Practices, 2007). Non–modified-release

tablet formulations can be crushed and taken with soft foods or put into suspensions (APS, 2003). Modified-release tablets; however, should not be cut, crushed, or chewed because this destroys the release mechanisms and risks severe overdose by releasing the half-day or full-day dose all at once. Modified-release medications in capsules may be opened and sprinkled on soft food, such as applesauce, but should not be chewed or allowed to dissolve (APS, 2003). Small amounts of food should be used to ensure consumption of the entire dose.

Disadvantages of the Oral Route

Two major disadvantages of the oral route are that it has a slow onset of action (typically 30 to 45 minutes) (APS, 2003) and a relatively delayed peak time (60 to 120 minutes after ingestion, and longer in the case of some of the modified-release tablets) (Hanks, Cherny, Fallon, 2004). As a result of these kinetics, the oral route is not ideal when it is imperative to get severe pain under control quickly, such as for pain crisis related to malignancy or myocardial infarction (Moryl, Coyle, Foley, 2008).

Although opioids tend to have a longer duration of action orally than parenterally, intervals between doses of short-acting preparations are relatively brief—commonly 4 hours. This requires the patient to take six to eight doses a day, a regimen that can interfere with patient activities, such as sleeping. The patient must remember to take all doses to maintain a constant level of analgesia.

A potential disadvantage for those opioids with active metabolites is that the ratio between the metabolite concentration and the parent compound is much higher when the drug is given orally and subjected to a larger first-pass effect through the liver than when it is given parenterally. This is true for morphine and its glucuronidated metabolites, for example (Lotsch, 2005). In most patients, this difference between oral and other routes is not clinically significant, but for some, particularly those with renal insufficiency, the relative concentration of the metabolites could be high enough to cause adverse effects.

The oral route is not an option for patients who are NPO (nothing by mouth), such as immediately after surgery. Some patients cannot tolerate the oral route because of GI obstruction or difficulty swallowing (Fine, Portenoy, 2007). Absorption by the oral route can be altered by a number of factors, including presence of food, gastric emptying time, and GI motility. Modified-release preparations appear to be less affected by the presence of food than short-acting preparations (see individual drugs later in this chapter, and see Chapter 13 for more).

The effectiveness of the oral route depends on patient compliance. Patients who must self-administer their medications but cannot adhere to the dosing regimen necessary to maintain stable effects are not good candidates for the oral route unless they are able to take formulations designed for once-a-day dosing (Lehne, 2004).

Finally, some oral medications, especially those in tablet or liquid form, have a bitter or unpleasant taste, to which most patients object. After administration, "chasers" of applesauce or lemon drops may be helpful in reducing the bitterness (Gardner-Nix, 1996).

Selected Oral Opioid Formulations

As mentioned, all of the first-line mu opioids except fentanyl are available in short-acting oral formulations, and several modified-release formulations exist. Opioids available in oral modified-release formulations in the United States include morphine (MS Contin, Oramorph SR, Kadian, Avinza, and generics), oxycodone (OxyContin), oxymorphone (Opana ER), hydromorphone (Exalgo), and tramadol (Ultram ER). Codeine is available as a modified-release product outside of the United States. Of the modified-release preparations, MS Contin has the smallest tablet, which is an important consideration in patients who have difficulty swallowing. MS Contin tablets are color-coded according to dose, as are Kadian and Avinza capsules, which may help prevent errors in dosing.

The modified-release opioid preparations have rendered the oral route more convenient than in the past by requiring only once- or twice-daily dosing. This may improve patient adherence to medication regimens and may also decrease the patient's sense of being sick (APS, 2003; Fine, Portenoy, 2007; Gallagher, Welz-Bosna, Gammaitoni, 2007). These preparations simplify the regimen necessary to maintain relatively stable blood levels of the drug, potentially increasing their effectiveness for continuous pain (APS, 2003). Although unproven, some experts recommend modified-release products as one of the treatment strategies for patients at risk of opioid abuse because they may be less reinforcing of some drug-related behaviors and may be less likely to cause euphoria (Webster, Dove, 2007).

Patients should be observed closely for the need to shorten the recommended dosing interval of the modified-release agent. For example, although MS Contin and Oramorph were designed for 12-hour dosing, it is not unusual for patients to experience some end-of-dose failure (pain at the end of the dosing interval), which can be eliminated by switching to 8-hour dosing (Argoff, 2007). An observational cohort study found that 86% and 91% of patients taking modified-release morphine or oxycodone, respectively, required dosing more frequently than that recommended by the product's manufacturers (Gallagher, Welz-Bosna, Gammaitoni, 2007). This underscores the importance of systematic assessment to determine the optimal dose interval as well as a need to develop modified-release formulations that provide satisfactory and sustained analgesia throughout the recommended dosing interval.

Although further research is warranted, the time of day that patients take their once-daily opioid dose does not appear to matter. A multicenter, randomized, placebo-controlled, cross-over study of patients with advanced cancer found essentially the same pain intensities when the once-daily dose of modified-release morphine was taken in the morning as when it was taken in the evening (Currow, Plummer, Cooney, et al., 2007). Patients can be told to find the time that works best to keep their pain under control.

Following is a discussion of the various oral formulations of morphine, oxycodone, oxymorphone, and hydromorphone. Formulations designed to deter abuse are also discussed.

Oral Morphine

Morphine is available in 15 and 30 mg short-acting tablets, and in 2, 4, 10, and 20 mg/mL solutions. These dose forms are used primarily when opioid therapy is initiated and for breakthrough pain (see Chapter 12 for more on breakthrough pain). MS Contin and Oramorph SR, modified-release formulations of morphine, are available in 15, 30, 60, and 100 mg tablets; MS Contin also is available in a 200 mg tablet. There are also generic products available at varying strengths. The recommended dosing interval is every 12 hours and no less than every 8 hours. There are two other modified-release morphine formulations, Kadian and Avinza, supplied as capsules that contain pellets which release drug at different rates. Kadian is available in 10, 20, 30, 50, 60, 80, 100, and 200 mg capsules and can be given every 12 or 24 hours. Avinza is available in 30, 45, 60, 75, 90, and 120 mg capsules and is approved for once-daily dosing. The Avinza prescribing information contains a black box warning that alcohol is not to be ingested while taking Avinza, as there is a risk of the pellets dissolving and the full daily dose of morphine being released at once (King Pharmaceuticals, 2008a). Kadian does not require such a warning (Alpharma Pharmaceuticals, 2008; Johnson, Wagner, Sun, et al., 2008), but alcohol can have additive CNS effects when ingested by a person taking any opioid and should be used with great caution. See Patient Education Form IV-9 (pp. 562-563) on short-acting morphine (includes concentrate), Form IV-10 (pp. 564-565) on modified-release 12-hour morphine, and Form IV-11 (pp. 566-567) on modified-release 24-hour morphine at the end of Section IV.

The pharmacokinetics of the modified-release formulations are complex because the time to steady state is determined by the half-life of absorption rather than the terminal elimination half-life. All of the modified-release formulations approach steady state in a 2- to 3-day timeframe. Like other oral formulations, the drugs are not preferable for rapid titration to address severe pain. Although patients can be titrated using the modified-release drug, an accepted alternative approach is to titrate first to a stable dose of short-acting morphine, then switch to the modified-release formulation (APS, 2003).

Co-administration of a short-acting opioid for breakthrough pain is conventional practice during the treatment of patients with pain related to active cancer or other types of serious illnesses; it is implemented on a case-by-case basis during the treatment of persistent noncancer pain based on a separate analysis of risk and benefit (Fine, Portenoy, 2007). Availability of a short-acting drug during dose titration of the modified-release formulation may facilitate dose finding and the comfort of the patient; the modified-release dose can be titrated every 24 to 48 hours (Twycross, Wilcock, 2007). The short-acting dose may or may not be continued after a stable dose of the modified-release drug is found. One study randomized 40 patients with uncontrolled cancer pain to titration with short-acting oral morphine given every 4 hours or titration with modified-release morphine (Kapanol, Kadian) given once daily (Klepstad, Kaasa, Jystad, et al., 2003). The mean time to achieve adequate pain control was 2.1 days with short-acting morphine and 1.7 days with modified-release morphine, and those taking the latter reported feeling less tired at the end of titration. No other differences in adverse effects, health-related quality of life functions, or satisfaction with treatment were noted.

Although the various forms of modified-release morphine contain the same drug and are of the same dose strength, they may or may not be bioequivalent. MS Contin and Oramorph SR, for example, are pharmaceutically equivalent because they contain the same drug, have the same dose form, can deliver the same amount of drug, are both available in the same dose strengths, and are given by the same route; however, the two are not necessarily therapeutically equivalent because they use different modified-release mechanisms. This means that the same dose of each product may not affect the patient in the same way (McCaffery, Lochman, 1996). The FDA does not consider any of the modified-release dose forms to be therapeutically equivalent unless bioequivalence data have been submitted. Given the many choices now available, it is best not to assume that very similar products will behave the same in a given individual. It should be recognized, however, that the FDA and some state laws have allowed pharmacists, physicians and other prescribers, institutions, and health care plans to consider drugs containing the molecule to be therapeutically equivalent, even in the absence of confirmatory clinical data. If patients report a change in the outcomes associated with stable drug therapy, the clinician should assess whether the formulation may have been changed by the pharmacist (McCaffery, Lochman, 1996). Box 14-1 provides recommendations when switching from one pharmaceutically equivalent product to another.

The first modified-release morphine formulations were Oramorph and MS Contin. Oramorph contains a simple matrix system; GI fluid penetrates the tablet, hydrates the matrix, and forms a gel layer that breaks down and dissolves gradually over the dosing period (Amabile, Bowman, 2006). MS Contin tablets contain morphine in a dual-control (hydrophilic and hydrophobic) polymer matrix that controls the release of morphine (Amabile, Bowman, 2006). This sophisticated hydrophilic/hydrophobic relationship is reported to provide a more constant and predictable release of morphine from the system than is possible with the simpler Oramorph release mechanism (Amabile, Bowman, 2006).

Avinza is a capsule containing both fast-acting and modified-release beads of morphine. The primary advantage of this combination is that the fast-acting component allows the morphine concentration to plateau rapidly (within 30 minutes), and the modified-release component maintains the plasma concentration throughout the dosing interval (Amabile, Bowman, 2006). Most patients obtain adequate pain relief with either 12- or 24-hour dosing of the drug (Argoff, 2007). A comparative steady-state analysis of once-daily Avinza and twice-daily modified-release morphine (MS Contin) found that the two formulations provide similar total systemic exposure of morphine and its metabolites throughout a 24-hour period but have distinct pharmacokinetic profiles due to divergent technologies (Portenoy, Sciberras, Eliot, et al., 2002). Avinza maintains morphine concentrations at or greater than

Box 14-1 | Switching from One Pharmaceutically Equivalent Product to Another

- Examples of pharmaceutically equivalent products are MS Contin, Oramorph SR, and Kadian at 100 mg each.
- Assume that some difference may exist in therapeutic effects between the products.
- Completely switch from one product to the other. Avoid having patients take more than one product at a time (except during the transition phase), and avoid switching back and forth between products. The same formulation should be used if the patient is moved from hospital to home and vice versa.
- Advise the patient and family that the new drug may not have the same effect as the previous drug and that the dose may need to be adjusted.
- Monitor pain and sedation. Use a flow sheet for documentation so that problems can be detected early.
- Instruct the patient and family about the different products (e.g., Oramorph SR tablets are white and about the size of an aspirin; MS Contin tablets are smaller, and each strength is a different color). Tell the patient to question anyone who attempts to substitute one brand for another.

Drugs can be pharmaceutically equivalent without being therapeutically equivalent. This is because the drugs use different modified-release mechanisms. This means that the same dose of each product may not affect the patient in the same way. Box 4-11 lists examples of drugs that are pharmaceutically equivalent but not therapeutically equivalent and guidelines for switching from one to another.

From Pasero, C., & McCaffery, M. (2011). *Pain assessment and pharmacologic management*, p. 373, St. Louis, Mosby. Data from McCaffery, M., & Lochman, C. (1996). Controlled release morphine products. *Am J Nurs*, 96(4), 65. © 2011, Pasero C, McCaffery M. May be duplicated for use in clinical practice.

50% and 75% for a longer duration of time than MS Contin. This may help to explain why studies have shown that the two drugs appear to have similar efficacy, but that Avinza may offer some additional benefits. For example, Avinza produced analgesia and adverse effects comparable to MS Contin but with greater improvements in sleep in patients with osteoarthritis (OA) pain (Caldwell, Rapoport, Davis, et al., 2002; Rosenthal, Moore, Groves, et al., 2007). Another study in patients with a variety of types of noncancer pain showed improvements in pain

relief and both sleep and physical functioning over the 3-month study period with Avinza (Adams, Chwiecko, Ace-Wagoner, et al., 2006). Patients with noncancer pain of various origins (including neuropathic) that was unresponsive to short-acting opioid regimens experienced reduced pain and improvements in depressive symptoms and cognitive functioning after taking Avinza for 4 weeks (Panjabi, Panjabi, Shepherd, et al., 2008).

Once-daily Avinza has also been shown to produce more consistent opioid plasma concentrations with less frequent dosing compared with twice-daily modified-release oxycodone (OxyContin, see the paragraphs that follow) in healthy volunteers (Eliot, Geiser, Loewen, 2001). A multicenter study randomized 392 patients with persistent back pain (including some with neuropathic pain) to receive either Avinza every 24 hours or modified-release oxycodone every 12 hours; supplemental ibuprofen was allowed (Rauck, Bookbinder, Bunker, et al., 2006). Following a titration period, 174 patients took their study drug at a fixed dose for four weeks followed by a four-week period during which the dose could be changed as needed. Those taking Avinza experienced better pain control with a lower daily opioid dose, consumed fewer breakthrough doses, and had better sleep quality than those taking modified-release oxycodone. Adverse effects were similar. Patient surveys were used to evaluate physical function and revealed improvements in both groups but no significant differences between the two; however, fewer patients were unable to work due to illness or treatment in the Avinza group than in the modified-release oxycodone group (Rauck, Bookbinder, Bunker, et al., 2007).

Kadian, the other once-daily morphine formulation, is available in a capsule containing polymer-coated modified-release pellets of morphine (Alpharma Pharmaceuticals, 2008; Amabile, Bowman, 2006). If differs from Avinza in that it does not contain a fast-acting component. Its time to maximum serum level (tmax) is the longest (approximately 9.5 hours) of any of the modified-release morphine formulations (Rosielle, 2007). An analysis of data on nearly 1042 patients with noncancer pain who were started on Kadian once daily and could switch after two weeks to 12-hour dosing if necessary (Nicholson, Ross, Weil, et al., 2006) was undertaken to determine factors that influenced the patients' choice of dosing interval (Weil, Nicholson, Sasaki, 2009). At the end of the study, 56.8% were taking the drug once daily and 43.2% were taking it every 12 hours. Race and gender did not influence dosing, but those with higher baseline and 2-week pain intensities were more likely to switch to a 12-hour dosing schedule, and older patients were more likely to remain on the 24-hour dosing schedule. Those who switched to 12-hour dosing experienced improved pain control, and by week 4, efficacy was comparable between the two dosing schedules. A review of the data of 68 patients taking Kadian for persistent pain showed the drug to be safe and effective for long-term opioid therapy (mean treatment = 12 months) (Chao, 2005). Patients in the review had a variety of pain conditions including radiculopathy and neck, head, and back pain. The median daily dose was 60 mg (range 20 to 400 mg); pain intensity (0 to 10) was reduced from a mean baseline of 7.8 to 5.2; 29% were considered non-responders, but over one-third of the patients experienced a reduction to 2.9; and, as in the previous study, over one-half of the patients were maintained on once-daily dosing.

In summary, some studies have shown patient preference for one morphine product or another, but as long as one product is used consistently and titrated to effect, they should all provide equally effective analgesia with the same adverse effect profile (Rosielle, 2007). Key to this is ensuring that the optimal dosing interval is prescribed. As mentioned, a high percentage of patients require more frequent dosing intervals than are recommended by the manufacturer (Argoff, 2007; Gallagher, Welz-Bosna, Gammaitoni, 2007).

Oral Oxycodone

Oxycodone is used extensively by the oral route and is available in both short-acting and modified-release formulations. It is also available alone or in combination (2.5 to 10 mg) with varying amounts of acetaminophen, aspirin, or ibuprofen (see Table 13-9 on p. 351). Single-entity oxycodone is available in 5, 15, and 30 mg tablets (capsules in 5 mg) and in two solution strengths, 5 mg/5mL and a 20 mg/mL concentrate (see the safety considerations for liquid opioids earlier in the chapter). The short-acting dose forms typically are used for short-term acute pain and for breakthrough pain.

With the varying doses and dose types (tablet, capsule, liquid) available, there is potential for confusion on the part of both clinician and patient. Prescriptions must be carefully written for each individual, and it is prudent to have the patient bring in the prescription bottle if refills are needed.

A drawback to the use of oxycodone combinations is that the clinician must carefully monitor the dose of acetaminophen, aspirin, or ibuprofen to ensure that maximum safe levels are not exceeded. Increases in the dose of oxycodone for inadequate pain relief are limited by acetaminophen's and aspirin's recommended maximum daily dose of 4000 mg and ibuprofen's limit of 3200 mg (see Section III). At the time of publication, the United States Food and Drug Administration (U.S. FDA) was considering the need to restrict the availability of a maximum dose/tablet of acetaminophen to 325 mg and eliminate analgesics with fixed combinations of opioids-nonopioids (e.g., oxycodone plus acetaminophen [Percocet, Vicodin]) because of concerns of overdose and resultant liver failure (U.S. FDA, 2009b; Harris, 2008).

Single-entity preparations have allowed broader use of oxycodone. Oxycodone is one of four opioid analgesics that are available in the United States in 12-hour modified-release form (OxyContin) for twice daily dosing; it is also approved for 8-hour dosing for patients who do not maintain pain relief for 12 hours (see Tamper-Resistant and Abuse-Deferrent Oral Opioid Formations on p. 378). OxyContin is available in 10, 15, 20, 30, 40, 60, 80, and 160 mg tablets. Doses of 60, 80 and 160 mg or any single dose of greater than 40 mg are approved for opioid-tolerant patients only. These are small tablets that are color-coded according to dose. See Patient Education Form IV-14 (pp. 572-573) on oxycodone with acetaminophen, Form IV-12 (pp. 568-569) on short-acting oxycodone, and Form IV-13 (pp. 570-571) on modified-release oxycodone at the end of Section IV.

OxyContin exhibits a biphasic release profile, with an initial peak at approximately 0.6 hours and a second peak at approximately 6.9 hours (Purdue Pharma, 2007). Analgesic onset occurs in most patients within 1 hour of administration, sooner than that produced by the delivery system in MS Contin (Kalso, 2005). The rapid-release phase of OxyContin has a half-life of 37 minutes and releases 38% of the total dose; the slower phase has a half-life of 6.2 hours and accounts for the remaining 62% of the dose (De Pinto, Dunbar, Edwards, 2006). The rationale for this formulation was to provide an extended duration of analgesia without significantly compromising the brisk onset of analgesia inherent in conventional short-acting products (Davis, Varga, Dickerson, et al., 2003). Early clinical trials demonstrated that patients with cancer pain or noncancer pain could be converted from other opioids and titrated to comfort using modified-release oxycodone as readily as with a short-acting opioid (Salzman, Roberts, Wild, et al., 1999).

The bioavailability of modified-release oxycodone is similar to short-acting oxycodone, and it is as effective at 12-hour dosing as the equivalent dose of short-acting oxycodone taken at 4-hour intervals (Davis, Varga, Dickerson, et al., 2003). A morphine to oxycodone ratio of 1.5:1 is considered equianalgesic.

Modified-release oxycodone has been found to be effective for a wide variety of types of pain (Riley, Eisenberg, Muller-Schwefe, et al., 2008) (see research below). Like modified-release morphine, it is used for continuous cancer pain and non–cancer-related pain of all types. It also has been used for treatment of some types of acute pain. The extensive literature on OxyContin includes the following types of pain:

- Acute postoperative pain (Blumenthal, Min, Marquardt, et al., 2007; Cheville, Chen, Oster, et al., 2001; de Beer, Winemaker, Donnelly, et al., 2005; Dorr, Raya, Long, et al., 2008; Ginsberg, Sinatra, Adler, et al., 2003; Kampe, Warm, Kaufmann, et al., 2004) (See also Trend in Oral Analgesics for Postoperative Pain in paragraphs that follow.)
- Cancer pain (Gralow, 2002; Pan, Zhang, Zhang, et al., 2007; Reid, Martin, Sterne, et al., 2006).
- Persistent noncancer pain (Portenoy, Farrar, Backonja, et al., 2007; Roth, Fleischmann, Burch, et al., 2000)

- Acute exacerbation of noncancer pain (Ma, Jiang, Zhou, et al., 2008)
- Neuropathic pain (Eisenberg, McNicol, Carr, 2006; Furlan, Sandoval, Mailis-Gagnon, et al., 2006; Gimbel, Richards, Portenoy, 2003; Watson, Moulin, Watt-Watson, et al., 2003).

Among the controlled trials conducted with OxyContin have been several demonstrating the potential utility of combination therapy. One randomized study of 338 patients with painful diabetic neuropathy, for example, found that those who took a combination of modified-release oxycodone and gabapentin required less rescue medication, experienced significantly better pain relief and sleep, and were less likely to discontinue treatment due to lack of therapeutic effectiveness than those who took gabapentin plus placebo (Hanna, O'Brien, Wilson, 2008). This finding was not surprising given data from another controlled trial (N = 87) demonstrating that modified-release oxycodone was more effective than gabapentin for relief of acute pain of herpes zoster (Dworkin, Barbano, Tyring, et al., 2009). Similarly, oxycodone has been included in multimodal postoperative pain treatment plans (see later in this chapter for trends in the use of oral opioids for postoperative pain).

Oral Oxymorphone

Oxymorphone is available in short-acting (Opana) and modified-release (Opana ER) oral formulations. Short-acting oxymorphone is available in 5 and 10 mg tablets, and modified-release oxymorphone is available in 5, 7.5, 10, 15, 20, 30, and 40 mg tablets. The tablets are color-coded according to dose.

Oxymorphone is more lipophilic than morphine, which may account for the slightly faster onset of action of its short-acting formulation (30 to 45 minutes) (Smith, 2009). A mean time to peak effect of 30 minutes has been associated with all doses of short-acting oxymorphone (Smith, 2009). The oral bioavailability of oxymorphone is 10% (Prommer, 2006b), and consumption of food at the time of dosing, particularly food with a high fat content, can increase the plasma concentration of oral oxymorphone (short-acting and modified-release) by as much as 50%. Oxymorphone is extensively metabolized in the liver and produces clinically inert metabolites (Smith, 2009). Oxymorphone's half-life (7 to 11 hours) is longer than morphine's (2 to 4 hours) (Chamberlin, Cottle, Neville, 2007), and, as a consequence, the time required to approach steady state is longer (Smith, 2009). Oxymorphone is more potent than morphine and oxycodone, and has suggested oral conversion ratios of 3:1 and 2:1, respectively (Smith, 2009).

Depending on pain severity, the initial dose of short-acting oxymorphone usually is 5 to 10 mg in opioid-naïve patients (Endo, 2006). Because food can increase the plasma concentration of oral oxymorphone, the drug should be taken on an empty stomach (1 hour before or 2 hours after a meal), and alcohol should be avoided as co-ingestion can increase serum levels up to 270% (Chamberlin, Cottle, Neville, 2007; Guay, 2007; Smith, 2009). These are important considerations when selecting an opioid; oral oxymorphone would not be a good choice in those who are unable to follow these dosing restrictions.

The use of short-acting oral oxymorphone is similar to morphine, hydromorphone, and oxycodone formulations. It is most appropriate for treatment of acute pain, such as postoperative pain (Gimbel, Ahdieh, 2004), and cancer- and non–cancer-related breakthrough pain (Sloan, Slatkin, Ahdieh, 2005). A randomized, placebo-controlled, parallel-group trial in 331 patients following abdominal surgery demonstrated that oxymorphone 5 mg or 10 mg provided comparable pain relief to oxycodone 10 mg (Aqua, Gimbel, Singla, et al., 2007). Another randomized controlled trial administered 5 mg of short-acting oxymorphone or placebo hourly as needed for up to 8 hours to 122 patients with mostly moderate-intensity pain following outpatient knee arthroscopy (Gimbel, Walker, Ma, et al., 2005). Patients in the oxymorphone group had significantly better pain relief, required less rescue medication, and were more likely to rate their pain relief as very good or excellent.

Modified-release oxymorphone (Opana ER) was approved for use in the United States in 2006 for the treatment of moderate to severe persistent pain. Its unique formulation allows the release of oxymorphone dependent on the rate of penetration of water into a hydrophilic matrix. Modified-release oxymorphone is dosed every 12 hours, and, like short-acting oxymorphone, steady state is reached after 3 days of every-12-hour dosing (Smith, 2009). As mentioned, oxymorphone is more potent than oxycodone. One study explored the dose equivalency of modified-release formulations of oxymorphone and oxycodone and established an equianalgesic dose ratio of 2:1 (oxymorphone was twice as potent as oxycodone) (Gabrail, Dvergsten, Ahdieh, 2004). See Patient Education Form IV-15 (pp. 574-575) on short-acting oxymorphone and Form IV-16 (pp. 576-577) on modified-release oxymorphone at the end of Section IV.

Although it is common to titrate the opioid dose using the short-acting formulation, and then switch to the modified-release formulation, one study demonstrated that it is safe to start with the lowest modified-release oxymorphone dose (5 mg every 12 hours) in opioid-naïve patients with moderate to severe noncancer pain and titrate from there (Rauck, Ma, Kerwin, et al., 2008). Similar to other opioids, research has shown that fixed dosing and rapid titration resulted in a higher incidence of adverse effects than gradual titration of modified-release oxymorphone (Brennan, 2009).

Modified-release oxymorphone has been found to be effective in the treatment of a variety of types of persistent cancer and noncancer pain (Brennan, 2009; Prager,

Rauk, 2004; Sloan, Barkin, 2008; Sloan, Slatkin, Ahdieh, 2005; Slatkin, Tormo, Ahdieh, 2004). One study that evaluated modified-release oxymorphone in patients with persistent low back pain found that positive effects were less profound for those aspects of the pain likely to be neuropathic in origin (and described as cold, itchy, sensitive, tingling, and numb) than pains that were inferred to be nociceptive (and were described as sharp, aching, and deep) (Gould, Jensen, Victor, et al., 2009). This study lends support to the conclusion that is applied to all opioid drugs, i.e., that opioids are effective for neuropathic pain but may be relatively less effective for some pains of this type than pains conventionally considered to be nociceptive. (See Section I for more on nociceptive pain and neuropathic pain.)

The number of clinical trials that evaluate modified-release oxymorphone in diverse types of acute and persistent pain has been increasing. Studies have appeared in the following types:

- Cancer pain (Sloan, Slatkin, Ahdieh, 2005; Gabrail, Dvergsten, Ahdieh, 2004)
- Persistent low back pain (Gould, Jensen, Victor, et al., 2009; Hale, Ahdieh, Ma, et al., 2007; Hale, Dvergsten, Gimbel, 2005; Katz, Rauck, Ahdieh, et al., 2007; Penniston, Gould, 2009; Rauck, Ma, Kerwin, et al., 2008)
- OA pain (Kivitz, Ma, Ahdieh, et al., 2006; Matsumoto, Babul, Ahdieh, 2005; McIlwain, Ahdieh 2005; Rauck, Ma, Kerwin, et al., 2008)

Oxymorphone has been shown to be safe for long-term therapy (McIlwain, Ahdieh, 2005; Prager, Rauck, 2004; Rauck, Ma, Kerwin, et al., 2008). A multicenter, open-label, nonrandomized study (N = 126) evaluated opioid-naïve patients with noncancer pain during a 6-month gradual dose-titration and stabilization phase followed by a 5-month maintenance phase and found that modified-release oxymorphone provided effective, well-tolerated, and stable analgesia in 75% of the patients (Rauck, Ma, Kerwin, et al., 2008).

Although further research in special populations is needed, plasma concentrations of the drug and its metabolites have been shown to be 40% (mean) higher in older adults; therefore, initial low doses should be used in these patients, and titration should proceed cautiously (Smith, 2009). As with short-acting oxymorphone, Guay (2007) recommends beginning with the lowest dose of modified-release oxymorphone, 5 mg every 12 hours. Dose adjustments of oxymorphone are also likely to be necessary in patients with moderate renal and hepatic disease (Smith, 2009). Guay (2007) recommends avoiding oxymorphone entirely in patients with moderate to severe hepatic impairment. The drug was shown in one study to be removed by hemodialysis (Smith, 2009). There appears to be a low risk for interaction with concurrent medications that are metabolized by the CYP450 enzyme system, which may be a significant benefit in patients who are poor metabolizers or those who take multiple medications that rely on this enzyme system for metabolism, such as some antidepressants, beta blockers, antipsychotics, chemotherapeutic agents, and some other opioids (Adams, Pieniaszek, Gammaitoni, et al., 2005; Chamberlin, Cottle, Neville, 2007; McIlwain, Ahdieh 2005; Smith, 2009) (see Chapter 11 for more on cytochrome P450 enzymes and drug-drug interactions). The reader is referred to a 2009 journal supplement devoted to content on oxymorphone: *Pain Med* 10(Suppl 1).

Oral Hydromorphone

Oral short-acting hydromorphone is available in 2, 4, and 8 mg tablets and in a 1 mg/mL oral solution. Modified-release formulations of oral hydromorphone are available in Canada and Europe, and a once-daily formulation (Exalgo) (8, 12, and 16 mg tablets) was approved in the United States in 2010 (Gupta, Sathyan, 2007). The formulation uses a novel bilayer tablet system, the OROS® Push-Pull™ technology, to release hydromorphone at a relatively constant rate during a 24-hour period (Gardner-Nix, Mercadante, 2010). The bilayer core within the semipermeable tablet consists of a single drug layer (the "pull" layer) and a hydrophilic expanding compartment (the "push" layer). After tablet ingestion, fluid from the gastrointestinal (GI) tract forms a drug suspension and causes the push layer to expand. This exerts force on the pull layer and pushes the suspended drug out of the tablet through a laser-drilled orifice in the tablet shell membrane (Gardner-Nix, Mercadante, 2010).

Research in 31 healthy volunteers demonstrated that the pharmacokinetics of modified-release hydromorphone are linear and dose proportional (Sathyan, Xu, Thipphawong, et al., 2007a). Median peak concentration was noted between 12 and 16 hours with a mean terminal half-life of approximately 11 hours, both independent of dose. Steady state is reached after 48 hours of dosing (Gupta, Sathyan, 2007). The presence of food has little effect on the bioavailability of the drug (Sathyan, Xu, Thipphawong, et al., 2007b), and alcohol does not cause immediate release ("dose dumping") of the drug (Sathyan, Sivakumar, Thipphawong, et al., 2008). Drug release is independent of pH and agitation (Gupta, Sathyan, 2007).

A study of opioid-tolerant patients with persistent cancer pain (N = 73) or persistent noncancer pain (N = 331) stabilized the patients on their previous opioid, converted this dose to modified-release hydromorphone, then titrated to optimal dose using a stepwise approach, which was then maintained for 2 weeks (Palangio, Northfelt, Portenoy, et al., 2002). The majority of patients reached a stable dose of modified-release hydromorphone quickly (mean 12.1 days), and most required no or few steps to achieve it. The most common adverse effects were nausea and constipation. A morphine to hydromorphone conversion ratio of 5:1

was used, but the researchers reinforced the principle of decreasing the equianalgesic dose of the new opioid by 25% to 50% until research establishes differently (see Chapter 18). This study also suggested that direct conversion from another opioid to modified-release hydromorphone could be done without the intermediate step of titration with short-acting hydromorphone first. In other clinical trials, the once-daily hydromorphone has also been well tolerated with an adverse effect profile similar to other short- and modified-release opioid analgesics, such as morphine and oxycodone (Cousins, 2007; Gardner-Nix, Mercadante, 2010; Gupta, Sathyan, 2007; Hale, Tudor, Khanna, et al., 2007; Hanna, Thipphawong, 118 Study Group, 2008; Wallace, Thipphawong, 2007; Wirz, Wartenberg, Elsen, et al., 2006).

Long-term use of modified-release hydromorphone has been shown to be effective and safe. A multicenter open-label study (N = 388) administered modified-release hydromorphone for 274 days to patients with persistent cancer or noncancer pain (Wallace, Moulin, Rauck, et al., 2009). The median daily dose was 48 mg at 6, 9, and 12 months, with 75.9% of patients reporting overall treatment as good to excellent at 12 months. The most common adverse effects were nausea and constipation. A ratio of 5:1 (5 mg of morphine equivalents to 1 mg of hydromorphone) was used to convert opioid-tolerant patients with persistent noncancer pain from other oral opioids to modified-release hydromorphone without loss of efficacy or increase in adverse effects (Wallace, Rauck, Moulin, et al., 2007). (See Exalgo package insert for patient medication guide.)

Trend in Oral Analgesics for Postoperative Pain

With the current trend toward early discharge of patients after relatively major surgical procedures, consideration must be given to more aggressive pain treatment in the home setting than is possible with the traditional fixed combination opioid/nonopioid analgesics. The fixed dose of the nonopioid in these preparations limits the number of tablets that patients may take in a 24-hour period without exceeding the maximum safe daily dose (e.g., 4000 mg of acetaminophen). Single-entity opioids, such as morphine, oxycodone, and oxymorphone, are better choices if the anticipated severity or persistence of the pain increases the likelihood that dose titration will be needed.

Research has addressed the safety of early postoperative oral analgesia. A randomized controlled trial (N = 227) showed that early oral analgesia (first postoperative day) with scheduled 20 mg doses of short-acting morphine every 4 hours and an additional 10 mg dose every 2 hours PRN was safe and effective, producing similar analgesia as IV PCA with a basal rate after intraabdominal surgery (Pearl, McCauley, Thompson, et al., 2002). Others have found similar positive results with this approach following orthopedic surgery (Zaslansky, Eisenberg, Peskin, et al., 2006).

Modified-release opioids, used most often for patients with persistent cancer or noncancer pain, are increasingly prescribed in selected patients in the postoperative setting (Holt, Viscusi, Wordell, 2007; Pasero, McCaffery, 2007). The modified-release opioid formulations, e.g., MS Contin, OxyContin, and Opana ER, are FDA-approved for postoperative pain treatment in patients who were taking the particular opioid prior to surgery. They should also be considered for some opioid-naïve patients who are undergoing major surgeries that are associated with moderate to severe pain and are likely to require repeated doses of analgesics over several days. Modified-release opioids are not appropriate for pain that is mild or not expected to persist for an extended period of time.

Oxycodone (OxyContin) is the most widely studied modified-release opioid for treatment of postoperative pain. One study randomized 40 patients to receive either 20 mg of modified-release oxycodone or placebo preoperatively and every 12 hours postoperatively, in addition to IV morphine via PCA and IV acetaminophen (1 g) for 2 days following lumbar discectomy (Blumenthal, Min, Marquardt, et al., 2007). Those who received oxycodone consumed significantly less morphine; had significantly lower pain scores during rest, coughing, and with movement; experienced less nausea and vomiting and earlier recovery of bowel function; and reported higher satisfaction with their pain treatment than those who received placebo. Another study (N = 59) demonstrated that, compared with placebo, modified-release oxycodone given preoperative and every 12 hours postoperatively produced better pain relief, greater range of motion and quadriceps strength during physical therapy, and a shorter length of hospital stay by 2.3 days in patients following total knee arthroplasty (Cheville, Chen, Oster, et al., 2001). Others have found similar superior pain relief, reduced supplemental analgesic requirements, and cost savings with a range of doses (10 to 30 mg) of pre- and postoperative modified-release oxycodone following knee or hip replacement (de Beer, Winemaker, Donnelly, et al., 2005; Dorr, Raya, Long, et al., 2006) and breast surgery (Kampe, Warm, Kaufmann, et al., 2004).

Patients have been rapidly converted from IV opioids to modified-release oxycodone following major surgery. A multicenter, open-label study of 189 patients who were receiving IV PCA opioid for 12 to 24 hours following abdominal, orthopedic, or gynecologic surgery were given an initial dose of modified-release oxycodone at 12 hours postoperatively (Ginsberg, Sinatra, Adler, et al., 2003). The initial dose of oxycodone was calculated by multiplying the amount of IV morphine used in the previous 24 hours by a conversion factor of 1.2 to determine the daily dose of oxycodone, which was then divided by 2 to determine the every-12-hour dose of oxycodone (matched with available tablet strengths). This calculated amount of modified-release oxycodone plus breakthrough doses of NSAIDs or short-acting oxycodone every 4 hours PRN was well tolerated and provided satisfactory pain control for seven days postoperatively.

Though further research is needed, positive results were found with the use of modified-release oxymorphone for postoperative pain. One study randomized patients to receive modified-release oxymorphone 20 mg every 12 hours or placebo following knee arthroplasty (Ahdieh, Ma, Babul, et al., 2004). IV oxymorphone PCA was used for rescue analgesia. Patients who received modified-release oxymorphone had significantly better pain control and used significantly less rescue analgesia than those who received placebo. Treatment was well tolerated.

Tamper-Resistant and Abuse-Deterrent Oral Opioid Formulations

Several oral opioid formulations designed to be tamper-resistant and deter abuse were in various phases of investigation, development, and approval at the time of publication (Fleming, Noonan, Wheeler, et al., 2008; Jones, Johnson, Wagner, et al., 2008; Katz, Adams, Chilcoat, et al., 2007; Katz, Sun, Fox, et al., 2008; King Pharmaceuticals, 2008b; Medical News Today, 2008). A unique modified-release formulation (ALO-01, EMBEDA) contains pellets of morphine and sequestered naltrexone, an opioid antagonist (Johnson, Sun, Stuaffer, et al., 2007). Embeda was approved in 2009 and is available in capsules containing morphine/naltrexone in the following strengths: 20 mg/0.8 mg, 30 mg/1.2 mg, 50 mg/2 mg, 60 mg/2.4 mg, 80 mg/3.2 mg, and 100 mg/4 mg (King Pharmaceuticals, 2009). When taken as directed, the naltrexone remains sequestered in a pellet core and passes through the GI tract without significant absorption; however, if the product is crushed, chewed, or dissolved, the naltrexone is released and free to reverse opioid effects. A phase II multicenter, randomized-controlled, cross-over trial of 113 patients with moderate to severe OA pain was conducted to compare ALO-01 and modified-release morphine (Kadian) (Katz, Sun, Fox, et al., 2008). After a washout period to induce pain flare, patients were titrated to comfort with Kadian then randomized to receive either Kadian or ALO-01 for 14 days. Patients were then treated with Kadian for 7 days followed by a cross-over to the other study medication (either Kadian or ALO-01) for 14 days. Most of the patients (Kadian, 80% and ALO-01, 92%) rated the analgesics as good to excellent. Morphine exposure at steady state was similar, and plasma naltrexone levels were below quantification and had no effect on analgesia in those who took ALO-01. Adverse effects were similar and typical of opioids. A crossover study randomized 113 patients with moderate-to-severe OA pain to receive modified-release morphine (Kadian) or ALO-01 and demonstrated similar morphine exposure at steady state with the two formulations, and again the sequestered naltrexone had no effect on pain scores (Katz, Sun, Johnson, et al., 2009). When tested in recreational opioid users, crushed ALO-01 reduced euphoria due to naltrexone absorption and was no more desirable than intact morphine (Jones, Johnson, Wagner, et al., 2008).

OxyContin (12-hour modified-release oxycodone) is available in a novel abuse-deterrent formulation. The drug is contained within a hard gelatin capsule designed to resist tampering, such as crushing or dissolving in alcohol; other similar oxycodone formulations are in development (Fleming, Noonan, Wheeler, et al., 2008; Gordon, 2008; King Pharmaceuticals, 2008b). Research in healthy volunteers demonstrated that the technology successfully protected the drug from rapid release in various tampering simulations, such as chewing (Fleming, Noonan, Wheeler, et al., 2008). Plasma levels were lower when the drug was taken in a fasted state.

Oral Transmucosal

The oral mucosa functions similar to the skin as a barrier to dangerous substances. It differs from the skin in that it is significantly more vascular, more permeable to drugs with similar properties, and has a lower drug depot (storage) effect than the skin. Although mucosal drug absorption also involves hydrophilic pathways, absorption is optimized with drugs that are lipid soluble, such as fentanyl, buprenorphine, and methadone (Reisfield, Wilson, 2007). Three areas within the mouth can be used for oral transmucosal drug delivery: the sublingual, buccal, and gingival areas. These areas usually are regarded as separate routes of administration and are studied and discussed separately. Drug development for oral transmucosal routes of delivery has focused on acute pain management, primarily breakthrough pain, because a relatively rapid onset of effect can be achieved using these formulations.

Sublingual

Use of the sublingual route involves placing the drug under the tongue for absorption through the oral mucosa into the systemic circulation. Because the drug is absorbed directly into systemic circulation, the first-pass effect is avoided (Zhang, Zhang, Streisand, 2002). Of all the areas within the mouth for oral transmucosal drug administration, the sublingual area appears to be the highest in drug permeability. It is only 25% as thick as the buccal mucosa and, unlike the gingival mucosa, is nonkeratinized (Reisfield, Wilson, 2007). The sublingual route is an alternative when oral, parenteral, and rectal routes are unavailable or impractical (Reisfield, Wilson, 2007).

Few opioids have been administered by the sublingual route. Hospice nurses report success with morphine by the sublingual route (Robinson, Wilkie, Campbell, 1995), but it is thought that this is related to the fact that the drug is eventually swallowed; sublingual absorption of morphine and other hydrophilic drugs is poor (Hanks, Cherny, Fallon, 2004; Reisfield, Wilson, 2007).

The effects of lipid solubility, oral cavity pH, and drug contact time on sublingual absorption of various opioids and naloxone have been studied. Normal saliva pH is 6.5, but can vary with mouth breathing, nutritional status, food or beverage consumption, vomiting, stomatitis, and decreased salivary flow. Salivary pH also varies by region of the mouth (Reisfield, Wilson, 2007). Absorption of drugs is improved with high lipid solubility and an alkaline environment. Compared with morphine at pH 6.5 (18% absorption), the more lipophilic opioids—buprenorphine (55%), fentanyl (51%), and methadone (34%)—were absorbed to a significantly greater extent, whereas levorphanol, hydromorphone, oxycodone, heroin, and the opioid antagonist naloxone were not (Weinberg, Inturrisi, Reidenberg, et al., 1988). At a pH of 8.5, methadone absorption increased to 75%. Drug absorption was not affected by concentration, but was affected by contact time. Sixty percent of the maximum methadone and fentanyl absorption at 10 minutes was seen at 2.5 minutes of contact time; maximum buprenorphine absorption was complete by 2.5 minutes of contact time. Adverse effects were minor (bitter taste, burning sensation, lightheadedness), with fentanyl and buprenorphine associated with the lowest incidence.

Sublingual oxycodone and hydromorphone have been studied to a very limited degree (Reisfield, Wilson, 2007). An alkalinized oxycodone sublingual spray had a bioavailability of 70% in an animal model. Hydromorphone in healthy volunteers had a bioavailability of only 25%. The injectable forms of sufentanil and alfentanil have been used sublingually for breakthrough pain, but have not been studied (Gardner-Nix, 2001a; Hanks, Cherny, Fallon, 2004); with their high lipophilicity and potency (which exceeds fentanyl), they are a good theoretical choice, but the lack of commercially available products makes them impractical (Reisfield, Wilson, 2007). Fentanyl and methadone are well absorbed sublingually, but no preparations are commercially available (see the following discussion on oral transmucosal fentanyl) (Hanks, Cherny, Fallon, 2004); a sublingual fentanyl tablet now is available in some countries (Lennernas, Hedner, Holmberg, et al., 2005). A sublingual buprenorphine wafer has been approved for use in treatment of opioid addiction (Heit, Gourlay, 2008). A buprenorphine liquid product is available in other countries and may provide relief of mild to moderate pain. Sublingual buprenorphine absorption occurs within 3 to 5 minutes, bioavailability is 51%, and peak plasma concentrations generally occur at approximately 60 minutes (Johnson, Fudala, Payne, 2005).

An advantage of the sublingual route is that administration requires little expertise, preparation, or supervision (Reisfield, Wilson, 2007; Stevens, Ghazi, 2000). Unfortunately, the sublingual route currently has limited value for the administration of most opioids because formulations are lacking, absorption is poor for most opioids, and high doses cannot be given. In addition, proper administration is seldom possible because the drug must be in contact with the oral mucosa at least 5 minutes, a length of time most patients find intolerable (Reisfield, Wilson, 2007).

Buccal and Gingival

The buccal route of administration involves placement of the drug, usually in tablet form, inside the mouth between the mucosal surface of the cheek and the gum of the upper molars (see buccal fentanyl in following paragraphs). The gingival route involves placing the tablet form between the upper lip and the gum of the incisors. Of all areas in the mouth for oral transmucosal drug administration, the gingival route appears to be the lowest in drug permeability (Reisfield, Wilson, 2007). If the buccal or gingival routes must be used, the site should be rinsed with water to remove residues of the drug after absorption. If these routes are used repeatedly, the site should be rotated because irritation of the mucous membrane can occur.

Oral Transmucosal Fentanyl for Breakthrough Pain

Breakthrough pain (sometimes called *pain flare, episodic pain,* or *transient pain*) is defined as a transitory exacerbation of pain in a patient who has relatively stable and adequately controlled baseline pain (Portenoy, Forbes, Lussier, et al., 2004) (see Chapter 12 for a detailed discussion of breakthrough pain). The ideal medication for breakthrough pain has been described as one with a fast onset, relatively short duration of action, and minimal adverse effects (Zeppetella, 2008). Transmucosal delivery of a lipophilic and potent drug such as fentanyl meets these characteristics. Fentanyl had been incorporated into three products approved in the United States for the treatment of breakthrough cancer pain at the time of publication; numerous others are in development. Although indicated for cancer-related breakthrough pain, these products are widely used for breakthrough pain in noncancer pain syndromes as well (Prime Therapeutics, 2007).

Oral transmucosal fentanyl citrate (OTFC, Actiq®) is provided as a solid matrix or lozenge on a plastic stick (Figure 14-1, *A*). The medication is intended to be dissolved by saliva and absorbed through all oral mucosal surfaces. An effervescent fentanyl buccal tablet (FBT, Fentora®) is designed for placement against the buccal mucosa—between the upper gum and cheek—until it is dissolved (Figure 14-1, *B*). The newest formulation, BEMA (BioErodible MucoAdhesive; Onsolis) is a microadhesive polymer disk, about the size of a nickel, that contains fentanyl and is designed to stick to the oral mucosa (inside of the cheek) and dissolve within 15 to 30 minutes (Blum, Breithaupt, Hackett, et al., 2008).

The safety guidelines for the oral transmucosal products are strict, and the titration recommendations are conservative (see the following). Although safe use in

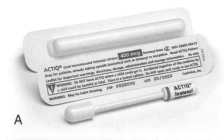

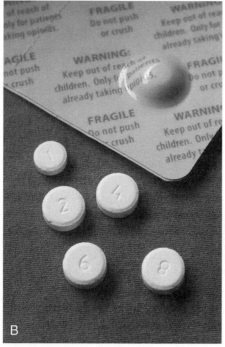

Figure 14-1 | **A,** Oral transmucosal fentanyl citrate (OTFC).
B, Fentanyl buccal tablet (FTB).

© 2011, Cephalon, Inc.

opioid-naïve patients with severe persistent noncancer pain has been described (Collado, Torres, 2008), these products have been approved for treatment of breakthrough pain in opioid-tolerant cancer patients only (Cephalon, 2007, 2008), and they should not be prescribed to patients with minimal or no existing opioid treatment unless appropriate monitoring is available. Titration usually should begin at the lowest dose (Cephalon, 2007, 2008). Despite using the same drug by a similar route, OTFC and FBT are not equivalent or interchangeable. These are important drugs for the treatment of breakthrough pain and are safe when used as directed; however, their potency must be respected, and clinicians, patients, and families must be well-versed in safe utilization.

OTFC is available in 200, 400, 600, 800, 1200, and 1600 mcg strengths (Cephalon, 2007). Individual titration, usually beginning with the lowest dose (200 mcg), is necessary. Dose adjustment on the basis of age alone is not required (Kharasch, Hoffer, Whittington, 2004), although elimination in older adults is prolonged (Gordon, 2006). To administer OTFC, the patient is

instructed to hold onto the stick and place the lozenge between the gum and cheek. The stick is used to move and twirl the lozenge around the oral mucosa, particularly between the gums and cheek and above and below the tongue, so that it dissolves in the saliva. Patients should be told not to suck on the lozenge as one would suck on a candy lollipop; this will result in much of the drug being swallowed (oral route), negating the benefits of exposure to direct systemic circulation that the oral transmucosal route offers. Further, clinicians should not refer to OTFC as a *lollipop, sucker,* or *popsicle,* as this is not only misleading but can result in family members, particularly children in the home, misunderstanding that this is a medication (not candy) that should be consumed by the patient only. Biting or chewing will cause a greater proportion to be swallowed, also resulting in decreased effectiveness. It has been suggested that the patient swish the fentanyl-containing saliva around the mouth prior to swallowing to enhance oral mucosal absorption (Gordon, 2006). If pain relief is insufficient after 15 to 25 minutes and the entire lozenge has been consumed, a second lozenge may be used; there are no published data about the use of more than two lozenges successively, and this is not recommended (Cephalon, 2007) (see Box 14-2 for complete dosing recommendations). See Patient Education Form IV-4 (pp. 551-552) on oral transmucosal fentanyl at the end of Section IV.

After administration, a portion of the fentanyl diffuses across the oral mucosa (25%) and the rest is swallowed and partially absorbed through the stomach and the intestine (75%). In total, OTFC has about 50% bioavailability (Mystakidou, Katsouda, Parpa, et al., 2005). The fentanyl absorbed from the mucosa rapidly crosses the blood-brain barrier to the CNS, its primary site of action (Mystakidou, Katsouda, Parpa, et al., 2005).

There is no predictable dose relationship between background opioid dose for persistent pain and an effective OTFC dose, and it may take several days to determine the optimal dose (Coluzzi, Schwartzberg, Conroy, et al., 2001). This observation, based on safety and efficacy trials, contradicts the usual assumption that an effective dose of breakthrough medication is a percentage of the total daily dose (see Chapter 12) (Mercadante, Villari, Ferrera, et al., 2007). A small study (N = 25) tested this conclusion with a fixed dose of OTFC based on the daily morphine dose. The results suggested that patients receiving more than 180 mg of oral morphine equivalents can be safely started at 600 mcg of OTFC (Mercadante, Villari, Ferrera, et al., 2007). It should be emphasized that this was a small, nonblinded study, but it is the first clinical trial to directly confront the issue of prolonged conventional titration.

Compared with oral (i.e., swallowed) fentanyl administration, OTFC yields higher and more rapidly attained plasma concentrations and greater bioavailability. These characteristics provide evidence that OTFC passes by mucosal transport directly into the systemic circulation without undergoing first-pass metabolism in the liver. Based on studies that show similar pharmacokinetics in single vs. multiple doses (Gordon, 2006), it appears that there is no depot effect in the mouth, in contrast to transdermally administered fentanyl. The clinical implications of this are that the onset of analgesia will be more consistent and rapid than by the oral or transdermal route of administration and adverse effects will dissipate quickly when administration is discontinued.

Although there is considerable variation in the time-action relationship following administration of a dose, OTFC usually has a more rapid onset, earlier peak effect, and shorter duration of action than a conventional short-acting oral opioid. With a typical onset of 30 to 45 minutes and a peak effect of 60 minutes or more, the oral drug has a profile that is likely to be poorly matched to the usual timing of a breakthrough pain episode (Zeppetella, 2008). Ashburn, Fine, and Stanley (1989) first reported effectiveness in the use of OTFC to manage breakthrough pain in a patient with metastatic carcinoma of the lung. They cited fentanyl's short duration (considered a drawback in the management of continuous pain) as an advantage in treating breakthrough pain because it allowed patients to avoid excessive sedation and other adverse effects associated with longer-acting oral opioids typically used for breakthrough cancer pain.

In clinical trials for OTFC in breakthrough pain, approximately 75% of patients were able to titrate to an effective transmucosal fentanyl dose, and these patients reported a faster onset than their usual oral breakthrough pain medication, with equal or better effectiveness, and acceptable adverse effects (Mystakidou, Katsouda, Parpa, et al., 2005; Mercadante, Villari, Ferrera, et al., 2007; Coluzzi, Schwartzberg, Conroy, et al., 2001). Analysis of the breakthrough pain experience of patients using OTFC concluded that OTFC had a positive impact on quality of life, particularly enjoyment of life and improvements in mood and ability to work (Taylor, Webster, Chun, et al., 2007). Another small study demonstrated that OTFC is an effective analgesic with no increase in adverse effects compared with placebo for burn patients during painful dressing changes (MacIntyre, Margetts, Larsen, et al., 2007).

Adverse effects include sedation, dizziness, nausea, constipation, and itching, all with an incidence of less than 15% (Bennett, Burton, Fishman, et al., 2005b). OTFC contains sugar and has been associated with dental caries. Patients should be instructed in good oral care, and diabetics should be informed that each OTFC lozenge contains 2 grams of sugar (Laverty, 2007; Gordon, 2006).

Potential cost benefits have been reported with the use of OTFC. Patients with non–cancer-related pain states who had a history of emergency department (ED) visits or hospitalizations for pain-control issues substituted OTFC for their usual breakthrough pain medication (Tennant, Herman, 2002). After 3 months, over 78% of the patients (N = 90) estimated that, based on previous experience, they had avoided at least one ED visit for pain control. Similar results have been found for cancer patients (Burton, Driver, Mendoza, et al., 2004) and sickle cell patients (Shaiova, Wallenstein, 2004).

Fentanyl Buccal Tablet (FBT)

An effervescent fentanyl tablet designed to rapidly dissolve when placed between the upper rear molar and cheek (buccal mucosa) approved for breakthrough cancer pain (fentanyl buccal tablet; FBT; Fentora) (see Figure 14-1, *B*) is available in 100, 200, 300, 400, 600, and 800 mcg tablets. Clinicians should not refer to FBT as a candy" as this is not only misleading but can result in family members, particularly children in the home, misunderstanding that this is a medication (not a candy) that should be consumed by the patient only.

FBT is clinically distinct from OTFC. Absorption through the oral mucosa is slightly faster, and the amount of fentanyl reaching the systemic circulation is higher with FBT. The effervescent design of the tablet increases pH, which enhances tablet dissolution and membrane permeability (Taylor, 2007). Fentora is twice the potency of OTFC, and titration of FBT usually should begin at the lowest dose (100 mcg). If pain relief is insufficient after 15 minutes and the entire tablet has been consumed, a second tablet may be used (Cephalon, 2008). Similar to OTFC, there are no data concerning a sequencing of more than 2 tablets, and it is not recommended. If a patient requires a higher dose, two tablets may be placed on each side of the mouth. It is estimated that a 30% smaller dose of FBT achieves systemic exposure equivalent to OTFC (Darwish, Kirby, Robertson, et al., 2007). It is, therefore, recommended that when switching from OTFC to FBT, the starting dose of FBT should be adjusted (Cephalon 2008) (see Box 14-3 for complete dosing recommendations and see Patient Education Form IV-3, pp. 549-550, on fentanyl buccal tablets).

Clinical trials with cancer patients with breakthrough pain have shown FBT to be superior to placebo in both pain intensity difference (pain score before and after intervention) and pain relief (Slatkin, Xie, Messina, et al., 2007; Blick, Wagstaff, 2006). One study evaluating FBT administered sublingually demonstrated nearly equivalent pharmacokinetics compared with buccal administration (Darwish, Kirby, Jiang, et al., 2008). It has not been subjected to a clinical trial, but sublingual may be an alternative route for some patients.

Adverse effects of FBT are similar to OTFC. The importance of correct prescribing and teaching patients proper use is stressed. The United States FDA issued an advisory about unsafe prescribing and use of Fentora® after serious toxicity and deaths had been reported (U.S. FDA 2007b).

Box 14-2 | Dosing of Oral Transmucosal Fentanyl Citrate (Actiq)[1]

INITIAL DOSE

1. The initial dose of Actiq to treat episodes of breakthrough pain is **200 mcg**.
2. Instruct the patient to place the Actiq unit in the mouth between the cheek and lower gum and to occasionally move the drug matrix from one side to the other using the handle. The Actiq unit should be sucked and not chewed. Chewing the matrix could result in lower peak concentrations and efficacy.
3. The Actiq unit should be consumed over a 15-minute period. Longer or shorter consumption times may produce less efficacy than reported in clinical trials.
4. Tell the patient that if pain relief occurs or signs of excessive opioid effects such as sedation appear before the unit is consumed, the dose unit should be removed from the patient's mouth immediately, disposed of properly (see below), and subsequent doses should be decreased.
5. From this initial dose, closely follow the patient and change the dose level until the patient reaches a dose that provides adequate analgesia using a single Actiq dose unit per breakthrough episode.
6. Ask patients to record their use of Actiq over several episodes of breakthrough pain and review their experience with their prescriber to determine if a dose adjustment is warranted.

REDOSING WITHIN A SINGLE EPISODE

Until the appropriate dose is reached, patients may find it necessary to use an additional Actiq unit during a single episode.

1. Redosing may start **15 minutes after** the previous unit has been completed (30 minutes after the start of the previous unit).
2. While patients are in the titration phase and consuming units that individually may be subtherapeutic, **no more than 2 units** should be taken for each individual breakthrough pain episode.

INCREASING THE DOSE

If treatment of several consecutive breakthrough pain episodes requires more than 1 Actiq per episode, consider an increase in dose to the next higher available strength.

At each new dose of Actiq during titration, it is recommended that 6 units of the titration dose be prescribed.

Evaluate each new dose of Actiq used in the titration period over several episodes of breakthrough pain (generally 1 to 2 days) to determine whether it provides adequate efficacy with acceptable adverse effects.

The incidence of adverse effects is likely to be greater during this initial titration period compared with later, after the effective dose is determined.

DOSE ADJUSTMENT

1. Increase the dose of Actiq when patients require more than 1 dose unit per breakthrough pain episode for several consecutive episodes.
2. When titrating to an appropriate dose, prescribe small quantities (6 units) at each titration step.
3. Once a successful dose has been found (i.e., average episode is treated with a single unit), patients should limit consumption to 4 or fewer units per day.

Continued

BioErodible MucoAdhesive (BEMA) Patch

At the time of publication, the most recently approved oral transmucosal fentanyl formulation in the United States was the BEMA patch. BioErodible MucoAdhesive (BEMA; Onsolis), is a bilayer polymer disk, about the size of a nickel, which contains fentanyl and is designed to stick to the oral mucosa (inside of the cheek) and dissolve within 15 to 30 minutes and provide rapid analgesia via systemic circulation (Blum, Breithaupt, Hackett, et al., 2008). The formulation was approved in July 2009 for the treatment of breakthrough cancer pain in opioid-tolerant individuals only (U.S. FDA, 2009a). It is available in 200, 400, 600, 800, and 1200 mcg strengths.

One benefit of this formulation is that the mucoadhesive polymer delivery system helps to control the mucosal surface application area and time in contact with the mucosa to optimize drug delivery. Two phase 1 open-label, randomized, crossover studies in 12 healthy volunteers evaluated the pharmacokinetics of BEMA (Vasisht, Stark, Finn, 2008). Absolute bioavailability was greater than 70% for both a single- and multi-unit (4 × 200 mcg) regimen, of which a high percentage (51%) of the fentanyl was absorbed through the oral mucosa.

Several clinical trials have demonstrated efficacy and safety of BEMA in patients with cancer pain (Blum, Breithaupt, Hackett, et al., 2008; Blum, Finn, 2008; North, Kapoor, Bull, et al., 2008; Slatkin, Hill, Finn, 2008). One study evaluated the breakthrough pain experience in 80 cancer patients on stable opioid doses who had participated in a previous double-blind, cross-over study in which their

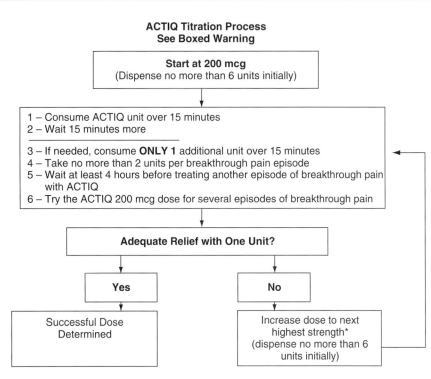

ACTIQ Titration Process
See Boxed Warning

Start at 200 mcg
(Dispense no more than 6 units initially)

1 – Consume ACTIQ unit over 15 minutes
2 – Wait 15 minutes more

3 – If needed, consume **ONLY 1** additional unit over 15 minutes
4 – Take no more than 2 units per breakthrough pain episode
5 – Wait at least 4 hours before treating another episode of breakthrough pain with ACTIQ
6 – Try the ACTIQ 200 mcg dose for several episodes of breakthrough pain

Adequate Relief with One Unit?

Yes

Successful Dose Determined

No

Increase dose to next highest strength*
(dispense no more than 6 units initially)

*Available dose strengths include: 200, 400, 600, 800, 1200, and 1600 mcg.

4. Consider increasing the around-the-clock opioid dose used for persistent pain in patients experiencing more than four breakthrough pain episodes daily.

Clinicians should not refer to OTFC as a lollipop, sucker, or popsicle as this is not only misleading but can result in family members, particularly children in the home, misunderstanding that this is a medication that should be consumed by the patient only.

This box describes the initial dosing, titration, and subsequent dosing of oral transmucosal fentanyl citrate (Actiq). See prescription information insert for other information, such as boxed warnings, contraindications, and storage. From Pasero, C., & McCaffery, M. (2011). *Pain assessment and pharmacologic management*, pp. 382-383, St. Louis, Mosby. Data from Cephalon. (2007). Actiq prescribing information. Cephalon Inc, Frazer, PA. Available at http://www.actiq.com/pdf/actiq_package_insert_4_5_07.pdf. Accessed April 13, 2008. © 2011, Pasero C, McCaffery M. May be duplicated for use in clinical practice.

optimal BEMA dose for breakthrough pain treatment was established (North, Kapoor, Bull, et al., 2008). After treatment with their optimal BEMA dose or placebo, patients recorded their pain intensity at multiple intervals for 60 minutes after administration during up to nine breakthrough pain episodes. BEMA demonstrated significantly greater pain relief than placebo at all time intervals and through 60 minutes. Other studies of patients with breakthrough pain have found only 10% of patients required additional rescue medication and 85% rated their breakthrough treatment with BEMA as "good" or better (North, Kapoor, Bull, et al., 2008). A double-blind, randomized, placebo-controlled, multiple cross-over study and an open-label study showed

that titration to optimal BEMA dose for breakthrough pain was well tolerated in cancer patients receiving concomitant long-term opioid therapy (Blum, Breithaupt, Hackett, et al., 2008). Adverse effects were typical of opioids: somnolence (6%), nausea (5.3%), dizziness (4.6%), and vomiting (4%). A multicenter, open-label study reported similar incidences of adverse effects (Slatkin, Hill, Finn, 2008). Three patients (1.4%) experienced mild stomatitis, which did not necessitate discontinuation of treatment. An abstract describing over 60,000 doses of BEMA taken for breakthrough pain in three different clinical trials reported a low incidence (4.6%) of application site reactions, including stomatitis (1.6%) (Blum, Finn, 2008).

Box 14-3 | Dosing of Fentanyl Buccal Tablet (Fentora)

INITIAL DOSE

1. For opioid-tolerant patients **not** being converted from Actiq, the initial dose of Fentora is **always 100 mcg.**
2. For patients being converted from Actiq, use the table below. The doses in the following table are starting doses and are not intended to represent equianalgesic doses to Actiq. **Patients must be instructed to stop the use of Actiq and dispose of any remaining units before switching to Fentora.**

INITIAL DOSING RECOMMENDATIONS FOR PATIENTS ON ACTIQ

Current Actiq Dose (mcg)	Initial Fentora Dose (mcg)
200	100 mcg tablet
400	100 mcg tablet
600	200 mcg tablet
800	200 mcg tablet
1200	2 × 200 mcg tablets
1600	2 × 200 mcg tablets

3. For patients converting from Actiq doses equal to or greater than 600 mcg, titration should be initiated with the 200 mcg Fentora tablet and should proceed using multiples of this tablet strength.
4. Administration technique: Instruct patient to place the entire tablet in the buccal cavity, above a rear molar, between the gum and cheek. Tablets should not be split.
5. Tell the patient not to suck, chew, or swallow the tablet as this will result in lower plasma concentrations and efficacy.
6. The tablet should be left in place between the gum and cheek until it disintegrates (usually 14 to 25 minutes).
7. After disintegration, if remnants of the tablet remain, they may be swallowed with water.
8. Tell the patient to alternate sides of mouth when administering subsequent doses.
9. In cases in which the breakthrough episode is not relieved after 30 minutes, patients may take **only one** additional dose using the same strength for that episode. Thus patients should take a maximum of two doses of Fentora for any episode of breakthrough pain.
10. Patients **must wait at least 4 hours** before treating another episode of breakthrough pain with Fentora.

TITRATION

1. From an initial dose, follow the patient closely and change the dose strength until the patient matches a dose that provides adequate analgesia with tolerable adverse effects.
2. Ask patients to record their use of Fentora over several episodes of breakthrough pain and discuss their experience to determine if a dose adjustment is warranted.
3. Patients whose initial dose is 100 mcg and who need to titrate to a higher dose can be instructed to use 2

Continued

Intranasal

The intranasal route has been used for centuries to administer a number of different drugs. It may be attractive as a noninvasive, rapid-onset, short-acting, and often convenient alternative to parenteral and oral opioids (Shelley, Paech, 2008).

The nasal mucosa has a surface area of 150 to 180 square centimeters of thin, permeable membrane with blood flow greater per cubic centimeter than muscle, brain, and liver (Shelley, Paech, 2008). This large surface area has uniform temperature and high permeability, and it provides easy access to extensive vasculature for rapid systemic absorption that eliminates the hepatic first-pass effect, potentially providing greater bioavailability compared with oral administration (Stoker, Reber, Waltzman, et al., 2008). In addition, there is evidence from animal studies that intranasal opioids may bypass the blood-brain barrier by a direct route to the brain via the olfactory nerve (Westin, Bostrom, Grasjo, et al., 2006).

Although the nasal mucosal surface provides a relatively large surface area, the volume of drug-containing fluid that can be administered per dose is limited (0.15 mL on each side). The drug needs to remain in contact with the mucosal surface long enough for absorption to occur. Chitosan, a naturally occurring substance that adheres to the mucosal surface and may enhance absorption, has been suggested as a vehicle for intranasal drug administration (Charlton, Davis, Illum, 2007; Pavis, Wilcock, Edgecombe, et al., 2002). A newer proprietary formulation uses pectin for the same purpose. Drug concentration and pH of the nasal environment also affect absorption (Dale, Hjortkjaer, Kharasch, 2002; Wolfe, 2007).

100 mg tablets (one on each side of the mouth in the buccal cavity) with their next breakthrough pain episode.

4. If this dose is not successful, the patient may be instructed to place two tablets on each side of the mouth in the buccal cavity (total of four 100-mcg tablets).

5. Titrate using multiples of the 200-mcg Fentora tablet for doses above 400 mcg (600 mcg and 800 mcg). Note: **Do not use more than 4 tablets simultaneously.**

6. In cases in which breakthrough pain is not relieved after 30 minutes, patients may take **only one** additional dose of the same strength for that episode. Thus patients should take a maximum of two doses of Fentora for any breakthrough pain episode.

7. During titration, one dose of Fentora may include administration of 1 to 4 tablets of the same dose strength (100 mcg or 200 mcg)

8. Patients **must wait at least 4 hours** before treating another episode of breakthrough pain with Fentora. To reduce the risk of overdose during titration, patients should have only one strength of Fentora tablets available at one time.

MAINTENANCE DOSING

1. Once titrated to an effective dose, patients should generally use only one Fentora tablet of the appropriate strength per breakthrough pain episode.

2. On occasion when the breakthrough pain episode is not relieved after 30 minutes, patients may take **only one** additional dose using the same strength for that episode.

3. Patients **must wait at least 4 hours** before treating another episode of breakthrough pain with Fentora.

4. Dose adjustment of Fentora may be required in some patients in order to continue to provide adequate relief of breakthrough pain.

5. Generally, the Fentora dose should be increased only when a single administration of the current dose fails to adequately treat the breakthrough pain episode for several consecutive episodes.

6. If the patient experiences more than four breakthrough episodes per day, consideration should be given to increasing the maintenance dose used to treat the persistent pain.

Clinicians should not refer to the fentanyl buccal tablet as a *candy* as this is not only misleading but can result in family members, particularly children in the home, misunderstanding that this is a medication that should be consumed by the patient only.

This box describes the initial dosing, titration, and subsequent dosing of buccal fentanyl citrate (Fentora). See prescription information insert for other information, such as boxed warnings, contraindications, and storage.

From Pasero, C., & McCaffery, M. (2011). *Pain assessment and pharmacologic management*, pp. 384-385, St. Louis, Mosby. Data from Cephalon. (2008). Fentora prescribing information. Cephalon Inc, Frazer, PA. Available at http://www.fda.gov/cder/foi/label/2008/021947s006lbl.pdf. Accessed April 13, 2008. © 2011, Pasero C, McCaffery M. May be duplicated for use in clinical practic.

The only intranasal opioid approved in the United States at the time of publication is the mixed agonist-antagonist butorphanol (Stadol NS), which has been used for migraine (Rapoport, Bigal, Tepper, et al., 2004) and for postoperative pain (Dale, Hjortkjaer, Kharasch, 2002). Other opioids have been used by this route for procedural (Finn, Wright, Fong, et al., 2004; Wolfe, 2007), dental (Christensen, Cohen, Mermelstein, et al., 2008; Wermeling, Grant, Lee, et al., 2005), postoperative (Mathieu, Cnudde, Engelman, et al., 2006; Stoker, Reber, Waltzman, et al., 2008), and breakthrough pain (Jackson, Ashby, Keech, 2002; Fitzgibbon, Morgan, Dockter, et al., 2003) and for prehospital use by emergency services (Rickard, O'Meara, McGrail, et al., 2007; Wolfe, 2007). It has also been suggested as an alternative to IV PCA (Miaskowski, 2005; Shelley, Paech, 2008). Intranasal opioids in use and under investigation include morphine, hydro-

morphone, butorphanol, sufentanil, alfentanil, and fentanyl.

As with other routes of administration, drug selection and proper technique are required for safety and efficacy. In clinical trials, nasal opioids have been administered using a simple mechanical device that delivers a metered-dose spray. In general, the more lipophilic opioids are better absorbed across mucosal surfaces, but this characteristic does not seem to apply to the nasal mucosa (Dale, Hjortkjaer, Kharasch, 2002).

Both morphine and hydromorphone have shown rapid absorption when administered intranasally. Hydromorphone has a peak time to effect of 20 minutes and is approximately 55% bioavailable (Cashman, 2008). A multicenter, open-label study compared single doses (2 mg, 4 mg, 6 mg, 8 mg, and 10 mg) of intranasal hydromorphone in the treatment of acute trauma pain in the ED and reported a mean decrease in pain intensity from baseline at 30 minutes of 24% in those who received 2 mg and 39% to 44% for those who received the higher doses (Wermeling, Clinch, Rudy, et al., 2009). Adverse effects were typical of opioids and of mild to moderate intensity. A randomized controlled clinical trial (N = 187) using an intranasal morphine-chitosan formulation (Rylomine) postoperatively following bunionectomy in 187 opioid-naïve patients demonstrated that the intranasal analgesic was comparable to IV morphine for both pain relief and systemic adverse effects (Stoker, Reber, Waltzman, et al., 2008). The minimally effective morphine dose was 7.5 mg, and 30 mg produced unacceptable adverse effects. The optimal dosing interval for 7.5 mg was 1 to 2 hours and for 15 mg was 2 to 3 hours. The researchers described the capacity of each nostril to hold only 150 to 200 microliters as a safety mechanism of this route of administration; it requires approximately 15 minutes for the drug to clear the nasal passages, and any attempt to instill additional drug would result in it being swallowed or dripping out of the nose.

A pilot study of a different morphine formulation administered intranasally (40 mg single dose) for breakthrough pain in cancer patients demonstrated meaningful pain relief at approximately 7 minutes (Fitzgibbon, Morgan, Dockter, et al., 2003). Intranasal fentanyl was shown to be comparable to IV morphine in a randomized controlled trial in a prehospital emergency setting (Rickard, O'Meara, McGrail, et al., 2007) and to produce the same or better analgesia than oral morphine in 75% of hospice patients in a pilot study (Zeppetella, 2000a). A randomized crossover study found that intranasal fentanyl produced equivalent pain relief as oral morphine for burn dressing changes in children (Borland, Bergesio, Pascoe, et al., 2005). Intranasal sufentanil has also been demonstrated in a randomized controlled clinical trial to provide effective postoperative pain relief (Mathieu, Cnudde, Engelman, et al., 2006). Intranasal hydromorphone has not been studied clinically, but pharmacokinetic studies have shown rapid absorption and good bioavailability (Rudy, Coda, Archer, et al., 2004). Similar results were found with methadone, but current formulations are probably too irritating for clinical applications (Dale, Hoffer, Sheffels, et al., 2002). Preliminary study of intranasal oxycodone suggests that it may have lower bioavailability than the oral oxycodone (Lugo, Kern, 2004). Anecdotal reports of intranasal alfentanil suggest it is effective for breakthrough pain but that patients may prefer the buccal route (Duncan, 2002).

Although studies of intranasal opioid delivery have produced promising results, many questions remain unanswered. Optimal formulations and delivery devices have yet to be determined. Patient selection, drug selection for specific indications, and safety and acceptability issues are still being defined (Dale, Hjortkjær, Kharasch, 2002). Bitter taste and transient nasal irritation are the most common local effects (Stoker, Reber, Waltzman, et al., 2008), which may be unacceptable to some patients.

Nebulized

Nebulized opioids, particularly morphine and fentanyl, have been used to treat dyspnea (Shirk, Donahue, Shirvani, 2006; Coyne, Viswanathan, Smith, 2002; Chandler, 1999) (see Chapter 20). Although the effectiveness of this route remains controversial, there has been interest in expanding its role to pain control. Published efficacy data are limited, but promising, and there are a few case studies. A study comparing placebo, IV morphine (4 mg) via 2 minute infusion, and either one (2.2 mg) or three (6.6 mg) inhaled doses of morphine over a period of 30 seconds to 2 minutes following bunionectomy showed that three doses of inhaled morphine compared favorably to IV morphine (Thipphawong, Babul, Morishige, et al., 2003). Nebulized morphine (20 mg in 3 to 5 mL buffered saline) was used to treat acute chest wall pain in 2 patients with sickle cell disease (Ballas, Viscusi, Epstein, 2004). Both patients reported significant pain relief, and treatment was continued for 10 days until the pain subsided. A prospective, cohort study, however, found that 0.2 mg/kg nebulized morphine was ineffective in treating acute pain in the emergency setting (Bounes, Ducasse, Bona, et al., 2009). Zeppetella (2000b) reported two cases of patients with advanced cancer. One patient, who was taking modified-release morphine for his pain, initially was started on inhaled fentanyl 25 mcg for dyspnea, but found that it relieved his pain more than his dyspnea. He subsequently used the same dose for breakthrough pain with significant relief within 15 minutes. A second patient, maintained on transdermal fentanyl, started on inhaled fentanyl 25 mcg and was titrated to good relief for pain on movement to 125 mcg.

The use of nebulized opioids for dyspnea is premised on the potential for local effects from drug binding to opioid receptors located in the airways or lungs, which may augment effects produced centrally following absorption through the lungs and into the systemic circulation (Shirk, Donahue, Shirvani, 2006). When used for pain, presumably the systemic effects are most relevant, unless the pain relates specifically to pulmonary pathology.

Morphine is absorbed rapidly by inhalation and reaches peak concentration in 10 minutes or less. Bioavailability is variable and is apparently a function of the efficiency of the delivery system rather than the capacity for absorption by the lung. Of the drug deposited in the lung, near 100% bioavailability of morphine and fentanyl are reached (Shirk, Donahue, Shirvani, 2006).

Adverse effects of nebulized opioids are typical of opioids in general: sedation, dizziness, nausea, and vomiting (Shirk, Donahue, Shirvani, 2006; Coyne, Viswanathan, Smith, 2002; Chandler, 1999). Airway irritation manifested by cough or bronchospasm have not been major problems but presumably can occur. Fentanyl is believed to be less likely to cause local irritation (Chandler, 1999). Clinicians sometimes cite concerns about the use of nebulized opioids in opioid-naïve patients with dyspnea; however, one prospective, nonrandomized study used transcutaneous carbon dioxide measurement and pulse oximetry and found that there was no higher risk of respiratory depression in opioid-naïve compared with opioid-tolerant palliative patients treated with nebulized morphine (Clemens, Quednauk, Klaschik, 2008).

Nebulized opioid administration is somewhat cumbersome because of the equipment required; some patients object to the mask needed to deliver the nebulized drug (Zeppettella, 2000a, 2000b), and some complain of a bitter taste (Chandler, 1999). Nonetheless, it is considered a possible alternative to IV administration because it is less expensive and invasive, and could be used more readily in the home than IV opioids (Shirk, Donahue, Shirvani, 2006). Significant improvements in equipment efficiency and portability may make the inhalation of opioids a viable alternative in the future.

Rectal

The rectal route offers an excellent, but frequently overlooked, alternative to the oral route. The rectum provides a large mucosal surface (although less than the upper GI tract) (Lugo, Kern, 2004) that permits passive diffusion of medications and absorption into the systemic circulation. Nurses and caregivers who care for the terminally ill often use the rectal route to administer medications. It is inexpensive and does not involve technical equipment or expertise to the extent that is required for parenteral administration. The rectal route is an alternative to the oral and parenteral routes for patients unable to swallow, experiencing nausea or vomiting, with a bowel obstruction, with a mental status change, or near death (Davis, Walsh, LeGrand, et al., 2002). (See Chapter 8 for rectal nonopioid analgesic administration in the perioperative setting.) It is particularly useful when other routes are unavailable and a delay is expected before the patient can be assessed for alternative treatment (Warren, 1996). The rectal route may be contraindicated in patients who are neutropenic or thrombocytopenic (platelet count of 50,000 per microliter or less) because of potential rectal bleeding from insertion of the suppository. Diarrhea, perianal abscess or fistula, and abdominoperineal resection are also relative contraindications (Davis, Walsh, LeGrand, et al., 2002).

Morphine, hydromorphone, and oxymorphone suppositories are commercially available. Custom-made capsules and suppositories containing methadone have been reported (Watanabe, Belzile, Kuehn, et al., 1996), as has the rectal administration of commercially available liquid preparations and modified-release formulations (Wiffen, McQuay, 2007; Mercadante, Arcuri, Fusco, et al., 2005; Davis, Walsh, LeGrand, et al., 2002; Walsh, Tropiano, 2002). All opioids may be compounded for rectal administration (Stevens, Ghazi, 2000). Oral tablets, oral solutions and suspensions, and injectable products have been administered rectally, sometimes without alteration of the medication, because of the lack of commercially available rectal preparations of opioids in various strengths. For example, intact oral tablets may be administered rectally, or they may be placed in an empty gelatin capsule for rectal insertion. From a pharmacoeconomic, convenience, and patient management perspective, modified-release preparations developed for oral administration are less expensive, provide for flexible dosing, and may be easier to use than suppositories (Walsh, Tropiano, 2002).

Rectal Anatomy and Drug Absorption

Understanding the anatomy of the rectum is important for effective use of the rectal route. The rectum makes up the last 15 to 19 cm of the large intestine. Minimal migration of rectal preparations occurs through the length of the rectum. Thus, the total surface area for drug absorption consists of a region approximately 6 to 8 cm long with no digestive enzymes. Three veins are responsible for blood return in the rectum. The middle and inferior rectal veins drain the remainder of the rectum into the inferior vena cava, bypassing the liver. The superior rectal vein drains the upper rectum into the portal vein, which transports the drug to the liver. However, there is no precise anatomic division that differentiates the rectal regions that drain to the different veins. Most drugs will, therefore, be absorbed by both systemic and hepatic circulation, with some degree of hepatic metabolism (Davis, Walsh, LeGrand, et al., 2002).

The bioavailability of rectal medications is affected by drug placement, rectal contents and tissue health, and degree of ionization of the medication (Fine, Portenoy, 2007; Davis, Rudy, Archer, et al., 2004). Morphine, including morphine in a modified-release delivery system (MS Contin) has 30% to 40% bioavailability (Stevens, Ghazi, 2000). Tradition and customary manufacturer recommendations are to insert rectal suppositories blunt end first to maximize absorption; however, a systematic review of the literature found that there is no research to support this recommendation or to guide correct suppository insertion procedure (Bradshaw, Price, 2007). Suppositories placed lower in the rectum may be better absorbed into the systemic circulation, while those higher in the rectum are absorbed into the portal circulation (Fine, Portenoy, 2007).

Contact time with the mucosal epithelium and moisture content of the rectum also influence absorption. The drug must dissolve in 1 to 3 mL of rectal fluid before being absorbed by the rectal mucosa. In addition, it may be necessary to remove rectal contents so that the medication can be placed against the rectal wall (Davis, Walsh, LeGrand, et al., 2002).

Given the variable influence of all these factors, it is not surprising that interindividual variability in response has been reported in relation to rectal drug administration (Davis, Rudy, Archer, et al., 2004; Lugo, Kern, 2004).

GUIDELINES

Box 14-4 Rectal Administration of Opioid Analgesics

1. Position the patient on the left side with the upper leg flexed or in knee-chest position.
2. Lubricate the dose form with a water-soluble lubricant or a small amount of water. If rectum is dry, instill 5 to 10 mL warm water with a syringe attached to a catheter before inserting tablets or capsules.
3. Do not crush modified-release preparations.
4. Gently insert the dose form approximately a finger's length into the rectum at an angle toward the umbilicus so that the medication is placed against the rectal wall. If a suppository is used, the blunted end should be introduced first.[1]
5. Keep liquid volumes of drug preparations at less than 60 mL to prevent spontaneous expulsion. Amounts of 25 mL are usually retained without difficulty. These may be injected into the rectal cavity with a lubricated rubber-tipped syringe or large-bore Foley catheter and balloon. Inflating the balloon may assist in retention.
6. Minimize the number of insertions. When administering multiple tablets for a single dose, enclose them in a single gelatin capsule.
7. Do not split or halve a suppository as this can cause errors in dosing. If it must be halved, cut it lengthwise.
8. After the finger is withdrawn, hold the buttocks together until the urge to expel has ceased.
9. Although rectal irritation is a concern, it need not be a limiting factor when administering commercially prepared suppositories, tablets, or capsules. Irritation

may be avoided or treated with lubrication, gentle insertion, and appropriate topical medications, such as cortisone ointment.

10. Prevent chronic rectal irritation. Avoid repeated rectal instillation of solutions of drugs with alcoholic vehicles or drugs that use glycols as solubilizing agents (parenteral forms of lorazepam, diazepam, chlordiazepoxide, and phenytoin).
11. Avoid rectal administration of enteric-coated tablets. The pH of the colon is alkaline, and these preparations require an acidic environment to be dissolved and the active drug to be released. The active drug would likely be expelled with the coating intact.

---

[1]Tradition and customary manufacturer recommendations are to insert rectal suppositories blunt end first to maximize absorption; however, a systematic review of the literature found that there is no research to support this recommendation or to guide correct suppository insertion procedure (Bradshaw, Price, 2007).

From Pasero, C., & McCaffery, M. (2011).*Pain assessment and pharmacologic management*, p. 388, St. Louis, Mosby. Data from Abd-El-Maeboud, K., el-Naggar, T., el-Hawi, E. M., et al. (1991). Rectal suppository: Common-sense and mode of insertion. *Lancet, 338*(8770), 798-800; Bradshaw, A., & Price, L. (2007). Rectal suppository insertion: The reliability of the evidence as a basis for nursing practice. *J Clin Nurs, 16*(1), 98-103; McCaffery, M., Martin, L., & Ferrell, B. R. (1992). Analgesic administration via rectum or stoma. *J Enterostomal Therapy Nurs, 19*(4), 114-121; Warren, D. E. (1996). Practical use of rectal medications in palliative care. *J Pain Symptom Manage, 11*(6), 378-387. © 2011, Pasero C, McCaffery M. May be duplicated for use in clinical practice.

Within-patient, dose-to-dose variability is a concern because of the difficulty in ensuring that tablet placement, contact time, and moisture level remain stable over time.

When administering a solution or suspension, the likelihood of spontaneous expulsion by the patient before the drug is absorbed can be prevented by administering volumes no greater than 60 mL (Warren, 1996). Even with caution, however, local irritation can develop over time, limiting the use of this route (Lugo, Kern, 2004). See Box 14-4 for guidelines on maximizing the rate and amount of drug absorption by the rectal route of administration and for minimizing complications.

Rectal Dosing

Acknowledging the concern about variability related to anatomy and other factors, the effective dose of opioids by the rectal route is, overall, approximately equal to oral dosing (Mercadante, Arcuri, Fusco, et al., 2005; Davis, Walsh, LeGrand, et al., 2002; Walsh, Tropiano,

2002). Nonetheless, when switching from the oral to the rectal routes, the starting dose typically is reduced by approximately 25%. In one study, 39 patients who were receiving MS Contin orally were switched to the same dose by the rectal route (Maloney, Kesner, Klein, 1989). All but 1 patient achieved adequate analgesia, but 28% required a decrease in the rectal dose because of excessive drowsiness.

A major disadvantage of the rectal route is that many individuals find it objectionable and are reluctant to use it. This can be especially problematic when family members must administer rectal medications and when medications must be administered several times a day. The need for frequent dosing can be mitigated by the use of a modified-release oral formulation. These oral formulations can be used rectally until the modified-release suppositories under development are commercially available (Walsh, Tropiano, 2002). The modified-release oral drugs demonstrate good rectal absorption and slow steady release compared with the rapid absorption and high peak effect of short-acting preparations. Compared with modified-release opioids given orally, studies show equal or greater systemic absorption, lower peak concentration, and a more prolonged time to peak by the rectal route. The apparent equivalence between the oral and rectal routes may be the result of a balance between slower rectal absorption but less first-pass effect (Davis, Walsh, LeGrand, et al., 2002). Modified-release oral formulations must not be crushed or dissolved.

In an early study, modified-release oral morphine tablets (Oramorph SR) were found to be safe and effective when administered every 12 hours by the rectal or vaginal routes to 8 patients with cancer pain (Grauer, Bass, Wenzel, et al., 1992). No consistent changes were found from the oral route in the frequency of adverse experiences, morphine requirements, or pain intensity ratings. Three of the eight patients reported better pain relief, and five reported the same relief as achieved with the oral route. Two small studies comparing the oral and rectal routes using modified-release morphine showed no differences in pain relief or pharmacokinetics between the groups (Wiffen, McQuay, 2007). In a study comparing liquid morphine administered orally versus rectally, pain relief was much faster in the rectal group and pain scores were better through 180 minutes (Wiffen, McQuay, 2007). Oxycodone tablets administered orally and rectally had similar bioavailability, but with great interindividual variability (Lugo, Kern, 2004).

Opioids that require extensive hepatic metabolism, such as codeine and tramadol, appear to be as effective rectally as when given by the oral route. This suggests a significant degree of absorption from the rectum into the hepatic circulation. These are drugs that would be at a disadvantage if not subjected to the first-pass effect (Davis, Walsh, LeGrand, et al., 2002).

Just as with the oral route, underdosing can occur with the rectal route. The most common reason for failure to achieve adequate analgesia is insufficient dose administration. It is best to control severe escalating pain rapidly with parenteral opioids, and then switch to rectal administration with scheduled ATC doses. Even severe pain that is stable can be managed by the rectal route if the principles of good pain management are followed (McCaffery, Martin, Ferrell, 1992).

Stomal

Treatment of a variety of cancers may include creation of an ostomy. Sigmoid colostomies (left-sided), which produce formed stool, are more likely than other ostomies to be an effective alternative route for administering opioids. Ostomies that are constructed of jejunum, ileum, ascending, transverse, and high descending colon (produce wet, liquid, or semisolid effluent) generally have rapid transit times. The constant pressure of the watery effluent from these ostomies will push out

---

GUIDELINES

Box 14-5 | Administering Medication Through a Stoma

1. Consider appropriateness of stoma (i.e., does it produce a formed stool?).
2. Ensure adequate hydration of the stomal mucosa. If it is dry, instill 10 mL warm water with a syringe attached to a catheter.
3. Determine bowel direction, and insert the drug form a finger's depth into the stoma.
4. Insert a foam stoma or colostomy plug. The plug may be left in place until bowel function occurs or until it is time for the next dose.
5. Ask the patient to recline for 15 to 30 minutes to prevent expulsion or loss as a result of gravity.

Information about the efficacy of stomal administration of opioids is limited; however, this route may be an effective alternative for some patients, at least temporarily.

From Pasero, C., & McCaffery, M. (2011). *Pain assessment and pharmacologic management*, p. 389, St. Louis, Mosby. Data from McCaffery, M., Martin, L., & Ferrell, B. R. (1992). Analgesic administration via rectum or stoma. *J Enterostomal Therapy Nurs, 19*(4), 114-121. © 2011, Pasero C, McCaffery M. May be duplicated for use in clinical practice.

---

the drug form before it can be dissolved and absorbed (McCaffery, Martin, Ferrell, 1992).

Colostomies usually are created in areas of the colon that are drained by vessels that go directly to the portal vein, subjecting drugs that are present to hepatic metabolism. Thus ostomy administration cannot be equated to rectal administration because it does not avoid the first-pass effect (Warren, 1996); however, the starting dose usually is the same as that for oral or rectal administration. Very limited information is available about the efficacy of stomal administration of opioids, but this route may be an effective alternative for some patients, at least temporarily. Box 14-5 presents guidelines for the administration of medications through a stoma.

Vaginal

Although opioid preparations for vaginal administration are not commercially available, opioids are absorbed by this route (Fisher, Stiles, Heim, et al., 2006). Anecdotally, many patients have reported using the vaginal route for opioid administration. Experience with the administration of other medications (i.e., misoprostol) suggests that vaginal pH may affect efficacy; the lower the pH (acidic), the faster the absorption and the lower the dose required to achieve effect (Abd-El-Maeboud, Ghazy, Nadeem, et al., 2008).

An early study showed that modified-release morphine (Oramorph SR) was safe and effective when administered every 12 hours by the vaginal route to patients with cancer pain (Grauer, Bass, Wenzel, et al., 1992). Patients in this study reported no consistent changes from the oral route in the frequency of adverse experiences, morphine requirements, or pain intensity ratings. In a case report, a patient achieved adequate analgesia using modified-release and short-acting morphine as well as morphine suppositories via the vaginal route as an alternative to IV PCA (Ostrop, Lamb, Reid, 1998). Unpredictable bioavailability was reported as a concern.

A more recent study examined the use of vaginal fentanyl in 4 patients with stable cancer pain (Fisher, Stiles, Heim, et al., 2006). The researchers compounded 50 mcg of fentanyl into a suppository with a water-soluble base and administered two suppositories 1.5 to 2 hours prior to the patients' regularly scheduled oral opioid. No plasma fentanyl was detected, and patients reported no discernable pain relief with this dose, so the researchers increased the dose to 200 mcg in the fourth patient. This patient reported transient mild dizziness 1 hour after administration, and although her pain intensity did not change, she required less breakthrough analgesia on that day. The researchers concluded that although their study showed that fentanyl is absorbed vaginally, a 200 mcg dose of fentanyl vaginally was at the low end of what would be needed for analgesic activity. As with any route or drug that has not been fully researched, other routes known to be safe and effective are preferred and recommended.

Transdermal

The oral and transdermal routes are generally the preferred routes of administration for long-term use of opioids. They are noninvasive and usually have high acceptability among patients. The transdermal route is particularly attractive for patients who are nauseated or have difficulty swallowing or for whom it is difficult to adhere to an oral regimen (Fine, Portenoy, 2007). The transdermal route avoids hepatic first-pass metabolism, which may pose an advantage for some patients. Drug is delivered at a relatively constant rate, which in some patients may reduce fluctuating effects associated with peak and trough plasma concentrations following oral administration. For some, adherence to the treatment regimen may be improved by the relatively long dosing interval possible with this route. The primary disadvantages of transdermal delivery compared with oral administration are that the skin and other tissues serve as both a barrier and a reservoir: there is significant lag time before the effects of the drug are felt after transdermal

application (see the section that follows), and the drug continues to enter the systemic circulation for a variable period after the patch is removed (Kaestli, Wasilewski-Rasca, Bonnabry, et al., 2008).

Two opioids are commercially available for transdermal administration: buprenorphine (Sittl, Likar, Nautrup, 2005; Skaer, 2004) (not released in the United States at time of publication) and fentanyl. Transdermal fentanyl patches are available in two delivery systems: a drug reservoir patch (e.g., Duragesic) and a matrix patch (e.g., Mylan transdermal system). Both these transdermal systems provide analgesia by passive diffusion of the fentanyl across the skin and into the systemic circulation (see discussion below). The equianalgesic ratio between transdermal buprenorphine and transdermal fentanyl has not been established. A retrospective study using a prescription database suggested a ratio of fentanyl 110 to 115:1 (fentanyl:buprenorphine) (Sittl, Likar, Nautrup, 2005).

A distinction should be made between transdermal and topical drug delivery. Transdermal medications are absorbed through the skin, enter the bloodstream, and then are transported throughout the body. They provide systemic analgesia and are an alternative to oral and IV administration. Topical medications may also be absorbed through the skin, but a much smaller percentage of the drug enters the circulation. Topical medications work locally (see Chapter 24 and Figure 24-1 on p. 685).

The outer layer of the skin, the stratum corneum, is the major barrier to absorption of medications through the skin. A lipid-rich intracellular pathway permits passive diffusion of highly lipophilic drugs through this and other layers. In addition to lipophilicity, other characteristics that enhance absorption include low molecular weight, solubility in water as well as oil, and a low melting point. Fentanyl meets all of these requirements. In contrast, morphine is very hydrophilic and is not absorbed across intact skin. Even when applied in a medium intended to increase absorption, quantifiable levels of morphine are not detectable in plasma (Paice, Von Roenn, Hudgins, et al., 2008).

Transdermal Fentanyl

The fentanyl transdermal patch (available in 12, 25, 50, and 100 mcg/h doses) is typically applied to the back or chest and left in place 48 to 72 hours (see application instructions below). The availability of a 12 mcg/hour-dose patch provides a better option than in the past for initiating therapy in patients who are opioid-naïve or have minimal prior opioid exposure; the availability of a lower starting dose in these patients reduces the risk of adverse effects when starting therapy (Mercadante, Villari, 2001).

Because of its lipophilicity, fentanyl is widely distributed in the body (Figure 14-2). A subcutaneous depot or reservoir is established in the skin near the patch, but following systemic uptake, the drug also redistributes into fat and muscle. At steady state, the level of drug in the

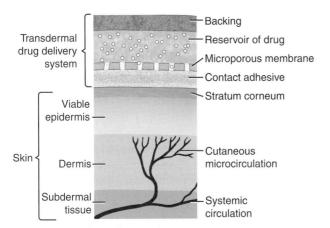

Figure 14-2 | Pathway of absorption from transdermal fentanyl. This image illustrates the pathway of absorption from transdermal fentanyl. The skin under the drug reservoir absorbs fentanyl, and depots of the drugs concentrate in the upper skin layers, fat, and skeletal muscles. From these depots, fentanyl is gradually released into systemic circulation.

From Pasero, C., & McCaffery, M. (2011). *Pain assessment and pharmacologic management*, p. 391, Mosby, Inc. May be duplicated for use in clinical practice.

blood represents the end result of absorption from the patch, movement into and out of these storage sites in various tissues, and drug elimination processes.

Conversion to transdermal fentanyl from another opioid is a multistep process that takes several days and requires close attention by the clinician. The starting dose of the patch may be determined using the dose conversion tables in the package inserts provided by the manufacturer or one of the conventional strategies developed by clinicians (see the paragraphs that follow). When the first patch is applied, 12 to 18 hours are required for clinically

relevant serum levels to be reached. A common approach is to provide a supplemental short-acting opioid along with the patch, at least during this titration period. This reduces the risk that both pain and withdrawal might occur in patients who are being switched from another opioid to transdermal fentanyl. This supplemental analgesia can be scheduled (not PRN) for the first 12 to 16 hours, with each dose equivalent to 10% to 15% of the total daily dose of the previous opioid (Skaer, 2006); a well-educated patient can be instructed to use the supplemental dose PRN, self-administering it in response to worsening pain or symptoms consistent with withdrawal.

As an alternative approach to transitioning from another drug and route (e.g., an oral modified-release opioid) to transdermal fentanyl, the patient can be instructed to overlap the administration of the last dose of the drug that is being discontinued with the placement of the first patch. Although it is still prudent to make available a supplemental short-acting opioid dose, at least during the transition period, there is less risk of pain flare or withdrawal if this overlap is instituted.

During the initial titration period, at least 24 hours should elapse before the fentanyl dose is increased; a 48-hour or 72-hour period reduces the risk of treatment-emergent adverse effects, but may be too long to wait if it is apparent that there are insufficient effects by the end of the first day. The increment in the dose depends on the existing dose, pain severity, and an assessment of medical factors associated with the risk of adverse effects. Similar to oral dosing, the usual increment is between 33% and 50%, and sometimes as high as 100%; when the dose is very low (e.g., 12 to 25 mcg/h), the dose is often doubled.

As noted, transdermal fentanyl patches are available in two delivery systems: a drug reservoir patch (e.g., Duragesic) (Figure 14-3, *A*) and a matrix patch (e.g.,

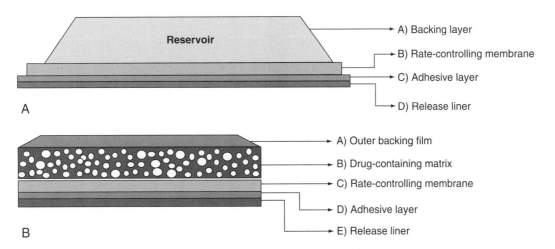

Figure 14-3 | Transdermal fentanyl drug delivery systems. **A,** Reservoir. **B,** Matrix.

From Marier, J. F., Lor, M., Potvin, D., et al. (2006). Pharmacokinetics, tolerability, and performance of a novel matrix transdermal delivery system of fentanyl relative to the commercially available reservoir formulation in healthy subjects. *J Clin Pharmacol, 46*(6), 642-653. As appears in Pasero, C., & McCaffery, M. (2011). *Pain assessment and pharmacologic management*, p. 391, Mosby, Inc. May be duplicated for use in clinical practice.

Mylan transdermal system) (see Figure 14-3, *B*). As the name implies, the reservoir patch has a fentanyl-gel reservoir that diffuses through a membrane to the skin. The fentanyl is incorporated into the adhesive of the matrix patch (Kaestli, Wasilewski-Rasca, Bonnabry, et al., 2008). There is the potential for leakage of the drug from a damaged reservoir patch; there is no such risk with the matrix patch. Although some patients report differences between the matrix and reservoir patches in terms of efficacy and patch adhesiveness, studies have shown they are bioequivalent and can be expected to produce similar analgesic efficacy and adverse effects (Hair, Keating, McKeage, 2008; Kress, Von der Laage, Hoerauf, et al., 2008; Marier, Lor, Morin, et al., 2006; Marier, Lor, Potvin, et al., 2006). A randomized controlled study also established similar efficacy and adverse effects when both transdermal fentanyl products and oral opioid formulations were compared (Kress, Von der Laage, Hoerauf, et al., 2008). Patients should be monitored closely when switching from one formulation to another to ensure ease of use, satisfactory analgesia, and tolerable and manageable adverse effects.

As with any modified-release opioid, concurrent administration of a supplemental, as-needed opioid may be provided for breakthrough pain (see Chapter 12) (Fine, Portenoy, 2007; Skaer, 2006). This is conventional practice for populations with pain due to active cancer or other serious illness; it is a strategy to be considered based on a separate assessment of potential benefit and risk in the population with persistent noncancer pain. If a decision is made to provide a supplement dose, this therapy can be transitioned simply from a supplemental dose given at the time of transitioning to the patch.

In the absence of an oral form of fentanyl, the typical breakthrough pain medication during treatment with transdermal fentanyl is one of the common oral opioids—morphine, hydromorphone, or oxycodone; alternatively, an oral or buccal transmucosal fentanyl formulation can be used. Some clinicians suggest an increase in the dose of the transdermal patch if a patient experiences more than three breakthrough episodes per day (Breitbart, Chandler, Eagle, et al., 2000), while others point out that the number of breakthrough doses that suggest inadequately controlled baseline pain varies widely and the decision to increase the dose of transdermal fentanyl (or any opioid) should be individualized to prevent an increase in unwanted adverse effects (Hewitt, 2000).

If pain consistently returns, or if more breakthrough medication is required on the third day of dosing, reducing the patch-application interval to 48 hours should be considered (Breitbart, Chandler, Eagel, et al., 2000). An observational cohort study found that 50% of patients taking transdermal fentanyl required dosing more frequently than the 72-hour interval recommended by the product's manufacturers (i.e., every 24 to 48 hours) (Gallagher, Welz-Bosna, Gammaitoni, 2007). Others have described a similar need for a shorter interval in

some patients (Sasson, Shvartzman, 2006). Patch changes more frequent than every 48 hours are not recommended, however (Breitbart, Chandler, Eagel, et al., 2000). Interindividual variation underscores the importance of systematic assessment to determine both the optimal dose and dose interval.

Converting to the fentanyl patch from another opioid requires calculating a safe starting dose (Fine, Portenoy, et al. 2009). The manufacturer provides a table of conversion values from oral morphine, but the morphine values constitute a fairly wide range at each dose interval, which can be confusing for the clinician. In addition, clinical experience has shown the values to be conservative, putting the patient at risk for pain and withdrawal and requiring a prolonged titration period (Skaer, 2006; Breitbart, Chandler, Eagel, et al., 2000). A more straightforward alternative method was proposed by Breitbart and colleagues (2000) using a morphine to fentanyl conversion ratio of approximately 2 mg/24 h:1 mcg/h (e.g., 60 mg/day of oral morphine provides analgesia approximately equal to a 25 mcg/h transdermal fentanyl patch). See Box 14-6 for calculation when switching from oral morphine to transdermal fentanyl. Clinical trials using this ratio have shown it to be safe and effective (Donner, Zenz, Tryba, et al., 1996; Mystakidou, Parpa, Tsilika, et al., 2004). Extensive clinical experience supports this approach (Carr, Goudas, 2000; Hewitt, 2000), or a somewhat more flexible guideline indicating that 100 mcg/h of transdermal fentanyl is equianalgesic to 2 to 4 mg/h of IV morphine or equivalent (Hanks, Cherny, Fallon, 2004; Fine, Portenoy, the Ad Hoc Expert Panel on Evidence Review and Guidelines for Opioid Rotation, 2009).

The use of parenteral fentanyl as an intermediate step in converting a patient to transdermal fentanyl is not recommended (Breitbart, Chandler, Eagle, et al., 2000); however, IV fentanyl may be helpful in controlling acute cancer-related pain. Patients (N = 9) experiencing an acute exacerbation of their continuous cancer pain were switched from transdermal fentanyl to IV fentanyl using a 1:1 conversion ratio (Kornick, Santiago-Palma, Schulman, et al., 2003). The median time to achieve mild levels of pain at rest was 1.5 days. Others have also used a 1:1 transdermal fentanyl-IV fentanyl conversion ratio during dose titration (Mercadante, Ferrera, Villari, et al., 2006).

Indications

Improper prescribing and use of transdermal fentanyl patches has resulted in serious toxicity and deaths (U.S. FDA, 2005, 2007c; Ross, Quigley, 2003). Transdermal patches should be used only by patients who have persistent cancer or noncancer pain and are able to follow application instructions (see the paragraphs that follow). It should not be used for acute or postoperative pain. In the United States, transdermal fentanyl is approved for opioid-tolerant patients only (see discussion on use

Box 14-6 | Converting from Oral Morphine to Transdermal Fentanyl

To convert a modified-release oral morphine dose to a starting transdermal fentanyl dose, consider morphine 2 mg/24 h orally to be approximately equianalgesic to fentanyl 1 mcg/h transdermally.[1]

SELECTING A STARTING DOSE

1. Calculate the patient's current 24-hour morphine dose.
   Example: If the patient is receiving 60 mg of oral modified-release morphine every 12 hours, the total 24-hour dose of morphine is 60 mg × 2 (doses per day) = 120 mg.
2. Determine the initial dose of transdermal fentanyl by dividing the 24-hour morphine dose by 2 (morphine:fentanyl conversion ratio of 2:1).
   Example: 120 mg of morphine ÷ 2 = 60 mcg/h of transdermal fentanyl
3. Round up or down to the available fentanyl patch strength based on the clinical status of the patient. There are three available patch strengths that provide options for starting transdermal fentanyl therapy in this patient example: 12 mcg/h, 50 mcg/h, and 75 mcg/h.
   a. If the patient has adequate pain relief from the current morphine dose, start with a 12 mcg/h patch plus a 50 mcg/h patch (62 mcg/h)
   b. If a more conservative starting dose is desired (e.g., in the frail older patient or a patient with a chronic pulmonary condition), start with the lower nearest patch strength (50 mcg/h).
   c. If the current morphine dose is not providing sufficient analgesia, start with the higher nearest patch strength (75 mcg/h).
4. Apply the first patch at the time the patient takes the last dose of modified-release morphine.
5. Monitor the patient for adequacy of pain relief and development of adverse effects.

TREATMENT OF BREAKTHROUGH PAIN DURING CONVERSION

1. The minimum amount of each rescue dose should be 25% of the total dose of the previous opioid the patient received in the past 24 hours.
   Example: Using oral morphine for breakthrough pain (see Boxes 14-2 and 14-3 for use of oral transmucosal fentanyl products)
   a. 120 mg of morphine was taken in the past 24 hours
   b. 120 mg × 0.25 (25%) = 30 mg
2. Provide PRN rescue doses in the amount of 30 mg every 3 to 4 hours PRN for breakthrough pain.
3. See Box 16-2 (p. 449) for long-term treatment of breakthrough pain.

TITRATION

1. Constant serum levels are achieved in 16 to 20 hours; steady state is attained at 72 hours of transdermal patch application.
2. After 24 to 30 hours (and always by 72 hours), determine if the patch dose is sufficient based on ongoing evaluation of pain relief and the requirement for breakthrough doses.
3. If breakthrough pain is persistent and frequent, the dose of transdermal fentanyl should be increased.[2]
4. The dose of transdermal fentanyl may be increased by 25% to 50%. At low doses such as in the example, the dose of the patch may be increased by 12 mcg/h to 50 mcg/h, depending on the severity of the pain.
5. In some patients, adjustment of dosing interval may be necessary. Patches should be changed every 48 hours in patients who have well controlled pain for only 48 hours and require more breakthrough doses on the third day of a 72-hour interval.
6. The number of patches that may be applied is limited only by dose requirement and body surface on which to apply and rotate the patches.

PRN, As needed.

[1]When studies that clarify equianalgesic dosing are lacking, such as is the case with fentanyl, various conversion formulas evolve. These formulas, and even the ones used in this text, are not necessarily comparable; different formulas lead to different answers. This conversion formula may be used to convert the patient from oral morphine to transdermal fentanyl and vice versa. The current recommendation by the manufacturer may be used only to convert from oral morphine to transdermal fentanyl, not vice versa, and the clinician should expect that approximately 50% of the patients will require additional analgesia.

[2]Some clinicians suggest an increase in the dose of the transdermal patch if a patient experiences more than three breakthrough episodes per day, while others point out that the number of breakthrough doses that suggest inadequately controlled baseline pain varies widely and the decision to increase the dose of transdermal fentanyl (or any opioid) should be individualized to prevent an increase in unwanted adverse effects.

in opioid-naïve patients in the paragraphs that follow). Despite a "black box" warning that reinforces its use in opioid tolerant patients only, it is sometimes prescribed as an initial drug. For example, a review of pharmacy data revealed that transdermal fentanyl was the most commonly prescribed formulation when opioid-naïve nursing home residents were started on a long-acting opioid (Dosa, Dore, Mor, et al., 2009).

Transdermal fentanyl has been shown to be effective for persistent cancer-related pain and various types of noncancer pain (see research below). Although a prospective study found no difference in the incidence of GI adverse effects with transdermal fentanyl compared with oral modified-release opioids (Wirz, Whittmann, Schenk, et al., 2009), several of the studies listed below demonstrated a lower incidence of opioid-induced adverse effects, particularly constipation (see Chapter 19). This and significant improvements in many of the indicators of quality of life (e.g., sleep, mood) may be primary reasons patients frequently express a preference for transdermal fentanyl over other modified-release formulations (Allan, Hays, Jensen, et al., 2001; Berliner, Giesecke, Bornhovd, 2007; Kornick, Santiago-Palma, Moryl, et al., 2003). The research that has demonstrated efficacy and effectiveness of transdermal fentanyl includes the following:

- Persistent cancer-related pain (Breitbart, Chandler, Eagel, et al., 2000; Mercadante, Porzio, Ferrera, et al., 2008; Mystakidou, Tsilika, Parpa, et al., 2003; Payne, Mathias, Pasta, et al., 1998; Vielvoye-Kerkmeer, Mattern, Uitendaal, 2000)
- Acute exacerbation of cancer pain (Kornick, Santiago-Palma, Schulman, et al., 2003)
- AIDS-related pain (Newshan, Lefkowitz, 2001)
- Pain associated with oral mucositis from chemotherapy (Cai, Huang, Sun, et al., 2008)
- Persistent postsurgical pain (Mystakidou, Parpa, Tsilika, et al., 2003)
- Osteoporosis (Mystakidou, Parpa, Tsilika, et al., 2003)
- OA pain (Collado, Torres, 2008; Langford, McKenna, Ratcliffe, et al., 2006)
- Rheumatoid arthritis (Berliner, Giesecke, Bornhovd, 2007; Collado, Torres, 2008)
- Persistent low back pain (Allan, Richarz, Simpson, et al., 2005; Collado, Torres, 2008)
- Persistent neck pain (Mystakidou, Parpa, Tsilika, et al., 2003)
- Multiple sclerosis (Mystakidou, Parpa, Tsilika, et al., 2003)
- Complex regional pain syndrome (Agarwal, Polydefkis, Block, et al., 2007; Mystakidou, Parpa, Tsilika, et al., 2003)
- Postamputation limb pain (Agarwal, Polydefkis, Block, et al., 2007)
- Trigeminal neuralgia (Collado, Torres, 2008)

- Ischemic vascular disease (Collado, Torres, 2008)
- Central pain (Collado, Torres, 2008)
- Neuropathic pain (variety) (Agarwal, Polydefkis, Block, et al., 2007; Collado, Torres, 2008; Mystakidou, Parpa, Tsilika, et al., 2003; Noble, Tregear, Treadwell, et al., 2008)

Transdermal Fentanyl in Opioid-Naïve Patients

Although transdermal fentanyl is approved in the United States as a second-line option in patients who require opioid analgesia for persistent pain (i.e., in opioid-tolerant patients only) (Kornick, Santiago-Palma, Moryl, et al., 2003), it has been used safely in opioid-naïve patients (Breitbart, Chandler, Eagel, et al., 2000). A large multicenter study randomized 680 patients with persistent low back pain to receive oral modified-release morphine (30 mg every 12 hours) or transdermal fentanyl (25 mcg/h every 72 hours) (Allan, Richarz, Simpson, et al., 2005). Starting doses were adjusted based on response. Pain relief was similar among the two groups, but those taking transdermal fentanyl experienced greater pain relief at rest and at night and less constipation. An open-label, prospective trial of 268 opioid-naïve and 321 opioid-tolerant (transferring from oral morphine) patients with cancer-related pain demonstrated improvements in pain and quality of life, high patient satisfaction, and no discontinuations due to adverse effects associated with the use of transdermal fentanyl for the 12-month study period (Mystakidou, Tsilika, Parpa, et al., 2003). An observational study of 215 opioid-naïve patients with noncancer pain found that transdermal fentanyl (starting dose, 12 mcg/h) administered for maintenance analgesia and OTFC (starting dose, 400 mcg) for breakthrough pain was well tolerated and produced sustained pain relief over the 6-month study period (Collado, Torres, 2008). Others have found similar results in patients with persistent cancer-related pain (Vielvoye-Kerkmeer, Mattern, Uitendaal, 2000). Breitbart and colleagues (2000) recommend beginning therapy in opioid-naïve patients with moderate to severe persistent pain with the lowest available dose of transdermal fentanyl (12 mcg/h) and providing a low-dose opioid-nonopioid (e.g., 5 mg oxycodone or hydrocodone plus acetaminophen) PRN every 4 hours for breakthrough pain.

Safety of Long-Term Use

Transdermal fentanyl has been shown to be safe for long-term opioid therapy. An observational study followed 73 cancer patients taking transdermal fentanyl for as long as 29 months after participating in a randomized clinical trial (Nugent, Davis, Brooks, et al., 2001). The median starting dose was 75 mcg/h, and the median final dose was 100 mcg/h. Treatment was well tolerated with a low incidence of adverse effects. Studies in populations with a variety of noncancer pain syndromes produced similar results (Milligan, Lanteri-Minet, Borchert, et al., 2001;

Mystakidou, Parpa, Tsilika, et al., 2003). A review of randomized controlled trials of individuals with long-standing low back pain could not identify a pattern of baseline pain (e.g., patient characteristics and severity of pain) that could be used to predict who would or would not respond to long-term opioid (transdermal fentanyl or morphine) therapy (Kalso, Simpson, Slappendel, et al., 2007). The researchers suggested that a one-month trial of opioid treatment would be sufficient to determine response and tolerability in most patients.

Patch Application and Disposal

The transdermal fentanyl patch may be placed on any intact, flat skin surface where adhesion can be maintained for 3 days; flank, back, chest, and upper arms are typically used. For example, skin folds should be avoided (see Patient Education Form IV-5 [pp. 554-555] on fentanyl transdermal system at the end of Section IV). Hair may be clipped but not shaved, and inflamed or irradiated skin should be avoided. The skin must be clean and dry, and soaps, oils, and alcohol should not be used on skin where a patch will be placed. Once in place, firmly rubbing the edges and the body of the patch will help to ensure that the patch sticks to the skin. Skin chemistry varies among patients, and some patches may need additional reinforcement with tape or an occlusive dressing (Skaer, 2004). Folding or cutting the patch in an attempt to reduce the dose of fentanyl will damage the drug-releasing mechanism of the reservoir system and is not recommended in either patch formulation, although a creative method for dose reduction by limiting the area of absorption using an occlusive dressing was proposed by a group of clinicians (Peng, Sun, Mok, 2005). Research is needed to confirm the safety and effectiveness of this approach. Patches are kept in place for 48 to 72 hours, and sites are rotated with each patch change to minimize skin irritation.

Nurses and caregivers are advised to wear plastic gloves prior to applying transdermal fentanyl patches to patients to avoid absorbing fentanyl. A case report described somnolence, weight loss, and depression in a woman who, without wearing gloves, applied transdermal fentanyl patches every 36 hours to her daughter who had persistent pain (Gardner-Nix, 2001b). After the use of gloves to change the patches was instituted, the mother experienced withdrawal symptoms, gradual resolution of somnolence, and regained most of her lost weight. The clinician who reported the case suggested that the situation was exacerbated by the concurrent use of steroid spray and cream to decrease the patient's skin irritation, which may have promoted absorption.

Proper disposal of medications has become a controversial topic because of the risk of misuse of prescription medications and environmental concerns about medications entering soil and drinking water. The U.S. federal government has issued medication disposal guidelines (Office of Drug Control Policy, 2007).

These guidelines confirm the Duragesic manufacturer's (Janssen, Ortho McNeil) recommendation that fentanyl patches should be folded in half (adhesive to adhesive) and disposed in the toilet. Some pharmacies and health systems and community household hazardous waste programs will also take used and unused medications for safe disposal.

Adverse Effects

The adverse effects seen with other opioids can be expected with fentanyl patches; however, there are data from observational studies that suggest a lower frequency of constipation (Fine, Portenoy, 2007; Kornick, Santiago-Palma, Moryl, et al., 2003; Malkin, Ackerman, Schein, et al., 2001; Staats, Markowitz, Schein, 2004; Tassinari, Sartori, Tamburini, et al., 2008). Despite the potential for less constipation, a bowel management regimen is recommended during any long-term opioid therapy in patients predisposed to this adverse effect. Nausea and vomiting may also be reduced compared with morphine (Skaer, 2006). Skin reactions such as rash and itching may occur (see Chapter 19 for treatment of opioid-induced adverse effects).

Local heat exposure can increase transdermal drug absorption and plasma concentrations by more than three-fold (Ashburn, Ogden, Zhang, et al., 2003). Patients should be instructed to avoid heating pads, electric blankets, hot tubs, and other sources of sustained heat, as these could increase the rate of absorption and lead to toxicity. This advisory applies to the care of patients receiving transdermal fentanyl in all settings. A case of overdose was reported when an upper body warming blanket was used to treat hypothermia during surgery in a patient who had a transdermal fentanyl patch on her chest for treatment of pre-existing persistent pain (Frolich, Giannotti, Modell, 2001). Patients with fever, which can also increase absorption of transdermal opioids, should be frequently assessed for opioid toxicity as well (Skaer, 2004).

Care must be taken to ensure that all hand-off communication (verbal and written) includes information about the analgesics patients are taking. A case of overdose and life-threatening respiratory depression was reported in a patient with a transdermal fentanyl patch in place for treatment of pre-existing persistent pain without the knowledge of the anesthesiologist who administered epidural opioid analgesia to the patient for postoperative pain control (Alsahaf, Stockwell, 2000). This reinforces the importance of communication regarding medication use across the continuum of care.

Despite changes in aging skin due to decreased water and lipid content, absorption of transdermal medications is not dramatically affected by age. The transdermal route is considered advantageous for older adults because no pills need to be swallowed; patch changes are typically every 2 to 3 days, obviating the need for frequent dosing; and stable plasma concentration reduces the risk of some adverse effects. Older adults are more likely to experience skin irritation, however (Kaestli, Wasilewski-Rasca, Bonnabry, et al., 2008). Warnings regarding improper prescribing of transdermal fentanyl (mentioned previously) should be emphasized when considering analgesic options for older adults.

As with all opioids, caution is recommended with the use of transdermal fentanyl in patients with underlying pulmonary conditions, such as emphysema or chronic obstructive pulmonary disease, as they are predisposed to hypoventilation (Kornick, Santiago-Palma, Moryl, et al., 2003). If respiratory depression occurs, the patient must be monitored closely for at least 24 hours after discontinuation of transdermal fentanyl. If naloxone is necessary, treatment will be needed for a prolonged period and the typical approach involves a naloxone infusion for 12 to 24 hours (see Chapter 19).

Nurses often express concern that transdermal fentanyl will not be effective in cachectic patients because they lack subcutaneous fat. Only one study could be found that addressed this issue. Ten normal-weight and 10 cachectic patients with cancer-related pain were recruited to evaluate whether or not absorption of transdermal fentanyl is affected by cachexia (Heiskanen, Matzke, Haakana, et al., 2009). A transdermal patch with a dose approximately equianalgesic to the patients' previous opioid dose was applied to each patient's upper arm and left in place for 3 days. Plasma concentrations at 48 and 72 hours were significantly lower in the cachectic patients. The researchers pointed out that absorption of transdermal fentanyl is governed by skin permeability and local blood flow, not by the amount of subcutaneous adipose tissue a patient has and that other factors, such as xerosis (abnormal dryness of the skin), may have been the cause. Although the researchers called for more studies to confirm their findings, they suggested that transdermal fentanyl may lead to inadequate analgesia in cachectic patients. Transdermal fentanyl may not be the best choice when initiating opioid therapy in a cachectic patient, and pain control must be closely monitored in patients who are already taking transdermal fentanyl and develop cachexia. If analgesia is inadequate, doses should be promptly increased or the patient switched to another opioid formulation.

Parenteral

The parenteral route includes the IM, SC, and IV routes of administration. Following is a discussion of these routes.

Intramuscular (IM)

Although commonly used, the IM route of administration is not recommended for pain management and should be abandoned (APS, 2003; Miaskowski, Cleary, Burney, et al., 2005). The IM route has numerous disadvantages

and essentially no advantages. Disadvantages include painful administration, unreliable absorption with a 30- to 60-minute lag time to peak effect, and a rapid drop in action compared with oral administration (APS, 2003). Chronic IM administration can result in sterile abscess and fibrosis of muscle and soft tissue. Other complications include nerve damage, hematoma, bleeding, cellulitis, tissue necrosis, and gangrene (Prettyman, 2005). The IM route is a particularly poor choice for older adults, who have decreased muscle mass, and children, who will endure severe pain rather than accept an IM injection (APS, 2003; Prettyman, 2005).

Early research demonstrated that the effects of IM meperidine vary considerably in different individuals and within the same individual (Austin, Stapleton, Mather, 1980b). IM administration of meperidine produced as much as a five-fold difference between individuals in the time to reach peak concentration. Any one patient given meperidine at different times of the day demonstrated a two-fold difference in time to peak concentration. At the dose given, pain control was poor during the first 4-hour dosing interval, and satisfactory pain control did not occur until the third or fourth dose. Pain control after an injection usually was not achieved until 45 minutes had passed, lasted only 75 to 90 minutes, and increased steadily to severe levels by the fourth hour after injection. Presumably, these results apply to any opioid given by the IM route.

In addition to being ineffective, the IM route of administration is dangerous, especially for opioid-naïve patients. Unreliable absorption makes it difficult to predict peak times of the opioid administered. As noted previously, typical IM meperidine doses may not result in satisfactory pain control until the third or fourth dose. If doses are administered at relatively short intervals, it is possible to overshoot the effective dose, a situation that is made more likely to occur by the delay in peak effect after IM injection. If injections are given in the setting of changing circulatory status (e.g., before or after a period of hypotension), the possibility that IM absorption can change further complicates decisions about the dosing interval and the monitoring required to reduce the risk of overshooting.

The unpredictability of the IM route warrants much closer monitoring of patients receiving opioids by this route than is customarily practiced. Careful nurse monitoring of respiratory status and sedation is critical to help ensure that clinically significant respiratory depression does not go undetected (see Chapter 19 for more on sedation and respiratory depression). Many institutions have established monitoring protocols for patients receiving IM opioids that are similar to those developed for IV PCA and epidural analgesia. For example, for postoperative patients, respiratory status and sedation level are assessed every hour for the first 12 hours, every 2 hours for the next 12 hours if stable, and then every 4 hours if stable after initiation of opioid therapy (Pasero, 2009b).

GUIDELINES

Box 14-7	Reducing the Discomfort of IM Injections

1. Match syringe size as closely as possible to volume injected.
2. Use a filter needle to draw up medication from vial or ampule.
3. If a prefilled syringe is used to draw up more medication, instill the complete dose into another syringe.
4. Change to a new dry, sterile needle before injecting.
5. If medication has dripped from the needle of a prefilled unit-dose syringe, wipe it clean with a dry, sterile pad before injecting.
6. Assess the amount of subcutaneous tissue at the site to determine needle length required to penetrate the muscle. Generally, use a 1.5-inch needle for adults and a 1-inch needle for children and infants as young as 4 months old and possibly as young as 2 months old.
7. Use the ventrogluteal site (Figure 14-4, *A*) as the primary site of injection for patients of any age. As an alternative, the vastus lateralis site (Figure 14-4, *B*) is preferred over the dorsogluteal site (Figure 14-4, *C*) because it contains no major nerves or vessels. The deltoid site (Figure 14-4, *D*) is associated with less site pain and fewer local adverse effects from vaccines compared with the vastus lateralis site.
8. Position patient correctly:
   - Side-lying: Flex knee of the side on which injection will be given, then pivot leg forward from the hip 20 degrees.
   - Supine: Flex knee of the side on which injection will be given.
   - Prone: Point toes in to internally rotate the femur.
   - Standing and using dorsogluteal site: Lean against a counter, put weight on side opposite injection site, and point toes on injection side toward opposite foot.
   - Prone or on side and using dorsogluteal site: Point toes inward to internally rotate femur and relax muscle.
9. Allow skin antiseptic to dry completely.
10. Use the Z-track method (Figure 14-5, *A*): Pull skin down or to one side, insert needle quickly and smoothly at a 90-degree angle, inject slowly (10 sec/mL), wait 10 sec before smoothly withdrawing the needle, and apply pressure at the site.
11. Limit volume of injection; if the muscle is large and healthy, up to 4 mL may be injected. If injections are to be given on an ongoing basis, consider concentrating the medication to reduce the volume.
12. Do not massage the site after injection.
13. Avoid using the same site twice in a row.

Sec, Second.
From Pasero, C., & McCaffery, M. (2011). *Pain assessment and pharmacologic management*, p. 397, St. Louis, Mosby. Data from Barnhill, B. J., Holbert, M. D., Jackson, N. M., et al. (1996). Using pressure to decrease the pain of intramuscular injections. *J Pain Symptom Manage, 12*(1), 52-58; Beecroft, P. C., & Kongelbeck, S. R. (1994). How safe are intramuscular injections? *AACN Clin Issues, 5*(2), 207-215; Beyea, S. C., & Nicoll, L. H. (1996). Back to basics: Administering IM injections the right way, *Am J Nurs, 96*(1), 34-35; Feldman, H. R. (1987). Practice may make perfect but research makes a difference. *Nursing, 87*(7), 82; Meissner, J. E. (1987). Using the vastus lateralis for injections. *Nursing, 87*(7), 82; Rettig, F. M., & Southby, J. (1982). Using different body positions to reduce discomfort from dorsogluteal injection. *Nurs Res, 31*, 219. © 2011, Pasero C, McCaffery M. May be duplicated for use in clinical practice.

Reducing the Discomfort of IM Injections

Although not recommended, IM injections continue to be used. Clinicians may lack the skill and knowledge required for delivering analgesics by other routes, such as the IV or epidural route, or the drug may be available only in the IM form, such as with immunizations. When the IM route cannot be avoided, pain and tissue trauma of injections may be reduced by improving the technique used to administer them. Topical local anesthetics should be applied whenever possible, particularly in patients who require repeated IM injections and when the solution being injected is viscous (see Chapter 28 for detailed discussion of topical local anesthetic creams). The site of the IM injection can influence the onset of analgesia, the analgesic plasma level, and injection discomfort. The ventrogluteal site is the primary site of IM injection, but the vastus lateralis is preferred because it contains no major nerves or blood vessels. Injection into the deltoid muscle, which is well-perfused, will provide a faster and higher plasma level than an injection into a less well-perfused muscle like the gluteal muscle (Buxton, 2006); however, because of the small size of the deltoid muscle and the proximity of major nerves and blood vessels, this site is appropriate only for small volumes of medications. Box 14-7 provides suggestions for reducing the discomfort of IM injections, and Figures 14-4 and 14-5 provides illustrations of the various injection sites.

The Z-track method for administering IM injections has been found to be less painful than the traditional injection technique (Beyea, Nicoll, 1996; Keen, 1986). The traditional IM technique allows leakage of the solution from the site, which can cause significant pain and irritation. The Z-track method involves pulling the skin down or to one side before the injection, then injecting slowly, removing the needle smoothly, and then allowing the skin to return to its original position (Figure 14-5, *A*). This prevents painful leakage by sealing the injected solution into the musculature.

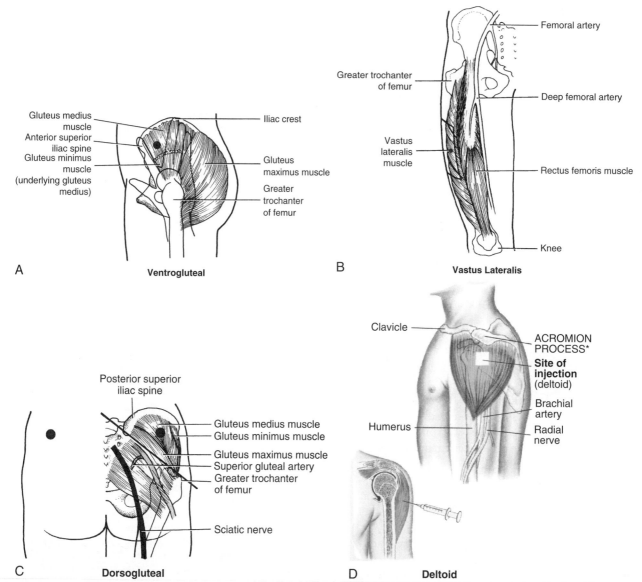

Figure 14-4 **A**, Ventrogluteal site for IM injections. To locate the ventrogluteal site, palpate the greater trochanter of the femur with the heel of the hand. The index and middle fingers are spread to form a V from the anterior superior iliac spine to just below the iliac crest. The triangle formed between the index finger, the middle fingers, and the crest of the ilium is the injection site. **B**, Vastus lateralis site for IM injections. The vastus lateralis site is the preferred site in patients of all ages. The belly of the muscle is one-third the distance between the greater trochanter and the knee. In adults, the site for injection is from one hand's breadth below the greater trochanter to one hand's breadth above the knee. The site is located on the medial outer aspect in the center third portion of the thigh in children. **C**, Dorsogluteal site for IM injections. To locate the dorsogluteal site for injection, draw an imaginary line from the posterior iliac spine to the greater trochanter of the femur. Because this line is lateral and parallel to the sciatic nerve, a site selected laterally and superiorly will be away from the nerve and the superior gluteal artery. **D**, Deltoid site for IM injections. To locate the densest area of the deltoid muscle and to avoid the radial nerve and deep brachial artery, locate the site 1 to 2 inches below the acromion process.

A-C, From Pagliaro, A. M., & Pagliaro, L. A. (1986). *Pharmacologic aspects of nursing*, St Louis, Mosby. **D,** From Wong, D. L. (1997). *Whaley and Wong's essentials of pediatric nursing*, ed 5, St Louis, Mosby.

A pinch-grasp technique has been shown to reduce the discomfort of IM injections into the deltoid muscle. This technique involves grasping the muscle, pulling it about ½ to 1 inch toward the person administering the injection, and applying a pinching pressure hard enough to cause mild discomfort. Resting the wrist about 3 inches from the site of injection, the injection is given at a 90-degree angle (Locsin, 1985) (Figure 14-5, *B*). Before pinching the skin, warn the patient and explain the purpose.

Manual pressure over the injection site may help reduce the pain associated with dorsogluteal IM injections of immune globulin in adults. In one study, investigators applied pressure over the injection site with the noninjecting thumb until resistance was felt, then maintained that

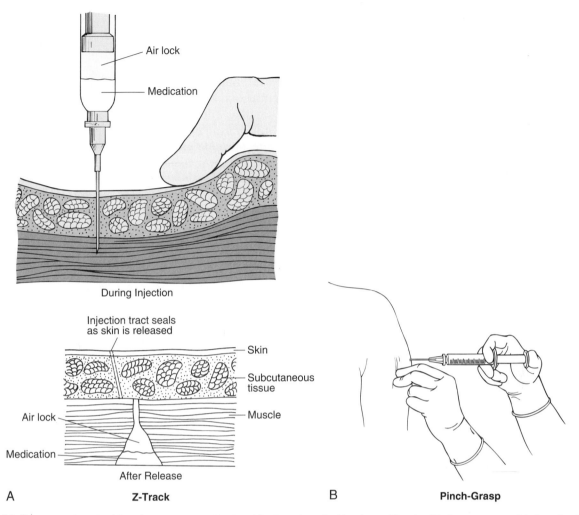

Figure 14-5 | **A,** Z-track method for administering IM injections. The Z-track method involves pulling the skin down or to one side, inserting the needle quickly and smoothly at a 90-degree angle, injecting slowly (10 sec/mL), and waiting 10 seconds before smoothly withdrawing the needle and applying pressure at the site. The Z-track left after injection prevents the deposit of medication through sensitive tissue. **B,** Pinch-grasp technique for administering IM injections. The pinch-grasp technique involves grasping the muscle, pulling it about ½ to 1 inch toward the person administering the injection, and applying a pinching pressure hard enough to cause mild discomfort. The injection is given at a 90-degree angle.

A, From Potter, P. A., & Perry, A. G. (1997). *Fundamentals of nursing,* ed 4, St Louis, Mosby. **B,** From Pasero, C., & McCaffery, M. (2011). *Pain assessment and pharmacologic management,* p. 399, St. Louis, Mosby. May be duplicated for use in clinical practice.

pressure for 10 seconds in patients in group 1 (Barnhill, Holbert, Jackson, et al., 1996). They applied no manual pressure over the injection sites of patients in group 2. For both groups, the skin at the injection site was held taut between the noninjecting thumb and index finger, and the immune globulin was injected over a period of 5 to 10 seconds. Patients in group 1 reported significantly less injection pain on injection compared with patients in group 2.

The use of cold in addition to manual pressure to reduce the pain of IM injection also has been studied (Hillman, Jarman, 1986). Ice and "slight" pressure applied to the IM injection site for 15 to 20 seconds before injection was found to reduce pain at deeper penetrations than without ice and pressure. Application of cold alone can be an effective pain reliever in some patients. A 5-minute ice massage to the site contralateral to that used for a bone

marrow aspiration reduced pain during the aspiration procedure (Hudziak, 1983). It seems likely that ice massage would be effective in reducing the pain of injection as well.

Even gentle slapping of the area before an IM injection can reduce its discomfort (Goodfriend, 1987). Obviously, before the slap, the patient should be warned and the reason explained.

Subcutaneous (SC)

The SC route can be used for continuous infusion (CI) of opioids, particularly in patients with persistent pain who are unable to take oral medications and who do not have central venous access (Mikkelsen, Butler, Huerta, et al., 2000; Stevens, Ghazi, 2000; Vascello, McQuillan, 2006). The SC route also can be used for repeated injections, and along with brief IV infusion or IV bolus, is preferred when this type of drug administration is required. Although it is a second-line route, it is a well accepted approach for medication delivery at end of life (Anderson, Shreve, 2004). The SC route obviates the need for normal GI function (Anderson, Shreve, 2004), and a trial of this route may be considered when patients experience dose-limiting adverse effects with oral opioids (Bourdeanu, Loseth, Funk, 2005), require a large number of tablets or patches for pain control, or require parenteral opioids because of bowel obstruction but have limited venous access (Miaskowski, Cleary, Burney, et al., 2005). Other candidates include patients with confusion or other mental status changes that make the oral route contraindicated because of the risk of aspiration (Miaskowski, Cleary, Burney, et al., 2005). The SC route is rarely used for acute pain management because onset is slow.

The most common opioid analgesics administered by SCCI are hydromorphone and morphine (Fine, Portenoy, 2007; Mikkelsen, Butler, Huerta, et al., 2000). Oxymorphone, fentanyl, and levorphanol also have been administered subcutaneously. A 6-day randomized, cross-over design study found SC fentanyl to be as effective with similar adverse effects and better bowel function compared with SC morphine (Hunt, Fazekas, Thorne, et al., 1999). The researchers suggested a conversion ratio of morphine 10 mg to fentanyl 150 mcg when given subcutaneously. Administration of methadone is more likely to produce irritation by the SC route and is not preferred for this reason (Fine, Portenoy, 2007); however, some suggest it can be managed by this route with low opioid concentrations, frequent site rotation, and co-administration of dexamethasone (Lynch, 2005). Others recommend flushing of the access site with normal saline to minimize irritation so that sites can be maintained for prolonged periods without the need for dose limitation or medications added to prevent irritation (Hum, Fainsinger, Bielech, 2007) See Chapter 15, for research on the stability and compatibility of many of the analgesics administered by SCCI.

Absorption and distribution vary depending on the placement of the needle and the patient's adipose tissue; however, cachexia is not a contraindication to SC analgesia. For conversion from oral morphine to SC morphine, a relative equivalency ratio of 3:1 is used, the same ratio used to calculate doses for the IV route (Coyle, Mauskop, Maggard, et al., 1986; Mikkelsen, Butler, Huerta, et al., 2000; Moulin, Johnson, Murray-Parsons, 1992). Although not contraindicated in older patients, this population may require a lower initial SC dose than younger adults (Aubrun, Bunge, Langeron, et al., 2003). An early study showed that patients prefer SC continuous infusion over IV infusion, citing greater and easier mobility and better pain control among the reasons (Bruera, Brennels, Michaud, et al., 1987).

SCCI administration is disliked by some patients, especially children. Although the technique of administration is relatively simple to master (see the paragraphs that follow), it does require a greater expertise than the oral route. Sterile technique is used to establish a site of infusion, and the patient and caregivers must become familiar and skilled in the use of needles, syringes, an infusion pump, and other equipment. The SC injection site must be changed at least weekly, and the potential for local tissue injury at the infusion site must be monitored.

High-concentration opioid formulations are used for SCCI infusion because infusion volumes are limited in most situations. Infusion pumps with the capability of delivering in tenths of a milliliter are necessary to accommodate the high-concentration/low-volume infusions. Most patients can absorb 2 or 3 mL/h, and some can absorb as much as 5 mL/h (Anderson, Shreve, 2004; Coyle, 1996). When necessary, some patients can even tolerate an infusion up to 8 mL/h for a few hours. Breakthrough doses may be provided as SC clinician-administered or PCA boluses (50% of hourly infusion administered as often as every 15 minutes) (Anderson, Shreve, 2004). Like other infusions, the need for bolus doses for breakthrough pain, if this is permitted, can be used to adjust the hourly dose (Anderson, Shreve, 2004). In patients requiring high infusion volumes, two sites can be used to deliver the required amount. For example, one site can be used for the infusion and one for breakthrough boluses. A four-way stopcock can be used to branch an infusion from one infusion pump to two sites (Gordon, 2008). As noted, most patients are able to tolerate the same site for seven days, and patients have been maintained on SC infusions for more than a year (Anderson, Shreve, 2004).

The volume of infusion during SCCI can be greatly increased by the addition of hyaluronidase to the infusate. Hyaluronidase typically is used for hypodermoclysis, or subcutaneous hydration. Although some authors recommend against this approach for the enhanced SC delivery of drugs (Anderson, Shreve, 2004), there is a favorable clinical experience, and the technique should be considered when an opioid is being delivered by SCCI and the required dose cannot be administered within the small volume of infusion. Hyaluronidase at a conventional dose of 150 units in 250 mL or 500 mL can routinely permit infusion rates greater than 100 mL/h (and significantly higher when needed) (see Figure 14-6 and Box 14-8 for guidelines on SC administration).

Successful SCCI administration in the home depends on the ability of the family and community health care system to manage the technology in the home (Anderson, Shreve, 2004). The cost and insurance coverage must be considered (Fine, Portenoy, 2007). Because an infusion device and supplies are necessary, SCCI administration usually is more expensive than oral administration.

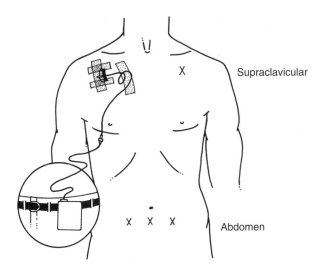

Figure 14-6 | Subcutaneous infusion needle placement. This image shows sites for SC infusion needle placement, which may be attached to an ambulatory infusion pump. X marks sites that interfere with mobility. Other sites to consider include upper arms and thighs. Sites should be rotated.

As appears in Pasero, C., & McCaffery, M. *Pain assessment and pharmacologic management*, p. 401, St. Louis, Mosby. © 2011, Pasero C, McCaffery M. May be duplicated for use in clinical practice.

Programmable portable pumps and disposable pumps are available; disposable infusion devices tend to be more expensive than the programmable infusion pumps (Moulin, Johnson, Murray-Parsons, 1992). Important points to address when establishing a plan for parenteral opioid analgesic infusion in the home include determining who will assume primary responsibility for the technologic aspects of the infusion, educating the patient and family regarding the infusion and pain and adverse effect assessment, and ensuring appropriate monitoring and follow-up (Coyle, Cherny, Portenoy, 1995) (see Box 14-8).

Intravenous (IV)

The IV route is most efficient when an immediate analgesic effect is required, such as for acute, severe escalating pain. It allows for rapid titration. The IV route is most commonly used for short courses of therapy in a hospitalized setting, where patients can be closely monitored because many who benefit from IV analgesia are opioid-naïve, such as surgical patients. The IV route may also be used temporarily for patients with cancer pain or noncancer pain who require rapid titration (Bourdeanu, Loseth, Funk, 2005). It is an alternative for patients who are unable to take oral opioid analgesics (Hanks, Cherny, Fallon, 2004; Miaskowski, Cleary, Burney, et al., 2005). In the terminally ill patient, bowel obstruction and dose-limiting adverse effects with other systemic opioids are common reasons for long-term IV infusion. Central lines are placed whenever possible for long-term IV infusion.

When patients are switched from oral dosing to parenteral administration, they typically report greater effectiveness with the IV route, but this should not be misconstrued. Opioids are not more effective when given by the IV route than by other routes; they are simply more bioavailable (100%) because first-pass hepatic metabolism is avoided (Stevens, Ghazi, 2000). A patient may very well feel less pain and fewer adverse effects, but this only reflects relatively higher plasma concentrations of the drug. The IV route may avoid certain adverse effects, such as nausea, caused when the drug is taken orally.

Methods of IV administration include bolus, continuous infusion (CI, basal rate), and PCA. A steady state is better maintained with a continuous infusion compared with the bolus method; however, continuous opioid infusions must be used with caution in opioid-naïve patients (Pasero, McCaffery, 2004) (see Chapter 17).

Duration of analgesia after an IV bolus is determined by the kinetics of the drug and the dose administered; the higher the dose, usually the longer the duration. Compared to equianalgesic doses by other routes, IV administration produces the highest peak concentration. Peak concentration is associated with toxicity (e.g., sedation, nausea), and it is therefore possible that adverse effects with repeated IV boluses are more severe than repeated boluses by other routes (Hanks, Cherny, Fallon, 2004). To decrease the peak effect and lower the level of toxicity, IV boluses may be administered more slowly (e.g., 10 mg of morphine over a 15-minute period) or smaller doses may be administered more often (e.g., 5 mg of morphine every 60 to 90 minutes).

There are drawbacks to the use of the IV route. IV administration depends on venous availability and ability to maintain patency. Sterile technique is required to prevent systemic infection. The IV route is generally more expensive and requires more expertise to use than the oral route (Vascello, McQuillan, 2006). If continuous IV infusion or IV PCA is used, equipment and tubings are required. Patients accustomed to the independence of oral analgesics may find adjusting to the IV route difficult.

Conclusion

This chapter presented the many routes of administration for opioid analgesics. The oral route is the most common for all types of pain. The oral and transdermal routes are first-line choices for long-term opioid therapy. The IV route is used when rapid analgesia is required. There are many second-line routes of administration, and it is often necessary to switch routes of administration during care, particularly in patients with advanced illness. For all types of pain, opioids should be administered by the least invasive and safest route capable of producing satisfactory analgesia.

GUIDELINES

Box 14-8 | Subcutaneous Infusion (SCCI)

BEFORE INITIATING SC THERAPY

- Convert current opioid dose to equianalgesic parenteral opioid dose (see Chapter 18 and Box 16-1 on p. 447)
- Calculate breakthrough dose (Box 16-2 on p. 449).
- → Breakthrough doses should be approximately 50% of hourly opioid requirement and offered as often as every 15 minutes.

SUPPLIES

- Nonsterile gloves (worn by person starting or discontinuing subcutaneous infusion)
- MiniMed Soft-set subcutaneous needle or 27-gauge butterfly needle
- Analgesic infusion pump that can deliver in tenths of a milliliter (0.1 mL/h). Pumps used to deliver continuous infusions or PCA are usually acceptable. Ideally, the pump should be portable and lightweight. Portable disposable infusion devices also are used for SC infusion.
- Subcutaneous infusion solution (prepared by pharmacy)
- Infusion administration set
- Transparent adhesive dressing or transparent tape (nonallergic tape if patient is sensitive)
- Chlorhexidine 2% + isopropyl alcohol 70% applicator
- 4-way stopcock and additional administration set if two sites will be used

PLACING SC NEEDLE AND INITIATING INFUSION

- → A single SC infusion site can usually accept 2 to 3 mL/h.
- → Highly concentrated solutions (e.g., hydromorphone 10 mg/mL or morphine 10 mg or more/mL are used for SC infusion; the pharmacy can prepare a parenteral morphine formulation by dissolving 50 mg in 1 mL of liquid.)
1. Connect solution to administration set; follow directions for loading and programming analgesic infusion pump.
- → Verify solution concentration and analgesic infusion pump programming by independent double-check process prior to initiation of therapy to help ensure accuracy.
2. Select site: Any area with a layer of SC fat is acceptable. Select the site that least interferes with mobility (ask patient about preferred sites and lying positions). Primary sites: left or right subclavicular anterior chest wall; left, right, or center abdomen. Other sites: upper arms, thighs, or buttocks. (Document why alternative sites are used.)
3. Prep skin: Clip excessive hair. Perform 30-second skin scrub with chlorhexidine applicator in circular motion from center outward. Do not wave, blow, or blow dry.
4. Needle insertion: Use a 27-gauge butterfly needle placed at a 45- to 90-degree angle, or use a Minimed Sof-set. (Be sure to remove introducer needle by grasping tip protruding from top of disk and pulling it straight out. The plastic catheter that surrounded the introducer needle is left in place.)
5. Dressing: Keep site as visible as possible for assessment purposes; cover with a moisture-responsive transparent adhesive dressing. Tape may be used if patient prefers or is allergic to transparent dressing. Make a loose loop of infusion tubing, and anchor with tape. Write date and time on small piece of adhesive tape, and place on edge of dressing.

DOCUMENTATION

Pain ratings; sedation levels; respiratory status; adverse effects; site; solution, including concentration and additives; biomedical number on pump if nondisposable pump is used (for risk management tracking purposes); infusion rate; PCA dose; delay; and pump history (therapy drug use). If PCA is not used, document short-acting opioid prescription for management of breakthrough pain.

MAINTAINING SC INFUSION

- Site should be checked every 2 hours for first 8 hours then at least twice daily (every 4 hours if the infusion rate is more than 1.7 mL/h). Home setting: Family can be instructed to check the site in the morning before the patient dresses and in the evening after undressing.
- Site inflammation, erythema, leakage, bruising, swelling, and burning indicate the need for a site change.
- Infusion site should be changed every 7 days or sooner if inflammation, leakage, or swelling occurs (rotate site in clockwise fashion, and use at least four distinct sites, if possible, to ensure healing).
- Change tubings and drug reservoirs according to institutional policy and procedure.

TROUBLESHOOTING

- Because the SC route has a slow onset, it is not acceptable for uncontrolled, severe escalating pain. The IV route must be used to control pain if necessary before SC infusion is initiated. Before discontinuing IV access, give an IV bolus dose equal to the hourly opioid dose the patient has been receiving to allow time for opioid absorption by the SC route and to prevent loss of pain control during the transition.

Continued

- If breakthrough pain occurs despite dose adjustments, poor absorption at the site may be the problem. Changing the infusion site may reestablish analgesia without increasing the dose.
- If possible, increase the concentration of the infusion solution when the required dose nears 2 mL/h.
- If the infusion is more than 2 mL/h, a four-way stopcock and two SC infusion sets can be used to branch the infusion from one infusion pump to two SC sites. The sites can be as close as 2 inches apart. In extreme cases (when switching to another route is not possible or death is imminent), this double-site method can be used to provide the mainstay opioid and a third site used for PCA bolus doses for management of breakthrough pain; however, the more sites used to deliver opioid, the fewer available sites for rotation. When multiple sites are used, more frequent assessment of sites is necessary (at least q 4 h).

PREPARING FOR DISCHARGE FROM THE HOSPITAL

- As soon as possible before discharge, determine whether SC infusion will be continued at home.
- If so, determine family's willingness to maintain SC infusion in the home because this is vital to successful therapy (see Patient Teaching below).
- Make necessary referrals and contacts (e.g., home health, hospice, home infusion company, insurance company) to arrange for appropriate level of home care after discharge.
- Make arrangements with local pharmacy/infusion service for infusion pump and preparation of drug reservoirs so that the family can pick up drug reservoirs and other supplies weekly.

PATIENT TEACHING

- Provide demonstrations and verbal and written instructions on needle placement, site care, pain and adverse effect assessment, management of breakthrough pain, pump management, and documentation.
- Allow patient and family time to practice working with supplies and pump under the guidance of a clinician.
- Remind family to keep extra batteries for portable pump at home. Routine battery changes can be done once the typical battery life for the patient is

determined (battery life depends on infusion rate and PCA demands).

- Provide instructions on how to obtain and store extra drug reservoirs.
- Provide family with name and number of 24-hour contact person.
- Reassure patient and family that another route can be substituted at any time if the SC route does not work.

DISCONTINUING SC ADMINISTRATION

1. Determine need for alternative analgesia. If patient will receive short-acting oral opioids, give the first scheduled dose 1 hour before stopping the SC infusion. If the patient will receive a modified-release opioid, give the first scheduled dose 2 hours before stopping the SC infusion.
2. Turn off pump.
3. Loosen dressing and pull infusion set straight out with a swift motion. Apply pressure for 30 seconds. If the skin is intact, a dressing is not needed. If the site is excoriated, dress with triple antibiotic cream and gauze until healed.
4. Discard unused opioid solution according to institutional policy and procedure.

---

q, Every; *SC*, subcutaneous.

The SC route of administration for the continuous infusion of opioids as opposed to intermittent injections is an alternative route for patients with persistent cancer pain who are unable to take oral medications and who do not have central venous access and for patients who experience dose-limiting adverse effects with oral opioids.

From Pasero, C., & McCaffery, M. (2011). *Pain assessment and pharmacologic management*, pp. 402-403, St. Louis, Mosby. Data from Anderson, S. L., & Shreve, S. T. (2004). Continuous subcutaneous infusion of opiates at end-of-life. *Ann Pharmacother*, 38(6), 1015-1023; Bruera, E., Brennels, C., Michaud, M., et al. (1987). Continuous SC infusion of narcotics using a portable disposable device in patients with advanced cancer. *Cancer Treatment Rep*, 71(6), 635-637; Capes, D., Martin, K., & Underwood, R. (1997). Performance of a restrictive flow device and an electronic syringe driver for continuous subcutaneous infusion. *J Pain Symptom Manage*, 14(4), 210-217; Chaiyakunapruk, N., Veenstra, D. L., Lipsky, B. A., et al. (2002). Chlorhexidine compared with povidone-iodine solution for vascular catheter-site care: A meta-analysis. *Ann Int Med*, 136(11), 792-801; Coyle, N. (1996). Cancer patients and subcutaneous infusions. *Am J Nurs*, 96(3), 61; Coyle, N., Mauskop, A., Maggard, J., et al. (1996). Continuous subcutaneous infusions of opiates in cancer patients with pain. *Oncol Nurs Forum*, 13(4), 53-57; University of Wisconsin Hospital & Clinics, Madison. (2009). Policy and procedure: Continuous subcutaneous opioid infusion. Madison, WI, University of Wisconsin Hospitals & Clinics. © 2011, Pasero C, McCaffery M. May be duplicated for use in clinical practice.

Chapter 15 Intraspinal Analgesia (Epidural and Intrathecal)

THE term *intraspinal* refers to the spaces or potential spaces surrounding the spinal cord or the nerve roots that constitute the cauda equina. Most often, the term is used when referring to the epidural and intrathecal spaces, each of which offers a route of administration for medications. The word *neuraxial* also is used to describe the group of spaces into which analgesic drugs can be administered. The word *spinal* is used interchangeably with the word *intrathecal* when referring to route of administration. It may also be used when referring generally to all of the routes of administration near or within the spinal meninges (Swarm, Karanikolas, Cousins, 2004). *Intrathecal* is often used synonymously with *subarachnoid,* but anatomically the intrathecal space includes the subdural space (Swarm, Karanikolas, Cousins, 2004) (see the following paragraphs on spinal anatomy). Table 15-1 shows some of the persistent misconceptions related to epidural analgesia. Box 15-1 presents patient selection guidelines and considerations for intraspinal analgesia.

Spinal Anatomy

The human spinal column consists of 33 individual vertebra referred to by their location: (1) 7 cervical, (2) 12 thoracic, (3) 5 lumbar, (4) 5 caudal or sacral (fused into one bone, the sacrum), and (5) 4 coccygeal (fused into one bone, the coccyx) (Figure 15-1).Vertebrae consist of an

Table 15-1 | Misconceptions: Epidural Analgesia

Misconception	Correction
Compared with opioid administration via IM injection and IV PCA, the incidence of respiratory depression is higher when opioids are administered by the epidural route.	The incidence of respiratory depression associated with the various pain control methods is not firmly established because of a lack of consensus on definitions and well-controlled research, but the incidence of respiratory depression with epidural analgesia is less than that of IM opioid injections and probably more consistent with that of IV PCA. A systematic review of the literature concluded that the mean reported incidence of opioid-induced respiratory depression varied between 0.8% and 37.0% for IM injection; 1.2% and 11.5% for IV PCA; and 1.1% and 15.0% for epidural analgesia (Cashman, Dolin, 2004). A study of the use of PCEA morphine with basal rate or IV PCA morphine with basal rate in 2696 patients after major surgery reported a higher incidence of respiratory depression with IV PCA (1.2%) than epidural analgesia (0.04%) (Flisberg, Rudin, Linner, et al., 2003). Clinically significant opioid-induced respiratory depression can be avoided in opioid-naïve patients by slow titration, careful nurse monitoring of sedation levels and respiratory status, and decreases in opioid dose when increased sedation is detected (see Chapter 19).
Patients receiving epidural analgesia must be cared for in intensive care settings where their respiratory status can be mechanically monitored.	Patients receiving epidural analgesia have been cared for safely outside of the intensive care setting for many years. Though mechanical monitoring is warranted in patients at high risk for respiratory complications (e.g., those with obstructive sleep apnea, chronic pulmonary disease), nurse assessment of sedation level and respiratory status is reliable and the most common method for monitoring most patients receiving epidural analgesia (see Chapter 19).
Epidural local anesthetics cause excessive and disabling sensory and motor blockade.	Local anesthetics are administered in low (subanesthetic) doses (e.g., 0.05% to 0.125% bupivacaine; 0.1% to 0.2% ropivacaine) for epidural analgesia. Higher doses are required to produce significant motor and sensory blockade (0.5% to 0.75% bupivacaine; 0.75 to 1.0% ropivacaine). Patients receiving epidural analgesia are able to ambulate and perform all the routine recovery activities expected of them to the extent their medical or surgical condition allows. The occasional occurrence of minor temporary numbness of lower extremities is resolved easily by decreasing the dose or removing the local anesthetic from the epidural analgesic solution.
Thoracic epidural catheter placement is technically more difficult and causes more damage than lumbar catheter placement.	The technique for placing a thoracic epidural catheter is quickly mastered by anesthesia providers. A review of 874 cases of high thoracic epidural analgesia provided over a 7-year period revealed no related neurologic complications (Royse, Soeding, Royse, 2007).

IM, Intramuscular; *IV,* intravenous; *PCA,* patient-controlled analgesia.
In spite of widespread use, misconceptions related to epidural analgesia persist. This table corrects some of these misconceptions.
From Pasero, C., & McCaffery, M. *Pain assessment and pharmacologic management,* p. 405, St. Louis, Mosby. Data from American Society of Anesthesiologists Task Force on Neuraxial Opioids. (2009). Practice guidelines for the prevention, detection, and management of respiratory depression associated with neuraxial opioid administration. *Anesthesiology, 110*(2), 218-230; Brown, D. L. (2005). Spinal, epidural, and caudal anesthesia. In R. D. Miller (Ed.), *Miller's anesthesia,* vol 2, ed 6, Philadelphia, Elsevier; Cashman, J. N., & Dolin, S. J. (2004). Respiratory and haemodynamic effects of acute postoperative pain management: Evidence from published data. *Br J Anaesth, 93*(2), 212-223; Cousins M. J., & Veering, B. T. (1998). Epidural neural blockade. In M. J. Cousins, & P. O. Bridenbaugh (Eds.), *Neural blockade in clinical anesthesia and management of pain,* Philadelphia, Lippincott-Raven; Dabu-Bondoc, S., Franco, S. A., & Sinatra, R. S. (2009). Neuraxial analgesia with hydromorphone, morphine, and fentanyl: Dosing and safety guidelines. In R. S. Sinatra, O. A. de Leon-Casasola, B. Ginsberg, et al. (Eds.), *Acute pain management,* Cambridge, NY, Cambridge University Press; Flisberg, P., Rudin, A., Linner, R., et al. (2003). Pain relief and safety after major surgery. A prospective study of epidural and intravenous analgesia in 2696 patients. *Acta Anaesth Scand, 47*(4), 457-465; Grape, S., & Schug, S. A. (2008). Epidural and spinal analgesia. In P. E. Macintyre, S. M. Walker, & D. J. Rowbotham (Eds.), *Clinical pain management. Acute pain,* ed 2, London, Hodder Arnold; Maalouf, D. B., & Liu, S. S. (2009). Clinical application of epidural analgesia. In R. S. Sinatra, O. A. de Leon-Casasola, B. Ginsberg, et al. (Eds.), *Acute pain management,* Cambridge, NY, Cambridge University Press; McCartney, C. J. L., & Niazi, A. (2006). Use of opioid analgesics in the perioperative period. In G. Shorten, D. B. Carr, D. Harmon, et al., (Eds.), *Postoperative pain management: An evidence-based guide to practice,* Philadelphia, Saunders; Royse, C. F., Soeding, P. F., & Royse, A. G. (2007). High thoracic epidural analgesia for cardiac surgery: An audit of 874 cases. *Anaesth Intensive Care, 35*(3), 374-377; Vascello, L., & McQuillan, R. J. (2006). Opioid analgesics and routes of administration. In O.A. de Leon-Casasola (Ed.), *Cancer pain. Pharmacological, interventional and palliative care approaches,* Philadelphia, Saunders. © 2011, Pasero C, McCaffery M. May be duplicated for use in clinical practice.

anterior body, the laminae that protect the lateral spinal cord, and spinous processes that project outwardly and posteriorly from the laminae. The vertebrae become larger as they descend in the vertebral column. The bones of the laminae are bound together by a number of ligaments (e.g., the dense ligamentum flavum) (Figure 15-2).

The spinal cord is located within and protected by the bony vertebral column and connective tissue (meninges). It is a continuous structure extending from the foramen magnum to approximately the first or second lumbar (L1 to L2) vertebral interspace. Below the tip of the spinal cord, which is called the *conus medullaris,* are the nerve

Box 15-1 | Use of Intraspinal Analgesia

PATIENT SELECTION

- Absence of contraindications to intraspinal needle or catheter placement (e.g., coagulopathies, abnormal clotting studies, immunocompromise, sepsis or signs of systemic infection [elevated white cells, pyrexia], infection in region of puncture site, history of multiple abscesses, patient refusal).
- For patients with persistent cancer or noncancer pain, pain is uncontrolled and/or adverse effects are unmanageable and intolerable with systemic analgesics.
- For patients with acute pain (e.g., surgery, trauma), the systemic routes have been considered and are not an option because they would produce unmanageable and intolerable adverse effects at the anticipated doses required for adequate analgesia.
- Patient has a painful condition or surgical procedure for which reduced morbidity and mortality is important but impractical or unattainable with other routes of administration. Such conditions include major thoracic, abdominal, and orthopedic surgery; intractable MI.
- Intraspinal preemptive analgesia could prevent or reduce the severity of a persistent postsurgical pain syndrome (e.g., phantom limb pain, postthoracotomy pain).
- Intraspinal route will be used to deliver anesthesia for surgery, and a single bolus dose before removal of needle or catheter will produce acceptable postoperative analgesia (e.g., preservative-free epidural morphine or extended-release epidural morphine for cesarean section or hip replacement).
- Patient has a pain syndrome that may be responsive to a specific intraspinal therapy such as local anesthetics, clonidine, or steroids (e.g., neuropathic pain unresponsive to systemic and topical adjuvant analgesics).
- In the patient with cancer or persistent noncancer pain who will receive long-term intraspinal opioid therapy, a reduction in pain in response to a trial dose of an intraspinally administered opioid has been experienced.

OTHER CONSIDERATIONS

- Appropriate equipment and supplies are available for therapy.

- Staff (or family) are trained to assess and manage epidural analgesia.
- Clinical support systems are available ATC if needed.

SURGICAL PROCEDURES FOR WHICH INTRASPINAL ANALGESIA IS COMMONLY PRESCRIBED

- Cesarean section
- Thoracotomy
- Aortic surgery
- Vascular surgery of the lower extremities
- Major joint replacement
- Limb amputation
- Whipple procedure
- Large open upper abdominal surgery (e.g., open cholecystectomy, pancreatectomy, nephrectomy, liver surgery, stomach surgery)
- Large open lower abdominal surgery (e.g., small bowel, mesentery, colon, radical prostate, total abdominal hysterectomy)
- Major breast reconstruction

MEDICAL CONDITIONS FOR WHICH INTRASPINAL ANALGESIA IS COMMONLY PRESCRIBED

- Intractable cancer pain
- Intractable neuropathic pain
- Myocardial ischemia unresponsive to conventional treatment

ATC, Around the clock; *MI,* myocardial infarction.

From Pasero, C., & McCaffery, M. *Pain assessment and pharmacologic management,* p. 406, St. Louis, Mosby. Data from Brown, D. L. (2005). Spinal, epidural, and caudal anesthesia. In R. D. Miller (Ed.), *Miller's anesthesia,* vol 2, ed 6, Philadelphia, Elsevier; Cashman, J. (2008). Routes of administration. In P. E. Macintyre, S. M. Walker, & D. J. Rowbotham (Eds.), *Clinical pain management. Acute pain,* ed 2, London, Hodder Arnold; Cousins, M. J., & Veering, B. T. (1998). Epidural neural blockade. In M. J. Cousins, & P. O. Bridenbaugh (Eds.), *Neural blockade in clinical anesthesia and management of pain,* Philadelphia, Lippincott-Raven; Swarm, R. A., Karanikolas, M., & Cousins, M. J. (2004). Anesthetic techniques for pain control. In D. Doyle, G. Hanks, N. I. Cherny, et al. (Eds.), *Oxford textbook of palliative medicine,* ed 3, New York, Oxford Press; Vascello, L., & McQuillan, R. J. (2006). Opioid analgesics and routes of administration. In O. A. de Leon-Casasola (Ed.), *Cancer pain. Pharmacological, interventional and palliative care approaches,* Philadelphia, Saunders; Wedel, D. J., & Horlocker, T. T. (2006). Regional anesthesia in the febrile or infected patient. *Reg Anesth Pain Med, 31*(4), 324-333. © 2011, Pasero C, McCaffery M. May be duplicated for use in clinical practice.

---

roots that exit the spine from below the L2 vertebra to the lower part of the sacrum. This tangle of roots is known as the *cauda equina.*

Moving from outside to inside the spine, the epidural space is first encountered. This is a potential space filled with vasculature, fat, and a network of nerve extensions. No fluid is in the epidural space; a true space is created when volume or air is injected into it (see Figure 15-2). The epidural space is outside of the dura, which is composed of the dura mater and the arachnoid membranes.

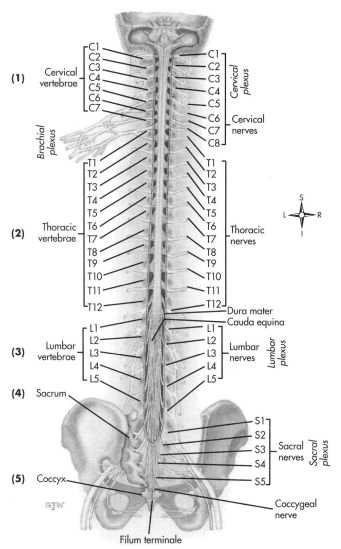

Figure 15-1 | Vertebral column. The human spinal cord consists of 33 individual vertebra referred to by their location: (1) 7 cervical, (2) 12 thoracic, (3) 5 lumbar, (4) 5 caudal or sacral (fused into one bone, the sacrum), and (5) 4 coccygeal (fused into one bone, the coccyx). At each vertebral body level, nerve roots exit from the spinal cord bilaterally. Specific skin areas are innervated by a single spinal nerve or group of spinal nerves.

From Thibodeau, G. A., & Patton, K. T. (1996). *Anatomy & physiology*, ed 3, St Louis, Mosby.

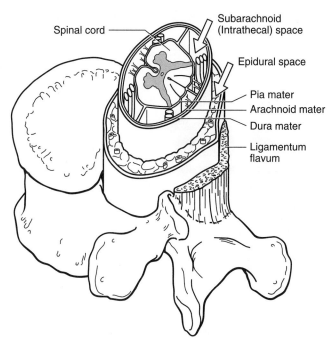

Figure 15-2 | Spinal anatomy. The spinal cord is a continuous structure extending from the foramen magnum to approximately the first or second lumbar (L1-L2) vertebral interspace. The subarachnoid space (also called the *intrathecal space* in the caudal part of the spine) surrounds the spinal cord, separated by the pia mater. The subarachnoid space is filled with cerebrospinal fluid that continuously circulates and bathes the spinal cord. The dura is composed of the arachnoid and dura mater membranes and separates the epidural space from the subarachnoid space. The epidural space is a potential space filled with vasculature, fat, and a network of nerve extensions.

From Salerno, E., & Willens, J. (1996). *Pain management handbook*, St Louis, Mosby.

The subarachnoid space (also called the *intrathecal space* in the caudal part of the spine) lies deep to the subarachnoid membrane, between this membrane and the spinal cord and cauda equina. The subarachnoid space is filled with clear, colorless cerebrospinal fluid (CSF) that continually circulates and bathes the spinal cord and nerve roots.

The fact that the epidural space is a potential space has clinical implications. Although injecting large amounts of air is not recommended, small amounts, such as tiny bubbles within the infusion tubing when therapy is initiated, are not considered dangerous. In addition, because the epidural catheter is in a space and not a blood vessel, a continuous epidural infusion may be stopped for hours and restarted without concern that the catheter has become occluded. However, crystallization of the saline within the epidural catheter can occur when catheters are unused for prolonged periods. In these cases, weekly or biweekly irrigation is recommended (DuPen, DuPen, 1998).

At each vertebral body level, nerve roots exit from the spinal cord bilaterally. A specific area of skin and subcutaneous tissue, known as a dermatome, is innervated by a single spinal nerve (Figure 15-3). The assessment of sensation in a dermatome is used to determine the integrity of the nerve root and subsequent pathway of innervation. Assessment of sensation in dermatomes is performed by anesthesia providers and others to determine the level of spinal anesthesia for surgical procedures and postoperative analgesia when epidural local anesthetics are used.

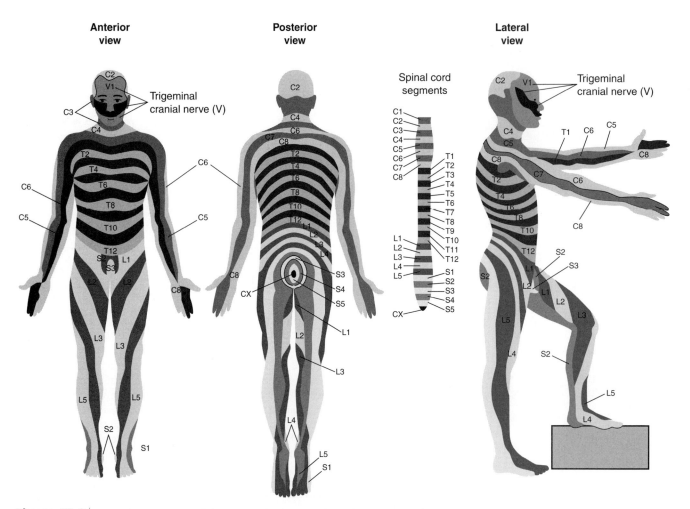

Figure 15-3 | Dermatomes. Segmental dermatome distribution of spinal nerves to the front, back, and side of the body. *C,* Cervical segments; *T,* thoracic segments; *L,* lumbar segments; *S,* sacral segments; *CX,* Coccygeal segment. Dermatomes are specific skin areas innervated by a single spinal nerve or group of spinal nerves. Dermatome assessment is done to determine the level of spinal anesthesia for surgical procedures and postoperative analgesia when epidural local anesthetics are used.

From Thibodeau, G. A., & Patton, K. T. (1996). *Anatomy & physiology,* ed 3, St Louis, Mosby.

Delivery of Intraspinal Analgesics

Delivery of analgesics by the intraspinal routes can be accomplished by inserting a needle into the subarachnoid space (for intrathecal analgesia) or the epidural space and injecting the analgesic, or threading a catheter through the needle and taping it in place temporarily for bolus dosing or continuous administration (Figures 15-4 to 15-6). Temporary catheters are used primarily for short-term acute pain management and are usually removed after 2 to 4 days. Intrathecal catheters for acute pain management are used more often for providing anesthesia and/or a single analgesic bolus dose.

For severe persistent cancer and noncancer pain, a catheter can be inserted then tunneled subcutaneously for intrathecal or epidural intermittent bolusing or continuous infusion or for patient-controlled epidural analgesia (PCEA) by an external ambulatory pump. The tunneling is done to decrease the incidence of infection and accidental displacement (Figure 15-7). These temporary tunneled catheters can be used for weeks to months to deliver analgesics. Temporary externalized intrathecal catheters are used less often than temporary epidural catheters primarily because of concerns about infection, although some clinicians report that such concerns may be unfounded (Vascello, McQuillan, 2006).

Although temporary tunneled epidural catheters continue to be useful for the management of intractable pain in some patients near end of life, totally implanted intrathecal infusion systems are preferred for long-term treatment of persistent pain (Deer, Krames, Hassenbusch, et al., 2007; Rathmell, Lake, Ramundo, 2006) (see Figure 15-7). Implanted catheters are less likely to dislodge and are associated with a lower infection rate than percutaneous catheters (Rathmell, Lake, Ramundo, 2006; Swarm, Karanikolas, Cousins, 2004) (see more on long-term intraspinal therapy later in the chapter).

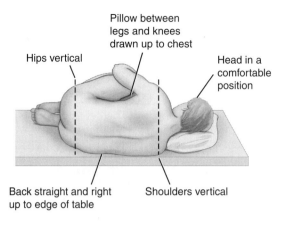

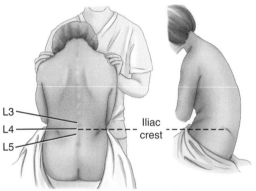

Figure 15-4 | Patient positioned for catheter placement. This figure shows two positions patients can assume for the epidural catheter placement procedure.

From Pasero C, McCaffery M: *Pain assessment and pharmacologic management*, p. 409, St. Louis, Mosby. May be duplicated for use in clinical practice.

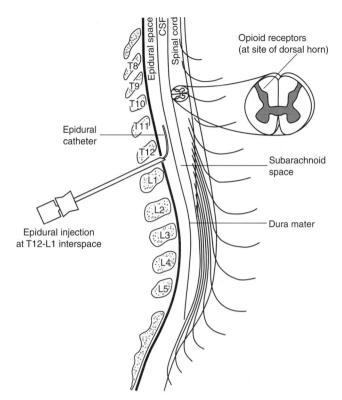

Figure 15-5 | Epidural needle and catheter placement. Delivery of analgesia by the interstitial routes can be accomplished by inserting a needle into the epidural space *(shown)* for epidural analgesia or the subarachnoid space for intrathecal analgesia and injecting the analgesic or threading a catheter through the needle and taping it in place temporarily for bolus dosing or continuous administration.

Modified from Sinatra, R. S., Hord, A. H., Ginsberg, B., et al. (Eds.). (1992). *Acute pain mechanisms and management*, St Louis, Mosby.

The level of nociceptive input (e.g., surgical site, site of injury, tumor location), the characteristics of the opioid being administered, and the goals of care (e.g., reduced stress response) are most important in determining the vertebral level at which the catheter is placed (Maalouf, Liu, 2009). For example, long-term catheters for treatment of cancer pain associated with spinal lesions can be placed in a location that avoids the tumor while providing necessary analgesia (DuPen, DuPen, 1998). Temporary epidural catheters for acute pain management usually are placed at the lumbar or thoracic vertebral level depending on surgical site (see the section on dermatomal spread and catheter placement later in the chapter). For example, the high thoracic level is preferred by several clinicians for coronary artery bypass surgery because placement at this level improves coronary perfusion, decreases heart rate and endogenous stress response, and reduces the risk for myocardial ischemia (Kessler, Neidhart, Bremerich, et al., 2002; Paiste, Bjerke, Williams, et al., 2001; Royse, Royse, Soeding, et al., 2000).

Percutaneous Intraspinal Catheterization

Intraspinal needle and catheter insertion is performed usually by an anesthesiologist or certified registered nurse

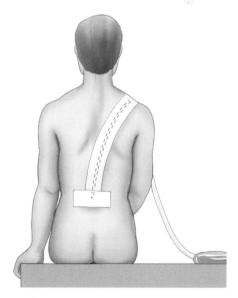

Figure 15-6 | Epidural catheter taped in place. This figure shows the catheter taped in place for continuous epidural infusion, patient-controlled epidural analgesia, or intermittent epidural blousing. Courtesy Astra Pharmaceuticals.

From Pasero C, McCaffery M. (2011). *Pain assessment and pharmacologic management*, p. 409, St. Louis, Mosby. May be duplicated for use in clinical practice.

External catheter and ambulatory infusion pump

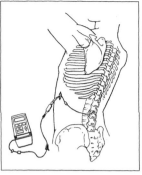

Implantable pump

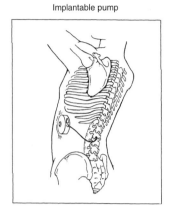

Implantable port and an ambulatory infusion pump

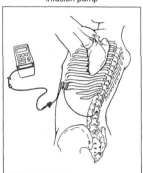

Figure 15-7 | Intraspinal delivery systems for persistent pain. This figure shows three intraspinal opioid delivery systems for treatment of persistent pain.

From St. Marie, B., & Williams, A. (1994). *Management of cancer pain with epidural morphine* (independent study module), St. Paul, MN, Sims Deltec Inc.

anesthetist (CRNA) or other advanced practice nurse. Nurses often assist with the procedure by preparing supplies and monitoring and supporting the patient during the procedure. Informed consent is obtained before the procedure.

The technique for placing a temporary percutaneous epidural catheter varies among practitioners; however, the points made in the Patient Example can be generalized to epidural catheter placement in all patients and may be helpful in reinforcing the anesthesia provider's explanation of the procedure to patients. The same principles apply to intrathecal needle and catheter placement.

Patient Example

Mr. Z. and his wife want to know everything about the epidural catheter placement procedure he is going to receive later today. His nurse reinforces the anesthesia provider's explanation by offering the following information: "You'll either be in a sitting position or lying on your side for the procedure. The doctor will be behind you facing your back. First he'll wash a small area on your back with a sponge. This may feel cool. Then he'll put drapes on your back to keep the area as clean as possible. You'll need to roll your shoulders inward and push your back out slightly. The doctor will use a local anesthetic to numb the place where the catheter will go. Sometimes injecting the local anesthetic produces a burning, stinging sensation that lasts less than a minute. It usually takes the doctor about 2 or 3 minutes to insert the needle into the epidural space. This will feel like dull pressure against your back. Next the doctor inserts the catheter through the needle into the epidural space, which usually takes less than a minute. As he inserts the catheter, you may feel some spark-like sensations in your legs and feet. These will go away very quickly. The doctor will remove the epidural needle and tape the catheter in place up your back to your shoulder. After the catheter is taped in place you'll be able to move and turn and lie on your back like you did before the procedure. The whole procedure usually takes less than 30 minutes. You may feel a very slight irritation for an hour or two after the procedure just at the site where the catheter goes into your back. If you feel any more discomfort in your back than that at any time while the catheter is in place, you'll need to let us know. Can I answer any questions?"

During intraspinal needle placement, most anesthesia providers are able to recognize when the point of the needle penetrates the dense ligamentum flavum (see Figure 15-2). In addition, entry into the epidural space exerts a negative pressure, which is registered by a loss of resistance in the syringe attached to the needle. Some anesthesia providers use the "hanging-drop" method whereby a drop of fluid at the needle hub is "sucked in" as soon as the needle tip passes the ligamentum flavum (Neruda, 2008); however, this method carries the risk of a small plug in the needle tip creating low or no negative pressure and is discouraged by some practitioners (Cousins, Veering, 1998). Once the ligamentum flavum is penetrated, the needle is not advanced if the epidural space is the desired location. If advanced further, the needle will penetrate the dura and enter the subarachnoid space. When in the subarachnoid space, free-flowing CSF can be aspirated. If a blood vessel is entered during placement, blood often can be aspirated.

Even when neither CSF nor blood is aspirated, epidural needle placement is often confirmed by injecting a test dose of lidocaine with epinephrine (if there is no contraindication to epinephrine; e.g., this approach is controversial in pregnant patients because of the potential difficulty in interpreting whether any variability in the woman's heart rate is in response to epinephrine or to uterine blood flow and contractions; see Birnbach, Browne, 2005). If the needle is in a blood vessel, the epinephrine will cause the patient's heart rate and blood pressure (BP) to increase suddenly and significantly; if in the subarachnoid space, the lidocaine will produce sensory anesthesia within 3 to 5 minutes (Covino, Wildsmith, 1998). If the patient exhibits neither of these changes, the needle is thought to be in the epidural space and the catheter is threaded through the needle.

Anesthesia providers turn the bevel of the intraspinal needle upward to facilitate threading the catheter 4 to 6 centimeters in a cephalad (toward the head) direction. Although rarely necessary for routine temporary intraspinal catheter placement, the only way to confirm conclusively the exact location of an intraspinal catheter is radiographically using contrast dye. When percutaneous catheters are to be used in the home setting, some clinicians recommend an epiduragram to confirm catheter position before patient discharge (DuPen, DuPen, 1998). (The reader is referred to a detailed explanation of epidural and intrathecal catheter placement techniques in the following two references: Brown, D. L. (2005). Spinal, epidural, and caudal anesthesia. In R. D. Miller (Ed.), *Miller's anesthesia*, vol 2, ed 6, pp. 1653-1683, Philadelphia, Elsevier; and Cousins, M. J., & Veering, B. T. (1998). Epidural neural blockade. In M. J. Cousins, & P. O. Bridenbaugh (Eds.), *Neural blockade in clinical anesthesia and management of pain*, pp. 243-321, Philadelphia, Lippincott-Raven.

Intraspinal Analgesia for Persistent Cancer and Noncancer Pain

A systematic review of the literature in 2000 by a panel of experts revealed widespread acceptance of long-term intraspinal analgesia therapy despite a lack of scientific evidence to support it (Bennett, Serafini, Burchiel, et al., 2000). The need for more well-controlled research of this therapy continues today; most studies are retrospective and underpowered (Simpson, Jones, 2008). Another systematic review found reports of improvements in pain and function, but also remarked on methodologic problems with the studies in the review (Turner, Sears, Loeser, 2007). Another systematic review identified just 8 evaluable studies (177 patients) on long-term intraspinal analgesia, and all of the studies were described as low quality (Noble, Tregear, Treadwell, et al., 2008).

An early consensus guideline on long-term intrathecal analgesic drug delivery recommended morphine as the mainstay analgesic for long-term intrathecal pain management based on its long history of use, the panel's extensive clinical experience with the drug, and responses to an online survey of physicians providing long-term intrathecal analgesia (Bennett, Burchiel, Buschser, et al., 2000). The survey revealed a usual starting morphine dose of 0.2 mg/day to 20 mg/day and an average maximum long-term infusion dose of 21.1 mg/day. Updated reviews of the literature and development of algorithms and dosing guidelines for the

therapy were published in 2004 (Hassenbusch, Portenoy, Cousins, et al., 2004) and again in 2007 (Deer, Krames, Hassenbusch, et al., 2007). The 2007 recommendations list morphine, hydromorphone, and ziconotide as first-line options. Second-line choices included fentanyl alone, and combinations of morphine/hydromorphone plus ziconotide, or morphine/hydromorphone plus bupivacaine/clonidine. (See Section V for a detailed discussion of ziconotide and other agents administered for long-term intraspinal analgesia.) Table 15-2 provides concentrations and dosing recommendations from the most recent consensus guideline (Deer, Krames, Hassenbusch, et al., 2007).

The above-mentioned online survey found that drug and dose adjustments were common and that one-half of patients receiving long-term intrathecal pain management who began on a single drug eventually received polytherapy, indicating a common need to adjust therapy to improve pain control or reduce adverse effects (Hassenbusch, Portenoy, Cousins, et al., 2004). A review of the literature found that 6.3% of patients withdrew from clinical trials of long-term intrathecal therapy because of adverse effects, and 10.5% withdrew because of insufficient pain relief (Noble, Tregear, Treadwell, et al., 2008).

Some publications provide insight into the pros and cons of the therapy. A summary of responses to a questionnaire administered to 36 patients with persistent low back pain receiving long-term intrathecal opioid treatment (mean 4.38 years) revealed significant improvements in pain after spinal implantation and a nonsignificant

Table 15-2 | Concentrations and Doses of Intrathecal Agents Recommended by the Polyanalgesic Consensus Panelists, 2007

Drug	Maximum Concentration	Maximum Dose/Day
Morphine	20 mg/mL	15 mg
Hydromorphone	10 mg/mL	4 mg
Fentanyl	2 mg/mL	No known upper limit
Sufentanil	50 mcg/mL (not available for compounding)	No known upper limit
Bupivacaine	40 mg/mL	30 mg
Clonidine	2 mg/mL	1.0 mg
Ziconotide	100 mcg/mL	19.2 mcg

From Pasero, C., & McCaffery, M. *Pain assessment and pharmacologic management,* p. 411, St. Louis, Mosby. Data from Deer, T., Krames, E. S., Hassenbusch, S. J., et al. (2007). Polyanalgesic consensus conference: Recommendations for the management of pain by intrathecal (intraspinal) drug delivery; report of an interdisciplinary expert panel. *Neuromodulation, 10*(4), 300-328. © 2011, Pasero C, McCaffery M. May be duplicated for use in clinical practice.

trend toward enhanced quality of life (Raphael, Southall, Gnanadurai, et al., 2002). The majority (88%) thought the therapy was quite or very worthwhile, and only 1 patient (3%) responded that it was not worthwhile. A systematic review of six articles on effectiveness and four others on complications associated with programmable intrathecal opioid delivery systems for persistent noncancer pain concluded that the therapy produced improvements in pain and functioning, but the typical opioid-induced adverse effects and device complications, such as mechanical failure and catheter migration, were relatively common (Turner, Sears, Loeser, 2007). A Cochrane Collaboration Review concluded that controlled research is lacking on neuraxial analgesia for cancer treatment, and although the therapy is often effective for cancer pain that is unresponsive to systemic analgesia, intraspinal catheter complications frequently occur (Ballantyne, Carwood, 2005).

An excellent review of the literature identified complications associated with programmable intrathecal opioid delivery systems, which include infection (e.g., wound infection, meningitis), hardware problems (e.g., mechanical failure, catheter occlusion), and opioid-related adverse effects (Turner, Sears, Loeser, 2007). Life-threatening complications were rare. The most common adverse effects were nausea (33%), pruritus (26%), and urinary retention (24%). Only two studies evaluated effects on sexual function and reported a variety, including amenorrhea and erectile dysfunction. One case of opioid withdrawal syndrome from catheter disconnection was reported. See later in this chapter for a detailed discussion of complications during intraspinal therapy.

Cost is a major consideration when implanted pumps are used in patients who are terminally ill; according to an early cost-benefit study, an implanted infusion pump was more favorable when survival times exceeded 3 months (Bedder, Burchiel, Larson, 1991). Some consider the intrathecal route to be more efficient, capable of providing a better distribution of medication, and less expensive for cancer pain (Vascello, McQuillan, 2006). An important aspect of care is helping the patient and the patient's family weigh all of the risks and benefits of long-term intraspinal analgesia therapy prior to initiation.

Stability and Compatibility of Agents for Analgesic Infusion Therapy

Research has established the stability and compatibility of admixtures of many of the commonly used agents for intraspinal and other infusion therapies. (For a discussion of microbiologic research on solutions, see the research list following this paragraph.) The reader is also referred to the Polyanalgesic Consensus Conference 2004 publication (Hassenbusch, Portenoy, Cousins, et al., 2004) for discussion of stability and compatibility of intraspinal analgesics. See the 2007 Polyanalgesic Consensus Conference recommendations for a detailed review of the research on the various drugs used for long-term intrathecal analgesia (Deer, Krames, Hassenbusch, et al., 2007).

- Baclofen (Alvarez, de Mazancourt, Chartier-Kastler, et al., 2004; Goodwin, Kim, Zuniga, 2001)
- Bupivacaine (Allen, Stiles, Wang, 1993; Classen, Wimbish, Kupiec, 2004; Hildebrand, Elsberry, Deer, 2001b; Nitescu, Hultman, Appelgren, et al., 1992; Rudich, Peng, Dunn, et al., 2004; Tu, Stiles, Allen, 1990; Wulf, Gleim, Mignat, 1994)
- Buprenorphine (Nitescu, Hultman, Appelgren, et al., 1992)
- Clonidine (Alvarez, de Mazancourt, Chartier-Kastler, et al., 2004; Classen, Wimbish, Kupiec, 2004; Goodwin, Kim, Zuniga, 2001; Hildebrand, Elsberry, Anderson, 2001b; Vranken, van Kan, van der Vegt, 2006; Wulf, Gleim, Mignat, 1994)
- Dexamethasone with ketamine (Watson, Lin, Morton, et al., 2005)
- Fentanyl (Allen, Stiles, Tu, 1990; Allen, Stiles, Wang, 1993; Chapalain-Pargade, Laville, Paci, et al., 2006; Nitescu, Hultman, Appelgren, et al., 1992; Tu, Stiles, Allen, 1990)
- Hydromorphone (Hildebrand, Elsberry, Anderson, 2001b; Rudich, Peng, Dunn, et al., 2004; Walker, Law, DeAngelis, 2001)
- Ketamine (Schmid, Koren, Klein, et al., 2002; Walker, Law, DeAngelis, 2001; Watson, Lin, Morton, et al., 2005)
- Meperidine (Nitescu, Hultman, Appelgren, et al., 1992; Vranken, van Kan, van der Vegt, 2006)
- Morphine (Classen, Wimbish, Kupiec, 2004; Hildebrand, Elsberry, Hassenbusch, 2003; Nitescu, Hultman, Appelgren, et al., 1992; Schmid, Koren, Klein, et al., 2002; Trissel, Pham, 2002; Trissel, Xu, Pham, 2002; Vermiere, Remon, 1999; Wulf, Gleim, Mignat, 1994)
- Ropivacaine (Sanchez del Aguila, Jones, Vohra, 2003)
- Sufentanil (Boitquin, Hecq, Evrard, et al., 2004; Chapalain-Pargade, Laville, Paci, et al., 2006)
- Tramadol with halodroperidol (Negro, Martin, Azuara, et al., 2005)

Methods for Administering Intraspinal Analgesia

The three methods for administering intraspinal analgesia are: (1) bolus (administered by the clinician), (2) continuous infusion or basal rate (administered by a pump), and (3) PCEA (administered by the patient usually using a pump).

Clinician-Administered Bolus Method

Clinicians can provide analgesia by administering a single intrathecal or epidural bolus injection, or the catheter can be left in place for intermittent bolus injections. The duration of the patient's pain usually determines which bolus method is used.

For some surgical procedures, a single intraspinal morphine bolus provides sufficient pain control for several hours. For example, an epidural or intrathecal bolus of morphine often is administered to manage pain that does not warrant placement of a catheter, such as after cesarean section and some gynecologic, orthopedic, and urologic procedures (Dabu-Bondoc, Franco, Sinatra, 2009). A single epidural morphine dose is capable of providing analgesia for up to 24 hours to 48 hours depending on the formulation used (see the paragraphs that follow). After this period of time, pain usually can be controlled with oral or IV analgesics. Single bolusing is also used when continuous epidural infusions are contraindicated such as in some patients who require anticoagulant therapy (Dabu-Bondoc, Franco, Sinatra, 2009).

When moderate to severe pain is expected to be constant for more than 24 hours, the epidural catheter can be left in place to provide intermittent analgesic bolus doses; however, this method is rarely used today with advances in infusion devices by which to administer therapy that is required for more than 24 hours. As mentioned, when the intrathecal route is used for acute pain, analgesia is administered most often by single bolus; however, implanted subcutaneous ports can be accessed to deliver intermittent boluses for long-term intraspinal pain management. When an intrathecal catheter is implanted for long-term pain control, analgesia usually is provided by continuous infusion.

The major drawback of the intermittent epidural bolus method is that a steady analgesic level is difficult to maintain, especially when bolus doses are administered PRN. Relatively large doses of the opioid are given, and a "peak and trough" effect occurs. Patients experience adverse effects at the peak (highest analgesic concentration level) and pain at the trough (lowest analgesic concentration level). Rather than a PRN approach to epidural dosing, it may be preferable to consider smaller scheduled around-the-clock (ATC) doses. A dosing frequency of less than every 6 hours is not recommended (DuPen, DuPen, 1998) (see Box 15-2 for guidelines for administering intermittent boluses through a temporary epidural catheter).

Continuous Infusion

The principle of providing continuous pain control with intraspinal analgesia can be accomplished by using an external (for acute pain and for persistent pain) or implanted (for persistent pain) infusion pump to deliver a continuous infusion (also called *basal rate*) of an analgesic solution. Supplemental bolus doses are prescribed for breakthrough pain and can be administered using the clinician-administered bolus mode available on most external infusion pumps or as outlined in Box 15-2. When implanted ports are used to deliver continuous infusion and/or intermittent boluses, meticulous aseptic precautions should be taken to protect the port from bacterial contamination (DuPen, DuPen, 1998; Holmfred, Vikerfors, Berggren, et al., 2006).

Continuous epidural analgesia has been shown to have more positive impact than IV PCA on some but not all patient outcomes following major surgery. One double-blind study randomized 60 patients undergoing radical prostatectomy to receive low thoracic (T10-T12) epidural ropivacaine (0.1%) plus fentanyl (2 mcg/mL) at 10 mL/h or IV PCA morphine (1 mg every 6 minutes) (Gupta, Fant, Axelsson, et al., 2006). Although there were no differences in hospital length of stay, those who received epidural analgesia had significantly better pain relief and expiratory muscle function than those who received IV PCA. Additionally, at 1 month, patients in the epidural group had better scores in emotional role, physical functioning, and general health. However, superior analgesia afforded by a continuous epidural infusion of bupivacaine and morphine in 60 older adults post–hip fracture surgery did not translate into improved rehabilitation in another randomized controlled study (Foss, Kristensen, Kristensen, et al., 2005). A prospective study showed similar results in 18 patients who received either epidural analgesia or IV PCA following mastectomy with immediate transverse rectus abdominis musculocutaneous (TRAM) flap breast reconstruction; continuous epidural analgesia produced better pain control and a 25-hour shorter hospital stay but no difference in time to first ambulation, first bowel sounds and flatus, tolerance of oral nutrition, and incidence of adverse effects (Correll, Viscusi, Grunwald, et al., 2001).

Patient-Controlled Epidural Analgesia (PCEA)

PCEA permits patients to treat their pain by self-administering doses of epidural analgesics to meet their individual analgesic requirements. A randomized controlled study compared fentanyl (4 mcg/mL) plus bupivacaine (0.125%) via PCEA (with basal rate) or continuous epidural infusion after colon resection and found that pain scores were similarly low but significantly fewer nurse/physician interventions for uncontrolled pain (e.g., epidural top-ups, systemic analgesia) were necessary, and patient satisfaction was significantly higher in those who received PCEA (Nightingale, Knight, Higgins, et al., 2007). Another randomized controlled study found that significantly less fentanyl-bupivacaine solution was consumed with PCEA (without basal rate) than with continuous epidural infusion following total knee arthroplasty (Silvasti, Pitkanen, 2001). Compared with nurse-administered PRN intermittent epidural bolus doses of meperidine (maximum of 50 mg/2 h), PCEA meperidine (25 mg PCEA dose with 10 minute lockout) resulted in better pain scores and a trend toward earlier return to activities of daily living and care for the newborn in women following cesarean section (Lim, Wilson, Katz, 2006). Although patient satisfaction was similar among the two groups, nurse satisfaction was higher with PCEA.

Box 15-2	Intermittent Boluses via a Short-Term Epidural Catheter

- Administer only preservative-free solutions that are labeled safe for intraspinal use.
- Before injecting, verify with another RN that the preservative-free drug, dose, and volume are in accordance with anesthesia provider's order.
- Before injecting, verify that the catheter to be injected is the epidural catheter. (Most catheters are color-coded to prevent errors, but this should always be checked prior to injection.)
- To prevent exerting too much pressure on injection, administer analgesic in at least a 10 mL syringe.
- The use of indwelling epidural filters depends on institutional policy (see text). A filter straw or needle should be used to draw solutions from glass ampules; if solutions are drawn unfiltered from glass ampules, they always should be injected through a 0.22 micron filter.
- Maintain sterility of the epidural system when removing catheter port cap, attaching syringes, and replacing port cap. (Some institutions require disinfecting connection before removing port cap. Use only nonneurotoxic agents to disinfect intraspinal catheter connections or ports [alcohol often is used to cleanse skin of secretions, but should not be used to disinfect catheter connections or ports].)
- Before injecting analgesic, gently aspirate catheter; allow time for fluid/air to travel up catheter[1]:
  - Minimal fluid return (e.g., less than 0.5 mL) or an air bubble in the syringe indicates catheter is in the epidural space.
    - → Steadily (speed of injection depends on resistance met during injection) inject analgesic through catheter filter (if filter is used).
  - Free-flowing clear fluid (CSF) return indicates catheter may be in the intrathecal space.
    - → Do not administer analgesic; notify anesthesia provider.
  - Bloody aspirate indicates catheter may be in a blood vessel.
    - → Do not administer analgesic; notify anesthesia provider.

- Do not inject analgesic if patient reports pain on steady injection; notify anesthesia provider.
- Some resistance during injection is normal, but if strong resistance is met during injection, reposition the patient so that the spine is flexed. If resistance continues, stop and notify anesthesia provider.
- Do not flush epidural catheter after injecting analgesic unless specifically ordered to do so.

CSF, Cerebrospinal fluid.

[1]Some anesthesia providers require the administration of a small test dose of local anesthetic (e.g., bupivacaine or ropivacaine) containing epinephrine to rule out intravascular or intrathecal migration prior to bolus administration; check with the state board of nursing before performing this function (also see Box 15-4 on p. 433).

When moderate to severe pain is expected to be constant for more than 24 hours, the epidural catheter is sometimes left in place to provide intermittent analgesic bolus doses. A majority of patients require epidural opioid bolus doses every 8 hours. Patients should be assessed systematically as frequency varies depending on analgesic requirement and opioid characteristics; some patients may require dosing more often, e.g., every 6 hours, while others may require boluses every 12 to 24 hours.

A retrospective review of the medical records of 245 patients who received PCEA (opioid plus local anesthetic) or IV PCA following lumbar spine surgery revealed that PCEA produced superior pain relief with less need for rescue analgesia (Cata, Noguera, Parke, et al., 2008). A randomized controlled study of older patients (N = 70) following major surgery observed better pain relief, higher patient satisfaction, and faster return of bowel function with PCEA (opioid plus local anesthetic) than with IV PCA (Mann, Pouzeratte, Boccara, et al., 2000). Although the incidence of postoperative delirium was similar among the two groups (24% to 26%), epidural

analgesia was associated with improved mental status on the fourth and fifth day.

When PCEA is administered, a basal rate usually provides most of the patient's analgesic requirement and the PCEA bolus doses are used to manage breakthrough pain. If a basal rate is not provided, it is especially important to remind patients to "stay on top of the pain," to maintain a steady neuraxial analgesic level and self-administer bolus doses before pain is severe and out of control. Research has shown that this type of patient teaching is critical to successful therapy (Cywinski, Parker, Xu, et al., 2004). PCEA is safe and effective in older adults (Ishiyama,

Iijima, Sugawara, et al., 2007; Mann, Pouzeratte, Boccara, et al., 2000), but the need for proper patient selection and frequent follow up to ensure appropriate PCEA use are emphasized (Silvasti, Pitkanen, 2001). See an example of a patient information brochure about PCEA on pp. 542-543 at the end of Section IV; see Chapter 12 for discussion of PCA principles and safeguards, such as patient-only use of PCA; and see Chapter 17 for discussion of PCA pump features and Table 17-2 on p. 469 for interventions for patients receiving PCEA.

Combined Spinal-Epidural Anesthesia/Analgesia (CSEA)

Although used less often than epidural analgesia, "combined spinal-epidural anesthesia/analgesia" (CSEA) is sometimes administered for labor and delivery and during and after cesarean section and other surgical procedures. CSEA involves placing an epidural needle (typically, 16- or 18-gauge Touhy) into the epidural space, and then passing a much smaller gauge and longer spinal needle (e.g., 29-gauge Quincke needle) through the epidural needle into the subarachnoid space. Subarachnoid placement is confirmed by aspiration of CSF. Opioid and/or local anesthetic is injected into the subarachnoid space, producing rapid and profound anesthesia/analgesia. The subarachnoid needle is removed, and an epidural catheter is inserted to administer supplemental doses as needed to prolong the block and provide ongoing analgesia (Cousins, Veering, 1998; Dabu-Bondoc, Franco, Sinatra, 2009).

The rationale for combining the routes is to minimize the shortcomings of both intrathecal and epidural analgesia while taking advantage of their benefits (Dabu-Bondoc, Franco, Sinatra, 2009; Teoh, Thomas, Tan, 2006). Intrathecal anesthesia has a rapid onset and produces dense neuraxial blockade, and epidural analgesia provides prolonged anesthesia and postoperative analgesia (Grape, Schug, 2008). For this reason, it has been suggested as an option for longer surgical procedures associated with significant postoperative pain, such as lower extremity surgery (Grape, Schug, 2008). CSEA improved intraoperative analgesia and reduced pain with cough better than an intermittent epidural bolus technique following major abdominal surgery in a prospective, randomized study (N = 160) (Stamenkovic, Geric, Slavkovic, et al., 2008) and produced faster motor recovery than single-shot spinal anesthesia following cesarean section in another prospective, randomized study (N = 62) (Lew, Yeo, Thomas, 2004). Because the CSEA technique uses the intrathecal route, lower doses of local anesthetic are possible for laboring patients, and less motor block is produced. The epidural route is used for low-dose supplemental analgesic boluses, and with appropriate assessment, patients have been able to safely and comfortably ambulate during labor while receiving CSEA (Brownridge, Cohen, Ward, 1998; Gautier, Debry, Fanard, et al., 1997).

Drug Bioavailability by the Intraspinal Routes

In contrast to drugs administered systemically, drugs administered intraspinally are more potent (i.e., small doses are effective) because distribution of the drug brings it close to the action site (opioid receptors in the dorsal horn of the spinal cord). This is particularly true when opioids are delivered by the intrathecal route where they are carried by the CSF to the dorsal horn. After epidural administration, drugs are distributed by three main pathways: (1) neural diffusion through the dura into the CSF then into the spinal cord directly to the receptors, (2) vascular uptake by the vessels in the epidural space into systemic circulation, and (3) uptake by the fat in the epidural space; a drug depot is created from which the drug enters the systemic circulation (Maalouf, Liu, 2009).

More direct delivery of opioids to the site of analgesic action explains why the dose of an opioid by the intraspinal routes is smaller than that required by the parenteral route to produce equal analgesia (i.e., the closer the opioid is delivered to the opioid receptors, the lower the required analgesic dose). For example, research has shown that epidural morphine provides superior analgesia at a lower dose compared with IV or IM morphine; the relative potency of epidural morphine compared with morphine by self-titrated IV PCA was 10:1 following orthopedic surgery (Maalouf, Liu, 2009). When converting opioid-tolerant patients from one route to another, the required dose of morphine is approximately three times less by the epidural route than by the IV route (ratio may vary for other opioids), and the dose required by the intrathecal route is approximately 10 times less than required by the epidural route to produce equal analgesia (DuPen, DuPen, 1998) (see Chapter 18 for switching to different routes of administration).

Drug Solubility

Drug solubility and the ability of the drug to traverse diffusion barriers (e.g., the dura mater) influence drug absorption and bioavailability by the intraspinal routes. The more lipid-soluble (readily dissolved in fatty tissue) the drug, the more readily it moves through membranes, resulting in faster absorption. For example, when administered by single epidural injection, lipid-soluble opioids, such as fentanyl, rapidly traverse the dura into the CSF, and then exit the aqueous CSF and easily penetrate the lipid-rich spinal tissue as well as surrounding vasculature (Maalouf, Liu, 2009; Dabu-Bondoc, Franco, Sinatra, 2009). This contributes to fentanyl's fast onset of action (5 minutes) (Grape, Schug, 2008). In contrast, hydrophilic opioids (readily dissolved in aqueous solution), such as morphine and hydromorphone, have more difficulty traversing the dura to reach the aqueous CSF. By either the epidural or intrathecal route, once in the aqueous CSF, hydrophilic drugs prefer to remain there. Eventually, high enough concentrations of morphine are reached in the CSF, and the drug moves into the spinal cord to the opioid receptors. This helps to explain intraspinal morphine's slow onset of action (30 to 60 minutes) (Dabu-Bondoc, Franco, Sinatra, 2009).

An opioid's duration of action when administered by the intraspinal routes is determined in large part by the amount of the drug that remains in the CSF. Because morphine is hydrophilic, it tends to remain within the aqueous CSF. This ensures continued opioid receptor binding by replenishing molecules that dissociate and are cleared from the spinal action sites and helps to explain morphine's large volume of distribution, high bioavailability, and exceptionally long duration of analgesia from a single intraspinal bolus dose (e.g., 12 to 24 hours). On the other hand, the highly lipid-soluble opioids such as fentanyl traverse membranes readily and are easily removed by vasculature or remain trapped within the fat of the epidural space (Dabu-Bondoc, Franco, Sinatra, 2009). This causes a rapid decline in drug concentration at action sites and results in a short duration of analgesia (2 hours). The highly lipid-soluble opioids are administered by continuous infusion to prolong their limited duration of activity if extended relief is desired. When steady state is reached by continuous infusion, the various opioids differ little in terms of duration.

Dermatomal Spread and Epidural Catheter Placement

An opioid drug deposited into the CSF, or diffusing into the CSF from the epidural space, distributes throughout the neuraxis with the movement of the CSF (Bernards, 2000; Maalouf, Liu, 2009). The extent to which the drug moves rostrally toward the brain, or caudally toward the lower end of the thecal sac, depends on the drug's clearance rate (Bernards, 2000). Hydrophilic drugs such as morphine and hydromorphone tend to remain in the CSF and produce a broad spread of analgesia across many dermatomes (Dabu-Bondoc, Franco, Sinatra, 2009). The opposite is true of lipophilic opioids such as fentanyl and sufentanil, which are rapidly cleared from the CSF, tend to be transported for shorter distances, and produce what is called *segmental* analgesia. By rapidly leaving the CSF and redistributing into spinal cord tissue, epidural fat, and vasculature, these lipophilic opioids have little rostral spread (Dabu-Bondoc, Franco, Sinatra, 2009).

Particularly when using the lipophilic opioids, it is important to put the tip of the catheter at the spinal level where there is a high level of nociceptive input (Grape, Schug, 2008). Research has shown that placement of the catheter tip at the spinal level congruent with the dermatomes where the incision is performed provides superior analgesia, helps to reduce adverse effects, and is associated with decreased morbidity compared with placement at other spinal levels (Maalouf, Liu, 2009; Wu, 2005).

As noted, appropriate placement of the catheter is especially important if lipophilic drugs are used. Whereas hydrophilic opioids ascend in the CSF and are likely to cover the spinal segments receiving input from the incisional dermatomes irrespective of catheter placement, lipophilic opioids such as fentanyl and sufentanil may not ascend to the necessary spinal level, leading to a situation in which the analgesia is produced largely by systemic redistribution (movement of the dose from the CSF into the bloodstream and then back to sites of action in the brain and spinal cord) rather than by local action of the drug at the spinal cord level (Dabu-Bondoc, Franco, Sinatra, 2009; Wu, 2005). Some studies indicated that lumbar epidural fentanyl infusions are equivalent to IV fentanyl infusions, suggesting that spinal fentanyl may in fact produce most of its analgesia through this systemic redistribution (McCartney, Niazi, 2006). Even lumbar administration of dilute lipophilic solutions at high infusion rates may result in plasma concentration levels equal to parenterally administered opioids. Given the rapid redistribution of lipophilic opioids and the need for appropriate placement of catheters to obtain the intended segmental analgesic effects, it is recommended that the tip always be placed at the thoracic level (T10 or higher) for lipophilic drugs such as fentanyl so that the spinal cord is adjacent to the entry site of the drug (Dabu-Bondoc, Franco, Sinatra, 2009). For practitioners choosing lumbar placement of epidural catheters, especially to treat upper-abdominal and thoracic nociceptive input, morphine or hydromorphone may be the best choice of drug (McCartney, Niazi, 2006; Wu, 2005).

Thoracic Epidural Catheter Placement

There is a trend toward thoracic epidural catheter placement in general and particularly for major thoracoabdominal surgeries (Grape, Schug, 2008). For certain types of surgery, such as cardiac surgery, thoracic epidural anesthesia and analgesia clearly have more advantages than lumbar epidural anesthesia and analgesia (Bracco, Hemmerling, 2008). Thoracic epidural analgesia has been associated with improved dynamic pain relief, minimal lower extremity motor blockade, enhanced mobility and functional exercise capacity, better cardiac perfusion and tissue oxygen tension, and less urinary retention and hypotension (Bauer, Hentz, Ducrocq, et al., 2007; Brodner, Van Aken, Hertle, et al., 2001; Buggy, Doherty, Hart, et al., 2002; Carli, Mayo, Klubein, et al., 2002; Grape, Schug, 2008; Kabon, Fleischmann, Treschan, et al., 2003; Kessler, Neidhart, Brenerich, et al., 2002; Mayer, Boldt, Schellhaafs, et al., 2007; Paiste, Bjerke, Williams, et al., 2001; Priestley, Cope, Halliwell, et al., 2002; Wu, 2005). A meta-analysis of 33 randomized controlled trials (2366 patients) showed that thoracic epidural analgesia reduced the incidence of perioperative acute renal failure, the time on mechanical ventilation, and the composite endpoint mortality and myocardial infarction (MI) in patients undergoing cardiac surgery (Bignami, Landoni,

Biondi-Zoccai, et al., 2010). Another meta-analysis revealed that compared with nonepidural analgesia, epidural analgesia resulted in a lower incidence of postoperative MI, and subgroup analysis showed that thoracic epidural placement was superior to lumbar placement in this regard (Beattie, Badner, Choi, 2001). A Cochrane Collaboration Review comparing systemic opioid analgesia with epidural analgesia following abdominal aortic surgery concluded that, regardless of regimen, thoracic epidural analgesia provided better pain relief, particularly during movement, for up to 3 postoperative days, reduced duration of mechanical ventilation and tracheal intubation time by 20%, and was associated with fewer cardiovascular (CV), gastrointestinal (GI), and renal complications (Nishimori, Ballantyne, Low, 2006). Others have found similar excellent results with epidural analgesia following this type of major surgery (Park, Thompson, Lee, et al., 2001). Whereas epidural analgesia appears to improve outcomes for cardiac surgical patients, a meta-analysis of 24 randomized controlled trials (1106 patients) concluded that spinal analgesia did not improve clinically relevant outcomes in patients undergoing cardiac surgery and discouraged further research on this method in these patients (Zangrillo, Bignami, Biondi-Zoccai, et al., 2009).

Thoracic epidural analgesia may provide solutions for the challenge of managing postoperative pain in individuals at risk for pulmonary complications. One study found that thoracic epidural analgesia with bupivacaine (0.25%) was safe and efficacious in patients with severe end-stage chronic obstructive pulmonary disease following thoracotomy (Gruber, Tschernko, Kritzinger, et al., 2001).

Some anesthesia providers may be reluctant to attempt thoracic catheter placement and prefer to insert lumbar catheters because the spinal cord becomes smaller as it progresses distally and the lumbar spinous processes are angulated posteriorly and farther apart making epidural catheter placement easier in the lumbar area. When placed below the spinal cord, the risk of trauma to the spinal cord is eliminated; however, it is a common misconception that thoracic epidural catheter placement is technically more difficult and causes more neurologic damage than lumbar catheter placement (Grape, Schug, 2008; Wu, 2005). It is a technique that is quickly mastered by anesthesia providers. A review of 874 cases of high thoracic epidural analgesia provided over a 7-year period revealed no related neurologic complications (Royse, Soeding, Royse, 2007).

Selected Analgesics Administered by the Intraspinal Routes

The two main types of drugs administered intraspinally to treat acute pain are opioids and local anesthetics. Other drugs used for the treatment of persistent pain are the calcium channel blocker ziconotide, the alpha$_2$-adrenergic agonist clonidine, and less often, the N-methyl-D-aspartate (NMDA) antagonist ketamine. Intraspinal clonidine is also used for acute pain treatment. Baclofen (Lioresal), a muscle relaxant and antispastic agent, is administered intraspinally for treatment of spasticity (see Section V for a detailed discussion of all of these agents). These drugs can be given alone or in combination with each other. The rationale for combining drugs is that they work synergistically to provide better analgesia and fewer adverse effects at lower doses.

Opioids

The mu agonist opioids morphine, fentanyl, and hydromorphone are the most common opioids administered by the intraspinal route; sufentanil, methadone, and meperidine (Demerol) are administered less often. Table 15-3 provides a summary of the characteristics of selected opioids administered intraspinally, and Table 15-4 provides dosing recommendations for the various neuraxial opioids. Following is a discussion of selected opioids.

Morphine

Morphine was the first opioid to be administered intraspinally for the relief of pain in humans (Wang, Nauss, Thomas, 1979) and the first to receive FDA approval for intraspinal administration. It is an excellent choice of opioid for intraspinal analgesia because it produces spinal-mediated analgesia by the epidural and intrathecal routes and can be given by all of the intraspinal delivery methods. It is ideal for single-bolus dose intraspinal administration because it has a particularly long duration of action (up to 24 hours in the opioid-naïve patient; see the section on extended-release epidural morphine later in the chapter) (Dabu-Bondoc, Franco, Sinatra, 2009; Wu, 2005). Several studies have demonstrated superior postoperative analgesia with single-dose epidural morphine compared with parenteral opioids for a wide variety of surgical procedures (Dabu-Bondoc, Franco, Sinatra, 2009). As discussed, another advantage is that morphine spreads rostrally, which makes the vertebral location of intraspinal administration less critical than when administering lipophilic opioids for acute postoperative pain. For example, intraspinal morphine can be administered in the lumbar region to produce analgesia after thoracic surgery (Chaney, Furry, Fluder, et al., 1997; Wu, 2005) and in the thoracic region for oral and facial pain treatment (Sakuramoto, Kanai, Matoba, et al., 1996).

With bolus injection in the opioid-naïve patient, intraspinal morphine has a slow onset of analgesia (30 to 60 minutes) and a peak effect of approximately 90 minutes (Wu, 2005). Additional analgesia usually is required until morphine takes effect. For example, some clinicians administer an epidural dose of a faster-acting lipophilic opioid analgesic, such as fentanyl (onset 5 minutes), at the time of the single epidural morphine bolus or initiation of infusion therapy to provide analgesia until morphine

Table 15-3 | Summary of Characteristics of Selected Intraspinal Opioids

Analgesic	Onset[1] (min)	Peak[1] (min)	Duration[1-3] (h)	Half-life (h)	Solubility	Dermatomal spread	Comments
Morphine	30-60 (EA); 30-60 (IA)	90-120 (EA); 60 (IA)	Up to 24 (EA); up to 24 (IA) 48 (EREM)	2-3	Hydrophilic (soluble in aqueous solution)	Wide	Standard for comparison; can be administered by all intraspinal methods of delivery; ideal for single bolus dose but with risk of late respiratory depression (6 to 12 h); wide rostral spread; drug of choice if lumbar placement. Extended-release formulation available for analgesia for up to 48 hours after a single lumbar epidural bolus.
Fentanyl	5-15 (EA); 5 (IA)	10-20 (EA); 10 (IA)	2-4 (EA); 2-4 (IA)	3-4	High lipid (soluble in fat)	Narrow; segmental	Because of short duration, continuous infusion preferred to intermittent boluses; catheter location important due to segmental analgesia. At steady state, slow elimination from tissues can result in a long half-life (up to 12 h) and accumulation leading to late and prolonged sedation and respiratory depression.
Hydromorphone (Dilaudid)	15-30 (EA)	45-60 (EA)	6-7; up to 18 (EA)	2-3	More lipid soluble (10 times) than morphine; less lipid soluble than meperidine and fentanyl	Less than morphine; more than meperidine and fentanyl	Similar to morphine in analgesia and adverse effects. Can be administered by all intraspinal delivery modalities.

Meperidine (Demerol)	5-30 (EA); 10 (IA)	30 (EA); 15 (IA)	6-8 (EA); 6-16 (IA)	2-3	More lipid soluble than morphine and hydromorphone; less lipid soluble than fentanyl	Less than morphine and hydromorphone; more than fentanyl	Toxic metabolite, normeperidine, can cause CNS irritability, seizures regardless of route of administration; metabolite half-life is 15 to 20 h. Local anesthetic properties. Contraindicated in older adults and patients with impaired renal function.
Sufentanil	5-10 (EA); 5 (IA)	10 (EA); 15-20 (IA)	2-4 (EA); 2-4 (IA)	2-4	Very high lipid solubility (2 times more lipid soluble than fentanyl)	Narrow; segmental	Because of short duration, continuous infusion is preferred to intermittent boluses; catheter location important; analgesia and adverse effects similar to fentanyl.

EA, Epidural analgesia (single bolus dose); *EM,* epidural morphine; *ER,* extended release; *IA,* intrathecal analgesia (single bolus dose).

[1]Onset, peak, and duration are based on single bolus administration.

[2]Duration of analgesia is dose dependent; the higher the dose, usually the longer the duration.

[3]When steady state is reached by continuous infusion, the various opioids differ little in terms of duration.

From Pasero, C., & McCaffery, M. *Pain assessment and pharmacologic management*, pp. 418-419, St. Louis, Mosby. Data from American Society of Anesthesiologists Task Force on Neuraxial Opioids. (2009). Practice guidelines for the prevention, detection, and management of respiratory depression associated with neuraxial opioid administration. *Anesthesiology, 110*(2), 218-230; Brown, D. L. (2005). Spinal, epidural, and caudal anesthesia. In R. D. Miller (Ed.), *Miller's anesthesia*, vol 2, ed 6, Philadelphia, Elsevier; Cashman, J. N., & Dolin, S. J. (2004). Respiratory and haemodynamic effects of acute postoperative pain management: Evidence from published data. *Br J Anaesth, 93*(2), 212-223; Cousins, M. J., & Veering, B. T. (1998). Epidural neural blockade. In M. J. Cousins, & P. O. Bridenbaugh (Eds.), *Neural blockade in clinical anesthesia and management of pain*, Philadelphia, Lippincott-Raven; Dabu-Bondoc, S., Franco, S. A., & Sinatra, R. S. (2009). Neuraxial analgesia with hydromorphone, morphine, and fentanyl: Dosing and safety guidelines. In R. S. Sinatra, O. A. de Leon-Casasola, B. Ginsberg, et al. (Eds.), *Acute pain management*, Cambridge, NY, Cambridge University Press; Grape, S., & Schug, S. A. (2008). Epidural and spinal analgesia. In P. E. Macintyre, S. M. Walker, & D. J. Rowbotham (Eds.), *Clinical pain management. Acute pain*, ed 2, London, Hodder Arnold; Kedlaya, D., Reynolds, L., & Waldman, S. (2002). Epidural and intrathecal analgesia for cancer pain. *Best Prac Res Clin Anaesth, 16*(4), 651-665; Maalouf, D. B., & Liu, S. S. (2009). Clinical application of epidural analgesia. In R. S. Sinatra, O. A. de Leon-Casasola, B. Ginsberg, et al. (Eds.), *Acute pain management*, Cambridge, NY, Cambridge University Press; McCartney, C. J. L., & Niazi, A. (2006). Use of opioid analgesics in the perioperative period. In G. Shorten, D. B. Carr, D. Harmon, et al. (Eds.), *Postoperative pain management: An evidence-based guide to practice*, Philadelphia, Saunders; Vascello, L., & McQuillan, R. J. (2006). Opioid analgesics and routes of administration. In O. A. de Leon-Casasola (Ed.), *Cancer pain. Pharmacological, interventional and palliative care approaches*, Philadelphia, Saunders; Wu, C. L. (2005). Acute postoperative pain. In R. D. Miller (Ed.), *Miller's anesthesia*, vol 2, ed 6, Philadelphia, Elsevier. © 2011, Pasero C, McCaffery M. May be duplicated for use in clinical practice.

Table 15-4 | Dosing of Neuraxial Opioids

Drug	Intrathecal or Subarachnoid Single Dose	Epidural Single Dose[1]	Epidural Continuous Infusion
Fentanyl	5-25 mcg	50-100 mcg	25-100 mcg/h
Sufentanil	2-10 mcg	10-50 mcg	10-20 mcg/h
Alfentanil	–	0.5-1 mg	0.2 mg/h
Morphine	0.1-0.3 mg	1-5 mg	0.1-1 mg/h
Hydromorphone	–	0.5-1 mg	0.1-0.2 mg/h
Meperidine	10-30 mg	20-60 mg	10-60 mg/h
Methadone	–	4-8 mg	0.3-0.5 mg/h

Data from Miller, R. D. (Ed.). (2005). *Miller's anesthesia*, vol 2, ed 6, Philadelphia, Churchill Livingstone. As appears in Pasero, C., & McCaffery, M. *Pain assessment and pharmacologic management*, p. 420, St. Louis, Mosby. © 2011, Pasero C, McCaffery M. May be duplicated for use in clinical practice.

Table 15-5 | Recommended Doses of Intrathecal Morphine and Epidural Bolus Dose Morphine for Postoperative Analgesia

Surgical Procedure	Intrathecal Dose	Epidural Bolus Dose
Vaginal hysterectomy, cesarean section	0.15-0.2 mg	2-3 mg
Hip and knee surgery	0.2-0.5 mg	2-5 mg
Lower abdominal surgery	0.2-0.4 mg	3-5 mg
Upper abdominal surgery	0.4-0.6 mg	5-7 mg
Nephrectomy	0.4-0.6 mg	5-7 mg
Cholecystectomy	0.4-0.6 mg	5 mg
Abdominal aortic aneurysm	0.4-0.6 mg	5-8 mg
Whipple procedure	0.5-0.6 mg	5-8 mg
Retroperitoneal lymph node dissection	0.5-0.6 mg	6-8 mg
Thoracotomy	0.6-1.0 mg	6-10 mg

Data from Sinatra, R. S., de Leon-Casasola, O. A., Ginsberg, B., et al. (Eds.). (2009). *Acute pain management*, Cambridge, NY, Cambridge University Press. As appears in Pasero, C., & McCaffery, M. *Pain assessment and pharmacologic management*, p. 420, St. Louis, Mosby. © 2011, Pasero C, McCaffery M. May be duplicated for use in clinical practice.

takes effect. Table 15-5 provides recommended intraspinal morphine bolus doses for pain management following various surgical procedures. See also Table 15-4.

When continuous epidural morphine is administered to surgical patients, a loading epidural morphine bolus dose (2 to 5 mg), usually combined with ropivacaine (0.2%) or bupivacaine (0.25%), is given preincision

followed by initiation of the epidural morphine infusion at the end of the surgical procedure (Dabu-Bondoc, Franco, Sinatra, 2009). Although a solution concentration of 60 mcg/mL is reported to produce more reliable analgesia, a 40 mcg/mL concentration at a rate of 4 to 10 mL/h is recommended to reduce adverse effects, such as nausea and pruritus (Dabu-Bondoc, Franco, Sinatra, 2009).

Morphine by PCEA has been used for many years in surgical patients (Pasero, Portenoy, McCaffery, 1999). It is less popular, however, than hydromorphone and fentanyl, which are easier to titrate and associated with fewer adverse effects by this modality (Dabu-Bondoc, Franco, Sinatra, 2009). Table 15-6 contains common PCEA prescription ranges for opioid-naïve patients.

Because of slow rostral spread in the CSF, large-volume bolus doses (more than 5 mg) of epidural morphine have been known to produce late respiratory depression (approximately 6 to 12 hours after lumbar injection, corresponding with the rate of CSF flow from the spinal level to the brainstem) (Angst, Ramaswamy, Riley, et al., 2000; McCartney, Niazi, 2006). Earlier respiratory depression at 5 to 10 minutes and before 2 hours also can occur due to vascular uptake of morphine. Monitoring the opioid-naïve patient's level of sedation and respiratory status every hour for 12 hours after a clinician-administered intraspinal bolus of morphine is recommended (American Society of Anesthesiologists, 2009) (see Chapter 19 for more on sedation and respiratory depression).

Fear of late respiratory depression has caused some clinicians to avoid using epidural morphine in opioid-naïve patients; however, rostral spread and late respiratory depression are uncommon when epidural morphine is administered in smaller, more frequent bolus doses or by continuous infusion or PCEA. Continuous administration leads to less fluctuation of drug levels, which reduces the risk of peak concentration toxicity (Gianino, York, Paice, 1996). Continuous epidural

Table 15-6 | Common PCEA Prescription Ranges for Opioid-Naïve Adults

Drug	Loading Dose	PCEA Dose	Lockout (Delay) (min)	Basal
Morphine	2-4 mg	0.2-0.3 mg	10	0-0.8 mL/h
Morphine 40 mcg/mL + 0.05-0.1% bupivacaine	2-4 mg	1-2 mL	15	2-8 mL/h
Hydromorphone 10 mcg/mL + bupivacaine 0.06%	ND	4 mL	10	4 mL/h
Hydromorphone 10-20 mcg/mL + bupivacaine 0.05% or less	0.5-1.5 mg (intraoperative)	1-3 mL	6-8	6-10 mL/h
Hydromorphone 15-30 mcg/mL + bupivacaine 0.0625-0.125%	0.5-1.0 mg (intraoperative)	1-4 mL	10	4-10 mL/h
Fentanyl	25-50 mcg	10-15 mcg	10	0-100 mcg/h
Fentanyl 2-4 mcg/mL + bupivacaine 0.05%-0.1%	50-100 mcg	1-3 mL	6	6-10 mL/h
Fentanyl 5 mcg/mL + 0.0625% bupivacaine	ND	3-4 mL	10	4-6 mL/h
Fentanyl 5 mcg/mL + ropivacaine 0.1%-0.2%	ND	2 mL	20	5 mL/h
Sufentanil	2.5-5 mcg/kg	2-4 mcg	10	0-10 mcg/kg/h
Sufentanil 0.5 mcg/mL + bupivacaine 0.125%	6 mL	2-3 mL	12	3-5 mL/h

ND, No data; *PCEA,* patient-controlled epidural analgesia.
PCEA prescribing habits vary widely. This table provides some of the common PCEA prescription ranges for opioid-naïve adults.
From Pasero, C., & McCaffery, M. *Pain assessment and pharmacologic management,* p. 421, St. Louis, Mosby. Data from Dabu-Bondoc, S., Franco, S. A., & Sinatra, R. S. (2009). Neuraxial analgesia with hydromorphone, morphine, and fentanyl: Dosing and safety guidelines. In R. S. Sinatra, O. A. de Leon-Casasola, B. Ginsberg, et al. (Eds.), *Acute pain management,* Cambridge, NY, Cambridge University Press; Maalouf, D. B., & Liu, S. S. (2009). Clinical application of epidural analgesia. In R. S. Sinatra, O. A. de Leon-Casasola, B. Ginsberg, et al. (Eds.), *Acute pain management,* Cambridge, NY, Cambridge University Press; McCartney, C. J. L., & Niazi, A. (2006). Use of opioid analgesics in the perioperative period. In G. Shorten, D. B. Carr, D. Harmon D, et al. (Eds.), *Postoperative pain management: An evidence-based guide to practice,* Philadelphia, Saunders; Wu, C. L. (2005). Acute postoperative pain. In R. D. Miller (Ed.), *Miller's anesthesia,* vol 2, ed 6, Philadelphia, Elsevier. © 2011, Pasero C, McCaffery M. May be duplicated for use in clinical practice.

morphine infusions with or without PCEA have been found to be highly effective and safe in opioid-naïve patients (Dabu-Bondoc, Franco, Sinatra, 2009).

As with more lipophilic drugs, when a continuous epidural infusion of morphine is discontinued, the concentration of opioid declines and adverse effects (e.g., sedation, respiratory depression) decrease, not increase. IV lines, if otherwise unnecessary, can be removed, and routine monitoring (e.g., every 4 to 8 hours in stable patients) of level of sedation and respiratory status is customary.

Consensus guidelines recommend morphine as the first-choice opioid for long-term intrathecal pain treatment (Deer, Krames, Hassenbusch, et al., 2007). When combined with bupivacaine for intrathecal administration with or without PCA capability, morphine has been shown to be highly effective for the management of refractory cancer pain (Vascello, McQuillan, 2006). Morphine and local anesthetics work synergistically, providing excellent pain relief with significantly smaller doses than are possible when administered epidurally. Advances in technology allow patients the benefits of neuraxial infusion therapy in the home setting (Vascello, McQuillan, 2006).

Extended-Release Epidural Morphine (EREM). EREM (Depodur™) is distinguished from conventional epidural morphine (e.g., Astramorph, Duramorph) by its

unique delivery system called DepoFoam™, which consists of multiple microscopic, liposomal (fat-based) particles (Pasero, McCaffery, 2005b). The liposomes contain aqueous chambers that encapsulate preservative-free morphine (Carvalho, Riley, Cohen, et al., 2005). After epidural injection, the liposomes slowly release morphine over a period of 48 hours by erosion or reorganization of the lipid membranes (Heitz, Viscusi, 2009). It should be administered in the lumbar epidural space only. Primary advantages of this formulation are that it allows up to 48 hours of pain relief without the use of an indwelling catheter, which can pose a risk of infection, impede mobility, and raise concerns about postoperative anticoagulant therapy (Pasero, McCaffery, 2005b; Viscusi, Martin, Hartrick, et al., 2005) (see Table 15-8 on p. 439). Further, concerns regarding infusion device programming errors are eliminated with this approach (see later in chapter for more on operator errors).

An open-label study of 39 patients undergoing total hip arthroplasty compared a 5 mg dose of conventional epidural morphine with 10 to 30 mg doses of EREM and found that the median time to request for first analgesia was three to six times longer, supplemental analgesia consumption was less, and patient satisfaction was better in patients who received EREM (Viscusi, Kopacz, Hartrick, et al., 2006). Another study of patients post hip

Box 15-3 | Care of the Patient Receiving Extended-Release Epidural Morphine (EREM)

- Ensure that staff is adequately trained regarding EREM before introducing therapy in the institution.
- Develop a standardized, preprinted order set that includes:
  - EREM dose and time of administration
  - Monitoring parameters
  - Activity, ambulation
  - IV access (e.g., heparin lock) for 24 hours
  - Management of breakthrough pain
  - Treatment of adverse effects
  - When to notify anesthesia provider (e.g., unrelieved pain, excessive adverse effects)
  - Implement measures that alert staff that EREM has been administered (e.g., colorful patient wristband or brightly-colored label on medical record or bed).
- Assess pain with every new report of pain; assess well-controlled pain at least every 4 hours.
- Monitor sedation and respiratory status q 1 h × 12 h, q 2 h × 12 h, then q 4 h if stable after EREM injection,

then every 4 hours for the next 24 hours, then per routine in stable patients (see Pasero Opioid-Induced Sedation Scale [POSS] in Box 19-4 on p. 510).
- Monitor other vital signs every 4 hours for 48 hours then per routine in stable patients (evaluate need to monitor blood pressure more often in some patients).
- Be aware that many of the drugs commonly used to treat opioid-induced adverse effects, such as antihistamines for pruritus and antiemetics for nausea, can produce an additive sedating effect (see Chapter 19 for better alternatives).

h, Hour; *q,* every

From Pasero, C., & McCaffery, M. *Pain assessment and pharmacologic management,* p. 422, St. Louis, Mosby. Data from Pasero, C., Eksterowicz, N., Primeau, M., et al. (2007). ASPMN position statement: Registered nurse management and monitoring of analgesia by catheter techniques. *Pain Manage Nurs, 8*(2), 48-54; Pasero, C., & McCaffery, M. (2005). Extended-release epidural morphine (Depodur™). *J PeriAnesth Nurs, 20*(5), 345-350. © 2011, Pasero C, McCaffery M. May be duplicated for use in clinical practice.

arthroplasty (Viscusi, Martin, Hartrick, et al., 2005) found similar positive results as did research following knee arthroplasty (Hartrick, Martin, Kantor, et al., 2006), cesarean section delivery (Carvalho, Riley, Cohen, et al., 2005), and lower abdominal surgery (Gambling, Hughes, Martin, et al., 2005). EREM produced lower pain scores on the first postoperative day but more nausea, vomiting, and pruritus than spinal anesthesia alone in patients undergoing total hip arthroplasty (Kahl, Parvizi, Viscusi, 2010).

Adverse effects associated with EREM are similar to conventional epidural morphine, with nausea and pruritus reported as most common (Hartrick, Hartrick, 2008; Pasero, McCaffery, 2005b). These appear to be at their worst during the first 24 hours after EREM administration (Gambling, Hughes, Martin, et al., 2005; Viscusi, Martin, Hartrick, et al., 2005). Administration of the lowest effective dose of EREM is critical; 10 to 15 mg is recommended (Heitz, Viscusi, 2009). This is facilitated when EREM is administered as part of a multimodal analgesic regimen, e.g., with an NSAID and acetaminophen (Hartrick, Hartrick, 2008). Higher doses (e.g., 20 to 25 mg) have been associated with clinically significant respiratory depression requiring naloxone administration (Hartrick, Hartrick, 2008; Pasero, McCaffery, 2005b). A meta-analysis of three randomized controlled trials concluded that, although EREM produced effective postoperative pain control for up to 48 hours, it was associated with a significantly higher risk of respiratory depression than IV PCA (Sumida, Lesley, Hanna, et al., 2009). See Box 15-3 for guidelines in the care of patients receiving EREM, and Chapter 19 for treatment of adverse effects.

Fentanyl

Epidural fentanyl has been used extensively for anesthesia and to provide postoperative analgesia (Finucane, Ganapathy, Carli, et al., 2001; Pasero, Portenoy, McCaffery, 1999; Wu, 2005). Single intraspinal doses of fentanyl provide analgesia for just 2 to 4 hours (Wu, 2005), making this method of administration appropriate only for very short-term pain control, such as following ambulatory surgery and when rapid analgesia is desired (onset is 5 to 15 minutes). Diluting the epidural dose (e.g., 50 to 100 mcg) in 10 mL of preservative-free normal saline helps to prolong analgesia and increase the initial spread and diffusion of the drug (Wu, 2005). Because lipid-soluble opioids such as fentanyl have such a short duration, administration by continuous infusion or PCEA, rather than intermittent bolus dosing, is preferred for extended pain control (Wu, 2005) (see Table 15-3).

As discussed, the concentration of fentanyl that can be measured in the blood after epidural delivery is very close to that attained from the same IV dose, suggesting that much of fentanyl's action is the result of systemic uptake from the vasculature in the epidural space. Although some research shows better analgesia with epidural fentanyl compared with parenteral fentanyl, the advantages also have been reported to be marginal (Wu, 2005). This may help to explain why fentanyl is administered epidurally most often in combination with a local anesthetic, such as ropivacaine or bupivacaine; however, whereas hydrophilic opioids and local anesthetics work synergistically to provide improved analgesia, such a relationship between the lipophilic opioids and local anesthetics is less clear and the benefit of this combination compared with the administration of a local anesthetic alone has been questioned (McCartney, Niazi, 2006). Nevertheless, this approach continues to be widely used (Grape, Schug, 2008), and fentanyl is a primary drug for continuous infusion and PCEA following major surgery. As with other pain management therapies, a variety of factors influence fentanyl PCEA dose requirements. A 3-year prospective study of almost 2000 patients found that the type of surgical procedure had more influence on PCEA (fentanyl 1 mcg/mL plus 0.625% bupivacaine with basal rate) dose requirements than patient demographic variables (e.g., sex, height, weight); patients who had thoracic or abdominal surgery consumed higher doses than those who had lower-extremity surgery (Chang, Dai, Ger, et al., 2006) (see Table 15-4 and Table 15-6 for dosing recommendations).

After repetitive dosing or continuous infusion of fentanyl, a steady state is approached. In this condition, the terminal half-life of fentanyl depends on how much is taken into tissue for storage and how quickly it is released. Although fentanyl is reported to have a terminal half-life of approximately 3 to 4 hours, at steady state, slow removal of fentanyl from storage sites can result in a longer terminal half-life (up to 12 hours). This prolongation of half-life as the fat stores are saturated can lead to accumulation effects during the period of initial dosing and dose titration, as well as prolonged duration of sedation and respiratory depression. As a rule, however, early-onset respiratory depression is more common than delayed with epidural fentanyl. This reflects vascular uptake of the opioid and occurs most often within an hour of initial injection (McCartney, Niazi, 2006).

Hydromorphone

Hydromorphone has gained wide acceptance as a first-line opioid for intraspinal administration. Its lipid solubility is intermediate between morphine and fentanyl. Because it is 10 times more lipophilic than morphine, its onset of analgesia (15 to 30 minutes) is faster and its duration of action (6 to 7 hours) is shorter (Dabu-Bondoc, Franco, Sinatra, 2009) (see Table 15-3). This makes single bolus doses of the drug suitable for short-stay surgical patients who will be transitioned to oral analgesics within 5 to 12 hours after surgery (Dabu-Bondoc, Franco, Sinatra, 2009). Hydromorphone is capable of spreading rostrally and can produce delayed respiratory depression after large epidural bolus administration, but it is reported to produce less sedation, nausea, and pruritus than epidural morphine (Dabu-Bondoc, Franco, Sinatra, 2009; Rockford, DeRuyter, 2009).

Hydromorphone has metabolites, and although all of their effects have not been clearly defined, they are not believed to be clinically relevant during short-term

epidural administration. Because hydromorphone has a short half-life (2 to 3 hours) and no clinically relevant metabolites by this route, it may be a better drug than morphine for patients with renal insufficiency. Hydromorphone also is a good alternative to morphine when high concentrations of drug are required, because epidural hydromorphone is more potent than epidural morphine; however, consensus guidelines recommend caution when converting patients from morphine to hydromorphone during intraspinal therapy because the exact potency ratio is unknown (Deer, Krames, Hassenbusch, et al., 2007). The switch to any new opioid should be done slowly with appropriate monitoring as described in Chapter 18 (Switching to Another Opioid).

Hydromorphone has been used for many years via continuous infusion and PCEA to provide effective analgesia following major surgery (Parker, White, 1992; Parker, Holtmann, White, 1997; Parker, Sawaki, White, 1992; Rapp, Egan, Ross, et al., 1996; Singh, Bossard, White, et al., 1997) (see Tables 15-4 and 15-6 for dosing recommendations). One early study showed that hydromorphone by PCEA provided satisfactory pain relief with three to four times less hydromorphone than when given by IV PCA (Parker, White, 1992). Others found similar results (Liu, Carpenter, Mulroy, et al., 1995), which prompted increased use of the drug (Dabu-Bondoc, Franco, Sinatra, 2009). Modifications in dosing protocols have evolved over the years to the current recommendations to infuse a lower concentration (e.g., from 50 to 30 mcg/mL previously to the current 10 to 20 mcg/mL) delivered at higher hourly infusion rates (e.g., from 2 to 5 mL/h previously to the current 10 to 12 mL/h). Local anesthetics (e.g., bupivacaine, ropivacaine) are often added to the infusion. Improved dosing regimens have produced greater efficacy and fewer adverse effects, and the drug has become the primary choice in many institutions for continuous infusion (Dabu-Bondoc, Franco, Sinatra, 2009). A detailed account of experience with thousands of patients at Yale-New Haven Hospital that includes dosing guidelines, drug preparation, assessment, and management of adverse effects and complications can be found in Dabu-Bondoc, S., Franco, S. A., & Sinatra, R. S. (2009). Neuraxial analgesia with hydromorphone, morphine, and fentanyl: Dosing and safety guidelines. In R. S. Sinatra, O. A. de Leon-Casasola, B. Ginsberg, et al (Eds.), *Acute pain management*, Cambridge, NY, Cambridge University Press.

There is limited research on the use of intrathecal hydromorphone for acute pain, and it is recommended for this type of pain only in patients who cannot tolerate intrathecal morphine (Dabu-Bondoc, Franco, Sinatra, 2009). Consensus guidelines for long-term intrathecal administration, however, recommend hydromorphone as a first-choice opioid with morphine and ziconotide (Deer, Krames, Hassenbusch, et al., 2007) (see Chapter 23 for a discussion on ziconotide).

Meperidine

Meperidine (Demerol) is administered by the epidural route less often than morphine, fentanyl, and hydromorphone in the United States and the United Kingdom; however, it is frequently used in Australia for treatment of post–cesarean section pain (Parris-Piper, 2008) (see Table 15-4 for dosing recommendations). Clinicians who prefer meperidine by this route cite the potential advantages of less vascular uptake than more lipophilic opioids such as fentanyl, a faster onset of analgesia (5 to 30 minutes) than less lipophilic opioids such as morphine, and an intermediate dermatomal spread that allows lumbar administration regardless of the site of nociceptive input (Slinger, Shennib, Wilson, 1995). Meperidine has been shown to produce local anesthetic effects (Armstrong, Morton, Nimmo, 1993), a characteristic that could have a favorable impact on analgesia and has not posed problems in terms of motor block when the drug is administered epidurally for pain control (Parris-Piper, 2008) (see Table 15-3).

Some experienced clinicians perceive that epidural meperidine produces fewer adverse effects than morphine (Parris-Piper, 2008), but there are very few comparative data. A randomized controlled trial (N = 37) found that subarachnoid morphine provided better pain relief than meperidine PCEA but with more nausea, pruritus, and sedation following cesarean section (Paech, Pavy, Orlikowski, et al., 2000). The addition of meperidine (10 mg) to intrathecal bupivacaine prolonged post–cesarean section analgesia but with a higher incidence of nausea and vomiting than without it (Yu, Ngan Kee, Kwan, 2002). Epidural meperidine and IV meperidine were found to produce similar satisfactory analgesia and adverse effects in patients following major abdominal surgery, but 33% less meperidine was required during the first 24 hours of therapy in patients who received the drug epidurally (Chen, Cheam, Ma, et al., 2001).

The primary potential disadvantage of using meperidine epidurally is its toxic metabolite normeperidine. Reports of normeperidine toxicity associated with epidural meperidine are rare, possibly because low doses are administered over a brief period of time; however, research shows that meperidine is more likely than other opioid drugs to cause delirium in postoperative patients of all ages (Fong, Sands, Leung, 2006). Meperidine plasma levels higher than 350 ng/mL and normeperidine plasma levels of more than 400 ng/mL are reported to cause CNS irritability (Kaiko, Foley, Grabinski, et al., 1983). In a case-control study (N = 91 with 1 to 2 controls), meperidine more than doubled the risk of delirium when given either epidurally or IV (Marcantonio, Juarez, Goldman, et al., 1994). In another early study comparing epidural with IV meperidine, plasma normeperidine levels were the same for both routes, despite the fact that the total meperidine dose was much less by the epidural route (Slinger, Shennib, Wilson, 1995). CNS irritability (shakiness and tremors) was noted when normeperidine plasma levels reached > 300 ng/mL, and the peak mean normeperidine plasma level after 72 hours of continuous epidural meperidine infusion was 573 ng/mL. No patients had seizures in this study, but 40% experienced CNS irritability. If meperidine is used epidurally, administering it by PCEA without a continuous infusion rather than by continuous infusion alone has been shown to reduce total meperidine consumption (Etches, Gammer, Cornish, 1996) and lower normeperidine plasma levels (Paech, Moore, Evans, 1994). The addition of bupivacaine also may allow a reduced dose and lower serum concentrations of meperidine (St. Onge, Fugere, Girard, 1997), but this combination may be associated with hypotension, oliguria, and excessive motor or sensory blockade (Etches, Gammer, Cornish, 1996). See Chapter 13 for more on meperidine and the assessment of normeperidine toxicity.

Intrathecal meperidine is rarely used. A study undertaken to determine if intrathecal meperidine would provide a long duration of anesthesia was discontinued after enrollment of 34 patients because of significant nausea and vomiting (Booth, Lindsay, Olufolabi, et al., 2000). Consensus guidelines for long-term intrathecal administration list meperidine as a fifth-line opioid because the data supporting its safety and efficacy are limited (Deer, Krames, Hassenbusch, et al., 2007).

Methadone

Methadone is a lipophilic opioid and, like other lipophilic opioids, produces less rostral spread than morphine when administered intraspinally. It has a fast onset of analgesic action (10 to 20 minutes), and because it is cleared rapidly from the CSF, it has a relatively short duration (4 to 8 hours) by the intraspinal routes (Kedlaya, Reynolds, Waldman, 2002). Methadone may be an option for patients with cancer pain who require continuous intraspinal pain treatment, but the concerns discussed in Chapter 13 about its long half-life (12 to 130 hours) and accumulation with repetitive dosing and continuous infusion apply. Consensus guidelines for long-term intrathecal administration describe methadone as a "promising alternative neuraxial agent for chronic pain", but the data supporting its safety and efficacy are limited (Deer, Krames, Hassenbusch, et al., 2007). This suggests it should be at least a fourth-line option.

Although rarely used for postoperative pain management, some studies have demonstrated that epidural methadone can be effective and safe in this setting (see Table 15-4 for dosing recommendations). Ninety patients undergoing abdominal or lower limb surgery were randomized to receive methadone by continuous infusion (up to 12 mg over 24 hours) or intermittent boluses of 3 to 6 mg every 8 hours for 72 hours (Prieto-Alvarez, Tello-Galindo, Cuenca-Pena, et al., 2002). Pain relief was similar among the groups. No plasma accumulation was observed in either group, although plasma concentrations were higher in the bolus group. Miosis was also more frequent in this group. The drug also has been delivered via PCEA for postoperative pain. A randomized controlled trial compared methadone by IV PCA or PCEA in 30 patients following thoracic surgery (Parramon, Garcia, Gambus, et al., 2003). Patients were given an IV or epidural methadone loading dose of 0.05 mg/kg depending on the modality to which they were assigned. IV PCA or PCEA therapy was initiated with a basal rate of 0.5 mg/h, and patients could self-administer 0.5 mg every 10 minutes to a maximum of 4 doses/h. Pain relief was similar, but analgesia was achieved in less time and at a lower dose in patients receiving methadone by PCEA. Adverse effects were few and similar among the groups. Another study described the safe use of methadone plus bupivacaine (0.5%) via continuous epidural infusion in 136 patients after liver resection (Matot, Scheinin, Eid, et al., 2002).

Epidural methadone has also been used for the palliative treatment of dyspnea. Nine patients with emphysema-related dyspnea received a thoracic level epidural infusion of methadone (6 mg/24 h) and demonstrated significant improvement in their symptoms within one week (Juan, Ramon, Valia, et al., 2005). Continued improvements in respiratory function, exercise capacity, and health-related quality of life were noted after one month of treatment.

Sufentanil

Sufentanil is used less frequently than other opioids for epidural analgesia, most likely because it is more costly. It is two times more lipid-soluble than fentanyl. Pain relief by the epidural route is detected within 3 minutes of injection and duration (2 to 4 hours) is similar to fentanyl. Research shows that the quality of analgesia is similar to fentanyl as well (Lilker, Rofaeel, Balki, et al., 2009). When given epidurally, its analgesic effect is largely systemic rather than spinally mediated. This characteristic has led some to suggest its use is probably unwarranted (Maalouf, Liu, 2009). Another study found no clinically or statistically significant differences between morphine and sufentanil epidural analgesia in patients undergoing abdominal and urologic surgery (Delvecchio, Bettinelli, Klersy, et al., 2008).

Although there are no comparative data supporting its selection over other drugs, sufentanil has been included in intraspinal anesthesia protocols (Buyse, Stockman, Coumb, et al., 2007; Chen, Qian, Fu, et al., 2009; Kaya, Buyukkocak, Basar, et al., 2008; Parpaglioni, Baldassini, Barbati, et al., 2009). It is used occasionally for the intraspinal management of labor pain (Buyse, Stockman, Coumb, et al., 2007; Lilker, Rofaeel, Balki, et al., 2009); one study found epidural sufentanil to be superior to epidural fentanyl for this type of pain (Lilker, Rofaeel, Balki, et al., 2009). It has been administered both epidurally (Kaya, Buyukkocak, Basar, et al., 2008) and intrathecally (Chen, Qian, Fu, et al., 2009) for cesarean section delivery.

In combination with local anesthetics, sufentanil produces dose-sparing effects and enhances epidural analgesia (De Cosmo, Congedo, Lai, et al., 2008; Parpaglioni, Baldassini, Barbati, et al., 2009). For example, a randomized controlled study of 60 patients undergoing major abdominal surgery found that the addition of sufentanil to ropivacaine or bupivacaine improved pain relief during coughing and reduced local anesthetic requirements (Pouzeratte, Delay, Brunat, et al., 2001). There were no major adverse effects in any of the groups. A retrospective study of 171 patients after major abdominal or urological surgery compared 5 mL/h continuous epidural infusions of morphine (0.03 mg/mL) plus ropivacaine 0.2% to sufentanil (0.75 mcg/mL) plus ropivacaine 0.2% and reported comparable analgesia and use of PCEA but faster onset of analgesia with sufentanil (Delvecchio, Bettinelli, Klersy, et al., 2008). Nevertheless, the authors concluded that morphine should be the standard for neuraxial use.

Sufentanil also has been administered via PCEA. A prospective study of 58 patients following lumbar anterior-posterior fusion found that sufentanil (1 mcg/mL at 14 mL/h) plus ropivacaine (0.125%) via PCEA (14 mL/h basal rate, 5 mL bolus, 15 minute lockout) provided better pain relief at rest and during activity and greater patient satisfaction than IV PCA morphine (3 mg bolus, 15 minute lockout) (Schenk, Putzier, Kugler, et al., 2006); however, it is unknown if the addition of a basal rate and the use of smaller PCA bolus doses in patients receiving IV PCA might have improved pain control in that group. (See Tables 15-4 and 15-6 for dosing recommendations.)

Intraspinal Opioid Adverse Effects

Opioid adverse effects by the intraspinal routes are the same as by other routes of administration and include nausea, vomiting, pruritus, sedation, and respiratory depression, among others. The treatment of the various intraspinal opioid adverse effects is presented in Chapter 19.

Local Anesthetics

Low ("subanesthetic") doses of local anesthetics are combined with intraspinal opioids for the treatment of acute or persistent pain because the two work synergistically to provide better analgesia at lower doses than would be possible with either drug alone (Jorgensen, Wetterslev, Moiniche, et al., 2001; Meek, 2004; Pouzeratte, Delay, Brunat, et al., 2001; Vascello, McQuillan, 2006). Local anesthetics are rarely used as a sole agent for postoperative pain management because a higher dose would be required to relieve pain, which would increase the likelihood of associated adverse effects, such as motor deficit and hypotension (Grape, Schug, 2008; Maalouf, Liu, 2009). Similarly, opioids alone are associated with an increase in adverse effects. However, in combination, the two agents allow a reduction in the doses of both the local anesthetic and the opioid, which results in a lower incidence of adverse effects of both agents (Ashburn, Caplan, Carr, et al., 2004; Doss, Ipe, Crimi, et al., 2001). In addition to improved analgesia and fewer adverse effects, adding local anesthetics to epidural opioids has been shown to improve GI function, suppress the stress response, and reduce CV, pulmonary, and infectious complications in postoperative patients (Basse, Hjort Jakobsen, Billesbolle, et al., 2000; Basse, Raskov, Hjort Jakobsen, et al., 2002; Jorgensen, Wetterslev, Moiniche, et al., 2001; Kehlet, 2005; Maalouf, Liu, 2009; Vadalouca, Mavromati, Goudas, et al., 2000). These benefits have the potential to reduce perioperative morbidity and mortality (Maalouf, Liu, 2009).

Low concentrations of the lipid-soluble, amide-type local anesthetics bupivacaine (Marcaine) (e.g., 0.05% to 0.125%) and ropivacaine (Naropin) (e.g., 0.05% to 0.2%) are used most often for epidural analgesia (see Table 15-6 for combinations used for PCEA). Levobupivacaine (0.1% to 0.125%) is used outside of the United States (Burlacu, Buggy, 2008; De Cosmo, Congedo, Lai, et al., 2008; Mendola, Ferrante, Oldani, et al., 2009). Ropivacaine in low concentrations may produce less motor blockade compared with low-dose bupivacaine (Maalouf, Liu, 2009), and the drug appears to have less CNS and cardiac toxicity than equipotent doses of bupivacaine (Covino, Wildsmith, 1998; Kedlaya, Reynolds, Waldman, 2002). Levobupivacaine may be less cardiotoxic than ropivacaine, but is used less often than ropivacaine, perhaps because ropivacaine is thought to produce less motor blockade (Grape, Schug, 2008). Compared with other local anesthetics, these are better able to block nerve fibers that transmit noxious stimuli with minimal effect on sensory and motor fibers ("differential sensory and motor blockade") (Covino, Wildsmith, 1998; Gianino, York, Paice, 1996). Bupivacaine and ropivacaine are moderate to fast acting (onset within 5 to 20 minutes) and have a long duration of action (bupivacaine epidural block up to 12 hours; ropivacaine has a slightly shorter duration) (Covino, Wildsmith, 1998).

There appears to be no consensus on optimal drug, dose, concentration, and volume of local anesthetic used for postoperative epidural analgesia. Dose is an important factor in determining effectiveness of therapy (Kehlet, Dahl, 2002), but a wide variety of dosing regimens and local anesthetic concentrations are used, making it difficult to draw conclusions about the comparative efficacy of the various epidural local anesthetics (see Table 15-6). Concentrations of 0.05% and 0.01% of bupivacaine and ropivacaine via thoracic PCEA were found to be equipotent, producing equivalent analgesia and motor block in a randomized, double-blind study of 40 patients following abdominal surgery (Hodgson, Liu, 2001). Another randomized study found no differences in patient outcomes (pain, motor block, ability to walk, time to first flatus) among 60 women who received epidural 0.2% bupivacaine or 0.2% ropivacaine for abdominal hysterectomy except that

those who received ropivacaine required significantly more ketorolac postoperatively (Jorgensen, Fomsgaard, Dirks, et al., 2000). A double-blind study randomized 60 patients undergoing major abdominal surgery to receive thoracic PCEA (all with a basal rate) of bupivacaine (0.125%) plus sufentanil (0.5 mcg/mL), ropivacaine (0.125%) plus sufentanil (0.5 mcg/mL), or ropivacaine (0.2%) alone and found that the addition of sufentanil improved pain relief during coughing and reduced local anesthetic requirements, but the bupivacaine combination produced more effective results than both concentrations of ropivacaine (Pouzeratte, Delay, Brunat, et al., 2001). There were no major adverse effects in any of the groups. Another study randomized 30 women undergoing major abdominal surgery to receive thoracic PCEA (all with a basal rate) bupivacaine (0.125%) plus sufentanil (0.5 mcg/mL) or ropivacaine (0.375%) plus sufentanil (0.5 mcg/mL) and observed comparable efficacy and incidence of adverse effects between the two groups (Gottschalk, Freitag, Burmeister, et al., 2002). Similarly, three different combinations of volumes and concentrations of levobupivacaine (0.5%, 0.25%, and 0.15%) combined with sufentanil (2.6 mcg/h) did not yield differences in sensory and motor block, pain scores, analgesic rescue dose requirements, patient satisfaction, or adverse effects in a randomized controlled trial of 150 patients postthoracotomy (Mendola, Ferrante, Oldani, et al., 2009).

An early study demonstrated that 0.2% ropivacaine plus fentanyl 4 mcg/mL produced a more intense motor block compared with ropivacaine 0.1% plus fentanyl 2 mcg/mL and ropivacaine 0.05 % plus fentanyl 1 mcg/mL, but the three treatments produced equivalent analgesia and similar mild adverse effects leading the authors to recommend the lower concentrations (0.05%, 0.1%) for low thoracic and lumbar PCEA (Liu, Moore, Luo, et al., 1999). Another randomized controlled study administered lumbar PCEA with concentrations of 0.05%, 0.075%, or 0.1% of ropivacaine, all combined with 4 mcg/mL fentanyl, to 312 women undergoing lower abdominal gynecologic surgery and found similar results (Iijima, Ishiyama, Kashimoto, et al., 2007). All three solutions produced comparable analgesia, motor blockade, GI motility, and mild adverse effects, which led the researchers to suggest the lowest ropivacaine concentration (0.05%) for lumbar PCEA.

Local anesthetics administered intrathecally (spinally) act faster than when administered epidurally because they are delivered in the immediate vicinity of the spinal cord and spinal nerve roots (action sites), and because such minute amounts are used when drugs are administered intrathecally, they also have a shorter duration of action (Covino, Wildsmith, 1998). Bupivacaine, lidocaine, and mepivacaine are administered most often for spinal anesthesia/analgesia. Bupivacaine and ropivacaine are the most common local anesthetics administered for long-term intrathecal therapy (Deer, Krames, Hassenbusch, et al., 2007). A small retrospective study reported the addition of intrathecal bupivacaine restored pain control and improved activity level, quality of life, and mental health in 17 patients with persistent noncancer pain (Kumar, Bodani, Bishop, et al., 2009).

Mechanism of Action

The sites of action of intraspinal local anesthetics are in the spinal cord and at the level of the spinal nerve roots, and they block both afferent and efferent signals to and from the spinal cord (Maalouf, Liu, 2009). As discussed in Sections I and V, local anesthetics are sodium blocking agents. They bind to sodium channels in nerve fibers and reduce action potential and subsequent nerve transmission of noxious stimuli (Maalouf, Liu, 2009; Strichartz, Berde, 2005). They also inhibit various potassium and calcium channels and other ion-gated channels, such as substance P receptors (Strichartz, 1998). Epidural local anesthetics are carried in the CSF to the dorsal root ganglion of the spinal nerve fibers immediately adjacent to their site of administration (see Figures 15-3 and 15-5). This results in segmental analgesia, which is influenced by the location of catheter placement as well as dose and volume of the local anesthetic.

The size of a nerve fiber influences its sensitivity to local anesthetics (Maalouf, Liu, 2009). As discussed in Section I, there are three categories of nerve fibers: (1) A fibers are myelinated somatic nerves, (2) B fibers are myelinated autonomic nerves, and (3) C fibers are unmyelinated nerves. A fibers are further divided into alpha, beta, gamma, and delta fibers. The thinnest of the A fibers are in the fast-conducting delta (δ) group. The smaller diameter A-δ and C nerve fibers carry pain impulses. This is fortuitous because local anesthetics block nerve conduction in small nerve fibers faster and at lower concentrations than in large fibers (Maalouf, Liu, 2009). Therefore it is possible to give very low doses intraspinally to block the impulses on the A-δ and C fibers without blocking the larger fibers that affect sensory and motor function (Gianino, York, Paice, 1996; Maalouf, Liu, 2009).

Lipid solubility of the local anesthetic determines its ability to cross membranes and access receptors (Lagan, McLure, 2004). Being lipid-soluble, bupivacaine and ropivacaine penetrate deeply into the spinal cord tissue (Strichartz, 1998). This characteristic also accounts for their rapid onset of action, especially by the intrathecal route (Covino, Wildsmith, 1998). The catheter is placed as close as possible to the dermatomes that, when blocked, will produce the most effective spread of analgesia for the site of nociceptive input (e.g., surgical site, site of injury, tumor location) (see Figure 15-3).

Adverse Reactions

Allergy to local anesthetics is uncommon, and the doses of local anesthetic used for intraspinal analgesia rarely result in blood concentrations sufficient to cause systemic effects. However, vascular uptake or injection or infusion of local anesthetic directly into the systemic circulation can result in adverse reactions related to high blood levels of local anesthetic, although there are reports of no adverse effects following accidental IV infusion of epidural doses of local anesthetics (Allegri, Baldi, Pitino, et al., 2009). CNS signs of systemic toxicity include ringing in ears, metallic taste, slow speech, irritability, twitching, and seizures. Signs of cardiotoxicity include circumoral tingling and numbness, bradycardia, cardiac dysrhythmias, acidosis, and CV collapse (Covino, Wildsmith, 1998).

Unwanted Effects

The goal of adding low-dose local anesthetics to epidural opioids for pain management is to provide analgesia, not to produce anesthesia. Patients should be able to ambulate if their condition allows, and epidural analgesia should not hamper this important recovery activity. However, many factors, including location of the epidural catheter, local anesthetic dose, and variability in patient response, can result in patients experiencing motor and sensory deficits and other unwanted local anesthetic effects. Because epidural local anesthetics produce a sympathetic blockade, vasodilation occurs, and minor hypotension, including orthostatic hypotension, is relatively common (Maalouf, Liu, 2009). The combination of opioid and local anesthetic may have an additive hypotensive effect. A randomized controlled trial of 155 patients undergoing colonic surgery compared ropivacaine 0.2% epidural infusions with and without fentanyl 2 mcg/mL (Finucane, Ganapathy, Carli, et al., 2001). Although the addition of fentanyl resulted in decreased infusion rates and better pain control, hypotension was more common, and time to discharge was approximately 1 day longer in the group receiving the opioid. This is not always the case, however. Other studies have shown that the addition of an opioid allows a lower dose of local anesthetic and less hypotension. For example, a minidose of bupivacaine (4 mg) with fentanyl (20 mcg) provided effective spinal anesthesia with less hypotension than 10 mg of bupivacaine alone and nearly eliminated the need for vasopressor support of BP during surgical repair of hip fracture in 20 patients ages 70 years and older (Ben-David, Frankel, Arzumonov, et al., 2000). CV adverse effects of spinal local anesthetics include hypotension as well as bradycardia, particularly when blockade is higher than T5 (Grape, Schug, 2009). Hypotension is much more common with the administration of spinal (33%) than with epidural (0.7% to 6%) local anesthetics (Grape, Schug, 2009) (see Chapter 19 for more on hypotension).

Intraspinal opioids are associated with a higher incidence of urinary retention than systemic opioids, and the addition of local anesthetics intraspinally can compound this adverse effect. However, urinary retention is seen less often in patients receiving thoracic than lumbar epidural analgesia, which indicates dermatomal level of the neuraxial blockade is a possible contributing factor

(Dabu-Bondoc, Franco, Sinatra, 2009; Wu, 2005). (See Chapter 19 for further discussion of urinary retention during neuraxial analgesia.)

Studies show that thoracic placement of epidural catheters for administration of local anesthetics is associated with less sympathetic block of the lower extremities than lumbar-placed catheters and may reduce several postoperative adverse effects and complications, including urinary retention, postoperative ileus, orthostatic hypotension, and difficulty ambulating (Carli, Trudel, Belliveau, 2005; Wu, 2005). Thoracic rather than lumbar epidural administration of local anesthetics is recommended, especially when early postoperative ambulation is expected to be a priority.

Unwanted local anesthetic effects often can be corrected with simple treatment. For example, hypotension frequently is corrected with hydration, and a change in

position may relieve temporary sensory loss in an extremity. Treatment of urinary retention and minor extremity weakness usually includes decreasing the epidural infusion rate slightly to reduce the local anesthetic dose. Patients are asked to remain in bed until muscle weakness resolves. A nonopioid can be given ATC to provide additional pain relief while the epidural analgesic dose is decreased. Sometimes removing the local anesthetic from the analgesic solution is necessary, such as when signs of local anesthetic toxicity are detected or simple treatment of hypotension, urinary retention, or motor and sensory deficits has been unsuccessful. In any case, care of the patient receiving epidural analgesia includes taking safety precautions and reporting unwanted effects of epidural local anesthetics to the anesthesia provider. Table 15-7 describes the assessment of some of the effects of epidural local anesthetics.

GUIDELINES

Table 15-7 | Assessment of Unwanted Effects of Epidural Local Anesthetics

Unwanted Effect	Cause and Comments	Assessment	What to Report
Sensory and/or motor deficit	Many factors, including vertebral location of the epidural catheter, local anesthetic dose, and variability in patient response, can result in patients experiencing unwanted sensory and/or motor deficit. The lower the level of intraspinal catheter placement, the lower the affected dermatome.	Sensory deficit: Every shift, ask patients to point to numb and tingling skin areas (numbness and tingling at the incision site is common and usually normal). An alcohol swab may be brushed lightly on the skin to determine level of sensation as well. Motor deficit: Every shift, ask patients to bend their knee and lift the buttocks off the mattress. Most are able to do this without difficulty. Determine patients' ability to bear weight and ambulate. Ask patients to remain in bed if they are unable to bear weight. Provide assisted ambulation PRN.	• Complete loss of sensation in a skin area • Muscle weakness, inability to move extremities or bear weight • Numbness and tingling in areas distant to the nociceptive site • Changes in sensory or motor deficit from last assessment (e.g., a lower location or increased intensity) • Unresolved deficits after changes in therapy have been made
Urinary retention	Epidural analgesics are delivered close to the micturation center, located in the lower segments of the spinal cord. The combination of epidural local anesthetics and opioids can cause relaxation of the detrusor muscle. An opioid-induced increase in sphincter tone can make urination difficult. The central effects of opioids and motor and sensory blockade can interfere with perception of bladder fullness and the patient's attention to bladder stimuli.	Regularly assess for bladder distention; in and out or Foley catheterization if needed.	• Persistent urinary retention

Continued

Table 15-7 | Assessment of Unwanted Effects of Epidural Local Anesthetics—cont'd

Unwanted Effect	Cause and Comments	Assessment	What to Report
Local anesthetic toxicity	Toxicity can result from vascular uptake or injection or infusion of local anesthetic directly into the systemic circulation. Older adults may be at higher risk for toxicity from accumulation because most have a decreased ability to clear local anesthetics.	Every shift, assess for and ask patients about signs of local anesthetic toxicity: circumoral tingling and numbness, ringing in the ears, metallic taste, slow speech, irritability, twitching, seizures, and cardiac dysrhythmias. Stop local anesthetic administration if signs are present.	• Signs of local anesthetic toxicity
Adverse hemodynamic effects	Because local anesthetics block nerve fibers, they affect the sympathetic nervous system and cause vasodilation. Mild hypotension is common. Some patients receiving intraspinal local anesthetics experience significant hypotension and bradycardia, especially when rising from a prone position or after large dose increases or boluses. Thoracic placement of the epidural catheter is associated with fewer hemodynamic disturbances.	Regular assessment of HR and BP, including orthostatic BP before ambulation until dose is stabilized and it is clear that bradycardia and hypotension are not problems.	• Symptomatic hypotension and/or bradycardia • Persistent hypotension and/or bradycardia • Symptomatic orthostatic hypotension

BP, Blood pressure; *HR*, heart rate.
Epidural local anesthetics can produce some unwanted effects. This table lists the causes of some of these effects, as well as how to assess and when to report them.
From Pasero, C., & McCaffery, M. *Pain assessment and pharmacologic management*, pp. 428-429, St. Louis, Mosby. Data from Brown, D. L. (2005). Spinal, epidural, and caudal anesthesia. In R. D. Miller (Ed.), *Miller's anesthesia*, vol 2, ed 6, Philadelphia, Elsevier; Cousins, M. J., & Veering, B. T. (1998). Epidural neural blockade. In M. J. Cousins, & P. O. Bridenbaugh (Eds.), *Neural blockade in clinical anesthesia and management of pain*, Philadelphia, Lippincott-Raven; Dabu-Bondoc, S., Franco, S. A., & Sinatra, R. S. (2009). Neuraxial analgesia with hydromorphone, morphine, and fentanyl: Dosing and safety guidelines. In R. S. Sinatra, O. A. de Leon-Casasola, B. Ginsberg, et al. (Eds.), *Acute pain management*, Cambridge, NY, Cambridge University Press; Grape, S., & Schug, S. A. (2008). Epidural and spinal analgesia. In P. E. Macintyre, S. M. Walker, & D. J. Rowbotham (Eds.), *Clinical pain management. Acute pain*, ed 2, London, Hodder Arnold; Kedlaya, D., Reynolds, L., & Waldman, S. (2002). Epidural and intrathecal analgesia for cancer pain. *Best Prac Res Clin Anaesth*, 16(4), 651-665; Maalouf, D. B., & Liu, S. S. (2009). Clinical application of epidural analgesia. In R. S. Sinatra, O. A. de Leon-Casasola, B. Ginsberg, et al. (Eds.), *Acute pain management*, Cambridge, NY, Cambridge University Press; McCartney, C. J. L., & Niazi, A. (2006). Use of opioid analgesics in the perioperative period. In G. Shorten, D. B. Carr, D. Harmon, et al. (Eds.), *Postoperative pain management: An evidence-based guide to practice*, Philadelphia, Saunders; Vascello, L., & McQuillan, R. J. (2006). Opioid analgesics and routes of administration. In O. A. de Leon-Casasola (Ed.), *Cancer pain. Pharmacological, interventional and palliative care approaches*, Philadelphia, Saunders; Wu, C. L. (2005). Acute postoperative pain. In R. D. Miller (Ed.), *Miller's anesthesia*, vol 2, ed 6, Philadelphia, Elsevier. © 2011, Pasero C, McCaffery M. May be duplicated for use in clinical practice.

Local Anesthetic Neurotoxicity

Although controlled studies have not shown neurotoxicity to be a significant complication of intrathecal local anesthetic infusion (Kedlaya, Reynolds, Waldman, 2002), some clinicians have raised concerns (Chabbouh, Lentschener, Zuber, et al., 2005; Grape, Schug, 2008; Hodgson, Neal, Pollock, et al., 1999; Rohm, Boldt, 2006). Case reports describe the occurrence of transient neurologic symptoms, such as various paresthesias and unilateral or bilateral lower extremity pain, in 4% to more than 30% of patients 12 to 24 hours following spinal anesthesia and lasting 6 hours to 4 days, after which the symptoms resolve spontaneously (Grape, Schug, 2008).

A serious complication that has been linked to local anesthetic toxicity is cauda equina syndrome, which is the acute loss of neurologic function below the termination (conus) of the spinal cord as a result of damage to the spinal nerve roots. The cauda equina consists of nerves that are partially unmyelinated, and their increased surface area makes them prone to contact with neurotoxic agents (Neal, 2008). Local anesthetic toxicity is concentration-dependent and can occur at concentrations lower than those used in the clinical setting. Maldistribution and excessive local anesthetic dose concentration in the CSF are thought to be causes of cauda equina syndrome (Birnbach, Browne, 2005; Neal, 2008). Neal (2008) summarizes that neuraxial local anesthetics are remarkably safe in the majority of patients, but that a rare patient may be vulnerable to local anesthetic neurotoxicity even in "normal" clinical situations. See later in this chapter for more on complications of intraspinal analgesia.

Alpha$_2$-Adrenergic Agonists (Clonidine and Dexmedetomidine)

The alpha$_2$-adrenergic agonist clonidine is some-times added in small doses to intraspinal analgesia to improve pain control, produce dose-sparing effects, and prolong analgesia (Andrieu, Roth, Ousmane, et al., 2009; Forster, Rosenberg, 2004; Huang, Lin, Huh, et al., 2007; Schug, Saunders, Kurowski, et al., 2006). A systematic review of 22 randomized tri-als concluded that clonidine prolonged the analgesic action and sensory and motor blockade of a variety of intrathecal local anesthetics in a dose-dependent manner, but was unable to establish the optimal dose of clonidine for these effects (Elia, Culebras, Mazza, et al., 2008) (see Chapter 22 for a detailed discussion of the underlying mechanisms and adverse effects of the alpha$_2$-agonists). Although rarely used as a sole agent, clonidine administered alone epidurally produced signif-icant improvements in pulmonary function in patients undergoing lung resection in one randomized controlled trial (Matot, Drenger, Weissman, et al., 2004).

Clonidine does not produce respiratory depression, nausea, pruritus, or urinary retention, which adds to its appeal as an adjuvant for intraspinal therapy (Grape, Schug, 2008); however, problems can occur with the tendency of alpha$_2$-agonists to produce sedation and hypotension. In combination with opioids, clonidine may exacerbate these adverse effects. A prospective trial randomized 100 patients to receive general anesthesia supplemented by IV fentanyl or general anesthesia pre-ceded by intrathecal clonidine (75 mcg), bupivacaine (15 mg), and morphine (0.2 mg) for radical prostatec-tomy (Brown, Hofer, Patterson, et al., 2004). Those who received intrathecal clonidine required more IV fluids and vasopressors intraoperatively but had lower pain scores, consumed less supplemental IV morphine postoperatively, and were discharged from the hospital significantly ear-lier (3 days compared with 5 days).

The timing of administration may be an important fac-tor in determining efficacy of intraspinal clonidine. A single dose of epidural clonidine administered before abdominal surgery resulted in a greater opioid dose-sparing effect, better pain scores at 6 and 24 hours, and less sedation than epidural clonidine administered at the end of colorec-tal surgery (Persec, Persec, Bukovic, et al., 2007).

Another alpha$_2$-adrenergic agonist, dexmedetomidine, given in low doses (3 mcg), prolonged bupivacaine spi-nal blockade in a similar fashion as clonidine (30 mcg) when administered for transurethral resection of prostate or bladder tumor (Kanazi, Aouad, Jabbour-Khoury, et al., 2006). Further research and clinical experience with dex-medetomidine in this setting is needed to define a role in epidural analgesia.

Prevention of Persistent Postsurgical Pain

Clonidine may have a role in preventing persistent post-surgical pain as well. A randomized controlled study found that intrathecal clonidine (300 mcg) given intra-operatively was more effective than intrathecal bupiva-caine or placebo given intraoperatively in influencing several postoperative outcomes in patients undergoing colonic surgery (De Kock, Lavand'homme, Waterloos, 2005). For example, patients in the clonidine group had a longer time to first request for analgesia, lower pain scores and supplemental analgesic consump-tion, and a lower incidence of persistent postsurgical pain at 6 and 12 months compared with those in the other groups. No adverse events occurred in any of the groups. Intraoperative hemodynamic adverse effects, e.g., hypotension and bradycardia, occurred most often in the clonidine group but were corrected without incident. No one experienced excessive sedation. (See Section I and Section V for more on persistent postsur-gical pain.)

Complications Associated with the Intraspinal Routes of Administration

Randomized controlled trials have demonstrated that intraspinal analgesia is associated with reduced mor-bidity and mortality (Rodgers, Walker, Schug, et al., 2000); however, the therapies are not without risk, and these must be considered when determining the appropriateness of therapy (Ballantyne, 2004; Choi, Bhandari, Scott, et al., 2003). Following is a discus-sion of the complications that can occur: postdural puncture headache; intraspinal catheter migration, and neurologic complications from trauma to neural tissue; injection or infusion of neurotoxic agents; infection; and hematoma.

Dural Puncture and Postdural Puncture Headache

Obviously the dura is punctured when intrathecal analge-sia is administered. Microcatheters were used in the early 1990s for continuous spinal anesthesia, which helped to minimize dural puncture-related symptoms but were with-drawn from the market in the United States after multiple reports of cauda equina syndrome (Grape, Schug, 2008). Some practitioners use epidural catheters for continuous spinal anesthesia but with the disadvantage of producing a large dural leak and the risk of subsequent postdural puncture headache (PDPH); large needles (and catheters) produce larger dural punctures and carry a higher risk of PDPH (Turnbull, Shepherd, 2003).

Inadvertent dural puncture, often referred to as "wet tap," can occur during placement of an epidural cath-eter. It is the most common complication from epidural catheter placement with an incidence between 0.32% and 3% (Grape, Schug, 2008; Maalouf, Liu, 2009).

The incidence is influenced by the experience of the anesthesia provider as well as the technique used to place the needle, the size and orientation of the needle, and the thickness of the dura (Meek, 2004; Turnbull, Shepherd, 2003). A study of 547 women in labor demonstrated that the use of air alone with the loss of resistance technique for epidural needle placement (see earlier in this chapter) was associated with a higher incidence of dural punctures than when the technique was used with lidocaine alone or with lidocaine plus air (Evron, Sessler, Sadan, et al., 2004). However, rarely, more serious complications can occur from a dural puncture, such as infection (Turnbull, Shepherd, 2003) and pneumocephalus if air is used in the loss of resistance technique; the use of saline is recommended to prevent pneumocephalus (Maalouf, Liu, 2009; Nafiu, Bullough, 2007). Orientation of the needle bevel parallel to the dural fibers is reported to reduce dural puncture (Turnbull, Shepherd, 2003). Perforation in thick areas of the dura may be less likely to result in CSF leak, and the thickness of the dura varies among individuals (Turnbull, Shepherd, 2003). The anesthesia provider usually knows when a dural puncture has occurred and will attempt needle placement at a higher vertebral interspace.

The exact mechanism underlying the development of PDPH is not clear (Turnbull, Shepherd, 2003). Some patients experience no symptoms after a dural puncture, yet for others, the leakage of CSF through the hole created in the dura causes a dull, aching, or throbbing headache. The headache may be frontal, occipital, or diffuse in location. It usually is moderate to severe in intensity and may be accompanied by neck or back soreness or stiffness, photophobia, visual disturbances, nausea, and vomiting. The decrease in CSF pressure as a result of the dural puncture is thought to be the reason patients routinely report that the headache worsens when they move into a sitting or standing position and improves when they lie down (Grape, Schug, 2008).

After a dural puncture, the anesthesia provider usually alerts the nursing staff to assess the patient for headache. Sometimes the headache appears during epidural analgesia after a decrease in the epidural continuous infusion rate or when the epidural catheter is removed. Most commonly, the headache occurs 1 to 5 days after the dural puncture and persists for approximately 7 days. On rare occasions, a PDPH lasts for months and even years (Turnbull, Shepherd, 2003). The development of a headache between 5 and 14 days after the dural puncture should be reported promptly to the anesthesia provider as this may be a sign of more serious complications, including death (Turnbull, Shepherd, 2003).

Treatment of PDPH

Treatment of PDPH usually is symptomatic and conservative, consisting of administration of oral opioid and nonopioid analgesics and reassuring the patient that the headache will most likely resolve within a week. Nondrug interventions may be helpful. For example, concentrated CSF can worsen symptoms, so fluid intake is encouraged. Ice packs also may be helpful. Abdominal binders and bedrest have shown little value in reducing symptoms; patients should be told to sit and lie in positions that are most comfortable to them (Turnbull, Shepherd, 2003).

Although the effectiveness of caffeine in the treatment of PDPH is disputed (Halker, Demaerschalk, Wellik, et al., 2007), some clinicians use 300 to 500 mg of oral or IV caffeine, which is thought to relieve symptoms by producing cerebral vasoconstriction (Turnbull, Shepherd, 2003) (see Section III and Table 9-2, p. 242, for oral nonopioid analgesics that contain caffeine and Table 9-1, p. 241, for nutritional sources of caffeine). Sumatriptan, used for migraine headaches, has been administered as well but has not been shown to be particularly effective (Connelly, Parker, Rahimi, et al., 2000). Another novel treatment for PDPH is the IV infusion of adenocorticotropic hormone (ACTH). Patients with PDPH unresponsive to conservative treatment were given a single IV infusion of ACTH, 1.5 units/kg in 250 mL normal saline over a 30-minute period (Kshatri, Foster, 1997). Headache resolved within 2 to 6 hours. The exact mechanism of analgesic action of ACTH in patients with PDPH is unknown but is thought to result from its adrenal (release of hormones) or extra-adrenal (metabolic) physiologic actions.

Blood Patch. The observation that "bloody taps" resulted in a reduced incidence of headache led to the use of blood patches to treat PDPH (Turnbull, Shepherd, 2003). A blood patch consists of withdrawing the patient's blood from the antecubital vein and injecting it into the epidural space. The blood is distributed both caudally and cephalad and forms a clot over the dural puncture site (Turnbull, Shephard, 2003). This has been described as similar to plugging a hole with a cork. There is no consensus on the ideal amount of blood to use for a blood patch, but 20 to 30 mL is reported to produce the best results; 2 to 3 mL is inadequate, and large volumes (e.g., 60 mL) have been associated with spontaneous intracranial hypotension (Turnbull, Shepherd, 2003). Patients are asked to lie still for 2 hours after the blood patch and then are allowed activity as tolerated.

A cohort study of 79 patients observed better success in relieving PDPH symptoms when the blood patch was performed at an early stage (i.e., at onset of severe headache) rather than waiting to see if the symptoms will subside (Vilming, Kloster, Sandvik, 2005). Clinical observations of effectiveness are often dramatic with rapid headache relief in many patients after blood patch; however, research is lacking. A Cochrane Collaboration Review could find only three randomized controlled trials (77 participants) comparing epidural blood patch and no blood patch in the prevention or treatment of PDPH and summarized that more well-controlled research is needed to draw conclusions about the efficacy of blood patch for PDPH (Sudlow, Warlow, 2001).

Complications from the blood patch procedure are very rare and include epidural infection and nerve root compression. Patients may report a minor backache after the injection of blood into the epidural space. Contraindications to the procedure are similar to those of epidural analgesia (see Box 15-1).

Dextran 40 in saline has also been injected epidurally for the treatment of PDPH. The rationale is that its high molecular weight and viscosity slows its removal and allows spontaneous closure of the puncture site, but there is no research to support the practice (Turnbull, Shepherd, 2003). In Sweden, a patient was treated with Dextran 40 when a PDPH persisted despite two consecutive blood patches (Reynvoet, Cosaert, Desmet, et al., 1997). Symptoms were relieved after 25 mL of Dextran 40 was injected into the epidural space and followed by a 3 mL/h infusion of Dextran 40 in saline through an epidural catheter. Informed consent is recommended because Dextran 40 in saline is not approved for epidural administration.

Surgical closure of the dural perforation has been performed for refractory PDPH. This is a last-resort treatment (Turnbull, Shepherd, 2003).

Catheter Displacement

Displacement of temporary catheters during epidural analgesia therapy is a relatively common occurrence (6%) and is often caused by patients accidentally pulling catheters out during activity (Heid, Piepho, Stengel, et al., 2009). Proper taping of the catheter and teaching patients to avoid tugging on the catheter helps to minimize the incidence of displacement. A variety of methods for dressing the epidural catheter sites are described in the literature, and some may be more effective than others in preventing catheter displacement and migration (Burns, Cowan, Barclay, et al., 2001). Catheters may also knot if they have been threaded too deep into the epidural space; a depth of 4 to 6 cm is recommended (Maalouf, Liu, 2009).

Catheter displacement can result in analgesic gaps and should be attended to promptly. When patients report inadequate pain relief during epidural analgesia continuous infusion or PCEA, the entire epidural line from the infusion pump to the epidural catheter site should be checked. Inadequate pain relief may be due to a number of mechanical and technical factors, including incorrect loading of the pump, a disconnection of the catheter from the infusion pump tubing, an empty drug reservoir, a disconnected PCEA button, a malfunctioning pump or tubing, or the epidural catheter may have been inadvertently pulled out.

When bolus doses and increases in the epidural analgesic dose do not yield satisfactory pain control or produce "patchy" analgesia (e.g., one-sided) and the epidural catheter appears to be in place, the infusion line connected, and the infusion pump infusing correctly, the anesthesia provider or the pain service is notified. The epidural catheter can be checked for optimal location by administering a concentrated dose of local anesthetic through the catheter. Optimal catheter placement would produce a bilateral sensory block of the desired dermatomes; lack of such a block would indicate that the catheter location is not optimal (see below and Box 15-4). If location is less than optimal, the epidural catheter should be removed and alternatives considered.

Catheter Migration

Catheter migration can occur at any time during epidural analgesia therapy and despite correct catheter placement. Epidural catheters can migrate out of the epidural space through the dura into the subarachnoid space or into the vascular system through an epidural blood vessel. The incidence of intrathecal migration of an epidural catheter during epidural analgesia is 0.15% to 0.18% and intravascular migration is 0.18% (Maalouf, Liu, 2009).

Early signs of intravascular or intrathecal epidural catheter migration during continuous infusion or PCEA are likely to be subtle and noted most often by a change in the patient's pain control or adverse effects since the last assessment. Signs and symptoms of epidural catheter migration are more pronounced when analgesia is administered by the bolus method. Intrathecal injection of an epidural dose of local anesthetic or opioid can result in a high block and life-threatening respiratory depression requiring aggressive intervention and support. The epidural catheter can be tested with the administration of a small dose of epinephrine-containing local anesthetic before administration of an epidural bolus to rule out intravascular or intrathecal migration (Maalouf, Liu, 2009).

A case report described an intervertebral foraminal catheter migration during implanted intrathecal drug therapy (Ko, Ferrante, 2006). Three months after implantation, the patient reported new-onset radicular pain (low-back pain that radiated to the right lateral thigh and terminated in the right foot) without bowel or bladder symptoms. The migration was confirmed by MRI and CT scan and corrected surgically (right lumbar hemilaminectomy with dissection of epidural scar tissue). The patient recovered rapidly without sequelae. This case reinforces the importance of systematic assessment and attention to the patient's response to therapy and particularly to any change in symptoms. See Box 15-4 and the Patient Example that follows.

Patient Example: Intrathecal Migration of Epidural Catheter

Mr. E. had a nephrectomy yesterday morning and is receiving a continuous epidural infusion of morphine and bupivacaine for his postoperative pain. During previous assessments, Mr. E. has been alert, comfortable with a pain rating no higher than 4 on a scale of 0 to 10, and ambulating without assistance. This time, Mr. E. rates his pain as 0. He is oriented but very drowsy with a respiratory rate of 18 breaths/min. The nurse knows that the only sedating medication Mr. E. is receiving is the epidural morphine, and Mr. E. confirms that he has taken only the medications the nurse has given him. The nurse checks the epidural infusion pump and finds it is programmed correctly and functioning properly. Mr. E. tells the nurse that he cannot ambulate because his "legs are numb." The nurse suspects the epidural catheter has migrated into the subarachnoid space. (Intrathecal infusion of an epidural dose of opioid would explain the increase in Mr. E.'s sedation level, and intrathecal infusion of an epidural dose of bupivacaine would explain Mr. E.'s report of lower extremity sensory loss.) The nurse stops the epidural infusion and takes Mr. E.'s BP, which is 120/70, only slightly lower than his baseline. The nurse stays with Mr. E. and takes vital signs every 5 minutes (the high dose of opioid could cause respiratory depression and the high dose of bupivacaine could cause adverse hemodynamic effects) and asks a co-worker to notify the pain service. The pain service nurse arrives and easily aspirates 5 mL CSF from the catheter confirming that it is in the subarachnoid space. The catheter is removed, and Mr. E. recovers without difficulty.

GUIDELINES

Box 15-4 | Intraspinal Catheter Displacement or Migration

Promptly report any of the following to the anesthesia provider:

INDICATIONS OF A DISPLACED INTRATHECAL OR EPIDURAL CATHETER

- Inadequate pain relief (e.g., a previously comfortable patient reports loss of pain control)
- No pain reduction with increase in opioid dose

INDICATIONS OF AN INTRATHECAL MIGRATION OF AN EPIDURAL CATHETER

- Unexplained increase in opioid-induced adverse effects (e.g., a previously alert patient is excessively sedated or nauseated)
- Sensory and/or motor block (possible if solution contains local anesthetics)
  → Confirmed by aspiration of CSF from epidural catheter and/or sensory blockade when local anesthetic test dose is administered

INDICATIONS OF AN INTRAVASCULAR MIGRATION

- Inadequate pain relief (e.g., a previously comfortable patient reports loss of pain control)
- Unexplained increase in opioid-induced adverse effects (e.g., a previously alert patient is sedated or nauseated [increase in adverse effects is possible even though the patient is being underdosed after intravascular migration because the opioid is being delivered systemically])

- Signs and symptoms of local anesthetic toxicity (e.g., metallic taste, ringing ears, circumoral numbness, slow speech, irritability [possible if solution contains local anesthetics])
  → Confirmed by aspiration of free-flowing blood from catheter and/or transient tachycardia when small test dose of local anesthetic (e.g., bupivacaine, ropivacaine) containing epinephrine is injected

---

CSF, Cerebrospinal fluid.

Displacement of temporary intraspinal catheters during analgesic therapy is a common occurrence and is often caused by patients accidentally pulling them out. Catheter migration can occur at any time during epidural analgesia therapy and despite correct catheter placement. Epidural catheters can migrate out of the epidural space through the dura into the subarachnoid space or into the vascular system through an epidural blood vessel.

From Pasero, C., & McCaffery, M. *Pain assessment and pharmacologic management,* p. 433, St. Louis, Mosby. Data from Grape, S., & Schug, S. A. (2008). Epidural and spinal analgesia. In P. E. Macintyre, S. M. Walker, & D. J. Rowbotham (Eds.), *Clinical pain management. Acute pain,* ed 2, London, Hodder Arnold; Maalouf, D. B., & Liu, S. S. (2009). Clinical application of epidural analgesia. In R. S. Sinatra, O. A. de Leon-Casasola, B. Ginsberg, et al. (Eds.), *Acute pain management,* Cambridge, NY, Cambridge University Press; Pasero, C., Eksterowicz, N., Primeau, M., et al. (2007). ASPMN position statement: Registered nurse management and monitoring of analgesia by catheter techniques. *Pain Manage Nurs,* 8(2), 48-54. © 2011, Pasero C, McCaffery M. May be duplicated for use in clinical practice.

Direct Needle or Catheter Trauma

Trauma to neural tissue from intraspinal needles and catheters is extremely rare (0.0005%). Case reports suggest that direct spinal cord trauma is most often the result of excessively caudad termination of the spinal cord or inaccurate determination of bony landmarks (Neal, 2008). Nerve root trauma is also rare and usually is indicated by patient reports of pain that is severe, sharp, and radiating along a nerve when the needle is placed.

Trauma from the indwelling intraspinal catheter is more common with long-term intraspinal analgesia treatment for persistent pain than with short-term intraspinal analgesia for acute pain management. For example, tissue fibrosis around the indwelling epidural catheter tip can occur with long-term use (Simpson, Jones, 2008). This can lead to spinal cord compression producing neurologic impairment of varying degrees. Tissue fibrosis rarely occurs with intrathecal catheters; factors limiting the occurrence include infusing solutions without additives, keeping drug solutions at pH 5, and using polyurethane or silicone catheters (Simpson, Jones, 2008).

Catheter Tip Granulomas

Catheter tip granulomas are one of the most serious adverse effects and risks of long-term intrathecal drug delivery (Deer, Krames, Hassenbusch, et al., 2007). Progressive motor and sensory deficits are usually permanent despite surgical intervention. A review of the literature revealed 41 cases between 1990 and 2000, but the researchers suggested that the condition may be underreported (Turner, Sears, Loeser, 2007). Granulomas have been reported with the use of all drugs except sufentanil and rarely with fentanyl (Deer, Krames, Hassenbusch, et al., 2007). Contributing factors are the dose and concentration of the drug, catheter position, and low CSF volume.

Injection or Infusion of Neurotoxic Agents

Generally local anesthetics and opioids administered in clinically-recommended doses are safe in the majority of patients; however, even under "normal" circumstances, some patients will be susceptible to neuraxial injury from neurotoxicity related to the administration of these agents (Neal, 2008). High concentrations of local anesthetics can cause neurotoxicity as can a number of preservative agents and antitoxins, including alcohol, phenol, formaldehyde, and sodium metabisulfite (Paice, Williams, 1995). Other agents that have resulted in significant neurologic damage after accidental epidural infusion include antibiotics, potassium chloride, and total parenteral nutrition. All agents and solutions injected or infused intraspinally must be sterile, preservative-free, and regarded safe for intraspinal administration. Epidural infusion lines that are color-coded and do not have injection ports should be used to prevent errors (Box 15-5).

GUIDELINES

Box 15-5 | Prevention of Intraspinal Neurotoxicity

The following measures may be helpful in preventing inadvertent intraspinal injection or infusion of neurotoxic agents:

- Do not use agents from a multiple-dose vial; it is wise to assume that all multiple-dose vials contain preservatives that may be harmful.
- Use only nonneurotoxic agents to disinfect intraspinal catheter connections and ports (e.g., alcohol often is used to cleanse skin of secretions, but should not be used to disinfect catheter connections or ports).
- Use color-coded infusion lines made specifically for epidural analgesia.
- Do not use infusion lines with injection ports for epidural analgesia; if such tubing must be used, tape over every injection port.
- Boldly label indwelling epidural catheters used for intermittent analgesic bolusing.
- Label all infusion lines when patients have several.
- Double-check the labels of epidural analgesia drug reservoirs for wording that indicates the solution is both preservative-free and prepared for intraspinal use.
- Return to the pharmacy drug reservoirs and agents that are unclearly labeled, cloudy, or contain particulate matter.

Neurologic complications can result from injection or infusion of neurotoxic agents. This box lists precautions that can be taken to prevent this from happening.

From Pasero, C., & McCaffery, M. *Pain assessment and pharmacologic management*, p. 434, St. Louis, Mosby. © 2011, Chris Pasero. © 2011, Pasero C, McCaffery M. May be duplicated for use in clinical practice.

Infection

Intraspinal infection, such as an epidural abscess, arachnoiditis, or bacterial meningitis, is a very rare but serious complication of neuraxial analgesia (Grape, Schug, 2008; Maalouf, Liu, 2009). A 6-year review of data from a hospital's experience with 8100 patients who received epidural analgesia revealed just 6 cases of epidural abscess and 3 of meningitis (Christie, McCabe, 2007). Another review of the data of 8210 patients who received epidural analgesia over a 16-year period also revealed only 6 patients with epidural abscess (Cameron, Scott, McDonald, et al., 2007).

Intraspinal infection is thought to be more common when catheters are left in place for a prolonged time (Rathmell, Lake, Ramundo, 2006). Although data are lacking on the incidence of infection during long-term intraspinal therapy (Turner, Sears, Loeser, 2007), the longer the catheter is left in place, the greater the risk of infection, and the incidence of infection with externalized tunneled epidural systems is higher than with totally implanted drug delivery systems (Rathmell, Lake, Ramundo, 2006). The risk of infection in patients receiving epidural therapy for more than 70 days is 15%, but the incidence of infection extending to the epidural space (deep infection) is about 1% (Rathmell, Lake, Ramundo, 2006). An extensive review of postmarketing and medical device reporting data, meta-analyses, and other publications related to infection associated with implanted spinal cord stimulators and drug delivery systems revealed an overall infection rate of 5% (Follett, Boortz-Marx, Drake, et al., 2004) (see the section on symptoms and treatment later in the chapter).

Predisposing factors to intraspinal infection are immunocompromised state, diabetes, HIV infection, malignancy, steroid use, difficult insertion, and longer catheterization time (e.g., more than 3 days for short-term epidural analgesia) (Christie, McCabe, 2007; Grape, Schug, 2009; Horlocker, Wedel, 2006). Most clinicians recognize septicemia as a contraindication to intraspinal catheterization, although single-injection technique is sometimes used in patients with systemic infection (Grape, Schug, 2009). Some clinicians suggest that regional anesthesia may be acceptable if appropriate antibiotic therapy is initiated and the patient has shown response to antibiotic therapy before dural puncture (Wedel, Horlocker, 2006).

Causes of intraspinal infection include spontaneous infection, hematogenous spread during episodes of bacteremia, and infection as a result of poor aseptic technique. However, most epidural abscesses are thought not to be related to epidural catheter placement but to infections of the skin, soft tissue, spine, or hematogenous spread to the epidural space instead (Wedel, Horlocker, 2006). The importance of using aseptic techniques during the placement of epidural catheters is often stressed as an important preventive measure, but there are limited data on what practices are essential (Hebl, 2006). The recommendations for surgical hand washing should be applied to regional anesthesia techniques including intraspinal catheter placement; alcohol-based solutions containing 2% to 4% chlorhexidine appear to have the best extended antimicrobial activity; chlorhexidine is recommended as the first-choice antiseptic for regional anesthetic techniques (Hebl, 2006). Wearing a surgical mask during intraspinal needle and catheter placement to prevent droplet transmission of nasal and oropharyngeal flora is recommended (Institute for Safe Medication Practices, 2010). The reader is referred to Hebl's (2006) excellent review of the research regarding aseptic technique and the variety of factors that may influence the incidence of infection during regional anesthesia, including the use of artificial nails; removal of jewelry; and donning of mask, cap, and gown.

Localized skin infection at the intraspinal needle or catheter entry site also can occur. The incidence of this may be influenced by level of insertion; one review reported an incidence of 2.8% and 0.8% in thoracic and lumbar level insertions, respectively, but the researchers pointed out that the thoracic catheters were in place longer than the lumbar catheters in this study (Cameron, Scott, McDonald, et al., 2007).

Localized bacteria are known to track down the catheter from the skin entry site to the epidural or intrathecal space (Wheatley, Schug, Watson, 2001). Bacterial migration was found to be the most common route of epidural catheter colonization in one study of 105 patients who received postoperative epidural analgesia (Yuan, Zuo, Yu, et al., 2008). Contamination of the intrathecal or epidural system can occur during drug reservoir preparation, catheter placement, refilling implanted reservoirs, or administration of the analgesic. When an external infusion pump is used to deliver intraspinal analgesia, contamination can also occur while loading the pump, connecting the catheter to the infusion, or changing the drug reservoir. Even the infusion pumps are a potential source of bacteria. A one-month study of all reusable analgesia infusion pumps at one hospital found 45% of the PCA buttons (pendants) and 46% of the keypads grew bacteria with the most common organism being coagulase-negative staphylococcus; the simple intervention of cleaning the devices with 70% isopropyl alcohol reduced contamination by 6% and 4%, respectively (Rothwell, Pearson, Wright, et al., 2009). The implementation of a vigorous, systematic cleaning process is recommended.

Symptoms and Treatment of Intraspinal Infection

Early signs and symptoms of an intraspinal infection can be difficult to detect. Systematic assessment is essential. Skin site infection and fever are not always present (DuPen, DuPen, 1998). The cardinal signs of deep intraspinal infection are increasing diffuse back pain or tenderness or pain or paresthesia on intraspinal injection (radicular symptoms). These occur most often approximately 5 days after epidural catheterization (Grape, Schug, 2009), although late presentation is also reported (Bussink, Gramke, van Kleef, et al., 2005; Rohm, Boldt, 2006). Bowel or bladder dysfunction may be present. Any one of these signs should immediately arouse suspicion and further investigation. The risk of neurologic deficit from epidural abscess is nearly 50% because of late recognition (Grape, Schug, 2009; Wheatley, Schug, Watson, 2001). Formation of an epidural abscess can cause spinal cord compression or sepsis and, in extreme cases, paralysis, which occurs rapidly after the onset of motor weakness (Wedel, Horlocker, 2006). Intraspinal abscess is confirmed by magnetic resonance imaging (MRI) or computed tomography (CT), and a neurology or neurosurgery consultation is requested.

Although practice varies (Christie, McCabe, 2007), it is recommended that percutaneous epidural catheters be removed whenever there are signs of local infection (e.g., local erythema or discharge) (Wedel, Horlocker, 2006). Many clinicians culture the catheter tip; however, one study cultured the catheter tips of 1443 patients who had received short-term epidural analgesia and found at least one type of microorganism in 28.8%, but no epidural space infections were identified, which led the researchers to suggest that a routine culture of an epidural catheter tip is clinically irrelevant and not a good predictor of the presence of an epidural catheter infection

(Simpson, Macintyre, Shaw, et al., 2000). To decrease the risk of hematogenous spread to the subarachnoid or epidural space, intraspinal catheters are also often removed when infection occurs outside the intrathecal or epidural space. Removal of implanted catheter systems sometimes can be avoided when superficial infections are treated early and aggressively with local wound care and antibiotics; however, deep infections warrant mandatory removal of the system (Rathmell, Lake, Ramundo, 2006).

Certain precautions to prevent intraspinal infection and regular assessment for signs of infection are essential nursing functions in caring for patients who receive any intraspinal analgesia technique (Pasero, Eksterowicz, Primeau, et al., 2007) (Box 15-6). Because the signs of intraspinal infection can occur after patients are released from the hospital and can occur even if the course of intraspinal analgesia was short and uneventful, it is imperative that discharge teaching include the signs and symptoms and to report them immediately if detected. Patients should know that it may be necessary to remind the primary care provider that they received intraspinal analgesia during hospitalization as this sometimes is overlooked as a possible cause of symptoms.

Epidural Catheter Disconnection

Occasionally epidural catheters become disconnected during therapy, which leaves the system open to the introduction of bacteria. The anesthesia provider must then determine whether or not to repair the line and continue therapy or remove the epidural catheter. Research is lacking regarding the correct action to take when this occurs, but one in vitro study demonstrated that 8 hours after contamination of an epidural catheter, no bacteria were detected more than 20 cm from the catheter hub, provided the fluid within the catheter remained static (i.e., no displacement of fluid toward the patient from the disconnected end) (Langevin, Gravenstein, Langevin, et al., 1996). If these conditions can be met (i.e., a recognized disconnect within 8 hours and a static fluid column), the anesthesia provider may immerse the catheter 10 inches from the disconnected end in povidone iodine for 3 minutes and allow it to dry completely. (Research has not been conducted on other antiseptic solutions, such as chlorhexidine, for this purpose.) The catheter should then be cut with a sterile instrument in the center of this area and reconnected with a sterile connector. However, if the disconnection was unwitnessed or the distal meniscus appears to have migrated more than 5 inches from the disconnected end (i.e., a nonstatic fluid state), the catheter should be removed (Hebl, 2006; Langevin, Gravenstein, Langevin, et al., 1996).

When a disconnection is detected, the nurse should wrap the end of the catheter with a sterile 4 × 4, taking care not to introduce any new bacteria, and contact the anesthesia provider immediately. The anesthesia provider makes the decision as to how to proceed in all cases. Repair of epidural catheter should be performed only by those who are trained in the procedure and supported by institutional policy and procedure.

Infusion Therapies: Solution and Tubing Changes

Although there are no guidelines to direct the frequency with which IV and percutaneous epidural analgesia infusion systems (solution and tubing) should be changed (also called *hang time*), the literature and clinical practice over the years support maintaining the integrity of the infusion system after therapy is initiated (Brooks, Pasero, Hubbard, et al., 1995; Dawson, Rosenfeld, Murphy, et al., 1991; Langevin, 2000; Sevarino, Pizarro, Sinatra, 2000; Strong, 1991; Waldman, 1991). This means that every effort should be made to minimize entry into the system to prevent inadvertent introduction of bacteria.

Because there are no guidelines, practice varies widely with regard to analgesic infusion hang time. Many institutions change main IV solutions and infusion tubing every 24 hours but extend the hang time for the IV PCA system; others change the solution but not the tubing every 24 hours, and still others maintain a closed system until the PCA reservoir is empty. Typically, epidural systems are not entered unless the reservoir is empty and a new one must be added. A survey of nurses who subscribed to the American Pain Society and American Society for Pain Management Nursing [ASPMN] e-mail list serve in 2007 yielded 48 responses to a question asking how often IV PCA solution and tubing were changed in their institutions (Pasero, unpublished data). Their responses reflected IV PCA hang times of 24 hours (12%), 48 hours (52%), and 72 hours (36%). Responses to the same question regarding epidural analgesia revealed hang times of 72 hours (88%), 96 hours (10%), and "whenever the drug reservoir runs dry" (2%). The difference in the hang times between the two therapies is not surprising given that most clinicians appreciate the need to keep the epidural infusion system closed to reduce inadvertent introduction of bacteria and the potential devastating consequences of an epidural abscess or meningitis.

Microbiologic research is lacking, but one early study established the safety of once-monthly filter and drug reservoir changes during long-term intrathecal analgesia infusion (Nitescu, Hultman, Appelgren, et al., 1992). Another study showed that fentanyl and sufentanil possess significant antimicrobial activity in solutions used for PCA delivery systems (Chapalain-Pargade, Laville, Paci, et al., 2006). For research on the stability and compatibility of various agents used for analgesic infusion therapies, see p. 412.

Bacterial Filters. There are no data to support the use of bacterial filters during short-term epidural or perineural catheter infusions (e.g., days) (Hebl, 2006). However, they are often used during therapy of a longer duration. A time-dependent study established a significant correlation between the incidence of catheter hub colonization and the frequency of epidural catheter filter changes during tunneled epidural therapy, prompting the researchers to recommend an extended interval of at least 60 days between filter changes during this long-term epidural therapy (De Cicco, Matovic, Castellani, et al., 1995).

Epidural Hematoma

Perhaps the most dreaded and serious adverse events of neuraxial analgesia are bleeding complications, such as an epidural hematoma, with resultant permanent spinal cord damage (Grape, Schug, 2009). Epidural hematomas occur as a result of epidural vessel puncture (Maalouf, Liu, 2009). The incidence of punctured vessels during needle and catheter placement is 3% to 12% of attempts, but these usually do not cause problems (Maalouf, Liu,

---

GUIDELINES

Box 15-6 | Prevention of Intraspinal Infection

- Use thorough hand washing prior to placement and manipulation of an intraspinal catheter.
  → Remove jewelry before hand washing.
  → Use the alcohol-based antiseptic solution chlorhexidine for hand washing, skin preparation, and other similar functions.
  → Use surgical gloves as a supplement, not a replacement, for hand washing.
- Although data are lacking, the use of surgical masks during placement and manipulation of an intraspinal catheter will maximize sterile barrier precautions.
- Minimize the number of times the intraspinal infusion system is entered (e.g., avoid frequent and unnecessary drug reservoir and tubing changes).
- Use strict aseptic technique when handling supplies used for intraspinal catheter placement, when placing intraspinal catheters, and when connecting drug reservoir to infusion tubing, administering supplemental boluses, and refilling reservoirs.[1]
- Report intraspinal system disconnects immediately to the anesthesia provider:
  → Wrap the free end of the intraspinal catheter with a sterile 4 × 4
  → Anesthesia provider will determine whether the catheter is to be removed or repaired and the infusion continued (see text for decision making).
  → Obtain an order for interim analgesia.
- Regularly assess intraspinal catheter entry site, implanted port, or pump site (usually as often as IV sites are assessed).
- Monitor patient's temperature (usually q 4 h).
- Immediately report to anesthesia provider signs and symptoms of infection, including infection thought to be unrelated to intraspinal catheterization (e.g., wound, urinary, and pulmonary infections).
- Immediately report unexplained changes in sensory or motor deficit since last assessment, particularly increases in spite of decreases in the analgesic infusion rate.

SIGNS AND SYMPTOMS OF INFECTION

Skin infection at intraspinal catheter entry site, implanted port, or pump site
- Inflammation, edema, drainage, warmth at intraspinal catheter entry site, implanted port or pump site.

- Patient reports soreness around intraspinal catheter entry site, implanted port, or pump site.

Epidural or intrathecal space infection[2]
- Constant diffuse back pain or tenderness.
- Pain or paresthesia during bolus injection.
- Decreased pain relief despite no decrease in analgesic.
- Sensory and/or motor deficit (particularly unexplained changes since last assessment).
- Bowel and bladder dysfunction may or may not be present.
- Skin infection of intraspinal catheter entry site may or may not be present.
- Fever may or may not be present.

Signs of acute bacterial infection[2]
- Fever
- Headache
- Nuchal rigidity
- Brudzinski's and Kernig's signs
- Altered mental status
- Convulsions

---

h, hour; *q*, every.

[1]Use only nonneurotoxic agents to disinfect intraspinal catheter connections or ports. Alcohol may be used to cleanse skin of secretions, but should not be used to disinfect catheter connections or ports.

[2]Because the signs of intraspinal infection can occur after patients are released from the hospital, it is imperative that discharge teaching include the signs and symptoms of intraspinal infection and what to do if these are detected.

Intraspinal infection is rare, and early signs and symptoms can be difficult to detect. This box lists the signs and symptoms of intraspinal infection and precautions that can be taken to prevent intraspinal infection in patients who receive intraspinal analgesia. See text for discussion.

From Pasero, C., & McCaffery, M. *Pain assessment and pharmacologic management*, p. 437, St. Louis, Mosby. Data from Hebl, J. R. (2006). The importance and implications of aseptic techniques during regional anesthesia. *Reg Anesth Pain Med, 31*(4), 311-323; Pasero, C., Eksterowicz, N., Primeau, M., et al. (2007). ASPMN position statement: Registered nurse management and monitoring of analgesia by catheter techniques. *Pain Manage Nurs, 8*(2), 48-54. © 2011, Pasero C, McCaffery M. May be duplicated for use in clinical practice.

2009). The exact incidence of symptomatic epidural hematoma is unknown but thought to be extremely rare (Christie, McCabe, 2007; Grape, Schug, 2009). A review of the data of 8210 patients who received epidural analgesia over a 16-year period revealed only two spinal hematomas, and neither required surgical removal or resulted in adverse sequelae (Cameron, Scott, McDonald, et al., 2007). Concurrent anticoagulation therapy is a primary risk factor for spinal-epidural hematoma (Wilson, 2009). The American Society of Regional Anesthesia and Pain Medicine published a consensus guideline on neuraxial anesthesia and anticoagulation, and their recommendations are outlined in Table 15-8.

Like epidural infection, early detection of epidural hematoma is difficult because symptoms often are obscure. Patients may report inadequate or uneven (better on one side than the other) pain relief. The cardinal signs of epidural hematoma are increasing diffuse back pain or tenderness or pain or paresthesia on epidural injection (radicular symptoms). Bowel or bladder dysfunction may also be present. As the hematoma increases in size, sensory or motor deficit develop. Any one of these signs should immediately arouse suspicion and further investigation. Patient recovery without neurologic injury from a major bleeding complication related to neuraxial analgesia depends on early recognition and aggressive treatment (Butterworth, Douglas-Akinwande, 2007). Although paraplegia is extremely rare with intraspinal analgesia, when it does occur, it is most often caused by epidural hematoma, and it occurs rapidly after the onset of motor weakness (Wedel, Horlocker, 2006). Epidural hematoma is confirmed by MRI or CT, and a neurology or neurosurgery consultation is requested. Epidural hematomas usually are treated by immediate surgical removal of the hematoma.

Patient Example: Possible Epidural Hematoma

Mrs. U. has been receiving a continuous epidural infusion of hydromorphone and bupivacaine for the last 36 hours for her postoperative hysterectomy pain. Her epidural site is clean and dry without edema, redness, or drainage. Mrs. U. says that the area around the epidural site in her back is "tender." She also reports numbness and tingling of her thighs. She has been afebrile and all of her vital signs have been stable since surgery. Her pain rating is 2 on a scale of 0 to 10. Mrs. U.'s nurse knows that early signs of an epidural abscess or hematoma often are subtle. The cardinal sign of both of these complications is diffuse back pain or tenderness. Although

lumbar epidural administration of bupivacaine can cause temporary numbness and tingling of the lower extremities, they could be signs of neurocompression caused by an epidural abscess or hematoma. The nurse asks the anesthesia provider to assess Mrs. U. as soon as possible. The anesthesiologist's examination is negative. Mrs. U.'s back tenderness resolves without treatment and her thigh numbness and tingling resolves with a slight decrease in the epidural infusion rate.

Regular patient assessment of motor and sensory function and reporting to the anesthesia provider abnormal blood clotting studies and orders for anticoagulants before and during intraspinal analgesia may help to prevent epidural hematoma and are essential nursing functions (Pasero, Eksterowicz, Primeau, et al., 2007). Because the signs of epidural hematoma can occur after patients are released from the hospital and can occur even if the course of intraspinal analgesia was short and uneventful, it is imperative that discharge teaching include the signs and symptoms and to report them immediately if detected. Patients should know that it may be necessary to remind the primary care provider that they received intraspinal analgesia during hospitalization as this sometimes is overlooked as a possible cause of symptoms.

Operator Errors

Operator (human) errors, particularly incorrect loading and misprogramming of infusion pumps, have been identified as a major cause of significant patient injuries and deaths over the years (Hicks, Heath, Sikirica, et al., 2008; Institute for Safe Medication Practices, 2003a, 2003b, 2004b; Macintyre, Coldrey, 2008). The use of devices that are not approved for pain management is another potential source of patient injury. Both issues are discussed here.

Misprogramming Analgesic Infusion Pumps

The administration of the wrong dose as a result of incorrect pump programming was by far the most common error (38.9%) identified in an analysis of data submitted to MEDMARX and the USP Medication Errors Reporting Program between 1998 and 2003 (United States Pharmacopeia, 2004). To help prevent these types of errors, staff must be trained in the proper use of analgesic infusion devices, both through initial training and annual competency checks (Pasero, Eksterowicz, Primeau, et al., 2007). Institution policy and procedure should mandate that all analgesic infusion device programming be independently double-checked at specified times, such as before the initiation of analgesic infusion therapy, at the time of any adjustments in prescription, and during the nursing hand-off communication

Table 15-8 | Overview of the American Society of Regional Anesthesia and Pain Medicine's Consensus Guideline on Neuraxial Anesthesia and Anticoagulation

Agent	Recommendation
Antiplatelet medications	• No contraindication with NSAIDs; COX-2 selective NSAIDs have no effect on platelet aggregation and should be considered in patients who require anti-inflammatory therapy in the presence of anticoagulation. • Discontinue ticlodipine 14 days and clopidogrel 7 days in advance. • GP IIb/IIIa inhibitors exert a profound effect on platelet aggregation and are contraindicated within 4 weeks of surgery; time to normal platelet aggregation is as long as 48 hours depending on agent; avoid neuraxial technique until platelet function recovers.
Unfractionated heparin SC	• No contraindication during SC mini-dose. • Consider delaying heparin until after block if technical difficulty is anticipated.
Unfractionated heparin IV	• Combining neuraxial techniques with intraoperative heparinization is acceptable. • Heparinize 1 hour after neuraxial technique. • Remove catheter 2 to 4 hours after last heparin dose. • Reheparinization should occur 1 hour after catheter removal. • No mandatory delay if traumatic.
Preoperative LMWH	• Patients receiving LMWH can be assumed to have altered coagulation. • At least 12 hours should elapse following standard doses and 24 hours after higher doses before neuraxial technique is attempted.
LMWH, twice-daily dosing	• The first dose of LMWH should be administered no earlier than 24 hours after surgery and only if adequate hemostasis is present. • Indwelling catheters should be removed the night before initiation of LMWH therapy. • Remove neuraxial catheter 2 hours before the first LMWH dose.
LMWH, single-daily dosing	• The first dose of LMWH should be administered no earlier than 6 hours after surgery. • The second dose should be administered no earlier than 24 hours after the first dose. • Neuraxial catheter may be safely maintained. • Catheter should be removed a minimum of 10 to 12 hours after the last dose of LMWH and 2 to 4 hours prior to the next dose. • Postpone LMWH 24 hours if traumatic.
Warfarin	• Stop oral anticoagulants prior to neuraxial technique (ideally 4 to 5 days prior). • Document normal INR after discontinuation of oral anticoagulants (prior to neuraxial technique). • Remove catheter when INR is 1.5 or lower (initiation of therapy). • Neurologic testing of sensory and motor function should be routinely performed during epidural analgesia for patients receiving oral anticoagulants. • Withhold or reduce dose of warfarin if INR higher than 3 in patients with indwelling neuraxial catheters. • ASRA makes no recommendation for removal of catheters in patients with therapeutic levels of anticoagulation during neuraxial catheter infusion.
Thrombolysis	• No data on safety interval for performance of neuraxial technique or catheter removal. • Avoid neuraxial technique in patients receiving or who are likely to receive fibrinolytic and thrombolytic drugs. • Guidelines detailing original contraindications for thromboembolytic drugs suggest avoidance of these drugs for 10 days following puncture of noncompressible vessels. • Neurologic monitoring at least every 2 hours is recommended in patients who have received neuraxial block at or near the time of fibrinolytic and thrombolytic therapy. • Following fibrinogen level (one of the last clotting factors to recover) may be helpful in determining optimal time for catheter removal.
Herbal therapy	• No evidence for mandatory discontinuation prior to neuraxial technique. • Be aware of potential drug interactions.

ASRA, American Society of Regional Anesthesia; *GP, glucoprotein*; *INR*, international normalized ratio; *LMWH*, low molecular weight heparin.
This table provides the ASRA recommendations for management of neuraxial anesthesia and analgesia during anticoagulation therapy with the goal of reducing bleeding complications. From Pasero, C., & McCaffery, M. *Pain assessment and pharmacologic management*, p. 439, St. Louis, Mosby. Data from Grape, S., & Schug, S. A. (2008). Epidural and spinal analgesia. In P. E. Macintyre, S. M. Walker, & D. J. Rowbotham (Eds.), *Clinical pain management. Acute pain*, ed 2, London, Hodder Arnold; Horlocker, T. T., Benzon, H., Enneking, K. F., et al. (2004). Regional anesthesia in the anticoagulated patient: Defining the risks. *Reg Anesth Pain Med, 29*(2), 1-11; Horlocker, T. T., Wedel, D. J., Benzon, H., et al. (2003). Regional anesthesia in the anticoagulated patient: Defining the risks (the second ASRA consensus conference on neuraxial anesthesia and anticoagulation). *Reg Anesth Pain Med, 28*(3), 172-197. © 2011, Pasero C, McCaffery M. May be duplicated for use in clinical practice.

processes. An independent double-check consists of having another clinician (e.g., nurse, physician, pharmacist) compare the analgesic solution's drug and concentration and the pump's programmed prescription against the patient's written prescription to ensure accuracy without prompting from the person administering the analgesic or anyone else. Distractions during programming and double-checks are identified as being factors contributing to errors (Hicks, Heath, Sikirica, et al., 2008), so clinicians must take steps to avoid being interrupted.

The concept of the 6 Rights (6 Rs) of medication safety (right patient, right drug, right dose, right time, right route, right documentation) forms the basis of safe analgesic therapies and is the responsibility of everyone on the health care team (Institute for Safe Medication Practices, 2004c). A concerted multidisciplinary effort that includes appropriate prescribing; the highest standard of drug-reservoir preparation, storage, and dispensation; uninterrupted attention during programming and double-checking; and careful patient monitoring during therapy are essential. Readers are encouraged to subscribe to the Institute for Safe Medication Practices newsletters, in which safety information on a variety of medications is regularly published (*http://www.ismp.org*). (See also Chapter 19 for transfer of care and hand-off communications.)

Use of Unapproved Infusion Devices for Analgesic Therapy

It goes without saying that the devices used to infuse analgesic therapies should be approved for that purpose. A surprisingly common practice, particularly in laboring patients, is to infuse epidural analgesia via an IV infusion pump that is not approved for epidural infusion. This practice has the potential for significant patient harm and is not recommended. Risk management personnel are encouraged to evaluate whether or not this practice exists in their institutions and facilitate the actions necessary to ensure approved devices are available for analgesic therapies in all clinical units.

Tapering and Cessation of Epidural Analgesia

For patients with acute pain who are receiving epidural analgesia, plans are necessary for smoothly weaning the patient as pain decreases or the patient is able to use a less invasive route of administration. Although most patients experience less pain as the days pass after surgery, it should not be assumed that all patients will follow this pattern. For example, the duration of postoperative pain tends to be longer in older patients (Melzack, Abbott, Zackon, et al., 1987). It is best to evaluate patients individually and taper analgesic doses on the basis of patients' reports of pain and ability to perform recovery activities rather than a preconceived notion of when epidural analgesics should be discontinued.

In preparation for discharge, transition to oral analgesia should be started as soon as the patient is able to retain fluids and pain is well controlled. As function returns and pain lessens, the epidural opioid dose can be reduced by 25% once or twice daily. To make the transition from epidural analgesia to oral analgesia as smooth as possible, the characteristics of the epidural opioid are considered before discontinuing it. When patients are receiving lipophilic epidural opioids (short duration; e.g., fentanyl, sufentanil), the oral analgesic can be administered before discontinuing epidural analgesia so that patients remain comfortable during the transition. Because analgesia tends to last longer after discontinuing hydrophilic epidural opioids (e.g., morphine, hydromorphone), these patients can be informed of the availability of oral analgesia and reminded to ask for it as soon as they feel pain return and before it becomes severe. Many nurses encourage patients to take their oral analgesic before sleep on the evening that epidural analgesia is discontinued to prevent them from waking up in severe pain. In all cases, patients should be comfortable before epidural analgesia is discontinued. Frequent pain assessment (every 1 to 2 hours) during the transition provides an opportunity to evaluate and adjust the new analgesic regimen. (See Chapter 18 for patient examples that involve switching from the epidural route to the IV route of administration and from the oral route to the epidural route of administration in opioid tolerant patients.)

Epidural Catheter Removal

Removing short-term epidural catheters is within the scope of practice for registered nurses in most states in the United States. Most state boards of nursing have approved this activity by registered nurses who possess the knowledge and skill to do so and where institutional policy and procedure support it. The ASPMN issued a consensus paper defining and supporting the nurse's role in the care of the patient receiving analgesia by catheter techniques, which includes the discontinuation and removal of catheters used to deliver analgesia (Pasero, Eksterowicz, Primeau, et al., 2007). The procedure for removing epidural catheters varies, but Box 15-7 lists important steps and considerations that can be generalized to all situations. See also Table 15-8 before performing intraspinal catheter removal.

Conclusion

Intraspinal analgesia is an extremely effective method for managing a variety of types of pain. It is a primary method for some types of postoperative pain and may provide relief for some patients with refractory persistent pain. This chapter discussed the many different agents administered intraspinally as well as their most common adverse effects and the complications of the therapy.

Box 15-7 | Removal of Short-Term Epidural Catheters

REQUIREMENTS OF NURSE REMOVAL OF AN EPIDURAL CATHETER

- Institutional policy and procedure and state board of nursing that supports removal of epidural catheters by the registered nurse.
- Knowledge and skills necessary to remove an epidural catheter gained by completing institutional competency requirements.
- Prescriber's order to remove the epidural catheter.

CONSIDERATIONS *BEFORE* REMOVAL OF AN EPIDURAL CATHETER

- If warranted (e.g., if patient is receiving or received anticoagulants during epidural therapy), blood clotting studies have been checked and abnormal findings reported to anesthesia provider. See Table 15-8.
- Signs of infection have been reported to anesthesia provider.
- Pain is under control.
- Adequate oral analgesia has been given to the patient who is receiving epidural analgesia from short-duration opioid (e.g., fentanyl, sufentanil) so that pain control is maintained when epidural analgesia is discontinued.
- The procedure has been explained to the patient, including the oral analgesic regimen that will replace the epidural analgesia.

CONSIDERATIONS RELATED TO REMOVING AN EPIDURAL CATHETER

- Epidural catheters are considered hazardous waste, so universal precautions are warranted.

- Removal of the epidural catheter is facilitated when the patient assumes a position similar to the one suggested for catheter placement (i.e., sitting or side-lying with the back arched out toward the person removing the catheter). This position helps to spread the vertebrae apart.
- Although gentle traction is necessary to remove the catheter, it should come out easily and painlessly. If resistance is met or the patient reports pain or unusual sensations (e.g., tingling or a "catch in the back"), the procedure is terminated and the anesthesia provider is notified.
- After the catheter is removed, the catheter tip is checked for the presence of a black or blue mark. This indicates that the catheter was removed intact. If the tip has no mark, notify anesthesia provider.
- After cleaning the entry site and surrounding skin with the institution's recommended solution (usually mild soap and water), some nurses cover the epidural catheter site with a Band-Aid, others leave it open to air.
- Signs of catheter entry site infection are reported to the anesthesia provider.

DOCUMENTATION

Patient tolerance of the procedure, presence of mark on catheter tip, condition of epidural catheter entry site and surrounding area, and specifics of a difficult or unusual removal.

From Pasero, C., & McCaffery, M. *Pain assessment and pharmacologic management*, p. 441, St. Louis, Mosby. Data from Pasero C, Eksterowicz N, Primeau M, Cowley C. (2007). ASPMN position statement: Registered nurse management and monitoring of analgesia by catheter techniques. *Pain Manage Nurs, 8*(2), 48-54. © 2011, Pasero C, McCaffery M. May be duplicated for use in clinical practice.

Chapter 16 Initiating Opioid Therapy

INITIATION of the opioid treatment plan is individualized to meet each patient's unique characteristics and condition. After the opioid and route of administration are determined, multiple factors, including the patient's age, previous exposure to opioids, and pain intensity are considered in selection of the initial dose. The initial dose is then titrated up or down based on the patient's response (pain relief and adverse effects).

Selecting an Analgesic and Route of Administration

As a rule, treatment of moderate-to-severe cancer pain and persistent noncancer pain is started with just one opioid analgesic at a time by one route of administration.

For example, the same drug and route are usually used for the short-acting opioid for breakthrough pain and for the around-the-clock (ATC) long-acting opioid. Starting with one drug and route at a time allows for simpler interpretation of adverse effects, if they occur, and presumably lowers the risk for additive toxicity. Notwithstanding those considerations, there are circumstances that may support the initiation of opioid therapy with more than one drug or route concurrently. For example, the emerging role of the oral transmucosal, rapid-onset fentanyl formulations for breakthrough pain was discussed in Chapter 14; these are often administered with transdermal or oral opioids for persistent pain. With close monitoring, the concomitant administration of a parenteral opioid for breakthrough pain may ensure very rapid onset of relief while a baseline drug is administered orally.

During planned long-term therapy, opioid selection is highly individualized, and treatment is usually initiated with a short-acting opioid, which can be titrated to effective analgesia more rapidly than a long-acting opioid (Fine, Mahajan, McPherson, 2009). As discussed in previous chapters, patients with persistent pain are commonly switched to a long-acting opioid to provide consistent pain relief and improve sleep and function. Initiating an opioid regimen in addition to an adjuvant analgesic is often warranted. For example, it may be necessary to use an opioid initially to control moderate to severe pain associated with a persistent noncancer pain syndrome for which the appropriate mainstay analgesic is an adjuvant that requires gradual titration over days or weeks before becoming effective (see Section V). In this case, it would be inhumane to expect the patient to endure severe pain while the adjuvant analgesic takes effect. As soon as the moderate to severe pain is resolved, the opioid can be tapered and discontinued if thought to be unnecessary to the treatment plan.

In contrast to the planned long-term management of persistent pain, the treatment of acute pain often requires beginning with more than one route and more than one analgesic. This is because there is not enough time to evaluate patients' responses to one analgesic at a time. Therefore, decisions about postoperative analgesics are made on the basis of research findings and clinical experience. The intensity of pain is anticipated, and multimodal analgesic regimens are planned preoperatively whenever possible. For example, in addition to an ATC oral or intravenous (IV) nonsteroidal anti-inflammatory drug (NSAID) and acetaminophen for some major surgeries, an epidural catheter may be placed preoperatively for continuous infusion of opioid and local anesthetic to control anticipated severe postoperative pain.

Occasionally, two different routes of administration at the same time may be appropriate for postoperative pain. For example, continuous peripheral nerve blockade is often administered in conjunction with oral opioid analgesics or IV patient-controlled analgesia (PCA) (see Chapter 26 for continuous peripheral nerve blockade); however, the practice of using two different parenteral routes of administration at the same time or parenteral and intraspinal routes at the same time to administer opioids must be carried out with caution and appropriate monitoring. In particular, the administration of intramuscular (IM) opioids to opioid-naïve patients receiving IV or intraspinal analgesia can result in excessive sedation and clinically significant respiratory depression (see Chapter 19).

Selecting an Opioid Dose

Traditionally, age and weight have been used to determine opioid dose; however, studies have shown that there is no correlation between weight and analgesic requirements (Burns, Hodsman, McLintock, et al., 1989; Ginsberg, Cohen, Ossey, et al., 1989; Monk, Parker, White, 1990). A study comparing remifentanil pharmacokinetics in 12 obese and 12 lean patients undergoing surgery demonstrated no significant differences between the two groups (Egan, Huizinga, Gupta, et al., 1998). The researchers preferred dosing regimens based on ideal body weight, or lean body mass, as opposed to those based on total body weight.

Age, on the other hand, is a valid consideration (Hanks, Cherny, Fallon, 2004; Keita, Tubach, Maalouli, et al., 2008; Mercadante, Ferrera, Villari, et al., 2006). Starting doses should be adjusted for patients at the extremes of the age spectrum, such as neonates and infants, who have incomplete organ development; and older adults, who have increased sensitivity to drug effects. For both the very young and the very old, initial doses are adjusted downward and a longer interval between doses is anticipated. For example, a common recommendation is to lower the recommended starting dose for adults in older individuals (older than 70 years) by 25% to 50% (American Pain Society [APS], 2003). It is important to remember, however, that numerous factors, including genetics (Argoff, 2010; Chou, Wang, Liu, et al., 2006; Fillingim, 2005; Landau, 2006; Nielsen, Stubhaug, Price, et al., 2008; Pasternak, 2005, 2010); underlying pathology and medical condition (Hanks, Cherny, Fallon, 2004; Soares, Martins, Uchoa, 2003); surgical procedure and incision site (Chang, Dai, Ger, et al., 2006); opioid tolerance (Davis, Johnson, Egan, et al., 2003; Hanks, Cherny, Fallon, 2004; Patanwala, Jarzyna, Miller, et al., 2008; Rozen, DeGaetano, 2006);

and pain intensity (Dahmani, Dupont, Mantz, et al., 2001), also contribute to wide variability in pain reports and dose requirements among patients.

Although pain intensity is obviously a very important factor to consider, selecting a dose based on a specific pain intensity can be dangerous and is strongly discouraged (Blumstein, Moore, 2003; Gordon, Dahl, Phillips et al., 2004; Lucas, Vlahos, Ledgerwood, 2007; Vila, Smith, Augustyniak, et al., 2005). The most important principle is to select a safe starting dose and be prepared to titrate to individualize the dose while monitoring patient response. No matter what method is used to predict analgesic requirements, the starting doses of opioid treatments are merely estimates. When starting doses are given, they are titrated up or down according to patient response (Fine, Mahajan, McPherson, 2009).

Using the Equianalgesic Chart

The term *equianalgesia* means approximately equal analgesia and is used when referring to the doses of various opioid analgesics that provide approximately the same amount of pain relief. Using the equianalgesic chart in Table 16-1 as an example, note that the chart provides a list of analgesics at doses, both oral and parenteral (with other routes such as rectal as appropriate), that are approximately equal to each other and theoretically interchangeable in their ability to provide pain relief in opioid-naïve patients. These doses are also referred to as equianalgesic dose units. Most of the doses in equianalgesic charts are made on the basis of single-dose studies, commonly conducted in surgical patients and using morphine, 10 mg IM, for comparison (Knotkova, Fine, Portenoy, et al., 2009). The parenteral doses listed are typical of IM doses given approximately every 3 to 4 hours. Equianalgesic dose calculation provides a basis for selecting the appropriate starting dose when changing from one opioid drug or route of administration to another. However, these calculations are just estimates and vary with repeated dosing and with opioid rotation (Knotkova, Fine, Portenoy, 2009; Shaheen, Walsh, Lasheen, et al., 2009). The optimal dose for the patient is always determined by titration (Fine, Portenoy, 2007).

A patient's pain intensity (see previous discussion) and the equianalgesic chart are practical tools that can be used to determine an appropriate opioid dose for an opioid-naïve patient. To become familiar with the equianalgesic chart, note that it has several columns. The first column lists the common opioid analgesics. Morphine is listed first because it has been the standard for comparison, and the others follow in alphabetical order. The remaining doses are equianalgesic to the doses listed for morphine. The second column lists the equianalgesic doses of opioids by the oral route. The third column lists the equianalgesic doses of opioids by the parenteral (IM, subcutaneous [SC], and IV) routes. The last four columns provide pharmacokinetic information about specific opioids.

Table 16-1 | Equianalgesic Dose Chart

A Guide to Using Equianalgesic Dose Charts*

- *Equianalgesic* means approximately the same pain relief.
- The equianalgesic chart is a guideline for selecting doses for opioid-naïve patients. Doses and intervals between doses are titrated according to individuals' responses.
- The equianalgesic chart is helpful when switching from one drug to another or switching from one route of administration to another.[1]
- Doses in this equianalgesic chart suggest a ratio for comparing the analgesic effects of one drug to those of another.
- The longer a patient has been receiving an opioid, the more conservative the starting dose of a new opioid should be. (See discussion of conversion charts in Chapter 11.)

Opioid	Oral (PO) (over ~4 h)	Parenteral (IM/SC/IV) (over ~4 h)	Onset (min)	Peak (min)	Duration (h)[2]	Half-life (h)
Mu Agonists						
Morphine	30 mg	10 mg	30-60 (PO)	60-90 (PO)	3-6 (PO)	2-4
			30-60 (MR)[3]	90-180 (MR)[3]	8-24 (MR)[3]	
			30-60 (R)	60-90 (R)	4-5 (R)	
			5-10 (IV)	15-30 (IV)	3-4 (IV)[2,4]	
			10-20 (SC)	30-60 (SC)	3-4 (SC)	
			10-20 (IM)	30-60 (IM)	3-4 (IM)	
Codeine	200 mg NR	130 mg	30-60 (PO)	60-90 (PO)	3-4 (PO)	2-4
			10-20 (SC)	ND (SC)	3-4 (SC)	
			10-20 (IM)	30-60 (IM)	3-4 (IM)	
Fentanyl		100 mcg IV 100 mcg/h of transdermal fentanyl is approximately equal to 4 mg/h of IV morphine[5]; 1 mcg/h of transdermal fentanyl is approximately equal to 2 mg/24 h of oral morphine[5]	5 (OT)[6] 5 (B)[6] 3-5 (IV) 10-15 (IM) 12-16 h (TD)	15 (OT)[6] 15 (B)[6] 15-30 (IV) 30-60 (IM) 24 h (TD)	2-5 (OT)[6] 2-5 (B)[6] 2 (IV)[2,4] 2-3 (IM) 48-72 (TD)	3-4[7] >24 (TD)
Hydrocodone (as in Vicodin, Lortab)	30 mg[8] NR	—	30-60 (PO)	60-90 (PO)	4-6 (PO)	4
Hydromorphone (Dilaudid)	7.5 mg	1.5 mg[9]	15-30 (PO)	30-90 (PO)	3-4 (PO)	2-3
			15-30 (R)	30-90 (R)	3-4 (R)	
			5 (IV)	10-20 (IV)	3-4 (IV)[2,4]	
			10-20 (SC)	30-90 (SC)	3-4 (SC)	
			10-20 (IM)	30-90 (IM)	3-4 (IM)	
Levorphanol (Levo-Dromoran)	4 mg	2 mg	30-60 (PO)	60-90 (PO)	4-6 (PO)	12-15
			10 (IV)	15-30 (IV) 4-6 (IV)[1,3]	4-6 (SC)	
			10-20 (SC)	60-90 (SC)	4-6 (IM)	
			10-20 (IM)	60-90 (IM)		
Meperidine (Demerol)	300 mg NR	75 mg	30-60 (PO)	60-90 (PO)	2-4 (PO)	2-3
			5-10 (IV)	10-15 (IV)	2-4 (IV)[2,4]	
			10-20 (SC)	15-30 (SC)	2-4 (SC)	
			10-20 (IM)	15-30 (IM)	2-4 (IM)	

Table 16-1 | Equianalgesic Dose Chart—cont'd

Opioid	Oral (PO) (over ~4 h)	Parenteral (IM/SC/IV) (over ~4 h)	Onset (min)	Peak (min)	Duration (h)[2]	Half-life (h)
Mu Agonists						
Methadone (Dolophine)	(See Chapter 13, pp. 339-350, and Table 13-8 and Box 13-3)					
Oxycodone (as in Percocet, Tylox)	20 mg	—	30-60 (PO) 30-60 (MR)[10] 30-60 (R)	60-90 (PO) 90-180 (MR)[10] 30-60 (R)	3-4 (PO) 8-12 (MR)[10] 3-6 (R)	2-3 4.5 (MR)[10]
Oxymorphone	10 mg (10 mg R)	1 mg	30-45 (PO) 15-30 (R) 5-10 (IV) 10-20 (SC) 10-20 (IM)	30-90 (PO) 60 (MR)[11] 120 (R) 15-30 (IV) ND (SC) 30-90 (IM)	4-6 (PO) 12 (MR)[11] 3-6 (R) 3-4 (IV)[2,4] 3-6 (SC) 3-6 (IM)	7-11 2 (parenteral)
Propoxyphene[12] (Darvon)	—	—	30-60 (PO)	60-90 (PO)	4-6 (PO)	6-12
Agonist-Antagonists						
Buprenorphine[13] (Buprenex)	—	0.4 mg	5 (SL) 5 (IV) 10-20 (IM)	30-60 (SL) 10-20 (IV) 30-60 (IM)	3 (SL) 3-4 (IV)[2,4] 3-6 (IM)	2-3 5-6
Butorphanol[13] (Stadol)	—	2 mg	5-15 (NS)[14] 5 (IV) 10-20 (IM)	60-90 (NS) 10-20 (IV) 30-60 (IM)	3-4 (NS) 3-4 (IV)[2,4] 3-4 (IM)	3-4
Dezocine (Dalgan)	—	10 mg	5 (IV) 10-20 (IM)	ND (IV) 30-60 (IM)	3-4 (IV)[2,4] 3-4 (IM)	2-3
Nalbuphine[13] (Nubain)	—	10 mg	5 (IV) <15 (SC) <15 (IM)	10-20 (IV) ND (SC) 30-60 (IM)	4-6 (IV)[2,4] 4-6 (SC) 4-6 (IM)	5
Pentazocine[13] (Talwin)	50 mg	30 mg	15-30 (PO) 5 (IV) 15-20 (SC) 15-20 (IM)	60-180 (PO) 15 (IV) 60 (SC) 60 (IM)	3-4 (PO) 3-4 (IV)[2,4] 3-4 (SC) 3-4 (IM)	2-3

*This table provides equianalgesic doses and pharmacokinetic information about selected opioid drugs. Characteristics and comments about selected mu opioid agonist drugs can be found in Table 13-1, pp. 326-327.

ATC, Around-the-clock; *h*, hour; *IM*, intramuscular; *IV*, intravenous; *MR*, oral modified-release; *ND*, no data; *NR*, not recommended; *NS*, nasal spray; *OT*, oral transmucosal; *PO*, oral; *R*, rectal; *SC*, subcutaneous; *SL*, sublingual; *TD*, transdermal.

[1]An expert panel was convened for the purpose of establishing a new guideline for opioid rotation and recently proposed a two-step approach (Fine, Portenoy, Ad Hoc Expert Panel on Evidence Review and Guidelines for Opioid Rotation, 2009). The approach presented in the text for calculating the dose of a new opioid can be conceptualized as the panel's Step One, which directs clinicians to calculate the equianalgesic dose of the new opioid based on the equianalgesic table. Step Two suggests that clinicians perform a second assessment of patients to evaluate the current pain severity (perhaps suggesting that the calculated dose be increased or decreased) and to develop strategies for assessing and titrating the dose as well as to determine the need for breakthrough doses and calculate those doses (see Box 16-2). The specific steps provided in the examples in the text reflect the panel's two-step approach (see Fine, Portenoy, the Ad Hoc Expert Panel on Evidence Review and Guidelines for Opioid Rotation, 2009).

[2]Duration of analgesia is dose dependent; the higher the dose, usually the longer the duration.

[3]As in, e.g., MS Contin and Oramorph (8 to 12 hours) and Avinza and Kadian (12 to 24 hours).

[4]IV boluses may be used to produce analgesia that lasts nearly as long as IM or SC doses; however, of all routes of administration, IV produces the highest peak concentration of the drug, and the peak concentration is associated with the highest level of toxicity (e.g., sedation). To decrease the peak effect and lower the level of toxicity, IV boluses may be administered more slowly (e.g., 10 mg of morphine over a 15-min period); or smaller doses may be administered more often (e.g., 5 mg of morphine every 1 to 1.5 hours).

Continued

Table 16-1 | Equianalgesic Dose Chart—cont'd

[5]This is the ratio that is used clinically.

[6]The delivery system for transmucosal fentanyl influences potency, e.g., buccal fentanyl is approximately twice as potent as oral transmucosal fentanyl (see Chapter 14).

[7]At steady state, slow release of fentanyl from storage in tissues can result in a prolonged half-life (e.g., 4 to 5 times longer).

[8]Equianalgesic data are not available.

[9]The recommendation that 1.5 mg of parenteral hydromorphone is approximately equal to 10 mg of parenteral morphine is based on single-dose studies. With repeated dosing of hydromorphone (as during PCA), it is more likely that 2 to 3 mg of parenteral hydromorphone is equal to 10 mg of parenteral morphine (see Chapter 13).

[10]As in, e.g., OxyContin.

[11]As in Opana ER.

[12]65 to 130 mg = approximately ⅙ of all doses listed in this chart.

[13]Used in combination with mu agonist opioids, this drug may reverse analgesia and precipitate withdrawal in opioid-dependent patients.

[14]In opioid-naïve patients who are taking occasional mu agonist opioids, such as hydrocodone or oxycodone, the addition of butorphanol nasal spray may provide additive analgesia. However, in opioid-tolerant patients such as those receiving ATC morphine, the addition of butorphanol nasal spray should be avoided because it may reverse analgesia and precipitate withdrawal.

From Pasero, C., & McCaffery, M. *Pain assessment and pharmacologic management*, pp. 444-446, St. Louis, Mosby. Data from American Pain Society (APS). (2003). *Principles of analgesic use in the treatment of acute pain and chronic cancer pain*. Glenview, IL, APS; Breitbart, W., Chandler, S., Eagel, B., et al. (2000). An alternative algorithm for dosing transdermal fentanyl for cancer-related pain. *Oncology, 14*(5), 695-705. See discussion in same issue, pp. 705, 709-710, 712, 17; Coda, B. A., Tanaka, A., Jacobson, R. C., et al. (1997). Hydromorphone analgesia after intravenous bolus administration. *Pain, 71*(1), 41-48; Donner, B., Zenz, M., Tryba, M., et al. (1996). Direct conversion from oral morphine to transdermal fentanyl: A multicenter study in patients with cancer pain. *Pain, 64*(3), 527-534; Dunbar, P. J., Chapman, C. R., Buckley, F. P., et al. (1996). Clinical analgesic equivalence for morphine and hydromorphone with prolonged PCA. *Pain, 68*, 226-270; Fine, P. G., Portenoy, R. K., & Ad Hoc Expert Panel on Evidence Review and Guidelines for Opioid Rotation. (2009). Establishing best practices for opioid rotation: Conclusions of an expert panel. *J Pain Symptom Manage, 38*(3), 418-425; Gutstein, H. B., & Akil, H. (2006). Opioid analgesics. In L. L. Brunton, J. S. Lazo, & K. L. Parker (Eds.), *Goodman & Gilman's The pharmacological basis of therapeutics*, ed 11, New York, McGraw-Hill; Hanks, G., Cherny, N. I., Fallon, M. (2004). Opioid analgesic therapy. In D. Doyle, G. Hanks, N. I. Cherny, et al (Eds.), *Oxford textbook of palliative medicine*, ed 3, New York, Oxford Press; Johnson, R. E., Fudala, P. J., & Payne, R. (2005). Buprenorphine: Considerations for pain management. *J Pain Symptom Manage, 29*(3), 297-326; Kaiko, R. F., Lacouture, P., Hopf, K., et al. (1996). Analgesic onset and potency of oral controlled release (CR) oxycodone CR and morphine. *Clin Pharmacol Ther, 59*(2), 130-133; Knotkova, H., Fine, P. G., & Portenoy, R. K. (2009). Opioid rotation: The science and limitations of the equianalgesic dose table. *J Pain Symptom Manage, 38*(3), 426-439; Lawlor, P., Turner, K., Hanson, J., et al. (1997). Dose ratio between morphine and hydromorphone in patients with cancer pain: A retrospective study. *Pain, 72*(1, 2), 79-85; Manfredi, P. L., Borsook, D., Chandler, S. W., et al. (1997). Intravenous methadone for cancer pain unrelieved by morphine and hydromorphone: Clinical observations. *Pain, 70*, 99-101; Portenoy, R. K. (1996). Opioid analgesics. In R. K. Portenoy, & R. M. Kanner (Eds.), *Pain management: Theory and practice*, Philadelphia, FA Davis; Sittl, R., Likar, R., & Nautrup, B. P. (2005). Equipotent doses of transdermal fentanyl and transdermal buprenorphine in patients with cancer and noncancer pain: Results of a retrospective cohort study. *Clin Ther, 27*(2), 225-237; Skaer, T. L. (2004). Practice guidelines for transdermal opioids in malignant pain. *Drugs, 64*(23), 2629-2638; Skaer, T. L. (2006). Transdermal opioids for cancer pain. *Health Qual Life Outcomes, 4*, 24; Vogelsang, J., & Hayes, S. R. (1991). Butorphanol tartrate (Stadol). A review. *J Post Anesthes Nurs, 6*(2), 129-135; Weinberg, D. S., Inturrisi, C. E., Reidenberg, B., et al. (1988). Sublingual absorption of selected opioid analgesics. *Clin Pharmacol Ther, 44*, 335-342; Wilson, J. M., Cohen, R. I., Kezer, E. A., et al. (1995). Single and multiple-dose pharmacokinetics of dezocine in patients with acute and chronic pain. *J Clin Pharmacol, 35*, 395-403. © 2011, Pasero C, McCaffery M. May be duplicated for use in clinical practice.

GUIDELINES

Box 16-1 | Selection of an Opioid Starting Dose

1. Use an equianalgesic chart and your patient's pain intensity (among other factors[1]) to determine an appropriate opioid dose.
2. Locate the prescribed opioid in column one in the equianalgesic chart (e.g., morphine).
3. Move horizontally from column one to column two if the opioid is to be given by the oral route or to column three if by the parenteral route.
4. This is the appropriate starting dose for an opioid-naïve patient with severe pain (e.g., 30 mg of PO morphine every 3 to 4 hours).
5. If the patient has moderate pain, calculate a dose that is 50% of the dose for severe pain: Severe pain dose × 0.5 (50%) = appropriate starting dose for patient with moderate pain (e.g., 15 mg of PO morphine every 3 to 4 hours).
6. If the patient has mild pain, calculate a dose that is 25% of the dose for severe pain: Severe pain dose × 0.25

(25%) = appropriate starting dose for patient with mild pain (e.g., 7.5 mg of PO morphine every 3 to 4 hours).

Note: A patient's pain intensity and the equianalgesic chart are practical tools to use to determine an appropriate opioid starting dose for an opioid-naïve patient. This box demonstrates how to combine these two tools to determine starting doses for opioid-naïve patients with mild, moderate, or severe pain intensity. The initial opioid dose is merely an estimate. At all times, the opioid dose is titrated up or down based on patients' responses (pain relief and adverse effects).

PO, Oral.

[1]The appropriateness of an opioid dose is considered after careful assessment of other factors, such as the patient's co-morbidities, previous exposure to opioids, and sedation and respiratory status. A dose is never selected based solely on a specific pain intensity (see text for discussion).

From Pasero, C., & McCaffery, M. *Pain assessment and pharmacologic management*, p. 446, St. Louis, Mosby. © 2011, Pasero C, McCaffery M. May be duplicated for use in clinical practice.

All of the opioid doses listed in the equianalgesic chart were developed in controlled trials that were conducted in opioid-naïve postoperative patients or in cancer patients with little or no prior exposure to opioids. For this reason, they may be considered a starting point for determining appropriate initial doses given about every 4 hours for opioid-naïve adults with severe pain. Percentages of these doses are used to determine the appropriate starting dose for moderate and mild pain, pain in patients at the extremes of age, and pain in patients who are medically frail or otherwise predisposed to the adverse effects of opioids. For example, the European Association for Palliative Care (EAPC) has recommended a starting dose of 5 mg of short-acting oral morphine every 4 hours in opioid-naïve patients and 10 mg in patients already being treated with "weak" opioids (Hanks, De Conno, Cherny, et al., 2001). This recommendation is more conservative than the dose that would be calculated from the equianalgesic dose table, but it recognizes the medical frailty of patients with advanced illness.

In contrast to the patient who is medically compromised, a healthy patient with severe pain who is to receive parenteral morphine might be prescribed as much as 10 mg of morphine parenterally every 4 hours. If, instead of severe pain, the patient has moderate pain, the starting dose would be 50% of 10 mg (5 mg) of morphine, and for mild pain, 25% of 10 mg (2.5 mg) (Box 16-1). When administered by the IV route, the total dose is given in smaller boluses over the 4-hour interval. Bolus doses over a 4-hour period are usually calculated by dividing the 4-hour dose by 4. In other words, the bolus dose is one-fourth of the 4-hour dose.

As discussed earlier in this section, mild pain may not require an opioid. A nonopioid, such as ibuprofen or acetaminophen, may be appropriate. If an opioid is indicated, mild pain can be treated with a low dose of any of the opioids or with an opioid-nonopioid combination, such as hydrocodone or oxycodone compounded with acetaminophen. In opioid-tolerant patients, these doses may be used as starting doses with the awareness that the dose will probably have to be titrated upward quickly.

Patient Example: PACU IV Starting Dose

Three opioid-naïve patients have just been admitted to the PACU. All three will be managed with IV boluses of hydromorphone (Dilaudid). Pain intensity and the equianalgesic chart are used to determine appropriate starting doses for each patient (see text for other factors to consider). Pain intensity is assessed by using a 0-to-10 numeric rating scale. The following steps are taken to determine appropriate starting doses.

PATIENT NO. 1

1. Hydromorphone is located in the first column of the equianalgesic chart.
2. Moving horizontally from hydromorphone to column 3 (parenteral route), the appropriate dose for severe pain is located (1.5 mg).
3. Patient No. 1 reports a pain rating of 8/10, or severe pain.
4. The appropriate starting dose for patient No. 1 is 1.5 mg of IV hydromorphone over 4 hours.
5. The calculation for the first bolus is 1.5 mg ÷ 4 (¼ of the 4-h dose) = approximately 0.4 mg (0.375 mg), titrating up or down using larger or smaller doses depending on the patient's responses (pain intensity and adverse effects).

PATIENT NO. 2

1. Steps 1 and 2 outlined for patient No. 1 are followed.
2. Patient No. 2 reports a pain rating of 5/10, or moderate pain.
3. The appropriate starting dose for moderate pain is 50% of the starting dose for severe pain. The calculation is 1.5 mg × 0.50 (50%) = 0.75 mg.
4. The appropriate starting dose for patient No. 2 is 0.75 mg of hydromorphone by the IV route over 4 hours.
5. The calculation for the first bolus is 0.75 mg ÷ 4 (¼ of the 4-h dose) = approximately 0.2 mg, titrating up or down using larger or smaller boluses depending on the patient's responses (pain intensity and adverse effects).

PATIENT NO. 3

1. Steps 1 and 2 outlined for patient No. 1 are followed.
2. Patient No. 3 reports a pain rating of 3/10, or mild pain.
3. The appropriate starting dose for mild pain is 25% of the starting dose for severe pain. The calculation is 1.5 mg × 0.25 (25%) = 0.375 mg.
4. The appropriate starting dose for patient No. 3 is approximately 0.4 mg of hydromorphone by the IV route over 4 hours.
5. The calculation for the first bolus is 0.4 mg ÷ 4 (¼ of the 4-h dose) = approximately 0.1 mg, titrating up or down using larger or smaller boluses depending on the patient's responses (pain intensity and adverse effects).

As mentioned, the doses in the equianalgesic chart are made on the basis of a 4-hour dosing schedule. To determine the appropriate starting dose when the dosing schedule is other than every 4 hours, different calculations are necessary.

Patient Example: Cancer Pain

Mr. H. has cancer pain. Until now he has been controlling his pain with two Percocet (oxycodone, 5 mg, plus acetaminophen, 325 mg per tablet) q 4 h ATC. He reports that his pain has been increasing. He rates his pain as 6/10. The decision is made to begin treatment with oral modified-release oxycodone. Mr. H.'s starting dose is calculated as follows:

10 mg oxycodone (2 Percocet) × 6 doses/day = 60 mg/day

60 mg ÷ 2 (number of doses/24 h with 12-h dosing) = 30 mg

Mr. H. is started on 30 mg modified-release oxycodone q 12 h. Acetaminophen is continued ATC. This will provide the same analgesia at more convenient dosing intervals for the opioid. Percocet 1 to 2 tablets can be taken every 4 hours for breakthrough pain (see Box 16-2 for how to calculate breakthrough doses). Mr. H. should be assessed regularly for the need for an increase in the oxycodone dose, which is based on the amount of breakthrough analgesic he requires over 24 hours.

Note: This approach to managing Mr. H.'s pain is logical and conservative. Other approaches may be used (e.g., starting at a higher dose [40 mg] of modified-release oxycodone).

Continuous Infusions

In patients with cancer pain and in opioid-naive postoperative or trauma patients in the intensive care unit (ICU) who require parenteral opioids, a maintenance continuous infusion is initiated after pain is controlled by IV or SC boluses (Coyle, Cherny, Portenoy, 1995). As mentioned, additional boluses offered every 15 to 30 minutes may be prescribed for the management of breakthrough pain (see Breakthrough Doses, discussed next, and Chapter 17 for continuous infusions in opioid-naïve patients outside of the ICU).

Patient Example: ICU Continuous Infusion

Ms. D. has been admitted directly to the ICU after an automobile accident and emergency abdominal surgery. In addition to abdominal surgery, she has deep face, neck, and chest cuts and contusions. She is opioid-naïve, is on a ventilator, and is somewhat disoriented and restless. She is unable to provide self-reports of pain yet but, based on Ms. D.'s pathology, the nurse assumes that she has moderate to severe pain. Her pain is to be controlled with a continuous IV infusion of morphine. The following calculation of the starting dose is necessary:

- Morphine is located in the first column of the equianalgesic chart.
- Moving horizontally from morphine to column 3 (parenteral route), the appropriate starting dose for severe pain is located (10 mg over a 4-hour period).

Because Ms. D. is opioid naïve and is expected to have moderate to severe pain, an appropriate conservative starting dose for her is 5 mg (50% of 10 mg) of morphine IV over a 4-hour period.

Ms. D. is to receive a continuous IV infusion, so an hourly dose must be calculated: 5 mg ÷ 4 h = approximately 1.3 mg/h.

The nurse suspects that Ms. D.'s restlessness may be related to unrelieved pain, so she administers a loading IV bolus equal to the starting hourly dose (1.3 mg) and begins the opioid infusion immediately. Within 45 minutes, Ms. D. is no longer restless, and her vital signs are stable.

Breakthrough Doses

The term *breakthrough dose* is used interchangeably with the terms *supplemental dose* or *rescue dose*. It is now conventional practice to offer all patients with pain related to active cancer or other serious illnesses who are receiving ATC opioid analgesics access to doses of a fast-acting mu agonist opioid analgesic to treat breakthrough pain (see Chapter 12 for a detailed discussion of breakthrough pain). The use of these short-acting supplemental doses for breakthrough pain should not be considered conventional practice in the large and heterogeneous population with persistent noncancer pain. In this population, the decision to provide such a treatment should be made after a careful risk-to-benefit analysis that assesses both the risk of pharmacologic adverse effects such as peak concentration sedation and the risk of problematic drug-related behaviors that may be consistent with abuse or addiction. Well-controlled research is needed to inform decisions on breakthrough pain in this diverse population (Devulder, Jacobs, Richarz, et al., 2009; Fine, Portenoy, 2007).

For patients taking oral opioids, the recommended amount of opioid for breakthrough doses is within a range of approximately 5% to 15% of the total daily dose of the ATC opioid analgesic; however, some clinicians prefer to use 10% to 15% unless there are circumstances that suggest a conservative calculation (5%) should be made, for example, in the case of a frail patient or a patient older than 70 years (Box 16-2). This calculation is used consistently, regardless of the total daily dose of opioid. For example, the range of a given breakthrough dose for a patient receiving a total daily dose of 8000 mg of modified-release morphine would be 800 mg (10%) to 1200 mg (15%).

Patient Example: Oral Breakthrough Dose

Mr. H. is receiving 30 mg of modified-release oxycodone twice daily. The breakthrough dose range is determined by calculating 10% to 15% of the total daily dose. The calculation is as follows:

- 30 mg × 2 = 60 mg/day
- 60 mg × 0.10 (10%) = 6 mg
- 60 mg × 0.15 (15%) = 9 mg

Mr. H.'s breakthrough dose range is approximately 5 to 10 mg (closest available dose strengths) of short-acting oxycodone q 1 h PRN for breakthrough pain.

Box 16-2 Calculation of Breakthrough Doses[1]

The formula for calculating rescue doses usually is 5% to 15% of the total daily dose. However, some clinicians prefer to use 10% to 15% unless there are circumstances that suggest a conservative calculation (5%) should be made, for example, in the case of frail patients or patients older than 70 years. Whenever possible, rescue doses should be the same opioid and route as the ATC drug (e.g., use oral short-acting morphine as rescue for modified-release morphine).

- Short-acting and modified-release oral morphine, oxycodone, or oxymorphone. Example: Calculate the breakthrough dose of short-acting oral morphine for patients taking 180 mg/24 h oral morphine as follows:
  - Total daily dose × 0.10 (10%), e.g., 180 mg × 0.1 = 18 mg
  - Total daily dose × 0.15 (15%), e.g., 180 mg × 0.15 = 27 mg

    The range of the breakthrough doses of short-acting oral morphine that can be taken every 1 to 2 hours PRN is 20 to 30 mg (closest available dose strengths).

    To calculate a breakthrough dose that is 5% of the total daily dose, the following calculation, using the same example, is needed:
  - Total daily dose × 0.05 (5%), e.g., 180 mg × 0.05 = 9 mg

    The breakthrough dose of short-acting oral morphine that is 5% of the total daily dose and that can be taken every 1 to 2 hours PRN is 10 mg (the closest available strength).

- Transdermal fentanyl
  - Oral transmucosal fentanyl citrate (Actiq); buccal fentanyl (Fentora); or a short-acting oral mu agonist opioid, such as morphine or oxycodone, may be used to treat breakthrough pain in patients taking transdermal fentanyl. (See Box 14-2 for dosing of oral transmucosal fentanyl [Actiq] and Box 14-3 for dosing of buccal fentanyl [Fentora].)
  - Oral short-acting opioid for breakthrough pain in patients who are already established on transdermal fentanyl: Research shows 1 mcg/h of transdermal fentanyl is approximately equianalgesic to 2 mg/day of oral morphine (i.e., 25 mcg/h of transdermal fentanyl [closest available dose strength] is approximately equianalgesic to 60 mg/day of oral morphine [closest available dose strength]).[2,3] Example: Calculate the breakthrough dose of short-acting oral morphine for patients taking 200 mcg/h of transdermal fentanyl as follows:

    Total mcg/h of fentanyl × 2 = approximate equianalgesic total daily dose of oral morphine, e.g., 200 × 2 = 400 mg of oral morphine

Approximate total daily dose of oral morphine × 0.10 (10%), e.g., 400 mg × 0.10 = 40 mg

Approximate total daily dose of oral morphine × 0.15 (15%), e.g., 400 mg × 0.15 = 60 mg

The range of the breakthrough doses of short-acting oral morphine that can be taken every 1 to 2 hours PRN is 40 to 60 mg.

To calculate a breakthrough dose that is 5% of the total daily dose, the following calculation using the same example is needed:

Total daily dose × 0.05 (5%), e.g., 400 mg × 0.05 = 20 mg

The breakthrough dose of short-acting oral morphine that is 5% of the total daily dose and that can be taken every 1 to 2 hours PRN is 20 mg of short-acting oral morphine.

- The recommended rescue dose for patients receiving continuous parenteral or epidural opioid infusions is 25% to 50% of the hourly opioid dose. Rescue doses should be offered at least every 15 to 30 minutes to patients receiving continuous parenteral infusions without PCA.

ATC, Around-the-clock; *IV*, intravenous; *PO*, oral.

[1]Whenever the dose of the baseline opioid is increased, the efficacy of the breakthrough pain dose should be reevaluated and recalculated as needed.

[2]100 mcg/h of transdermal fentanyl is considered to be approximately equianalgesic to 4 mg/h of IV morphine or equivalent (Hanks, Cherny, Fallon, 2004).

[3]A ratio of 1:1 has been used to convert patients from transdermal fentanyl to IV fentanyl during opioid titration (Mercadante, Ferrera, Villari, et al., 2006) (see text).

All patients who receive ATC opioid analgesics should have access to rescue (supplemental) doses of a fast-acting mu agonist opioid analgesic to treat breakthrough pain. This box provides guidelines for calculating rescue doses for various opioid formulations and routes of administration.

From Pasero, C., & McCaffery, M. *Pain assessment and pharmacologic management*, p. 449, St. Louis, Mosby. Data from American Pain Society (APS). (2003). *Principles of analgesic use in the treatment of acute and cancer pain*, ed 5, Glenview, IL, APS; Breitbart, W., Chandler, S., Eagel, B., et al. (2000). An alternative algorithm for dosing transdermal fentanyl for cancer-related pain. *Oncology*, 14(5), 695-705. See discussion in same issue, pages 705, 709-710, 712, 17; Donner, B., Zenz, M., Tryba, M., et al. (1996). Direct conversion from oral morphine to transdermal fentanyl: A multicenter study in patients with cancer pain. *Pain*, 64(3), 527-534; Hanks, G., Cherny, N. I., & Fallon, M. (2004). Opioid analgesic therapy. In D. Doyle, G. Hanks, N. I. Cherny, et al. (Eds.), *Oxford textbook of palliative medicine*, ed 3, New York, Oxford Press; McCaffery, M. (1996). How to calculate a rescue dose. *Am J Nurs*, 96(4), 65-66; Mercadante, S., Ferrera, P., Villari, P., et al. (2006). Opioid escalation in patients with cancer paIn The effect of age. *J Pain Symptom Manage*, 32(5), 413-419. © 2011, Pasero C, McCaffery M. May be duplicated for use in clinical practice.

The recommended breakthrough dose for patients receiving continuous parenteral opioid infusions is 25% to 50% of the hourly opioid dose (see Box 16-2). (Although 5% to 15% of the 24-hour dose can be used to calculate breakthrough doses for parenteral opioid treatment, hourly percentages are simpler when using continuous parenteral opioid infusions, and the results are essentially the same.) The total number of parenteral breakthrough doses given in 1 hour may be equal to but ordinarily do not exceed the hourly opioid dose. The need for breakthrough doses greater than the hourly opioid dose indicates a need to increase the hourly opioid dose. For example, an opioid-tolerant patient receiving 6 mg/h of IV morphine could be given a 3-mg breakthrough dose every 30 minutes but ordinarily should not repeatedly be given more than two 3-mg boluses in 1 hour. If more than two boluses are required, the continuous infusion should be increased.

Patient Example: IV Breakthrough Dose

Ms. D. is receiving a continuous IV infusion of morphine at 1.3 mg/h after an automobile accident and abdominal surgery. The IV breakthrough dose range is calculated as follows:

- 1.3 mg × 0.25 (25%) = approximately 0.3 mg
- 1.3 mg × 0.50 (50%) = approximately 0.7 mg

Ms. D.'s IV morphine breakthrough dose range could be 0.3 mg to 0.7 mg (not to exceed approximately 1.3 mg total in breakthrough doses in 1 hour) of IV morphine provided q 15 to 30 minutes PRN for breakthrough pain.

Dose Titration

Titration of the opioid dose usually is required at the beginning of therapy and repeatedly during the course of treatment (Vascello, McQuillan, 2006). Whereas patients with cancer pain most often are titrated upward over time for progressive pain, patients with acute pain, particularly postoperative pain, are eventually titrated downward as pain resolves.

As discussed, considerable variation exists in the amount of opioid individuals require for comfort (APS, 2003). For example, research has established that as much as a tenfold difference exists among patients in opioid requirements during the postoperative period (Myles, 2004). Even greater differences are noted in patients with persistent pain (Hanks, Cherny, Fallon, 2004). This wide variability reinforces the need for prompt and individualized attention to unrelieved pain. At all times, inadequate pain relief is addressed by gradual escalation of the opioid dose until adequate analgesia is reported, or until intolerable and unmanageable adverse effects occur. The absolute opioid dose is unimportant as long as the balance between pain relief and adverse effects is favorable (Hanks, Cherny, Fallon, 2004). The goal of titration is to use the smallest dose that provides satisfactory pain relief with the fewest adverse effects. Clinicians new to titrating opioid doses in opioid-tolerant patients are often uncomfortable with the high doses sometimes required; seeking the assistance of a clinician experienced with providing opioids for opioid-tolerant patients may be helpful.

Identifying the Need for an Opioid Dose Increase

The first sign that an increase in opioid dose is needed is most commonly a decrease in the duration of analgesia for a given opioid dose. For example, patients receiving IV PCA may repeatedly attempt to self-administer PCA doses before the programmed lockout (delay) interval elapses (see Chapter 17), or patients taking a modified-release opioid may report breakthrough pain occurring invariably toward the end of the continuous analgesic dosing interval, such as in the eleventh hour of a 12-hour dosing schedule. Patients also may report the need for an increased number of breakthrough doses. As a rule of thumb, two or more breakthrough doses during a 12-hour period (four to six daily) should alert the clinician that the opioid regimen for cancer or persistent noncancer pain needs to be re-evaluated. Six doses a day approximates every-4-hour dosing and defeats the purpose of using modified-release formulations.

When an increase in the opioid dose is necessary, it can be done by percentages. When a slight improvement in analgesia is needed, a 25% increase in the total daily opioid dose may be sufficient; for a moderate effect, a 50% increase, and for a strong effect, such as for the treatment of severe pain, a 100% increase may be indicated. The time at which the dose should be increased is typically determined by considering the onset or peak effect of the opioid. For example, titration of IV opioid doses may occur as often as every 5 to 15 minutes (depending on the lipid solubility of the drug) (see the following patient example), whereas titration of oral modified-release opioids may occur every 24 to 48 hours. Increases in the ATC analgesia may need to be accompanied by proportional increases in the breakthrough dose, so that the size of breakthrough doses remains an effective percentage of the fixed dose. Whenever the dose of the baseline opioid is increased, the efficacy of the breakthrough pain dose should be re-evaluated and adjusted as needed (see Box 16-2).

Patient Example: IV Titration

Ms. L. is in outpatient PACU after a laparoscopy. Her pain is 6/10. She has an order for titration with 20 to 60 mcg IV fentanyl boluses q 15 min PRN. Her nurse gives her 20 mcg of IV fentanyl, and approximately 15 minutes later Ms. L. reports her pain as 5/10. Her nurse decides to increase the amount of the bolus dose by 50% and gives 30 mcg this time (20 mg × 0.50 [50%] = 10 mg; 20 mg + 20 mg = 30 mg [50% increase in the dose of the last bolus]). Within 15 minutes, Ms. L. says she is comfortable and has a pain rating of 3/10. At that time she is given two Vicodin (5 mg hydrocodone and 500 mg acetaminophen), which is prescribed for her pain control at home. She is discharged 75 minutes later, alert and with a pain rating of 3/10.

Another method of increasing opioid doses is possible when patients are receiving ATC opioids and taking breakthrough doses. If the combination of the ATC dose and the breakthrough doses provide satisfactory pain relief, the ATC dose can be increased to the amount of opioid provided by the current ATC dose plus breakthrough doses. This may allow elimination or a considerable decrease in the number of breakthrough doses required (see the following patient examples).

Patient Example: SC Titration

Mr. K. has been receiving a continuous SC infusion of 1 mg/h of hydromorphone at home. He has required SC breakthrough doses of 0.5 mg of hydromorphone q 30 to 45 minutes, with a total of 18 boluses required during the last 24-hour period to maintain an acceptable comfort level (4/10). The decision is made to increase the dose of hydromorphone provided by continuous infusion on the basis of his total 24-hour requirement.

- 1 mg/h × 24 h = 24 mg/day (continuous infusion)
- 0.5 mg × 18 = 9 mg/day (bolus doses)
- 24 mg + 9 mg = 33 mg
- 33 mg ÷ 24 = 1.4 mg/h

Mr. K.'s hydromorphone dose by continuous SC infusion is increased to 1.4 mg/h.

The new breakthrough dose range is calculated (see Box 16-2, p. 449):

- 1.4 mg × 0.25 (25%) (or 1.4 mg ÷ 4) = approximately 0.4 mg
- 1.4 mg × 0.50 (50%) (or 1.4 mg ÷ 2) = 0.7 mg

Mr. K.'s breakthrough dose range is approximately 0.4 mg to 0.7 mg of SC morphine q 15 to 30 minutes PRN for breakthrough pain.

The next day Mr. K. reports that his comfort level is 2/10 and he has required only two breakthrough doses since the increase in his continuous infusion.

Patient Example: Oral Titration

Mrs. R. is reporting inadequate relief of her cancer pain after a period of stable dosing with 30 mg of short-acting oral morphine q 4 h. She has required an increased number of breakthrough doses (from 2 doses to about 5 doses of 10 mg short-acting oral morphine/day), and most of the time the breakthrough doses are needed during the last hour of the dosing interval. She is finding it increasingly difficult to work and sleep. She rates her pain as moderate (5/10) most of the day. Mrs. R. would like to try twice-daily modified-release morphine with a 25% increase in the opioid dose.

- 30 mg × 6 doses = 180 mg/day (ATC dose)
- 10 mg × 5 = 50 mg/day (breakthrough doses)
- 180 mg + 50 mg = 230 mg/day
- 230 mg × 0.25 (25%) (or 230 mg ÷ 4) = approximately 60 mg
- 230 mg + 60 mg = 290 mg (25% increase in opioid dose)
- 290 mg ÷ 2 (q 12 h doses) = 145 mg modified-release morphine q 12 h
- Modified-release morphine (12-h) is available in 15, 30, 60, 100, and 200 mg tablets. Mrs. R. will take 1 15, 1 30, and 1 100 mg tablet q 12 h.

The new breakthrough dose is calculated (see Box 16-2):

- 290 mg × 0.10 (10%) = approximately 30 mg
- 290 mg × 0.15 (15%) = approximately 45 mg
- Mrs. R.'s new breakthrough dose range is 30 to 45 mg q 1 h PRN for breakthrough pain. Because a lag period occurs before the onset of modified-release morphine, Mrs. R. takes 30 mg of short-acting morphine when she takes the first dose of modified-release morphine. Two days later Mrs. R. reports that she is able to work and sleep better and has a pain rating of 2/10 most of the day, without the need for breakthrough doses.

Patients should be involved in the decision to increase the opioid dose. Valuable information is obtained by asking patients to describe the patterns of pain they are experiencing. For example, patients commonly take more breakthrough doses during the times when they are active than when they are resting. Patients with cancer pain or persistent noncancer pain who work or are particularly active frequently take more than 2 breakthrough doses during a 12-hour period. Many patients would prefer to administer additional doses during these periods of activity rather than risk increased sedation that can accompany an increase in the ATC opioid dose. Some postoperative patients receiving PCA prefer less than complete pain relief rather than risk nausea with an increased dose.

Inadequate Pain Relief During Analgesic Infusion Therapies

When patients report inadequate pain relief during analgesic infusion therapies, such as IV PCA or epidural analgesia, the entire infusion system, from the infusion pump to the IV site or epidural catheter site, should be checked. Inadequate pain relief may be caused by a number of mechanical and technical factors, including incorrect loading of the pump, disconnection of the catheter from the infusion pump tubing, an empty drug reservoir, a disconnected PCA button, or a malfunctioning pump or tubing. In patients receiving epidural analgesia, the epidural catheter may have been inadvertently pulled out.

When bolus doses and increases in the epidural analgesic dose do not yield satisfactory pain control or produce patchy (e.g., one-sided) analgesia, and the epidural catheter appears to be in place, the infusion line connected, and the infusion pump infusing correctly, the anesthesia provider or pain service is notified. The epidural catheter can be checked for optimal location by administering a concentrated dose of local anesthetic through the catheter. Optimal catheter placement would produce a bilateral sensory block of the desired dermatomes; lack of such a block would indicate that the catheter location is not optimal. If location is less than optimal, the epidural catheter should be removed and alternatives considered (see Chapter 15 for more on epidural analgesia).

Titration in Patients with Cancer Pain

As noted previously, the conventional approaches to titration of the opioid dose involve either an increase by percentages or an increase based on the usage of breakthrough pain medication during the past day or more. The typical percentage increase is 25% to 50% (Hanks, Cherny, Fallon, 2004), with the proviso that some patients with severe pain should be considered for a larger increase, as much as 100% if the pain is severe and the increment appears to be safe. The approach that involves summing the medication used for breakthrough pain and increasing the baseline dose by an equivalent amount has the advantage of a high likelihood that the increment is safe, given that the patient has taken a comparable amount prior to the change. The EAPC recommends a modification of the latter approach as the simplest method, suggesting that a short-acting opioid analgesic be administered every 4 hours and the same dose offered as needed for breakthrough pain as often as every hour (Hanks, De Conno, Chery, et al., 2001). The mainstay opioid dose can then be increased based on the amount of breakthrough medication the patient requires.

The provision of appropriate starting doses may influence the need for dose titration in some cancer patients. The EAPC recommends a starting dose of 5 mg of short-acting oral morphine every 4 hours in opioid-naïve patients and 10 mg in patients already being treated with "weak" opioids (Hanks, De Conno, Cherny, et al., 2001) (see Chapter 12, WHO Ladder). A multicenter study enrolled 159 consecutive patients with cancer pain and established that these dosing recommendations resulted in significant pain reduction and the need for minimal dose escalation (Ripamonti, Campa, Fagnoni, et al., 2009). The presence of neuropathic pain was associated with the need for higher opioid doses. Similarly, 40 cancer patients with uncontrolled pain were converted from nonopioid-opioid analgesics to oral short-acting morphine administered on a fixed schedule, and they achieved adequate pain control within 2.3 days; patients were then converted to an equivalent dose of modified-release morphine (Klepstad, Kaasa, Skauge, et al., 2000). The mean daily morphine dose during titration was 97 mg, adverse effects were essentially unaltered, and 82% were satisfied or very satisfied with treatment. A later study by these same researchers randomized 40 patients with uncontrolled cancer pain to titration of short-acting oral morphine given every 4 hours or titration of a modified-release morphine (Kapanol, Kadian) given once daily (Klepstad, Kaasa, Jystad, et al., 2003). The mean time to achieve adequate pain control was 2.1 days with short-acting morphine and 1.7 days with modified-release morphine. Those taking the latter reported feeling less tired at the end of titration. No other differences in adverse effects, health-related quality-of-life functions, or satisfaction with treatment were noted.

As discussed, the starting dose should be reduced in older patients. An interesting study of opioid titration in cancer patients found that although older patients required lower doses, opioid effects—as evaluated by dose escalation, number of opioids, or routes of administration to obtain a balance between analgesia and adverse effects—did not differ among age groups (Mercadante, Ferrera, Villari, et al., 2006). The researchers cautioned against labeling older patients as more responsive to opioids, either for analgesia or adverse effects, and emphasized the need for careful, individualized titration in this population, as is recommended in all patients.

Cancer Pain Crisis

The concept of pain emergency is poorly defined in the literature but is useful clinically. Some patients with cancer pain experience severe, and usually increasing, pain associated with high levels of distress and, in some cases, autonomic changes, such as tachycardia and hypertension. At some threshold, the treatment of these patients should be considered an emergency (Miaskowski, Cleary, Burney, et al., 2005; Soares, Martins, Uchoa, 2003). This designation may justify admission to the hospital and usually provides a rationale for a switch to an IV opioid. Although the level of pain can be managed with oral or SC opioid titration (Klepstad, Kaasa, Jystad, et al., 2003; Klepstad, Kaasa, Skauge, et al., 2000), IV opioids have advantages: much faster peak effects occur (e.g., 15 minutes for morphine); repeated doses can be given more frequently; and analgesia is achieved more rapidly (Miaskowski, Cleary, Burney, et al., 2005). In patients who are already taking an opioid, the APS recommends a dose that is 10% to 20% of the total daily dose of their current opioid regimens (Miaskowski, Cleary, Burney, et al., 2005) (see Chapter 18 for conversion from oral to IV route). If the patient is not taking an opioid, management of severe pain should begin with 2 to 5 mg of IV morphine or an equivalent short-acting opioid (again, less than the dose indicated on the equianalgesic dose table in recognition of the medical co-morbidities common in patients with cancer).

After the initial bolus, pain should be reassessed in 5 to 20 minutes and the same dose repeated. If repeated doses are necessary, and there appears to be no somnolence or other adverse effects, the size of the bolus can be increased, usually by 25% to 50%. Repeated boluses continue until pain is reduced by at least 50% or unmanageable and intolerable adverse effects occur.

The principle underlying this repeated-bolus approach to the management of severe pain is to repeat the dose after enough time has elapsed to observe the peak effect of the prior dose. If the oral route is used for rapid titration, the dose may be repeated in 60 to 90 minutes, and if the SC route is used, the interval typically is approximately 45 minutes.

When IV morphine is used to deliver repeated bolus injections, it is best to wait for 15 to 20 minutes between doses because this period is required to observe the peak effect. Shorter intervals can be used, but they require careful monitoring because of the risk for overshooting when additional injections are given prior to the peak effects of those that were administered earlier. IV morphine doses administered at 2-minute intervals achieved pain control in a mean time of 9.7 minutes in 45 patients admitted to an inpatient palliative care unit for severe cancer pain (Mercadante, Villari, Ferrera, et al., 2002). Patients'

effective doses were converted to oral morphine doses, which were initiated 4 hours after IV titration had been completed. This rapid conversion to oral morphine allowed early discharge back to the home setting.

For acute severe pain in patients with advanced cancer who are relatively opioid-naïve, Davis (2004) recommends IV treatment with 1 mg morphine (20 mcg fentanyl or 0.2 mg of hydromorphone may be substituted), repeated every 5 minutes until (1) the initial onset of analgesia; (2) opioid toxicity; or (3) a total of 30 mg of morphine (or the equivalent) over 45 minutes. This is followed by parenteral-maintenance morphine at one quarter of the titrated loading dose infused per hour; the breakthrough dose should equal the hourly dose. To calculate an oral morphine maintenance dose, the total effective titrated IV dose is calculated as the 4-hourly parenteral dose of morphine, then multiplied by 3. For example, if a 10-mg bolus morphine dose was necessary to achieve onset of analgesia, the conversion would be 30 mg of short-acting oral morphine every 4 hours or the equivalent dose in modified-release formulation (Davis, 2004).

In contrast to morphine, which is hydrophilic and requires many minutes to cross the blood-brain barrier and yield peak effects, more lipophilic opioids cross into the brain very quickly and produce peak effects almost immediately. IV fentanyl was used successfully to provide rapid analgesia for severe cancer pain in 18 patients admitted to the emergency department (ED) (Soares, Martins, Uchoa, 2003). The patients' oral morphine doses were converted to IV morphine equivalents using a 3:1 ratio (average daily oral morphine dose was 276 mg). This amount was then converted to IV fentanyl using a ratio of 1:100. An IV fentanyl bolus dose equivalent to 10% of the total IV morphine daily dose taken in the previous 24 hours was administered and repeated every 5 minutes, with a 50% increase in dose if necessary to reduce patients' pain intensity score to less than 4/10. Vital signs were monitored during titration and for 6 hours afterward. All 18 patients achieved pain control in an average of 11 minutes without significant adverse effects, although 5 patients experienced slight sedation. The mean dose of IV fentanyl required for pain control was 214 mcg.

Continuous IV infusions are also used to treat pain crises. This can be accomplished by converting the existing dose into the infusion rate and adding breakthrough doses equal to 50% to 200% of the hourly infusion rate available every 15 minutes as needed (Miaskowski, Cleary, Burney, et al., 2005).

These strategies for managing cancer pain crises require rapid decision making and sometimes very large opioid doses. If the clinician is not familiar with this approach, it may be advisable to contact another clinician or a prescriber who has had experience with these situations and can either demonstrate the strategy in person or be available by telephone to offer assurance and advice.

Fear of causing opioid-induced respiratory depression can pose a barrier to the use of aggressive titration, which led researchers to evaluate changes in respiratory parameters during IV opioid (morphine, hydromorphone, or fentanyl in various doses) titration in 25 opioid-tolerant and 5 opioid-naïve patients with severe uncontrolled cancer pain (Estfan, Mahmoud, Shaheen, et al., 2007). Several of the patients had compromised respiratory function resulting from a variety of sources, but none were receiving oxygen supplementation. Oxygen saturation remained above 92% during IV titration, and transcutaneous carbon dioxide levels never exceeded 50 mm Hg in any of the patients. Two opioid-naive patients experienced transient, self-resolving decreases in respiratory rate to 8 to 9 breaths/minute. No patient required arterial blood gas evaluation due to hypercapnia or hypoxia. Mean pain scores were reduced from 6.8 to 1.9.

After pain has been controlled by aggressive titration, a thorough evaluation of the underlying causes of acute or sudden worsening of pain is recommended (Davis, 2004). Such events may indicate complications, such as bone fractures, hemorrhage into tumor, infarction thrombosis, obstructed viscus, nerve compression, inflammation, or infection.

Titration in Patients with Persistent Noncancer Pain

There is a lack of research regarding opioid titration in patients with persistent noncancer pain. A retrospective study of 206 patients experiencing a variety of types of noncancer pain, including neuropathic pain, found that older patients, regardless of type of pain, demonstrated the need for increased opioid doses at significantly lower rates (two times) than younger patients over the 2-year study period (Buntin-Mushock, Phillip, Moriyana, et al., 2005). A slower rate of dose escalation was required in patients with neuropathic pain than in patients who had nociceptive pain. Portenoy and colleagues (2007) studied patients taking modified-release oxycodone for a variety of types of noncancer pain and reported a modest need for dose escalation during the 3-year study period.

Titration in Patients with Severe Acute Pain

Providing effective pain control while minimizing opioid-induced adverse effects presents special challenges for clinicians who work in outpatient surgery settings, postanesthesia care units (PACUs), and ICUs, because they must deal also with the additional central nervous system (CNS) depression caused by the sedative and anesthetic agents that are administered intraoperatively and sometimes throughout care in the ICU. Rapid analgesia must be provided to patients who are in a nonsteady state, and that adds to the complexity of titration (Berde, Brennan, Raja, 2003). Furthermore, many of these patients are opioid-naïve, which places them at greater risk for adverse opioid-induced effects, particularly excessive sedation and respiratory depression.

Less difficulty is experienced when a multimodality approach is used in patients with acute pain (Pasero, 2003; Pasero, McCaffery, 2007). As discussed earlier in this section, combinations of analgesics improve pain relief with lower analgesic doses; lower doses result in fewer adverse effects. If an NSAID was not given preoperatively and is not relatively contraindicated, it can be started as soon as the patient reaches the PACU or ICU; epidural opioids are usually combined with long-acting local anesthetics to reduce the opioid dose. Acetaminophen may be added to any treatment plan (see Section III).

Before a trauma or postoperative patient becomes oriented enough to provide self-reports of pain, the nurse should assume that pain is present by the fact that sufficient noxious stimuli are present (see Chapter 20 for discussion of opioid use and dose selection in critically ill patients who cannot report pain). As soon as it is safe to do so, an IV bolus of an opioid can be administered and then repeated as described previously to titrate rapidly against adverse effects (e.g., 2 to 3 mg morphine every 10 to 15 minutes [see subsequent material]). Patients must be observed closely for adverse effects, particularly sedation and respiratory depression (see Chapter 19) (Aubrun, Monsel, Langeron, et al., 2001; Lovovschi, Aubrun, Bonnet, et al., 2008). Epidural bolus doses may be given for uncontrolled pain in patients who are receiving epidural analgesia. The presence of other signs of pain, such as moaning, facial grimacing, or elevated vital signs, may be considered in the assessment of pain, but it is important that clinicians remember that their absence does not necessarily mean the absence of pain. Do not assume that sleeping means adequate pain control (see Section II).

Opioid Selection for Initial Titration in Patients with Acute Pain

The mu agonist opioids—morphine, hydromorphone, and fentanyl—are most commonly used for initial titration in patients with severe acute pain, but nurses often ask which one is the best choice. Important patient characteristics to consider when selecting an opioid for titration are discussed in detail in Chapter 13 and include, for example, previous exposure to and tolerance of opioids, current organ function, and hemodynamic stability. For example, fentanyl is favored in patients with any type of end-organ failure. It also produces minimal hemodynamic effects, which adds to its appeal for patients with unstable blood pressure.

In addition to patient characteristics, the pharmacokinetics of the opioids and the goals of treatment are considered when deciding which opioid is best for titration in particular patients. As discussed, morphine is hydrophilic and requires several minutes to cross the blood-brain barrier and yield peak effects after IV administration; the more lipophilic opioids such as fentanyl cross into the brain very quickly and produce peak effects almost immediately when given intravenously. Hydromorphone is less hydrophilic than morphine so has an intermediate effect. These pharmacokinetics help to explain why fentanyl is often selected when the goal is to control severe, rapidly escalating pain quickly (e.g., severe pain on admission to the ED or PACU) (see speed of injection, later in this chapter). Although IV fentanyl's short duration is an advantage when short patient stays are expected, it can be a drawback when pain is expected to be continuous. For example, fentanyl tends to be a first-choice opioid for procedural pain and is a logical selection in an ambulatory surgery PACU where the goal is to transition patients quickly to the oral analgesic that the patients will take after discharge. However, research has shown that the use of fentanyl does not result in faster discharge times because patients require additional analgesia to control pain (Claxton, McGuire, Chung, et al., 1997). In addition, frequent dosing is necessary when fentanyl is used for ongoing continuous pain. For example, a short lockout (delay) interval (e.g., 5 minutes) and a basal rate are often prescribed when fentanyl is used for IV PCA; however, the lockout interval is 8 to 10 minutes when morphine is used for acute pain, and it is often administered without a basal rate (see Chapter 17).

For patients who have undergone major surgery, some PACU nurses like to administer a few doses of fentanyl, then follow with either hydromorphone or morphine for longer lasting analgesia. However, although it makes sense to use a fast-onset opioid such as fentanyl in patients presenting with severe, escalating pain, it may not be necessary and can complicate the assessment process in those with less severe pain; when opioids are combined and adverse effects occur, it is difficult to interpret which one might be the culprit. Therefore, a general principle of initial titration in patients with acute pain is to keep in mind the patients' ongoing pain treatment plan. As an example, consider the patient who is admitted to the PACU and will have hydromorphone IV PCA for ongoing postoperative pain management. Unless the patient has severe, rapidly escalating pain on admission, it makes sense to begin titration with hydromorphone so that the effects (both pain relief and adverse effects) of the drug that will be used for the next day or so can be evaluated more easily. In all cases, the time it takes an opioid to reach its analgesic action site is always considered when determining dose and how often to administer it during titration; adequate time must be allowed to assess response to one dose before administering another (Loetsch, Dudziak, Freynhagen, et al., 2006).

Titration Protocols in the Emergency Department

Some studies have shown that standard practices related to titration in patients with acute pain may lead to undertreated pain. The use of adequate starting doses in the titration protocols appears to be critical. For example, although weight is not recommended for the calculation of opioid doses in adults, most guidelines for titration in patients with severe pain in the ED setting call for a starting dose based on weight; i.e., 0.1 mg/kg of IV morphine

(approximately 7 mg in a 150-lb person) followed by titration until adequate pain relief is achieved (Ungar, Brandes Reinoehi, et al., 1999); however, a prospective study of 119 patients showed that this starting dose resulted in 67% of the patients' experiencing less than 50% pain relief within 30 minutes; no patient required an opioid antagonist (Bijur, Kenny, Gallagher, 2005). A later randomized controlled study (N = 280) found that 0.15 mg/kg (approximately 10 mg in a 150-lb person) provided pain relief superior to 0.1 mg/kg in the ED (Birnbaum, Esses, Bijur, et al., 2007). This higher dose was supported in another study of 621 patients with severe pain in the ED; 3-mg increment doses of IV morphine (2 mg in older patients) were administered every 5 minutes to comfort or sleep and resulted in adequate pain relief in 82% of the patients (Lovovschi, Aubrun, Bonnet, et al., 2008). The mean morphine dose administered was 10.5 mg (0.16 mg/kg); the median time of titration was 15 minutes; and the median number of boluses was 3. Nausea and vomiting were the most common adverse effects (4.2%), and mild respiratory depression (slight decreases in respiratory rates and oxygen saturations) occurred in 2.6%. These researchers stressed the need to use flexible rather than fixed (mg/kg) dosing during titration. Although no serious adverse events were reported, it was unclear if sleep might have actually been excessive sedation in this study. It is important to remember that sedation can occur before pain is completely relieved and that sleep during opioid titration is usually not normal sleep but primarily the result of the sedative effects of the opioid (see Chapter 19). This type of rapid dosing always carries the risk for excessive sedation and respiratory depression; these parameters must be watched closely during titration and for at least 3 hours after the peak of the last dose administered (APS, 2003) (see Chapter 19).

A patient-driven titration procedure dubbed the *1 + 1 hydromorphone protocol* may provide an alternative to traditional procedures. The protocol involved the administration of 1 mg of hydromorphone to 223 patients in the ED who had severe pain. That was followed by assessment and the offer of another 1 mg dose 15 minutes later (Chang, Bijur, Campbell, et al., 2009). This led to adequate analgesia in 95% of the patients. A follow-up study (N = 224) comparing this protocol to physician-driven management, which was described as being reflective of current practice and consisted of the administration of an IV opioid dose with no offer of additional analgesia, found that the 94% of the patients in the 1 + 1 group achieved adequate analgesia within 60 minutes of protocol initiation and had significantly greater decreases in pain than did the physician-driven group (Chang, Bijur, Davitt, et al., 2009). Just 10% of the patients in the physician-driven group were given a follow-up dose of analgesia. Adverse effects were similar in the groups, and no one required naloxone.

Another protocol, which called for the administration of 2 mg of IV hydromorphone over 2 to 3 minutes, relieved pain effectively and rapidly (within 5 minutes) in the ED but resulted in one or more periods of desaturation in 26% of the patients in 1 prospective study (Chang, Bijur, Napolitano, et al., 2009). The researchers appropriately concluded that 2 mg of IV hydromorphone is too much opioid to be given routinely to opioid-naïve patients as a single initial dose.

A common and recommended practice is to store a specified number of PCA pumps, drug reservoirs, and infusion tubings (number is dependent on the size of the institution) in the ED so that the therapy can be initiated without delay in patients who are admitted for treatment of severe pain crises. As discussed in Chapter 17, the clinician-administered bolus mode on most PCA pumps can be used to administer doses during titration.

Titration Protocols in the Postanesthesia Care Unit

Although opioid-induced adverse effects are dose related and have been identified as a limiting factor during titration in postoperative patients (Berde, Brennan, Raja, 2003), some suggest that the customary doses used to manage immediate postoperative pain are well tolerated and that an exaggerated fear of adverse effects may pose the greater threat (Larijani, Goldberg, 2004). A placebo-controlled study of 88 patients following abdominal hysterectomy or prostatectomy found that a single IV bolus dose of 7.5 mg of morphine did not cause any clinically significant cardiovascular (CV) or respiratory adverse effects but provided only slight relief of moderate to severe pain in the PACU (Larijani, Goldberg, Gratz, et al., 2004).

A large prospective, nonrandomized study illustrated the challenges of finding a balance between comfort and adverse effects in the immediate postoperative period by evaluating four different dosing regimens (Aubrun, Monsel, Langeron, et al., 2001). Each regimen consisted of administering 2 to 3 mg IV morphine boluses until patients experienced pain relief or adverse effects. SC morphine was given to all of the patients following IV bolus titration. The regimens were as follows. Group 1: boluses given every 10 minutes to a limit of five boluses (N = 400); group 2: boluses given every 5 minutes to a limit of five boluses (N = 400); group 3 and 4: boluses given in unlimited numbers every 5 minutes (N = 400 each group). Groups 1, 2, and 3 received SC morphine 4 hours after IV titration, and group 4 received SC morphine 2 hours after IV titration. Group 4 had the highest percentage of pain relief (73%) at the end of the PACU period, but sedation was dose-related and was highest in groups 3 (62%) and 4 (61%), both of which received an unlimited number of IV boluses compared with group 1 (27%), which received the more conservative regimen of IV boluses every 10 minutes up to a maximum of five boluses.

Titration in Older Adults with Severe Acute Pain

As discussed, age is an important consideration during opioid titration, and a common recommendation is to reduce the initial dose in older patients; however, one study (N = 224; 68% young, 32% old) showed that the dose of IV morphine required during postoperative titration to achieve adequate pain relief was not significantly different in older (0.14 mg/kg) compared with younger (0.15 mg/kg) patients (Aubrun, Bunge, Langeron, et al., 2003). Higher pain intensity was associated with higher morphine requirements; no patients required naloxone. It is important to note that the lack of difference noted in this research was assessed after normalizing for body weight, which was lower in the older patients. An earlier study (N = 875 young, 175 old) by these same researchers also found no differences in morphine requirements in age groups after doses were normalized for body weight (Aubrun, Monsel, Langeron, et al., 2002).

Other factors have been found to influence analgesic requirements. One study (N = 4317; 54% male, 46% female) observed that sex, but not age, was a predictor of severe pain and higher morphine requirements in postoperative patients (Aubrun, Salvi, Coriat, et al., 2005). Women experienced more severe postoperative pain than men and required higher opioid doses; however, an interesting finding in this study was that sex-related differences disappeared in the older patients. A prospective study of 149 surgical patients found that the patients' initial pain-intensity ratings, rather than age, predicted morphine requirements in the PACU (Dahmani, Dupont, Mantz, et al., 2001). Nevertheless, conservative initial opioid doses, along with careful monitoring during titration, continue to be recommended in the older adult population; doses should be increased based on patients' responses rather than specific age. An observational study (N = 418) demonstrated the safety of a postoperative protocol for patients older than 65 in whom IV morphine was started at a dose one third less than for younger patients (Keita, Tubach, Maalouli, et al., 2008). This method was found to be as safe and efficacious for the older patients at the lower dose (2 mg) as for younger patients at the higher dose (3 mg).

Dosing to a Specific Pain Intensity

Research has shown that the relationship between visual analog scale (VAS) pain intensity scores and dose requirement during and after titration in postoperative patients is not linear, suggesting that many factors influence pain and its relief and that there is no specific dose that will relieve pain of a specific intensity (Aubrun, Riou, 2004; Blumstein, Moore, 2003). Pain was assessed in a study of more than 3000 patients admitted consecutively to the PACU, and those with a VAS score above 30 were titrated with 3 mg of IV morphine every 5 minutes until their VAS scores were below 30 (Aubrun, Langeron, Quesnel, et al., 2003). The mean morphine requirement to obtain pain relief was 12 mg. A VAS score of 70 or higher was indicative of severe pain based on the need for a morphine dose of more than 0.15 mg/kg, which corresponds with the 10-mg morphine dose suggested by other research as being appropriate for some patients with severe pain. However, when VAS scores were analyzed, a sigmoid rather than linear relationship between morphine requirement and pain intensity was noted, as demonstrated by pain intensities that changed little with initial doses and then decreased rapidly with the final incremental dose. Although this study has noted limitations (Aubrun, Riou, 2004; Larijani, Goldberg, 2004; Myles, 2004), it underscores the importance of individualized selection of analgesic doses and systematic assessment of response during titration.

An interesting prospective, observational study evaluated patients' desire for pain medication in 104 patients with acute pain and found that no single pain intensity can reliably predict a given patient's analgesic requirements or desire for additional analgesia (Blumstein, Moore, 2003). As mentioned previously, dosing to a specific pain intensity can be dangerous and is strongly discouraged (Blumstein, Moore, 2003; Gordon, Dahl, Phillips et al., 2004; Lucas, Vlahos, Ledgerwood, 2007; Vila, Smith, Augustyniak, et al., 2005). Numerous other factors, such patient co-morbidities, previous opioid exposure, desire for pain medication, and the presence of adverse effects, particularly excessive sedation and respiratory depression, must be considered when selecting an opioid dose (see Chapter 19).

Transfer of Care: Hand-off Communication

Pain control should be included in the criteria for discharge from one area of care to another. Some EDs, short-stay units, outpatient surgery units, and PACUs establish a comfort-function goal of at least 4/10 before discharge (see Section II); however, the expectation that all patients must be discharged from these areas with pain ratings below an arbitrary number can lead to the unsafe administration of further opioid doses to patients who are excessively sedated (Blumstein, Moore, 2003; Lucas, Vlahos, Ledgerwood, 2007). Instead, achieving optimal pain relief is best viewed on a continuum, with the primary objective being to provide both effective and safe analgesia. Although it is not always possible to achieve a patient's comfort-function goal within the short time the patient is in these areas, the comfort-function goal provides direction for ongoing care. Important information to give to the nurse assuming care of the patient is the patient's comfort-function goal, how close the patient is to achieving it, what has been done thus far to achieve it (analgesics, doses, and times of administration), and how well the patient has tolerated the administration of analgesics (adverse effects) (see Chapter 19).

The transferring nurse should also alert staff on the receiving clinical unit of a patient's risk factors for respiratory depression so that appropriate monitoring can be initiated (see Box 19-5 on p. 516). For example, opioid-naïve patients who require high opioid doses (e.g., more than 10 mg of IV morphine or its equivalent) during titration for acute pain are at higher risk for respiratory depression (Dahan, Aarts, Smith, 2010) and must be watched closely for at least 3 hours after the peak concentration of the last dose has passed (APS, 2003); the highest risk for respiratory depression is during the entire first 24 postoperative hours. Mechanical monitoring is warranted in patients with diagnosed or suspected obstructive sleep apnea or pulmonary disease. Providing the postoperative patient's American Society of Anesthesiologists Patient Status Classification is recommended as a simple way to further communicate the patient's risk for respiratory depression (see Chapter 19 for a detailed discussion and risk factors for sedation and respiratory depression).

Speed of Intravenous Injection

Too-rapid injection of IV medications can cause significant patient harm (Institute for Safe Medication Practices, 2003c). Chest wall rigidity and subsequent difficult ventilation is a potential complication of opioid administration and is most likely to occur with rapid IV administration of relatively high doses of lipophilic opioids such as the fentanils (Fukuda, 2005; Lalley, 2005). The injection time of opioid analgesics varies according to the opioid and the dose (i.e., the larger the dose, the longer the injection time); lower doses (e.g., 2 to 3 mg of morphine) may be given by steady injection over 2 or 3 minutes. Some clinicians dilute opioids with normal saline to reduce the likelihood of injecting too rapidly. It may be appropriate to administer large doses of opioids via piggyback infusion using an infusion device. During injection, the patient should be watched closely for effect, and injection must be stopped if adverse effects occur. Pharmacies are encouraged to make information readily available to clinicians about the maximum safe injection rate (mg/min) of the various drugs they administer (Institute for Safe Medication Practices, 2003c).

Clinician-Administered Boluses via the Infusion Pump

If IV PCA is used for pain control, the clinician-administered bolus mode on the infusion pump can be used in the PACU or ED to administer doses during the titration process and whenever they are needed on the clinical unit. This eliminates the time-consuming task of drawing up and administering opioid boluses from a separate syringe.

Supplemental clinician-administered epidural boluses also may be given via the analgesic infusion pump to patients receiving epidural analgesia (see the following patient example). This can help to avoid the need for IV opioid boluses and the sedation they can produce. Administration of epidural analgesic bolus doses is within the scope of practice for nurses in the United States. As discussed, the American Society for Pain Management Nursing (ASPMN) position paper endorses this practice as essential to registered nurses' role in the management of pain by catheter techniques (Pasero, Eksterowicz, Primeau, et al., 2007) (see Chapter 19 for more about intraspinal analgesia).

Patient Example: Titration via Infusion Pump

Mr. M. is awake, responding, and knows where he is when admitted to the PACU after a colon resection. He has an epidural catheter in place with a continuous infusion of hydromorphone (20 mcg/mL) and 0.05% bupivacaine at 10 mL/h (200 mcg/h of hydromorphone). He reports moderate to severe incisional pain (6/10) and his comfort-function goal is 3/10 to cough and deep breathe. He has no nausea, and his respiratory status is acceptable, with a rate of 16/minute and oxygen saturation of 98% on room air. The anesthesiologist's order calls for titration with epidural boluses of 50% to 100% of the hourly opioid dose for patients with moderate to severe pain. At 10:30, Mr. M.'s nurse administers a 5-mL epidural bolus (50% of hourly dose by continuous infusion = 10 mL × 0.50 = 5 mL, or 200 mcg × 0.50 = 100 mcg) using the clinician-administered bolus mode on the pump. At 10:45, Mr. M. reports that his pain is somewhat relieved but continues to be moderate (5/10). He is more alert now and his vital signs are stable. The nurse administers another 5-mL epidural bolus (100 mcg of hydromorphone) through the infusion pump. At 10:55 Mr. M. reports a pain rating of 3/10 and no adverse effects. He is transferred to the nursing unit at 11:15 with his epidural continuous infusion of hydromorphone and bupivacaine at 10 mL/h and a pain rating of 2/10.

Opioid Range Orders

Opioid range orders are medication orders in which the selected dose varies over a prescribed range according to the patient's situation and status (Manworren, 2006). These orders have been used for decades to manage pain (Pasero, Manworren, McCaffery, 2007) and are considered essential to its effective management (Gordon, Dahl, Phillips, et al., 2004).

Support for Opioid Range Orders

The ASPMN and the APS developed a consensus statement advocating the use of range orders in 2004. It states that "a registered nurse who is competent in pain assessment and analgesic administration can safely interpret and implement properly written 'as needed' or PRN range orders for analgesic medications." (p. 1, ASPMN, 2004). Similarly, The Joint Commission (TJC), an independent organization that accredits health care facilities in the United States, approves of the use of range orders, provided policies and procedures are in place and nurses are educated in their implementation (Manworren, 2006).

The ASPMN/APS task force that developed the consensus statement on range orders provided a list of considerations for writing and interpreting PRN opioid range orders

in its publication of the statement (Gordon, Dahl, Phillips, et al., 2004). Among the considerations was the recommendation of a reasonable range, which was described as one with a maximum dose that is at least two times, but generally no larger than four times, the smallest dose in the range. Other important considerations are whether patients are opioid-naïve or opioid-tolerant; their previous responses to opioid analgesics; their ages, organ function, and co-morbidities; the severity of their pain; and the concomitant administration of sedating analgesics. The task force also emphasized the large inter- and intraindividual differences in responses to analgesics and that analgesics should be started at low doses and titrated gradually.

The lack of a predictable relationship between an opioid dose and pain relief underscores the danger of prescribing and administering predetermined doses based on specific pain intensities (Gordon, Dahl, Phillips, et al., 2004). For example, the practice of prescribing IV morphine boluses of 2 mg for mild pain, 4 mg for moderate pain, and 6 mg for severe pain should be avoided. As discussed, nurses must evaluate more than pain intensities when selecting opioid doses (Blumstein, Moore, 2003; Lucas, Vlahos, Ledgerwood, 2007; Taylor, Kirton, Staff, et al., 2005; Taylor, Voytovich, Kozol, 2003). Using the same example, it would be unsafe to administer a 6 mg IV morphine bolus to a patient with severe pain who is excessively sedated (see patient scenarios mentioned later).

Research conducted in two large academic settings to determine which factors nurses consider when implementing a range order revealed that there is wide variability in how nurses interpret such orders (Gordon, Pellino, Higgins, et al., 2008). The nurses in this study were asked to participate in a self-administered online survey that required them to read four vignettes about patients with acute postoperative pain and determine the appropriate dose and timing of dose administration. For example, the first vignette required the nurses to determine how soon a dose could be given to a patient with severe pain following an initial ineffective and safe 2-mg dose from a range order of 2 to 8 mg of IV morphine every 2 hours PRN. Although the majority (68%) responded appropriately, saying that they would administer a dose after 15 to 30 minutes (past peak time), 23% chose to make the patient wait the full 2-hour time period before giving another dose. Responses to another vignette revealed that only 25% of the nurses appeared to recognize that administration of more opioid to a patient experiencing excessive sedation following an initial dose is dangerous (see Chapter 19 for more information about sedation). Clearly, nursing education must precede the use of opioid-range orders in institutions.

Development of a Range Order Protocol

A protocol for implementing opioid range orders that is developed with input from nursing, medicine, and pharmacy may help to ensure more consistent interpretation of range orders and meet TJC requirements. Box 16-3

| **Box 16-3** | Establishment and Implementation of Intravenous Opioid Range Order Protocols |

- Develop guidelines for initial opioid titration.
- Provide prescribers with range order guidelines.
  - When selecting a dose range, consider among other factors the patient's pain intensity, age, co-morbidities (including underlying persistent pain and opioid tolerance), previous response to analgesics, and concomitant medications.
  - Avoid frequency ranges; if they are prescribed, the lowest frequency in the range should be applied; e.g., every 2 hours if every 2 to 4 hours is prescribed.
  - The maximum dose in the range should be at least two times but no more than four times the minimum dose in the range.
  - The range order should include the drug, route of administration, minimum and maximum dose, total time interval, and indication, e.g., morphine 2 to 8 mg IV every 2 hours PRN pain.
  - If the frequency of individual doses is not specified, a frequency of as often as every 10 minutes can be applied.
  - Use a multimodal analgesic approach whenever possible. The addition of nonopioid analgesics, such as acetaminophen and an NSAID, to the opioid regimen will produce better analgesia at lower doses than is possible with any single agent alone.
- Provide recommendations for the interpretation of range orders and demonstrate with examples; the following protocol is described using the example of a range order of morphine 2 to 8 mg IV every 2 hours PRN pain.
  - The nurse will administer an opioid dose if the patient has a sedation level of less than 3 (see POSS, Box 19-4, p. 510) and reports pain that is above the comfort-function goal or if pain is anticipated (e.g., during dressing changes, ambulation, turning, suctioning).
  - The nurse will initiate the order by giving the lowest dose in the range (2 mg).
  - Additional doses equal to the previous dose (2 mg) or 50% of the previous dose (2 mg × 0.50 = 1 mg)—if the nurse considers that repeating the previous dose is unnecessary or potentially unsafe—may be given as often as every 10 minutes until the range order maximum dose is reached within the specified time interval (8 mg in a 2-h period).
  - Total time intervals (2 h) are established according to the time of the first dose administered[1] or according to each individual dose (rolling clock),[2] depending on institutional policy.
  - If the patient's pain ratings are above the comfort-function goal and the patient has a sedation level of

2 or less (see Box 19-4, p. 510) after the first time interval (i.e., the first 2 hours), the initial dose may be increased by 50% (2 mg × 0.50 = 1 mg; 1 mg + 2 mg = 3 mg) to the maximum amount (8 mg) allowed in the range order.
  - The maximum dose (8 mg) is not to be exceeded during any time interval (2 h).
  - Contact the prescriber if either of the following occurs:
    Satisfactory and safe pain relief cannot be accomplished with the dosing parameters of the range order and the institutional protocol; consider alternative methods such as IV PCA or oral ATC analgesia.
    The patient experiences intolerable or unmanageable adverse effects.
- Ensure that sedation level and respiratory status are monitored q 1 h × 12 h, q 2 h × 12 h, then q 4 h if stable (see Chapter 19).
    Perform comprehensive respiratory assessments and use valid and reliable sedation scale to assess sedation levels (see POSS, Box 19-4, p. 510).
- Consider using capnography during parenteral opioid therapy in high-risk patients, such as those with obstructive sleep apnea or chronic obstructive pulmonary disease and those who are very young or very old (see Chapter 19 and Box 19-5, p. 516).
- Develop an education program that ensures nurses' competency in pain assessment and opioid titration.
- Create a quality improvement plan that monitors nurses' performances in the implementation of range orders.

---

[1]The total time period is defined according to the time at which the first dose is given (see text).

[2]The total dose amount cannot be exceeded within the specified time interval, starting at each individual dose, rather than at the first dose (see text).

ATC, Around-the-clock; *IV,* intravenous; *PCA,* patient-controlled analgesia; *POSS,* Pasero Opioid-Induced Sedation Scale; *PRN,* as needed; *q,* every.

From Pasero, C., & McCaffery, M. *Pain assessment and pharmacologic management,* p. 459, St. Louis, Mosby. Data from Gordon, D. B., Dahl, J., Phillips, P., et al. (2004). The use of as-needed range orders for opioid analgesics in the management of acute pain; A consensus statement from the American Society for Pain Management Nursing and the American Pain Society. *Pain Manage Nurs, 5*(2), 53-58; Manworren RCB. (2006). A call to action to protect range orders. *Am J Nurs, 106*(7), 30-33; Pasero, C., Manworren, R. C. B., & McCaffery, M. (2007). IV opioid range orders for acute pain management. *Am J Nurs, 107*(2), 52-59. © 2011, Pasero C, McCaffery M. May be duplicated for use in clinical practice.

provides considerations for protocol development that are based on the principles of IV PCA. Fundamental to successful treatment by both IV PCA and range orders is an understanding that patients should be given access to as much analgesia as the prescription allows, administered in a way that maintains a balance between pain relief and adverse effects (Pasero, Manworren, McCaffery, 2007) (see the following patient examples).

Patient Example: Increase in Dose

Ms. U. has acute pain associated with kidney stones. Her pain rating on admission to the clinical unit is 3/10 after receiving ketorolac and 50 mcg of IV fentanyl in the ED. Her comfort-function goal is 3/10 to visit with her family. She has a range order for fentanyl 10 to 40 mcg IV every hour PRN pain. An hour after admission, Ms. U. reports a pain rating of 4/10. She is alert and her respiratory status is satisfactory. The nurse administers 10 mcg of IV fentanyl. In 15 minutes, Ms. U. rates her pain as 1/10 and she is just slightly drowsy and has a satisfactory respiratory status. An hour later, Ms. U. reports a pain rating of 4/10 and requests analgesia again. Again, she is alert and her respiratory status continues to be satisfactory. The nurse decides to increase the initial dose by 50% (per protocol; see Box 16-3) and administers fentanyl 15 mcg IV (10 mcg × 0.50 [50%] = 5 mcg; 10 mcg + 5 mcg = 15 mcg). Thereafter, Ms. U. experiences stable pain control and no adverse effects with 15 mcg doses of IV fentanyl approximately every 2 hours.

Patient Example: Decrease in Dose

Mr. E. is an alert 82-year-old patient with postoperative pain. He has a range order of morphine 2 to 8 mg IV every 2 hours PRN and is receiving ATC acetaminophen and celecoxib. His comfort-function goal is 4/10 to ambulate to the bathroom. After admission to the clinical unit, his pain rating is 7/10 and his nurse administers 2 mg of IV morphine, but 10 minutes later, his pain rating is essentially the same at 6/10 with no change in sedation or respiratory status, so the nurse repeats the 2-mg morphine dose. Although this reduces Mr. E.'s pain to 2/10 and his respiratory status remains stable, he is excessively sedated and drifts off to sleep during conversation (see Chapter 19). The nurse assigns a nursing technician to monitor

his sedation and respiratory status every 10 to 15 minutes until his sedation level improves. Within 1 hour, Mr. E. is drowsy but no longer excessively sedated, and his pain rating is 2/10. About 2 hours later he reports a pain rating of 4/10 with satisfactory sedation and respiratory status. The nurse wants to maintain good pain control but is concerned that 2 mg of morphine could produce excessive sedation again, so she administers 1 mg (50% decrease in previous dose per protocol; see Box 16-3) (2 mg × 0.50 [50%] = 1 mg; 2 mg − 1 mg = 1 mg). This dose given approximately every 2 hours plus the nonopioid analgesics produced pain ratings of 2/10 with stable sedation levels and respiratory status.

Dose Frequency

One source of confusion regarding range order implementation is related to how often a nurse can administer doses within a range. Using IV PCA as a point of reference, consider that the recommended delay (lockout) interval for acute pain is 5 to 10 minutes (APS, 2003). Although a frequency of 5 to 10 minutes for nurse-administered IV doses may not be realistic in a busy clinical unit, it can be used as a framework for practice. That is, the protocol can state that unless the frequency is prescribed otherwise, nurses may administer subsequent IV doses within a range order as often as every 10 minutes. It may not always be possible to repeat a dose in 10 minutes, but such a protocol allows for those times when it is necessary, safe, and possible (Pasero, Manworren, McCaffery, 2007).

Total Time Interval

Another source of confusion is related to what is called the total time interval, which is the time in which the maximum dose in the range may be administered (Pasero, Manworren, McCaffery, 2007). There are at least two ways to define the total time interval: either according to the time the first dose was given; or according to a "rolling-clock" method whereby the total dose amount cannot be exceeded within a specified time interval, starting at the time of each individual dose, rather than the first dose. Consider a range order for 2 to 8 mg of IV morphine every 2 hours PRN. Clinicians who believe that the total time interval is defined by the time of the first dose would proceed as follows: if a dose is given at 0800, the patient may receive up to 8 mg between 0800 and 1000; the next time interval would begin at 1000 and the patient can be given another 8 mg between 1000 and 1200. Using this same range order example, clinicians who use the rolling-clock approach must be sure the dose about to be administered does not cumulatively exceed the maximum amount (8 mg) in the previous 2-hour period. There is no research or consensus about which method is best; therefore, it is recommended that each institution define the total time interval so that range orders in that institution are interpreted consistently, taking into consideration the potential for error and the time required to calculate the time interval prior to administering a dose (Pasero, Manworren, McCaffery, 2007). Regardless of how the total time interval is defined, it is essential to train nurses to select the appropriate doses and give them at safe intervals on the basis of patients' status and the pharmacokinetics of the opioids. The use of opioid range orders is not recommended in institutions in which this level of training and the establishment of quality-improvement processes that monitor the safety of range order administrations are not possible. Following are two examples; one describes a scenario that applies the total time interval based on first dose; the second describes the same scenario but applies the total time interval based on the rolling clock, starting from each dose.

Patient Example: Total Time Interval Based on the Rolling-Clock Method

Mrs. R. has a range order for 1 to 2 Percocet (oxycodone 5 mg/acetaminophen 325 mg/tablet) every 4 hours PRN pain. She is alert and her condition is stable. She has a pain rating of 4/10 and requests pain medication. The nurse administers 1 Percocet at 1000 (establishing the time interval of 1000 to 1400). An hour later Mrs. R. says her pain has not changed much and rates it 4/10. She continues to be alert. The nurse administers another Percocet tablet (at 1100, establishing a new time interval of 1100 to 1500). An hour later, Mrs. R. reports she is comfortable with a pain rating of 2/10. At 1400 Mrs. R. tells the nurse her pain has returned and is 4/10 again and requests pain medication. The nurse can give 1 Percocet now, or wait 60 minutes for the next time interval to start (1500) and give 2 Percocet, or call Mrs. R.'s physician for additional orders. The nurse knows that 2 Percocet are needed to control Mrs. R.'s pain, so the nurse contacts the physician who orders 2 Percocet to be given now and q4h PRN pain thereafter.

Patient Example: Total Time Interval Based on First Dose

Mrs. R. has a range order for 1 to 2 Percocet (oxycodone 5 mg/acetaminophen 325 mg/tablet) every 4 hours PRN for pain. She is alert and her condition is stable. She has a pain rating of 4/10 and requests pain medication. The nurse administers 1 Percocet at 1000 (establishing the time interval from 1000 to 1400). An hour later Mrs. R. says her pain has not changed much and rates it 4/10. She continues to be alert. The nurse administers another Percocet tablet (at 1100). An hour later, Mrs. R. reports she is comfortable with a pain rating of 2/10. At 1400 Mrs. R. tells the nurse her pain has returned and is 4/10 again and requests pain medication. The nurse administers 2 Percocet at 1400 (establishing a new time interval from 1400 to 1800).

Conclusion

Selection of the initial opioid dose is based on many factors, including patient age, co-morbidities, previous exposure to opioids, and current pain status. Although pain intensity is an important consideration, selection of a dose based solely on a specific pain intensity is dangerous and strongly discouraged. No matter what method is used to predict analgesic requirements, the starting doses of opioid treatments are merely estimates. When starting doses are given, they are titrated up or down according to patient responses. The goal of titration is to use the smallest dose that provides satisfactory pain relief with the fewest adverse effects. It is clear that more research is needed to determine the best titration regimens and how aggressive titration affects the adverse-effect profiles of patients after discharge from areas like the ED and PACU. The best course of action is for clinicians and patients to view the achievement of optimal pain relief as occurring on a continuum, with the primary objective being to provide both effective and safe analgesia.

Chapter 17 Intravenous Patient-Controlled Analgesia

PCA pumps are used to administer opioids by the SC, IV, and epidural routes. Their use requires prescribing a number of parameters (Box 17-1), many of which are safety features to help prevent overdosing; however, it is important for clinicians to appreciate that the safety of PCA depends on appropriate patient selection, initial and ongoing patient/family and staff teaching and goal setting, patient-only use, systematic assessment of responses, and adjustments in therapy as needed (Macintyre, Coldrey, 2009). The reader is referred to an in-depth discussion and comparison of the various analgesic infusion devices used to administer PCA in Sherman, B., Enu, I., & Sinatra, R. S. (2009). Patient-controlled analgesia devices and analgesic infusion pumps. In R. S. Sinatra, O. A. de Leon-Casasola, B. Ginsberg, et al. (Eds.), *Acute pain management*, Cambridge, NY, Cambridge University Press. Included are desirable pump features and general purchasing considerations.

The focus of this chapter is primarily on the clinical use of IV PCA. See Chapter 12 for the underlying principles and research on the efficacy of PCA, Chapter 15 for epidural patient-controlled analgesia (PCEA), and Section V for PCRA.

Initial Intravenous Patient-Controlled Analgesia (PCA) Prescription

The starting prescription for IV PCA in an opioid-tolerant patient is based on the patient's current total daily opioid dose. If the patient is switched from one opioid or route to another, this initial prescription is an estimate and must be adjusted according to the patient's pain and adverse effect profile. The starting PCA prescription for an opioid-naive patient is also just an estimate of a patient's opioid requirement and must be titrated on the basis of patient response. Table 17-1 provides guidelines for selecting an initial IV PCA prescription for opioid-naive patients and Form 17-1 provides an example of a PCA order set. See an example of a patient information brochure about IV PCA on pp. 544-545 at the end of Section IV.

P ATIENT-CONTROLLED analgesia (PCA) is an interactive method of pain management that permits patients to treat their pain by self-administering doses of analgesics. It has been used to manage all types of pain, most commonly acute pain and less often cancer pain because most cancer pain can be managed by oral or transdermal opioid analgesics. Although patients with pain often self-administer their oral analgesics, the term *PCA* is usually applied when opioids are administered by the intravenous (IV); subcutaneous (SC); continuous peripheral nerve block (patient-controlled regional analgesia [PCRA]; epidural; or intranasal routes of administration. The PCA approach recognizes that only the patient can feel the pain, and only the patient know how much analgesic will relieve it (Pasero, McCaffery, 1993; Pasero, Portenoy, McCaffery, 1999). By allowing patients to determine dosing, PCA addresses the significant variations in analgesic requirements between individuals (Grass, 2005; Lehmann, 2005).

- Drug concentration: Concentration of drug per milliliter solution in the drug reservoir.
- Drug reservoir volume: Amount of solution in drug reservoir.
- PCA bolus dose: Amount patient will receive each time a bolus is self-administered.
- Lockout (delay) interval: Amount of time that must elapse between PCA doses administered.
- Basal rate: Amount of the continuous infusion. This feature is optional.
- Hour limit: The maximum amount the patient can receive in 1 hour or 4 hours by PCA bolus doses and basal rate. This feature is optional on many pumps.
- Important history available in most PCA pumps:
  - PCA attempts: Number of times patient presses the PCA button
  - PCA injections: Number of times patient successfully self-administers a PCA dose
  - Volume given
  - Volume remaining in drug reservoir

PCA, Patient-controlled analgesia.
From Pasero, C., & McCaffery, M. *Pain assessment and pharmacologic management*, p. 463, St. Louis, Mosby. © 2011, Pasero C, McCaffery M. May be duplicated for use in clinical practice.

Bolus Dose and Lockout Interval

To a great extent, the success of IV PCA depends on prescribing an adequate bolus dose that can be self-administered frequently enough for patients to manage their pain effectively. Small doses of analgesia (e.g., 1 mg of morphine or equivalent) and short lockout (delay) intervals (e.g., 5 to 10 minutes) are best for opioid-naïve patients so as to prevent excessive sedation at peaks (the highest blood levels of opioid) and to prevent breakthrough pain at troughs (the lowest blood levels of opioid); however, if the dose is too small, patients may have difficulty maintaining analgesia (Macintyre, Coldrey, 2008). Larger bolus doses at lockout intervals of 15 to 30 minutes are commonly required and are usually well tolerated by opioid-tolerant patients with cancer or persistent noncancer pain. The optimal dose should provide consistent, satisfactory analgesia without excessive or dangerous adverse effects (Macintyre, Coldrey, 2008).

There is surprisingly little research to guide selection of an optimal PCA bolus dose for an opioid-naïve patient. An early randomized controlled trial found comparable efficacy, morphine consumption, and adverse effects with PCA doses of 1 mg every 6 minutes, 1.5 mg every 9 minutes, and 2 mg every 12 minutes (Badner, Doyle, Smith, et al., 1996). PCA attempts, successful injections, missed injections, and dose adjustments were greatest in the group receiving 1 mg; however, one patient in the group receiving 1.5 mg and one in the group receiving 2 mg required naloxone for respiratory depression. The researchers

GUIDELINES

Table 17-1 | Starting IV PCA Prescription Ranges for Acute Pain in Opioid-Naïve Adults[1]

Drug	Typical Concentration	Loading Dose	PCA Dose	Lockout (delay) (min)	Basal Rate[2]
Morphine	1 mg/mL	2.5 mg, may repeat PRN	0.5-2 mg	8	0-0.5 mg/h
Hydromorphone	0.2 mg/mL	0.4 mg, may repeat PRN	0.1-0.4 mg	6-8	0-0.1 mg/h
Fentanyl	10-20 mcg/mL	25 mcg, may repeat PRN	5-25 mcg	5-6	0-5 mcg/h
Oxymorphone	0.25 mg/mL	0.4 mg, may repeat PRN	0.25-0.5 mg	8-10	0-0.25 mg/h
Meperidine[3]	10 mg/mL	20 mg, may repeat PRN	5-20 mg	5-10	NR[4]

h, Hour; *mcg,* microgram; *mg,* milligram; *min,* minute; *mL,* milliliter; *NR,* not recommended; *PRN,* as needed.
[1]Prescription ranges in this table are calculated for severe acute pain. Ranges can be reduced by percentages for less severe pain (e.g., 50% reduction, see Chapter 16).
[2]Basal rates in opioid-naïve patients should be used with caution. If used, the amount should be low (e.g., 0.5 mg/h of morphine or less), and patients must be watched closely for advancing sedation and respiratory depression. The basal rate should be discontinued promptly if excessive sedation is detected (see Chapter 19).
[3]Should be used for very brief course (e.g., no more than 48 hours), in patients who are allergic to and intolerant of the other opioids listed in this chart. Maximum daily amount should not exceed 600 mg (see Chapter 13 for assessment of normeperidine toxicity).
[4]Accumulation of normeperidine can cause toxic central nervous system effects, such as irritability and seizures, and is more likely to occur when meperidine is administered by continuous infusion.

To save time and prevent errors, tables containing PCA prescription ranges commonly used in opioid-naïve patients can be developed in advance. This table is an example of a table used in cases of for severe pain.
From Pasero, C., & McCaffery, M. *Pain assessment and pharmacologic management*, p. 463, St. Louis, Mosby. Data from American Pain Society (APS). (2003). *Principles of analgesic use in the treatment of acute and cancer pain*, ed 5, Glenview, IL, APS; Cashman, J. (2006). Patient-controlled analgesia. In G. Shorten, D. B. Carr, D. Harmon, et al. (eds). *Postoperative pain management: An evidence-based guide to practice*, Philadelphia, Saunders; Macintyre, P. E., & Coldrey, J. (2008). Patient-controlled analgesia. In P. E. Macintyre, S. M. Walker, & D. J. Rowbotham (Eds.), *Clinical pain management. Acute pain*, ed 2, London, Hodder Arnold; Macintyre, P. E., & Coldrey, J. (2009). Intravenous patient-controlled analgesia. In R. S. Sinatra, O. A. de Leon-Casasola, B. Ginsberg, et al. (Eds.), *Acute pain management*, Cambridge, NY, Cambridge University Press. © 2011, Pasero C, McCaffery M. May be duplicated for use in clinical practice.

1. Discontinue previous analgesia orders; no other opioids or sedatives are to be given except as ordered here.

2. Administer PCA therapy via antireflux y-tubing with maintenance IV.

3. Label PCA button with Patient-Use Only sticker.

4. Drug and concentration:
   ___ Morphine sulfate 1 milligram (**mg**)/mL
   ___ Hydromorphone HCl (Dilaudid) 0.2 milligram (**mg**)/mL
   ___ Fentanyl 10 micrograms (**mcg**)/mL
   ___ Other: _____

   Meperidine (Demerol) is not recommended, especially in patients older than 65 years of age and those with renal impairment, or for therapy lasting longer than 72 hours, because of its metabolite, normeperidine, which can produce central nervous system irritability, seizures, and death. References available upon request.

5. Complete prescription:

Suggested Initial Dosing Regimens

Opioid	Morphine 1 mg/mL	Hydromorphone (Dilaudid) 0.2 mg/mL	Fentanyl 10 mcg/mL
Loading bolus dose	2-8 mg (2.5 mg)____	0.4-1.6 mg (0.4 mg)____	25-100 mcg (25 mcg)____
PCA bolus dose	0.5-2 mg (1 mg)____	0.1-0.4 mg (0.2 mg)____	5-25 mcg (10 mcg)____
Lockout	5-10 min (8 min)____	5-10 min (6 min)____	4-8 min (5 min)____
Continuous (basal) rate (use with caution in opioid-naive patients)	0-1 mg/h (0.5 mg/h)____	0-0.2 mg/h (0.1 mg/h)____	0-10 mcg/h (5 mcg/h)____

6. Unrelieved pain (contact prescriber for pain unrelieved by the following):
   ___ Repeat loading dose × 2 prn if pain rating is more than 3/10 and sedation level is lower than 3 (see POSS in Box 19-4, p. XXX).
   ___ Increase PCA dose by 25% to 50% if pain rating is more than 3/10 and sedation level lower than 3 (see POSS in Box 19-4, p. XXX).

7. Laxative (one recommended for all patients):
   ___ Docusate sodium 50 mg + senna 8.6 mg PO qd
   ___ Bisacodyl 5 mg PO or PR qd

8. Nonopioid (**one** NSAID + acetaminophen recommended ATC for all postoperative patients unless contraindicated):
   ___ Ketorolac 15 mg IV q 8 h × 48 h for patients <60 years of age
   ___ Ketorolac 7.5 mg q 8 h × 48 h for patients ≥60 years of age
   (Do not give ketorolac if hypovolemia, renal dysfunction, peptic or gastric ulcers, or bleeding problems are present)
   ___ Ibuprofen 400 mg IVPB infusion over 30 min q 6 h
   ___ Ibuprofen 400 mg PO or PR q 6 h (give PR if NPO or nauseated)
   ___ Celecoxib 400 mg PO qd (consider CV risk; see Chapter 19)
   ___ Acetaminophen 650 mg PO or PR q 6 h (may be given at same time as NSAID; give PR if patient is nauseated)

9. Monitoring and documentation (use 24-Hour Pain Management Flow Sheet in Chapter 3):
   • Sedation level (see POSS in Box 19-4, p. 510) and respiratory status q 1 h × 12 h, q 2 h × 12 h, then q 4 h if stable for duration of therapy; pain rating q 4 h if pain is stable
   • Other vital signs q 4 h
   • PCA pump history q 4 h and whenever prescription changes are made

10. Side-effect management (contact prescriber for side effects unrelieved by the following):
    • Pruritus (itching): Stop basal rate. If patient has no basal rate and pain is acceptable, reduce PCA bolus dose 25%. In addition, give:
      ___ Ondansetron 4 mg IV q 8 h
      ___ Diphenhydramine 12.5 mg IV q 4 h prn
      ___ Diphenhydramine 25 mg PO
      ___ (Diphenhydramine can cause excessive sedation; do not give if POSS >2)
      ___ Other: _____
    • Nausea/vomiting: Stop basal rate. If patient has no basal rate and pain is acceptable, reduce PCA bolus dose 25%. Give:
      ___ Droperidol 0.625 mg IV q 6 h
         Dexamethasone 8 mg IV × 1
      ___ Ondansetron 4 mg IV q 8 h
      ___ Other: _____
    • Increasing sedation (POSS = 3): (1) Stop basal rate. If patient has no basal rate, reduce PCA bolus dose by 50%; (2) hold other CNS depressants, including diphenhydramine, and (3) monitor LOS, respiratory status, and pain rating q 15 min until LOS is less than 3.
    • Excessive sedation (POSS = 4) or respiratory depression (respiratory rate 8/min or less): (1) *Stop PCA pump*; stimulate patient, support respirations as needed; (2) call Rapid Response Team; (3) ask coworker to notify primary physician immediately; (4) give IV dilute naloxone (0.4 mg of naloxone per 10 mL normal saline) 0.5 mL over 2 minutes; repeat this dose until POSS is less than 4 and respirations are more than 8/minute (see Box 19-6, p. 521); (5) monitor LOS, respiratory status, and pain rating q 15 min until LOS is less than 3 for more than 1 hour.

Signature_____   Date_____

Form 17-1 | Example Order Set: Opioid-Naïve Adult IV PCA

CNS, Central nervous system; *CV,* cardiovascular; *hs,* at sleep; *IV,* intravenous; *IVPB,* IV piggyback; *LOS,* level of sedation; *PO,* oral; *POSS,* Pasero Opioid-Induced Sedation Scale; *PR,* per rectum; *PRN,* as needed; *q,* every.

From Pasero, C., & McCaffery, M. *Pain assessment and pharmacologic management,* p. 464, St. Louis, Mosby. © 2011, Pasero C, McCaffery M. May be duplicated for use in clinical practice.

concluded that 1 mg every 6 minutes represents appropriate titration but may result in lower patient satisfaction. Another study concluded similarly that 0.5 mg of IV morphine was not large enough to control pain, and 2 mg was associated with adverse effects, but 1 mg was an optimal bolus dose for postoperative pain in opioid-naïve patients (Owen, Plummer, Armstrong, et al., 1989). A randomized controlled study of IV fentanyl use during burn dressing changes showed that PCA bolus doses of 30 to 40 mcg of fentanyl with a lockout of 5 minutes produced better analgesia and demand/delivery ratios than did 10-mcg and 20-mcg bolus doses (Prakash, Fatima, Pawar, 2004). No research could be found on the optimal PCA bolus dose or lockout interval for hydromorphone, the other opioid commonly used for IV PCA; however, 0.1 to 0.2 mg of IV hydromorphone is considered roughly equal to 1 mg of IV morphine in this setting (Knotkova, Fine, Portenoy, 2009).

There is also very little research on the optimal lockout (delay) interval for IV PCA (Macintyre, Coldrey, 2008). The length of the lockout interval should allow for adequate analgesic coverage during times when patients need the most opioid. For example, postoperative patients should be able to activate PCA before and frequently during potentially painful activities, such as ambulation, self-care, and physical therapy or respiratory therapy treatments. The lockout interval also should be long enough for a patient to appreciate the effect of one bolus before self-administering another (Macintyre, Coldrey, 2008). The characteristics of the opioid, such as the onset and peak times, are primary determinants of the length of the lockout interval. The American Pain Society (APS, 2003) recommends a lockout interval of between 5 and 10 minutes for most of the IV opioids used for acute pain. For example, commonly used lockout intervals are 5 to 6 minutes for IV fentanyl and 6 to 8 minutes for IV PCA morphine and hydromorphone for acute pain management.

The customary adult starting dose should be reduced by 25% to 50% for opioid-naïve older patients because research has shown that analgesia requirements decrease with increasing age (Gagliese, Jackson, Ritvo, et al., 2000; Macintyre, Coldrey, 2009). In a review of more than 6000 patients aged 65 and older who had received IV PCA, bolus doses greater than 1 mg/dose and intraabdominal surgery were cited as risk factors for hypoxemia and respiratory depression during IV PCA (Sidebotham, Dijkhuizen, Schug, 1997). Also, the lockout interval is sometimes increased to 10 minutes in this population.

Hour Limit

The hour limit is the maximum amount of opioid a patient has access to in an hour-limit time period. Most PCA pumps can be programmed for a 1-hour or 4-hour limit, and some pumps allow this parameter to be bypassed altogether. If an hour limit has been programmed and the patient consumes the programmed amount before the time period has expired, the pump denies the patient any further PCA bolus doses until the next hour-limit time period begins. The programmed hour limit includes the number of PCA bolus doses and the basal rate (if one is programmed). Some PCA pumps also include clinician-administered bolus doses in the hour-limit amount.

There is no consensus about whether hour limits should be used. Those who choose not to use them do so because they think patients should have access to as much opioid as they need to manage their pain, restricted only by the amount of the dose and the length of the lockout interval. Those who choose to use an hour limit do so because they think it offers an additional safeguard against overdosing; however, this thinking may provide false reassurance; the only built-in safeguard of PCA is patient-only use (see discussion of PCA by proxy later in this chapter). A benefit of programming an hour limit is that it alerts caregivers that increased doses might be necessary. Hour limits seem to be used more commonly in opioid-naïve than in opioid-tolerant patients. If used, a 1-hour limit is preferable to a 4-hour limit for at least two reasons: (1) caregivers are alerted to the need for an increase in the opioid dose sooner (i.e., within 1 hour instead of within 4 hours); and (2) it eliminates a scenario in which an increase in dose is neglected in patients who use the 4-hour amount in less than 4 hours (i.e., a patient who uses the 4-hour amount in 2 hours and is left for 2 hours without analgesia). In an analysis of data submitted to MEDMARX and the United States Pharmacopeia (USP) Medication Errors Reporting Program between 1998 and 2003, the USP identified this scenario as a common PCA-related underdosing error (USP, 2004). It is essential that the hour limit be adjusted up or down as necessary on the basis of patient response. If used, the APS (2003) recommends that the hour limit be set at 3 to 5 times the projected hourly IV requirement for at least the first 24 hours.

Continuous Infusion (Basal Rate)

The purpose of a continuous infusion (basal rate) is to help maintain a stable analgesic level (American Society of Anesthesiologists [ASA], 2004; Flisberg, Rudin, Linner, et al., 2003). It has the advantage of letting the patient sleep without frequent interruptions by pain. If a continuous infusion is not added, patients must self-administer the PCA dose often enough to maintain a stable analgesic level. When IV PCA is used to manage cancer or persistent noncancer pain in opioid-tolerant patients, the continuous infusion usually provides the larger part of the patient's total opioid requirement, with PCA doses being used as breakthrough doses (APS, 2003). Although continuous infusion is recommended and is commonly used for opioid-tolerant patients, the addition of continuous infusion to IV PCA bolus doses for opioid-naïve patients outside of a monitored setting such as the intensive care unit (ICU) is controversial (APS, 2003; Pasero, McCaffery, 2004). The primary safeguard in PCA therapy is that a patient must be awake to self-administer a PCA dose. Patients who are excessively sedated are likely to drop the PCA button, thereby preventing further sedation and clinically significant respiratory depression (Pasero, McCaffery, 2004). Herein lies the controversy. The patient has no control over the delivery of a continuous infusion, so the built-in safeguard is gone. The APS (2003) recommends extreme caution in using basal rates for acute pain management in opioid-naïve patients.

Studies have produced mixed findings in terms of the effectiveness and safety of adding continuous infusions to IV PCA in opioid-naïve patients. Early research showed that the addition of a continuous infusion did not improve analgesia, produced excessive adverse effects, and resulted in consumption of greater amounts of opioid drugs (Parker, Holtmann, White, 1991; Russell, Owen, Ilsley, et al., 1996; Smythe, Zak, O'Donnell, 1996). A more recent study of 35 patients following open heart surgery found no differences in pain intensity scores or adverse effects between patients who received PCA with or without a basal rate and concluded that no benefit could be found in adding a basal rate to PCA therapy (Dal, Canback, Cagler, et al., 2003). There was no excessive sedation or clinically significant respiratory depression. Another study of 60 patients after cardiac surgery reported that a basal rate with PCA increased morphine consumption but improved pain relief without increasing adverse effects (Guler, Unlugenc, Gundogan, et al., 2004). There were no episodes of respiratory depression or hypoxemia. Others have also found less fluctuation in sedation and better pain control and have recommended the addition of a basal rate to IV PCA for some patients (Hansen, Noyes, Lehman, 1991; Rayburn, Smith, Woods, 1989). A prospective study of more than 1000 patients receiving IV PCA morphine with basal rates after major surgery reported that respiratory depression occurred in 13 patients (1.2%) (Flisberg, Rudin, Linner, et al., 2003). Interestingly, a study of 178 postoperative patients who were monitored using continuous pulse oximetry (oxygen saturation) and capnography (end-tidal CO_2) while receiving IV PCA demonstrated that despite consuming approximately two times more opioid, those who were receiving PCA with a continuous basal rate (1 mg/h morphine equivalent) had lower incidences of bradypnea (32% vs. 53%) and desaturation (8% vs. 17%) than did those who were receiving PCA bolus doses without a basal rate (Overdyk, Carter, Maddox, et al., 2007) (see Chapter 19 for discussion of mechanical monitoring).

An important finding in an early study by Parker and colleagues (1991) is noted in the percentages of patients in the various groups in the study who required changes in morphine PCA therapy or discontinuation of therapy entirely because of adverse effects. The lowest was 10% of the group receiving a 0.5 mg/h basal rate followed by 11% of those with no basal rate, 14% of those with a 1 mg/h basal rate, and 66% of those receiving a 2 mg/h basal rate (Parker, Holtmann, White, 1991). During the first 2 days of the study, the pain ratings were lowest in the group receiving the 0.5 mg/h basal rate. These findings reinforce the rationale that the adverse effects of opioids are dose related and that basal rates greater than 1 mg/h are not well tolerated and may be unsafe; however, a basal rate of 0.5 mg/h can be safe and may improve analgesia for some patients.

Clinical experience indicates that the addition of a continuous infusion to IV PCA can be done safely and may benefit some patients (ASA, 2004; Pasero, McCaffery, 2004). A cautious approach and one that is supported by research is to begin PCA without a basal rate, and then add one later if a patient has difficulty maintaining satisfactory pain control, especially after sleep (Pasero, Portenoy, McCaffery, 1999) (see the following patient example). Initiating therapy without a basal rate may be particularly appropriate in older patients. As mentioned, PCA requirements tend to decrease with increasing age (Macintyre, Coldrey, 2008; Sidebotham, Dijkhuizen, Schug, 1997); however, the decision to add a continuous infusion to IV PCA for older opioid-naïve patients should be made on the basis of patients' responses rather than on a preconceived notion that they cannot tolerate continuous infusions.

Absolutely essential to the safe use of continuous infusions in opioid-naïve patients is close monitoring by nurses of sedation and respiratory status and prompt decreasing of the opioid dose if increased sedation is detected (Pasero, 2009b). The use of mechanical monitoring (e.g., pulse oximetry, capnography) may be appropriate in some patients receiving IV PCA (see Chapter 19 for more information about monitoring sedation and respiratory depression). If careful monitoring of sedation and respiratory status is not possible, the use of continuous opioid infusions in opioid-naive patients is not recommended (Pasero, McCaffery, 2004).

Patient Example: Opioid Naïve

After total hip replacement, Mrs. G. is managing her pain with IV PCA hydromorphone. She has been stable since surgery 7 hours earlier. She is alert and has a respiratory rate of 16 breaths/minute. She has self-administered an average of four PCA doses every hour since PCA was started in the PACU. She rates her pain 4/10, has a comfort-function goal of 2/10 to turn and deep breathe, and says that she is unable to fall asleep and is afraid that if she does, her pain will become out of control. Adding a basal rate to her PCA therapy may provide the solution. Mrs. G. self-administers a PCA dose of 0.2 mg about 4 times/h, so her hourly requirement is 0.2 mg × 4 = 0.8 mg/h. A conservative basal rate of 0.1 mg is started. The nursing staff monitors Mrs. G.'s sedation level and respiratory status every hour during infusion. Later that day Mrs. G. reports that she is able to rest much better, is no longer worried about losing pain control, and does not have to "work so hard" to keep her pain under control. (She now averages one to two PCA doses/h.) She notes that her present pain rating of 2/10 is better than it was before the basal rate was added. Her respiratory status has been stable, and she has experienced no more than mild sedation.

PCA in Opioid-Tolerant Patients

For patients with cancer or persistent noncancer pain who are receiving continuous opioid infusions, PCA offers an independent means of managing breakthrough pain (see the following patient example). In these opioid-tolerant patients, the continuous infusion provides most of the opioid requirements. The PCA bolus doses are larger, usually allowing patients to double the dose provided by the continuous infusion, and lockout intervals are longer than in opioid-naïve patients (APS, 2003). For example, a PCA bolus dose usually is 25% to 50% of the hourly continuous-infusion dose, and the lockout interval usually is set at 15 to 30 minutes.

Patient Example: Opioid Tolerant

Mrs. S. has been receiving a subcutaneous (SC) infusion of morphine 30 mg/h to control her cancer pain. While in the hospital, the nurses offer her SC breakthrough bolus doses every 2 hours. Often, Mrs. S. has been tolerating pain rather than asking the nurses for breakthrough doses. Her family is concerned that this pattern will continue at home. Her nurse discusses the concept of PCA with Mrs. S. and her family. They are receptive to the idea of using SC PCA to control Mrs. S.'s breakthrough pain. Her PCA bolus dose is calculated at 8 mg (approximately 25% of the hourly morphine dose) with a lockout interval of 15 minutes. Mrs. S. self-administers doses readily, reports better pain control, and is significantly more satisfied with her pain treatment plan once she has PCA. She remains alert and her activity level improves.

Loading Dose

A key principle of PCA therapy is that it be initiated in a patient who has reasonably well-controlled pain. Before the PCA button is handed to the patient for self-management,

loading doses are administered to establish analgesia (Cashman, 2006). A common and recommended practice is to store a specified number of PCA pumps, drug reservoirs, and infusion tubings (number is dependent on the size of the institution) in the emergency department [ED] so that the therapy can be initiated without delay in patients who are admitted for treatment of severe pain crises. Loading doses can be administered using the clinician-administered bolus mode on most PCA pumps (see Chapter 16 for titration in patients with severe acute pain and loading-dose recommendations in Table 17-1).

Initiating PCA in the Postanesthesia Care Unit and Patient Transfer to the Clinical Unit

When IV PCA is prescribed for postoperative patients, it should be initiated when the patients arrive in the postanesthesia care unit (PACU) (Krenzischek, Wilson, 2003). Initiating IV PCA in the PACU rather than in the nursing unit allows the health care team to evaluate patient responses to the therapy early in the postoperative period and prevents delays in analgesia (analgesic gaps) in the nursing unit. A particularly dangerous scenario that is to be avoided is that of patients receiving intramuscular (IM) injections of opioid in the clinical unit while waiting for IV PCA to be initiated (see Chapter 14 for more on the dangers of IM injections).

The PACU nurse can save time by using the PCA pump to administer loading doses and establish satisfactory analgesia. Then the PCA button should be given to patients as soon as they are awake and alert enough to manage their own pain. At that time, pain management plans can be reviewed with patients, including which actions to take when pain relief is inadequate. PACU nurses can reinforce information about the safety mechanisms of the PCA pump and about how to use the PCA button correctly, reminding patients that it is for their use only.

Some PACUs establish discharge goals that include acceptable pain ratings for patients, usually 4/10 or less (Pasero, McCaffery, 2003) (see Section II); however, the expectation that all patients must be discharged from the PACU with pain ratings below an arbitrary number can lead to the unsafe administration of further opioid doses to patients who are excessively sedated (Blumstein, Moore, 2003; Lucas, Vlahos, Ledgerwood, 2007). Instead, achieving optimal pain relief is best viewed on a continuum, with the primary objective being to provide both effective and safe analgesia. Although it is not always possible to achieve the patient's comfort-function goal within the short time the patient is in an area like the PACU, the comfort-function goal provides direction for ongoing care. Important information to give to the nurse assuming care of the patient in the clinical unit is the patient's comfort-function goal, how close the patient is to achieving it, what has been done thus far to achieve it (analgesics, doses, and times of administration), and how well the patient has tolerated the administration of analgesics (adverse effects) (see Chapter 19 for more on transfer of care and hand-off communication).

Patient Example: PACU

Mrs. B. is in the PACU after a total abdominal hysterectomy. She will be managing her postoperative pain with IV PCA morphine. Mrs. B.'s nurse has attached the PCA pump to Mrs. B.'s IV line and will use the clinician-administered bolus mode on the pump to deliver IV boluses of morphine until Mrs. B. can manage her own pain. The equianalgesic chart that can be used to calculate appropriate clinician-administered IV boluses for titration in the PACU is as follows:

- Morphine is located in the first column of the equianalgesic chart.
- Moving horizontally from morphine to column number 3 (parenteral route), the appropriate dose for severe pain is located (10 mg).
- Mrs. B. reports a pain rating of 9/10, or severe pain, so the appropriate starting dose for her is 10 mg of morphine IV over a 4-hour period (approximately 2.5 mg/h).
- The nurse decides to administer the starting hourly dose and titrate upward or downward by using larger or smaller boluses according to institutional protocol, depending on patient response (pain intensity and adverse effects).

Mrs. B. requires three boluses of 2.5 mg within a 45-minute period to reduce her pain to 4/10, which is acceptable to her. She is only slightly drowsy, is reporting mild nausea requiring no treatment, and is ready to manage her own pain. Because Mrs. B. is opioid-naïve, her starting PCA prescription is selected using the equianalgesic chart and her pain intensity before titration, which was 9/10, or severe:

- The amount of morphine appropriate for Mrs. B. is 10 mg over a 4-hour period.
- The projected hourly requirement for Mrs. B. is 10 mg ÷ 4 h = 2.5 mg.
- The average lockout interval for morphine is 8 minutes. With an 8-minute lockout, the number of times Mrs. B. can self-administer a PCA dose in 1 hour is calculated: 60 minutes ÷ 8 = approximately 7 times.
- The PCA dose is calculated as 2.5 mg ÷ 7 times/h or approximately 0.4 mg/PCA dose. The decision is made to start with PCA only and no basal rate. Her starting IV PCA prescription is PCA dose 0.5 mg (morphine PCA doses are usually prescribed in 0.5-mg increments); lockout interval 8 minutes; no basal rate.

The nurse reviews with Mrs. B. how to use the PCA pump to manage her pain, then discharges her from the PACU mildly sedated, comfortable with a pain rating of 4/10, and self-administering PCA without difficulty.

To save time and prevent errors, tables containing prescription ranges of PCAs commonly used in opioid-naïve patients can be developed in advance (see Table 17-1). These tables can be posted in areas where prescribers write orders for PCA. Preprinted order sets with the appropriate starting IV PCA prescriptions for the most commonly used opioids guide prescribers to select individualized doses on the basis of their patients' unique characteristics (see Form 17-1).

Titration of IV PCA

As discussed, initial PCA prescriptions are estimates of the amounts of opioid patients will require. It is crucial that patients be evaluated regularly and titrated when necessary to maintain adequate analgesia and tolerable and manageable adverse effects. Patients reporting inadequate pain relief with the use of PCA require prompt evaluation. The need for readjustment of the parameters of PCA is signaled by pain ratings above the identified comfort-function goal or by unmanageable and intolerable adverse effects. Pain ratings and the incidence of adverse effects, in addition to the patient's account and the PCA history retained in the pump's memory, provide valuable information about the pain and should be used to guide the various approaches to titration. For example, approaches differ between patients who are not activating PCA before painful activity (incident pain) and those who make multiple unsuccessful attempts to obtain a PCA dose. Table 17-2 provides interventions for patients receiving IV PCA or epidural analgesia.

The use of PCA does not absolve nurses from their roles as patients' primary pain managers. Simply telling a patient to "press the PCA button" does not constitute acceptable pain management. Likewise, concluding that a patient is using too much opioid or pressing the PCA button too often (e.g., when a patient self-administers the maximum programmed amount [hour limit] in less than 1 hour) has no scientific basis and creates an adversarial relationship between patient and caregiver. More importantly, it presents a tremendous barrier to providing acceptable pain treatment and improving patient outcome.

PCA by Proxy

PCA by proxy is the *unauthorized* administration of a PCA dose by another person. This has the potential to produce significant patient harm because it circumvents an important safeguard of PCA; that is, the excessively sedated patient will drop the PCA button, thereby preventing further opioid administration and subsequent respiratory depression (Pasero, McCaffery, 2005a). Over the years, there have been reports of the dangers of PCA by proxy. One early report evaluated 3785 patients who

Table 17-2 | Improvement of Pain Control and Reduction of Adverse Effects Associated with IV PCA and Epidural Analgesia

Problem	Intervention
No pain relief and no adverse effects	1. Check that infusion system is patent and functioning from pump to patient access site. 2. Check that pump is loaded and programmed correctly. 3. Check that PCA (PCEA) button is attached to pump. Review PCA (PCEA) history (see disproportionate injection/attempt ratio, below). 4. Check that lockout (delay) interval is appropriate (see text). 5. Relieve pain by administering supplemental boluses (see text). 6. Increase the opioid dose 25% to 100%. For patient with continuous epidural infusion (basal rate) only, increase basal rate. For opioid-tolerant patient, increase basal rate with proportional increase in the PCA (PCEA) bolus dose. For opioid-naïve patient, increase PCA bolus dose or shorten lockout interval. Addition of a basal rate should be considered if patient is unable to rest adequately; however, this must be used with extreme caution (see text). 7. If hour limit is used, increase it proportionately.
No pain relief with adverse effects	1. Complete intervention steps 1 through 4 for the first problem in this box (above). 2. Treat with adverse-effect medication. 3. Add or increase nonopioid or appropriate adjuvant. 4. Decrease opioid dose 25% (in opioid-naïve patients receiving basal rate with IV PCA, stop basal rate first). 5. Monitor pain and adverse effects closely; contact provider for orders if pain or adverse effects continue.
Pain relief with adverse effects	1. Treat with adverse-effect medication. 2. Decrease opioid dose by 25% to 50%; larger decreases or discontinuation of therapy may be necessary to treat excessive sedation and respiratory depression. In opioid naïve patients receiving a basal rate with IV PCA, stop basal rate first. 3. Monitor pain and adverse effects closely; contact provider for orders if pain control is lost or adverse effects continue.
Pain relief with adverse effects occurring just after PCA (PCEA) dose administration (e.g., excessive sedation after self-administration of PCA [PCEA] dose)	1. Treat with adverse-effect medication. 2. In opioid naïve patients receiving a basal rate with IV PCA, stop basal rate first. To decrease the peak effect and lower the level of toxicity associated with PCA dose administration, give smaller doses more often (i.e., decrease the PCA [PCEA] bolus dose 25% to 50% and shorten the lockout interval). 3. Monitor pain and adverse effects closely; contact provider for orders if pain control is lost or adverse effects continue.
Pain relief except during activity; no adverse effects	Remind patient to self-administer PCA (PCEA) before activity (e.g., 2 to 3 minutes for IV PCA and 5 to 10 minutes for PCEA), then continue to self-administer as needed during activity.
Maximum programmed amount used (1- or 4-hour limit reached)	In this situation, the infusion pump will not allow the patient to self-administer anymore PCA (PCEA) bolus doses until the PCA hour elapses. Patients may or may not be in pain, but the need to assess and consider increasing the dose is the same for all who reach their hour limits. If patient is in pain and has tolerable and manageable adverse effects, relieve pain by administering supplemental boluses (see text). All patients: 1. Check to see whether lockout interval and hour limit are appropriate (see text) and are programmed correctly. 2. Increase the opioid dose 25% to 100% if patient is in pain and has tolerable and manageable adverse effects. For opioid-tolerant patient, increase the basal rate with a proportional increase in the PCA (PCEA) bolus dose and hour limit; for opioid-naïve patient, increase PCA (PCEA) bolus dose; the addition of a basal rate may be appropriate; however, this must be used with extreme caution (see text). 3. Increase hour limit proportionately.

Continued

Table 17-2 | Improvement of Pain Control and Reduction of Adverse Effects Associated with IV PCA and Epidural Analgesia—cont'd

Problem	Intervention
Somnolence, respiratory depression	1. In opioid-naïve patient, stop opioid; in opioid-tolerant patient, consider decreasing opioid dose by 75% instead of stopping opioid, to maintain enough opioid to prevent withdrawal. 2. Consider administering naloxone (follow steps in Box 19-6 on p. 521). 3. Add nonsedating nonopioid. 4. Monitor closely until sedation level and respiratory status are acceptable; use mechanical monitoring if indicated by patient status (see Chapter 19 and POSS, Box 19-4, on p. 510). 5. Resume opioid with 50% reduction in opioid dose when sedation level and respiratory status acceptable. 6. Continue to monitor sedation and respiratory status every 1 to 2 hours.

Disproportionate number of injections and attempts (injection/attempt ratio)	1. Check that patient is the only one pressing the PCA (PCEA) button (often, when another person [e.g., family member] is activating PCA [PCEA] for the patient, a significantly disproportionate injection/attempt ratio is found) (see PCA by proxy in text).
	2. Determine ratio of injections to attempts.
	  • If ratio is 1 injection for less than 2 or 3 attempts and patient has no pain, do nothing.
	  • If ratio is 1 injection to less than 2 or 3 attempts and patient has pain and tolerable and manageable adverse effects, relieve pain by administering supplemental boluses and increase opioid dose 25% to 100%.
	  • If ratio is 1 injection to more than 3 attempts and patient has pain and tolerable and manageable adverse effects, relieve pain by administering supplemental boluses and remind patient to "press the button to give yourself a dose of pain medicine before pain is severe, then put the button down and wait long enough (e.g., the length of lockout interval) to evaluate the effect of the dose before pressing the button again."

PCA, Patient-controlled analgesia; *PCEA,* patient-controlled epidural analgesia.
Initial PCA prescriptions are estimates of the doses patients will require. Patients reporting inadequate pain relief or adverse effects with the use of PCA require prompt evaluation. The need for upward or downward titration of PCA is signaled by pain ratings above the identified comfort-function goal or by unmanageable and intolerable adverse effects.

From Pasero, C., & McCaffery, M. (2011). *Pain assessment and pharmacologic management,* pp. 469-470, St. Louis, Mosby. © 1999, Pasero C. May be duplicated for use in clinical practice.

received IV PCA and reported 14 critical events, 3 of which involved unauthorized family members pressing the PCA button (Ashburn, Love, Pace, 1994). A review of nearly 6000 patients who had received IV PCA with no basal rate identified unauthorized PCA delivery to sleeping patients by relatives as the cause of 2 of 14 cases of respiratory depression (Sidebotham, Dijkhuizen, Schug, 1997).

These types of reports prompted The Joint Commission (TJC), an independent accrediting body of health care facilities in the United States, to issue a "sentinel event alert" on unauthorized PCA administration. This alert identified 460 PCA-related adverse events over a 5-year period; 15 of these events were the result of unauthorized family or staff members pressing the PCA button (TJC, 2004). Others have echoed concerns regarding this phenomenon (Institute for Safe Medication Practices, 2003a, 2003b).

Given the risks associated with PCA by proxy, TJC now expects to see proof that institutions have taken steps to minimize the potential for this outcome. These include patient education about the use of PCA prior to initiation of therapy and the use of verbal and written instructions warning against individuals other than the patient pressing the PCA button (see Box 12-3 on p. 316). The observation that most PCA by proxy is initiated by well-intentioned family members who want to ensure that their loved one is comfortable underscores the importance of frequent assessment of patients during PCA therapy to identify those who are unable to manage their own pain effectively as well as telling family members to contact staff if they have concerns about the patient's pain.

Authorized Agent-Controlled Analgesia

When patients are unable or unwilling to self-administer analgesics, another individual may be authorized to manage the patient's pain using the PCA technology. For example, family-controlled analgesia (FCA) or caregiver-controlled analgesia (CCA) designates *one* person to be the patient's primary pain manager, with the responsibility of pressing the PCA button (on the face of the pump or pendant attached to the pump) (Pasero, McCaffery, 1993; Pasero, Portenoy, McCaffery, 1999). With nurse-activated dosing (NAD) (also called *nurse-controlled analgesia*), the patient's primary nurse has that responsibility. These methods have collectively been called "authorized agent-controlled analgesia" (AACA) (Wuhrman, Cooney, Dunwoody, et al., 2007) and have been safely and effectively used for many years in patients of all ages. AACA is supported by a position paper with clinical practice recommendations developed by the American Society for Pain Management Nursing (Wuhrman, Cooney, Dunwoody, et al., 2007) and endorsed by other nursing specialty organizations such as the Oncology Nursing Society and the Hospice and Palliative Care Nurses Association (see Chapter 12 for a more detailed discussion and Box 12-4 on p. 318 for guidelines for the use of AACA).

Operator Errors: Misprogramming Analgesic Infusion Pumps

Operator (human) errors, particularly incorrect loading and misprogramming of PCA pumps, have been identified as a major cause of significant patient injuries and deaths over the years (Hicks, Heath, Sikirica, et al., 2008; Institute for Safe Medication Practices, 2003a, 2003b, 2004b; Macintyre, Coldrey, 2008). Administration of the wrong dose as a result of incorrect pump programming was by far the most common error (38.9%) identified in an analysis of data submitted to MEDMARX and the USP Medication Errors Reporting Program between 1998 and 2003 (United States Pharmacopeia, 2004).

To help prevent these types of errors, staff must be trained in the proper use of analgesic infusion devices (initial training and annual competency checks) (Pasero, Eksterowicz, Primeau, et al., 2007). Institution policy and procedure should mandate that all analgesic infusion device programming be independently double-checked at specified times, such as prior to the initiation of analgesic infusion therapy, at the time of any adjustments in prescription, and during the nursing hand-off communication processes. An independent double-check consists of having another clinician (e.g., nurse, physician, or pharmacist) compare the analgesic solution's drug and concentration and the pump's programmed prescription against each patient's written prescription to ensure accuracy without prompting from the person administering the analgesic or anyone else. Distractions during programming and double-checks are identified as being factors contributing to errors (Hicks, Heath, Sikirica, et al., 2008), so clinicians must take steps to avoid being interrupted.

The concept of the 6 Rights (6 Rs) of medication safety (right patient, right drug, right dose, right time, right route, right documentation) forms the basis of safe analgesic therapies and is the responsibility of everyone on the health care team (Institute for Safe Medication Practices, 2004c). A concerted multidisciplinary effort that includes appropriate prescribing; the highest standard of drug-reservoir preparation, storage, and dispensation; uninterrupted attention during programming and double-checking; and careful patient monitoring during therapy are essential. Readers are encouraged to subscribe to the Institute for Safe Medication Practices newsletters, which regularly publish safety information on a variety of medications (http://www.ismp.org). (See also Chapter 19 for transfer of care and hand-off communications.)

Infusion Solution and Tubing Changes

There are no national guidelines to direct the frequency with which IV PCA infusion systems (solution and tubing) should be changed (also called "hang time"), and microbiologic research is lacking on this therapy. As a result, practices vary widely with regard to this aspect of care. For a more in-depth discussion as well as research on the stability and compatibility of various agents used for analgesic infusion therapies, see Chapter 15.

Tapering and Cessation of Parenteral Analgesia

For patients with acute pain who are receiving parenteral analgesia, plans are necessary for smoothly weaning the patient as pain decreases or the patient is able to use a less invasive route of administration. Although most patients experience less pain as the days pass after surgery, it should not be assumed that all patients will follow this pattern. For example, the duration of postoperative pain tends to be longer in older patients (Melzack, Abbott, Zackon, et al., 1987). It is best to evaluate patients individually and taper analgesic doses on the basis of patients' reports of pain and ability to perform recovery activities rather than a preconceived notion of when parenteral analgesics should be discontinued.

In preparation for discharge, transition to oral analgesia should be started as soon as the patient is able to retain fluids and pain is well controlled. As function returns and pain lessens, the parenteral opioid dose can be reduced 25% once or twice daily. Table 17-3 provides helpful dosing guidelines that can be used to make a smooth transition from IV to oral opioid analgesia using analgesics found on most hospital formularies. The table can be posted in clinical areas where analgesic orders are written so that clinicians may use it for a quick reference guide.

Table 17-3 | Making the Transition from IV to PO Analgesia*: An Example Based on a Typical Hospital's Formulary

Daily Dose IV Analgesia		Suggested Daily PO Dose (mg)†
Morphine	**Hydromorphone (Dilaudid)**	
15 mg	2.2 mg	Hydrocodone 5/APAP 500 (Vicodin) 1 tab q 4 h (8 tabs maximum‡)
20 mg	3 mg	Hydrocodone 7.5/APAP 500 (Lortab) 1 tab q 4 h (8 tabs maximum) or Oxycodone 5/APAP 325 (Percocet 5/325) 1 tab q 4 h (12 tabs maximum)
25 mg	3.75 mg	Hydrocodone 10/APAP 325 (Norco) 1 tab q 4 h (12 tabs maximum) or Percocet 5/325 1 or 2 tabs q 4 h (12 tabs maximum)
30 mg	4.5 mg	Percocet 5/325 2 tabs q 4 h (12 tabs maximum) or Percocet 7.5/325 1 tab q 4 h (12 tabs maximum) or Oxycodone controlled release (OxyContin) 20 q 12 h plus Percocet 5/325 1 tab q 4 h PRN (12 tabs maximum)
35 mg	5.25 mg	Percocet 5/325 2 tabs q 4 h (12 tabs maximum) or OxyContin 20 q 12 h plus Percocet 5/325 1 tab q 4 h PRN (12 tabs maximum)
45 mg	6.75 mg	OxyContin 20 q 12 h plus Percocet 7.5/325 1 or 2 tabs q 4 h PRN (12 tabs maximum)
50 mg	7.5 mg	OxyContin 20 q 12 h plus Percocet 10/325 1 tab q 4 h PRN (12 tabs maximum) or OxyContin 30 q 12 h plus Percocet 7.5/325 1 tab q 4 h PRN (12 tabs maximum)

APAP, Acetaminophen.
*Equianalgesic doses: morphine 10 mg IV = hydromorphone 1.5 mg IV = hydrocodone 30 mg PO = oxycodone 20 mg PO (suggested dose may be reduced if a nonsteroidal anti-inflammatory drug is added).
†In calculating the oral dose, acetaminophen is given the following opioid values:
acetaminophen 325 mg = hydrocodone 2.5 mg or oxycodone 1.5 mg
acetaminophen 650 mg = hydrocodone 5 mg or oxycodone 3 mg
For example, Vicodin (hydrocodone 5 mg/acetaminophen 500 mg) = hydrocodone 7.5 to 8 mg.

‡Maximum acetaminophen dosage is 4000 mg/day. For some patients, such as older adults or heavy consumers of alcohol, the dosage should be 2000 mg or less per day.
Note: Recommend a laxative to patients on daily opioids.
This table provides a guideline to help ensure approximately the same pain relief when switching from IV to oral opioid analgesia. It can be posted in clinical units where opioid orders are written for the clinician's quick reference.
As appears in Pasero, C., & McCaffery, M. (2011). *Pain assessment and pharmacologic management*, p. 472, St. Louis, Mosby. © 2003, McCaffery M. May be duplicated for use in clinical practice.

Conclusion

IV PCA is an effective, interactive method that allows patients to manage their own pain. A built-in safeguard of the therapy is patient-only activation of the PCA button. Close monitoring by nurses of sedation and respiratory status is critical to the safe use of a continuous infusion with IV PCA. Optimal PCA therapy is dependent on adequate initial prescriptions, the administration of loading doses to establish satisfactory analgesia prior to initiation of PCA, and PCA prescription adjustments based on patients' responses to the therapy.

Chapter 18 Switching to Another Opioid or Route of Administration

WITH few exceptions, analgesia is dose-related rather than opioid-related. Thus unrelieved pain per se is not a sound reason for switching to another opioid. Other options for improving analgesia should be tried, such as increasing the opioid dose, providing a nonsteroidal anti-inflammatory drug (NSAID) around the clock (ATC), or adding local anesthetic to epidural opioids. Adverse effects that are intolerable and unmanageable are more likely to be an appropriate reason to switch to another opioid (Knotkova, Fine, Portenoy, 2009). Because of great interindividual variability, even opioids that bind to the same receptor site can produce adverse effects of different intensities in patients. The development of toxic effects from metabolite accumulation is a common reason for opioid rotation during long-term opioid therapy, and some recommend multiple switches if the first change in drug does not relieve symptoms (Hanks, Cherny, Fallon, 2004; Knotkova, Fine, Portenoy, 2009) (see Table 18-1 for options when analgesia from opioids is limited by adverse effects). Although switching to another opioid is common and recommended under these circumstances, a Cochrane Collaboration Review concluded that randomized controlled research is lacking and the practice is based largely on anecdotal or observational and uncontrolled studies (Quigley, 2004).

Patient difficulty in adhering to an analgesic regimen may be a sound reason to switch to another opioid. Sometimes another opioid allows a reduction in pills or liquid volume needed for pain relief. Fewer or smaller doses may be possible, making it easier for some patients to comply with the pain treatment regimen.

There is no good evidence that analgesic efficacy is dependent on route of administration; morphine is equally efficacious when given in appropriate doses by the oral, parenteral, or intraspinal routes (Hanks, Cherny, Fallon, 2004). However, occasionally switching from one opioid or route to another opioid or route is done to reduce the cost of long-term opioid treatment (Knotkova, Fine, Portenoy, 2009). For example, in one case the cost of opioid treatment was reduced from $1000 per day to less than $25 per day when a patient was switched from parenteral hydromorphone to oral methadone (Thomas, Bruera, 1995). The cost of the 10-day hospital stay required during the conversion process was not included in the cost analysis. Thus several factors must be considered when switching opioids to reduce costs.

When switching an opioid-tolerant patient to an alternative opioid drug, it is wise to assume that cross-tolerance will be incomplete (Knotkova, Fine, Portenoy, 2009). This means that a patient who has developed tolerance to one opioid analgesic may not be equally tolerant to another. In such cases, the starting dose of the new opioid must be reduced by at least 25% to 50% of the calculated equianalgesic dose to prevent overdosing (see Chapter 13, pp. 339-350, for the recommended approach when converting to methadone); otherwise, the full calculated equianalgesic dose of the new opioid could lead to effects such as sedation that would be greater than expected (Fine, Portenoy, the Ad Hoc Expert Panel on Evidence Review and Guidelines for Opioid Rotation, 2009; Knotkova, Fine, Portenoy, 2009; Indelicato, Portenoy, 2002; Vadalouca, Moka, Argyra, et al., 2008). Even with this approach, some patients will experience underdosing and some will experience overdosing because of individual sensitivities.

Table 18-1 | Options When Analgesia from Opioids Is Limited by Adverse Effects

Option	Approaches
Reduce systemic opioid requirement	
Pharmacologic techniques	Adjuvant analgesics
	Intraspinal opioids
Nonpharmacologic techniques	Cognitive-behavioral methods
	Physical methods (ice, TENS)
	Exercise programs
	Rehabilitation programs
	Anesthetic therapies (e.g., blocks)
	Surgical treatment (e.g., cordotomy)
Identify an opioid with a more favorable balance between analgesia and adverse effects	Sequential opioid trials
Improve the tolerability of the opioid regimen to allow further dose escalation	More aggressive adverse effect management (e.g., psychostimulant for somnolence)

TENS, Transcutaneous electrical nerve stimulation.
From Pasero, C., & McCaffery, M. *Pain assessment and pharmacologic management*, p. 474, St. Louis, Mosby. Modified from Portenoy, R. K. (1998). Adjuvant analgesics in pain management. In D. Doyle, G. Hanks, & N. MacDonald (Eds.), *Oxford textbook of palliative medicine*, ed 2, New York, Oxford University Press. © 2011, Pasero C, McCaffery M. May be duplicated for use in clinical practice.

It is also best not to abruptly discontinue the present opioid and convert to the new opioid in one step. This could cause a significant overdose that precipitates undesirable adverse effects or an underdose that precipitates severe pain. Instead, it is best to make the transition with 50% of the current opioid dose combined with 50% of the projected dose for the new opioid for several days. From this starting point, gradual increases in the new opioid drug and decreases in the old drug can be made until the switch is complete. The higher the dose of the current opioid, the more important it is to make the transition using 50/50 dosing (see Box 18-1 for guidelines when switching from one opioid to another).

The principles described above underscore the importance of careful dose selection and monitoring during opioid rotation (see Chapter 11 for more on cross-tolerance and the use of conversion charts, Box 14-6 on p. 393 for guidelines on switching from oral morphine to transdermal fentanyl, and Box 13-3 on p. 345 for guidelines on switching to methadone). It requires the clinician to have an understanding of opioid pharmacology and a commitment to tailoring the choice of opioid and dose to the patient's individual characteristics and response (Shaheen, Walsh, Lahsheen, et al., 2009).

An expert panel was convened for the purpose of establishing a new guideline for opioid rotation and recently proposed a two-step approach (Fine, Portenoy, the Ad Hoc Expert Panel on Evidence Review and Guidelines for Opioid Rotation, 2009). The approach presented in this chapter for calculating the dose of a new opioid can be conceptualized as the panel's *Step One*, which directs the clinician to calculate the equianalgesic dose of the new opioid based on the equianalgesic table. *Step Two* suggests that the clinician perform a second assessment of the patient to evaluate the current pain severity (perhaps suggesting that the calculated dose be increased or decreased) and to develop a strategy for assessing and titrating the dose as well as determining the need for a breakthrough dose and calculating that dose (see Box 16-2 on p. 449). The specific steps of patient examples given in this chapter reflect the panel's two-step approach (see Fine, Portenoy, the Ad Hoc Expert Panel on Evidence Review and Guidelines for Opioid Rotation, 2009). Following are several patient examples of conversions from one opioid to another, one route of administration to another, and combinations of both. The equianalgesic dose chart in Table 16-1 on pp. 444-446 is used for the necessary conversion calculations.

| **Box 18-1** | Switching from One Opioid to Another[1] |

NOTE: See Chapter 14 and Box 14-6 (p. 393) for switching to transdermal fentanyl; see Chapter 13 and Box 13-3 (p. 345) and Table 13-8 (pp. 346-347) for switching to methadone. For all other opioid analgesics, use the equianalgesic dose chart in Table 16-1 on pp. 444-446 and follow the steps listed below, which provide direction for switching from one oral opioid to another oral opioid, using the example of oral short-acting morphine to oral short-acting oxycodone:

1. Determine the total daily dose of the current opioid (e.g., morphine, 30 mg, taken q 4 h PO: 30 mg × 6 doses/day = 180 mg/24 h).

2. Locate the dose of the current opioid by the current route listed in the equianalgesic dose chart (e.g., 30 mg).

3. Determine the number of equianalgesic dose units in the 24-hour dose by dividing the 24-hour dose by the equianalgesic dose (e.g., 180 mg ÷ 30 mg = 6 units).

4. Locate the dose of the new opioid by the route of the new opioid listed on the equianalgesic dose chart (e.g., oxycodone 20 mg).

5. Determine the 24-hour dose of the new opioid by multiplying the equianalgesic dose of the new opioid by the equianalgesic dose units of the current opioid (e.g., 20 mg × 6 units = 120 mg/24 h of oxycodone).

6. Divide the 24-hour dose of the new drug by the number of doses to be given each 24 hours (e.g., 120 mg/24 h of oxycodone ÷ 6 doses = 20 mg of oxycodone q 4 h).

7. If the patient is opioid tolerant and has been taking a high dose of opioid, it is best to reduce the calculated dose of the new opioid by 25% to 50% (e.g., for 25% reduction: 20 mg oxycodone × 0.25 = 5 mg; 20 – 5 mg = 15 mg; for 50% reduction: 20 mg oxycodone × 0.50 = 10 mg).

8. It is also important not to abruptly discontinue the current opioid and convert to the new in one step. This could lead to an overdose, causing undesirable adverse effects, or an underdose, precipitating severe pain. Instead, in these cases, make the transition starting with 50% of the current opioid dose (e.g., 30 mg of morphine × 0.50 = 15 mg of morphine) combined with 50% of the projected dose for the new opioid (e.g., 15 mg of oxycodone × 0.50 = 7.5 mg of oxycodone, or 10 mg of oxycodone × 0.50 = 5 mg). Gradual increases in the new opioid drug and decreases in the old one can be made until the switch is complete over a period of several days. For example, in the case of a 25% reduction (see step 7),

start by giving oxycodone 7.5 mg PO q 4 h and morphine 15 mg PO q 4 h. In the case of a 50% reduction (see step 7), start by giving oxycodone 5 mg PO q 4 h and morphine 15 mg PO q 4 h. It may be necessary to adjust the dose of the new opioid (i.e., maintain the 50% dose of the old opioid and increase the new opioid for insufficient pain relief). Once the combined doses provide good pain control, drop the old opioid dose and double the new one.

9. After all calculations are made, perform a second assessment of pain severity, patient response, and medical and other characteristics to determine whether to apply an additional increase or decrease of 15% to 30% to enhance the likelihood that the initial dose will be effective for pain, or conversely, unlikely to cause withdrawal or opioid-related adverse effects.

10. Have a strategy to frequently assess initial response and titrate the dose of the new opioid regimen to optimize outcomes.

11. If a supplemental dose is used for titration, see Box 16-2 (p. 449) for calculation; if oral transmucosal formulation is used, see Boxes 14-2 (pp. 382-383) and 14-3 (pp. 384-385).

---

h, Hour; *hs,* at sleep; *PO,* oral; *q,* every.

[1]An expert panel was convened for the purpose of establishing a new guideline for opioid rotation and recently proposed a two-step approach (Fine, Portenoy, the Ad Hoc Expert Panel on Evidence Review and Guidelines for Opioid Rotation, 2009). The approach presented in the text for calculating the dose of a new opioid can be conceptualized as the panel's *Step One,* which directs the clinician to calculate the equianalgesic dose of the new opioid based on the equianalgesic table. *Step Two* suggests that the clinician perform a second assessment of the patient to evaluate the current pain severity (perhaps suggesting that the calculated dose be increased or decreased) and to develop strategies for assessing and titrating the dose as well as determining the need for a breakthrough dose and calculating that dose (see Box 16-2 on p. 449). The specific steps of patient examples given in the text reflect the panel's two-step approach (see Fine, Portenoy, the Ad Hoc Expert Panel on Evidence Review and Guidelines for Opioid Rotation, 2009).

Occasionally, during opioid treatment it is necessary to switch from one opioid to another. Calculating the equianalgesic dose of the new opioid increases the likelihood that patients will tolerate the switch to a new opioid without loss of pain control or excessive adverse effects. This box provides calculations for equianalgesic dosing.

From Pasero, C., & McCaffery, M. (2011). *Pain assessment and pharmacologic management,* p. 475, St. Louis, Mosby. Data from Fine, P. G., Portenoy, R. K., & Ad Hoc Expert Panel on Evidence Review and Guidelines for Opioid Rotation. (2009). Establishing best practices for opioid rotation: Conclusions of an expert panel. *J Pain Symptom Manage, 38*(3), 418-425. © 2011, Pasero C. May be duplicated for use in clinical practice.

Patient Example: Switching from One Oral Opioid to Another Oral Opioid

For the last two months, Mrs. N. has been taking 30 mg of PO modified-release oxycodone every 12 hours plus 10 mg of short-acting oxycodone for breakthrough pain about twice daily for severe osteoarthritis pain. Although her pain is well-controlled with pain ratings between 1/10 and 3/10, she has experienced severe nausea that has been unresponsive to all treatment efforts since the oxycodone was started. Her nurse practitioner thinks she will respond more favorably to a different opioid. She will be switched to PO modified-release oxymorphone. The following calculations are necessary (use the equianalgesic dose chart, Table 16-1, on pp. 444-446):

1. Determine the total 24 h dose of PO oxycodone:

$$30 \text{ mg} \times 2 \text{ doses}/24 \text{ h} = 60 \text{ mg}/24 \text{ h}$$

$$10 \text{ mg} \times 2 \text{ breakthrough doses}/24 \text{ h} = 20 \text{ mg}/24 \text{ h}$$

$$60 \text{ mg} + 20 \text{ mg} = 80 \text{ mg}/24 \text{ h of oxycodone}$$

2. Locate the equianalgesic dose of PO oxycodone in the equianalgesic chart (20 mg).
3. Determine the number of equianalgesic dose units in the 24-hour dose by dividing the 24-hour dose of PO oxycodone by the equianalgesic dose of PO oxycodone: 80 mg ÷ 20 mg = 4 units/24 h of oxycodone.
4. Locate the dose of PO oxymorphone in the PO dose column of the equianalgesic dose chart (10 mg) that is approximately equal to 20 mg of PO oxycodone.
5. Determine the 24-hour dose of PO oxymorphone by multiplying the equianalgesic dose of PO oxymorphone (10 mg) by the equianalgesic units of PO oxycodone (4 units): 10 mg × 4 units = 40 mg/24 h of oxymorphone.
6. Mrs. N. is opioid tolerant, so the dose of the new opioid will be reduced by 25%; 40 mg × 0.25 = 10 mg; 40 mg – 10 mg = 30 mg/24 h of oxymorphone.
7. Mrs. N. may have developed some tolerance to oxycodone, but she may not be equally tolerant to oxymorphone, therefore, the complete transition is done slowly. To avoid significant overdosing or underdosing, Mrs. N. will be transitioned by continuing to take 50% of her previous opioid, oxycodone, plus 50% of her new opioid, oxymorphone. The two calculations are as follows:
   a. 50% of oxycodone: 80 mg × 0.50 = 40 mg oxycodone/24 h, divided into 2 doses = 20 mg oxycodone q 12 h

   b. 50% of oxymorphone: 30 mg × 0.50 = 15 mg oxymorphone/24 h, divided into 2 doses = 7.5 mg oxymorphone q 12 h
8. Breakthrough doses equal to 10% to 15% of the total daily oxymorphone dose are calculated as follows (see Box 16-2 on p. 449):

$$30 \text{ mg} \times 0.10 \, (10\%) = 3 \text{ mg}$$

$$30 \text{ mg} \times 0.15 \, (15\%) = 4.5 \text{ mg}$$

Mrs. N.'s breakthrough dose is approximately 5 mg (closest available dose strength) of short-acting oxymorphone q 1 h PRN for breakthrough pain.

After 3 days on the combined opioids and a breakthrough dose of 5 mg about twice a day, Mrs. N.'s nausea is significantly less and her pain never goes above 3/10. She is then completely converted to oxymorphone by doubling the current dose of oxymorphone to 15 mg q 12 h and continuing the breakthrough dose of 5 mg. Within two days, her nausea completely subsides and her pain ratings range from 1/10 to 3/10.

Patient Example: Switching from One IV Opioid to Another IV Opioid

Mr. T. has been receiving a continuous IV infusion of morphine 4 mg/h, with 2 mg breakthrough bolus doses q 2 h PRN since his admission to the ICU 15 days ago after an automobile accident. He uses about 3 breakthrough doses a day. His pain is well-controlled with pain ratings varying from 2/10 to 4/10, but tremors and twitching are noted during assessment and thought to be due to morphine metabolite accumulation. He will be switched to a continuous IV infusion of hydromorphone. The following calculations are necessary (use the equianalgesic dose chart, Table 16-1, on pp. 444-446):

1. Determine the total daily dose of morphine from continuous infusion and breakthrough bolus doses:

$$4 \text{ mg} \times 24 \text{ h} = 96 \text{ mg}$$

$$2 \text{ mg} \times 3 \text{ breakthrough boluses in the last 24 h} = 6 \text{ mg}$$

$$96 \text{ mg} + 6 \text{ mg} = 102 \text{ mg}/24 \text{ h}$$

2. Locate the dose of IV morphine listed in the equianalgesic chart (10 mg).
3. Determine the number of equianalgesic dose units in the 24-hour morphine dose: 102 mg ÷ 10 mg = 10.2 units.
4. Locate the dose of IV hydromorphone listed in the parenteral column in the equianalgesic chart (1.5 mg) that is approximately equal to 10 mg of morphine IV.
5. Determine the 24-hour equianalgesic dose of IV hydromorphone: 1.5 mg hydromorphone × 10.2 units of morphine = 15.3 mg/24 h of IV hydromorphone.
6. Determine the hourly IV hydromorphone dose: 15.3 mg ÷ 24 = approximately 0.6 mg/h.
7. Because Mr. T. has been receiving morphine for several days, he may have developed some tolerance to its analgesia; however, he may not be equally tolerant to hydromorphone. Therefore, Mr. T. will be started on 50% of the equianalgesic dose of IV hydromorphone: 0.6 mg × 0.50 (50%) = 0.3 mg/h.
8. Breakthrough doses of 0.15 mg (50% of the hourly opioid dose) IV hydromorphone q 30 min PRN are prescribed for breakthrough pain (see Box 16-2 on p. 449).
9. For the first day, Mr. T.'s tremors and twitching decreased, but he used 10 breakthrough doses and on two occasions awoke with pain 5/10. The 24-hour dose and the breakthrough dose were recalculated as follows:
   a. The total of 10 breakthrough doses of 0.15 mg = 0.15 ×10 = 1.5 mg hydromorphone.
   b. 1.5 mg of hydromorphone is added to the current 24-hour dose (0.3 mg x 24 h) of 7.2 mg = 8.7 mg/24 h.
   c. The new 24-hour dose of hydromorphone, 8.7 mg, is divided by 24 = approximately 0.4 mg/h of IV hydromorphone.
   d. The new breakthrough dose is calculated by taking 50% of the hourly opioid dose, 0.4 mg, and dividing by 2 = 0.2 mg IV hydromorphone q 30 min.

For the next two days, Mr. T. used only 2 breakthrough doses, his pain remained at 2/10, and no further twitching or tremors were noted.

Patient Example: Switching from One SC Opioid to Another SC Opioid

For the last 2 months, Mrs. Q. has been receiving a continuous SC infusion of morphine, 25 mg/h with 5 mg breakthrough bolus doses q 15 min PRN. She has developed unmanageable sedation and confusion. Her physician would like to switch her to an equianalgesic continuous SC infusion of hydromorphone. The following calculations are necessary (use the equianalgesic dose chart, Table 16-1, on pp. 444-446):

1. Determine the total daily dose of morphine from continuous infusion and breakthrough bolus doses:

$$25 \text{ mg} \times 24 \text{ h} = 600 \text{ mg}$$

$$5 \text{ mg} \times 4 \text{ breakthrough boluses in the last 24 h} = 20 \text{ mg}$$

$$600 \text{ mg} + 20 \text{ mg} = 620 \text{ mg}/24 \text{ h}$$

2. Locate the dose of parenteral morphine listed in the equianalgesic chart (10 mg).
3. Determine the number of equianalgesic dose units in the 24-hour morphine dose: 620 mg ÷ 10 mg = 62 units.
4. Locate the dose of parenteral hydromorphone listed in the equianalgesic chart (1.5 mg) that is approximately equal to 10 mg of morphine.
5. Determine the 24-hour equianalgesic dose of parenteral hydromorphone: 1.5 mg × 62 units = 93 mg of hydromorphone/24 h.
6. Determine the hourly hydromorphone dose: 93 mg ÷ 24 h = approximately 4 mg/h.
7. Because Mrs. Q. has been receiving morphine for several weeks, she may have developed some tolerance to its analgesia; however, she may not be equally tolerant to hydromorphone. Therefore the starting hourly equianalgesic dose of hydromorphone will be reduced by 50%: 4 mg × 0.50 (50%) = 2 mg /h of hydromorphone
8. Breakthrough doses of 1 mg (50% of hourly requirement = 2 mg × 0.50 [50%] = 1 mg) SC hydromorphone PRN q 30 min are prescribed for breakthrough pain (see Box 16-2 on p. 449).

Because Mrs. Q. has been receiving a high dose of opioid for a long period of time, it is best to make the transition to the new opioid slowly. To do this, she is started on 50% of the new opioid dose (hydromorphone 2 mg/h × 0.50 [50%] = 1 mg/h) while taking 50% of the old opioid dose (morphine 25 mg/h × 0.50 [50%] = 12.5 mg/h) for several days. Gradual increases in the hydromorphone dose and decreases in the morphine dose are made until the switch to hydromorphone is complete. Inadequate pain relief is treated with breakthrough doses of hydromorphone and increases in the hourly hydromorphone dose. Within 9 days, the switch to hydromorphone is complete without loss of pain control, and Mrs. Q. is much less sedated and confused.

Switching from Epidural to IV Opioid Analgesia

Occasionally, a patient must be switched from epidural opioids to IV opioids before the transition to oral analgesia can be made (e.g., when the epidural catheter is accidentally pulled out or analgesia is unsatisfactory because the epidural catheter location is less than optimal). When this happens, conversion ratios usually are used as guidelines for selecting starting IV doses. Studies are lacking and controversy exists over the correct ratios to use when switching opioid-naïve patients from the various epidural opioids to parenteral opioids (see Chapter 15 for selecting starting epidural opioid doses). Most often, a conversion ratio of 1:10 is used to determine a starting dose when switching opioid-naïve patients from epidural morphine to IV morphine (Maalouf, Liu, 2009) (see the following patient example). Many clinicians use a ratio of 1:5 for switching from epidural hydromorphone to IV hydromorphone and a ratio of 1:3 for switching from epidural fentanyl to IV fentanyl.

Patient Example: Switching from an Epidural Opioid to an IV Opioid

Mrs. J. had a Whipple procedure 2 days ago. Her postoperative pain has been well-controlled (3/10) with PCEA morphine (basal rate = 0.1 mg/h; PCEA dose = 0.1 mg; lockout interval = 10 minutes). While ambulating this morning, Mrs. J.'s epidural catheter was accidentally pulled out. Mrs. J. is NPO with an NG tube, so she is unable to take oral analgesia and will be given IV PCA morphine instead. Because Mrs. J. will continue with the same opioid (morphine) and the same method of administration (PCA), the calculation for determining an equianalgesic starting prescription for the IV route is relatively simple. The ratio of 1:10 is used to calculate starting doses when changing from the epidural morphine to IV morphine:

1. Determine the equianalgesic IV PCA morphine dose: 0.1 mg (PCEA dose) × 10 = 1 mg for the PCA dose q 10 min.
2. The lockout (delay) interval of 10 minutes is acceptable for both IV PCA and PCEA morphine.

Mrs. J. is 78 years old and rarely required a PCEA dose while receiving epidural analgesia, so IV PCA is started without a basal rate and will be added if she is unable to maintain comfort and rest adequately. She manages her pain effectively with IV PCA only for the remainder of therapy.

Switching from IV to Oral Opioid Analgesia

Most often switching to another route of administration is done when acute pain subsides and the opioid-naïve patient is switched from IV opioids to oral opioids as described in the following patient example. Equianalgesic doses increase the likelihood that the transition to the oral route will be done without loss of pain control.

Patient Example: Switching from an IV Opioid to an Oral Opioid

Mrs. J. had a Whipple procedure 4 days ago. She has been managing her postoperative pain using IV PCA morphine for the last 2 days; the first 2 days were managed with epidural analgesia. Her condition has improved to the point that she presses her PCA button just once or twice an hour. She is tolerating oral fluids. Her surgeon wants to discontinue PCA and has prescribed 1 Percocet (oxycodone, 5 mg, plus acetaminophen, 325 mg per tablet) q 4 h PRN for pain. To be sure this prescription is comparable to what Mrs. J. has been taking to control her pain with IV PCA, her nurse calculates Mrs. J.'s analgesic requirements as follows (use the equianalgesic dose chart, Table 16-1, on pp. 444-446):

1. Determine Mrs. J.'s current total 24-hour dose of morphine by adding the number of times she self-administered morphine during the last 24 hours (29 times) and multiplying it by the PCA dose (1 mg). The total 24-hour dose of morphine is: 1 mg × 29 times = 29 mg. (If Mrs. J. had been receiving a basal rate during the past 24 hours, the amount of the basal rate would need to be added into her total 24-hour dose.)
2. Locate the equianalgesic dose of morphine by the IV route in the equianalgesic chart (10 mg).
3. Determine the number of equianalgesic dose units in the 24-hour dose of morphine by dividing the total 24-hour dose (29 mg) by the equianalgesic dose (10 mg): 29 mg ÷ 10 = 2.9 dose units.
4. Locate the equianalgesic dose of PO oxycodone in the equianalgesic chart (20 mg).
5. Determine the 24-hour dose of PO oxycodone that will be required by multiplying the equianalgesic dose of oxycodone (20 mg) by the equianalgesic dose units of morphine (2.9 units): 20 mg × 2.9 = 58 mg of PO oxycodone/24 h.
6. Determine the number of doses that would be equianalgesic to what Mrs. J. is currently taking by dividing the total 24-hour dose of oxycodone

(58 mg) by the number of doses that may be taken as prescribed each 24-hour (6 doses): 58 mg ÷ 6 doses = approximately 9.7 mg oxycodone/dose.

7. Determine whether the prescription the surgeon has written is equianalgesic. Because Percocet has just 5 mg of oxycodone per tablet, Mrs. J. would need to take 2 tablets, not 1, q 4 h to achieve the level of pain relief provided by IV PCA morphine. The acetaminophen (325 mg/tablet) will provide some additional analgesia, but not enough. The prescription the surgeon has written is not equianalgesic to the previous dose. Rather, it is about one-half the previous dose and probably will not provide adequate relief for Mrs. J.

Mrs. J.'s nurse first faxes her calculations to the surgeon who is in the clinic today and follows with a telephone call to discuss her calculations. The surgeon agrees that the prescription needs to be changed to 2 Percocet q 4 h. (See Table 17-3 on p. 472. This table can be posted in the clinical units to facilitate equianalgesic conversions from IV to oral analgesics.)

Switching from Oral to IV Opioid Analgesia

Sometimes a patient's condition worsens and analgesia is no longer possible by the oral route making it necessary to switch to IV analgesia (see the following patient example). Equianalgesic doses increase the likelihood that the transition will be done without loss of pain control.

Patient Example: Switching from Oral to IV Opioid Analgesia

Ms. R. has advanced ovarian cancer and has been taking PO modified-release oxymorphone 60 mg q 12 h and short-acting oxymorphone 10 mg q 2 h PRN for breakthrough pain with satisfactory pain control until now. She has just been admitted to the ED with a possible bowel obstruction. She is to be switched to IV oxymorphone. The following calculations are necessary (use the equianalgesic dose chart, Table 16-1, on pp. 444-446):

1. Determine the total 24-hour dose of PO oxymorphone:

$$60 \text{ mg} \times 2 \text{ doses}/24 \text{ h} = 120 \text{ mg}/24 \text{ h}$$

$$10 \text{ mg} \times 2 \text{ breakthrough doses}/24 \text{ h} = 20 \text{ mg}/24 \text{ h}$$

$$\text{Total 24 h dose} = 120 \text{ mg} + 20 \text{ mg} = 140 \text{ mg}/24 \text{ h}$$

2. Locate the equianalgesic dose of PO oxymorphone in the equianalgesic chart (10 mg).
3. Determine the number of equianalgesic dose units in the 24-hour dose by dividing the 24-hour dose of PO oxymorphone by the equianalgesic dose of PO oxymorphone: 140 mg ÷ 10 mg = 14 units.
4. Locate the dose of IV oxymorphone in the equianalgesic dose chart (1 mg) that is approximately equal to 10 mg of PO oxymorphone.
5. Determine the 24-hour dose of IV oxymorphone by multiplying the equianalgesic dose of IV oxymorphone by the equianalgesic units of PO oxymorphone: 1 mg × 14 units = 14 mg/24 h.
6. Divide the 24-hour dose of IV oxymorphone by the number of doses to be given each 24 hours: 14 mg ÷ 24 doses = approximately 0.6 mg/h.
7. Breakthrough doses are 0.3 mg (50% of the hourly dose). Because she is opioid tolerant, most of her pain control will come from the IV continuous infusion, and she will be allowed to double her hourly IV dose if necessary with boluses of IV oxymorphone q 30 min PRN for breakthrough pain.

Ms. R. tolerates the transition from oral oxymorphone to IV oxymorphone with pain ratings no higher than 3/10 and no adverse effects. A bowel obstruction is confirmed, but she decides against surgery; she will continue to receive IV oxymorphone for pain control.

Patient Example: Switching from One Opioid and Route to Another Opioid and Route

Mr. X., previously at home, had satisfactory pain control with 120 mg of PO modified-release oxycodone q 12 h and did not require breakthrough doses. He has been admitted for initiation of a hydromorphone SC infusion because he can no longer swallow. He finds the rectal route of administration highly objectionable, and he had a severe dermal reaction to the transdermal fentanyl patch, so these methods of pain control are not options. To determine the dose of SC hydromorphone that is approximately equal to the dose of PO oxycodone Mr. X. is taking, the following calculations are necessary (use the equianalgesic dose chart, Table 16-1, on pp. 444-446):

1. Determine the total 24-hour dose of oxycodone: 120 mg × 2 doses/24 h = 240 mg/24 h.
2. Locate the equianalgesic dose of PO oxycodone in the equianalgesic chart (20 mg).
3. Determine the number of equianalgesic dose units in the 24-hour dose by dividing the 24-hour dose of oxycodone by the equianalgesic dose of PO oxycodone: 240 mg ÷ 20 = 12 units.
4. Locate the dose of SC hydromorphone listed in the equianalgesic chart (1.5 mg) that is approximately equal to 20 mg of PO oxycodone.
5. Determine the 24-hour dose of SC hydromorphone by multiplying the dose of SC hydromorphone by the equianalgesic dose units of oxycodone: 1.5 mg × 12 units = 18 mg/24 h.
6. Divide the 24-hour dose of hydromorphone by the number of doses to be given each 24 hours: 18 mg ÷ 24 doses = approximately 0.8 mg/h.
7. Because Mr. X. is opioid tolerant, he is started on 50% of the equianalgesic dose of hydromorphone: 0.8 mg × 0.50 (50%) = 0.4 mg/h SC.
8. His breakthrough SC bolus doses are calculated as 50% of his hourly infusion = 0.2 mg q 30 min.

In Mr. X.'s situation, it is not possible to make the transition using a combination of 50% oxycodone and 50% hydromorphone. Therefore when the oxycodone is discontinued and the hydromorphone is started, he is watched closely for adverse effects and the number of breakthrough bolus doses he requires. He tolerates the transition without difficulty and only requires 2 to 3 bolus doses/24 h.

Switching from Multiple Opioids and Routes to One Opioid and Route

Sometimes patients are taking multiple opioid prescriptions by more than one route to control their pain. For example, they may be taking an IM opioid to control their ongoing pain and using a combination opioid and nonopioid, such as Percocet, for breakthrough pain. To switch a patient from multiple opioids and routes to one opioid and one route, the total daily dose of all of the opioids must be calculated. The following patient examples explain how this is done.

Patient Example: Switching from Multiple Opioids and Routes to One Opioid and Route

Mrs. V. is admitted to hospice care. She has been taking 2 Norco 10/325 (hydrocodone 10 mg, and acetaminophen 325 mg/tablet) plus 2 Percocet 5/325 (oxycodone 5 mg, and acetaminophen 325 mg/tablet) every 4 hours ATC for pain control. Although she has had good pain control, the amount of acetaminophen she is taking (7800 mg/day) is well above the maximum recommended daily amount of 4000 mg (see Section III). She will be switched to PO once-daily modified-release morphine. The following calculations are necessary (use the equianalgesic dose chart, Table 16-1, on pp. 444-446):

1. Determine the 24-hour dose of hydrocodone (2 Norco q 4 h = 12 doses): 10 mg × 12 doses = 120 mg/24 h
2. Determine the equianalgesic dose units of hydrocodone orally (although equianalgesic data are unavailable for hydrocodone, 30 mg is used as an amount approximately equal to the other opioid doses listed in the equianalgesic chart): 120 mg ÷ 30 = 4 units.
3. Determine the 24-hour dose of oxycodone: 5 mg × 12 doses = 60 mg.
4. Determine the equianalgesic dose units of oxycodone: 60 mg ÷ 20 = 3 units.
5. Determine the 24-hour total equianalgesic dose units: 4 + 3 = 7 units.
6. Determine the 24-hour dose of morphine by multiplying the dose units/24 h by the equianalgesic dose of oral morphine (30 mg): 30 mg × 7 = 210 mg oral morphine.
7. Because Mrs. V. is opioid tolerant, she is started on 50% of the equianalgesic dose of morphine: 210 mg × 0.50 (50%) = 105 mg/24 h. A 100 mg strength capsule of modified-release morphine (Kadian) would approximate a dose of 105 mg/24 h. A 10 mg strength capsule is also available and would allow a dose of 110 mg/24 h. The decision is made to start Mrs. V. on 100 mg of PO modified-release morphine taken once daily, provide adequate breakthrough doses (see below), and adjust the dose of PO modified-release morphine as needed.
8. Breakthrough doses of PO short-acting morphine are used for breakthrough pain (see Box 16-2 on p. 449):

$$105 \text{ mg} \times 0.10 \,(10\%) = \text{approximately } 10 \text{ mg}$$

$$105 \text{ mg} \times 0.15 \,(15\%) = \text{approximately } 15 \text{ mg}$$

In Mrs. V.'s case, combining the old with the new opioid during transition is not feasible. Therefore, when the previous opioids are discontinued and the modified-release morphine is started, she is watched closely for pain and adverse effects.

Mrs. V. is given 15 mg of short-acting morphine with the first dose of modified-release morphine. Breakthrough doses of 10 mg to 15 mg are provided hourly as needed during the transition. Ibuprofen 400 mg is administered q 8 h ATC to compensate for the nonopioid doses of acetaminophen she was taking previously. During the first 24 hours of the transition to modified-release morphine, Mrs. V. required 3 10 mg breakthrough doses and rated her pain as acceptable at 3/10 most of the day. No changes were made in the starting dose of modified-release morphine at that time.

Patient Example: Switching from Multiple Opioids and Routes to One Opioid and Route

Mr. C. has been admitted to the hospital from a skilled nursing facility for diagnostic tests and evaluation of his rheumatoid arthritis pain. His long-standing prescription for pain control is 50 mg IM meperidine q 4 h PRN and 1 to 2 Vicodin 5/500 (hydrocodone, 5 mg, and acetaminophen, 500 mg/tablet) PO q 4 h PRN. He has required an average of 6 doses of meperidine and 12 Vicodin per day for the last 5 days. He rates his pain as 4/10 most of the day, which is acceptable for him. His physician would like to discontinue the meperidine and Vicodin and switch Mr. C. to modified-release oxymorphone. The total 24-hour dose of opioid is calculated as follows (use the equianalgesic dose chart, Table 16-1, on pp. 444-446):

1. Determine the 24-hour dose of meperidine: 50 mg × 6 doses = 300 mg/24 h.
2. Locate the equianalgesic dose of parenteral meperidine (75 mg).
3. Determine the equianalgesic dose units of meperidine: 300 mg ÷ 75 = 4 units.
4. Determine the 24-hour dose of hydrocodone: 5 mg × 12 doses = 60 mg.
5. Determine the equianalgesic dose units of hydrocodone (although equianalgesic data are unavailable for hydrocodone, 30 mg is used as an amount approximately equal to the other opioid doses listed in the equianalgesic chart): 60 mg ÷ 30 = 2 units.
6. Determine the 24-hour total equianalgesic dose units: 4 + 2 = 6 units.
7. Determine the 24-hour dose of oxymorphone by multiplying the dose units/24 h by the equianalgesic dose of oral oxymorphone (10 mg): 10 mg × 6 = 60 mg.
8. Because Mr. C. is opioid tolerant, he is started on 50% of the equianalgesic dose of oxymorphone: 60 mg × 0.50 (50%) = 30 mg/24 h.
9. Determine the q 12 h starting dose of modified-release oxymorphone: 30 mg ÷ 2 = 15 mg.
10. Determine the breakthrough dose of PO short-acting oxymorphone (see Box 16-2 on p. 449):

$$30 \text{ mg} \times 0.10 \,(10\%) = 3 \text{ mg}$$

$$30 \text{ mg} \times 0.15 \,(15\%) = \text{approximately } 5 \text{ mg}$$

In Mr. C.'s case, combining the old with the new opioid during transition is not feasible. Therefore, when the previous opioids are discontinued and the modified-release oxymorphone and breakthrough doses are started, he is watched closely for pain and adverse effects. Mr. C. is given his breakthrough dose of 5 mg of short-acting oxymorphone with the first dose of 30 mg of modified-release oxymorphone. Breakthrough doses are offered hourly during the transition. Ibuprofen 400 mg is administered q 8 h ATC to substitute for the nonopioid acetaminophen he was receiving. During the first 24 hours of the transition to modified-release oxymorphone, Mr. C. required just two breakthrough doses and rated his pain 2/10 most of the day. He reported being able to sleep through the night for the first time in a week. No changes were made in his starting oxymorphone dose. He was discharged back to the skilled nursing facility 72 hours later with a pain rating of 2/10.

Switching from an Oral Opioid to Epidural Analgesia in Opioid-Tolerant Patients

Initiating epidural analgesia in opioid-tolerant patients involves initial opioid dose conversion followed by titration. As discussed above, studies are lacking and controversy exists over the correct conversion ratio to use when switching opioid-tolerant patients from oral or parenteral opioids to epidural opioids. When switching from parenteral morphine to epidural morphine, a conversion ratio of 10:1 is recommended (Swarms, Karanikolas, Cousins, 2004). A more aggressive approach uses a 3:1 parenteral/epidural ratio that considers the influence of pain severity, patient's age, previous systemic opioid dose, and the presence of neuropathic pain (DuPen, DuPen, 1998). A 10:1 ratio is used to switch from an epidural opioid dose to an intrathecal opioid dose (Swarms, Karanikolas, Cousins, 2004).

As discussed previously, ratios are used only for calculating starting doses and then the dose is titrated to achieve acceptable analgesia and tolerable adverse effects. It is recommended that epidural analgesia in opioid-tolerant patients be initiated in a setting where the patient can be observed closely for adverse effects until the opioid dose is stabilized (DuPen, DuPen, 1998). The conversion begins with calculating the total 24-hour dose of oral or parenteral opioid as described in the following patient example.

Patient Example: Switching from an Oral Opioid to Epidural Analgesia in Opioid-Tolerant Patients

Mrs. W. has cancer pain and has experienced intolerable and unmanageable adverse effects with oral oxymorphone, oral oxycodone, and SC hydromorphone. Until about 10 days ago, she was taking 160 mg of oral modified-release morphine q 12 h and had not required any breakthrough doses for several days. She had no adverse effects, and her pain was well-controlled, usually at 2/10 to 3/10. She then began to have escalating nociceptive and neuropathic pain with pain ratings up to 7/10 despite increasing doses of morphine. Yesterday she took 600 mg of modified-release morphine q 12 h and 6 breakthrough doses of 120 mg short-acting morphine with pain ratings of 7/10 to 9/10. Her neuropathic pain, which was being treated with gabapentin 3600 mg/day and despiramine 150 mg/day, was unresponsive to noninvasive management. She refuses to take methadone. Her escalating pain is due in part to increased metastasis.

Mrs. W. will be switched to morphine via patient-controlled epidural analgesia (PCEA) today since she has had no uncontrollable adverse effects from morphine. An advantage of this route is that a local anesthetic can be added to the epidural solution if morphine alone does not control her pain. To calculate her epidural dose of morphine, her current oral morphine dose will need to be converted to parenteral morphine and then to epidural morphine. An aggressive approach using a ratio of 3:1 (instead of 10:1) will be employed because she is relatively young (50 years old) and is experiencing severe pain, some of which is neuropathic pain. Further, she is tolerant to morphine, which

will be used epidurally. What epidural morphine starting dose would be appropriate for Mrs. W? (Use the equianalgesic dose chart, Table 16-1, on pp. 444-446.)

1. Determine the total 24-hour dose of oral morphine:
   a. 600 mg modified-release morphine q 12 h = 600 × 2 doses/24 h = 1200 mg/24 h of modified-release morphine.
   b. 120 mg short-acting morphine × 6 doses/24 h = 720 mg/24 h of short-acting morphine.
   c. 1200 mg + 720 mg = 1920 mg oral morphine/24 h
2. Determine the number of equianalgesic dose units in the 24-hour dose of oral morphine by dividing the 24-hour dose by the equianalgesic dose unit of oral morphine (30 mg): 1920 mg ÷ 30 mg = 64 units.
3. Determine the 24-hour dose of parenteral morphine by multiplying the equianalgesic dose of parenteral morphine (10 mg) by the equianalgesic dose units: 10 mg × 64 units = 640 mg/24 h of parenteral morphine.
4. Determine the 24-hour epidural morphine dose by using the ratio of 3:1. This is accomplished by dividing the 24-hour parenteral dose of morphine by 3: 640 mg ÷ 3 = approximately 213 mg/24 h.
5. Determine the hourly epidural morphine dose by dividing the total 24-hour epidural morphine dose by 24 hours: 213 mg ÷ 24 = approximately 9 mg/h of epidural morphine.
6. To avoid overdosing with this aggressive conversion approach, Mrs. W. is started on a basal rate of 50% of the calculated starting epidural morphine dose: 9 mg/h × 0.50 (50%) = 4.5 mg/h. In addition, she is provided with PCEA doses that allow her to double her epidural dose every hour: 2.25 mg PCEA doses q 15 min.

Based on the number of PCEA doses needed every 24 hours to achieve a pain rating of 3/10 or better, gradual increases in the basal rate and decreases of the PCEA doses were made until most of Mrs. W.'s pain relief was provided by the basal rate with only 2 to 3 PCEA doses required per 24 hours. Within 5 days, Mrs. W. was very comfortable with pain ratings of 3/10 or less without adverse effects on 7.5 mg/h of epidural morphine and occasional PCEA doses of 2 mg. The gabapentin and despiramine were continued as well.

Conclusion

Pain relief is almost always dose related rather than opioid related. Although unrelieved pain per se is not a sound reason for switching to another opioid or route of administration, there are times when this may be necessary. Application of the principles of equianalgesia and consideration of opioid tolerance as described in accepted guidelines increase the likelihood that the transition from one opioid or route to another opioid or route will be done without loss of pain control or the introduction of opioid adverse effects.

Chapter 19 Management of Opioid-Induced Adverse Effects

IN opioid-naïve patients, common opioid adverse effects include constipation, nausea and vomiting, sedation, pruritus, and mental confusion and clouding. Respiratory depression is less common but is the most feared adverse effect. As the patient becomes opioid tolerant, these adverse effects, except for constipation, tend to subside. Other less common opioid adverse effects include urinary retention, dry mouth, sweating, orthostatic hypotension, delirium, myoclonic jerks, and seizures. The underlying mechanisms of opioid adverse effects, even the most common, are not completely understood (Hanks, Cherny, Fallon, 2004). A number of factors influence the development of opioid adverse effects including patient age, co-morbidities, prior opioid exposure, concurrent administration of other drugs, and route of administration (Hanks, Cherny, Fallon, 2004). This explains why there is great individual variation in their development, and why most must be managed by using an individualized approach.

Prevention rather than treatment of opioid adverse effects is an important principle of pain management. Most adverse effects are dose dependent (Sinatra, 2009; Zhao, Chung, Hanna, et al., 2004). Therefore a practical approach includes the use of nonsedating analgesics that have an opioid dose-sparing effect, such as nonopioids and local anesthetics, so that the lowest effective opioid dose can be given. For some patients, simply decreasing the opioid dose is sufficient to eliminate or make an adverse effect tolerable (Pasero, McCaffery, 2003). Based on clinical experience, a decrease of 25% usually is sufficient to initiate a meaningful reduction in an adverse effect; if this dose change can be tolerated without severe pain, it is reasonable to attempt it. Again, based on clinical observation, a trial of a lower dose is least effective as a strategy for addressing constipation, presumably because the dose that produces constipation is approximately 4-fold less than the analgesic dose (Yuan, 2005) and because the symptom is so commonly multidetermined (see the discussion that follows).

The following is a discussion of many of the opioid adverse effects. Table 19-1 is a guide to preventing and

managing the common ones. See Table 11-1 on p. 285 for information on the specific opioid receptor binding sites of each adverse effect.

Constipation

Opioids work in both the peripheral and central nervous systems to suppress neuronal excitability and inhibit neurotransmitter release from enteric neurons that innervate the secretory glands. This can result in delayed gastric emptying, slowed bowel motility, and decreased peristalsis (Murphy, 2006; Thomas, 2008; Wood, 2005). The

GUIDELINES

Table 19-1 | Prevention and Management of Opioid-Induced Adverse Effects

Adverse Effect	Management
Constipation[1]	1. Begin all patients receiving ATC opioids with a combined stool softener and mild peristaltic stimulant (start on postoperative patients as soon as permissible). The use of fiber bulking agents requires abundant fluid intake, which is a problem for many patients so should be avoided, particularly in patients with advanced illness who often have fluid deficits. Gum chewing may be effective (see text). • Docusate sodium 50 mg + senna 8.6 mg (Senokot-S) 1 tab qd to 4 tabs tid 2. If no BM in any 48 h period, add *one to two* of the following to above: • Senna (Senokot) 8.6 mg 2 tabs hs to 4 tabs tid • Bisacodyl (Dulcolax) 5 mg PO hs to 15 mg PO tid • Milk of magnesia 30 to 60 mL qd or bid • Lactulose (10g/15 mL) 15 to 60 mL qd or bid; response may take 2 to 4 days. • Polyethylene glycol (Miralax) 17 g (1 heaping tsp) in 120 to 240 mL of fluid PO qd. Response may take 2 to 4 days (maximum dose 34 g/d). 3. If no BM by 72 h, perform rectal examination to rule out impaction. If not impacted, go to step 4. If impacted, go to step 5. 4. If not impacted, try *one* of the following[2]: • Bisacodyl (Dulcolax) suppository 10 mg • Magnesium citrate 8 oz PO • Senna extract (X-prep liquid) 2.5 oz PO • Mineral oil 30 to 60 mL PO • Milk of magnesia 25 mL + cascara 50 mg (5 mL) suspension • Fleet enema 5. If impacted: • Administer rescue analgesic if indicated before disimpaction (anxiolytic may be necessary in some cases). • Manually disimpact if stool is soft enough. • If not, soften with glycerin suppository or oil retention enema, then disimpact manually. • Follow up with enema (tap water, soapsuds) until clear. • Increase daily bowel regimen and monitor laxation patterns closely. 6. In patients with refractory constipation, use the opioid antagonist methylnaltrexone, which is approved for the treatment of opioid-induced constipation in patients with advanced illness; SC doses of 8 mg every other day for patients weighing 38 to 62 kg, and no more than 8 mg in a 24-hour period is recommended (see text for research).

Continued

Table 19-1 | Prevention and Management of Opioid-Induced Adverse Effects—cont'd

Adverse Effect	Management
Postoperative Ileus	Prevent with the use of multimodal approach. Strategies include the following: • Continuous thoracic epidural analgesia with local anesthetics with or without low-dose opioids • Opioid-sparing analgesic techniques • Peripheral mu opioid antagonists, i.e., alvimopan (Entereg), which is approved for the acceleration of the time to upper and lower GI recovery following partial large or small bowel resection with primary anastomosis; 12 mg 30 minutes to 5 hours prior to surgery, then 12 mg twice daily for up to 7 days for a maximum of 15 doses is recommended (see text). • Laparoscopic surgical techniques • Avoidance of routine NG tube, fluid excess, and immobility • Gum chewing

Nausea, vomiting	1. Consider prophylactic antiemetic therapy in:
	  • Patients beginning long-term opioid therapy who have a history of severe opioid-induced nausea and vomiting
	  • Postoperative patients with moderate to high risk for PONV (see Box 19-1 on p. 493); use 1 to 2 interventions for moderate risk; 2 or more for high risk (see text)[3]
	  • Patients at risk for medical sequelae from vomiting (i.e., patients with wired jaws or increased intracranial pressure or who are having fundoplication surgery)
	2. Titrate opioid doses slowly and steadily.
	  • Add or increase nonopioid or adjuvant for additional pain relief so that the opioid dose can be reduced.
	  • If analgesia is satisfactory, reduce opioid dose by 25%.
	  • Avoid adding a basal rate to IV PCA in opioid naïve patients with moderate to high risk; discontinue basal rate if one has been added and nausea occurs.
	3. Drug treatment of nausea and vomiting differs according to the cause.
	  • If caused by stimulation of the chemoreceptor trigger zone (common cause of vomiting), try one or more[3] of the following:
	    • Most effective:
	      a. Corticosteroid, e.g., dexamethasone (Decadron) 4-8 mg IV
	      b. Droperidol in doses less than 1.25 mg
	      c. Serotonin receptor antagonists, e.g., dolasetron (Anzemet), granisetron (Kytril), ondansetron (Zofran), palonosetron (Aloxi)
	      d. IV propofol rescue doses in PACU
	    • Less effective:
	      a. Prokinetic with dopamine antagonist properties, e.g., metoclopramide (Reglan), prochlorperazine (Compazine)
	      b. Neuroleptics, e.g., haloperidol (Haldol), olanzapine (Zyprexa)
	      c. Antihistamines, e.g., diphenhydramine (Benadryl), hydroxyzine (Vistaril)
	      d. Benzodiazepine, e.g., lorazepam (Ativan)
	  • If caused by slowed GI motility, try a prokinetic, e.g., metoclopramide 10 mg q 8 h PO, IV, or SC
	  • For enhanced vestibular sensitivity (nausea associated with motion, often accompanied by vertigo), try dimenhydrinate (Dramamine), transdermal scopolamine patch.[4]
	4. For chronic nausea in advanced cancer:
	  • Give metoclopramide 10 mg q 4 h SC, IV, or PO.
	  • If nausea persists, add dexamethasone 10 mg bid.
	  • If nausea persists, add other antiemetics.

Continued

Table 19-1 | Prevention and Management of Opioid-Induced Adverse Effects—cont'd

Adverse Effect	Management
	5. Other suggestions for chronic refractory nausea: • Haloperidol (Haldol) 0.5 mg tid up to 15 mg/day + antihistamine + dexamethasone + ondansetron. • Dronabinol 2.5 mg PO q 12 h. • Risperidone 1 mg PO qd. • Apply a nicotine patch. • Switch to another opioid. • Switch to an intraspinal route. • Use an anesthetic or neurosurgical technique to allow drug reduction. 6. Support use of nondrug interventions such as relaxation techniques and acustimulation (see text).
Pruritus[5]	Postoperative treatment: 1. If analgesia is satisfactory, reduce opioid by 25%. 2. Add or increase nonopioid or nonsedating adjuvant for additional pain relief so that the opioid dose can be reduced. 3. Pharmacologic treatment according to severity: • Ondansetron 4 mg IV prophylactically prior to intraspinal opioid administration. • Gabapentin 1200 mg PO prophylactically 2 hours prior to intraspinal opioid administration; can be tried also for refractory itch associated with advanced illness. • Ondansetron 0.1 mg/kg IV (first choice for established pruritus). • IV propofol 10 mg IV bolus; MR in 5 minutes. • Topical local anesthetics for localized itch. • Diphenhydramine (Benadryl) 12.5 to 25 mg IV or 25 to 50 mg PO may be given to alleviate symptoms, but is sedating; monitor sedation closely (see text and sedation below). • Naloxone IV bolus (0.04 to 0.08 mg) or IV infusion (0.4 to 0.8 mg/1000 mL at 100 mL/h or 1 to 2 mcg/kg/h) is generally used only for severe pruritus; monitor pain closely.
Myoclonus	Mild myoclonic jerks may resolve as tolerance develops. Primary treatment: • Consider all possible causes. • If the patient is receiving meperidine, immediately change to another opioid since myoclonus may be a result of accumulation of normeperidine, a neurotoxic metabolite (see Chapter 13). • Attempt to control pain with lower opioid doses after ruling out the (rare) possibility that the myoclonus could be a sign of opioid withdrawal (see text); add or increase adjuvant analgesics. • Try a benzodiazepine or an anticonvulsant; clonazepam (Klonopin), 0.25 mg to 0.5 mg orally two or three times daily may help but is sedating. Treatment of more severe symptoms: • Opioid rotation; methadone is often the opioid of choice if not contraindicated (see Chapter 13). • Anesthetic procedures may be indicated in some patients. • IV midazolam titrated until myoclonic jerks disappear (1 to 2 mg/h). • IV diazepam provides transient relief. • IV dantrolene (Dantrium). • Valproic acid 500 mg/day may help. • Rehydration to facilitate renal elimination of metabolites. • Dialysis may be necessary in some patients.

Continued

Table 19-1 | Prevention and Management of Opioid-Induced Adverse Effects—cont'd

Adverse Effect	Management

Mental confusion, clouded consciousness, delirium, hallucinations, paranoia in patients receiving long-term opioid therapy	1. Assess using valid and reliable tool (see text and Form 19-1 on p. 504).
	2. Evaluate all potential causes with consideration of baseline cognitive status and the role of primary therapy.
	  • Exclude sepsis or metabolic derangement.
	  • Exclude CNS involvement by tumor.
	3. If thought to be related to opioid use, reassure patient that mild mental confusion following initiation of opioids or an increase in dose is common and usually resolves within days to a couple of weeks.
	4. Eliminate nonessential CNS-acting medications, e.g., steroids.
	5. If analgesia is satisfactory, reduce opioid by 25%.
	  • Do not administer naloxone, even if delirium is thought to be due to the opioid.
	6. If delirium persists, consider:
	  • Trial of neuroleptic (e.g., haloperidol 0.5 to 1 mg PO bid or tid or 0.25 to 0.5 mg IV or IM)
	  • Switch to another opioid.
	  • Switch to an intraspinal route with or without local anesthetic.
	  • Consider use of an anesthetic or neurosurgical technique/procedure to allow drug reduction.
	  • Use benzodiazepines with caution as they can exacerbate sedation and acute confusion.

Postoperative confusion and delirium	1. Assess using valid and reliable tool (see text and Form 19-1). 2. Evaluate all potential causes with consideration of risk factors and baseline cognitive status (see Box 19-2). 3. Eliminate nonessential CNS-acting medications, e.g., benzodiazepines, antihistamines. 4. Optimize pain control; add or increase nonsedating adjuvant or nonopioid analgesics. Reduce opioid dose by 25%, if an opioid dose reduction is necessary. • Do not administer naloxone even if opioid is thought to be the cause. 5. Ensure patient safety. 6. Ask family or someone with whom patient is familiar to stay with patient. 7. Haloperidol 0.25 to 0.5 mg IV. For severe symptoms: 1. Monitor closely; transfer to unit where close nursing observation and aggressive pharmacologic management are possible. 2. Monitored setting: haloperidol 2 to 10 mg IV q 20 to 30 minutes, and then 25% of loading dose every 6 hours.

Sedation during long-term opioid therapy	1. Titrate opioids based on patient response.
	2. Determine whether sedation is due to the opioid. It is most likely due to the opioid therapy if there has been a recent increase in dose; reassure patient that tolerance usually develops. Correct underlying cause if unrelated to opioid.
	3. If due to opioid and analgesia is satisfactory, reduce opioid dose by 10% to 25%; add or increase nonopioid or nonsedating adjuvant for additional pain relief so that the opioid dose can be reduced.
	4. Eliminate nonessential CNS depressant medications.
	5. Add simple stimulants during the day, e.g., caffeine (see Section III).
	6. If analgesia is unsatisfactory or dose reduction is not viable, consider one of the following:
	  • Give a lower opioid dose more frequently to decrease peak concentration.
	  • Add a psychostimulant, e.g., methylphenidate (Ritalin) 2.5 to 5 mg in morning (or beginning of patient's awake time); increase dose if necessary to maintain effects until bedtime (see Section V for more on psychostimulants).
	  • Add donepezil 5 mg daily.
	7. If excessive sedation persists, consider one of the following:
	  • Switch to another opioid.
	  • Switch to an intraspinal route.
	  • Use an anesthetic or neurosurgical technique/procedure to allow dose reduction.

Continued

| Table 19-1 | Prevention and Management of Opioid-Induced Adverse Effects—cont'd |
| | |

Adverse Effect	Management
Sedation during short-term opioid therapy in opioid-naïve patients (e.g., postoperative)	1. Titrate opioids based on patient response. 2. Administer the lowest effective opioid dose, accomplished with a multimodal pain management approach initiated before or at the initiation of opioid therapy. For example, unless contraindicated, add nonsedating nonopioid analgesics such as acetaminophen and an NSAID. 3. Eliminate nonessential CNS depressant medications. 4. Assess sedation using a scale that is valid and reliable for assessment of sedation during opioid administration for pain management (see POSS, Box 19-4 on p. 510) (see text for frequency). 5. If analgesia is satisfactory, reduce opioid dose by 25% to 50% for level 3 on POSS; stop opioid for level 4 on POSS (see respiratory depression below). 6. Increase nurse monitoring until sedation level is less than 3 on POSS and respiratory status is stable.
Respiratory depression during short-term opioid therapy in opioid-naïve patients (e.g., postoperative)	1. All steps in the above discussion of sedation during short-term opioid therapy apply here. 2. Perform comprehensive respiratory assessments (depth, regularity, rate, and noisiness) (see text for technique and frequency). 3. Consider mechanical monitoring in high-risk patients[6] (see Box 19-5 on p. 516). 4. If patient is minimally responsive or unresponsive to stimulation, stop opioid administration and consider administering naloxone (Narcan). Box 19-6 on p. 521 outlines naloxone administration technique. 5. Increase nurse monitoring until sedation level is less than 3 on POSS and respiratory status is stable; consider use of mechanical monitoring, e.g., continuous capnography or pulse oximetry[6], or transfer to monitored setting depending on severity of respiratory depression and responsiveness to treatment. 6. Monitor pain closely, continue nonopioid analgesics ATC, and resume opioid analgesia at reduced dose when sedation level is less than 3 on POSS and respiratory status is stable.

bid, Twice daily; *BM*, bowel movement; *cap*, capsule; *CNS*, central nervous system; *GI*, gastrointestinal; *hs*, at sleep; *IM*, intramuscular; *IV*, intravenous; *MR*, may repeat; *oz*, ounce; *PO*, oral; *POSS*, Pasero Opioid-Induced Sedation Scale; *q*, every; *qd*, once daily; *SC*, subcutaneous; *tab*, tablet; *tid*, three times daily.

[1]Some of the suggestions for oral treatment of constipation in this table may cause electrolyte imbalance; systematic assessment for signs of imbalance is recommended.
[2]For acute treatment; rectal therapies are not generally recommended for long-term management of constipation.
[3]Preventive multimodal antiemetic therapy is recommended for the management of patients at moderate to high risk for PONV. In such cases, combinations of drugs, such as dexamethasone plus droperidol, may be used.
[4]Remove after 72 hours and if confusion is noted.
[5]For treatment of pruritus related to advanced disease, see Pittelkow, M. R., & Loprinzi, C. L. (2004). Pruritus and sweating in palliative medicine. In D. Doyle, G. Hanks, N. I. Cherny, et al. (Eds.), *Oxford textbook of palliative medicine*, ed 3, New York, Oxford Press.
[6]Pulse oximetry is an unreliable method of monitoring in patients receiving supplemental oxygen as it can produce false high oxygen concentration readings (see text for more on mechanical monitoring).

From Pasero, C., & McCaffery, M. (2011). *Pain assessment and pharmacologic management*, pp. 484-488, St. Louis, Mosby. Data from Amador, L. F., & Goodwin, J. S. (2005). Postoperative delirium in the older patient. *J Am Coll Surg, 200*(5), 767-773; Berardi, R. R., Kroon, A. L., McDermott, J. H., et al. (2006). *Handbook of nonprescription drugs*. An interactive approach to self care, ed 15, Washington DC, American Pharmacists Association; Casarett, D. J., & Inouye, S. K. (2001). Diagnosis and management of delirium near the end of life. *Ann Intern Med, 135*(1), 32-40; Fine, P., & Portenoy, R. K. (2007). A clinical guide to opioid analgesia. New York, Vendome Group, LLC; Gan, T. J., Meyer, T., Apfel, C. C., et al. (2003). Consensus guidelines for managing postoperative nausea and vomiting. *Anesth Analg, 97*(1), 62-71; Gan, T. J., Meyer, T., Apfel, C. C., et al. (2007). Society for Ambulatory Anesthesia guidelines for the management of postoperative nausea and vomiting. *Anesth Analg, 105*(6), 1615-1628; Golembiewski, J. A., Chernin, E., & Chopra, T. (2005). Prevention and treatment of postoperative nausea and vomiting. *Am J Health-Syst Pharm, 62*(5), 1247-1262; Dabu-Bondoc, S., Franco, S. A., & Sinatra, R. S. (2009). Neuraxial analgesia with hydromorphone, morphine, and fentanyl: Dosing and safety guidelines. In R. S. Sinatra, O. A. de Leon-Casasola, B. Ginsberg, et al. (Eds.), *Acute pain management*, Cambridge, NY, Cambridge University Press; Harris, J. D., & Kotob, F. (2006). In O. A. de Leon-Casasola (Ed.), *Cancer pain. Pharmacological, interventional and palliative care approaches*, Philadelphia, Saunders; Goodheart, C. R., & Leavitt, S. B. (2006). Managing opioid-induced constipation in ambulatory-care patients. *Pain Treatment Topics*. Available at http://pain-topics.org/pdf/ Managing_Opioid-Induced_Constipation.pdf#search="constipation". Accessed July 28, 2007; Hagen, N. A., & Swanson, R. (1997). Strychnine-like multifocal myoclonus and seizures in extremely high-dose opioid administration: Treatment strategies. *J Pain Symptom Manage, 14*(1), 51-58; Hanks, G., Cherny, N. I., & Fallon, M. (2004). Opioid analgesic therapy. In D. Doyle, G. Hanks, N. I. Cherny, et al. (Eds.), *Oxford textbook of palliative medicine*, ed 3, New York, Oxford Press; Jacobi, J., Fraser, G., Coursin, D., et al. (2002). Clinical practice guidelines for the sustained use of sedatives and analgesics in the critically ill adult. *Crit Care Med, 30*(1), 119-141; Kehlet, H. (2005). Preventive measures to minimize or avoid postoperative ileus. *Sem Colon Rec Surg, 16*(4), 203-206; Kehlet, H., & Holte, K. (2001). Review of postoperative ileus. *Am J Surg, 182*(5A Suppl), 3S-10S; Kehlet, H., & Wilmore, D. W. (2008). Evidence-based surgical care and the evolution of fast-track surgery. *Ann Surg, 248*(2), 189-198; Mercadante, S., Ferrera, P., Villari, P., et al. (2009). Frequency, indications, outcomes, and predictive factors of opioid switching in an acute palliative care unit. *J Pain Symptom Manage, 37*(4), 632-641; Okamoto, Y., Tsuneto, S., Matsuda, Y., et al. (2007). A retrospective chart review of the antiemetic effectiveness of risperidone in refractory opioid-induced nausea and vomiting in advanced cancer patients. *J Pain Symptom Manage, 34*(2), 217-222; Slatkin, N., Rhiner, M., & Bolton, T. M. (2001). Donepezil in the treatment of opioid-induced sedation: Report of six cases. *J Pain Symptom Manage, 21*(5), 425-438; Thomas, J. (2008). Opioid-induced bowel dysfunction. *J Pain Symptom Manage, 35*(1), 103-113; Portenoy, R. K., Thomas, J., Moehl Boatwright, M. L., et al. (2008). Subcutaneous methylnaltrexone for the treatment of opioid-induced constipation in patients with advanced illness: A double-blind, randomized, parallel group, dose-ranging study. *J Pain Symptom Manage, 35*(5), 458-468; Sheen, M. J., Ho, S. T., Lee, C. H., et al. (2008). Preoperative gabapentin prevents intrathecal morphine-induced pruritus after orthopedic surgery. *Anesth Analg, 106*(6), 1868-1872; Vaurio, L. E., Sands, L. P., Wang, Y., et al. (2006). Postoperative delirium: The importance of pain and pain management. *Anesth Analg, 102*(4), 1267-1273; Waxler, B., Dadabhoy, Z. P., Stojiljkovic, L., et al. (2005). Primer of postoperative pruritus for anesthesiologists. *Anesthesiology, 103*(1), 168-178; Yuan, C. S. (Ed.). (2005). *Handbook of opioid bowel dysfunction*. New York, Haworth Medical Press.

result is slow-moving, hard stool that is difficult to pass. At its worst, GI dysfunction can result in unresolved ileus, fecal impaction, and obstruction (Kehlet, 2005; Wood, 2005). GI dysfunction is worsened by the presence of other conditions of advanced disease, such as ascites or tumors (Thomas, 2008).

Constipation is the most common opioid adverse effect and the one that is most often persistent (Gutstein, Akil, 2006; Hanks, Cherny, Fallon, 2004). It requires a preventive approach, regular assessment, and aggressive management if symptoms are detected. Factors contributing to the problem of constipation in patients taking opioids include advanced age, immobility, abdominal disease, and concurrent medications (Hanks, Cherny, Fallon, 2004; Hinrichs, Huseboe, 2001). Most patients placed on ATC opioid analgesics should be directed to take laxatives regularly. Although some clinicians do not endorse prophylactic treatment of a subpopulation that has no other risk factors and is younger, active, and well-nourished, there is general acceptance of the value of prophylaxis in others. A coadministered laxative usually must be continued as long as the patient takes opioids.

The goals of prophylactic treatment of constipation are to maximize stool volume, keep stool soft, and enhance peristalsis (Thomas, 2008). Although it has been suggested that a complete bowel movement at least every 3 days without difficulty is ideal (Goodheart, Leavitt, 2006), the frequency of defecation is less important than comfortable evacuation (Yuan, 2005). Attention to diet and exercise in addition to providing for privacy and convenience for patients are important aspects of bowel management but are insufficient alone to prevent opioid-induced constipation. Natural fiber and large amounts of fluid are a preferred strategy unless intrinsic bowel disease (usually partial obstruction) increases the risk associated with more intraluminal volume, the approach increases adverse effects such as bloating, or the patient finds this strategy unpalatable. Bulk laxatives, such as psyllium (Metamucil), are relatively contraindicated unless fluid intake is adequate, because of an increased risk of fecal impaction and obstruction (Thomas, 2008).

Stool softeners alone appear inadequate, and the usual initial therapy is a combination of stool softener and mild peristaltic stimulant, such as senna (e.g., Senokot-S) (Hanks, Cherny, Fallon, 2004; Thomas, 2008). Stool softeners are detergents and allow better water penetration into stool; stimulant laxatives induce peristalsis (Thomas, 2008).

The simple activity of chewing gum also seems to stimulate bowel motility (Schuster, Grewal, Greaney, et al., 2006). In a small prospective study, 34 patients undergoing elective open sigmoid resections were randomized into two groups: gum chewing or a control group. The patients chewing sugarless gum three times a day for one hour passed flatus, had their first bowel movement, and were discharged significantly sooner than the control group. More studies are needed, but gum chewing appears harmless and may help with constipation.

Other tips on managing constipation are listed in Table 19-1. Tables containing the various classifications and properties of laxatives and the amount of fiber in common foods can be found in Curry, C. E., & Butler, D. M. (2006). Constipation. In R. R. Berardi, A. L. Kroon, J. H. McDermott, et al. (Eds.), *Handbook of nonprescription drugs. An interactive approach to self care*, ed 15, pp. 299-326, Washington DC, American Pharmacists Association. Tools with established reliability and validity for assessment of bowel function and constipation (Downing, Kuziemsky, Lesperance, et al., 2007; Goodman, Low, Wilkinson, 2005; Hinrichs, Huseboe, 2001; McMillan, Williams, 1989) are available. Figure 19-1 provides the Victoria Bowel Performance Scale (BPS), a simple-to-use 9-point tool. See also Form IV-1 on p. 546 at the end of Section IV. It contains valuable information that should be given to all patients receiving opioid therapy.

Opioid Antagonists for Bowel Dysfunction

Although receptors in the central nervous system (CNS) are involved in the pathophysiology of opioid-induced constipation, the effect appears to be mediated predominantly by GI mu opioid receptors (Thomas, Karver, Cooney, et al., 2008). This observation led to a search for a peripherally acting mu opioid antagonist that could specifically reverse opioid-induced bowel dysfunction without reversing analgesia (Thomas, 2008).

When taken orally, the opioid antagonists naloxone, naltrexone, and nalmefene are absorbed systemically, and although they can effectively reverse bowel dysfunction, they can cross the blood-brain barrier, reverse central opioid receptors and analgesia, and produce withdrawal symptoms (Becker, Galandi, Blum, 2007; Goodheart, Leavitt, 2006; Liu, Wittbrodt, 2002; Thomas, 2008). This outcome is least likely to occur with naloxone, which has a very limited oral bioavailability (around 3%). Although there is a risk of systemic absorption with associated return of pain and withdrawal, the risk with this drug is low, and oral naloxone (20 to 40 mg) has been used clinically for refractory constipation (Meissner, Leyndecker, Mueller-Lissner, et al., 2009).

In contrast to these other antagonists, methylnaltrexone (Relistor) and alvimopan (Entereg) have the potential to block opioid actions mediated by peripheral opioid receptors while sparing actions mediated by opioid receptors in the CNS (Portenoy, Thomas, Moehl Boatwright, et al., 2008). Methylnaltrexone has approval in the United States for the treatment of opioid-induced constipation in patients with advanced illness (Wyeth Pharmaceuticals, 2009), and alvimopan is approved for acceleration of the time to upper and lower GI recovery following partial large or small bowel resection with primary anastomosis (GlaxoSmithKline, 2009). Methylnaltrexone is given subcutaneously (8 mg for patients weighing 38 to 62 kg every other day and no more than one dose in a 24-hour period), and alvimopan is taken orally (12 mg 30 minutes to 5 hours prior to surgery, then 12 mg twice daily for up

-4	-3	-2	-1	BPS Score 0	+1	+2	+3	+4
← Constipation						Diarrhea →		
Characteristics								
Impacted or Obstructed ± small leakage	Formed Hard with pellets	Formed Hard	Formed Solid	Formed Soft	Unformed Soft	Unformed Loose or Paste-like	Unformed Liquid ± mucus	Unformed Liquid ± mucus
Pattern								
No stool produced	Delayed ≥3 days	Delayed ≥3 days	Pt's Usual	Pt's Usual	Pt's Usual	Usual or Frequent	Frequent	Frequent
Control								
Unable to defecate despite maximal effort or straining	Major effort or straining required to defecate	Moderate effort or straining required to defecate	Minimal or no effort required to defecate	Minimal or no effort to defecate	Minimal or no effort required to control urgency	Moderate effort required to control urgency	Very difficult to control urgency and may be explosive	Incontinent or explosive — unable to control or unaware

Downing, Watson, Carter (© Victoria Hospice Society)

Instructions for use

1. BPS is a nine-point numerical scale. It is a single score, based on the overall "best vertical fit" among the above three parameters (characteristics, pattern, and control) and is recorded, for example, as: BPS +1, BPS –3, or BPS +2.
2. Look vertically down each BPS level to become familiar with how the three parameters of characteristics, pattern, and control change in gradation from constipation to diarrhea.
3. The "usual" bowel pattern for a patient may be in the 0, –1, or +1 columns. For any of these, the actual frequency of bowel movements may vary among patients from one or more times daily to once every 1–2 days but the patient states as being their usual pattern.

4. Patients with a surgical intervention (colostomy, ileostomy, and short loop bowel) may have a more frequent "usual" bowel pattern than above. BPS is still overall graded by combining all three parameters (e.g., +2 or +3 with ileostomy) to ascertain a "best fit."
5. Patients may use different words than above to describe their bowel activity. One must use clinical judgment in deciding which boxes are most appropriate.
6. In potential confounding cases, determination of the most appropriate BPS score is made using the following methods:
   - Two vertically similar parameters generally outweigh the third;
   - Single priority weighting among parameters is characteristics > pattern > control.

Figure 19-1 | Victoria Bowel Performance Scale (BPS).

From Downing, G. M., Kuziemsky, C., Lesperance, M., et al. (2007). Development and reliability testing of the Victoria Bowel Performance Scale (BPS). *J Pain Symptom Manage, 34*(5), 513-522.

to 7 days for a maximum of 15 doses). Methylnaltrexone is not approved for IV use but has been used by this route for treatment of nausea, pruritus, and urinary retention (Gold Standard Clinical Pharmacology, 2009).

A systematic review of 20 studies that were conducted on the use of methylnaltrexone and alvimopan for treatment of constipation concluded that further research with larger numbers of patients and varying types of pain are required (Becker, Galandi, Blum, 2007). Another analysis of 22 studies concluded that there is insufficient evidence for the safety and efficacy of naloxone or nalbuphine for the treatment of opioid-induced bowel dysfunction and that further research is needed to fully assess the role of alvimopan and methylnaltrexone in therapy (McNicol, Boyce, Schumann, et al., 2008). Following is a discussion of some of the research on methylnaltrexone. See pp. 491-493, Postoperative Ileus, for more on alvimopan.

One of the first studies conducted on methylnaltrexone was a double-blind study of 22 adults who were enrolled in a methadone maintenance program and had methadone-induced constipation (Yuan, Foss, O'Connor, et al., 2000). The subjects were randomized to receive either IV methylnaltrexone (up to 0.365 mg/kg) or placebo infusion over 9 minutes. All of the subjects who received methylnaltrexone had abdominal cramping followed by laxation on day 1 or day 2; none of those who received placebo had these effects. The effects of methadone maintenance were not reversed in this study.

A 2-week double-blind trial randomized 133 patients with incurable cancer or other end-stage disease who had been taking stable doses of opioid analgesics for 2 or more weeks to receive either SC methylnaltrexone (0.15 mg/kg) or placebo (Thomas, Karver, Cooney, et al., 2008). The median dose of morphine equivalent the patients were taking was 100 mg and 150 mg in the methylnaltrexone and placebo groups, respectively, and the patients were constipated at baseline. Laxation occurred within 4 hours of the first study dose in 48% of those who received methylnaltrexone compared with 15% of those who received placebo, and 52% had laxation without a rescue laxative within 4 hours after two or more of the first four study doses compared with 8% in the placebo group. Adverse effects were mild or moderate (e.g., abdominal pain, flatulence, nausea, increased body temperature, and dizziness) in 8% and 13% of those in the methylnaltrexone and placebo groups, respectively. Life-threatening adverse events were assessed as related to the primary illness. Eighty-nine of the patients in this study entered a 3-month, open-label extension study in which methylnaltrexone was administered to all of them. The response rate in those who had received methylnaltrexone and placebo in the double-blind phase was 45% to 58% and 48% to 52%, respectively. Similar adverse effects occurred in the open-label phase as in the double-blind phase. Analgesia was maintained throughout both phases of this study.

Methylnaltrexone was studied in a randomized, parallel-group, repeated dose, dose-ranging trial that included a one-week double-blind phase followed by an open-label phase for up to 3 weeks (Portenoy, Thomas, Moehl Boatwright, et al., 2008). The patients (N = 33) in this study had terminal or end-stage diseases and were receiving palliative care and long-term opioid therapy with stable doses for at least 2 weeks (mean and median opioid morphine equivalent dose = 289.9 mg and 180 mg, respectively) and reported ongoing constipation. They were randomized to receive 1, 5, 12.5, or 20 mg of SC methylnaltrexone. Doses between 5 mg and 20 mg (0.05 to 0.5 mg/kg) induced a bowel movement within 4 hours of drug administration significantly more often than a dose of 1 mg (less than 0.05 mg/kg), and there was no dose-response relationship above 5 mg/day. Approximately 50% of the patients responded with doses 5 mg or more within 4 hours and maintained favorable effects with repeated doses. These doses produced effective and rapid relief of constipation without producing pain flare or opioid withdrawal symptoms. All of the patients in this study experienced at least one adverse effect related to treatment; however, most were mild and not related to the dose of methylnaltrexone; abdominal pain was the most common. More recent research (N = 52) showed methylnaltrexone (0.15 mg/kg) given SC every other day for 2 weeks to patients with advanced illness resulted in a higher percentage of patient-rated improvements in bowel status, prompt and predictable laxation, and less use of other laxation techniques (e.g., laxatives and enemas) compared with placebo (Chamberlain, Cross, Winston, et al., 2009) (see Table 19-1).

Postoperative Ileus

Postoperative ileus is the temporary impairment of GI motility following surgery (Moore, Kalff, Bauer, 2005). Kehlet (2005) defines it as the time from surgery until passage of flatus or stool and tolerance of diet and describes it as part of the normal pathophysiologic response to surgical injury with multiple underlying mechanisms. As such, it requires a multimodal approach to preventing and treating it (Gannon, 2007; Kehlet, 2005). It is characterized by delayed gastric emptying, dilation of the small bowel and colon, loss of normal propulsive contractile patterns, and inability to pass gas or stool (Moore, Kalff, Bauer, 2005). Unresolved ileus is a postoperative complication that can cause significant discomfort, pulmonary morbidity, delayed rehabilitation, prolonged hospitalization, and increased cost of care (Kehlet, 2005; Mythen, 2005).

The effectiveness of traditional measures to reduce the incidence of postoperative ileus, such as nasogastric (NG) tube drainage and avoidance of early fluid and food intake, have been questioned (Mythen, 2005; Viscusi, Gan, Leslie, et al., 2009; Wilmore, Kehlet, 2008). A systematic review of the literature concluded that routine NG decompression after abdominal surgery did not accomplish any of the intended goals, patients with ileus recovered earlier without an NG tube, and the practice of routine NG decompression should be abandoned in favor of selective use (Nelson, Tse, Edwards, 2005). When used, NG tubes should be removed as soon as possible to avoid adverse effects including fever, atelectasis, and pneumonia (Holte, Kehlet, 2002; Kehlet, 2005; Saclarides, 2006).

Oral intake is traditionally restricted in the early postoperative period, and although a Cochrane Collaboration Review found early feeding to be safe, no significant difference in postoperative ileus could be found between early and delayed oral fluids and food after major abdominal surgery (Charoenkwan, Phillipson, Vutyavanich, 2007). Nevertheless, research is ongoing regarding its impact on ileus (Saclarides, 2006), and postoperative rehabilitation protocols that include early feeding have produced impressive results (Wilmore, Kehlet, 2001). Oral intake has been successfully initiated as early as 6 hours after colonic surgeries that use an anastomosis (Basse, Hjort Jakobsen, Billesbolle, et al., 2000; Basse, Raskov, Hjort Jakobsen, et al., 2002; Muller, Zalunardo, Hubner, et al., 2009).

Gum chewing has been suggested as a novel and inexpensive approach to reducing ileus. More research with larger numbers of patients are needed to clarify a role (Gannon, 2007), but one randomized controlled trial (N = 34) found patients who chewed gum after open sigmoid resection experienced a significantly faster return of GI function and shorter length of stay than those who did not chew gum (Schuster, Grewal, Greaney, et al., 2006). An earlier smaller study (N = 19) of patients undergoing laparoscopic colectomy found similar results (Asao, Kuwano, Nakamura, et al., 2002).

Fluid excess can be detrimental to GI motility and should be avoided during and after colorectal surgery (Kehlet, 2005). Further research is needed to clarify the optimal amount and composition of fluid that should be administered for the various surgical procedures (Wilmore, Kehlet, 2008).

Randomized controlled trials demonstrate a reduction in duration of ileus from approximately 5 days to 3 days with the use of laparoscopic surgery (Kehlet, 2005). More randomized controlled research is needed to confirm the impact of laparoscopic techniques, but the additional benefits of reduced pain and opioid requirements can be expected to improve bowel function (Kehlet, 2005; Schwenk, Haase, Neudecker, et al., 2005).

Although early ambulation has not been shown to reduce the duration of ileus, immobility may lead to other complications, so aggressive mobilization is recommended as part of the overall strategy to reduce postoperative ileus (Kehlet, Holte, 2001). To this end, effective pain management is critical. Opioids slow bowel motility and contribute to ileus (Wood, 2005); therefore, administration of the lowest effective opioid dose (or, in some cases, avoiding opioids entirely) during the perioperative period is an important strategy in patients at high risk for ileus, such as those having open colorectal surgery. Continuous epidural analgesia with local anesthetics provides effective pain management for these types of surgeries, produces a positive effect on the stress response, and reduces postoperative ileus (Jorgensen, Wetterslev, Moiniche, et al., 2001). Because inhibitory neural reflexes are mediated through the sympathetic enteric nervous system and contribute to postoperative ileus, mid-to-low thoracic epidural catheter placement is essential (Kehlet, 2005). Very low thoracic and lumbar epidural analgesia and epidural opioids have no positive effects on ileus (Holte, Kehlet, 2002; Kehlet, 2005); however, low-dose opioid (e.g., morphine less than 1 mg/h) added to a sufficient amount of local anesthetic (e.g., bupivacaine 0.25%) epidurally will improve analgesia and preserve the ileus-reducing effect of epidural analgesia (Kehlet, 2005). Epidural analgesia should be provided for 2 to 3 days following major surgery.

For many years, the only effective pharmacologic agent for treatment of ileus was the prokinetic agent cisapride, but it was removed from the market because of potential cardiac adverse effects (Kehlet, 2005; Holte, Kehlet, 2002). Metoclopramide has been used as well but has not been shown to reduce postoperative ileus (Kehlet, Holte, 2001). There are no randomized controlled studies evaluating the use of laxatives to reduce ileus.

Opioid Antagonists for Management of Ileus

A major advance in the management of postoperative ileus is the approval of alvimopan (Entereg) for the acceleration of the time to upper and lower GI recovery following partial large or small bowel resection with primary anastomosis (GlaxoSmithKline, 2009). Alvimopan is a synthetic peripherally acting mu opioid receptor antagonist taken orally (12 mg 30 minutes to 5 hours prior to surgery, then 12 mg twice daily for up to 7 days for a maximum of 15 doses) (Kraft, 2007). Randomized controlled trials have shown that the drug can reduce ileus, shorten hospital length of stay, and is well tolerated with adverse effects similar to placebo after major abdominal surgery (Becker, Blum, 2009; Leslie, 2005; Neary, Delaney, 2005; Sinatra, 2006; Viscusi, Gan, Leslie, et al., 2009; Viscusi, Goldstein, Witkowski, et al., 2006). Methylnaltrexone, another peripherally acting mu opioid antagonist, has also been shown to reduce ileus (Viscusi, Gan, Leslie, et al., 2009) but is approved and used most often for the treatment of opioid-induced constipation in patients with advanced illness (see previous discussion earlier in the chapter). The opioid antagonists naloxone and nalmefene are not selective for the mu opioid receptors in the GI tract and should not be used for the prevention or treatment of ileus (Kraft, 2007).

In summary, postoperative ileus has multiple underlying mechanisms and is influenced by a number of factors. Management requires the implementation of a multimodal approach that focuses on prevention. Strategies include continuous thoracic epidural analgesia, opioid-sparing analgesic techniques, peripheral mu opioid antagonists, laparoscopic surgical techniques, and avoidance of routine NG tube, fluid excess, and immobility (see Table 19-1).

Nausea and Vomiting in Patients Receiving Long-Term Opioid Therapy

Initiating or increasing opioid therapy may cause nausea through both peripheral and central mechanisms that stimulate the chemoreceptor trigger zone in the brain, slowing GI mobility, and sensitizing the labyrinth vestibular system (needed for balance and equilibrium) (Gibbison, Spencer, 2009; Hanks, Cherny, Fallon, 2004; Pleuvry, 2009). Nausea is most common with the initial opioid dose and usually subsides within weeks of opioid therapy (Fine, Portenoy, 2007). In some patients, nausea is persistent and severe. Intractable nausea and vomiting in terminally ill patients have a significant negative impact on quality of life and function (Wood, Shega, Lynch, et al., 2007). Further investigation is warranted if it is suspected that factors other than opioid therapy are the cause.

The incidence and severity of nausea does not justify prophylactic treatment, with the possible exception of those patients who have a history of severe opioid-induced nausea and vomiting (Fine, Portenoy, 2007; Hanks, Cherny, Fallon, 2004). However, nausea should be treated aggressively once it occurs. Once controlled, the antiemetic can be tapered after a week to determine if the patient has developed tolerance to the emetogenic effects of the opioid. If not, treatment should be resumed and another tapering trial attempted again in one week (Fine, Portenoy, 2007).

A variety of antiemetics is available to treat nausea and can be selected based on assumptions concerning the underlying mechanism (see Table 19-1). A dopamine antagonist, such as prochlorperazine, is most often selected, but the occurrence of nausea immediately after eating, or nausea associated with early satiety and bloating, suggests the occurrence of delayed gastric emptying, which in turn, supports a trial of a prokinetic drug, such as metoclopramide (Reglan) (Fine, Portenoy, 2007). A retrospective chart review led researchers to recommend risperidone 1 mg daily for refractory nausea and vomiting in advanced cancer patients (Okamoto, Tsuneto, Matsuda, et al., 2007). When nausea occurs in patients with medical illness and is both severe and presumably determined by several causes, combination therapy should be considered. For example, a prospective, multicenter, phase II clinical trial administered daily IV granisetron (Kytril) (3 mg) and dexamethasone (Decadron) (8 mg) to 24 patients with intestinal obstruction who were refractory to previous antiemetic treatment (Tuca, Roca, Sala, et al., 2009). This regimen controlled nausea and vomiting in 86.9% of the patients.

Slow and steady opioid titration helps to reduce nausea. Eliminating nonessential drugs that may be contributing to nausea may be helpful as well (Fine, Portenoy, 2007). Adjustments in diet and activity plus the use of relaxation techniques can also be effective remedies (Coyle, Cherny, Portenoy, 1995). Table 19-1 outlines approaches commonly used to treat opioid-induced nausea and vomiting.

Postoperative Nausea and Vomiting (PONV)

Nausea and vomiting are among the most unpleasant of the adverse effects associated with surgery and are the cause of low patient satisfaction and higher cost of care in patients who have them compared with those who do not (Habib, Gan, 2004; Watcha, 2000). Many patients consider postoperative nausea and vomiting (PONV) to be as debilitating as the pain associated with the surgery. A questionnaire administered to postoperative patients revealed that they place high value on not having PONV and are willing to pay a significant amount for an effective antiemetic (Gan, Sloan, de L Dear, et al., 2001). PONV also is associated with detrimental effects, including aspiration of vomitus, tension on sutures, increased intracranial and intraocular pressure, and fluid and electrolyte imbalance. Not only does PONV have a negative impact on patient outcomes, but it can increase the burden on nursing staff (Miaskowski, 2009). It was once described as the "big little problem" by clinicians who manage it (Watcha, White, 1995).

| **Box 19-1** | Risk Factors for Postoperative Nausea and Vomiting (PONV) in Adults |

PATIENT-SPECIFIC RISK FACTORS

- Female sex
- Nonsmoking status
- History of PONV/motion sickness

ANESTHETIC RISK FACTORS

- Use of volatile anesthetics within 0 to 2 hours
- Nitrous oxide
- Use of intraoperative and postoperative opioids

SURGICAL RISK FACTORS

- Duration of surgery (each 30-minute increase in duration increases PONV risk by 60%, so that a baseline risk of 10% is increased by 16% after 30 minutes)
- Type of surgery (laparoscopy, ear-nose-throat, neurosurgery, breast, strabismus, laparotomy, plastic surgery)

From Pasero, C., & McCaffery, M. (2011). *Pain assessment and pharmacologic management*, p. 493, St. Louis, Mosby. Data from Gan, T. J., Meyer, T., Apfel, C. C., et al. (2003). Consensus guidelines for managing postoperative nausea and vomiting. *Anesth Analg, 97*(1), 62-71; Apfel, C. C., Laara, E., Koivuranta, M., et al. (1999). A simplified risk score for predicting postoperative nausea and vomiting. *Anesthesiology, 91,* 693-700; Sinclair, D. R., Chung, F., & Mezei, G. (1999). Can postoperative nausea and vomiting be predicted? *Anesthesiology, 91,* 109-118. Koivuranta, M., Laara, E., Snare, L., et al. (1997) A survey of postoperative nausea and vomiting. *Anaesthesia, 52,* 443-449; Apfel, C. C., Katz, M. H., Kranke, P., et al. (2002). Volatile anaesthetics may be the main cause of early but not delayed postoperative vomiting: A randomized controlled trial of factorial design. *Br J Anaesth, 88,* 659-668; Sukhani, R., Vazquez, J., Pappas, A. L., et al. (1996). Recovery after propofol with and without intraoperative fentanyl in patients undergoing ambulatory gynecologic laparoscopy. *Anesth Analg, 83,* 975-981; Apfel, C. C., Kranke, P., Eberhart, L. H., et al. (2002). Comparison of predictive models for postoperative nausea and vomiting. *Br J Anaesth 88,* 234-240; Moiniche, S., Romsing, J., Dahl, J. B., et al. (2003). Nonsteroidal antiinflammatory drugs and the risk of operative site bleeding after tonsillectomy: A quantitative systematic review. *Anesth Analg, 96,* 68-77; Polati, E., Verlato, G., Finco, G., et al. (1997). Ondansetron versus metoclopramide in the treatment of postoperative nausea and vomiting. *Anesth Analg, 85,* 395-399; Fabling, J. M., Gan, T. J., El-Moalem, H. E., et al. (2000). A randomized, double-blinded comparison of ondansetron, droperidol, and placebo for prevention of postoperative nausea and vomiting after supratentorial craniotomy. *Anesth Analg, 91,* 358-361; Gan, T. J., Ginsberg, B., Grant, A. P., et al. (1996). Double-blind, randomized comparison of ondansetron and intraoperative propofol to prevent postoperative nausea and vomiting. *Anesthesiology, 85,* 1036-1042. © 2011, Pasero C. May be duplicated for use in clinical practice.

Opioids are among a number of factors that increase the incidence of PONV. Box 19-1 lists the primary risk factors. A review of the literature described other factors in addition to this established list, including history of migraine, presence of preoperative anxiety, and the use of longer-acting versus shorter-acting opioids (Gan, 2006). It is important to note that postoperative pain, particularly incident pain, is associated with a higher incidence of postoperative vomiting (Chia, Kuo, Liu, et al., 2002; Ho, Gan, 2009).

Despite being listed as a risk factor in accepted guidelines (see Box 19-1), there is controversy about whether or not the type of surgical procedure influences the incidence of PONV (Habib, Gan, 2010; Scuderi, 2010). Researchers conducted a retrospective review of oncology surgeries from their electronic database to evaluate the impact of type of surgery on antiemetic administration within the first 2 hours of PACU admission and found that patients who underwent neurologic, head or neck, and abdominal surgeries received significantly more antiemetic in the PACU than patients who underwent integumetary-musculoskeletal (e.g., puncture procedures of the skin or muscles) and superficial (e.g., breast or axillary, endoscopic) surgeries (Ruiz, Kee, Frenzel, et al., 2010). In a commentary about this research, Habib and Gan (2010) discuss several limitations of this study and problems with methodology, and they conclude that large well-designed studies are needed to firmly establish the type of surgery as a risk factor (Habib, Gan, 2010).

Consensus guidelines present a number of recommendations for the management of PONV (Gan, Meyer, Apfel, et al., 2003, 2007). Algorithms that incorporate guideline recommendations are available (American Society of PeriAnesthesia Nurses, 2006; Gan, Meyer, Apfel, et al., 2007), and the December 2006 focus issue of the *Journal of PeriAnesthesia Nursing* is devoted entirely to content on PONV. Below is a summary of the major guideline recommendations in adults followed by a more detailed discussion of various antiemetics and strategies for treatment of PONV (see Table 19-1).

- Identify patients at high risk for PONV (see Box 19-1). There is no consensus on how many risk factors a patient must have to warrant the designation of high risk (Apfel, Kranke, Eberhart, et al., 2002; Gan, Meyer, Apfel, et al., 2003; van den Bosch, Kalkman, Vergouwe, et al., 2005). A simple scoring system (the Apfel risk score) developed by Apfel and colleagues (1999) is widely used and has been shown to be reliable and valid for this purpose. It is based on four predictors: female gender, prior history of motion sickness or PONV, nonsmoking status, and the use of postoperative opioids. If no or only one factor is present, the incidence of PONV varies from 10% to 21%. If two or more are present, the risk rises to 39% to 78% (Apfel, Laara, Koivuranta, et al., 1999).
- Reduce baseline risk factors, e.g., implement multimodal analgesic strategies to treat postoperative pain so that no opioid or the lowest effective dose of opioid can be given. This may also include the use of effective nonpharmacologic strategies such as

relaxation techniques, acupuncture, and acupressure (Lee, Done, 1999; Nunley, Wakim, Guinn, 2008; Roscoe, Bushunow, Jean-Pierre, et al., 2009). Although nondrug interventions may be helpful, the mainstay of PONV treatment is pharmacologic (Wilhelm, Dehoorne-Smith, Kale-Pradhan, 2007). The use of regional rather than general anesthesia is widely recommended to reduce PONV, although some surgical procedures (e.g., cesarean, some major orthopedic surgeries) are associated with a high incidence of PONV despite using regional anesthesia (Borgeat, Ekatodramis, Schenker, 2003).

- Administer PONV prophylaxis using one to two interventions to patients at moderate risk for PONV. For example, administer dexamethasone (Decadron) before anesthesia induction and a serotonin receptor antagonist (e.g., ondansetron [Zofran]) at the end of surgery. It is important to consider that research has shown that single-drug prophylaxis has a high failure rate and is associated with a resultant increased cost of care (Gan, Meyer, Apfel, et al., 2007; Watcha, 2000), so combinations of two antiemetics rather than a single antiemetic prophylactically are preferred.
- Administer PONV prophylaxis using two or more interventions (multimodal approach) to patients at high risk for PONV. For example, administer dexamethasone before anesthesia induction, IV total anesthesia (IVTA) propofol (Diprivan), a serotonin receptor antagonist at the end of surgery, and IV propofol rescue doses in the PACU. A prospective study of 376 patients at high risk for PONV revealed that the administration of three or more prophylactic antiemetics produced the largest reduction in PONV, but despite this aggressive treatment, 30% still experienced symptoms severe enough to interfere with function (White, O'Hara, Roberson, et al., 2008). A prospective observational study concluded similarly that compared with lower Apfel risk scores, a high Apfel risk score (see above) was associated with a higher incidence of emetic sequelae in the first 24 hours after surgery despite the prophylactic administration of multiple antiemetics (White, Sacan, Nuangchamnong, et al., 2008).
- Do not administer prophylactic antiemetic treatment to low-risk patients as this is not supported by current practice (Apfel, Korttila, Abdalla, et al., 2004; Gan, Meyer, Apfel, et al., 2003, 2007); however, provide antiemetic treatment to patients with PONV who did not receive prophylaxis or in whom prophylaxis failed.

Antiemetics

There are numerous antiemetic drug options available (Carlisle, Stevenson, 2006), and selection should be based on evidence of efficacy and safety as well as consideration of cost (see Table 19-1). A systematic review concluded that no one antiemetic agent is superior to another (Wilhelm, Dehoorne-Smith, Kale-Pradhan, 2007). A multicenter study of over 4000 patients at high risk for PONV (greater than 40% risk per Apfel risk scoring system [Apfel, Laara, Koivuranta, et al., 1999]) and undergoing a variety of types of surgeries were randomized to receive one of the following interventions: ondansetron (4 mg IV) or no ondansetron; dexamethasone (4 mg IV) or no dexamethasone; droperidol (Inapsine) (1.25 mg IV) or no droperidol; propofol or a volatile anesthetic (i.e., isoflurane, desflurane, or sevoflurane); nitrogen or nitrous oxide; and remifentanil or fentanyl. Because propofol has been shown to reduce PONV (see the paragraphs that follow), twice as many patients were assigned to the propofol group to ensure adequate power to compare treatments. All of the antiemetics were similarly effective; ondansetron, dexamethasone, and droperidol reduced risk by approximately 26%, propofol by 19%, and nitrogen by 12%. Droperidol, which has a "Black Box" warning for potential QTc prolongation and torsades de pointes, was safe (see later in the chapter for more on droperidol). The researchers pointed out that the clinical implication of their findings is that, because the interventions were similarly effective, the safest and least expensive treatment should be used first.

The glucocorticoid dexamethasone is an excellent choice antiemetic because numerous studies have shown it to be effective, safe, and inexpensive (Gan, Meyer, Apfel, et al., 2007) (see Table 19-1). It may be given prophylactically before induction of anesthesia as well as for established PONV (Golembiewski, Chernin, Chopra, 2005) and has been shown to have similar efficacy to the serotonin antagonist tropisetron, which is not available in the United States (Wang, Ho, Uen, et al., 2002). Dexamethasone is administered as a single 4 mg to 8 mg IV bolus dose most often and has been combined in multimodal treatment plans with a number of other agents including ondansetron (Zofran) (Paech, Rucklidge, Lain, et al., 2007; Pan, Lee, Harris, 2008), granisetron (Kytril) (Fujii, Saitoh, Tanaka, et al., 1999; Gan, Coop, Philip, et al., 2005), dolasetron (Anzemet) (Coloma, White, Markowitz, et al., 2002; Rusch, Arndt, Martin, et al., 2007), droperidol (Sanchez-Ledesma, Lopez-Olaondo, Pueyo, et al., 2002), metoclopramide (Reglan) (Wallenborn, Gelbrich, Bulst, et al., 2006), and haloperidol (Haldol) (Chu, Shieh, Tzeng, et al., 2008; Rusch, Arndt, Martin, et al., 2007). Adverse effects are rare with short-term use (Gan, Meyer, Apfel, et al., 2007).

The serotonin receptor antagonists dolasetron, granisetron, and ondansetron are most effective when administered at the end of surgery (Gan, Meyer, Apfel, et al., 2007) (see Table 19-1). The newest serotonin antagonist palonosetron (Aloxi) is approved for prevention of chemotherapy-induced nausea and has been shown to significantly decrease PONV in a dose-related manner (0.075 mg IV significantly better than 0.025 mg IV) when administered immediately prior to anesthesia

induction (Candiotti, Kovac, Melson, et al., 2008). The serotonin receptor antagonists are often combined with other antiemetics in multimodal PONV prophylaxis regimens. This practice is supported by a meta-analysis of 33 randomized controlled trials (3447 patients), which concluded that various combinations of a serotonin antagonist with dexamethasone or droperidol were equally effective with similar adverse effects, and the combinations were more effective than a serotonin antagonist alone (Habib, El-Moalem, Gan, 2004). A 2001 systematic review of the literature found that the serotonin antagonists available at the time were similarly effective for treatment of established PONV and that lower doses were as effective as higher doses, so the lowest dose in the dosing range was recommended (Kazemi-Kjellberg, Henzi, Tramer, 2001).

The serotonin antagonists are reported to prevent postoperative vomiting better than nausea (Gan, Meyer, Apfel, et al., 2007; Kazemi-Kjellberg, Henzi, Tramer, 2001); however, an analysis of data from 5161 patients concluded that ondansetron prevents both symptoms equally well (Jokela, Cakmakkaya, Danzeisen, et al., 2009). Ondansetron 8 mg twice daily is effective in an orally disintegrating tablet formulation (Zofran ODT) (Gan, Franiak, Reeves, 2002; Grover, Mathew, Hegde, 2009; Hartsell, Long, Kirsch, 2005). The most common adverse effect of the serotonin antagonists is headache (Kazemi-Kjellberg, Henzi, Tramer, 2001).

The anticholinergic scopolamine delivered via a transdermal patch (Transderm-Scop, Transderm-V) has been shown to prevent PONV with minimal adverse effects when applied preoperatively (White, Tang, Song, et al., 2007) (see Table 19-1). One patch (1.5 mg) should be applied behind the ear preoperatively, taking into account its 2- to 4-hour onset of action, and it can provide relief for up to 72 hours. A second patch may be applied after the first is removed at 72 hours. Transdermal scopolamine may be combined with other antiemetics in a multimodal treatment plan (Kranke, Morin, Roewer, et al., 2002). A randomized study of 126 patients undergoing cosmetic surgery found that the transdermal scopolamine patch combined with IV ondansetron (4 mg) was more effective in reducing PONV than ondansetron plus a placebo patch (Sah, Ramesh, Kaul, et al., 2009). Another study also found the combination to be more effective than ondansetron alone (Gan, Sinha, Kovac, et al., 2009). Transdermal scopolamine has also been used to reduce nausea and vomiting associated with intrathecal morphine post–cesarean section (Harnett, O'Rourke, Walsh, et al., 2007). Adverse effects include dry mouth, sedation, and visual disturbances; older patients may be more sensitive to CNS adverse effects, such as dizziness and agitation (Golembiewski, Chernin, Chopra, 2005).

Research in the 1990s demonstrated that the IV sedative hypnotic propofol at subhypnotic doses (5 to 10 mg IV push q 4 to 6 h or 0.5 to 1 mg/kg per hour continuous infusion) reduced the overall incidence of PONV in patients at high risk for PONV without untoward sedative or cardiovascular (CV) effects compared with placebo (Ewalenko, Janny, Dejonckheere, et al., 1996). Since then, the drug has gained in popularity as a component of multimodal approaches designed to reduce PONV (Eberhart, Mauch, Morin, et al., 2002; Scudieri, James, Harris, et al., 2000) (see Table 19-1). A randomized controlled study administered 90 patients undergoing laparoscopic cholecystectomy one of the following regimens: (1) a multimodal management strategy that involved the use of TIVA propofol plus droperidol and ondansetron, (2) IV propofol at induction followed by inspired isoflurane/nitrous oxide-based anesthesia, droperidol, and ondansetron, or (3) TIVA with no other antiemetic prophylaxis (Habib, White, Eubanks, et al., 2004). The droperidol (0.625 mg) was administered at induction and ondansetron (4 mg) was administered at the end of surgery in groups 1 and 2. Complete response rate (no PONV and no rescue antiemetic) at 2 hours and 24 hours after surgery was 90% and 80% in group 1, 63% and 63% in group 2, and 66% and 43% in group 3. Patient satisfaction was also higher in group 1. The researchers noted, however, that the higher cost of propofol compared with volatile anesthetics and its short-lived antiemetic effect (limited to early postoperative period) makes it suitable for use only in patients at very high risk for PONV.

Droperidol and the "Black Box" Warning

Since its approval for use in general anesthesia in the 1970s, the butyrophenone droperidol (Inapsine) has been used to effectively and cost-efficiently treat PONV (White, 2002). In 2001, the United States Food and Drug Administration (U.S. FDA) issued a "Black Box" warning that described the drug's potential to cause prolonged QTc interval and torsade de pointes, a life-threatening cardiac dysrhythmia (Martinez, Moos, Dahlen, 2006). However, citing a lack of documentation of cardiac adverse events, the FDA warning has been widely criticized by anesthesia experts (Gan, White, Scuderi, et al., 2002; White, 2002). A review of the 273 reported adverse events involving the use of droperidol at doses of 1.25 mg or less (customary for treatment of PONV) revealed extensive use of the drug (over 11 million ampules sold in 2001) (Habib, Gan, 2003). Of the 273 adverse events, 74 and 17 were cases of possible cardiac events and torsades de pointes or prolonged QTc interval, respectively. The researchers concluded that there was no evidence of a cause-and-effect relationship between the occurrence of arrhythmias and small-dose droperidol (1.25 mg or less). A later randomized controlled trial of 120 patients undergoing outpatient surgery found no statistically significant increase in QTc interval compared with placebo during general anesthesia and no evidence of any droperidol-induced QTc prolongation after surgery (White, Song, Abrao, et al., 2005). The drug is recommended in doses less than 1.25 mg as a first-line option in evidence-based PONV management guidelines (Gan, Meyer, Apfel, et al., 2003, 2007) (see Table 19-1).

Novel Approaches to the Management of PONV

Some novel and relatively inexpensive approaches have been tried for the management of PONV. Researchers applied nicotine patches to patients undergoing laparoscopic cholecystectomy under general anesthesia based on research that shows cigarette smoking reduces risk of PONV (Ionescu, Badescu, Acalovschi, 2007). Patients in this study (N = 75) were randomized according to their cigarette smoking status: (1) nonsmokers, (2) patients who had stopped smoking at least 5 years prior and received one 16.6 mg nicotine patch, and (3) patients who currently smoked. There was a 20% reduction in PONV in patients in group 2 compared with group 1 and no difference between group 2 and group 3.

Intraoperative supplemental oxygen has been suggested as a strategy to reduce PONV, but research is conflicting. One early study showed that the incidence of PONV was significantly reduced in patients following laparoscopic gynecologic surgery who received 80% supplemental intraoperative oxygen (22%) and those who received 8 mg of ondansetron at induction (30%) compared with patients who received 30% supplemental oxygen intraoperatively (44%) (Goll, Akca, Grief, et al., 2001). However, a later study showed that neither 30% nor 80% intraoperative oxygen administration reduced PONV in 100 patients undergoing ambulatory gynecologic laparoscopy (Purhonen, Turunen, Ruohoaho, et al., 2003). Intraoperative supplemental oxygen did not decrease the incidence of PONV post–cesarean section delivery with neuraxial anesthesia either (Phillips, Broussard, Sumrall, et al., 2007).

Studies have shown that wrist acustimulation/acupressure (acupuncture point P6 [pericardium 6]) (ReliefBand®) reduces PONV (Gan, Jiao, Zenn, et al., 2004; Lee, Fan, 2009; Nunley, Wakim, Guinn, 2008; Roscoe, Bushunow, Jean-Pierre, et al., 2009) and that when combined with ondansetron (4 mg), the response rate to acustimulation is increased and quality of recovery and patient satisfaction are improved (Coloma, White, Ogunnaike, et al., 2002; White, Issioui, Hu, et al., 2002). The optimal time to administer acustimulation for antiemetic prophylaxis is after surgery (White, Hamza, Recart, et al., 2005). Figure 19-2 shows the location of acupuncture point P6.

A meta-analysis of research on gum chewing during the early postoperative period following colectomy concluded that the practice may enhance GI recovery and reduce length of stay (Purkayastha, Tilney, Darzi, et al., 2008). Improved GI recovery may contribute to a lower incidence of PONV.

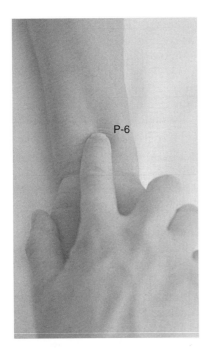

Figure 19-2 | Wrist acustimulation for PONV: Location of acupuncture point P-6.

From Focks, C. (2008). *Atlas of acupuncture*, Philadelphia, Churchill Livingstone.

Effective, Safe, and Inexpensive Treatment

By far, the most effective, safest, and least expensive way to treat PONV is to reduce the opioid dose whenever possible. Postoperative opioid orders should include the expectation that nurses will consider decreasing the opioid dose by 25% prior to or in conjunction with pharmacologic treatment of moderate-to-severe PONV (see following patient example and Form 17-1 on p. 464 for an example of how decreases in opioid dose can be included in opioid order sets). Decreasing the opioid dose is facilitated by adding or increasing a nonopioid, such as an NSAID or acetaminophen, or adding a local anesthetic to the epidural opioid solution to provide additional pain relief. If patients are too nauseated to take oral nonopioids, they may be given rectally (see Section III and Chapter 14 in this section for more on rectal administration).

Patient Example

Mr. F. is receiving IV ketorolac and IV PCA hydromorphone for management of his pain after radical prostatectomy. His prescription is: PCA dose 0.2 mg; lockout interval 6 minutes; no basal rate. His pain rating is 0/10. He reports feeling nauseated for a few minutes after he presses his PCA button. He has been given an antiemetic twice without relief and dislikes feeling "sleepy" after the antiemetic is given. The nurse practitioner has left orders to decrease the opioid dose 25% to 50% for minor adverse effects. Because Mr. F. is completely comfortable and slightly drowsy, his nurse decides to decrease his PCA dose by 50%: 0.2 mg × 0.50 (50%) = 0.1 mg. (Mr. F.'s report that nausea occurs only after he administers a PCA dose means he is experiencing toxicity at the peak concentration of the PCA dose. The best treatment for this is smaller PCA doses. Had Mr. F. been receiving a basal rate, it would be appropriate to discontinue the basal rate and consider also decreasing the PCA dose [see Table 17-2 on pp. 469-470].) Within an hour, Mr. F. is less drowsy and reports that nausea no longer occurs when he administers PCA. His pain rating is 3/10, which is acceptable to him.

Approaches with Little or No Effectiveness

In their 2007 guidelines, the American Society for Ambulatory Anesthesia concluded that there is a lack or limited evidence of a prophylactic effect for metoclopramide (10 mg IV), ginger root, and cannabinoids for PONV (Gan, Meyer, Apfel, et al., 2007). Metoclopramide is reported to be no more effective than placebo for its treatment (Gan, 2002); however, one randomized controlled study (N = 3140) found doses of 25 to 50 mg of metoclopramide in combination with dexamethasone administered intraoperatively reduced the frequency of PONV without a high incidence of adverse effects (Wallenborn, Gelbrich, Bulst, et al., 2006). Doses this high are not recommended; the drug has been reported to produce extrapyramidal symptoms, even in low doses (i.e., 10 mg) (Moss, Hansen, 2008).

Although promethazine (Phenergan) has been used for many years and has efficacy for the treatment of established PONV (Habib, Breen, Gan, 2005; Gan, Meyer, Apfel, et al., 2007; Habib, Reuveni, Taguchi, et al., 2007; Moser, Caldwell, Rhule, 2006), it is associated with significant adverse effects, including excessive sedation, respiratory depression, dysphoria, dystonia, and extrapyramidal symptoms (McGee, Alexander, 1979; Sheth, Verrico, Skledar, et al., 2005). Further, significant tissue damage can occur when promethazine is given intravenously (Institute for Safe Medication Practices, 2006a, 2006b). A "Black Box" warning added to promethazine prescribing information describes these injuries and the risk of unintentional intraarterial injection and recommends deep IM injection of the drug; SC injection is contraindicated (U.S. FDA, 2009c). It is common practice to administer promethazine based on the belief that it will enhance opioid analgesia; however, early research dispelled this misconception (McGee, Alexander, 1979), and the practice is discouraged (Pasero, Portenoy, McCaffery, 1999). If promethazine is used, low doses are recommended, particularly in older adults (Habib, Breen, Gan, 2005; Moser, Caldwell, Rhule, 2006). Doses of 6.25 mg were found to be as effective as higher doses (e.g., 12 mg) (Habib, Reuveni, Taguchi, et al., 2007).

Prochlorperazine (Compazine) provided better relief of nausea and vomiting than promethazine in patients in the emergency department (ED) (Ernst, Weiss, Park, et al., 2000). Prochlorperazine has a faster onset and causes less sedation than promethazine as well (Golembiewski, Chernin, Chopra, 2005).

Another commonly used drug is hydroxyzine (Vistaril), but the doses that would be required to produce analgesia create significant risk of respiratory depression that is not reversible by naloxone (Gordon, 1995). IM hydroxyzine is especially irritating to the muscle and soft tissue and can produce sterile abscesses, so this practice is discouraged as well. Other older drugs—dimenhydrinate (Dramamine) (Kothari, Boyd, Bottcher, et al., 2000) and diphenhydramine (Benadryl)—are occasionally used for PONV but can cause significant sedation and dizziness. Antiemetics with better efficacy and safety should be considered before these drugs are used for treatment of PONV (Gan, Meyer, Apfel, et al., 2007) (see Table 19-1).

The routine use of NG tubes during surgery as a means of reducing PONV is not recommended. A large case control study (N = 4055) evaluated the association between NG tube use and the incidence of nausea, emesis, and overall PONV and showed no reduction in the incidence of these three outcome measures; the incidence of PONV was 44.4% with intraoperative NG tube versus 41.5% in controls (Kerger, Mascha, Steinbrecher, et al., 2009).

Biliary Spasm

Opioids increase smooth muscle tone in the biliary tract, especially in the sphincter of Oddi, which regulates the flow of bile and pancreatic fluids. This can result in a decrease in biliary and pancreatic secretions and a rise in bile duct pressure (Fukuda, 2005). Patients may experience epigastric distress and occasionally biliary spasm from this effect.

All opioids are capable of causing constricture of the sphincter of Oddi and the biliary tract ("biliary spasm") and do so in a drug- and dose-dependent manner (Fukuda, 2005). This effect is complex with multiple underlying mechanisms (Helm, Venu, Geenen, et al., 1988). Research on this response is somewhat conflicting with regard to differences between the various opioids. The research that has been done has never shown much clinical relevance in humans (Lee, Cundiff, 1998; Spiegel, 2001). Meperidine produces a dual effect on the biliary tract (Fukuda, 2005); at low concentrations it inhibited the response of the common bile duct to electrical stimulation, and in higher concentrations it produced an excitatory effect and increased spontaneous contractions in guinea pigs (Goldberg, Vatashsky, Haskel, et al., 1987). A common misconception is that meperidine causes less constricture of the sphincter of Oddi than other opioids, but research does not support this (see the paragraphs that follow).

Early research showed morphine increased bile duct pressure in animals (Coelho, Runkel, Herfarth, et al., 1986) and humans (Zsigmond, Vieira, Duarte, et al., 1993). A study of 36 patients without common bile duct stones or anatomic abnormalities who were undergoing cholecystectomy demonstrated that morphine increased the frequency of sphincter of Oddi motility more than meperidine (Thune, Baker, Saccone, et al., 1990); however, an earlier study showed fentanyl, meperidine, morphine, and pentazocine caused a rise in bile duct pressure of 99.5%, 61.3%, 52.7%, and 15.1%, respectively in humans (Radnay, Brodman, Mankikar, et al., 1980). In other words, morphine produced less of a rise than both fentanyl and meperidine. Although pentazocine produced the smallest rise in this study, it causes dysphoria, anxiety, nightmares, depersonalization, and hallucinations, has an analgesic ceiling, and is not recommended for the management of any type of pain (see Chapter 13).

Later randomized controlled research showed fentanyl and sufentanil had no effect on common bile duct diameter in 17 patients during cholecystectomy, and the researchers recommended fentanyl and sufentanil in patients in whom spasm of the common bile duct should be avoided (Vieira, Zsigmond, Duarte, et al., 1994). Remifentanil, another lipophilic, short-acting mu opioid, was shown to cause a shorter delay in biliary tract drainage into the duodenum in 6 healthy volunteers than had been previously reported in studies of morphine and meperidine (Fragen, Vilich, Spies, et al., 1999).

The agonist-antagonist opioids (in addition to pentazocine above) have also been researched for their effect on the sphincter of Oddi. One early study showed that fentanyl, morphine, and meperidine increased common bile duct pressure more than butorphanol or placebo in 50 patients undergoing cholecystectomy (Radnay, Duncalf, Novakovic, et al., 1984). Later research found no differences between butorphanol, nalbuphine, and placebo in patients undergoing cholecystectomy (Vieira, Zsigmond, Duarte, et al., 1993); however, a more recent study found that nalbuphine caused a significant stimulatory effect on the sphincter of Oddi in 17 patients with suspected sphincter of Oddi dysfunction when used as a premedication for endoscopy; the researchers recommended against its use for endoscopic diagnosis of this condition (Madacsy, Bertalan, Szepes, et al., 2003). As discussed in Chapter 13, the agonist-antagonists are not recommended as first-line opioid analgesics for the treatment of pain.

The Meperidine Misconception

Although institutional quality improvement initiatives have resulted in a significant decline in the use of meperidine over the years (Gordon, Jones, Goshman, et al., 2000), the drug continues to be a first-choice analgesic of many prescribers (Seifert, Kennedy, 2004). This is particularly true for the management of pain during GI procedures and in patients with pancreatitis or cholecystitis; however, there are many disadvantages to the use of meperidine for pain management, including accumulation of its toxic metabolite with repeated dosing and its inappropriateness in older adults (Latta, Ginsberg, Barkin, 2002) (see Chapter 13).

A review of the literature concluded that morphine may be of more benefit than meperidine by offering analgesia without the risks associated with meperidine and that there are no studies or evidence to indicate morphine is contraindicated for use in acute pancreatitis (2001). Low-dose transdermal fentanyl (12.5 to 25 mcg) caused no significant changes in sphincter of Oddi pressure in patients with pancreatitis in one study and was described as the ideal analgesic for treatment of pancreatitis pain (Koo, Moon, Choi, et al., 2009). An interesting letter to the editor suggested that the choice of meperidine over other opioids is not based on evidence and persists because of the perpetuation of the misconception that meperidine has no effect on the sphincter of Oddi (Lee, Cundiff, 1998). The authors equated this to the "medical equivalent of an urban legend." The best course of action is to avoid meperidine for all types of pain, including procedural pain and pancreatitis pain, and rely instead on other mu agonist opioids, such as morphine, hydromorphone, or fentanyl.

Pruritus

Pruritus (itching) is an adverse effect, not an allergic reaction to opioids (Ho, Gan, 2009). Its incidence ranges from 18% to 40% in the postoperative setting depending on the route of opioid administration and opioid administered (Wheeler, Oderda, Ashburn, et al., 2002). It is one of the most common adverse effects when opioids are delivered by the intraspinal routes (Ganesh, Maxwell, 2007; Wheeler, Oderda, Ashburn, et al., 2002) and is more common with intraspinal morphine than hydromorphone and fentanyl (Dabu-Bondoc, Franco, Sinatra, 2009).

Pruritus is sometimes generalized all over the body but usually is localized to the face, neck, or upper thorax (Ho, Gan, 2009). It rarely is accompanied by a rash. It can range from being annoying to so severe that it interferes with sleep, accomplishment of daily activities, and quality of life (Pittelkow, Loprinzi, 2004).

Pruritus, like pain, is transmitted via unmyelinated C-fiber nociceptors from the periphery (skin) to the CNS (dorsal horn of the spinal cord) where they synapse with itch-specific secondary neurons (Waxler, Dadabhoy, Stojiljkovic, et al., 2005) (see Section I). Secondary neurons then transmit the signal to the thalamus and sematosensory cortex. Opioids reduce tonic inhibition of this itch-specific pathway and allow spontaneous activity of central itch neurons (Ho, Gan, 2009). This pathway is the only one identified so far, but others are likely to exist, and further research is needed to more clearly understand

all of the underlying mechanisms of pruritus (Waxler, Dadabhoy, Stojiljkovic, et al., 2005).

Although itch is transmitted by a subset of C-fibers that are different from those that transmit pain, the two sensations seem to be interrelated; painful stimuli can inhibit itching, and inhibition of pain processing may enhance itching. Several substances have been identified as mediators of itch, including histamine, prostaglandins, and serotonin (Waxler, Dadabhoy, Stojiljkovic, et al., 2005). When applied into the epidermis, histamine stimulates histamine receptors on the itch-specific C-fibers, which can cause the itching sensation. There are two types of histamine receptors in the skin (H_1 and H_2), and clinicians have taken advantage of this in treating some types of pruritus. This may explain why the combination of the H_1 antagonist cetirizine (Zyrtec) and the H_2 antagonist cimetidine (Tagamet) was significantly more effective than diphenhydramine (Benadryl) and placebo for burn-related pruritus (Baker, Zeller, Klein, et al., 2001).

Pruritus associated with advanced illness may be caused by multiple factors related to the disease process and is particularly challenging to treat. The reader is referred to an excellent overview of the anatomy and physiology and treatment options for pruritus in patients with advanced disease in Pittelkow, M. R., & Loprinzi, C. L. (2004). Pruritus and sweating in palliative medicine. In D. Doyle, G. Hanks, N. I. Cherny, et al. (Eds.), *Oxford textbook of palliative medicine,* ed 3, pp. 573-587, New York, Oxford Press. The treatment options presented in this chapter are used primarily for postoperative pruritus.

Assessment of Pruritus

The use of a self-report tool to assess pruritus may be helpful, particularly in cases of intractable pruritus. A 4-point verbal rating scale (VRS-4) and an 11-point verbal numeric rating scale (VNRS-11) are used most often (Jenkins, Spencer, Weissgerber, 2009). The VRS-4 matches a score to the patient's description of itch intensity: 0 = no itching; 1 = mild itching; 2 = moderate itching; 3 = severe itching; the VNRS-11 is used similarly to the numerical rating scale (NRS) for pain intensity assessment: 0 = no itch and 10 = the worst imaginable level of itching. A study of 50 parturients demonstrated a strong correlation between the two scales, leading the researchers to conclude that each verbal descriptor on the VRS-4 could be substituted with a quantifiable range on the VNRS-11, i.e., 1 to 3 = mild itching; 4 to 7 = moderate itching; and 8 to 10 = severe itching (Jenkins, Spencer, Weissgerber, 2009).

Pharmacologic Management of Pruritus

Antihistamines such as diphenhydramine relieve only itch caused by histamine release, such as insect bites, urticaria, and allergic skin reactions. Although they are widely used, there is no strong evidence that antihistamines relieve opioid-induced pruritus (Grape, Shug, 2008). Some suggest that they may be more effective for pruritus caused by systemic opioids than neuraxial opioids, but research is lacking (Waxler, Dadabhoy, Stojiljkovic, et al., 2005). Patients may report being less bothered by itching after taking an antihistamine, but this is likely the result of sedating effects (Ho, Gan, 2009). Sedation can be problematic in those already at risk for excessive sedation, such as postoperative patients, as this can lead to life-threatening respiratory depression (Anwari, Iqbal, 2003) (see later in this chapter). Thus careful monitoring of sedation levels is recommended when antihistamines are combined with opioid administration, and they should not be administered if patients are excessively sedated.

Prostaglandins do not elicit pruritus when applied to the skin, but they do act synergistically with histamine to potentiate the histamine-elicited itch (Waxler, Dadabhoy, Stojiljkovic, et al., 2005). Topical ketorolac tromethamine has been shown to relieve ocular itching, most likely through its inhibition of prostaglandin synthesis (Donshik, Pearlman, Pinnas, et al., 2000) (see Section III).

It is thought that serotonin (5-HT) acts on 5-HT$_3$ receptors to generate the sensation of pruritus (Waxler, Dadabhoy, Stojiljkovic, et al., 2005). This helps to explain why the serotonin receptor antagonists have been used to successfully treat pruritus caused by intraspinal opioids. A prospective study randomized 105 patients to receive ondansetron 4 mg, dolasetron 12.5 mg, or placebo 30 minutes before spinal morphine and bupivacaine anesthesia (Iatrou, Dragoumanis, Vogiatzaki, et al., 2005). Patients in both treatment groups experienced significantly less pruritus during the first 8 postoperative hours than the placebo group, and severe pruritus was noted only in those who received placebo. Others have reported similar results with ondansetron for prevention of pruritus from intrathecal morphine (Yeh, Chen, Lin, et al., 2000) and fentanyl (Gurkan, Toker, 2002). However, no benefit was found with the combination of dexamethasone (8 mg) and ondansetron (4 mg) for prevention of intrathecal morphine-induced pruritus (Szarvas, Chellapuri, Harmon, et al., 2003). Ondansetron orally disintegrating tablets (ODT) 8 mg, ondansetron IV 4 mg, or placebo was administered prior to intrathecal morphine in 150 men undergoing surgery, and although there were no significant differences in PONV, the incidences of pruritus were 56%, 66%, and 86% in the ODT, ondansetron IV, and placebo groups, respectively (Pirat, Tuncay, Torgay, et al., 2005).

Established pruritus is responsive to treatment with ondansetron as well. A randomized controlled study of 80 women with moderate to severe pruritus following intrathecal morphine for cesarean section were given ondansetron (4 mg) or placebo (Charuluxananan, Somboonviboon, Kyokong, et al., 2000). Relief was achieved in 80% of those who received ondansetron

compared with 36% of those who received placebo. The recurrence rates within 4 hours after administration were 12% and 70% for ondansetron and placebo, respectively. Nausea and vomiting were also significantly less in the ondansetron group. A case report described the treatment of intractable pruritus with 4 mg of IV ondansetron following spinal fentanyl and bupivacaine anesthesia (Henry, Tetzlaff, Steckner, 2002).

An interesting study found that gabapentin (Neurontin) was effective in reducing the incidence of intrathecal morphine-induced pruritus (Sheen, Ho, Lee, et al., 2008). Patients (N = 86) were randomized prior to limb surgery to receive 1200 mg of gabapentin or placebo orally 2 hours prior to surgery. The incidence of pruritus was 47.5% in the gabapentin group and 77% in the placebo group. The severity of pruritus was greater, its onset shorter, and duration longer in the placebo group. The researchers suggested that the effectiveness of gabapentin may be related to its action on central neurons and the fact that intrathecal morphine-induced pruritus is a "neurogenic itch." Anticonvulsants such as gabapentin are used to treat pruritus associated with advanced illness as well (Pittelkow, Loprinzi, 2004).

Subanesthetic doses of IV propofol (e.g., 10 mg) have been shown to relieve pruritus associated with intrathecal morphine and are suggested as a second-line option after administration of a serotonin receptor antagonist (Grape, Schug, 2008). One study randomized 50 postoperative patients who had intrathecal morphine-induced pruritus to receive 10 mg of IV propofol or placebo; a dose was repeated 5 minutes later in patients who had a pruritus score of more than 2 on scale of 0 to 5 (Borgeat, Wilder-Smith, Saiah, et al., 1992). Treatment failure was defined as the persistence of a pruritus score of greater than 2 at 5 minutes after treatment. The success rate was 86% and 16% in the propofol and placebo groups, respectively. In contrast, a later randomized controlled study of 29 women with intrathecal morphine-induced pruritus following cesarean section found no difference between propofol 10 mg IV and placebo (Beilin, Bernstein, Zucker-Pinchoff, et al., 1998).

Topical local anesthetics such as EMLA or lidocaine patch 5% may provide relief of pruritus in some patients. These preparations are not convenient for generalized pruritus, but may be helpful for localized areas that are particularly bothersome (Pittelkow, Loprinzi, 2004).

Opioid Antagonists for Pruritus

Opioid antagonists, such as naloxone and naltrexone, are sometimes used to treat pruritus; however, this practice risks reversal of analgesia if the doses administered are too high. Ultra low-dose IV naloxone boluses (0.04 to 0.08 mg) or infusions (0.4 to 0.8 mg/liter IV fluid at 100 mL/h or 0.1 to 0.2 mcg/kg/h) or naltrexone (6 to 9 mg orally) may be effective in some patients with severe pruritus (Dabu-Bondoc, Franco, Sinatra, 2009; Grape, Schug, 2008) (see Table 19-1). The agonist antagonist opioid nalbuphine 4 mg IV given prior to intrathecal morphine for cesarean section for prevention of pruritus had a better success rate (20%) than ondansetron 4 mg IV (13%), ondansetron 8 mg (12%), or placebo (6%) (Charuluxananan, Kyokong, Somboonviboon, et al., 2003). Pain must be monitored closely when opioid antagonists are used.

The peripherally-acting opioid antagonist, methylnaltrexone, indicated for treatment of opioid-induced constipation, was shown to reduce the sensation of skin itch in healthy volunteers who were given IV morphine (Yuan, Foss, O'Connor, et al., 1998). Clinical research and more options from this group of drugs are needed, but these agents may have a role in the management of a variety of opioid-induced adverse effects in the future (Bates, Foss, Murphy, 2004).

Switching to Another Opioid

Switching to another opioid may relieve pruritus but is usually reserved for patients with pruritus that has been unresponsive to other treatments. A case report described intractable itching that began when morphine was initiated in a patient with small round cell tumor of the pelvis and was not improved when the patient was switched to fentanyl and then to hydromorphone (Tarcatu, Tamasdan, Moryl, et al., 2007). Diphenhydramine and hydroxyzine also had no effect. When oxycodone and a low-dose naloxone infusion (0.25 mcg/kg/h) were started, the patient's pruritus dramatically improved. Pain control was achieved with titrated doses of oxycodone (60 mg every 3 hours) and IV hydromorphone PRN. Naloxone was discontinued seven days later with no recurrence of itching. The authors suggested that the resolution of pruritus was because the oxycodone created a balance between mu and kappa opioid receptors through a predominantly kappa agonist effect. (Morphine, hydromorphone, and fentanyl bind primarily to mu opioid receptors.) Further, the authors discounted a singular role for naloxone since itching did not recur after it was discontinued.

Effective, Safe, and Inexpensive Treatment

A common clinical observation is that patients with postoperative opioid-induced pruritus have well-controlled pain. This may be because, as mentioned, the two sensations of pain and itch seem to be interrelated; painful stimuli can inhibit itching, and inhibition of pain processing may enhance itching. This helps to explain why a small decrease in the opioid dose is such an efficient solution to opioid-induced pruritus. Opioid dose reduction is by far the single most effective, safest, and least expensive treatment for pruritus. Postoperative opioid orders should include the expectation that nurses will decrease the opioid dose by 25% prior to or in conjunction with pharmacologic treatment of moderate-to-severe pruritus (see Form 17-1 on p. 464 for an example of how decreases in opioid dose can be included in opioid order sets). Patients usually tolerate this small reduction in opioid dose without any loss of analgesia and experience a significant reduction or complete resolution of their pruritus. Decreasing the opioid dose is facilitated by adding or increasing a nonopioid, such as an NSAID or acetaminophen, or adding a local anesthetic to the epidural opioid solution to provide additional pain relief.

In summary, pruritus should be treated according to its severity or prevented based on its expected severity (see Table 19-1). The use of a self-report pruritus assessment scale is recommended to help determine severity and effectiveness of treatment in patients with intractable pruritus. Intraspinal opioid-induced pruritus should be prevented with administration of a serotonin antagonist, particularly when a single-bolus intraspinal technique is used. Serotonin antagonists may be helpful for established pruritus as well. Mild facial and chest pruritus may be relieved by cold compresses. The easiest and most effective treatment for pruritus is to decrease the opioid dose if possible. Opioid agonist-antagonists and opioid antagonists should be reserved for severe pruritus, and the patient should be watched closely for any increase in pain if these are used.

Hypotension

Research studies vary widely in their definitions of hypotension, so the reported incidences vary widely. Some studies do not provide any definition, but most describe hypotension as a systolic arterial pressue of less than 80 mm Hg to less than 100 mm Hg and/or a greater than 20% decrease in arterial pressure. The overall rate of hypotension related to postoperative pain management is thought to be 4.7%, with the lowest incidence associated with IV PCA and the highest with epidural analgesia (Cashman, Dolin, 2004). An audit of over 2500 patients cared for by an acute pain service who had received a variety of analgesic techniques reported hypotension in just 4 patients due to bupivacaine and fentanyl, all with a sensory block higher than T5 (Tsui, Irwin, Wong, et al., 1997) (see Chapter 15 for discussion of thoracic epidural analgesia).

Opioids have no effect on myocardial contractility or output and, therefore, do not produce severe hemodynamic instability (i.e., severe hypotension); however, they can produce dose-related, asymptomatic bradycardia (Harris, Kotob, 2006; Ho, Gan, 2009). This is thought to be related to stimulation of the vagal nuclei in the medulla (Ho, Gan, 2009). The exception to this is meperidine, which has intrinsic antimuscarinic properties and can increase resting heart rate. Morphine can indirectly cause hypotension through the release of histamine, which causes vasodilation (Harris, Kotob, 2006), and this effect varies among individuals (Ho, Gan, 2009).

The opioid doses commonly used for pain management rarely cause hypotension (Ho, Gan, 2009). Cashman and Dolin (2004) appropriately point out that research shows that many factors other than analgesic technique (e.g., surgical factors) influence hypotension. When it does occur, it is more likely to be in individuals with high sympathetic tone, such as those with pain or poor cardiac function, or in patients who are hypovolemic. In fact, addressing pain is important because it may be contributing to hemodynamic instability. In other words, opioids should not be withheld for fear of causing hypotension.

When hypotension is a concern, it can be minimized by administering the opioid slowly, keeping the patient supine, and optimizing intravascular volume (Harris, Kotob, 2006; Ho, Gan, 2009). Therapy can begin with a small dose while closely observing patient response. Administration of opioids via slow IV infusion may be appropriate in some patients (Harris, Kotob, 2006).

Caution is recommended when administering morphine and any other histamine-releasing opioid to patients with cor pulmonale as deaths have been reported with their use in this population (Harris, Kotob, 2006). Opioids that do not release histamine are fentanyl and sufentanil (Ho, Gan, 2009). See Chapter 15 and Table 15-7 on pp. 428-429 for discussion and treatment of hypotension as an unwanted effect of intraspinal local anesthetics.

Urinary Retention

Opioids increase smooth muscle tone in the bladder and ureters and can cause bladder spasm and urgency (Hanks, Cherny, Fallon, 2004). An opioid-induced increase in sphincter tone can make urination difficult. The central effects of opioids may reduce a patient's attention to bladder stimuli, which can result in urinary retention. Urinary retention is not a common adverse effect of opioids but is observed most often in older-aged men (Hanks, Cherny, Fallon, 2004). A review of the literature revealed an incidence of urinary retention requiring catheterization to be 23% in the postoperative setting (Dolin, Cashman, 2005).

Neuraxial opioids are associated with a higher incidence of urinary retention than systemic opioids, and intrathecal opioid administration has the highest reported incidence of urinary retention (35.6%) (Wheeler, Oderda, Ashburn, et al., 2002). Although the mechanism is not fully understood, urinary retention from neuraxial opioids is thought to be the result of spinally-mediated inhibition of parasympathetic outflow (Bates, Foss, Murphy, 2004; Dabu-Bondoc, Franco, Sinatra, 2009). The addition of local anesthetic to the opioid intraspinally can compound urinary retention. It is seen less often in patients receiving thoracic than lumbar epidural analgesia, so dermatomal level of the neuraxial blockade has been cited as a possible contributing factor (Dabu-Bondoc, Franco, Sinatra,

2009; Wu, 2005). It is likely that there are multiple causes and risk factors including age, type of surgery, lack of ambulation, and abnormal voiding history. The incidence of urinary retention in the PACU (16%) was influenced only by amount of intraoperative fluids and bladder volume on entry to the PACU in one study (Keita, Diouf, Tubach, et al., 2005).

Low-dose naloxone has been used to treat urinary retention but can reverse analgesia and is not recommended (Dabu-Bondoc, Franco, Sinatra, 2009; Wang, Pennefather, Russell, 1998). A double-blind study found that both naloxone (0.01 mg/kg IV) and the peripheral opioid antagonist methylnaltrexone (0.3 mg/kg IV) reversed remifentanil-induced urinary retention in 13 male volunteers; however, whereas methylnaltrexone appeared to work via peripheral mechanisms, naloxone reversed central opioid effects (Rosow, Gomery, Chen, et al., 2007). Clinical research is needed to determine the role of the peripheral opioid antagonists in the treatment of opioid-induced urinary retention.

In and out bladder catheterization may be necessary and sufficient to relieve urinary retention in postoperative patients. For refractory urinary retention and for urinary retention in patients with persistent pain, indwelling catheterization is recommended rather than repeated catheterizations if the opioid dose cannot be reduced.

The common practice of using indwelling urinary catheters in patients receiving thoracic epidural analgesia has been questioned. A prospective study of 100 consecutive patients receiving continuous thoracic epidural analgesia for colon resection demonstrated that removal of indwelling urinary catheters 24 hours after surgery was well tolerated with just 8 patients requiring a single in and out catheterization and 1 requiring indwelling recatheterization (Basse, Werner, Kehlet, 2000). A later study of 49 patients receiving thoracic PCEA removed indwelling urinary catheters within 12 to 48 hours after surgery and found just 5 patients (10%) required recatheterization (Ladak, Katznelson, Muscat, et al., 2009). Others have found similar results (Chia, Wei, Chang, et al., 2009). If urinary catheters are used, removing them as soon as possible after surgery to reduce pain, improve mobility, and prevent infection is recommended (Pasero, Belden, 2006; Wilmore, Kehlet, 2008).

Tolerance to opioid-induced urinary retention does develop. As with the other opioid-induced adverse effects, decreasing the opioid dose, if possible, is the most effective treatment.

Myoclonus

Myoclonus is sudden, brief, involuntary muscle contractions arising from the CNS (Harris, Kotob, 2006). They can be multifocal, occurring in different places in the body. Mild and infrequent myoclonus is common in patients taking opioids with a prevalence of

83% (Glare, Walsh, Sheehan, 2006) and may resolve as tolerance develops (Coyle, Cherny, Portenoy, 1995); however, occasionally they are severe and can cause increased breakthrough pain during myoclonic episodes (Hanks, Cherny, Fallon, 2004). Myoclonic jerks usually are experienced only by patients receiving high doses of opioids (Hagen, Swanson, 1997; Han, Arnold, Bond, et al., 2002; Okon, George, 2008). Although all opioids can produce myoclonus, the effect is most prominent with meperidine, presumably from normeperidine accumulation (Hagen, Swanson, 1997) (see Chapter 13). One case report suggested that the patient's myoclonus might have been related to opioid withdrawal, underscoring the need to consider all possible causes for symptoms to determine the appropriate treatment (Han, Arnold, Bond, et al., 2002).

If the patient is taking meperidine, switching to another opioid should be done immediately to prevent further possible accumulation of normeperidine and subsequent seizures. For other opioids, primary treatment includes attempts to control pain with lower opioid doses and by adding or increasing adjuvant analgesics (Coyle, Cherny, Portenoy, 1995; Hanks, Cherny, Fallon, 2004). A benzodiazepine or anticonvulsant may be tried (Hanks, Cherny, Fallon, 2004). For example, clonazepam (Klonopin) 0.25 mg to 0.5 mg orally two or three times daily may help to control jerking, but patients may dislike the sedation it produces.

Rotation to a new opioid is instituted if symptoms worsen despite primary treatment (Mercadante, Ferrera, Villari, et al., 2009) (see Chapter 18). The muscle relaxant dantrolene (Dantrium) has been used to reduce symptoms (Mercadante, 1995), and anesthetic procedures may be indicated in some patients (Coyle, Cherny, Portenoy, 1995). A series of five case reports described treatment of severe toxicity and myoclonus. Carbamazepine (Tegretol) and phenytoin (Dilantin) were ineffective, valproic acid 500 mg/day was of uncertain benefit, and large doses of diazepam (Valium) provided only transient relief; however, cessation of the offending opioid, rotation to a new opioid, and midazolam infusion, titrated upward until myoclonic jerks disappeared (1 to 2 mg/h), successfully controlled severe myoclonus in 2 patients (Hagen, Swanson, 1997). Rehydration to facilitate renal elimination of metabolites is recommended (Morita, Tei, Tsunoda, et al., 2002). Dialysis may be necessary (Hagen, Swanson, 1997) (see Table 19-1).

Mental Status Changes

Confusion, disorientation, and cognitive impairment are among the most feared of opioid-induced adverse effects for patients and families. It occurs in 28% to 83% of patients near the end of life, depending on the population studied and criteria used to define it (Casarett, Inouye, 2001). Mild cognitive impairment

and occasional hallucinations may occur when opioid therapy is initiated and with significant dose increases (Hanks, Cherny, Fallon, 2004). Patients can be reassured that these are transient and will resolve within days to a couple of weeks. Unresolved delirium may necessitate switching to another opioid. An open-label trial described switching patients experiencing delirium related to morphine toxicity to transdermal or parenteral fentanyl (Morita, Takigawa, Onishi, et al., 2005). Others have advocated the use of methadone in this situation (Mercadante, Ferrera, Villari, et al., 2009) (see Chapter 13). Table 19-1 outlines treatment options. See also Chapter 20 for more on cognitive effects during long-term opioid therapy.

Delirium in the terminally ill has a variety of manifestations, including hallucinations, disorientation, clouding consciousness, fear, and paranoia. Opioids usually are not a cause but may be a contributing factor. Terminally ill patients with delirium tend to be taking higher opioid doses than those who do not have delirium (Gagnon, Allard, Masse, et al., 2000), but a higher dose requirement could be related to underlying pathologic processes that contribute to delirium as well. Other potential causes of delirium are major organ failure, neoplastic involvement of the CNS, sepsis, hypoxia, and electrolyte disorders, such as hypercalcemia (Hanks, Cherny, Fallon, 2004).

Up to half of delirium episodes are not noted by clinicians, underscoring the importance of a careful history and thorough evaluation that includes an accurate assessment of the patient's baseline status (Casarett, Inouye, 2001). A variety of tools are available for the assessment of delirium (Schuurmans, Deschamps, Markham, et al., 2003; Timmers, Kalisvaart, Schuurmans, et al., 2004). The Confusion Rating Scale allows evaluation of observable behaviors, and the Neecham Confusion Scale includes vital signs and oxygen saturation levels, which may provide early signs of delirium (Williams, 1991). The Delirium Observation Screening (DOS) Scale (Schuurmans, Shortridge-Baggett, Duursma, 2003) (Form 19-1) is a simple screening tool that can be easily integrated into routine care (Gagnon, Allard, Masse, et al., 2000). The Confusion Assessment Measure (CAM) (Inouye, van Dyck, Alessi, et al., 1990) is often used to confirm the diagnosis of delirium (Gagnon, Allard, Masse, et al., 2000; Schuurmans, Shortridge-Baggett, Duursma, 2003; Vaurio, Sands, Wang, et al., 2006). (See templates for some of the tools at http://www.clintemplate.org/groups/15/) (see Table 19-1).

Postoperative Delirium

The reported incidence of postoperative delirium is 10% to 60%, and it is most frequent in older adults (Vaurio, Sands, Wang, et al., 2006). This number is likely to increase as more old than young adults have surgery (Amador, Goodwin, 2005). Delirium is associated with

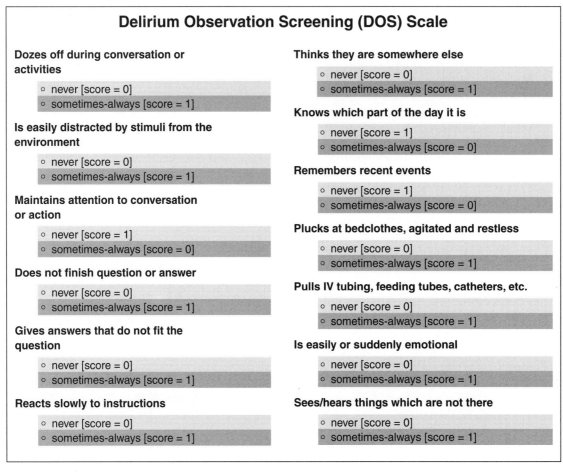

Delirium Observation Screening (DOS) Scale

Dozes off during conversation or activities
- never [score = 0]
- sometimes-always [score = 1]

Is easily distracted by stimuli from the environment
- never [score = 0]
- sometimes-always [score = 1]

Maintains attention to conversation or action
- never [score = 1]
- sometimes-always [score = 0]

Does not finish question or answer
- never [score = 0]
- sometimes-always [score = 1]

Gives answers that do not fit the question
- never [score = 0]
- sometimes-always [score = 1]

Reacts slowly to instructions
- never [score = 0]
- sometimes-always [score = 1]

Thinks they are somewhere else
- never [score = 0]
- sometimes-always [score = 1]

Knows which part of the day it is
- never [score = 1]
- sometimes-always [score = 0]

Remembers recent events
- never [score = 1]
- sometimes-always [score = 0]

Plucks at bedclothes, agitated and restless
- never [score = 0]
- sometimes-always [score = 1]

Pulls IV tubing, feeding tubes, catheters, etc.
- never [score = 0]
- sometimes-always [score = 1]

Is easily or suddenly emotional
- never [score = 0]
- sometimes-always [score = 1]

Sees/hears things which are not there
- never [score = 0]
- sometimes-always [score = 1]

Form 19-1 | Delirium Observation Screening (DOS) Scale. Maximum DOS score is 13. A score of less than 3 = not delirious; a score of 3 or more = probably delirious (contact primary provider).

From Schuurmans, M. J., Shortridge-Baggett, L. M., & Duursma, S. A. (2003). The delirium observation screening scale: A screening instrument for delirium. *Res Theory Nurs Pract, 17*(1), 31-50.

prolonged hospital stay, greater use of hospital resources, and increased cost of care (Demeure, Fain, 2006). Despite this, there is little well-controlled research on the incidence and prevention of delirium in the hospitalized patient (Siddiqi, Holt, Britton, et al., 2007).

Similar to the terminally ill, delirium tends to be underdiagnosed in the postoperative setting (Amador, Goodwin, 2005). It is characterized by alterations in orientation, consciousness, memory, thought processes, and behavior (Demeure, Fain, 2006). Patients may demonstrate either hyperactivity or hypoactivity and may be lucid at times, but typically the symptoms are worse at night ("sundowning"). A variety of delirium screening and diagnostic tools are available (see previous discussion and Form 19-1). Table 19-1 provides treatment suggestions.

Opioids are often blamed for the occurrence of postoperative confusion; however, little research supports the assertion that they are a major cause. In fact, pain and other factors, such as sleep disturbance, type of surgery, choice of opioid, and method of administering opioids, have been directly linked to postoperative cognitive

impairment. As described in the terminally ill, the importance of an accurate assessment with consideration of the patient's baseline cognitive status is critical in the confused postoperative patient; many patients undergoing surgery have pre-existing confusion and cognitive impairment and should be assessed as "at risk" for postoperative confusion. Box 19-2 lists the risks associated with postoperative delirium.

Poorly managed pain appears to be an important risk factor for postoperative delirium. Early research showed that a decline in mental status was linked to poor pain control in patients aged 50 to 80 in one study (Duggleby, Lander, 1994). Pain, not analgesic intake, predicted mental decline. More recently, a study was conducted in 330 consecutively admitted patients (age 65 years or older) scheduled for cardiac surgery (Vaurio, Sands, Wang, et al., 2006). Interviews and baseline assessments of neurologic, functional, and cognitive status and pain were completed within 48 hours before surgery and repeated at 24 and 48 hours after surgery. Both the presence of postoperative pain and increased pain postoperatively were found to be independent predictors of

Older age (e.g., 65 years or older[1])
Cognitive impairment
Functional impairment
Decreased postoperative hemoglobin
Markedly abnormal sodium, potassium, or glucose
Alcohol abuse
Noncardiac thoracic operation
History of delirium
Preoperative use of narcotic
Low postoperative oxygen saturation
History of cerebrovascular disease
Untreated or poorly managed pain

---

[1]There is no consensus on what age constitutes "older" age; some cite it as 65 years or older, and others cite it as older than 75 years. It is important to consider the patient's general health and condition in addition to age.

From Pasero, C., & McCaffery, M. (2011). *Pain assessment and pharmacologic management*, p. 505, St. Louis, Mosby. Data from Amador, L. F., & Goodwin, J. S. (2005). Postoperative delirium in the older patient. *J Am Coll Surg, 200*(5), 767-773; Wang, S. G., Lee, U. J., Goh, E. K., et al. (2004). Factors associated with postoperative delirium after major head and neck surgery. *Ann Otol Rhinol Laryngol, 113*, 48-51; Litaker, D., Locala, J., Franco, K., et al. (2001). Preoperative risk factors for postoperative delirium. *Gen Hosp Psychiatry, 23*, 84-89; Weed, H. G., Lutman, C. V., Young, D. C., et al. (1995). Preoperative identification of patients at risk for delirium after major head and neck cancer surgery. *Laryngoscope, 105*, 1066-1068; Marcantonio, E. R., Goldman, L., Mangione, C. M., et al. (1994). A clinical prediction rule for delirium after elective noncardiac surgery. *JAMA, 271*, 134-139; Bucerius, J., Gummert, J. F., Borger, M. A., et al. (2004). Predictors of delirium after cardiac surgery delirium: Effect of beating-heart (offpump) surgery. *J Thorac Cardiovasc Surg, 127*, 57-64; Marcantonio, E. R., Goldman, L., Orav, E. J., et al. (1998). The association of intraoperative factors with the development of postoperative delirium. *Am J Med, 105*, 380-384; Lynch, E. P., Lazor, M. A., Gellis, J. E., et al. (1998). The impact of postoperative pain on the development of postoperative delirium. *Anesth Analg, 86*, 781-785. © 2011, Pasero C. May be duplicated for use in clinical practice.

Russo, Urquhart, Sharrock, et al., 1992). In contrast, fewer complications, including mental confusion, were found in older adult men receiving IV PCA morphine compared with those receiving IM morphine (Egbert, Parks, Short, et al., 1990).

The choice of opioid used to control pain also may influence the incidence of mental confusion, but research demonstrating differences among the various opioids is lacking. One exception is meperidine, which is more likely than other opioid drugs to cause delirium in postoperative patients of all ages (Fong, Sands, Leung, 2006). In a case control study (N = 91 with 1 to 2 controls), meperidine more than doubled the risk of delirium when given either epidurally or IV (Marcantonio, Juarez, Goldman, et al., 1994). It has also been shown to be the only opioid to have a negative impact on mood (Latta, Ginsberg, Barkin, 2002), sometimes the first sign of neurotoxicity. Early research found that IV PCA fentanyl produced less depression of postoperative cognitive function than IV PCA morphine (Herrick, Ganapathy, Komar, et al., 1996). IV PCA morphine and IV PCA hydromorphone provided similar analgesic efficacy, adverse effects, mood, and cognitive function in another study (Rapp, Egan, Ross, et al., 1996). Although the patients receiving hydromorphone experienced improved mood, they also demonstrated poorer cognitive performance than those receiving morphine.

In summary, these research findings reinforce that factors other than dose of opioid, such as quality of pain control, play a more important role in the development of delirium. Studies and clinical observations suggest that improvement in pain management practices, including the administration of appropriate doses of opioids, is one way to reduce confusion after surgery. The common reaction of many clinicians to abruptly discontinue the opioid when a patient develops confusion may worsen the confusion and is not recommended. After careful evaluation of all potential causes, a better approach is to add or increase a nonopioid or nonsedating adjuvant analgesic and decrease the opioid dose if a decrease is thought to be necessary (see Table 19-1).

postoperative delirium in these patients and to have a greater impact on the development of delirium than any of the other factors evaluated (e.g., age, type of anesthesia, postoperative medications, and preoperative cognitive status). There was also an ordered relationship between levels of postoperative pain and risk of delirium; those with severe pain were at a greater risk of developing delirium than those with moderate pain. An important finding was that neuraxial analgesia and IV PCA carried the same risk despite the lower opioid doses given neuraxially. Similarly, an earlier study reported no difference in the incidence of delirium between IV fentanyl and epidural fentanyl analgesia for pain following total knee replacement (Williams-

Sedation or Cognitive Impairment During Long-Term Opioid Therapy

Most patients experience sedation at the beginning of opioid therapy and whenever the opioid dose is increased significantly (Hanks, Cherny, Fallon, 2004). The incidence of sedation in patients receiving oral morphine for cancer pain is 20% to 60% (Cherny, Ripamonti, Pereira, et al., 2001), and it is often cited as a reason for inability to titrate an opioid to pain relief (Harris, Kotob, 2006). The underlying mechanisms of opioid-induced sedation or cognitive impairment are unclear, but are thought to be related to their effects on cholinergic pathways that modulate cortical arousal and information processing (Harris, Kotob, 2006). Opioids inhibit REM sleep and other aspects of normal sleep due to anticholinergic activity (Slatkin, Rhiner, Bolton, 2001; Young-McCaughan, Miaskowski, 2001). They also depress sensitivity of central and peripheral chemoreceptors to carbon dioxide, which has the potential to diminish wakefulness (Slatkin, Rhiner, Bolton, 2001). Sometimes patients experience persistent sedation during long-term opioid treatment if other sedating drugs are taken or there are underlying conditions that cause sedation, such as metabolic disturbances (Coyle, Cherny, Portenoy, 1995). Care must be taken not to confuse sedation with exhaustion and the need to "catch up" on sleep when poorly controlled pain is finally controlled (Coyle, Cherny, Portenoy, 1995).

Although a disturbing adverse effect, especially for patients on long-term opioid therapy, they can be reassured that tolerance to sedation and cognitive impairment usually develops over a period of days to weeks (Hanks, Cherny, Fallon, 2004). The clinical presentation ranges from drowsiness to somnolence, and the degree of sedation is used to guide its treatment (Pasero, 2009b; Young-McCaughan, Miaskowski, 2001). If possible, the opioid dose is decreased to treat sedation. If opioid dose reduction cannot be done or is unsuccessful, adding a psychostimulant is an option. Modafinil (Provigil) 200 mg in the morning, or methylphenidate (Ritalin) at 2.5 mg to 5 mg in the morning and repeated midday are the most commonly selected psychostimulants (see Chapter 31). Doses can be titrated upward. A report of 6 cases also described the use of the acetylcholinesterase inhibitor donepezil (Aricept) 5 mg daily in patients taking the equivalent of 200 mg/day of oral morphine and experiencing excessive sedation and unstable pain control (Slatkin, Rhiner, Bolton, 2001). Patients demonstrated improved alertness after donepezil was started, which allowed the clinicians to better optimize the pain management regimen.

If significantly impaired, patients should be discouraged from performing dangerous activities, such as driving or operating complicated mechanical equipment, until sedation subsides (see the section that follows for more on driving during long-term opioid therapy). Severe sedation precedes respiratory depression, and if sedation is severe or is worsening, it should be addressed promptly, typically either by dose reduction or a switch to a different opioid (Harris, Kotob, 2006) (see Chapter 18). Alternative methods of pain control, such as intraspinal opioids and/or local anesthetics, must be considered if the effect cannot be mitigated with systemic therapy (Coyle, Cherny, Portenoy, 1995). Table 19-1 provides treatment suggestions for patients receiving long-term opioid therapy.

Opioids and Driving Ability

For many people, driving an automobile is a daily activity that is a key element to maintaining their independence, engaging in employment, and remaining socially active. They are essentially disabled if they are deprived of the freedom to drive. As the use of long-term opioid therapy gains greater favor, especially in the care of patients with persistent noncancer pain, it is of great importance to the patient, physician, and public to determine their ability to drive safely.

This problem has been studied since the early 1960s when methadone maintenance therapy was introduced (Dole, Nyswander, 1965). One of the first studies compared the driving records of 401 patients before and after methadone maintenance therapy with 182 drivers selected at random (Gordon, 1973). During methadone treatment, patients did not differ significantly from the comparison group in rates of accidents or in convictions for driving offenses. Interestingly, while using heroin the patients had had fewer accidents, a finding that had no satisfactory explanation. (Of interest, another similar study found that heroin users had a slightly better driving record on heroin than they did on methadone [Maddux, Williams, Ziegler, 1977]). Gordon's conclusion was the same as many studies to follow: that taking an opioid (methadone in this case) on a long-term basis does not have a significant detrimental effect on the ability to drive.

Before embarking on an exploration of the effects on driving ability of long-term opioid therapy for persistent pain, it is important to point out that those patients who take opioids short-term, those in whom long-term opioid therapy is being initiated, and those on long-term therapy in whom opioid doses are being increased are different circumstances. Studies of the psychomotor and cognitive effects of opioids in these groups are generally different from those discussed in relation to long-term stable opioid therapy.

Extensive reviews of the literature have examined studies on the effects of a single opioid dose or an increased dose of opioid in patients on long-term therapy (Chapman, Byas-Smith, Reed, 2002; Zacny, 1996). These reviews reveal that this is a complex topic and that results of various studies are inconclusive. Results depend upon a multitude of factors such as type of opioid administered, dose of opioid, use of other medications, and whether or not the patient is in pain. For example, it appears that in opioid-naïve, healthy volunteers without pain, psychomotor and cognitive functioning are impaired more by some opioids (e.g., mixed-agonist-antagonists such as buprenorphine and pentazocine) than others (e.g., codeine and morphine). However, this may have little relevance to patients with pain, since pain itself impairs cognition (Lorenz, Beck, Bromm, 1997), and pain relief may improve cognitive functioning (Jamison, Schein, Vallow, et al., 2003). For example, treatment of neuropathic pain with both low and high doses of levorphanol resulted in improvement in some measures of cognitive performance (Rowbotham, Twilling, Davies, et al., 2003).

In a landmark study of patients with cancer, the cognitive effects of stable doses of opioids compared with changes in opioid dose in patients on long-term opioid therapy was conducted by Bruera and others (Bruera,

Macmillan, Hanson, et al., 1989). Twenty inpatients with cancer who had increased their opioid dose by at least 30% in the 3 days before testing were compared with 20 other inpatients who had been on a stable opioid dose for at least 7 days. A variety of opioids were used. Compared with the group on a stable opioid dose, the group taking the recently increased dose reported more drowsiness after the dose, and significantly more cognitive impairment occurred 45 minutes after opioid administration compared with several hours afterwards.

The immediate cognitive effects following a dose of opioid are often observed by clinicians and are supported by other studies. The immediate effects of 130 mg of dextropropoxyphene showed impairment was greater when measured 2 hours after than 4 hours after a dose (Saarialho-Kere, Julkunen, Mattila, et al., 1988). Thinking that the immediate effects of an opioid will persist seems to cause some clinicians to fear long-term use of opioids. In correcting this misconception, an explanation of the effects of tolerance may be helpful.

Cognitive performance was examined in a study comparing 6 female patients with persistent noncancer pain before and after being treated with modified-release morphine (Lorenz, Beck, Bromm, 1997). The first testing was before initiation of morphine, and the second examination was after the patients reported sufficient pain relief and had been on a stable dose for at least 3 days. Doses ranged from 30 to 150 mg of modified-release morphine per day. During the second testing session, behavioral and physiologic indicators of vigilance and cognitive function revealed lack of sedation and improved alertness. The authors suggested that these effects might be due in part to the possibility that pain relief made it unnecessary to constantly shift attention between pain and other activities.

The above studies and others have resulted in the recommendation that after a person's stable opioid dose is increased, caution should be exercised during the first few hours after taking the dose and until the patient has been on a stable dose for 7 days. Cognitive performance during the first few days of opioid use and during the first few hours after a given dose seems likely to be worse. However, after about 7 days of stable opioid dosing, cognitive effects such as sedation seem to subside.

Effects of long-term opioid therapy on driving ability were studied by comparing 16 patients with persistent noncancer pain on opioids for 6 months or longer with 327 cerebrally compromised patients from another study who had off-road and on-road testing for driving ability (Galski, Williams, Ehle, 2000). In the study of the cerebrally impaired patients, certain off-road tests were found to predict success or failure in the on-road evaluation. The patients on opioids were given the off-road tests, and the results were compared with those of the cerebrally impaired patients who had undergone the same evaluation and then passed or failed the on-road evaluation. Generally the patients on opioid therapy performed better than the cerebrally compromised patients

who passed the on-road test. Patients on long-term opioid therapy had faster reaction times and did not manifest any major problems with coordination, but they had greater difficulty following instructions and a tendency toward impulsivity, that is, hurrying and sacrificing accuracy for speed. Nevertheless, the results give general support for the ability of patients on long-term opioid therapy to pass actual on-road driving tests.

Twenty-nine patients with persistent noncancer pain (primarily low back pain) on long-term modified-release oxycodone were compared with 90 healthy volunteers to assess their driving ability (Gaertner, Radbruch, Giesecke, et al., 2006). Attention reaction, visual orientation, motor coordination, and vigilance were evaluated. This included a test battery that followed the German national recommendations on tests to determine driving ability. Permission to drive is usually denied if the score is below the sixteenth percentile. Using this definition of driving ability, there was no significant difference between the patients receiving modified-release oxycodone and the control group. The authors concluded that long-term treatment with modified-release oxycodone did not prohibit driving. However, they recommended individual assessment.

Another study using the German national recommendations on tests to determine driving ability compared 90 healthy controls with 21 patients with noncancer pain who had been treated with transdermal fentanyl for at least 4 weeks without a dose change in the last 12 days (Sabatowski, Schwalen, Rettig, et al., 2003). The median dose of transdermal fentanyl was 50 mcg/h with a range of 25 to 400 mcg/h. Of the 21 patients on transdermal fentanyl, all but 1 considered themselves fit to drive while the one "didn't know." Based on test results, the authors concluded that patients with noncancer pain on a stable dose of transdermal fentanyl do not have any clinically significant impairment of psychomotor or cognitive function that would prevent them from driving a car.

Of note is the fact that in the above study all patients except 1 correctly assumed they were able to drive. This suggests the wisdom of asking patients about their ability to drive and also of comparing these answers in future studies to actual ability to drive.

Driving performance, cognition, and balance were also studied before and after adding transdermal fentanyl to treatment regimens for 23 patients with persistent noncancer pain (Menefee, Frank, Crerand, et al., 2004). After patients were stabilized on a dose for 1 month, the tests were repeated. The median dose was 50 mcg/h. Once the dose of transdermal fentanyl had stabilized, it did not have a negative effect on driving performance, reaction time, or cognition. In fact, there was improvement on some measures of cognitive performance.

A poster presentation (Furlan, Lakha, Yegneswaran, et al., 2007) reported on the results of a literature search for controlled studies of long-term opioid use and the effect on driving. Although 1720 studies were located, only 31 were usable. They found that only one study tested driving on the road and two on a driving simulator and that, in these studies, stable opioid doses did not impair driving ability. In all 31 studies, there were 79 evaluations, and 27 found impairment, but no details about this impairment were given. The authors concluded that the quality of the studies was very low, but stated, "stable doses of opioids do not affect driving performance in a chronic pain population" (p. 127).

A structured evidence-based review, which is different from a meta-analysis, was conducted to examine whether long-term stable opioid dosing caused impairment in driving ability (Fishbain, Cutler, Rosomoff, et al., 2003). A literature search revealed 209 references, but only 48 were relevant to addressing driving abilities of patients on stable doses of opioids. These articles were reviewed in detail and then sorted and tabulated in several topic areas such as psychomotor abilities, cognitive functioning, and motor vehicle violations. Based on guidelines developed by the Agency for Health Care Policy and Research (AHCPR), the studies were categorized according to various levels of evidence, from well-designed controlled studies to case reports, and then categorized as to their strength and consistency of evidence. Following are the results of this evidenced-based review of studies of patients on long-term stable doses of opioids:

1. Psychomotor abilities—moderate, generally consistent evidence for no impairment
2. Psychomotor abilities immediately after being given new, additional doses of opioids—strong consistent evidence on multiple studies for there being no impairment of psychomotor abilities
3. Cognitive abilities—inconclusive evidence to support there being no cognitive impairment
4. Incidence of motor vehicle violations/motor vehicle accidents in the general population versus comparable controls of opioid-maintained patients—strong consistent evidence for no greater incidence in motor vehicle violations/motor vehicle accidents
5. Impairment as measured in driving simulators or off/on road driving as compared to controls—consistent evidence of no impairment in opioid-maintained patients

The authors of the above study concluded that overall the majority of studies appeared to indicate that patients on stable doses of long-term opioid therapy are not impaired in regard to driving skills. The authors also pointed out that the most relevant evidence were those studies that showed that opioid-tolerant patients appear to perform driving skills as well as controls, as stated in number 5 above. Nevertheless, they recommended that the decision to drive be made on an individual basis and specified the recommendations in Box 19-3.

A structured evidence-based literature review using methodology similar to the above study was conducted to determine if there was evidence of an association between opioid use and intoxicated driving, motor vehicle accidents (MVA), and MVA fatalities (Fishbain, Cutler, Rosomoff,

GUIDELINES

Box 19-3 | Addressing Driving Ability with Patients on Long-Term Opioid Therapy

When a patient is on long-term opioid therapy or it is being initiated, some recommendations to the prescriber regarding the patient driving an automobile are as follows:

1. Understand that being on long-term opioid therapy does not preclude driving.
2. Consider obtaining some form of informed consent that covers the risks of driving and perhaps some of the educational points below.
3. Educate the patient about maintaining driving safety when taking opioids long term. Explain the following to the patient:
   a. Whether you do or do not drive should be based on the information below and is your personal decision.
   b. Most of the research findings on driving ability in patients on a stable dose of opioid indicate that that they can drive safely.
   c. A stable dose means taking the same dose of opioid for 7 or more days.
   d. When opioid treatment begins or when a dose is increased, do not drive for 4 to 5 days until you become tolerant to the dose.
   e. Do not drive if you feel drowsy or dizzy.
   f. Report sedation or any other difficulties in thinking to the prescriber so that the dose can be reduced.
   g. Never drive after you have used alcohol or other illegal drugs such as marijuana and cocaine.
   h. Avoid taking any over-the-counter antihistamines as these may cause drowsiness.
   i. Do not make any changes in your opioid dose without consulting your prescriber.

From Pasero, C., & McCaffery, M. (2011). *Pain assessment and pharmacologic management*, p. 508, St. Louis, Mosby. Modified from Fishbain, D. A., Lewis, J. E., Cole, B., et al., (2007). Medicolegal rounds: Medicolegal issues and alleged breaches of standards of medical care in a patient motor vehicle accident allegedly related to chronic opioid analgesic therapy. *J Opioid Manage*, 3(1), 16-20. © 2011, Pasero C. May be duplicated for use in clinical practice.

et al., 2002). Except for those subjects identified as being on methadone maintenance therapy, no information was provided on how long the subjects had been taking opioids. The evidence indicated that opioids probably are not related to intoxicated driving, MVA, or MVA fatalities, supporting the recommendation that patients on opioids be allowed to drive. However, again, this decision should be made on an individual basis.

Compared with patients with noncancer pain on long-term opioid therapy, determining if patients with cancer on long-term opioid therapy are able to drive is a more complex matter (Brandman, 2005). Patients with cancer often have co-morbidities, neurologic changes, other medications, and advancing disease, causing their driving ability to change over time. The reader is referred to the specific guidelines given in the Brandman (2005) article for helping patients and physicians determine safe driving ability in patients with cancer on long-term opioid therapy. Some of these suggestions include asking occupational therapists to perform a driving assessment of the patient and considering the use of a CNS stimulant such as methylphenidate or modafinil for patients who report drowsiness.

In a medicolegal case report that presented the details of the case of a patient with persistent low back pain on long-term opioid therapy, the authors submitted some recommendations on how pain physicians should approach the problem of whether patients should be allowed to drive while on long-term opioid therapy (Fishbain, Lewis, Cole, et al., 2007). Although their literature review indicated that such patients could drive safely once they had developed a tolerance to the sedating effects of opioids, they offered specific guidelines such as suggesting that some form of informed consent concerning the risks of driving while on long-term opioid therapy should be obtained. Specific points they felt should be discussed with the patient on long-term opioid therapy included advising the patient of the current literature on driving while on this therapy, that whether or not to drive was their own personal decision, and that if they decided to drive they should obey certain rules. Some of these rules were not to drive for 4 to 5 days after beginning opioid treatment, not to drive if they felt sedated, and not to use alcohol or other illicit drugs before driving. The reader is referred to this article for information on other recommendations. Similar recommendations are available in Fishbain, Cutler, Rosomoff, et al., 2003 (see Box 19-3).

Not only patients and their families but also policy-makers should be informed that the majority of the current literature shows that driving ability is not necessarily impaired in patients on stable doses of opioids. Without this knowledge, those responsible for enacting laws related to driving may restrict patients taking opioids. For example, in 1995 a guide was distributed to the British medical community recommending that people taking morphine-like opioids should not drive (as reported in Zacny, 1996). Zacny (1996) pointed out that the science of opioids and functioning should be used when making policy decisions, rather than hearsay and speculation.

In summary, whether or not a patient taking opioid analgesics can drive must be decided on an individual basis. Some patients will be able to drive safely, but others may be impaired by opioids. Impairment may be brief such as at the beginning of opioid therapy or following significant increases in dose. Some opioids cause more impairment for an individual patient than others, and a change in opioid may remedy the situation. It seems

prudent to warn all patients that driving ability may be compromised and that they should not drive if they feel drowsy, dizzy, or impaired in any way.

It should be noted that the concern over effects of medication on driving ability should not be limited to opioids. Currently there seems to be a bias against the use of opioids that has helped fuel the concern about how these analgesics affect driving ability. However, other medication deserves attention too. Studies of older adults indicate that medications such as antidepressants or benzodiazepines (Ray, Fought, Decker, 1992), especially long–half-life benzodiazepines (Hemmelgarn, Suissa, Huang, et al., 1997) are at greater risk for motor vehicle crashes than those on opioids. Cognitive impairment was studied by comparing 13 patients taking benzodiazepines only with 13 patients taking opioids only (Hendler, Cimini, Long, 1980). The results showed that benzodiazepines were far more likely to produce cognitive impairment. In a study of 40 licensed drivers, age 25 to 44, the effects of fexofenadine (60 mg, Allegra), diphenhydramine (50 mg, Benadryl), alcohol (approximately 0.1% blood alcohol concentration), and placebo on driving performance were studied (Weiler, Bloomfield, Woodworth, et al., 2000). Driving performance was the poorest after taking diphenhydramine, impairing driving even more than alcohol.

Sedation During Short-Term Opioid Therapy in Opioid-Naïve Patients

Unfortunately, for patients receiving short-term opioid therapy, time does not allow for development of tolerance to sedation. In addition to affecting the patient's ability to participate in the recovery process, if left untreated, excessive sedation can progress to clinically significant opioid-induced respiratory depression in opioid-naïve patients (Mcintyre, Upton, 2008; Vila, Smith, Augustyniak, et al., 2005).

Sedation Assessment

The observation that excessive sedation precedes opioid-induced respiratory depression (Abou hammoud, Simon, Urien, et al., 2009; Taylor, Voytovich, Kozol, 2003) indicates that systematic sedation assessment is an essential aspect of the care of opioid-naïve patients receiving opioid therapy (Nisbet, Mooney-Cotter, 2009; Pasero, 2009b). The importance of monitoring sedation to prevent clinically significant respiratory depression cannot be overemphasized. As the American Pain Society (APS) (2003) succinctly states, "No patient has succumbed to (opioid-induced) respiratory depression while awake" (p. 35).

Nursing assessment of opioid-induced sedation is convenient, inexpensive, and takes minimal time to perform (Pasero, 2009b). To assess sedation, the nurse should ask the patient a simple question, such as "What did you have for breakfast today?" then observe the patient's ability to stay awake and answer the question. Patients who are

Box 19-4 | Pasero Opioid-Induced Sedation Scale (POSS) with Interventions*

S = Sleep, easy to arouse

Acceptable; no action necessary; may increase opioid dose if needed

1 = Awake and alert

Acceptable; no action necessary; may increase opioid dose if needed

2 = Slightly drowsy, easily aroused

Acceptable; no action necessary; may increase opioid dose if needed

3 = Frequently drowsy, arousable, drifts off to sleep during conversation

Unacceptable; monitor respiratory status and sedation level closely until sedation level is stable at less than 3 and respiratory status is satisfactory; decrease opioid dose 25% to 50%[1] or notify primary[2] or anesthesia provider for orders; consider administering a nonsedating, opioid-sparing nonopioid, such as acetaminophen or an NSAID, if not contraindicated; ask patient to take deep breaths every 15 to 30 minutes.

4 = Somnolent, minimal or no response to verbal and physical stimulation

Unacceptable; stop opioid; consider administering naloxone[3,4]; call Rapid Response Team (Code Blue), if indicated by patient status; stay with patient, stimulate, and support respiration as indicated by patient status; notify primary[2] or anesthesia provider; monitor respiratory status and sedation level closely until sedation level is stable at less than 3 and respiratory status is satisfactory.

---

*Appropriate action is given in italics at each level of sedation.

[1]Opioid analgesic orders or a hospital protocol should include the expectation that a nurse will decrease the opioid dose if a patient is excessively sedated.

[2]For example, the physician, nurse practitioner, advanced practice nurse, or physician's assistant responsible for the pain management prescription.

[3]See Box 19-6. For adults experiencing respiratory depression, mix 0.4 mg of naloxone and 10 mL of normal saline in syringe and administer this dilute solution very slowly (0.5 mL over 2 minutes) while observing the patient's response (titrate to effect). If sedation and respiratory depression occurs during administration of transdermal fentanyl, remove the patch; if naloxone is necessary, treatment will be needed for a prolonged period, and the typical approach involves a naloxone infusion (see text). Patient must be monitored closely for at least 24 hours after discontinuation of the transdermal fentanyl.

[4]Hospital protocols should include the expectation that a nurse will administer naloxone to any patient suspected of having life-threatening opioid-induced sedation and respiratory depression.

This box presents a reliable and valid scale for assessment of sedation during opioid administration for pain management (references for reliability/validity below).

From Pasero, C., & McCaffery, M. (2011). *Pain assessment and pharmacologic management*, p. 510, St. Louis, Mosby. Data from American Pain Society. (2003). Principles of analgesic use in the treatment of acute pain and chronic cancer pain, ed 5, Glenview, IL, The Society; Pasero, C. (2009). Assessment of sedation during opioid administration for pain management. *J PeriAnesth Nurs, 24*(3), 186-190; Pasero, C., & McCaffery, M. (2002). Monitoring sedation. *Am J Nurs, 102*(2), 67-69. Reliability and validity information for the POSS can be found in Dempsey, S. J., Davidson, J., Cahill, D., et al. (2008). Selection of a sedation assessment scale for clinical practice: Inter-rater reliability, ease of use, and applicability testing of the Richmond-Agitation-Sedation and Pasero Opioid-Induced Sedation Scale. Poster presentation, National Association of Orthopedic Nurses Congress, Tampa, FL, May 6-10; Nisbet, A. T., & Mooney-Cotter, F. (2009). Selected scales for reporting opioid-induced sedation. *Pain Manage Nurs, 10*(3), 154-164. © 1994, Pasero C. May be duplicated for use in clinical practice.

---

excessively sedated will typically have difficulty keeping their eyes open and will fall asleep while responding, usually in the middle of a sentence. Nursing technicians (and other health care team members, including ancillary staff such as pastoral care counselors and dieticians) should be trained to watch for and report these signs of excessive sedation if evident and to routinely observe how alert patients are every time they obtain vital signs. Touching the patient to provide care and even simply entering the room can arouse a patient, giving the false impression of an acceptable level of sedation. Therefore, it is essential that the nurse or nursing technician observe the patient without stimulation for long enough to ensure an accurate evaluation.

Sedation Scales

A simple, easy-to-understand sedation scale that includes what should be done at each level of sedation should be used to enhance accuracy and consistency of assessment and treatment, monitor trends, and communicate effectively between members of the health care team. The use of a scale to assess sedation during opioid pain management is common in hospitals in the United States; a 2006 survey of members of the APS and the American Society for Pain Management Nursing (ASPMN) email list serve revealed that all but one respondent (N = 64) used some type of sedation scale during opioid therapies, such as IV PCA and epidural analgesia (Pasero, unpublished data, 2006). The most commonly used scale among those surveyed was the Pasero Opioid-Induced Sedation Scale (POSS) (Box 19-4). A later survey (N = 92) conducted by the ASPMN of its members found a high use of sedation scales; however, the survey did not ask the respondents the purpose for using the selected scales, so it was not possible to evaluate whether the scales were being used appropriately (Pasero, unpublished data, 2009). For example, the Aldrete scale, which is used to determine readiness for discharge from the postanesthesia care unit (PACU) by scoring several criteria (including level of consciousness), was listed as the most commonly used scale (53.3%); the POSS, which is used for assessment of opioid-induced sedation during pain management, was the second most commonly used scale (45.5%).

Note in Box 19-4 that the POSS links nursing interventions to the various levels of sedation. Research has shown that nurses find this approach helpful in making the appropriate decisions on how to proceed with opioid treatment. A descriptive survey-based study compared three sedation scales, the Inova Sedation Scale (ISS) (the researchers' scale), Richmond Agitation and Sedation Scale (RASS) (Sessler, Gosnell, Grap, et al., 2002), and the POSS (Nisbet, Mooney-Cotter, 2008, 2009). This study invited nurses (N = 96) to participate in an online survey that presented a scenario describing a patient with excessive sedation during IV PCA therapy. The participants were asked to determine the patient's level of sedation using each of the sedation scales and select the course of action they would take. The percentage of correct sedation score responses with each scale was 46.9% (ISS), 76% (RASS), and 79.2% (POSS); however, the most important finding of this study was that when using the POSS, nurses selected the correct nursing action significantly more often (80.2%) than when using the RASS (68.8%) or the ISS (67.7%). Validity for the POSS and RASS for sedation assessment during pain management was established by a panel of experts for this study, but a lack of discrimination between scale items on the ISS prevented establishment of its validity. Reliability for the scales using Cronbach's alpha was 0.803 (ISS), 0.770 (RASS), and 0.903 (POSS). Another group of researchers found similar results when they compared the POSS and RASS in patients receiving opioids for pain management (Dempsey, Davidson, Cahill, et al., 2008). The POSS demonstrated reliability of 0.909 (Cronbach's alpha) in this study.

Sedation scales such as the RASS (Ely, Truman, Shintani, et al., 2003) and the Ramsay Scale (Ramsay, Savege, Simpson, et al., 1974; Olson, Lynn, Thoyre, et al., 2007) have been tested for assessment during goal-directed (purposeful) sedation during procedures and in ventilated critically ill patients but are not recommended for use during opioid administration for pain management because they incorporate assessment of other conditions in addition to sedation (Pasero, McCaffery, 2002; Pasero, 2009b). For example, most goal-directed sedation scales link anxiety or agitation to the scale (Peck, Down, 2009), which complicates assessment because agitation and anxiety are not indicators of increasing opioid-induced sedation. Patients may be either calm or anxious *and* sedated. Further, the scales used for purposeful sedation were not developed for assessment of unwanted sedation during opioid administration for pain management. Similarly, simple sedation scales such as the POSS were not developed for assessment of purposeful, goal-directed sedation. It is

recommended that institutions use two different sedation scales depending on the goal of treatment—one scale for assessment during purposeful sedation (the goal is to *produce* sedation) and a simpler scale for sedation assessment during opioid administration for pain management (the goal is to *prevent* sedation) (Pasero, 2009b). As mentioned, PACU nurses often use scoring systems (e.g., Aldrete) that include level of consciousness to determine readiness for discharge, which is acceptable for that area; however, a simple scale such as the POSS is more appropriate for ongoing assessment of opioid-induced sedation after transfer to the clinical unit. A review of sedation scales for assessment of goal-directed sedation can be found in: Odom-Forren, J. & Watson, D. (2005). *Practical guide to moderate sedation/analgesia.* St. Louis, Mosby. See Table 19-1 and later discussion of the frequency of monitoring sedation and respiratory depression.

Coadministration of Other Sedating Drugs

The administration of IM opioids to opioid-naïve patients receiving IV or epidural analgesia is unnecessary, can result in excessive sedation and clinically significant respiratory depression due to unpredictable absorption (see Chapter 14), and should be avoided. Instead, patients who are receiving IV or epidural opioid analgesia and experiencing uncontrolled pain should be carefully reevaluated. Clinician-administered IV or epidural supplemental doses and increases in the dose of the mainstay opioid usually are indicated (see Chapters 15 and 17).

Although not necessarily contraindicated with parenteral and intraspinal analgesia, muscle relaxants and anxiolytics can produce sedation. Therefore, prior to administering them, it is best to obtain approval for their administration from the prescriber responsible for the pain management plan (e.g., anesthesia provider with postoperative epidural analgesia). Antihistamines are often used to treat pruritus but also must be used with caution as they can be extremely sedating (see earlier discussion and Section V). Sedation can be problematic in those already at risk for excessive sedation, such as postoperative patients, as this can lead to life-threatening respiratory depression (Anwari, Iqbal, 2003). When these drugs are administered, increased monitoring of sedation is recommended, and they should not be administered if patients are excessively sedated.

Patients with Severe Pain and Excessive Sedation

It is important to note that the presence of sedation does not necessarily mean that patients are comfortable. Research shows that caring for patients with both severe pain and excessive sedation is common and presents major challenges to providing safe opioid therapy. In a time-course study of sedation and analgesia in 73 patients in the PACU after major surgery, 52 (73%) patients became sedated during titration necessitating discontinuation of titration; 21 remained awake, and titration was continued (Paqueron, Lumbroso, Mergoni, et al., 2002). Among those in whom titration was stopped because of sedation, 25% had a pain level higher than 50 on the VAS and only 50% had satisfactory pain relief (VAS less than 30). The findings of this study are important to consider when titrating opioids, i.e., that sedation can occur before pain is completely relieved and that sleep during opioid titration is not normal sleep but primarily the result of the sedative effects of the opioid.

Another time course study was conducted in 228 patients in the PACU following major orthopedic surgery who were titrated to either pain relief (VAS of 3 or less) or excessive sedation (Ramsay score higher than 2—a score of 3 indicates response to verbal commands only) (Abou Hammoud, Simon, Urien, et al., 2009). Titration was stopped when analgesia was achieved or an adverse effect occurred such as respiratory rate less than 12 breaths/min, oxygen saturation less than 95%, or sleep (sedation). Titration was stopped in nearly one half (45%) of the patients because of excessive sedation, but no serious adverse events (e.g., respiratory depression) occurred. The effectiveness of morphine was found to be increased in patients who had a decreased delay between extubation and titration, low initial VAS, and intraoperative multimodal analgesia (NSAID and/or acetaminophen administration). Analgesia was attained with a mean of 4 bolus doses and a mean morphine dose of 11 mg. The researchers emphasized that a multimodal approach is essential and that patients may benefit from earlier initiation of nonopioids (e.g., preoperatively). They proposed that higher amounts of bolus doses (e.g., 4 to 5 mg) rather than smaller bolus doses given at shorter intervals may be more effective in controlling severe pain, but appropriately pointed out that this could also increase adverse effects and compromise safety. An important finding was that 20 mg of titrated morphine was associated with a high incidence of excessive sedation, underscoring the need to use other approaches to manage pain that will allow lower opioid doses (i.e., multimodal analgesia). The effectiveness of stopping titration or reducing opioid dose when sedation is excessive is also demonstrated in this study by the lack of clinically significant respiratory depression.

A case control study demonstrated similar challenges in managing patients who have severe pain and also are excessively sedated. Patients in the PACU (N = 285) were titrated with IV morphine (2 to 3 mg) boluses every 5 minutes and then evaluated at 24 hours postoperatively (Lentschener, Tostivint, White, et al., 2007). PACU titration was discontinued when pain relief (VAS less than 3) was achieved or if adverse effects occurred such as excessive sedation (Ramsay score more than 3, sluggish or no response to loud voice or pain). Of the 285 patients, 26 were discharged from the PACU excessively sedated

(mean Ramsay score 4) with uncontrolled pain (mean VAS 6.5). These patients were matched with 52 patients who were discharged not excessively sedated with adequate pain relief. The sedated patients received significantly more morphine in the PACU (mean 12 mg vs. 5 mg), had a two-times longer stay in the PACU (mean 240 min vs. 120 min), more often recalled having moderate-to-severe pain in the PACU, and had poorer quality sleep and higher pain scores at 24 hours after surgery.

An observational study compared pain, oxygen saturation levels, and sedation levels in three groups of patients: those receiving conscious sedation for colonoscopy (N = 18), those receiving IV PCA for postoperative pain management (N = 15), and those receiving nurse-controlled analgesia (PRN schedule) (N = 20) (Taylor, Voytovich, Kozol, 2003). The researchers reported that the analgesics and sedatives given were chosen by surgeons or anesthesiologists and adjusted to optimize analgesia, sedation, and safety, but exact drugs and doses were not provided in the publication of this study. Patients in group 2 (PCA) had trends in sedation levels greater than or equal to patients in group 1 (conscious sedation) during the first 10 hours postoperatively, and 72.7% of those receiving PCA were excessively sedated within the first 4 hours after discharge from the PACU. The lowest level of sedation was in group 3 (nurse controlled). Of interest, oxygen saturation was well maintained in all groups throughout the study. Pain scores declined steadily during the study in patients in groups 1 and 2 (average mean maximal pain score = 6.5/10) and undulated in group 3 (average mean maximal pain score = 5.5).

These studies add to a growing body of research showing that sedation precedes analgesia and despite being sedated, some patients will report pain. Nevertheless, opioid doses should not be increased (titration should be stopped) in patients who are excessively sedated, and they should be watched closely until they are no longer sedated. The APS (2003) recommends close monitoring of sedation and respiratory status for at least 3 hours after the peak of the last dose administered. Other options to achieve comfort such as adding or increasing the dose of nonopioids should be implemented. See the following discussion and Table 19-1 for the recommended approach for prevention and treatment of sedation and respiratory depression in these complex patients.

Treatment of Excessive Sedation

Opioid-induced sedation is dose-related (Abou Hammoud, Simon, Urien, et al., 2009; Aubrun, Monsel, Langeron, et al., 2001); therefore, opioid orders and hospital protocols should include the expectation that nurses will stop titration or promptly decrease the opioid dose whenever excessive sedation is detected. For example, the opioid dose should be decreased by 25% to 50% in patients receiving PCA or epidural analgesia who have a sedation level of

3 on the POSS (see Box 19-4 and see Form 17-1 [p. 464] for an example of how decreases in dose can be included in opioid order sets). Monitoring of sedation level and respiratory status is then increased in frequency (e.g., every 15 to 30 minutes) until the sedation level is less than 3 and the respiratory status is stable (see p. 517 for respiratory assessment). Nonsedating nonopioid analgesics can be added or increased to facilitate opioid dose reduction. Routine administration of these agents as part of a multimodal approach initiated preoperatively or as soon as the patient is started on opioid therapy (e.g., admission to the PACU) is essential to help prevent excessive sedation from occurring later in the course of care. Giving less opioid more frequently to decrease peak concentration may be effective in reducing sedation in some cases. For example, large PCA doses and long lockout (delay) intervals can be reduced in patients who report excessive sedation following PCA injection. Catheter migration to either the intravascular or intrathecal space should be ruled out in patients receiving epidural analgesia who have a sudden change in sedation level (see Box 15-4 on p. 433). See the following patient example and Table 19-1 for treatment of opioid-induced sedation during short-term opioid therapy and the following section on prevention and treatment of clinically significant respiratory depression.

Patient Example

Mrs. P. is 4 hours post–abdominal hysterectomy. She is receiving oral acetaminophen and a continuous epidural infusion of fentanyl 5 mcg/mL with bupivacaine 0.0625% at 8 mL/h (40 mcg/h of fentanyl) for management of her postoperative pain. She rates her pain as 1/10 and has a sedation level of 3 (see POSS, Box 19-4), drifting off to sleep before completing a sentence. Over the last 2 hours, the depth of her respirations has become shallow and her hourly respiratory rate has decreased from 18 to 14 breaths/min. The anesthesiologist's orders call for a decrease in the epidural opioid dose (infusion rate) by 25% to 50% for a sedation level of 3. Since Mrs. P. has good pain control, her nurse decides to decrease the dose by 50%: 8 mL/h (40 mcg/h of fentanyl) × 0.50 (50%) = 4 mL/h (20 mcg/h of fentanyl). Mrs. P.'s nurse asks the nursing technician to check Mrs. P.'s sedation and respiratory status and to ask Mrs. P. to deep breathe every 15 minutes. Within 1 hour, Mrs. P. has a sedation level of 2 and is able to carry on a conversation without falling asleep. Her respiratory rate is 16 breaths/min, and her pain rating is unchanged at 1/10. Hourly monitoring of sedation and respiratory status is resumed.

Respiratory Depression

Respiratory depression is assessed on the basis of what is normal for a particular individual. Respiratory depression associated with opioid use usually is described as clinically significant when there is a decrease in the rate and depth of respirations from baseline, rather than just by a specific number of respirations per minute. This means that in some cases even patients breathing less than 10 breaths/minute may not have respiratory depression if they are breathing deeply (Pasero, Portenoy, McCaffery, 1999). Respiratory rates of less than 8 breaths/min have been described as severe respiratory depression (Dahan, Aarts, Smith, 2010). Oxygen (O_2) saturation and exhaled carbon dioxide (end-tidal [ET] CO_2) are increasingly used to define respiratory depression, particularly in research. Postoperative hypoxemia has been characterized as an oxygen saturation level of less than 90% and severe hypoxemia as less than 85% for more than 6 minutes per hour (Wheatley, Shepherd, Jackson, et al., 1992). It is important, however, for clinicians to understand that respiratory rate and oxygen saturation are surrogate indicators of ventilatory drive and provide little information about the effects of a drug on the ventilatory system (Dahan, Aarts, Smith, 2010). Arterial carbon dioxide and inspired minute ventilation are direct measures, but continuous monitoring of these is difficult in the clinical setting (Dahan, Aarts, Smith, 2010) (see later in this chapter for a discussion of mechanical monitoring).

Respiratory Depression During Long-Term Opioid Therapy

Clinically significant respiratory depression is the most feared of the opioid-induced adverse effects, but like sedation, tolerance to respiratory depression develops over a period of days to weeks and rarely occurs if opioids are titrated according to patient response (Hanks, Cherny, Fallon, 2004). The longer the patient receives opioids, the wider the margin of safety. Therefore, fear of respiratory depression in patients who have been receiving opioids for more than 1 week should not pose a barrier to administering adequate opioid doses (see later discussion of the postoperative opioid tolerant patient). Similar to opioid-naïve patients, when respiratory depression occurs in an opioid-tolerant individual, it is preceded by increased sedation; however, if appropriate steps are taken to address persistent sedation, respiratory depression is unusual in patients receiving long-term opioid therapy (Hanks, Cherny, Fallon, 2004).

Respiratory Depression in Opioid-Naïve Patients

The incidence of opioid-induced respiratory depression in opioid-naïve patients is unclear, mainly because of variations in the definition of respiratory depression used in research (Cashman, Dolin, 2004; Dahan, Aarts, Smith, 2010). This has resulted in reported incidences based on a variety of indicators, including respiratory rate, number of hypoxemic or hypercarbic episodes, and the need for treatment with naloxone (rescue) (Cashman, Dolin, 2004). The incidence of respiratory depression may be much higher than reported here because of the lack of consensus on definitions and uniform reporting as well as the reliance on retrospective data, the source of most published reports, which may not record the reasons for interventions (Etches, 1994).

Incidence of respiratory depression varies according to the method of opioid administration. A small study (N = 38) reported that no episodes of respiratory depression occurred in patients who were randomized to receive 10 mg of morphine by the IV or the IM route of administration (Tveita, Thoner, Klepstad, et al., 2008). A systematic review of IV PCA reported a range of respiratory depression of 0.6% to 15.2% when hypoventilation and oxygen desaturation were used as indicators (Walder, Schafer, Henzi, et al., 2001). Another systematic review of the incidences of respiratory depression associated with IM, IV PCA, and epidural opioids found wide variations in indicators resulting in wide ranges of incidences (Cashman, Dolin, 2004). Using hypoventilation and oxygen desaturation as indicators, the researchers reported mean incidences of between 0.8% to 37.0% (IM), 1.2% to 11.5% (IV PCA), and 1.1% to 15.1% (epidural). They concluded that an incidence of 1% or less (defined by a low respiratory rate) can be expected in patients receiving IV PCA or epidural analgesia and cared for by an acute pain service. They noted that if oxygen desaturation is used as a definer, a much higher percentage should be expected (see the discussion of respiratory assessment later in the chapter). In a review of the literature, Dahan and colleagues state that the many studies that have been conducted on patients receiving IV PCA yield an incidence of respiratory depression between 0.2% and 0.5% (Dahan, Aarts, Smith, 2010); however, it has been pointed out that many of the studies of IV PCA were published in the early 1990s before emphasis was placed on reducing patients' pain intensity ratings, and the incidence of oversedation and respiratory depression may actually be much higher today (Taylor, Voytovich, Kozol, 2003).

A prospective study of nearly 3000 patients receiving either PCEA morphine with basal rate (N = 1670) or IV PCA morphine with basal rate (N = 1026) after major surgery found a higher incidence of respiratory depression (defined as less than 8 breaths/min) in the IV PCA group (1.2%) than in the epidural group (0.04%) (Flisberg, Rudin, Linner, et al., 2003) (see Chapter 17 for safe use of a basal rate with IV PCA). In their neuraxial analgesia practice guidelines, the American Society of Anesthesiologists (ASA) reported an incidence of 0.01% to 7% with single-bolus intrathecal morphine and 0.08% to 3%

with single-bolus epidural morphine (ASA Task Force on Neuraxial Opioids, 2009). They suggested that the range of incidence for respiratory depression with single-bolus neuraxial opioids (0.01% to 7%) is similar to that of IM, IV, and IV PCA opioids and recommended continuous epidural opioids over parenteral opioids as a way of reducing the risk of respiratory depression.

A significantly higher incidence of respiratory depression than had been previously reported was found when continuous pulse oximetry (O_2 saturation) and capnography ($ETCO_2$) were utilized to evaluate respiratory depression in a study of 178 postoperative patients receiving morphine or meperidine by IV PCA (Overdyk, Carter, Maddox, et al., 2007). The incidence of oxygen desaturation (less than 90%) lasting 2 or more minutes was 21.4% and lasting 3 or more minutes was 11.8%; the incidence of bradypnea (rate less than 10 breaths/min) lasting 2 or more minutes was 58.4% and lasting 3 or more minutes was 41%. Only 1 patient (0.6%) required naloxone treatment. The researchers attributed the low need for naloxone rescue to the monitoring equipment's audible alarm that arouses a patient and summons a nurse, but they suggested that more research is needed to verify this (see p. 518 for a discussion of mechanical monitoring). An interesting finding in this study was that despite consuming approximately two times more opioid, patients receiving a basal rate with IV PCA had a significantly lower incidence of bradypnea (32% vs. 53%) and desaturation (8% vs. 17%) than those who did not have a basal rate. The reason for this was not clear.

Risk Factors for Opioid-Induced Respiratory Depression

There is no set dose of an opioid that is safe for all patients. All opioid-naïve patients are at risk for clinically significant respiratory depression when they receive their first dose of an opioid. Even opioid-tolerant patients have an elevated risk if they are given a significant amount of opioid in addition to their usual amount, for example, the patient who takes an opioid analgesic for persistent pain and receives several IV opioid bolus doses in the PACU followed by IV PCA with a basal rate for ongoing acute postoperative pain (Pasero, 2009b). Any patient who required a large amount of opioid in a relatively short period of time to achieve comfort (e.g., more than 10 mg morphine equivalent in an opioid-naïve patient in the PACU) is at risk for subsequent respiratory depression (Dahan, Aarts, Smith, 2010; Lotsch, Dudziak, Freynhagen, et al., 2006) and should be watched closely for at least 3 hours past the time of the expected peak analgesic blood concentration of the last opioid dose (APS, 2003) (see Table 16-1 on pp. 444-446). A study of morphine pharmacokinetics and pharmacodynamics in the immediate postoperative period found that 20 mg of IV morphine during titration was associated with a high likelihood of sedation (Abou Hammoud, Simon, Urien, et al., 2009). A disturbing case report supports this conclusion (Lotsch, Dudziak, Freynhagen, et al., 2006).

The first 24 hours after surgery is a particularly high-risk period for postoperative patients. A retrospective case control study examined 62 patients who experienced a respiratory event. It found that 77.4% had the respiratory event in the first 24 hours postoperatively, and 56.5% of these experienced the event within the first 12 hours postoperatively (mean time to event was 20.48 hours after the end of surgery) (Taylor, Kirton, Staff, et al., 2005). Risk factors for the event were identified as age greater than 65 years, coexisting chronic obstructive pulmonary disease, having one or more co-morbidities, and receiving hydromorphone. Morphine was described as a "protective factor." The researchers suggested that the elevated risk of respiratory depression with hydromorphone was due to its higher potency but did not provide dosing information, so it is unclear if equianalgesic opioid doses were administered (see Chapter 11 for a discussion of potency and equianalgesia). Randomized controlled trials have not demonstrated differences between morphine and hydromorphone in terms of the incidences of sedation and respiratory depression (Chang, Bijur, Meyer, et al., 2006; Hong, Flood, Diaz, 2008). A retrospective analysis of medical records compared adverse effects associated with IV PCA morphine, hydromorphone, and fentanyl and found no difference in sedation among the three opioids; an incidence of respiratory depression (respiratory rate less than 12 breaths/min or oxygen saturation less than 90%) of 8%, 7%, and 4%, respectively, was reported, but this was not statistically significant (Hutchison, Chon, Tucker, et al., 2006). One randomized controlled trial (N = 56) compared remifentanil and fentanyl administered by IV infusion for postoperative pain and reported three episodes of serious respiratory depression in patients who received remifentanil and none in those who received fentanyl; however, other causes for the episodes could not be ruled out (Choi, Koo, Nam, et al., 2008). More well-controlled research with large numbers of patients is needed to conclude differences in risk of respiratory depression among the various opioids; however, the time it takes an opioid to reach its analgesic site of action must be considered during titration (Lotsch, Dudziak, Freynhagen, et al., 2006).

Because pain stimulates respiration (Borgbjerg, Nielsen, Franks, 1996), patients in whom pain is controlled after a period of poor control are at risk for respiratory depression and should be watched closely until steady state is reached. As mentioned, others at risk for opioid-induced respiratory depression are older opioid-naïve patients (age 65 or older) and those who have coexisting conditions such as chronic pulmonary disease or major organ failure (Dahan, Aarts, Smith, 2010; Lucas, Vlahos, Ledgerwood, 2007; Taylor, Kirton, Staff, et al., 2005).

Individuals with obstructive sleep apnea (OSA) are at particularly high risk for opioid-induced respiratory depression (ASA, 2006; Dahan, Aarts, Smith, 2010) as are obese patients (body mass index [BMI] 35 kg/m^2 or more) with or without OSA (Overdyk, Ahmed, 2009).

One group of researchers recommends routine mechanical monitoring postoperatively in all patients undergoing bariatric surgery for obesity because of their elevated risk for severe and prolonged epiosodes of hypoxemia (Gallagher, Haines, Osterlund, et al., 2010). A high incidence of sleep-disordered breathing has been reported in patients receiving long-term opioid therapy, particularly in those taking methadone for pain management (Webster, Choi, Desai, et al., 2008). Clinicians are encouraged to establish processes in their insitutions that will help to identify patients with possible OSA before opioid therapy is initiated (e.g., preoperatively). The ASA provides a list of clinical signs that are suggestive of OSA, such as frequent snoring; neck circumference of 17 inches in men or 16 inches in women; and BMI 35 kg/m^2 or more, as well as recommendations for the management of OSA in the perioperative setting (ASA, 2006). All patients and family members should be asked on admission or as soon as possible thereafter about whether the patient snores, awakens spontaneously to take a deep breath, or has apneic episodes (even brief) during sleep (Pasero, 2009b). The family is especially important to query as many individuals who have these characteristics are often not aware that they do (see the discussion later in the chapter). If any of the signs of OSA are reported, further evaluation, such as a sleep study to diagnose OSA, may be warranted before surgery or administration of sedating agents. At the very least, the primary physician and anesthesia provider should be made aware of the findings.

As mentioned, some therapies are associated with a higher incidence of respiratory depression than others, such as neuraxial single-bolus dosing (ASA, 2006) and IV PCA with a basal rate (continuous infusion) (APS, 2003; Dahan, Aarts, Smith, 2010; Pasero, McCaffery, 2004) (see Chapter 17). It is important for nurses to increase sedation and respiratory status assessments in patients receiving opioid therapy and concomitant administration of sedating agents, such as benzodiazepines and anxiolytics. Patients who are given antihistamines for treatment of adverse effects, such as pruritus, should also be watched closely as these increase sedation and can lead to respiratory depression (Anwari, Iqbal, 2003). Box 19-5 lists these and other risk factors for opioid-induced respiratory depression.

Prevention of Opioid-Induced Respiratory Depression

Clinically significant opioid-induced respiratory depression in opioid-naïve patients can be prevented by careful opioid titration and close nurse monitoring of sedation (see Box 19-4) and respiratory status (Pasero, 2009b; Pasero, McCaffery, 2002) (see later in this chapter for a discussion of mechanical monitoring). A principle of safe pain management is to administer the lowest effective opioid dose necessary to achieve satisfactory pain control (Pasero, Portenoy, McCaffery, 1999). This is best accomplished with the use of a multimodal analgesic approach that combines drugs with different

| Box 19-5 | Risk Factors for Opioid-Induced Respiratory Depression |

Patient may have one or more of the following to be considered high risk:

- Opioid naïvety (patients who have not been taking regular daily doses of opioids for several days)
- Older age (e.g., 65 years or older[1])
- Obesity (e.g., BMI 35 kg/m² or more)
- Obstructive sleep apnea (OSA)[2]
- History of snoring (see text) or witnessed apneas[2]
- Excessive daytime sleepiness[2]
- Preexisting pulmonary disease or dysfunction, e.g., chronic obstructive pulmonary disease
- Major organ failure
- One or more co-morbidities
- Smoker
- ASA Patient Status Classification 3, 4, or 5 in surgical patients (level determined by anesthesia provider preoperatively):
  - Classification 3: A patient with severe systemic disease
  - Classification 4: A patient with severe systemic disease that is a constant threat to life
  - Classification 5: A moribund patient who is not expected to survive without the operation
- Increased opioid dose requirement
  - Opioid-naïve patients who require a high dose of opioid in a short period (e.g., 10 mg of IV morphine or equivalent in the PACU)[3,4] (see text)
  - Opioid-tolerant patients who are given a significant amount of opioid in addition to their usual amount, such as the patient who takes an opioid analgesic preoperatively for persistent pain and receives several IV opioid bolus doses in the PACU followed by high-dose IV PCA for ongoing acute postoperative pain[4]
- First 24 hours of opioid therapy (e.g., first 24 hours following surgery is a high risk period for surgical patients)
- Pain is controlled after a period of poor control
- Prolonged surgery
- Thoracic and other large incisions that may interfere with adequate ventilation
- Concomitant administration of sedating agents, such as benzodiazepines, anxiolytics, or antihistamines
- Large single-bolus techniques (e.g., single injection neuraxial morphine)
- Continuous opioid infusion in opioid-naïve patients, e.g., IV PCA with basal rate (background infusion) or epidural continuous infusion

- Naloxone administration: Patients who are given naloxone for clinically significant respiratory depression are at risk for repeated respiratory depression; another dose of naloxone may be needed as early as 30 minutes after the first dose because the duration of naloxone is shorter than the duration of most opioids (see Box 19-6).

[1]There is no consensus on what age constitutes "older" age; some cite it as 65 years or older and others cite it as older than 75 years. It is important to consider the patient's general health and condition in addition to age.

[2]Most people with OSA do not know they have the condition; therefore, all patients and particularly their family members should be asked on admission if the patient snores or has apneic episodes during sleep or is excessively sleepy during the day. Other risk factors for OSA should be assessed as well. See Table 1 on p. 1083 of American Society of Anesthesiologists (ASA). (2006). Practice guidelines for the perioperative management of patients with obstructive sleep apnea. *Anesthesiology* 104(5):1081-1093.

[3]Patients who require 20 mg or more of morphine are at very high risk for opioid-induced sedation and clinically significant respiratory depression (see Abou hammoud, Simon, Urien, et al., 2009).

[4]It is recommended that patients be watched closely for at least 3 hours past the peak concentration of the last opioid dose.

From Pasero, C., & McCaffery, M. (2011). *Pain assessment and pharmacologic management*, p. 516, St. Louis, Mosby. Data from Abou hammoud, H., Simon, N., Urien, S., et al. (2009). Intravenous morphine titration in immediate postoperative pain management: Population kinetic-pharmacodynamic and logistic regression analysis. *Pain*, 144(1-2), 139-146; American Pain Society. (2003). *Principles of analgesic use in the treatment of acute pain and cancer pain*, ed 5, Glenview, IL, The Society; American Society of Anesthesiologists (ASA) physical status classification system. Available at http://www.asahq.org/clinical/physicalstatus.htm. Accessed August 10, 2009; American Society of Anesthesiologists (ASA). (2006). Practice guidelines for the perioperative management of patients with obstructive sleep apnea. *Anesthesiology, 104*(5), 1081-1093; American Society of Anesthesiologists Task Force on Neuraxial Opioids. (2009). Practice guidelines for the prevention, detection, and management of respiratory depression associated with neuraxial opioid administration. *Anesthesiology, 110*(2), 218-230; Dahan, A., Aarts, L., Smith, T. W. (2010). Incidence, reversal, and prevention of opioid-induced respiratory depression. *Anesthesiology, 112*(1), 226-238; Overdyk, F., & Ahmed, Q. (2009). Postoperative monitoring of obese patients with obstructive sleep apnea. (Letter). *Anesth Analg, 108*(3), 1044-1045; Pasero, C. (2009). Assessment of sedation during opioid administration for pain management. *J PeriAnesth Nurs, 24*(3), 186-190; Pasero, C., & McCaffery, M. (2002). Monitoring sedation. *Am J Nurs, 102*(2), 67-69; Pasero, C., & McCaffery, M. (2004). Safe use of a continuous infusion with IV PCA. *J PeriAnesth Nurs, 19*(1), 42-45; Taylor, S., Kirton, O. C., Staff, I., et al. (2005). Postoperative day one: A high risk period for respiratory events. *Am J Surg, 190*(5), 752-756. © 2011, Pasero C. May be duplicated for use in clinical practice.

underlying mechanisms, such as acetaminophen, NSAIDs, and local anesthetics (see Chapter 12). Lower opioid doses have the potential to reduce the incidence and severity of adverse effects like sedation and respiratory depression. Unless contraindicated, the administration of acetaminophen, an NSAID, or both preoperatively or before opioid therapy is initiated (e.g., on admission to the PACU) is recommended in all patients receiving short-term opioid therapy for nociceptive pain (e.g., surgery).

In all patients with elevated risk, starting opioid doses should be decreased 25% to 50%. Mechanical monitoring may also be indicated in some patients with high risk factors or who develop excessive sedation during opioid therapy (see following discussion). The expectation that nurses will reduce opioid doses promptly whenever advancing sedation is detected and increase monitoring frequency is essential for safe opioid administration (see previous discussion of sedation assessment). These actions should be included in all opioid orders and hospital protocols and taught in nursing orientation and ongoing educational courses (see Form 17-1 on p. 464 for an example of how decreases in opioid dose can be included in opioid order sets).

Respiratory Assessment

Ventilation is driven by a balance between arterial partial pressure of oxygen (PaO_2) and arterial partial pressure of carbon dioxide ($PaCO_2$) (Cretikos, Bellomo, Hillman, et al., 2008). Respiratory rate reflects the body's attempts to maintain that balance (e.g., tidal volume is increased to correct hypoxemia and hypercarbia). This helps to explain why abnormal respiratory rate is often a predictor of serious adverse events and critical illness (Cretikos, Bellomo, Hillman, et al., 2008; McBride, Knight, Piper, et al., 2005; Ridley, 2005).

Efforts to improve the quality and documentation of respiratory assessment, such as rigorous education of staff and evaluation of performance, are needed in all health care settings (Cretikos, Bellomo, Hillman, et al., 2008; Hogan, 2006). Research shows that assessment of respiratory rate alone is inadequate for determining ventilatory adequacy and propensity for respiratory depression (Dahan, Aarts, Smith, 2010; Overdyk, Carter, Maddox, 2006). Further, clinical observation suggests that staff often do not actually count the number of times a minute a patient breathes, and if it is counted, it is not counted long enough to obtain an accurate respiratory rate. This is supported by research that showed that respiratory rate was assessed and recorded in just 30% (McBride, Knight, Piper, et al., 2005), 50% (Hogan, 2006), and 58% (Edwards, Murdin, 2001) of patients on general care nursing units. One study found that almost 77% of patients who suffered an adverse event, such as unexpected cardiac arrest, unplanned ICU admission, and unexpected death, had a high proportion of missing documentation of vital signs, with respiratory rate being documented the least (Chen, Hillman, Bellomo, et al., 2009). A retrospective analysis showed that even when the diagnosis was of a respiratory nature (e.g., asthma, chronic obstructive pulmonary disease), respiratory rate was not documented in 27% of admissions and in only 65% of patients with chest symptoms in the ED (Edwards, Murdin, 2001). The introduction of a new vital signs chart and an early modified warning score in one hospital improved documentation of respiratory rate from approximately 30% to nearly 70% (McBride, Knight, Piper, et al., 2005). Similar results were found in another study with this approach (Hogan, 2006).

Although respiratory rate is an important parameter to obtain (Cretikos, Bellomo, Hillman, et al., 2008), it is emphasized again that clinically significant respiratory depression is not defined by a specific number of breaths/minute. Rather, it is defined by several characteristics of a patient's respiratory status. A comprehensive assessment of respiratory status goes hand-in-hand with sedation assessment and constitutes more than counting a patient's respiratory rate over a 30- or 60-second period (Pasero, 2009b) (see the discussion of sedation earlier in the chapter). A proper respiratory assessment requires the nurse or nurse technician to watch the rise and fall of the patient's chest to determine rate, depth, and regularity of respirations (Stemp, Ramsay, 2005). Current rate and quality is compared with baseline, and trends are noted (Pasero, 2009b).

Snoring Is a Warning Sign. Listening to the sound of the patient's respiration is critical. Snoring indicates airway obstruction and must be attended to promptly with repositioning (Isono, Tanaka, Nishino, 2002) and, depending on the severity, a request for respiratory therapy consultation and further evaluation for the presence of obstructive sleep apnea (OSA) (ASA, 2006). Even subtle snoring can evolve into complete obstruction in a sedated patient, and so must be promptly addressed and monitoring increased (Pasero, 2009b).

Patients and family members often report that snoring is "normal" because the patient snores at home. This thinking can lead to fatal consequences. In the home setting, patients are usually awakened by their own snoring and ineffectual respiration, or a family member awakens them; however, in the context of opioid administration and perhaps other sedating medications, patients may be too sedated to self-arouse. Under these circumstances, snoring is an ominous sign and requires the nurse to arouse and further evaluate the patient to avert disaster (Pasero, 2009b) (see the discussion that follows).

Frequency of Sedation and Respiratory Assessment

Assessment of sedation level and respiratory status should be done together at the same frequency. The risk factors previously discussed in this chapter and in Box 19-5 are considered when determining the frequency of assessment. Although there is no set frequency for sedation and respiratory assessment that fits all patients, the most dangerous time for a patient in terms of developing respiratory depression is during the first 24 hours of opioid therapy for moderate-to-severe pain in opioid-naïve patients and others at risk for respiratory depression (Pasero, 2009b; Taylor, Voytovich, Kozol, 2003; Taylor, Kirton, Staff et al., 2005). Therefore, sedation and respiratory assessment should be performed every hour for the first 12 hours after opioid therapy is initiated, and, if stable, this may be followed by a frequency of every

2 hours for the next 12 hours of opioid therapy. Other vital signs may be obtained as required by the primary provider's routine orders (e.g., every 4 hours). The ASA recommends this same protocol for patients receiving neuraxial analgesic therapies except that frequency may be every hour for just 2 hours after a single bolus neuraxial dose of a lipophilic opioid, such as fentanyl (ASA Task Force on Neuraxial Opioids, 2009). After 24 hours of opioid therapy, most patients are able to go to every-4-hour sedation and respiratory assessments, but this must be individualized and based on the patient's condition.

Nurses are expected to evaluate each patient initially and on an ongoing basis during opioid therapy for the need for more or less frequent monitoring based on the patient's risk factors and current status. If a patient's condition warrants closer monitoring than can be provided on the current clinical unit, the patient should be promptly moved to a more closely monitored setting (Pasero, 2009b). Institutions are encouraged to establish protocols that support the nurse's role in ensuring patient safety during opioid administration (see Table 19-1).

Assessment of the Sleeping Patient. Nurses often ask if they should awaken sleeping patients to determine level of sedation. It is acceptable to allow a patient to sleep who has been receiving stable opioid doses and demonstrates optimal respiratory status determined by a comprehensive respiratory assessment as described above (ASA, 2009; Pasero, 2009b). However, patients must be aroused if there is any question about whether they are sleeping normally or are sedated. Research discussed earlier showed that sleep during morphine titration is mainly the result of the sedative effects of the opioid (Lovovschi, Aubrun, Bonnet, et al., 2008). It is important to realize that arousal will stimulate respiration; to obtain a more accurate picture of the patient's respiratory status, the comprehensive respiratory assessment should be performed before arousing the sleeping patient (ASA, 2009; Pasero, 2009b).

It is reassuring to know that patients who are sleeping normally and have well-controlled pain will fall back to sleep after they are aroused for a sedation assessment if one is necessary. Those who do not fall back to sleep require further evaluation because they may be experiencing pain and the need for additional analgesia. Note that patients who achieve pain control and fall asleep after a period of poor pain control should be carefully assessed to be sure that what seems to be normal sleep is not actually excessive sedation.

Mechanical Monitoring During Short-Term Opioid Therapy

The risk factors listed in Box 19-5 are considered when determining who might benefit from mechanical monitoring (e.g., pulse oximetry [O_2 saturation] or capnography [$ETCO_2$]) during opioid therapy. Having a risk factor for respiratory depression does not automatically mean the patient must receive mechanical monitoring; however, careful consideration of the severity of the factor and the patient's general health and current condition is essential to decision making. Mechanical monitoring should also be considered in patients who require naloxone administration for clinically significant respiratory depression until their condition is stable (see the discussion of reversing opioid-induced respiratory depression later in the chapter).

The most common technologies used for mechanically monitoring patients during opioid administration are pulse oximetry and capnography; however, research is lacking on their effectiveness in reducing episodes of clinically significant opioid-induced respiratory depression. As mentioned earlier, a low incidence of rescue naloxone (one patient, 0.6%) in a study of 178 patients who were monitored with capnography and pulse oximetry during IV PCA was attributed to the monitoring equipment's audible alarm that arouses a patient and summons a nurse, but the researchers suggested that more research is needed to verify this (Overdyk, Carter, Maddox, et al., 2007). A systematic review of randomized controlled trials that compared postoperative patients with and without pulse oximetry found that the incidence of hypoxemia in the PACU was 1.5 to 3 times less with pulse oximetry but could find no significant difference in postoperative complications between those who received pulse oximetry (10%) and those who did not (9.4%) (Pedersen, Moller, Pedersen, 2003).

Pulse Oximetry. Oxygen saturation monitoring via finger-sensor pulse oximetry is commonly used but has several drawbacks that can have significant consequences, particularly when used on clinical units (i.e., outside of PACU, ICU, and ED). Research shows that finger-sensor pulse oximetry is associated with a high incidence of technical false alarms from the loss of signal and poor signal quality when blood flow is low to the sensor area or when patients move (Eisenkraft, 2006; Reich, Timcenko, Bodian, et al., 1996). Forehead-sensor technology may provide a solution to the problem of technical false alarms but has not proven to be superior to finger-sensor technology (Agashe, Coakley, Mannheimer, 2006; Blaylock, Brinkman, Carver, et al., 2008). Nurses often do not respond to alarms, particularly if the alarm self-resolves within a short period of time (Overdyk, Carter, Maddox, et al., 2007). It is important for nursing staff to appreciate that alarm resolution does not necessarily mean the patient is safe—all alarms should be evaluated. Sometimes nurses disable alarms when repeated false alarms occur in some patients. Instead, when repeated false alarms occur, the patient's primary health care provider should be consulted to determine the need for mechanical monitoring. Patients often become annoyed and remove the oximetry sensor as well, so initial and ongoing patient teaching on the purpose of monitoring is required but not always provided.

Some institutions implement periodic pulse oximetry readings (spot checks) that are taken usually when the patient's vital signs are obtained; however, this practice may lead to inaccurate assumptions about the patient's respiratory status. The process of applying the pulse oximeter sensor is likely to stimulate the patient to take a deep breath, which can yield a higher oxygen saturation than the patient has when not stimulated. If mechanical monitoring is warranted, it should be done continuously (Pasero, 2009b).

Finally, as mentioned earlier, oxygen saturation is a measure of gas exchange rather than a direct indicator of ventilatory efficacy; it provides limited information on the effects of an opioid on ventilatory control (Dahan, Aarts, Smith, 2010). In addition, a primary disadvantage of pulse oximetry is that it will yield high oxygen saturation readings despite the presence of respiratory depression in patients who are receiving supplemental oxygen (Overdyk, Ahmed, 2009; Overdyk, Carter, Maddox, 2006). If a patient requires both supplemental oxygen and mechanical monitoring and pulse oximetry is the only mechanical monitoring available, the patient should be moved to a more closely monitored setting (Overdyk, Ahmed, 2009; Pasero, 2009b).

End-Tidal CO_2 Monitoring (Capnography). Expired CO_2 is considered a highly reliable measure of the quality of ventilation and, unlike pulse oximetry, is an early indicator of impending respiratory depression (Kopka, Wallace, Reilly, et al., 2007). The technology to monitor $ETCO_2$ is rapidly advancing and is likely to rival or replace pulse oximetry as the primary method for monitoring patients in the perioperative, procedural, critical care, and emergency settings. Current technology utilizes a nasal catheter to detect expired CO_2, but transcutaneous sensors have been researched (Kopka, Wallace, Reilly, et al., 2007). The latter may suffer the same drawbacks of pulse oximetry in terms of sensitivity to blood flow. Further research is needed.

Modular technology that links continuous capnography and pulse oximetry monitoring to analgesic devices, such as PCA pumps, is available. Such a device can be programmed to alarm and discontinue opioid administration whenever the device detects a reading outside of the set threshold (e.g., oxygen saturation less than 90% or end-tidal CO_2 more than 50 mm Hg or less than 30 mm Hg). Research is lacking regarding the safe minimal settings for these parameters and the effectiveness of this technology in reducing the incidence of clinically significant respiratory depression. Anecdotally, nurses report that this feature is frequently triggered for reasons unrelated to the patient's physiologic status, such as signal failure (discussed earlier in the chapter), and they cite the subsequent loss of pain control and difficulty regaining control as major drawbacks to the technology.

The use of capnography during opioid administration is evolving. The reader is referred to an excellent website (http://www.capnography.com) that provides extensive information and access to research about capnography including the physiology of capnography, clinical uses, and advances in technology.

Summary Points on Mechanical Monitoring. In summary, further research is needed to determine who will benefit from mechanical monitoring during opioid therapy. More data are needed to assess the clinical significance of the oxygen desaturation and hypercarbia that occur during opioid therapy. As technology improves, it is likely to become more commonplace, but it is extremely important to remind staff members that the use of mechanical monitoring does not absolve them of sedation and respiratory assessments (Pasero, 2009b). Mechanical monitoring can be an extremely valuable technology in some patients, but excessive use can lull staff into a false sense of security and a tendency to ignore alarms. Institutions are encouraged to form a multidisciplinary task force to establish guidelines for the rational use of mechanical monitoring during short-term opioid therapies. Clinician decision making about whether to use mechanical monitoring or not is enhanced when it is based on the patient's risk factors and current condition.

Transfer of Care: Hand-off Communication

Pain control should be included in the criteria for discharge from one area of care to another. Some EDs, short-stay units, outpatient surgery units, and PACUs establish a comfort-function goal of at least 4/10 before discharge (see Section II); however, the expectation that all patients must be discharged from these areas with pain ratings below an arbitrary number can lead to the unsafe administration of further opioid doses to patients who are excessively sedated (Blumstein, Moore, 2003; Lucas, Vlahos, Ledgerwood, 2007). Instead, achieving optimal pain relief is best viewed on a continuum, with the primary objective being to provide both effective and safe analgesia. Although it is not always possible to achieve a patient's comfort-function goal within the short time the patient is in these areas, the comfort-function goal provides direction for ongoing care. Important information to give to the nurse assuming care of the patient is the patient's comfort-function goal, how close the patient is to achieving it, what has been done thus far to achieve it (analgesics, doses, and times of administration), and how well the patient has tolerated the administration of analgesics (adverse effects).

The transferring nurse should also alert staff on the receiving clinical unit of a patient's risk factors for respiratory depression so that appropriate monitoring can be initiated (see Box 19-5). For example, opioid-naïve patients who require high opioid doses (e.g., more than 10 mg of IV morphine or its equivalent) during titration for acute pain are at higher risk for respiratory depression (Dahan, Aarts, Smith, 2010; Lotsch, Dudziak, Freynhagen, et al., 2006) and must be watched closely for at least 3 hours after the peak concentration of the last dose has passed (APS, 2003); the highest risk for respiratory depression is during the entire first 24 postoperative hours. Mechanical monitoring is warranted in patients with diagnosed or suspected obstructive sleep apnea or pulmonary disease. Providing the postoperative patient's ASA Patient Status Classification is recommended as a simple way to further communicate the patient's risk for respiratory depression.

Reversing Respiratory Depression: Naloxone Administration

The opioid antagonist naloxone has been used since the early 1970s to reverse respiratory depression related to opioid overdose (Buck, 2002). It is administered IV and has a rapid onset of action (2 minutes) with a peak concentration in 10 minutes, duration of 1 to 4 hours, and a half-life of 30 to 81 minutes (Leavitt, 2009). The extent and duration of naloxone reversal of opioid effects varies and is dependent on many factors, such as specific opioid used, opioid dose, method of administration, and concurrent medications (Dahan, Aarts, Smith, 2010).

If it is necessary to use naloxone to reverse clinically significant respiratory depression, it should be titrated very carefully (APS, 2003). Sometimes more than one dose of naloxone is necessary because naloxone has a shorter duration (1 hour in most patients) than most opioids (Dahan, Aarts, Smith, 2010); however, giving too much naloxone or giving it too fast can precipitate severe pain that is extremely difficult to control and increase sympathetic activity leading to hypertension, tachycardia, ventricular dysrhythmias, pulmonary edema, and cardiac arrest (Brimacombe, Archdeacon, Newell, et al., 1991; O'Malley-Dafner, Davies, 2000). Box 19-6 outlines the procedure for correctly administering naloxone to an adult. Hospital protocols and opioid orders should include the expectation that nurses will administer naloxone in accordance with the procedure outlined in Box 19-6 whenever a patient is found to have clinically significant opioid-induced respiratory depression.

In physically dependent patients, withdrawal syndrome can be precipitated by naloxone administration; patients who have been receiving opioids for more than 1 week may be exquisitely sensitive to antagonists (APS, 2003). If sedation and respiratory depression occurs during administration of transdermal fentanyl, the patch should be removed immediately, and if naloxone is necessary, treatment will be needed for a prolonged period and the typical approach involves a naloxone infusion over a 12- to 24-hour period (e.g., mix 0.8 mg of naloxone in 250 mL of IV solution and run at 9 to 20 mL/h to administer approximately 0.2 to 0.6 mg/h naloxone). The patient must be closely monitored for at least 24 hours after discontinuation of the transdermal fentanyl.

IV access for naloxone administration usually is maintained for 24 hours after a stable epidural opioid dose has been achieved. After that time, naloxone rarely is needed because most patients are alert and, in many cases, are ready for a decrease in the epidural opioid dose.

Although no formulation is commercially available in the United States, naloxone has been administered intranasally. One randomized controlled trial found an equally safe and favorable response within 10 minutes of administering 2 mg intranasally or intramuscularly in the prehospital setting for suspected heroin overdose (Kerr, Kelly, Dietze, et al., 2009). A retrospective study compared intranasal naloxone with IV naloxone for opioid overdose in the prehospital setting and found the mean time to clinical response was longer in those who received intranasal naloxone, but the researchers suggested that the response time was equivalent when the time required to prepare an IV injection of naloxone is considered (Robertson, Hendey, Stroh, et al., 2009). In both of these studies, patients who received intranasal naloxone were more likely to require an additional rescue dose of naloxone.

Patient Example

Ms. V. is receiving IV PCA morphine with a basal rate of 1 mg/h, PCA bolus dose of 1 mg, and a lockout interval of 8 minutes for postoperative pain after an exploratory laparotomy. She is found with a sedation level of 4 (see Box 19-4), but arouses with physical stimulation. Her respirations are shallow, and her respiratory rate is 6 breaths/min. The first actions the nurse who finds Ms. V. takes are to stop the PCA pump and call for help from other staff members. The nurse continues to vigorously arouse Ms. V., who is responsive to physical stimuli, and asks a coworker to bring a syringe of diluted naloxone (0.4 mg naloxone/10 mL saline, see Box 19-6). When the naloxone arrives, the nurse slowly administers it while observing Ms. V.'s response. After about 3 mL (0.12 mg), Ms. V. has a sedation level of 3, responds to questions appropriately, and is able to follow the nurse's instructions to deep breathe. The nurse stops administering naloxone after 0.12 mg because the desired effect is a reversal of Ms. V.'s sedation and respiratory depression without loss of pain control. The primary physician is notified and alternative analgesia (ketorolac, 15 mg IV) is given because PCA is discontinued. Ms. V.'s sedation and respiratory status are monitored every 10 to 15 minutes until her sedation level is stable at less than 3 and respiratory status is satisfactory. After about 90 minutes, Ms. V.'s sedation level is less than 3, her respiratory depth is adequate, and her respiratory rate is 12 breaths/min. Her pain rating is 2/10. Nurse-administered IV bolus doses of morphine 1 mg to 4 mg q 2 h PRN are prescribed for pain, and the ketorolac is continued q 6 h around the clock.

Box 19-6 | Naloxone Administration in Adults[1]

1. Patients who require naloxone (Narcan) usually meet all of the following criteria:
   - Minimal or no response to physical stimulation
   - Shallow respirations or respiratory rate less than 8 breaths/minute
   - Pinpoint pupils
2. Stop the administration of the opioid and any other sedative drugs. If given IV, maintain IV access.
3. Summon help. Call Rapid Response Team if indicated by patient status and ask a coworker to prepare naloxone (see No. 4) and bring it to you. Remain with the patient, continue to attempt to vigorously arouse him or her, and support respirations as indicated by patient status.
4. Ask coworker to mix 0.4 mg (1 ampule) of naloxone and 10 mL of normal saline in a syringe for IV administration.[2,3]
5. Administer the dilute naloxone solution IV very slowly (0.5 mL over 2 minutes)[3-5] while you observe the patient's response (titrate to effect).
6. The patient should open his or her eyes and talk to you within 1 to 2 minutes. If not, continue IV naloxone at the same rate up to a total of 0.8 mg or 20 mL of dilute naloxone. If no response, begin looking for other causes of sedation and respiratory depression.
7. Discontinue the naloxone administration as soon as the patient is responsive to physical stimulation and able to take deep breaths when told to do so. Keep the syringe nearby. Another dose of naloxone may be needed as early as 30 minutes after the first dose because the duration of naloxone is shorter than the duration of most opioids.
8. Assign a staff member to monitor sedation and respiratory status and to remind the patient to deep breathe every 1 to 2 minutes until the patient becomes more alert.
9. Notify the primary physician and pain service. Document your actions.
10. Provide a nonopioid for pain relief.
11. Resume opioid administration at one half the original dose when the patient is easily aroused and respiratory rate is more than 9 breaths/min.
12. Monitor sedation and respiratory status in accordance with the pharmacokinetics of the opioid administered.[5]

IV, Intravenous.

[1]Orders for opioids should include the administration of naloxone according to the APS recommendations, or a protocol incorporating the APS recommendations can be adopted for use by any nurse who suspects a patient is experiencing clinically significant opioid-induced respiratory depression.

[2]If naloxone is available only in a prefilled syringe, 10 mL of saline can be drawn into a 12 mL syringe, leaving enough room to accept the transfer of naloxone from the prefilled syringe. This procedure would ensure correct dilution.

[3]If IV route is inaccessible, administer undiluted naloxone, 0.4 mg, subcutaneously or intramuscularly. The patient should respond within 5 minutes. If not, repeat dose up to a total of 2 mg. Intranasal naloxone (2 mg) has been shown to be as safe and effective as intramuscular and IV naloxone in the treatment of opioid overdose with a favorable response within 10 minutes; however, an additional dose of naloxone was more likely when given intranasally (see text for discussion and references). More well-controlled research is needed to recommend this route of administration for naloxone.

[4]This is the recommended amount and rate for administering naloxone to reverse opioid-induced respiratory depression. Administering a larger amount in a shorter period of time than this risks reversing more than opioid-induced respiratory depression (e.g., analgesia).

[5]If sedation and respiratory depression occur during administration of transdermal fentanyl, remove the patch; if naloxone is necessary, treatment will be needed for a prolonged period after initial resuscitation, and the typical approach involves a naloxone infusion (see text). Patient must be closely monitored for at least 24 hours after discontinuation of the transdermal fentanyl.

This box provides the recommended titrate-to-effect procedure for administering naloxone (Narcan) to reverse clinically significant respiratory depression. Giving too much naloxone or giving it too fast can precipitate severe pain, which is extremely difficult to control, and increase sympathetic activity leading to hypertension, tachycardia, ventricular dysrhythmias, pulmonary edema, and cardiac arrest. In physically dependent patients, withdrawal syndrome can be precipitated; patients who have been receiving opioids for more than one week may be exquisitely sensitive to antagonists.

From Pasero, C., & McCaffery, M. (2011). *Pain assessment and pharmacologic management*, p. 521, St. Louis, Mosby. Data from American Pain Society (APS). (2003). *Principles of analgesic use in the treatment of acute and cancer pain*, ed 5, Glenview, IL, APS. © 2011, Pasero C. May be duplicated for use in clinical practice.

Inappropriate Use of Opioid Antagonists

More often than clinically significant respiratory depression, cancer patients receiving long-term opioid treatment may develop confusion and be somewhat sedated but remain easily aroused with an acceptable respiratory rate and depth. Great care must be taken to prevent the administration of an opioid antagonist drug to patients exhibiting such symptoms because the symptoms may be caused by disease progression rather than opioid overdose. This is not an emergency situation, and observation for a few hours is the best diagnostic and therapeutic approach (Manfredi, Ribeiro, Chandler, et al., 1996). If a terminally ill patient cannot be aroused and an opioid overdose is suspected, an opioid antagonist drug is warranted only if it is clear that this is not a natural progression of the disease. Only small doses are given very slowly because opioid-tolerant patients are extremely sensitive to an opioid antagonist and easily experience withdrawal symptoms and loss of pain control.

Conclusion

The most common opioid adverse effects include constipation, nausea and vomiting, sedation, pruritus, and mental confusion and clouding. Respiratory depression is less common but is the most feared effect. As the patient becomes opioid tolerant, these adverse effects, except for constipation, tend to subside. A number of factors influence the development of opioid adverse effects, including patient age, co-morbidities, prior opioid exposure, concurrent administration of other drugs, and route of administration. This underscores the need for an individualized approach to preventing and managing the effects. Prevention rather than treatment of opioid adverse effects is an important principle of pain management. Most adverse effects are dose dependent, which is why an effective and practical approach to treatment of these is to administer the lowest effective opioid dose.

Chapter 20 Unwarranted Withholding of Opioids

THIS chapter discusses pain management for patients in whom opioid analgesics are sometimes withheld. It will discuss the controversies, correct any misconceptions, and provide recommendations for pain treatment in these patients. (See also Chapter 13, p. 339 for care of the patient with sickle cell disease and p. 331 for care of the patient post craniotomy.)

Long-Term Opioid Use in Patients with Persistent Noncancer Pain

Of all the types of pain experienced by patients, the use of opioids is the most controversial in patients with persistent noncancer pain. Opioids are recognized as the mainstay of treatment for moderate to severe acute pain and moderate to severe cancer pain (American Pain Society [APS], 2003). Length of time on opioids seems to be the key issue. Acute pain is defined as being brief, subsiding as healing takes place. Cancer pain, on the other hand, is known to be both acute and persistent, lasting months. However, with newer cancer treatments, pain may last up to one or two years, even longer. The patients who may live the longest are those with persistent noncancer pain, and sadly, this is the group that may be denied pain relief if opioids are needed. Some patients with persistent noncancer pain who cannot obtain needed opioids have been known to say they wished they had terminal cancer so that they would be afforded pain relief.

Is withholding of opioids from patients with persistent noncancer pain warranted? Multiple reasons have been given for withholding opioids from this group of patients, including, fear of addiction, tolerance, limitations on activity such as driving, opioid-induced hyperalgesia, harm to the immune system, and opioid-induced hypogonadism. As will be seen in the discussion that follows, evidence does not support using these reasons for denying opioids to patients with persistent noncancer pain. Rather, the decision to implement a trial of long-term opioid therapy should be based on a careful assessment of potential benefits and burdens (Chou, Fanciullo, Fine, et al., 2009).

Addiction

The likelihood of a patient developing addictive disease as a result of being treated with opioids has already been discussed in Chapter 11. The risk of iatrogenic addiction after short-term exposure for postoperative pain is known to be less than 1%. The risk during long-term treatment is not clear, and is likely to be related to risk factors, the most important of which—a personal history of drug or alcohol abuse, or a family history of drug or alcohol abuse—underscore the importance of a genetic determinant for the disease of addiction.

A review of definitions related to conditions often confused with addiction will clarify some of the confusion about addiction. Following are the definitions proposed by the American Academy of Pain Medicine (AAPM), the APS, and the American Society of Addiction Medicine (ASAM) (2001):

- *Physical dependence* is a normal response that occurs with repeated administration of the opioid for more than 2 weeks and cannot be equated with addictive disease. It is manifested by the occurrence of withdrawal symptoms when the opioid is suddenly stopped or rapidly reduced or an antagonist such as naloxone (Narcan) is given. Withdrawal symptoms may be suppressed by the natural, gradual reduction of the opioid as pain decreases or by gradual, systematic reduction, referred to as *tapering*.
- *Tolerance* is also a normal response that occurs with regular administration of an opioid and consists of a decrease in one or more effects of the opioid (e.g., decreased analgesia, sedation, or respiratory depression). It cannot be equated with addictive disease. Tolerance to analgesia usually occurs in the first days to 2 weeks of opioid therapy but is uncommon after that. It may be treated with increases in dose. However, disease progression, not tolerance to analgesia, appears to be the reason for most dose escalations. Stable pain usually results in stable doses. Thus tolerance poses very few clinical problems.
- *Opioid addiction,* or addictive disease, is a chronic neurologic and biologic disease. Its development and manifestations are influenced by genetic, psychosocial, and environmental factors. No single cause of addiction, such as taking an opioid for pain relief, has been found. It is characterized by behaviors that include one or more of the following: impaired control over drug use, compulsive use, continued use despite harm, and craving.

In addressing the relationship between addictive disease and the use of opioids for persistent noncancer pain, the following two questions need to be considered:

- How many patients who are receiving opioids for persistent pain also have addictive disease? This is prevalence data. Based on their review of the literature, Nicholson and Passik (2007) found that some studies indicate that the rate of addiction to illicit drugs, prescribed opioids, and alcohol in this population is approximately the same as in the general population, which ranges from 6% to 10% (Savage, 2002).

- How many patients who receive opioids for persistent pain become addicted? This is a causal relationship and cannot be answered by prevalence data.

Very few studies have been conducted to examine the latter question. The appropriate research needs to start with patients who do not already have addictive disease and find out how many become addicted as a result of long-term use of opioids for pain. In a review of all available studies on the development of abuse, addiction, and aberrant drug-related behaviors in patients with persistent pain of noncancer origin who received opioids for pain, only four studies preselected patients for no previous or current history of abuse or addiction (Fishbain, Cole, Lewis, et al., 2008). In these studies, the percentage of patients who became addicted was calculated at 0.19%. A more recent registry study of patients who participated in controlled trials and therefore represented a population from which patients with a history of drug abuse were excluded demonstrated an incidence of 2.6% of drug misuse and no addiction during 3 years of follow-up (Portenoy, Farrar, Backonja, et al., 2007). These data suggest that patients who do not develop a pattern of misuse of psychoactive drugs are at very low risk of developing prescription drug abuse later. None of these data provide insight into the true risk of opioid addiction or abuse among the large population that has a history, or a family history, of alcohol or drug abuse and later receives an opioid for persistent pain.

Ability to Drive and Engage in Other Activities

The effect of opioids on performance of normal activities is sometimes given as reason for withholding opioids. Sometimes employers will not allow patients on opioids to continue their employment. Some prescribers have asked patients to sign agreements that stipulate "no driving" if opioids are taken on a long-term basis (Fishman, Bandman, Edwards, et al., 1999). These outcomes reduce the likelihood that a patient will agree to a trial of this treatment.

According to the opioid treatment guidelines developed by a panel for the APS and the AAPM, the evidence does not support universal prohibition of driving for patients on long-term opioid therapy (Chou, Fanciullo, Fine, et al., 2009). The ability to drive should be assessed in each patient and not prevented in all patients. This is discussed earlier in Chapter 19. Highlights of this discussion are repeated here, and the reader is referred to the earlier discussion for details.

In one study with findings similar to other research, driving tests based on German national recommendations were conducted on 90 healthy controls and 21 patients with noncancer pain who had been treated with transdermal fentanyl for at least 4 weeks without a dose change in the last 12 days (Sabatowski, Schwalen, Rettig, et al.,

2003). The median dose of transdermal fentanyl was 50 mcg/h, with a range of 25 to 400 mcg/h. Based on test results, the authors concluded that patients with noncancer pain on stable doses of transdermal fentanyl do not have any clinically significant impairment of psychomotor or cognitive function that would prevent them from driving a car. These results suggest that patients on long-term opioid therapy are probably also able to continue with many other activities. In fact, other drugs such as diphenhydramine (Benadryl) may impair persons more than opioids (Weiler, Bloomfield, Woodworth, et al., 2000).

Whether or not a patient taking opioid analgesics can drive or perform other activities must be decided on an individual basis. Some patients will be able to drive safely, but others may be impaired by opioids. Impairment usually is transient and occurs only at the beginning of opioid therapy or following significant increases in dose, but the reality that some patients have persistent problems requires a careful assessment on a case-by-case basis. Patients who report mental clouding or sedation, or who have signs of impairment on exam should be considered for a change in opioid. It seems prudent to warn all patients that driving ability may be compromised and not to drive if they feel drowsy, dizzy, or impaired in any way, and to advise them of the current literature on driving while taking opioids. In addition, some clinicians advocate asking patients on long-term opioid therapy to obey certain rules if they decide to drive. These rules and a consent form are discussed earlier in Chapter 19 and Box 19-3 on p. 508.

Opioid-Induced Hyperalgesia (OIH)

Hyperalgesia means increased sensitivity to pain. In opioid-induced hyperalgesia (OIH) increasing doses of opioid result in increasing sensitivity to pain (Compton, 2008). OIH has only recently been identified as a clinical reality (Mitra, 2008), but the extent to which it compromises treatment is unknown (Angst, Clark, 2006; Chu, Angst, Clark, 2008). OIH is discussed in more detail in Chapter 11, and the highlights of this discussion are repeated here.

OIH is suspected when increasing doses (usually high, rapidly escalating doses) of opioid fail to relieve pain and actually make pain worse at the original site of pain or at other sites (Chu, Angst, Clark, 2008; Mitra, 2008). OIH may involve unexplained pain, diffuse pain (even the whole body), and diffuse allodynia (Compton, 2008; Chu, Angst, Clark, 2008; Mitra, 2008). To assess the possible presence of OIH, other reasons for failure of the opioid to relieve pain must be ruled out. These include increase in pain pathology, opioid tolerance, opioid withdrawal, pseudoaddiction, and opioid addiction (Compton, 2008). Only when these are ruled out can a diagnosis of OIH be entertained. Table 11-3 (p. 296) gives a brief description of these conditions compared with OIH and suggests some distinguishing characteristics.

Treatment strategies may include opioid dose reduction, opioid rotation, use of N-methyl-D-aspartate (NMDA) receptor antagonists, and continued use of a COX-2 selective NSAID in persistent pain. Once OIH is established, the current opioid dose should be reduced, but the patient is also usually treated with other pain relief strategies as well.

Research has begun to identify potential approaches to preventing OIH. These include proper timing of COX-2 selective NSAIDs in postoperative patients, NMDA antagonists, opioid dose-sparing medications such as certain adjuvants, and avoidance of rapid opioid dose escalation when possible. Theoretically, continued use of COX-2 selective NSAIDs in persistent pain is not only opioid dose-sparing but also may help prevent OIH because these medications reduce the spinal release of excitatory neurotransmitters (Mitra, 2008).

Knowing that long-term opioid therapy, especially if doses escalate rapidly, might actually worsen pain for selected patients adds to the list of reasons to be cautious about this use of opioids. At present, the importance of this outcome is unknown, however, and its reality calls only for careful assessment of patients who do not appear to be improving when an opioid is prescribed.

Other Concerns

Many other concerns about using long-term opioid therapy for patients with persistent noncancer pain exist but are beyond the scope of this book. However, two others deserve at least brief mention: opioid effects on the immune system and opioid effects on the endocrine system in the form of opioid-induced hypogonadism.

A review of the literature by Page (2005) points out that the effect of opioids on immune function has been studied in animals and in humans in the absence of pain and found to suppress immune function. But, in the presence of acute pain, opioid administration in analgesic doses seems to be protective. However, much less is known about the effect on the immune system of prolonged opioid administration in the presence of persistent pain. To date, one small study of 10 patients with persistent pain receiving oral modified-release morphine for 12 weeks indicates that morphine does not influence immune function (Palm, Lehzen, Mignat, et al., 1998). The conclusion was that, at this point in our evidence, concern about opioid effect on immune function is not a reason to withhold opioids from patients with persistent pain. Page (2005) reasons that since it is well known that pain itself suppresses immune function, opioids in analgesic doses could provide relief of pain and thereby provide some relief of the immune suppression of pain.

Negative effects of opioids on the endocrine system have been known for years, but little is written about this. Most of the literature concerns opioid-induced hypogonadism, which is probably common in both male and female patients on long-term opioid therapy (Katz, Mazer, 2009). No standards for laboratory monitoring exist, but recommendations include testing for total and free testosterone (especially in men) and monitoring bone density. Symptoms include decreased libido, erectile dysfunction in men, depression, anxiety, and fatigue. Of course, these symptoms may be due to many other causes such as pain itself. Treatment considerations include opioid rotation and testosterone supplementation. Based on available information, it is not reasonable to withhold opioid therapy because of concerns about endocrine effects of long-term opioid use. These can be monitored and treated.

Treatment Guidelines

The first treatment guidelines developed by professional organizations and designed specifically for the use of long-term opioid therapy for persistent noncancer pain were published in 2009 by a panel convened by the APS and the AAPM (Chou, Fanciullo, Fine, et al., 2009). By contrast, treatment guidelines for cancer pain were published by the World Health Organization (WHO) in the 1980s (WHO, 1986), quickly followed by the APS (APS, 1987) guidelines for acute pain and cancer pain but not for persistent noncancer pain. The Agency for Health Care Policy and Research (AHCPR) then developed guidelines for acute pain (Acute Pain Management Guideline Panel, 1992) and cancer pain (Jacox, Carr, Payne, et al., 1994) but again, not for persistent noncancer pain. Notably, it was approximately 2 decades between the development of guidelines for acute and cancer pain and guidelines for the pharmacologic treatment of persistent noncancer pain. During those years and up to the present time, considerable controversy exists about the long-term use of opioids for persistent noncancer pain.

Despite this controversy, the use of opioids for persistent noncancer pain has increased considerably. Although evidence is limited, the APS-AAPM panel concluded that long-term opioid therapy can be effective with carefully selected patients with persistent noncancer pain. The guideline includes, among other things, a discussion of informed consent and opioid management plans, initiation and titration of long-term opioid therapy, and monitoring of patients.

This guideline is a step in the right direction but has been subject to some criticism, making it important to remember that guidelines are not rules—they are simply guides. Some recommendations are considered questionable since they were presented as "strong recommendation, low-quality evidence" (Leavitt, 2009).

Another criticism is related to a previously registered serious objection to the Washington State Agency Medical Directors' Group (2007) recommendation in their guidelines that doses greater than 120 mg/day of oral morphine or equivalents should rarely be given and only prescribed after consultation with a pain management expert (Fishman, Webster, 2009). Yet, based on low-level evidence, the APS-AAPM defined a "high" dose of opioid as greater than 200 mg/day of oral morphine

or its equivalent and stated that such doses require more intense monitoring.

Another guideline from the American Geriatrics Society (AGS) addresses the pharmacologic treatment of persistent noncancer pain in people 75 years or older (AGS, 2009). Previously, NSAIDs were recommended if acetaminophen did not relieve pain. However, new evidence has drawn attention to the dangerous adverse effects of NSAIDs, such as cardiovascular risk, nephrotoxicity, and gastrointestinal (GI) toxicity (see Section III). Since NSAIDs may result in life-threatening problems, opioids are suggested as a safer alternative in many older adults (AGS, 2009).

Regulatory Issues

The APS-AAPM panel points out that surveys show that prescribers have limited understanding of the laws, policies, and other matters that govern the prescribing of opioids, and that this may have an impact on the care patients receive (Chou, Fanciullo, Fine, et al., 2009). Our impression is that fear of regulatory scrutiny causes prescribers to be fearful of long-term prescribing of opioids and in turn causes them to be overly cautious of prescribing opioids. For their own protection and the patient's benefit, prescribers should find out about the numerous policy changes that have occurred in recent years. The Pain and Policy Studies Group, University of Wisconsin Database, provides information on state laws, regulations, and other official government policies, and is available at www.painpolicy.wisc.edu/matrix.htm.

Opioid Safety Regulations: Risk Evaluation and Mitigation Strategy (REMS)

A defining consideration in the approval of any drug by the United States Food and Drug Administration (U.S. FDA) is that the benefit of the drug must outweigh its risks. In the case of opioids, abuse potential and the consequent concerns for public health are receiving increasing attention in the review process for new drugs, while new regulations are being considered for some drugs already marketed.

In February of 2008, a new federal law gave the U.S. FDA expanded powers to regulate both new and established medications. One of the provisions authorizes the U.S. FDA to require that a drug manufacturer submit a Risk Evaluation and Mitigation Strategy (REMS). REMS typically include patient and prescriber education. Some may require restricted distribution through specified pharmacies and registries of approved patients, prescribers, and pharmacists. The most restrictive REMS requires that a courier deliver the prescription to the approved pharmacy and also deliver the medication to the patient (Biodelivery Sciences International, 2009) (See U.S. FDA, 2010 for approved REMS).

Manufacturers of methadone and all modified-release opioids were informed in early 2009 that they would be required to develop a REMS for each of their products. A "Draft Guidance" document for opioid REMS has been published (U.S. FDA, 2009d) but a final rule is unlikely before 2011. In the meantime, individual product REMS will be required for any newly approved opioid analgesic.

The REMS approach for opioid analgesics is controversial. Patient advocacy groups and professional societies have endorsed the goals of safe use and avoidance of abuse and diversion. However, they have expressed concerns about the potential unintended consequence of decreased access to appropriately prescribed opioids (American Pain Foundation, 2009; American Pharmacists Association, 2009; Inturrisi, 2009; Shane, 2010). There is broad consensus that patient and public safety must be considered at all levels of opioid development, approval, and clinical use. It will be some time before either positive or negative outcomes of opioid REMS are known.

Withholding Opioids from Patients with Addictive Disease

Opioids, if they are appropriate, should not be withheld from patients with pain who also have addictive disease. Unfortunately, when persons with addictive disease come to health care providers for help with their painful conditions, they may encounter disrespect and poor pain management. Abundant evidence suggests that pain in persons with addictive disease is undertreated (Iocolano, 2000; Nichols, 2003).

Clinicians often fear that by providing opioids for pain they are "feeding the addiction." No research shows that providing opioid analgesics to this person will worsen the disease. Conversely, there is no research to show that withholding opioid analgesics when needed will increase the likelihood of recovery (Compton, 1999; McCaffery, Vourakis, 1992). In fact, withholding opioids in this situation may cause significant pain, which can increase the patient's level of stress and lead to increased craving for drugs of abuse. The patient may make efforts to obtain the drug that has been abused, or a patient in recovery may relapse. In the inpatient setting, the patient may make efforts to bring in illicit drugs. Clearly, on many levels, providing pain relief to the patient with addictive disease, even when it includes opioids, is preferable to withholding opioids.

Nevertheless, persons with addictive disease and pain often encounter many biases in the health care system. In addition to the problem of inappropriately withholding opioids because of misguided information, the disease of addiction is often misdiagnosed. Section II on assessment discusses the definition of addictive disease, misconceptions that result in a "label" (not a diagnosis)

of addiction, and a warning about the use of the term *drug seeking,* which often erroneously implies addictive disease (see Chapter 2). The reader is asked to review this information. Many behaviors suggestive of addiction may be "pseudoaddiction," a situation of undertreated pain. When pain is adequately treated, the behaviors that suggested addiction subside.

Care of patients with addictive disease and pain is complex and ideally would be undertaken in a multidisciplinary manner, but this is not always possible. Since these patients may present in almost any clinical setting, all clinicians are encouraged to learn how to treat pain in actively using and recovering patients. Before attempting to manage pain in these patients, clinicians need to acknowledge their own biases about addictive disease and attempt to prevent them from interfering with their care of the patient. Rather than understanding that addiction is a chronic, neurobiologic disease, some clinicians may believe that addiction reflects a moral weakness, blaming the patient for not just stopping their drug use. In their eyes, the patient does not deserve care, or worse, is someone who should be punished. This often poses an ongoing challenge for clinicians. Openly discussing these attitudes with staff may assist all of those caring for the patient with addictive disease to more comfortably provide appropriate pain management.

An excellent guide to pain management in the patient with pain and addictive disease was developed by the American Society for Pain Management Nursing (ASPMN) in 2002. It is titled, "ASPMN Position Statement: Pain Management in Patients with Addictive Disease," available at http://www.aspmn.org/Organization/documents/addictions_9pt.pdf. It covers patients actively using alcohol or other drugs, patients in recovery, and those receiving methadone maintenance therapy (MMT) for opioid addictive disease. All of these conditions will be discussed briefly here.

The first sentence of the ASPMN paper states a belief that is crucial for clinicians to adopt, "...**patients with addictive disease and pain have the right to be treated with dignity, respect, and the same quality of pain assessment and management as all other patients**" (p. 1). It is a quote worth posting for all to see, including clinicians, patients, and families.

Patients with Pain and Active Addictive Disease

Patients who are actively using alcohol and other drugs may come to the inpatient or outpatient health care setting under the influence of these drugs. Treatment of pain may be difficult if the patient is unable to give consistent answers to questions about the pain or the drugs he or she has taken, sometimes causing a delay in treating pain. However, pain treatment should begin as soon as possible. If the patient is too sedated to safely receive opioids, the use of NSAIDs, regional anesthetic techniques,

Box 20-1 | Management of Pain in the Patient with Active Addictive Disease*

GENERAL GUIDELINES THAT APPLY TO ALL CLINICAL SETTINGS

1. If the patient acknowledges addiction or use of substances for nonmedical reasons, openly discuss this and encourage the patient to express any fears of how this may affect pain management and treatment by staff. Assure the patient that this will not have an adverse effect on his pain management; but if you suspect that it will, tell the patient to let you know if he or she experiences undertreated pain or any disrespectful treatment.
2. If it is true, reassure the patient that staff is committed to providing aggressive and effective pain relief.
3. Record and discuss with the patient any behavior that suggests inappropriate medication use. Do not simply be suspicious and talk only to co-workers, since this creates harmful rumors. Discuss it with the patient in a calm and respectful manner.
4. Accept and act on the patient's report of pain with appropriate assessment and treatment.
5. Request consultation from an addiction specialist and a pain specialist, if available, so that both patient and staff know that support and guidance are available if needed. A multidisciplinary approach is ideal.
6. Aggressively manage pain. Addiction treatment is not a priority when the patient has unrelieved pain. Be prepared to titrate opioid analgesics and benzodiazepines to doses higher than the usual patient requires.

7. Develop with the patient a treatment plan for pain management. If feasible, provide the patient with a written copy. Emphasize to the staff that consistency in the implementation of the plan is essential.
8. Remind staff that (a) prescription of opioids to a known addict for the management of pain is not illegal, (b) persons with addictive disease may be relatively pain intolerant, (c) detoxification alone is an ineffective treatment for addictive disease, (d) patients with addictive disease may require higher doses of opioid than most patients because of opioid tolerance and the possibility that drugs have caused an increased sensitivity of pain.
9. Begin with nonpharmacologic or nonopioid analgesia when pain is mild. However, if pain relief is inadequate, add opioids. Begin with opioids when pain is moderate to severe.
10. If the patient is physically dependent on opioids, *do not* administer mixed opioid agonist/antagonists for analgesia (e.g., nalbuphine) because withdrawal will be precipitated and pain will increase.
11. Avoid benzodiazepines, phenothiazines, and other sedating medications that do not relieve pain unless they are required for other medical conditions.
12. Use the oral route and modified-release opioids when possible.
13. If pain is present most of the time, provide modified-release analgesics for ATC pain control.
14. Assess the patient's motivation for drug treatment, and have treatment referral references on hand. If the patient is not interested, do not pursue the issue since this could result in an adversarial relationship.

Continued

adjuvant analgesics, or nonpharmacologic methods of pain control is recommended.

If the patient has been using opioids, naloxone or other opioid antagonists should not be administered for the purpose of decreasing the opioid's effect unless the patient's life is in danger. Opioid antagonists could increase the patient's pain and throw the patient into withdrawal.

As soon as possible, obtain information from the patient and family about which drugs the patient has been abusing and all medications that have been prescribed. Become familiar with signs of withdrawal from each of the drugs and how to minimize withdrawal symptoms, such as by an appropriate tapering of the drug or an appropriate substitute. Obtain protocols for assessing and treating withdrawal from opioids, other drugs, and alcohol (e.g., to assess symptoms of alcohol withdrawal, obtain a protocol from http://www.ncbi.nlm.nih.gov/books/bv.fcgi?rid=hstat5.table.4060; for clinical detoxification protocols, also see

http://www.ncbi.nlm.nih.gov/books/bv.fcgi?rid=hstat5.table.4060. Withdrawal from alcohol can be life-threatening if not assessed and treated properly.

Box 20-1 presents general guidelines for treating patients with addictive disease and pain in all clinical settings, and more specific guidelines for treating patients in the inpatient setting and in the outpatient setting.

Patients in Recovery from Addictive Disease

Most clinicians, persons with addictive disease, and their families expect complete abstinence from the drug of abuse and other drugs with abuse potential. However, it is not realistic to expect all patients recovering from addictive disease to be totally abstinent (Passik, Kirsh, 2004). Harm reduction may be a more realistic goal and should not be considered a failure. Some patients may find it possible to cut down on their drugs of abuse or find a less

INPATIENT SETTING

1. Consider IV PCA or PCEA as a method of administering opioid analgesics. PCA gives the patient more control and may reduce potentially confrontational interactions with staff. Monitor and adjust pump parameters because active addicts may require and safely receive larger doses than other patients.

2. Obtain protocols for assessing and treating withdrawal symptoms from all drugs potentially abused by the patient, including alcohol, and treat aggressively and symptomatically. Monitor at least q4h for emergence of withdrawal symptoms.

3. For persons physically dependent on alcohol, sedative-hypnotics, or opioids, provide long-acting formulations of substitution medications to prevent emergence of withdrawal symptoms.

4. When opioids are no longer needed for analgesia, taper them very slowly to minimize emergence of withdrawal symptoms; assess for presence of withdrawal symptoms at least q4h during analgesic taper; and treat the patient symptomatically. Initial symptoms of withdrawal are often described as "flu like," such as tearing, rhinorrhea, gooseflesh, tremor, vomiting, and diarrhea. The patient is also irritable and anxious.

OUTPATIENT SETTING

1. When opioid analgesics are required, select long-acting formulations such as transdermal fentanyl or modified-release morphine. Less frequent dosing may increase the patient's adherence to the treatment plan. Also, drugs with a slow onset tend to have a low street value.

2. Administer analgesics ATC; provide the specific times the patient should take the medications, e.g., "at 8 AM and 8 PM" rather than saying "two times a day."

3. Carefully document the treatment plan, and provide the patient with a copy.

4. Provide the patient with whatever written information is available such as hours of operation, policies, method of obtaining refills, and telephone number, especially when the facility is not open.

5. At each visit, assess the patient's analgesic use, pain severity and quality, level of function, and side effects. Record and discuss with the patient any behavior suggestive of inappropriate opioid use.

ATC, Around the clock; *h*, hour; *PCA*, patient-controlled analgesia; *PCEA*, patient-controlled epidural analgesia; *q*, every

*These guidelines are not comprehensive but are intended to help the clinician begin to focus on a plan of care for the patient with pain and addictive disease.

From Pasero, C., & McCaffery, M. *Pain assessment and pharmacologic management*, pp. 528-529, St. Louis, Mosby. Data from American Society or Pain Management Nurses (ASPMN). (2002). *ASPMN position statement: Pain management in patients with addictive disease*. Lenexa, KS, ASPMN; Compton, P. (1999). Substance abuse. In M. McCaffery, & C. Pasero. *Pain: Clinical manual*, ed 2, St. Louis, Mosby; May, J., White, H. C., Leonard-White, A., et al. (2001). The patient recovering from alcohol or drug addiction: Special issues for the anesthesiologist. *Anesth Analg, 92*(6), 1601-1608. © 2011, McCaffery M, Pasero C. May be duplicated for use in clinical practice.

harmful way to consume the drug, such as smoking heroin instead of sharing needles to give it IV. Others may need medically prescribed medications, such as opioids or benzodiazepines.

Alcoholics Anonymous (AA) published a pamphlet in 1984 to address the use of medications and other drugs while in recovery from alcoholism. They point out that while some members of AA believe that no one in AA should take any medication, this can be disastrous for some people. Those with depression, schizophrenia, manic depression, epilepsy, and others requiring medication may meet with serious consequences, such as suicide or seizures, if they do not take their prescribed medications, some of which admittedly carry the potential for abuse. This pamphlet may be ordered by writing AA World Services, Inc., Box 459, New York, NY 10163 or by contacting AA at 212-870-3400. Having this available is often reassuring and informative for staff as well as patients with addictive disease and their families. Nonetheless, whether or not to take opioids for pain relief is the patient's decision, not the clinician's.

Patients who are in recovery and are totally abstinent are often fearful of relapse, and clinicians should discuss any intent or recommendation to use opioids or other psychoactive medications in their treatment. Establish from the beginning that the patient can make the final decision about the use of opioids or other drugs. In the past, clinicians used to make this decision for the patient and simply withhold opioids. Assure the patient that this will not happen. Discuss alternative options, such as nonopioids (NSAIDs and acetaminophen), regional anesthetic techniques, adjuvant analgesics, and nonpharmacologic methods, with those who do not want to take an opioid for pain relief.

Address fear of relapse by encouraging patients to continue and increase their activities with their recovery program. Remember to include the patient's family in these discussions because they may be equally or even more fearful of relapse.

Some patients recovering from addiction to opioids may be receiving opioid agonist therapy with either methadone or buprenorphine. These patients are likely to be undertreated for acute pain due to several misconceptions (Alford, Compton, Samet, 2006). Some clinicians erroneously believe that the maintenance opioid dose will suffice to relieve pain, and, therefore, fail to take additional action to provide pain relief. Other misconceptions are that adding another opioid analgesic may result in addiction relapse or cause respiratory depression. If these misconceptions are not corrected, the patient with acute pain will likely suffer, and the patient's reports of pain may be seen as manipulation to obtain more opioids.

If the patient is receiving methadone maintenance therapy (MMT) a common approach is to continue the methadone maintenance dose and add short-acting opioids, titrating the dose upward until pain relief is achieved (Alford, Compton, Samet, 2006). MMT has been used for decades, but buprenorphine maintenance therapy was only approved in the United States in 2004. Research and clinical experience have not yet identified the most effective approach for relieving pain in buprenorphine-maintained patients. Four options were suggested by Alford, Compton, and Samet (2006). The simplest one consisted of continuing the buprenorphine maintenance therapy and titrating a short-acting opioid analgesic to a dose that relieves the pain. A similar approach was suggested by other researchers in which the maintenance dose is given in divided doses and an additional opioid agonist such as morphine is added and titrated to effect (Vadivelu, Hines, 2007). In a study of managing acute postpartum pain in one group of patients on MMT (N = 10) and the other maintained on buprenorphine (N = 8), ibuprofen was used along with adding an opioid agonist for both groups and appeared to be beneficial in relieving pain (Jones, O'Grady, Johnson, et al., 2009). Patients on either form of maintenance therapy are likely to require higher doses of opioid for pain relief than the usual opioid-naïve patient. Box 20-2 presents guidelines for the management of pain in the patient recovering from addictive disease.

Comments on the Treatment of Pain in Patients with Addictive Disease

This aspect of patient care, relieving pain when the patient has addictive disease, especially the active addict, is one of the most challenging situations clinicians encounter. Knowledge of pain, addictive disease, and regulations governing the prescribing of controlled substances are required. It takes courage—the clinician's fear of endangering his or her license is not unfounded. Extensive experience and considerable self-awareness are always helpful. And the clinician needs to be willing to spend the extra time these patients usually require. Too often patients recovering from addictive disease are dismissed from practice when any suggestion of relapse or abuse occurs, and this is understandable in view of the above demands on the

clinician. Hopefully, such patients are referred to others who are more prepared or willing to care for these patients. Unfortunately, an appropriate referral cannot always be made. So, who is going to be responsible for the care of these patients? This question has yet to be answered. Following is one response.

A pain specialist speaking about addictive disease to an audience of other pain specialists received this comment from a member of the audience, "These patients are too difficult, take up too much time, and put me in legal jeopardy. I simply have to discharge them from my practice." To this the speaker replied, "If we, the pain specialists, don't treat them, who will?"

Opioid Use During Pregnancy

Opioids have a long history of safely relieving pain during pregnancy, such as following surgery, traumatic injury, or painful conditions associated with the pregnancy itself. For example, pelvic girdle pain is common during pregnancy; 10% of women with this condition experience severe pain, and a large number of these have persistent pain and disability (Hess, Aleshi, 2008). Some pregnant women have chronic conditions, such as sickle cell disease or rheumatoid arthritis, for which they take regular doses of opioid analgesics. The mu opioid agonists, such as morphine, hydromorphone, fentanyl, oxycodone, hydrocodone, and methadone, are recommended when an opioid is needed during pregnancy. Meperidine is often prescribed for pregnant women, but this is discouraged. Meperidine is not recommended for any type of pain because of its toxic metabolite, normeperidine (see Chapter 13).

Research conducted over the years has looked at the incidence of teratogenic effects in babies born to mothers who took opioids during pregnancy. One large collaborative study found no congenital anomalies in infants whose mothers took hydrocodone, meperidine, methadone, morphine, or oxycodone during pregnancy (Heinomen, Slone, Shapiro, 1977). Anomalies were observed in the offspring of those who took codeine or propoxyphene, but with the exception of respiratory malformation associated with codeine use, the incidence was not statistically greater than in the general population (Viscomi, Rathmell, 1998). A more recent retrospective review of the data of 15 parturients with persistent pain who received regular doses of opioid analgesics during pregnancy revealed that opioids were safe in both the mothers and infants (Hadi, da Silva, Natale, et al., 2006).

There is surprisingly little research on the use of opioids during pregnancy. A Cochrane Collaboration Review searched for randomized controlled trials that enrolled "opiate-dependent pregnant women" and revealed just three studies. These were in women who took long-acting opioids for treatment of addictive disease: two studies compared methadone with buprenorphine, and

Box 20-2 | Management of Pain in the Patient Recovering from Addictive Disease*

1. Openly acknowledge the patient's history of addiction, and allow the patient to discuss fears of re-addiction.

2. Encourage the patient to contact or strengthen contact with his or her recovery program and/or sponsor for advice, information, and support. The patient's support system can be a powerful defense against relapse. Reassure the patient that even in programs with a "drug-free" philosophy, it is acceptable to take medications for medical reasons.

3. Convey respect and admiration for the patient's attempts to recover from addictive disease.

4. Explain any intent to use opioids or other psychoactive medications. Involve the patient in deciding whether or not to take these medications.

5. Respect the patient's right to decide whether or not to take opioid analgesics.

6. Explain health risks associated with unrelieved pain, including increased risk for relapse due to the stress of illness or unrelieved pain.

7. Offer nonpharmacologic and nonopioid analgesic and local anesthetic alternatives, for example, NSAIDs, acetaminophen, or topical lidocaine patch 5% or local anesthetic creams for localized pain; discuss the appropriateness of epidural analgesia or continuous peripheral nerve block for major surgery.

8. Explain to the patient that the known risk for addiction to opioids in the context of pain appears to be minimal.

9. Ensure that the patient understands differences between addiction and physical dependence.

10. Request consultation from an in-house addiction medicine specialist, so that the patient knows that professional support is available if needed.

11. Taper opioid analgesics *very* slowly to minimize emergence of withdrawal symptoms.

12. Assess for presence of withdrawal symptoms at least q4h during analgesic taper; treat symptomatically. Initial symptoms of withdrawal are often described as "flu like," such a tearing, rhinorrhea, gooseflesh, tremor, vomiting, and diarrhea. The patient is also irritable and anxious.

13. *If patient is on methadone maintenance treatment:*
    a. Initiate regular discussion with the methadone treatment providers about the pain management plan.
    b. Verify the methadone maintenance dose the patient is receiving, and continue that dose. Remember that the methadone maintenance dose does not relieve pain.
    c. Either add another opioid on an ATC basis for analgesia or give additional methadone doses for

pain relief. When methadone is used for pain relief, it must be given more often than once a day, e.g., q8h.
    d. Consult a clinician who has experience in managing pain in methadone-maintained patients.

14. *If patient is on buprenorphine maintenance:*
    a. Initiate a regular discussion with buprenorphine treatment providers about the pain management plan.
    b. Verify the buprenorphine maintenance dose the patient is receiving. Remember that this dose is not enough to provide pain relief.
    c. Consult a clinician who has experience in managing pain in buprenorphine maintained patients.
    d. Several approaches to relief of acute pain in buprenorphine-maintained patients have been suggested, but research and clinical experience have not yet established a preferred method. A simple suggestion is to continue the buprenorphine maintenance dose, perhaps in divided doses, and add a short-acting opioid agonist, titrating the dose until pain relief is achieved.

15. Include family in these discussions; family members are typically as concerned as patients about relapse.

16. If the patient is being treated with opioids on an outpatient basis or is being discharged from an inpatient setting with an opioid prescription, encourage the patient to establish a plan that will help prevent relapse. Such plans are extremely varied, but an example is for the patient's family member or sponsor to have possession of the full prescription and give the patient enough for one day at a time.

17. If relapse occurs, *do not* terminate pain care. Recovery efforts should be intensified or reevaluated.

ATC, Around the clock; *h,* hour; *q,* every.

*These guidelines are not comprehensive but are intended to help the clinician begin to focus on a plan of care for the patient with pain who is also recovering from addictive disease.

From Pasero, C., & McCaffery, M. *Pain assessment and pharmacologic management,* p. 531, St. Louis, Mosby. Data from Alford, D. P., Compton, P., & Samet, J. H. (2006). Acute pain management for patients receiving maintenance methadone or buprenorphine therapy. *Ann Int Med,* 144(2), 127-134; American Society or Pain Management Nurses (ASPMN). (2002). *ASPMN position statement: Pain management in patients with addictive disease.* Lenexa, KS, ASPMN; Compton, P. (1999). Substance abuse. In M. McCaffery, & C. Pasero. *Pain: Clinical manual,* ed 2, St. Louis, Mosby; May, J., White, H. C., Leonard-White, A., et al. (2001). The patient recovering from alcohol or drug addiction: Special issues for the anesthesiologist. *Anesth Analg,* 92(6), 1601-1608; Vadivelu, N., & Hines, R. L. (2007). Buprenorphine: A unique opioid with broad clinical applications. *J Opioid Manage,* 3(1), 49-58. © 2011, McCaffery M, Pasero C. May be duplicated for use in clinical practice.

one compared methadone with modified-release morphine (Minozzi, Amato, Vecchi, et al., 2008). The researchers could find no significant difference between the opioids in terms of abstinence from the use of heroin but underscored the urgent need for more randomized controlled trials with large numbers of patients to draw sound conclusions. They cited a number of benefits of treatment of addiction with the long-acting opioids, including prevention of repeated episodes of opioid withdrawal in the fetus, reduction in maternal illicit drug use, improved compliance with obstetric care, and improved infant birth weight. Other studies have demonstrated less prematurity, higher birth weights, and a lower rate of stillbirth in infants born of women with addictive disease who were maintained in addiction treatment programs compared with women who were not (Fajemirokun-Odudeyi, Sinha, Tutty, et al., 2006; Little, Snell, Van Beveren, et al., 2003). One study found no difference in the Apgar scores of infants of mothers in addiction treatment programs who took methadone, buprenorphine, or modified-release morphine during pregnancy and those who were not addicted and did not take any opioids (Ebner, Rohrmeister, Winklbauer, et al., 2007). The researchers observed that this finding is consistent with other research.

An interesting case report described a woman who had been taking transdermal fentanyl (25 mcg/h) for 2 years for systemic lupus erythematosus and fibromyalgia prior to becoming pregnant and who delivered a healthy baby with an Apgar score of 9 and who nursed readily after birth (Einarson, Bozzo, Taguchi, 2009). The infant required no special observation or treatment and was roomed in with his mother who monitored the baby for withdrawal symptoms (see the following paragraphs), which were not observed. Follow-up visits with the pediatrician revealed the baby to be healthy and achieving all developmental milestones.

Neonatal Abstinence Syndrome

Physical dependence can occur in an infant whose mother took opioids during pregnancy, and abrupt discontinuation of the opioid can result in withdrawal symptoms after birth. These symptoms are collectively called *neonatal abstinence syndrome* and are characterized by neuralgic excitability (e.g., tremor, irritability, hypertonicity, abnormal crying, insomnia, and rarely seizures); GI dysfunction (e.g., nausea, vomiting, diarrhea); and autonomic dysfunction (e.g., fever, chills, nasal congestion). It is important to understand that physical dependence is not addiction. Addiction implies the psychological dependence on a particular drug and a cause-and-effect mode of thinking. Infants are incapable of this higher-level cognitive recognition and therefore cannot become addicted (Stevens, 1999). (See Chapter 11 for the difference between addiction and physical dependence.)

Not all infants born of mothers who take opioids during pregnancy will exhibit neonatal abstinence syndrome, as noted in the case study described earlier (Einarson, Bozzo, Taguchi, 2009). Studies have consistently shown that approximately 40% of infants will not develop symptoms (Berghella, Lim, Hill, et al., 2003; Ebner, Rohrmeister, Winklbaur, et al., 2007). Research is conflicting regarding whether or not the dose of opioid the mother takes influences the severity of symptoms. Whereas one retrospective review showed that the higher the methadone dose the more likely it was that the infant would have withdrawal symptoms and the longer the duration of treatment (Lim, Prasad, Samuels, et al., 2009), another retrospective review showed no correlation between methadone dose and severity or duration of neonatal abstinence syndrome (Berghella, Lim, Hill, et al., 2003).

Expecting a newborn to endure neonatal abstinence syndrome without appropriate treatment is unethical, dangerous, and not recommended. Rather, symptoms are prevented with the administration and gradual tapering of a mu opioid over several days; oral morphine or tincture of opium is usually used for this purpose (Stevens, 1999). A Cochrane Collaboration Review found that opioids and supportive care compared with supportive care only for the treatment of neonatal abstinence syndrome reduced the time to regain birth weight and the duration of supportive care (Osborn, Jeffery, Cole, 2005a). Length of hospitalization was longer in those who were treated with morphine, but it was not clear if this was related to infant status. The review also revealed that oral morphine was associated with better outcomes than diazepam and prevented seizures better than phenobarbital. Another Cochrane Collaboration Review found that phenobarbital was more effective than diazepam for neonatal abstinence syndrome (Osborn, Jeffery, Cole, 2005b). Phenobarbital was associated with shorter hospital stays than oral morphine, but the researchers observed that this may have been related to the willingness of health care providers to discharge an infant with a prescription for phenobarbital but not with one for morphine (Osborn, Jeffery, Cole, 2005b). A study of the babies of women who attended an addiction treatment clinic found that oral morphine (0.05 to 0.1 mg/kg/dose PRN) was more effective than phenobarbital (5 to 10 mg/kg/day) for the treatment of neonatal abstinence syndrome, and unlike the previously mentioned study, found that morphine was associated with a significantly shorter treatment time (Ebner, Rohrmeister, Winklbaur, et al., 2007).

In summary, the current research suggests that oral morphine is the preferred drug for the prevention and treatment of neonatal abstinence syndrome. During administration, infants should be monitored closely, and other comfort measures, such as swaddling, massage, relaxation bathing, waterbeds, and pacifiers, should be provided (Osborn, Jeffery, Cole, 2005a).

Opioid Use During Breast-Feeding

Opioids taken by breast-feeding women are secreted in the breast milk, ingested by the nursing baby, and undergo hepatic metabolism. It is quite common for women to require an opioid during lactation, and guidelines and other publications have listed opioids as compatible with breast-feeding for several years (American Academy of Pediatrics, 2001; Dillon, Wagner, Wiest, et al., 1997). A case report described safe and successful breast-feeding of an infant born to a mother who took transdermal fentanyl (100 mcg/h) throughout pregnancy and lactation (Cohen, 2009). The baby's blood fentanyl levels were undetectable.

An exception to this is meperidine, which is associated with sedation, poor suckling, and neurobehavioral delay in the nursing baby (Bar-Oz, Bulkowstein, Benyamini, et al., 2003; Wilbeck, Schorn, Daley, 2008; Wittels, Glosten, Faure, et al., 1997). The U.S. FDA issued a warning that nursing mothers who are ultra-rapid metabolizers of codeine can transfer sufficient morphine to their breast-feeding infants to cause life-threatening or fatal adverse effects, so this drug should be avoided during breast-feeding as well, especially since few women know whether or not they are an ultra-rapid metabolizer of codeine (U.S. FDA, 2007a) (see Chapter 13 for more on codeine metabolism). A better choice would be oxycodone.

To minimize sedation during exposure to opioids in breast-feeding infants, mothers who are receiving IV PCA can be encouraged to self-administer a dose just after nursing. Intraspinal analgesia typically administers very low doses of opioid, and drug exposure is minimal (Rathmell, Viscomi, Ashburn, 1997).

The impact of labor epidural analgesia on breast-feeding has been studied and shown to have an opioid dose-dependent effect. Laboring women (N = 177) who had previous experience with breast-feeding a child and were recruited in the prenatal period were randomized to receive epidural analgesia with no fentanyl, intermediate-dose fentanyl (1 to 150 mcg), or high-dose fentanyl (more than 150 mcg) (plus 0.0625% to 0.125% bupivacaine in all groups) (Beilin, Bodian, Weiser, et al., 2005). On postpartum day 1, twice as many women who received high-dose fentanyl (N = 12) reported difficulty breast-feeding than those who received intermediate-dose fentanyl (N = 6) or no fentanyl (N = 6), although this number did not reach statistical significance. There were no significant differences among the groups based on the lactation consultant's evaluation. Neurobehavior scores were lowest in infants whose mothers received more than 150 mcg of fentanyl. An interesting finding was that at 6 weeks, significantly more women in the high-dose group (N = 10) had stopped breast-feeding than in the intermediate-dose fentanyl (N = 3) and no fentanyl (N = 1) groups. A randomized controlled trial evaluated women who received epidural fentanyl analgesia or no epidural analgesia during labor

and found a similar rate of initiation and duration of breast-feeding among the groups (Wilson, MacArthur, Cooper, et al., 2010). It is important to note that numerous factors influence a woman's decision and ability to breast-feed.

Opioid Use in the Critically Ill

Patient surveys indicate that the critically ill experience a high level of pain and other discomforts associated with underlying pathology and care activities while in the ICU (Nelson, Meier, Oei, et al., 2001; Puntillo, Pasero, Li, et al., 2009). This population is at particularly high risk for undertreated pain because many are unable to report their pain and discomforts using customary methods, such as the 0-to-10 numerical pain rating scale (Puntillo, Pasero, Li, et al., 2009) (see Section II).

Opioids have a long history as first-line analgesics for the management of pain in the critically ill and should be started before or concomitantly with sedatives (Erstad, Puntillo, Gilbert, et al., 2009). The recommended treatment approach in critically ill patients who cannot report their pain is to administer opioid analgesics based on the assumption that their underlying condition or disease process is associated with significant pain (see Section II).

Opioids are warranted also because tracheal intubation, mechanical ventilation, and the aftermath of care, such as chest physiotherapy and suctioning, are known to be extremely painful (Pasero, McCaffery, 2002). A multicenter study supported by the American Society of Critical Care Nurses of over 6000 acutely or critically ill patients ranging from the age of 4 to 97 years old evaluated pain and distress associated with six common procedures these patients would experience: turning, wound drain removal, tracheal suctioning, femoral catheter removal, placement of central venous catheter, and changing of non-burn wound dressing (Puntillo, White, Morris, et al., 2001). Simple turning was identified as the most painful and distressing of the procedures in adults ages 18 and older. Other research confirmed a high incidence of pain in 30 traumatically injured patients in the ICU; 96% reported pain in injured areas of their bodies, and 36% reported pain related to devices and tubings, such as chest tubes, Foley catheters, wound drains, and orthopedic fixation devices (Stanik-Hutt, Soeken, Belcher, et al., 2001). Again, turning was found to be very painful; resting pain intensity scores (mean 26.5) nearly doubled after turning (mean, 48.1).

These studies underscore the high prevalence of pain in the critically ill and the need for an aggressive approach to managing it. Mu agonist opioids are first-line analgesics in a multimodal treatment plan. The risk of adverse effects of the nonopioid and adjuvant analgesics must be carefully considered in the critical care population (Erstad, Puntillo, Gilbert, et al., 2009), but unless contraindicated, nonopioids (e.g., acetaminophen and an NSAID) and appropriate adjuvant analgesics (e.g., anticonvulsants for neuropathic pain, if thought to be likely), are added. Local anesthetics applied topically or given by continuous peripheral nerve block (e.g., for some orthopedic surgeries) or added to opioids for epidural administration (e.g., thoracotomy) should be considered in some patients. The reader is referred to a series of articles focusing on various aspects of pain in the critically ill published in the Postgraduate Corner of the journal of *Chest* (see volume 135, issues 4 to 6, 2009).

Selection of Opioid Doses in Patients Unable to Report Pain

Nurses often ask how to select a starting opioid dose and how to know if that dose is effective in patients who cannot report their pain. Chapter 16 discusses in detail the method used to determine opioid doses, and this method is applicable to patients who cannot report pain. In most cases, pain is assumed to be severe in critically ill patients based on the presence of significant pathology (Puntillo, Pasero, Li, et al., 2009), and doses are selected accordingly (e.g., 2.5 mg/h IV morphine or equivalent starting dose in an opioid-naïve adult; higher doses will be required for opioid tolerant patients). As in patients who can report pain, pain is also prevented prior to painful procedures with IV opioid bolus doses (e.g., 1 to 2 mg). If present, changes in behaviors after an opioid dose is administered or an opioid infusion is initiated are used to evaluate analgesic effectiveness. In patients who are unresponsive, no change in behavior will be evident to guide assessment of analgesic effectiveness; therefore, the optimized opioid dose is continued (Pasero, 2009a).

Weaning from the Mechanical Ventilator

When critically ill patients show improvement, they are weaned from mechanical ventilation. Often opioids are discontinued before beginning the weaning process out of a fear that opioids will produce adverse respiratory effects and impede weaning. However, the fear of respiratory depression, cited as the main reason for stopping opioids before weaning, usually is unfounded in critically ill patients. Most critically ill patients will receive opioids long enough for some tolerance to develop, and tolerance to respiratory depression develops relatively rapidly within days of regular dosing. Therefore, fear of respiratory depression should not be a barrier to continuing opioids for patients who have been receiving them for several days or longer (APS, 2003).

In addition, loss of pain control can cause ventilator weaning to fail. Unrelieved pain can contribute to pulmonary dysfunction (Ghori, Zhang, Sinatra, 2009; Jacobi,

Fraser, Coursin, et al., 2002). Even when the source of pain is remote from the thoracic and abdominal region, respiratory dysfunction can occur. Involuntary responses to pain cause reflex muscle spasm at the site of tissue damage and in muscle groups above and below the site. Patients with pain also voluntarily limit their thoracic and abdominal muscle movement in an effort to reduce the pain they are experiencing.

The measurable respiratory effects of severe pain are small tidal volumes and high inspiratory and expiratory pressures, as well as decreases in vital capacity, functional residual capacity, and alveolar ventilation (Ghori, Zhang, Sinatra, 2009). If adequate pain relief is not provided, these effects can progress to significant pulmonary complications, such as atelectasis and pneumonia.

Abrupt discontinuation of opioids can have other undesirable consequences besides loss of pain control. At the time of weaning, many critically ill patients have been receiving opioids long enough to have developed physical dependence. If the opioid is stopped abruptly for weaning, physically dependent patients will experience withdrawal syndrome. Signs of withdrawal include restlessness and agitation and may be confused with failed weaning or "ICU psychosis." The practice of abrupt discontinuation of opioids can result in inaccurate assessment of the patient's response and inappropriate treatment (e.g., benzodiazepines to sedate the patient).

If a reduced opioid dose is required for successful weaning, using a multimodal analgesic approach may make it easier to do so without compromising good pain control. If an NSAID is not contraindicated and is not being administered around the clock (ATC) already, one can be added before weaning to allow a reduced opioid dose. Acetaminophen can be given rectally for additional analgesia. Anticonvulsants, such as gabapentin, can be added to treat neuropathic pain and prevent the development of persistent pain. Other appropriate nonsedating adjuvants, such as local anesthetics via continuous peripheral nerve block or added to epidural opioids, should be considered.

The lack of a respiratory depressant effect with dexmedetomidine (Precedex) has implications for its use during weaning from mechanical ventilation and extubation. A study of patients who had failed previous attempts at ventilator weaning secondary to agitation unresponsive to traditional sedatives described successful extubation of 14 of the 20 patients who were given dexmedetomidine (Arpino, Klafatas, Thompson, 2008). Other positive results were a reduction in concomitant sedative and analgesic use and minimal adverse effects. Dexmedetomidine has also been reported to facilitate terminal weaning and withdrawal of ventilatory support at end of life in palliative care (Kent, Kaufman, Lowy, 2005) (see Section V for more on dexmedetomidine).

The intraspinal routes are frequently used to deliver opioids to the critically ill. One of the benefits of intraspinal analgesia in mechanically ventilated patients is excellent analgesia with lower opioid doses and less threat of respiratory depression during weaning. In addition, a number of studies have demonstrated improved pulmonary function with intraspinal analgesia (see Chapter 15 for research and detailed discussion of intraspinal analgesia). Continuous peripheral nerve blocks, which rely on local anesthetics for analgesia, may be ideal for some patients in the ICU (see Section V).

Managing Pain in the Terminally Ill

The American Nurses Association's 2003 position statement on Pain Management and Control of Distressing Symptoms in Dying Patients states:

> "In the context of the caring relationship, nurses perform a primary role in the assessment and management of pain and other distressing symptoms in dying patients. Therefore, nurses must use effective doses of medications prescribed for symptom control and nurses have a moral obligation to advocate on behalf of the patient when prescribed medication is insufficiently managing pain and other distressing symptoms. The increasing titration of medication to achieve adequate symptom control is ethically justified." (p. 1, American Nurses Association, 2003)

The American Medical Association (AMA) maintains its stand taken in a 1992 position paper stating that "the administration of a drug necessary to ease the pain of a patient who is terminally ill and suffering excruciating pain may be appropriate medical treatment even though the effect of the drug may shorten life" (AMA, 1992).

Despite these standards, pain in the terminally ill continues to be undertreated. The 1995 publication of a disturbing study of more than 9000 terminally ill hospitalized patients revealed that 50% of conscious seriously ill patients who died in the hospital experienced moderate to severe pain at least half of the time (SUPPORT, 1995). Four in 10 experienced severe pain; 59% preferred a treatment plan that focused on comfort, but 10% received care contrary to this (Lynn, Teno, Phillips, 1997). The SUPPORT publication spurred a number of initiatives, and one of the most notable was the Robert Wood Johnson Foundation Last Acts national campaign to promote improvements in care and caring near the end of life. In 2002, Last Acts conducted the first ever state-by-state evaluation of end-of-life care and found that, despite years of research, educational, and grass roots efforts, and millions of dollars of private philanthropy "... care for dying Americans is no better than mediocre." The entire Last Acts analysis can be found in the publication: *Means to a Better End. A Report on Dying in America Today* at http://www.rwjf.org/files/publications/other/meansbetterend.pdf. Last Acts completed its work in 2005. In response to its Report on Dying, many states initiated

comprehensive educational efforts to improve their performance (Virani, Malloy, Ferrell, et al., 2008) (also see ELNEC later in the chapter).

The underdosing of opioids in terminally ill patients is particularly tragic because it is usually based on the unfounded fear that the opioid will produce adverse respiratory effects and hasten death. However, most terminally ill patients have been receiving opioids long enough to have developed tolerance to the opioid's respiratory depressant effects. In fact, in an early study of patients from whom life support had been withdrawn or withheld, those who received analgesics and sedatives lived longer (2.2 hours) than those who did not receive analgesics and sedatives (Wilson, Smedira, Fink, et al., 1992). More recent research reports similar findings. A case note review of 238 consecutive patients who died in a palliative care unit observed that there were no significant differences in survival from admission or frequency of unexpected death between those who received a marked increase in opioids at end of life and those who needed no increase (Thorns, Sykes, 2000). A study of the use of sedatives at end of life also demonstrated that increased doses of sedatives in the last hours of life were not associated with shortened survival (Sykes, Thorns, 2003a). Another study found no evidence that opioids or benzodiazepines hastened death in critically ill patients after withdrawal of life support; in fact, for every 1 mg/h increase in benzodiazepine dose, time to death was increased by 13 minutes (Chan, Treece, Engelberg, et al., 2004). The same was found in terminally ill cancer patients (Morita, Tsunoda, Inoue, et al., 2001). A more recent multicenter, observational, prospective study evaluated overall survival in two cohorts of hospice patients, one submitted to palliative sedation (sedatives and analgesics) and the other managed by routine hospice practice (Maltoni, Pittureri, Scarpi et al., 2009). The median survival was 12 days and 9 days for those who received palliative sedation and those who received routine hospice care, respectively, which led the researchers to conclude that palliative sedation therapy does not shorten life when used to treat refractory symptoms. These studies suggest that the underlying disease, not the analgesics and sedatives, usually determines death (Brody, Campbell, Faber-Langendoen, et al., 1997).

An extensive analysis of data derived from the National Hospice Outcomes Project (Connor, Horn, Smout, et al., 2005) appropriately concluded that concern about hastening death does not justify withholding opioid therapy at end of life (Portenoy, Sibirceva, Smout, et al., 2006). Nevertheless, research shows that clinicians continue to be apprehensive about using high doses of analgesics and sedatives in the terminally ill even when deemed necessary and appropriate (Bendiane, Bouhnik, Favre, et al., 2007; Bilsen, Norup, Deliens, et al., 2006; Rocker, Heyland, Cook, et al., 2004; Sykes, Thorns, 2003a,b; Thorns, Sykes, 2000).

The enormous tolerance that patients develop to the respiratory depressant effects of opioids is illustrated by numerous accounts of opioid doses that have escalated over time. One of the earliest studies on pain and other symptoms in patients with advanced cancer reported that all 90 of the patients reviewed had pain, and almost 40% required increases in their opioid requirements by 25% during the last 4 weeks of life (Coyle, Adelhardt, Foley, et al., 1990). Total daily opioid doses in these patients ranged from 7 to 35,164 mg parenteral morphine equivalents. Five percent used an opioid dose of more than 900 mg parenteral morphine equivalents per day 4 weeks before death, and within 24 hours of death, this proportion increased to 9%. Even patients receiving the highest doses were titrated in the home setting. These findings reinforce that "high" doses of opioids are both appropriate and safe in terminally ill patients with pain.

Other recent research has shown similar findings. A retrospective medical record review of 661 home-care hospice patients noted that 66% received morphine for pain relief and that 91% of these received a dose of between 5 and 299 mg/day and 1.6% received doses of more than 600 mg/day (Bercovitch, Adunksy, 2004). A prospective Canadian study observed that morphine was the most commonly administered drug at end of life in critically ill patients, and the dose ranged from 2 to 450 mg; midazolam was the second most common with a range of 2 to 380 mg (Rocker, Heyland, Cook, et al., 2004). This study also surveyed the families of the patients and reported strong evidence of the staff's ability to convey a caring attitude; 92.3% of surveyed family members reported feeling "supported" or "very supported" by the health care team during their loved ones' dying process. This type of positive experience is not always the case (Teno, Clarridge, Casey, et al., 2004). The health care team often misses opportunities to facilitate family interactions and improve the family's involvement in decision making and understanding of the comprehensive treatment plan (Mularski, Puntillo, Varkey, et al., 2009).

Research shows that there is wide variation in the treatment of pain and other discomforts during withdrawal of life support in the ICU; the use of standardized protocols and guidelines are recommended as a way to improve the health care team's decision making and ultimately patient outcomes at end of life (Mularski, Puntillo, Varkey, et al., 2009). The implementation of a standardized order form for the withdrawal of life support in the ICU resulted in an increase in total doses of opioids and benzodiazepines, and there was no change in the median time from ventilator withdrawal pre- and post-implementation of the form (Treece, Engelberg, Crowley, et al., 2004).

Most patients with advanced illness lose the ability to communicate during the final days of life. This loss of communication should not be interpreted as loss of pain. As described above, higher doses at end of life suggest that pain often increases as death approaches. Patients who are confused, grimacing, moaning, agitated, or restless most likely are experiencing unrelieved pain and require an increase in the opioid dose (see Section II). Opioids should be continued at the optimized dose in patients who lose consciousness at the end of life.

Treatment of Dyspnea

Dyspnea is a very distressing symptom that can occur in both opioid-naïve and opioid-tolerant patients (Bruera, Currow, 2009). It is a common symptom in many cancer and noncancer-related chronic illnesses (Newton, Davidson, Macdonald, et al., 2008). It is often present at end of life and is an independent predictor for shorter survival among cancer patients (Bruera, Currow, 2009). An early prospective study of hospice patients in the last 6 weeks of life found that as many as 70% suffered from the condition (Reuben, Mor, 1986). There is no consensus on how to measure breathlessness (Bruera, Currow, 2009). Patients' subjective descriptions of dyspnea vary widely, for example, "difficult, labored, uncomfortable breathing" and "the sensation of breathlessness or air hunger" (American Thoracic Society, 1999). The condition is associated with significant patient distress and poor quality of life (Edmonds, Higginson, Altmann, et al., 2000). It often coexists with fatigue, depression, and anxiety (Bruera, Currow, 2009).

Clinical assessment of dyspnea is described as having four components: (1) obtaining a comprehensive history about onset and exacerbating and relieving factors; (2) performing a physical examination for causes; (3) assessing the intensity of unpleasantness of breathlessness with a scale (e.g., 0-to-10) to establish a baseline; and (4) tracking dyspnea along with other symptoms to evaluate its impact on quality of life (Bruera, Currow, 2009). A variety of medications and routes of administration have been used to treat dyspnea, although opioids have been the mainstay for treatment of dyspnea for many years (Pasero, Portenoy, McCaffery, 1999). A Cochrane Collaboration Review concluded that there was evidence to support the use of systemic (oral, parenteral) but not nebulized opioids to treat dyspnea (Jennings, Davies, Higgins, et al., 2001). The researchers encouraged more research with larger numbers of patients, the use of standardized protocols, and evaluation of quality of life measures. A later review of 20 articles with evaluable evidence reached similar conclusions (Joyce, McSweeney, Carrieri-Kohlman, et al., 2004). In their evidence-based guidelines on interventions to improve the palliative care of pain, dyspnea, and depression, the American College of Physicians recommended the use of opioids for both pain and dyspnea based on a history of proven effectiveness (Qaseem, Snow, Shekelle, et al., 2008).

Oxygen has been used for treatment of dyspnea, but a prospective study (N = 46) found no correlation between intensity of dyspnea and oxygen saturation in either hypoxic or nonhypoxic palliative care patients who received -oxygen (4 L/min) by nasal cannulation; opioids on the other hand, significantly reduced the intensity of the patients' dyspnea (Clemens, Quednau, Klaschik, 2009). A small randomized controlled, double-blind, crossover trial (N = 9) administered placebo or 5 mg of subcutaneous morphine to 7 opioid-naïve older adults and 3.5 mg of subcutaneous morphine in addition to their usual oral morphine doses to 2 older adults (all patients had cancer) and found that the subcutaneous morphine significantly improved the symptoms of dyspnea and did so without compromising respiratory effort or oxygen saturation (Mazzocato, Buclin, Rapin, 1999). Another small study (N = 6) found similar results in patients with terminal amyotrophic lateral sclerosis (Clemens, Klaschik, 2008a).

Clinicians are sometimes reluctant to use opioids to treat dyspnea, citing concern that adding another or more opioid to the opioid a patient is already receiving for analgesia, or starting an opioid in an opioid-naïve patient, increases the risk of opioid-induced sedation or respiratory depression. Studies have not confirmed this fear.

A randomized, double blind, placebo-controlled crossover trial found that oral modified-release morphine (20 mg) provided significant improvement in refractory dyspnea in 48 opioid-naïve patients (Abernethy, Currow, Frith, et al., 2003). Treatment was tolerated well with minimal adverse effects, and patients cited improved sleep as a major benefit of treatment. Hydromorphone has also been used for dyspnea. A small prospective study demonstrated that titrated doses of oral hydromorphone produced considerable and sustained improvement of moderate or severe dyspnea during both rest and mild activity in 14 palliative care patients (Clemens, Klaschik, 2008b). The mean single dose of hydromorphone was 2.5 mg (0.5 to 6.0 mg range). Half of the patients were opioid-naïve. An important finding was that there were no significant increases in carbon dioxide (CO_2) or decreases in oxygen (O_2) saturation. Treatment with hydromorphone was continued in all patients after the study was completed.

As mentioned earlier in the chapter, more well-controlled research is needed on the use of nebulized opioids (see Chapter 14). Nevertheless, morphine by this route has been used for many years to treat dyspnea. A prospective, nonrandomized study (N = 46) used transcutaneous CO_2 measurement and pulse oximetry (O_2 saturation) and found that there was no higher risk of respiratory depression in opioid-naïve compared with opioid-tolerant palliative patients treated with nebulized morphine (Clemens, Quednau, Klaschik, 2008). The patients experienced a significant decrease in the intensity of dyspnea and respiratory rate. These studies and clinical experience support the recommendation that carefully titrated doses of opioids for treatment of dyspnea should be administered to patients who are suffering from the distress of having to fight to breathe.

End-of-Life Nursing Education Consortium (ELNEC)

There have been numerous educational efforts directed toward improving the nurse's ability to manage pain and the other symptoms patients experience at the end of life. One of the most successful efforts is the End-of-Life Nursing Education Consortium (ELNEC), which began in 2000 and was funded initially by the Robert Wood Johnson Foundation and administered by the American Association of Colleges of Nursing (AACN) and the City of Hope in Duarte, California. Partnerships have developed with other organizations, such as the Oncology Nursing Society, Sigma Theta Tau International, and the National Cancer Institute, among many others, to fund and provide training (Malloy, Paice, Virani, et al., 2008). By the summer of 2009, almost 9000 nurses representing all 50 states in America had received ELNEC training through national courses and, as instructors, had extended that knowledge to countless other nurses and members of the health care team (AACN, 2009). There are international ELNEC courses as well. One oncology training program reported that participants had educated 26,000 nurses after attending the course (Coyne, Paice, Ferrell, et al., 2007). The ELNEC educational modules focus on palliative care in advanced practice nursing; pain and symptom management; communication; ethical issues; final hours of life; loss, grief, and bereavement; and achieving quality care at the end of life (Malloy, Paice, Virani, et al., 2008). Follow-up evaluation of ELNEC seminars reveal many successes as well as ongoing challenges, such as a lack of funds and minimal institutional support for educational efforts (Ferrell, Virani, Paice, et al., 2009). For information on ELNEC training, the reader is referred to the AACN website http://www.aacn.nche.edu/ELNEC/. For information on international ELNEC training, see http://www.aacn.nche.edu/elnec.

Conclusion

The undertreatment of pain as a result of the unwarranted withholding of opioids is particularly disturbing. Among the many patients at risk for this are those with persistent noncancer pain, individuals with addictive disease, women during pregnancy and breast-feeding, the critically ill, and individuals at the end of life.

Section IV | Conclusion

OPIOID analgesics remain first-line agents for the treatment of moderate-to-severe acute pain, persistent cancer pain, and some persistent noncancer pain states. For many patients with pain, particularly those in the palliative care settings, opioid drugs continue to be the mainstay of analgesia. Pain control is improved and adverse effects are reduced when they are given in combination with nonopioids and adjuvant analgesics as part of a multimodal pain treatment plan.

Documenting Pain Management

Documentation is a means for communicating pain assessments (e.g., pain ratings), interventions to manage the pain, and the patient's response (e.g., pain ratings and adverse effects). The more severe the pain, the more often it is assessed and documented. The use of opioid analgesics requires documentation, not only as an intervention but also for substance control purposes. When invasive therapies are used, such as epidural analgesia and PCA, special flow sheets are useful for ensuring that the patient's pain assessments, adverse effects, and use of opioids during therapy are documented. Use of a flow sheet helps to centralize and standardize documentation, avoid duplication of documentation, save time, meet substance control requirements, and provide an overall picture of the patient's pain experience during treatment. The reader is referred to Section II for a detailed discussion of documentation of pain and examples of a variety of flow sheets.

Patient Education

As discussed in Chapter 12, adherence to the pain treatment plan helps to ensure optimal pain control. A review of the literature revealed numerous reasons why patients do not adhere to a variety of medications prescribed for pain (Monsivais, McNeil, 2007). In addition to an introductory review of the literature, these authors examined 42 abstracts and 17 full-text articles. Some of the concerns revealed are pertinent to opioid analgesics and may be diminished by providing the patient with both verbal and written information about their medications. (See Patient Medication Education Forms for selected medications on pp. 547-579 at the end of this section.) A common reason for nonadherence was high levels of concern about the medication, such as adverse effects, "dependency," and questions about the real need for the medication. Patients also had misconceptions about how long it should take for the drug to be effective, and they would stop taking it if no benefits occurred by the expected time. Patients also feared tolerance, that is, that the medication might cease to work if taken on a regular basis.

An excellent synthesis of quantitative and qualitative research on the use of morphine for cancer pain treatment revealed key social, contextual, and physical concerns held by patients, caregivers, and health care professionals (Flemming, 2010). The synthesis showed that patients commonly perceive that the use of morphine is a balancing act and a trade-off between pain relief and adverse effects. For example, there is evidence that patients struggle with wanting pain relief but fearing that adverse effects would prevent them from maintaining functionality. Deep-seated concerns about the symbolism of morphine, addiction, and tolerance held by patients, caregivers, and health care professionals were shown to affect prescription, dispensation, and use of opioids. For many of the patients, the use of morphine was considered a "last resort" or "death sentence."

A superb qualitative study of the perspectives of patients receiving long-term opioid treatment for persistent noncancer pain revealed that desperation, humiliation, and thoughts of suicide were common before opioid treatment (Vallerand, Nowak, 2009). After treatment was initiated, patients described the challenge of maintaining a balance between pain, pain relief, and functionality as well as having to live a "secret life" (hiding medications) for fear that others would misunderstand the need for opioid treatment. An overriding theme of this research was the anticipation or dread of losing their treatment regimen and returning to a life of pain.

All of this research underscores the importance of initial and ongoing discussion about pain and opioid use with patients and their families and caregivers to ensure such fears and barriers are adequately addressed. It should be assumed that all patients share at least some of the feelings described in the research, so such discussion should be an integral part of care. Ensuring that patients obtain the maximum benefit from opioid analgesics requires education of the patient and family/caregiver. Teaching patients and families about addiction, tolerance, and physical dependence often fails to allay fears and change attitudes. Efforts to present the facts about such emotionally charged issues frequently are overshadowed by fiercely held beliefs. No proven method exists for breaking down such strong barriers to achieving effective pain control. Where one method may work with 1 patient, it may fail with another. Giving consistent and confident explanations about addiction and repeating information frequently provides reassurance for patients and their families. Table IV-1 provides considerations and

Table IV-1 | Talking with Patients and Families about Addiction

Issue	Approach
Concern about addiction. Patient is thinking, "I don't want to get hooked."	• Assume that all patients who take opioids and their families will have some concern about addiction. Don't wait for them to express concern. Initiate discussion with comments such as, "This pain medicine is sometimes called a narcotic, and lots of people wonder if taking a narcotic will cause addiction. This hardly ever happens. Do you have any concerns about this?" (Be sure to ask family caregivers this question.) • To encourage discussion, ask "What do you know about addiction? Have you known people with drug or alcohol problems?" • Assume that health care providers have expressed to patients and their families concerns about addiction. Ask, "What have other nurses and doctors said to you about addiction?" • If the patient has no questions, simply say, "There's no need to worry about addiction being caused by taking pain medication to be comfortable. Taking pain medication for pain relief is not the same thing as addiction. If you think of any questions, please let us know."
The word *narcotic* has a negative connotation. Patients may say, "Narcotics are what drug addicts take."	• Reinforce that pain medicines are "good" drugs by linking adequate pain control to achieving goals or improving quality of life. For example, equate an activity the patient values, such as walking the dog, with taking pain medicine to achieve a comfort goal of 3 on a 0 to 10 scale. • Avoid the words *narcotics* or *drugs*. • Use the words *pain medicine* or *pain medications*. • Refer to the analgesics by brand names, e.g., MS Contin rather than morphine. • "It's true that many addicts take narcotics, but that is a case of using medicine for the wrong reason. Taking a narcotic for pain relief is the right reason to use pain medicine. Any medicine can be used in the wrong way or the right way."
Confusion about addiction, tolerance, and physical dependence. Patients may say, "I don't want to be like those street addicts who get sick and crazy whenever they can't get a dose."	• "It's easy to confuse addiction with tolerance and physical dependence. Addiction to pain medicine would mean that your pain has gone away, but you still take medicine regularly when you don't need it, maybe just to 'escape from your problems.' I don't know any patients who do this. If the pain decreases, they take less pain medicine. If the pain stops, they stop taking pain medicine." • "Physical dependence means that you would go into withdrawal if you suddenly stopped taking the medicine. Physical dependence occurs with many medicines, such as cortisone, after they are taken regularly for weeks. Even caffeine can cause physical dependence. For example, if every day you consume several caffeine-containing beverages, such as coffee or soft drinks, and one day you don't drink any, you would probably experience withdrawal in the form of a headache. That's why we tell you not to suddenly stop taking your pain medication. If you take pain medicine regularly and you suddenly stop, you could develop withdrawal symptoms such as sweating, tearing, and diarrhea. To avoid withdrawal, the dose is decreased gradually over a few days so that your body can adjust to lower doses. Physical dependence is not the same thing as addiction, and does not cause addiction." • "Tolerance to pain medicine means that the dose no longer relieves as much pain. When this happens, it is easily handled by raising the dose. This is not the same thing as addiction and does not cause addiction." (See below.)

Continued

Table IV-1 | Talking with Patients and Families about Addiction—cont'd

Issue	Approach
Reluctance to begin opioid treatment for fear that the effectiveness of opioid analgesics will diminish over time. Patients may say, "If I take too much medicine, it will stop working." Or, "It won't work when I really need it later."	• "You don't need to save your pain medicine until your pain gets bad and you really need it. Pain medicine will not stop working. You can start taking pain medicine regularly every day when you hurt only a little. If you hurt more, the dose can be increased or other medicine can be added. Don't deny yourself pain relief now." • "Many people 'save' pain medicine for later, but you don't need to. There is no limit to the amount of pain medicine we can give you for pain relief." • "Although larger doses may be needed over time, the pain medicine does not stop working." • "It's not possible to 'use up' the pain-relieving effect of pain medicine." Use patient examples by drawing similarities when appropriate, e.g., "I am taking care of someone who, like you, wanted to hold off taking pain medicine. But he did start taking it after we assured him it would keep working. Last week his pain increased, and we were able to double his dose of pain medication and relieve his pain without any difficulty."
Misconception that the risk of addiction is high. Patients may say, "Look at all of the people on television who get addicted."	• Use descriptors (e.g., "Addiction **very rarely** happens in people who are taking pain medicine to relieve pain"). • Use graphics (e.g., pie charts, bar graphs) to show that addiction is rare. Simply draw a large circle and put a small dot in it to show those who become addicted. • Use patient examples, e.g., "I am caring for a woman right now who took the same pain medicine you are taking for several weeks. Because of successful surgery, her pain is gone. Now that she has no need for her pain medicine, she has found that she does not want it at all." Or, "I am taking care of several patients who are taking the same pain medicine you are, and not one is addicted to it." • "Headlines sometimes report that a movie star or rock star is addicted to pain relievers. This makes it sound like taking pain medicine causes addiction. Chances are that the star had problems with drugs in the past. Or, the person may have had a pain problem and was wrongly labeled an addict. Remember, thousands of people take pain medicine every day without becoming addicted."
Persistent fear that "if anybody gets addicted, it will probably be me."	• "Ask yourself, 'If I had no pain, would I still want to take this pain medicine? If I stopped hurting, would I lie to my doctor to get more pain medicine? Would I try to buy it in the streets?' If the answer is no, then you would be able to stop taking the medication if the pain stopped." • "I take care of many people who take pain medicine to stay comfortable, and none of them has become addicted." • Draw similarities to a specific patient similar to this patient. An example for a patient with chronic pain might be, "Not too long ago I cared for a man about your age. He had a tumor somewhat like yours, and his pain was right here over his chest, just like yours. We started him on the same medicine you're taking, and he did very well. It took us a week or so to hit exactly the right dose, but then he took it around the clock every day. He didn't get addicted. He started playing golf again and actually took a trip to visit his children." • For a patient with short-term pain, a patient example might be, "Last week I cared for a man who had his knee replaced. He was afraid of addiction and was reluctant to take his pain medicine after surgery. Because of this, he was in pain and not able to perform his exercises with the physical therapist. He ended up with a very stiff knee because he didn't control his pain effectively."

Continued

Table IV-1 | Talking with Patients and Families about Addiction—cont'd

Issue	Approach
Misconception that ATC dosing will lead to addiction; belief that pain medicine should be taken only when pain is present. Patients may say, "If I take it when I don't need it, it's like being addicted."	• "Certainly you need pain medicine when you feel pain, but you also need it to prevent pain." • "Pain needs to be kept under control just like we control diseases such as high blood pressure. We don't wait until a person with high blood pressure has a stroke before we give medicine to control his blood pressure. We ask the person to take blood pressure medicine at regular times every day to keep the blood pressure under control. The same logic applies to pain. We don't want to wait for the pain to return and become severe before giving pain medicine. We want you to take it regularly to keep the pain under control." • "Remember, we will be working with you and watching your doses carefully to be sure that you are taking what is safe and right for you." • "The purpose of pain medicine is to put you back in control of your life rather than let pain control your life. Right now, pain controls what you do. We want to put you back in charge. Taking pain medicine regularly in the right doses is how you get control again." • "People think that, like John Wayne, they should bite the bullet with pain. This makes a good movie, but it doesn't make a good life." • "Pain is harmful to your health. Sometimes we get so concerned about the possible harm from pain medicine that we forget that pain is also dangerous. Research shows that pain increases cancer growth and decreases your immune function so that you are more prone to other diseases and infections." • "Addiction *very rarely* occurs from taking pain medicine. Whether you take pain medicine regularly or occasionally does not change this."

From Pasero, C., & McCaffery, M. *Pain assessment and pharmacologic management,* pp. 539-541, St. Louis, Mosby. Data from Jacox, A., Carr, D. B., Payne, R., et al. (1994). Managing cancer pain: Consumer version. *Clinical practice guideline No. 9.* AHCPR Publication No. 94-0595, Rockville, MD, U.S. Public Health Service, AHCPR, March 1994; Lang, S. L., & Patt, R. B. (1994). *You don't have to suffer,* New York, Oxford University Press. © 2011, McCaffery M, Pasero C. May be duplicated for use in clinical practice.

examples of responses to the concerns patients and families often express about addiction. Using a variety of these approaches is recommended at the start and periodically during the course of treatment.

In addition to verbal explanations, providing written information reinforces explanations about method of opioid delivery, dose, dosing schedules, and other important points that the patient and family will need to remember. The information in the "Patient Medication Information" forms that follow is based on content from this section and the following five references:

1. Clinical Pharmacology Online. Gold Standard, Inc. Available at http://clinicalpharmacology.com.
2. Drug inserts, available online for each medication.
3. Fox Chase Cancer Center/Pain Management. *Patient Education Forms,* Philadelphia. (Codeine plus acetaminophen, 2007; Darvocet, 2007; extended-released morphine, 2008; fentanyl patch, 2008; hydrocodone, 2007; morphine concentrate, 2007; morphine sulfate tablets or capsules, 2007; oral transmucosal fentanyl citrate, 2007; oxycodone, 2007; oxycodone HCL modified-release tablets, 2008; oxycodone plus acetaminophen, 2008; time-released morphine, 2007; Tylenol with codeine, 2007.)
4. Clinical Pharmacology Online. Gold Standard, Inc. Available at http://clinicalpharmacology.com.
5. Lacy, C. F., Armstrong, L. L., Goldman, M. P., et al. (Eds.). (2009-2010). *Drug information handbook,* ed 18, Hudson, OH, American Pharmacists Association, Lexi-Comp.

Patient Information Brochure: Patient-Controlled Epidural Analgesia (PCEA)

HOW DOES PAIN AFFECT MY BODY?

- When you are injured, pain warns you to protect yourself and avoid further injury. However, unrelieved pain can be harmful, especially when you are sick or after surgery. Pain can make it difficult to take a deep breath and interferes with your ability to move and walk. This can result in complications and a long stay in the hospital.

HOW WILL OTHERS KNOW HOW MUCH PAIN I HAVE?

- Your nurses will check you often while you are receiving PCEA. They will ask you to rate your pain on a 0 to 10 scale. A rating of 0 means you feel no pain at all, 5 means you feel a moderate (medium) amount of pain, and 10 means you feel the worst pain you can imagine.

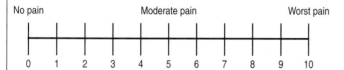

- Your comfort-function goal is _____. If you are unable to maintain this level of comfort, especially during activities such as physical therapy, let your nurse know. The dose of pain medicine usually can be increased to keep you as comfortable as possible.

WHAT ARE SOME OF THE GOALS OF PAIN MANAGEMENT WITH PCEA?

- To keep pain from becoming severe and out of control.
- To keep comfortable so that you can sleep, visit with others, and participate in your recovery.
- To decrease the length of time spent in the hospital.

HOW DOES PCEA WORK?

- Pain medicine will be given by a small pump through an epidural catheter, which is a tiny tube that will be put in your back before surgery.
- The pump will give you a small amount of pain medicine continuously.
- You also will have a PCEA button that is attached to the pump. You can press the PCEA button to give yourself a dose of pain medicine when you hurt.
- The recovery room nurse will manage your pain for you when you arrive in the recovery room, then give you the PCEA button as soon as you are awake enough to manage the pain yourself.

- It is difficult to treat pain when it is severe, so it is important to "stay on top" of your pain. When you begin to feel some discomfort, press the PCEA button, and then wait a few minutes to see if the dose helped to relieve the pain. If the pain has not been relieved, press the PCEA button again.

HOW IS THE EPIDURAL CATHETER PLACED?

- You will be positioned on your side or sitting up with your back arched out to the anesthesiologist.
- Your back will be washed with a cool soap solution.
- The anesthesiologist will inject local anesthetic to numb the area where the catheter will go. This will sting like a bee bite.
- You will feel pressure against your back while the anesthesiologist finds the epidural space.
- A very small catheter will be inserted through the needle into the epidural space, and then the needle will be removed.
- The catheter will be taped to your back and up to your shoulder where it will be connected to the pump.
- While the catheter is in place, you may lie on your back, turn, walk, and perform any activities your physician or nurse approves.

IS PCEA SAFE?

- The pump will be programmed to give you an amount of pain medicine that is typically safe for someone your sex, size, age, and diagnosis or type of surgery. If this is too much, the dose of the pain medicine can be reduced.
- The pump will be set with a safe time between doses so you cannot give yourself too much pain medicine too often.
- **PATIENT-ONLY USE!** You are the only person who will know when you are hurting and when it is necessary and safe to have a dose of pain medicine. Therefore *you are the only person who should press the PCEA button.* Your family, visitors, physicians, and hospital personnel are not to press the PCEA button. If you or they are concerned about your pain, let the nurse know.
- Let the nurse know before you take any other medicines, including the ones you usually take at home.

WHAT ARE THE SIDE EFFECTS OF PCEA?

- Itching is not an allergic reaction but is a fairly common adverse effect of pain medicine. Ask the nurse for medicine to relieve the itching when necessary.
- Nausea can occur from pain medicine, and it also can be treated with medicine that has been prescribed.
- Some patients have difficulty urinating while taking pain medicine. Reducing the dose of pain medicine helps relieve this adverse effect, and it usually resolves on its own within 48 hours.

Continued

- Pain medicine slows the bowel and can cause constipation. If your condition allows, the nurse will give you medicine to prevent constipation.
- Excessive drowsiness and respiratory depression are the most serious but least common adverse effects of pain medicine. It is rare for patients to experience these effects. These effects develop slowly, and nurses will be checking your sedation and breathing frequently. If these occur, both are easily treated and corrected by decreasing the dose of pain medicine. Let the nurse know if you feel too sleepy.
- Numbness and tingling from the epidural local anesthetic is normal in and around the surgery incision area. Let your nurse know if numbness or tingling occurs in other areas. *If you have difficulty feeling or moving your legs, stay in bed and call your nurse.* This usually can be corrected by reducing the dose of pain medicine. Be sure to ask someone to help you up the first few times you walk.

HOW LONG WILL PCEA BE USED?

- As your condition improves, your pain will decrease. You will find that you need to press the PCEA button less often as you improve.
- The dose of pain medicine will be decreased gradually until the pump is no longer necessary and you are able to use a different method for taking pain medicine.
- Your nurse will remove the epidural catheter. This is a simple and painless procedure.

In addition to talking with patients about opioids and their adverse effects, providing written information reinforces explanations about the method of opioid delivery and other important points the patient will need to remember. This box provides an example of a patient information brochure on PCEA.

From Pasero, C., & McCaffery, M. *Pain assessment and pharmacologic management*, pp. 542-543, St. Louis, Mosby. © 2011, McCaffery M, Pasero C. May be duplicated for use in clinical practice.

Patient Information Brochure: Intravenous Patient-Controlled Analgesia (IV PCA)

HOW DOES PAIN AFFECT MY BODY?

- When you are injured, pain warns you to protect yourself and avoid further injury. However, unrelieved pain can be harmful, especially when you are sick or after surgery. Pain can make it difficult to take a deep breath and interferes with your ability to move and walk. This can result in complications and a long stay in the hospital.

HOW WILL OTHERS KNOW HOW MUCH PAIN I HAVE?

- Your nurses will check you often while you are receiving IV PCA. They will ask you to rate your pain on a 0 to 10 scale. A rating of 0 means you feel no pain at all, 5 means you feel a moderate (medium) amount of pain, and 10 means you feel the worst pain you can imagine.

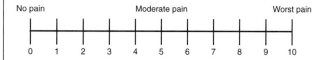

- Your comfort-function goal is _____ _____. If you are unable to maintain this level of comfort, especially during activities such as physical therapy, let your nurse know. The dose of pain medicine usually can be increased to keep you as comfortable as possible.

WHAT ARE SOME OF THE GOALS OF PAIN MANAGEMENT WITH IV PCA?

- To keep pain from becoming severe and out of control.
- To keep comfortable so that you can sleep, visit with others, and participate in your recovery.
- To decrease the length of time spent in the hospital.

HOW DOES IV PCA WORK?

- Pain medicine will be given by a small pump through your IV line. If you have surgery, this will be attached to your IV in the recovery room.
- You will have a PCA button that is attached to the pump. You can press the button to give yourself a dose of pain medicine when you hurt.
- The recovery room nurse will manage your pain for you when you arrive in the recovery room, then give you the PCA button as soon as you are awake enough to manage the pain yourself.

- It is difficult to treat pain when it is severe, so it is important to "stay on top" of your pain. When you begin to feel some discomfort, press the PCA button, and then wait a few minutes to see if the dose helped to relieve the pain. If the pain has not been relieved, press the PCA button again.
- If you have any trouble controlling your pain, let your nurse know. The dose of pain medicine may need to be increased, or you may be given oral pain medicine.

IS IV PCA SAFE?

- The pump will be programmed to give you an amount of pain medicine that is typically safe for someone your sex, size, age, and diagnosis or type of surgery. If this is too much, the dose of the pain medicine can be reduced.
- The pump will be set with a safe time between doses so you cannot give yourself too much pain medicine too often.
- **PATIENT-ONLY USE!** You are the only person who will know when you are hurting and when it is necessary and safe to have a dose of pain medicine. Therefore *you are the only person who should press the PCA button.* Your family, visitors, physicians, and hospital personnel are not to press the PCA button. If you or they are concerned about your pain, let the nurse know.
- Let the nurse know before you take any other medicines, including the ones you usually take at home.

WHAT ARE THE SIDE EFFECTS OF IV PCA?

- Itching is not an allergic reaction but is a fairly common adverse effect of pain medicine. Ask the nurse for medicine to relieve the itching when necessary.
- Nausea can occur from pain medicine, and it also can be treated with medicine that has been prescribed.
- Some patients have difficulty urinating while taking pain medicine. Reducing the dose of pain medicine helps relieve this adverse effect, and it usually resolves on its own within 48 hours.
- Pain medicine slows the bowel and can cause constipation. If your condition allows, the nurse will give you medicine to prevent constipation.
- Excessive drowsiness and respiratory depression are the most serious but least common adverse effects of pain

Continued

medicine. It is rare for patients to experience these effects. These effects develop slowly, and nurses will be checking your sedation and breathing frequently. If these occur, both are easily treated and corrected by decreasing the dose of pain medicine. Let the nurse know if you feel too sleepy.

HOW LONG WILL IV PCA BE USED?

• As your condition improves, your pain will decrease. You will find that you need to press the PCA button less often as you improve.

• The dose of pain medicine will be decreased gradually until the pump is no longer necessary and you are able to use a different method for taking pain medicine.

In addition to talking with patients about opioids and their adverse effects, providing written information reinforces explanations about the method of opioid delivery and other important points the patient will need to remember. This box provides an example of a patient information brochure on IV PCA.

From Pasero, C., & McCaffery, M. *Pain assessment and pharmacologic management,* pp. 544-545, St. Louis, Mosby. © 2011, McCaffery M, Pasero C. May be duplicated for use in clinical practice.

PATIENT MEDICATION INFORMATION

Constipation Caused by Opioids

Occurrence:
Opioids cause constipation in almost everyone who takes them for several doses or longer. Opioids cause stools to move more slowly along the intestinal tract, resulting in the stool becoming hard and difficult to pass.

Symptoms of Constipation:
Most people know when they are constipated. Following are some common symptoms:
• Less frequent bowel movements (BMs)
• More difficulty having BMs
• Abdominal bloating
• Rectal fullness or pressure
• Having the urge to have a BM but unable to do so

Prevention and Treatment of Constipation Caused by Opioids:
Constipation is such a common side effect of opioids that most patients need to start a bowel program at the same time they start taking opioids. Prevention of constipation is the key. The following bowel program is designed especially for patients who start taking opioids around the clock.

Medications used to prevent or treat constipation are usually a laxative to stimulate the bowels to move the stool more quickly plus a stool softener to draw moisture into the stool so that it moves more easily through the bowels. Examples are Senokot S (generic equivalent is docusate sodium 50 mg + senna 8.6 mg) or Peri-Colace (generic equivalent is docusate + casanthranol). Avoid bulk such as Metamucil (psyllium) because they increase the mass that must be moved through the bowels.

A Commonly Used Bowel Program:
Goal: To have a complete, easy, and comfortable BM at least every 3 days.
• Start with Senokot-S 2 tablets at bedtime. Continue with the following steps.
• If no BM in any 24-hour period, increase Senokot-S up to 3 to 4 tablets at bedtime or 2 tablets twice a day.
• If no BM in any 48-hour period, add 1 to 2 of the following:
  - Dulcolax (bisacodyl) 2-3 tablets at bedtime or 1 tablet 3 times a day. Take with food, milk, or antacids to avoid stomach irritation.
  - Miralax (polyethylene glycol) 1 heaping teaspoon in 4 to 8 oz of fluid orally. Response may take 2 to 4 days.
• If no BM in any 72-hour period, call your nurse or doctor to discuss your symptoms to determine if you are impacted. If not impacted, add 1 to 2 of the following:
  - Lactulose 1½ to 2 oz orally
  - Magnesium citrate 8 oz orally
  - Dulcolax suppository 1 rectally
  - Fleet enema 1 rectally

Precautions:
• If the above bowel program does not result in a BM in 3 days, call your doctor or nurse at once. You may have an impaction that needs to be removed.
• Once you have a BM, DO NOT stop taking your bowel medicines. Continue to use whatever bowel medicines you were taking. If this causes your BMs to be too frequent or too soft, you may need to reduce your bowel medicines by ¼ to ½ to maintain a level that results in a comfortable bowel movement every 1 to 2 days.
• If you experience diarrhea, stop your bowel medicines for 1 to 2 days. Start them again at a reduced dose.
• If your opioid dose increases, you probably will need to increase your bowel medicines.

Additional Things You Can Do to Help with Your Constipation:
• Exercise as much as you can.
• Drink plenty of fluids. Try to drink 8 to 10 cups of liquid each day.
• Try to have a BM whenever you have the urge.
• Do not strain or use extreme force to try to have a BM.

Form IV-1 | Constipation caused by opioids: patient information.

From Pasero, C., & McCaffery, M. *Pain assessment and pharmacologic management,* pp. 546, St. Louis, Mosby. © 2011, McCaffery M, Pasero C. May be duplicated for use in clinical practice.

PATIENT MEDICATION INFORMATION

Codeine with Acetaminophen (generic name)

BRAND NAME: Tylenol® with Codeine

TYPE OF PAIN MEDICINE: Opioid (narcotic) and nonopioid

DESCRIPTION: Tylenol® with codeine comes in tablet and liquid form.
- Tablets:
    Tylenol® with Codeine No. 3 contains acetaminophen 300 mg and codeine 30 mg
    Tylenol® with Codeine No. 4 contains acetaminophen 300 mg and codeine 60 mg
- Liquid: Each teaspoon contains acetaminophen 120 mg and codeine 12 mg

USES:
Relieves mild to moderate pain.
Sometimes used to control cough or shortness of breath.

DOSAGE AND ADMINISTRATION:
- Take only as directed.
- These directions may change.
- You should feel pain relief in 30 to 60 minutes.
- Usually 1 to 2 tablets may be taken every 4 hours up to a maximum of 12 tablets in 24 hours. Take at first sign of pain.
- May be taken alone or in addition to other pain medicines.
- May be taken with or without food.
- May be taken with other medicines.
- Do not take more than 4000 mg acetaminophen in 24 hours. Some patients should take less than 4000 mg; check with your nurse or doctor. Be aware that other medicines that you take such as certain cold medicines or sleep medicines may have acetaminophen in them.
- Tell your nurse or doctor if you are pregnant, plan to become pregnant, or are breast-feeding.
- Tell you doctor, nurse, and pharmacist about all medicines you take.

POSSIBLE SIDE EFFECTS:
- Constipation. Opioids block pain and block bowels. Constipation can be controlled with daily laxatives such as Senokot-S. Try to drink 8 large glasses of fluid a day. Increase your activity by walking or exercising. (For more helpful information, see Constipation Caused by Opioids form.)
- Nausea and vomiting. Take your medicine with food to lessen this. If nausea and vomiting continue, call your nurse or doctor. May be controlled with medicines.
- Drowsiness. May occur when starting Tylenol® with Codeine or increasing the dose. This usually goes away in about 2 to 3 days. Rest as needed.
- Confusion. This is less common than drowsiness. If this happens, call your nurse or doctor.

PRECAUTIONS:
- Be careful driving or using machinery such as lawn mowers, power tools, or saws. Do not do these things if you are drowsy.
- Be careful when drinking alcohol. Alcohol will increase drowsiness. Your medicine contains acetaminophen, and drinking alcohol with acetaminophen may increase risk of liver damage.
- Call your doctor or nurse if pain increases or if you do not get pain relief.

Continued

Form IV-2 | Patient medication information: codeine with acetaminophen.

As appears in Pasero, C., & McCaffery, M. (2011). *Pain assessment and pharmacologic management*, pp. 547-548, St. Louis, Mosby. Modified from Fox Chase Cancer Center/Pain Management, Philadelphia, 2007. May be duplicated for use in clinical practice.

PATIENT MEDICATION INFORMATION—cont'd

Codeine with Acetaminophen (generic name)

STOPPING MEDICATIONS: Do not suddenly stop taking your medicine. Opioids must be stopped gradually. Call your pharmacist, nurse, or doctor before you stop taking your medicine.

REMEMBER!
- Keep count of your medicine.
- Do not mix medicines in the same container.
- Do not run out of medicine.
- In some states prescriptions for this medicine cannot be <u>re</u>filled or phoned in to your pharmacy. Check with your doctor or nurse.
- Get a **<u>new</u>** prescription filled a few days before you will run out of medicine.
- **<u>Call</u>** your nurse or doctor if side effects occur or if pain changes or does not go away. Your medicine may need to be changed.
- Take unused, unneeded, or expired medicines out of their original containers and flush them down the toilet. Do not put them in the trash.

COMMENTS:

- <u>Warning:</u> Keep this medicine out of reach of children! A dose could be fatal to a child.
- <u>Be sure to keep this medicine in a safe place out of sight of others</u>. A locked box may be indicated to prevent someone else from taking this medicine.

Form IV-2 | Cont'd.

PATIENT MEDICATION INFORMATION

Fentanyl Buccal Tablet (FBT) (generic name)

BRAND NAME: Fentora®

TYPE OF PAIN MEDICINE: Opioid (narcotic)

DESCRIPTION: Available in white tablets: 100 mcg, 200 mcg, 300 mcg, 400 mcg, 600 mcg, 800 mcg (mcg = micrograms, sometime written as µg; mg = milligrams; mcg is not the same as mg)

USES:
Relieves breakthrough pain. Sometimes called a rescue dose. When other medicine is taken around the clock for persistent pain, a brief episode of additional pain may occur that is more severe. This is called a flare or breakthrough pain.

DOSAGE AND ADMINISTRATION:
- Take only as directed.
- These directions may change.
- To take Fentora, you should already be taking another opioid around the clock. You must continue to take your around the clock opioid medicine.
- Keep Fentora in blister packs until ready to use. Do not store in pillboxes. Peel back the foil on the blister pack to expose the tablet. Do not push the tablet through the foil because this could split or damage the tablet.
- Fentora is not flavored and is almost tasteless.
- As soon as the breakthrough pain occurs, place the entire tablet above a rear molar, between the gum and cheek. Do not split the tablet.
- Do not suck, chew, or swallow the tablet since this will reduce the amount of pain relief you receive.
- Leave the tablet in place between the gum and cheek until it crumbles (usually 14 to 25 minutes). If some pieces of the tablet remain after 30 minutes, they may be swallowed with water.
- Pain relief is usually felt within 15 minutes.
- If pain is not satisfactorily relieved after 30 minutes, your nurse or doctor may have told you to take one more dose. Place the second dose of Fentora on the other side of the mouth.
- Do not take more than two doses of Fentora for an episode of breakthrough pain.
- If you take Fentora and have trouble breathing, extreme drowsiness with slowed breathing, or feel very dizzy, spit out the tablet and do not take a second dose. Call your nurse or doctor, or get emergency help.
- If you have a dry mouth, you may drink some water before taking Fentora, but do not eat or drink anything while the Fentora tablet is in your mouth.
- After taking Fentora for one episode of breakthrough pain, you must wait 4 hours before taking any more Fentora.
- Try to record the time you take your doses of Fentora and your pain ratings for several episodes of breakthrough pain. This information can be used to adjust your dose, if needed.
- Adjustment of dose: This is done only under the direction of your nurse or doctor. If a higher dose of Fentora is needed, you may be told to take two of your Fentora tablets at the same time—one on each side of the mouth. The dose may be increased in this way until a dose is identified that adequately relieves your pain. Hopefully, after adjusting your dose, it will be necessary for you to take only one Fentora for each breakthrough pain episode.
- If you need to take Fentora for more than four breakthrough episodes a day, your doctor will probably increase the dose of your around the clock opioid.
- May be taken with other medicines.
- Tell your nurse or doctor if you are pregnant, plan to become pregnant, or are breast-feeding.
- Tell your doctor, nurse, and pharmacist about all medicines you take.

Continued

Form IV-3 | Patient medication information: fentanyl buccal tablet.

PATIENT MEDICATION INFORMATION—cont'd

Fentanyl Buccal Tablet (FBT) (generic name)

POSSIBLE SIDE EFFECTS:
- Constipation. If you have already been taking opioids, you may have worked out an effective way of preventing constipation. Continue with what has been working. Constipation seems to be less of a problem with fentanyl than with the other opioids, but it still occurs. If you have not been taking opioids and have no method of preventing constipation caused by opioids, constipation can be controlled with daily laxatives such as Senokot-S. Try to drink 8 large glasses of fluid a day. Increase your activity by walking or exercising. (For more helpful information, see Constipation Caused by Opioids form.)
- Nausea and vomiting. Try eating something right before you take Fentora. If nausea and vomiting continue, call your nurse or doctor. May be controlled with medicines.
- Drowsiness. May occur when starting Fentora or increasing the dose. This usually goes away in about 2 to 3 days. Rest as needed.
- Confusion. This is less common than drowsiness. Call your nurse or doctor if this occurs.
- Reactions in the mouth where you place Fentora. You may feel pain, irritation, numbness, inflammation of the mucosal lining, ulceration, or bleeding. This may occur early in treatment but usually goes away.

PRECAUTIONS:
- Be careful driving or using machinery such as lawn mowers, power tools, or saws. Do not do these things if you are drowsy.
- Avoid alcohol. Alcohol will increase your chance of getting side effects.
- Call your doctor or nurse if pain increases or if you do not get pain relief.

STOPPING MEDICATIONS: Do not suddenly stop taking your medicine. Opioids must be stopped gradually. Call your pharmacist, nurse, or doctor before you stop taking your medicine.

REMEMBER!
- Keep count of your medicine.
- Do not mix medicines in the same container.
- Do not run out of medicine.
- Prescriptions for this medicine cannot be <u>re</u>filled or phoned in to your pharmacy.
- Get a <u>**new**</u> prescription filled a few days before you will run out of medicine.
- Be sure your pharmacist does not substitute Actiq for Fentora.
- <u>**Call**</u> your nurse or doctor if side effects occur or if pain changes or does not go away. Your medicine may need to be changed.

COMMENTS:

- <u>Warning</u>: Keep this medicine out of reach of children! A dose could be fatal to a child.
- <u>Be sure to keep this medicine in a safe place out of sight of others</u>. A locked box may be indicated to prevent someone else from taking this medicine.
- Store at room temperature.
- Dispose of any unneeded Fentora by removing tablets from the blister packs and flushing the tablets down the toilet. Do not put them in the trash.

PATIENT MEDICATION INFORMATION

Oral Transmucosal Fentanyl Citrate (OTFC) (generic name)

BRAND NAME: Actiq®

TYPE OF PAIN MEDICINE: Opioid (narcotic)

DESCRIPTION: A plastic stick with a white lozenge on one end that contains the opioid fentanyl (referred to as a unit). Each Actiq comes in a blister package. It is supplied in micrograms (mcg, sometimes written as ug) in the following doses: 200 mcg, 400 mcg, 600 mcg, 800 mcg, 1200 mcg, 1600 mcg.

USES:
Relieves breakthrough pain. Sometimes called a rescue dose. When other medicine is taken around the clock for persistent pain, a brief episode of additional pain may occur that is more severe. This is called a flare or breakthrough pain.

DOSAGE AND ADMINISTRATION:
- <u>Take only as directed.</u>
- These directions may change.
- To take Actiq, you should already be taking another opioid around the clock.
- Actiq may be prescribed in small amounts, such as 6 units, until the right dose for you is determined.
- The usual dose is 1 Actiq for each episode of breakthrough pain. However, until the right dose for you is determined, you may need more than 1 Actiq for an occurrence of breakthrough pain. If so, the doctor may prescribe a higher dose of Actiq.
- Do not open the blister package of Actiq until you are ready to use it.
- When you are ready to use Actiq, open the package using scissors and remove the Actiq unit.
- Place Actiq in the mouth between the cheek and lower gum.
- Let Actiq be absorbed through the mouth. If possible, do not swallow it because you will get less pain relief.
- Actively suck on Actiq, and twirl the handle often. Do not suck on it as hard as you would suck on a lollipop because this could result in the medicine being swallowed.
- Move Actiq around in your mouth, especially along your cheeks and under the tongue.
- DO NOT BITE OR CHEW Actiq.
- Finish Actiq completely in 15 minutes. Do not finish it in less time or you will get less relief.
- If you begin to feel dizzy, sick to your stomach, or very sleepy before Actiq is completely dissolved, remove Actiq from your mouth. Dispose of it right away. Follow the directions below for proper disposal.
- Pain relief occurs in about 5 minutes and peaks at 15 minutes. It lasts about 2 hours.
- If 1 unit of Actiq does not provide enough pain relief, another unit may be taken 15 minutes after the previous unit has been completed.
- <u>No more than 2 units</u> should be taken for each episode of breakthrough pain, and no more than 4 units a day.
- You may drink some water before using Actiq but do not drink or eat anything while using Actiq.
- Call your doctor or 911 if any of the following occur because you have probably taken too much and these symptoms could be life-threatening:
  - Trouble breathing
  - Extreme drowsiness with slowed breathing
  - Slow, shallow breathing (chest does not move much when you breathe)
  - Feeling very dizzy or confused
- After you have used Actiq, you must <u>properly dispose of it</u> as follows, even if there is little or no medicine left on it:
  - If the medicine is totally gone, throw the handle away in a place that is out of reach of children and pets.
  - If any medicine remains on the handle after you have finished, place the handle under hot running water until the medicine is gone, and then throw the handle away in a place out of reach of children and pets.
- May be taken with other medicines.

Continued

Form IV-4 | Patient medication information: oral transmucosal fentanyl citrate.

From Pasero, C., & McCaffery, M. *Pain assessment and pharmacologic management*, pp. 551-552, St. Louis, Mosby. © 2011, McCaffery M, Pasero C. May be duplicated for use in clinical practice.

PATIENT MEDICATION INFORMATION—cont'd

Oral Transmucosal Fentanyl Citrate (OTFC) (generic name)

- Store Actiq at room temperature.
- Tell your nurse or doctor if you are pregnant, plan to become pregnant, or are breast-feeding.
- Tell your doctor, nurse, and pharmacist about all medicines you take.

POSSIBLE SIDE EFFECTS:

- Constipation. Opioids block pain and block bowels. Constipation can be controlled with daily laxatives such as Senokot-S. Try to drink 8 large glasses of fluid a day. Increase your activity by walking or exercising. (For more helpful information, see Constipation Caused by Opioids form.)
- Nausea and vomiting. Take your medicine with food to lessen this. If nausea and vomiting continue, call your nurse or doctor. May be controlled with medicines.
- Drowsiness. May occur when starting Actiq or increasing the dose. This usually goes away in about 2 to 3 days. Rest as needed.
- Each Actiq contains about ½ teaspoon of sugar and may cause cavities and tooth decay. Dry mouth may also occur. See your dentist to discuss proper care of your teeth.

PRECAUTIONS:

- Be careful driving or using machinery such as lawn mowers, power tools, or saws. Do not do these things if you are drowsy.
- Avoid alcohol. Alcohol will increase your chance of getting side effects.
- Call your doctor or nurse if pain increases or if you do not get pain relief.
- Do not refer to Actiq as a lollipop, sucker, or popsicle since this can result in family members, especially children, misunderstanding that it is candy and safe for them to take.

STOPPING MEDICATIONS: Do not suddenly stop taking your medicine. Opioids must be stopped gradually. Call your pharmacist, nurse, or doctor before you stop taking your medicine.

REMEMBER!

- Keep count of your medicine.
- Do not mix medicines in the same container.
- Do not run out of medicine.
- Prescriptions for this medicine cannot be refilled or phoned in to your pharmacy.
- Get a **new** prescription filled a few days before you will run out of medicine.
- **Call** your nurse or doctor if side effects occur or if pain changes or does not go away. Your medicine may need to be changed.
- Dispose of unused, unneeded, or expired Actiq blister packages and dispose of them as described below. Do not put them in the trash.
  1. Remove 1 Actiq unit from its blister package using scissors, and hold it by its handle over the toilet bowl.
  2. Using wire-cutting pliers, cut the medicine end off so that it falls into the toilet.
  3. Throw the handle away in a place that is out of reach of children.
  4. Repeat steps 1, 2, and 3 for each Actiq.
  5. Flush the toilet twice after 5 Actiq units have been cut. Do not flush more than 5 Actiq units at a time.

COMMENTS:

- Warning: Keep this medicine out of reach of children! A dose could be fatal to a child.
- Be sure to keep this medicine in a safe place out of sight of others. A locked box may be indicated to prevent someone else from taking this medicine.
- Actiq comes with a Welcome Kit to help you store Actiq and other medicines out of reach of children. If you were not offered a Welcome Kit when you received your medicine, call Cephalon Professional Services at 1-800-896-5855 to request one.

Form IV-4 | Cont'd.

PATIENT MEDICATION INFORMATION

Fentanyl Transdermal System (generic name)

BRAND NAME: Duragesic®

TYPE OF PAIN MEDICINE: Opioid (narcotic)

DESCRIPTION: Duragesic is a patch that adheres to the skin. It contains the opioid fentanyl, and fentanyl is gradually absorbed through the skin into the blood stream. Duragesic patches are supplied in 12 mcg, 25 mcg, 50 mcg, 75 mcg, and 100 mcg (mcg = micrograms; mg = milligrams; mcg and mg are not the same). The size of the patch differs depending on the dose of fentanyl.

USES:
Relieves persistent pain that occurs around the clock.

DOSAGE AND ADMINISTRATION:
- <u>Take only as directed.</u>
- These directions may change.
- Usually you start with wearing only one patch. More patches may be ordered later. Some patients need to wear three or more patches.
- The patch is usually changed every 72 hours. The nurse or doctor may decide some people need to change the patch every 48 hours.
- <u>Selecting a skin area where the patch will be applied:</u>
  - Avoid sensitive or irritated areas.
  - The patch should be applied to intact skin on the sides of the waist, back, chest, and upper arms. Sometimes other sites are used. Placing the patch over the site of pain is not harmful but is not recommended and has no advantage.
  - If the site, such as the chest, is hairy, the hair must be clipped but not shaved, because shaving can irritate the skin.
  - Avoid skin areas that move around a lot since the patch will tend to come loose. Avoid placing the patch on folds of skin.
  - When you remove an old patch, be sure to apply the new patch at a new site.
- <u>Preparing to apply the Duragesic patch</u>:
  - Select a time of day that will be convenient for you 2 to 3 days to remove the patch and apply another patch. Change patches at the same time of day if possible.
  - The area where the patch will be applied should be cleaned with clear water only. Pat it dry. Soaps, oils, and alcohol should not be applied to the area before the patch is placed.
  - Open pouch by folding and tearing at the slit, or cut the slit. Remove the patch when you are ready to apply it.
  - <u>Do not cut the patch</u>. Do not use a patch that is cut or damaged. This could increase release of fentanyl, causing a serious increase in side effects.
  - You or your caregivers may decide to put on plastic gloves prior to applying the patch to protect yourselves from absorbing fentanyl.
  - Peel off both parts of the protective liner from the sticky side of the patch. Touch the sticky side of the patch as little as possible.
  - Throw the clear plastic lining away.
- <u>Applying the patch to the skin</u>:
  - Always take off the old patch(es) when you apply new ones.
  - Press the patch onto the chosen skin site with the palm of your hand and hold it there for at least 30 seconds.

Continued

Form IV-5 | Patient medication information: fentanyl transdermal system.

PATIENT MEDICATION INFORMATION—cont'd

Fentanyl Transdermal System (generic name)

- Once in place, firmly rub the edges and the body of the patch to make sure it sticks well.
- Wash your hands when you have finished applying the patch.
- Trouble with the patch sticking:
  - If the patch falls off right away after applying it, put on a new patch at a different site. Prepare the new site as instructed above. Dispose of the old patch as described below.
  - The patch may not stick well on you or at all sites. You may need to check the patches often to make sure that they are sticking well to the skin.
  - If you have a problem with the patch sticking, place first aid tape on the edges of the patch.
  - If you continue to have problems with the patch sticking, you may cover the patch with Bioclusive or Tegaderm patches. These are see-through adhesive dressings. (Never cover the patch with any other type of bandage or tape.)
  - If the patch falls off later before 3 days of use, discard it properly (see below) and apply a new patch at a different site. Call your nurse or doctor to let them know this has happened. Do not replace this patch for 3 days.
- Disposing of a Duragesic patch:
  - Fold the used patch in half so that the sticky sides stick together.
  - Flush the used patch down the toilet right away. Do not put it in the trash.
  - Dispose of any left over patches in the same manner as above. Open each one, fold in half, and flush down the toilet. Do not flush the pouch or protective liner down the toilet.
- With your first patch application you will not begin to feel pain relief for about 12-18 hours. Your nurse or doctor may advise you to continue your previous medicine for a while, or if you have medicine for breakthrough pain (rescue doses) you may use this to treat your pain until this patch effectively relieves pain. The full effect may not be felt for 1 to 3 days. If pain returns before the next patch is due to be applied, call your doctor or nurse. Your patch dose or time between patches may need to be changed.
- You can bathe, swim, or shower while you are wearing a Duragesic patch. Do not take very hot baths or showers.
- Do not expose the site of the patch to direct heat sources, such as heating pads, electric blankets, heat lamps, saunas, hot tubs, heated water bed, or sunbathing. These situations could cause an increase in the dose of fentanyl and lead to side effects.
- If you have a fever greater than 104° F, this could cause an increase in the dose of fentanyl. Watch closely for an increase in side effects, and call your nurse or doctor if this occurs.
- If you are having an MRI, the patch will be removed before the test. Bring another patch with you to put on after the MRI. Do not replace this patch for 3 days.
- May be taken alone or in addition to other pain medicines.
- May be taken with other medicines.
- If you miss the time to apply your next patch, apply it as soon as possible. Remove the old patch(es) and apply the new patch(es). Do not double your dose. If you have medicine for breakthrough pain (rescue doses) you may use this to treat your pain until the new patch effectively relieves pain.

POSSIBLE SIDE EFFECTS:

- Constipation. If you have already been taking opioids, you may have worked out an effective way to prevent constipation. Continue with what has been working for you. Constipation seems to be less of a problem with fentanyl than with the other opioids, but it still occurs. If you have not been taking opioids and have no method of preventing constipation caused by opioids, constipation can be controlled with daily laxatives such as Senokot-S. Try to drink 8 large glasses of fluid a day. Increase your activity by walking or exercising. (For more helpful information, see Constipation Caused by Opioids form.)
- Nausea and vomiting. If this occurs call your nurse or doctor. May be controlled with medicines.

Continued

PATIENT MEDICATION INFORMATION—cont'd

Fentanyl Transdermal System (generic name)

- Drowsiness. May occur when starting or increasing dose or number of patches. This usually goes away in about 2 to 3 days. Rest as needed.
- Confusion. This is less common than drowsiness. If this happens, call your nurse or doctor.
- Skin irritation or itching under the patch: Call your nurse or doctor if the patch causes a rash. May be controlled with various medications.

PRECAUTIONS:
- Be careful driving or using machinery such as lawn mowers, power tools, or saws. Do not do these things if you are drowsy.
- Be careful when drinking alcohol. Alcohol will increase drowsiness.
- Call your doctor or nurse if pain increases or if you do not get pain relief.
- Always wash your hands after applying a Duragesic patch.

STOPPING MEDICATIONS:
- Do not suddenly stop wearing the patch. Opioids must be stopped gradually. Call your pharmacist, nurse, or doctor before you stop wearing your patch(es).
- When the Duragesic patch is removed it takes a long time for the effects of fentanyl to wear off. For example, over half of the fentanyl still remains in the body after 17 hours. If the patch has been removed because you were experiencing serious side effects, such as trouble breathing, someone must watch you closely for 24 hours after the patch is taken off. The effects will wear off slowly.

REMEMBER!
- Keep count of your patches.
- Do not mix patches of different doses in the same container.
- Do not run out of patches.
- Prescriptions for this medicine cannot be <u>re</u>filled or phoned in to your pharmacy.
- Get a <u>**new**</u> prescription filled a few days before you will run out of patches.
- Ask your pharmacist not to substitute any other brand of transdermal patch for Duragesic. The other patch may have the same dose of fentanyl in it but it may be released differently into your body.
- <u>**Call**</u> your nurse or doctor if side effects occur or if pain changes or does not go away. Your patches may need to be changed.
- Take unused, unneeded, or expired patches out of their original containers and flush them down the toilet (as described above). Do not put them in the trash.

COMMENTS:

- <u>Warning</u>: Keep the patches out of reach of children! A dose could be fatal to a child.
- <u>Do not refer to the patches as band aids</u>. Children may think they can play with the patches and apply them to themselves or others.
- <u>Be sure to keep this medicine in a safe place out of sight of others</u>. A locked box may be indicated to prevent someone else from taking this medicine.

Form IV-5 | Cont'd.

PATIENT MEDICATION INFORMATION

Hydrocodone with Acetaminophen (generic name)

BRAND NAMES: Vicodin®, Norco®, Lortab®, and others

TYPE OF PAIN MEDICINE: Opioid (narcotic) and nonopioid

DESCRIPTION: Vicodin®, Norco®, Lortab®, and other brands are made up of two medicines: hydrocodone and acetaminophen. Acetaminophen is the same as Tylenol®. There are several brands and combinations of hydrocodone and acetaminophen as well as generics. It comes in pills and liquid. Common examples are listed below.

Tablets/caplets:
- Vicodin 5/500—hydrocodone 5 mg and acetaminophen 500 mg
- Vicodin 7.5/500—hydrocodone 7.5 mg and acetaminophen 500 mg
- Vicodin 10/500—hydrocodone 10 mg and acetaminophen 500 mg
- Vicodin ES—hydrocodone 7.5 mg and acetaminophen 750 mg
- Vicodin HP—hydrocodone 10 mg and acetaminophen 660 mg
- Lortab 5/500—hydrocodone 5 mg and acetaminophen 500 mg
- Norco—comes in hydrocodone 5 mg, 7.5 mg, or 10 mg plus acetaminophen 325 mg

Liquid:
- hydrocodone 7.5 mg and acetaminophen 500 mg in 3 teaspoons.

USES:
Relieves pain.
Sometimes used to control cough or shortness of breath.

DOSAGE AND ADMINISTRATION:
- Take only as directed.
- These directions may change.
- You should feel pain relief in 30 to 60 minutes.
- Usually taken every 4 to 6 hours. Take at the first sign of pain.
- The maximum number of tablets/caplets allowed in any 24-hour period is limited by the amount of acetaminophen. Do not take more than 4000 mg acetaminophen in 24 hours. For example, do not take more than 8 Vicodin or 12 Norco in 24 hours. Some patients should take less than 4000 mg; check with your nurse or doctor. Be aware that other medicines that you take such as certain cold medicines or sleep medicines may have acetaminophen in them.
- May be taken alone or in addition to other pain medicines.
- May be taken with or without food.
- May be taken with other medicines.
- Tell your nurse or doctor if you are pregnant, plan to become pregnant, or are breast-feeding.
- Tell your doctor, nurse, and pharmacist about all medicines you take.

POSSIBLE SIDE EFFECTS:
- Constipation. Opioids block pain and block bowels. Constipation can be controlled with daily laxatives such as Senokot-S. Try to drink 8 large glasses of fluid a day. Increase your activity by walking or exercising. (For more helpful information, see Constipation Caused by Opioids form.)

Continued

Form IV-6 | Patient medication information: hydrocodone with acetaminophen.

PATIENT MEDICATION INFORMATION—cont'd

Hydrocodone with Acetaminophen (generic name)

- Nausea and vomiting. Take your medicine with food to lessen this. If nausea and vomiting continue, call your nurse or doctor. May be controlled with medicines.
- Drowsiness. May occur when starting hydrocodone and acetaminophen or increasing the dose. This usually goes away in about 2 to 3 days. Rest as needed.
- Confusion. This is less common than drowsiness. If this happens, call your nurse or doctor.

PRECAUTIONS:
- Be careful driving or using machinery such as lawn mowers, power tools, or saws. Do not do these things if you are drowsy.
- Be careful when drinking alcohol. Alcohol will increase drowsiness. Your medicine contains acetaminophen, and drinking alcohol with acetaminophen may increase risk of liver damage.
- Call your doctor or nurse if pain increases or if you do not get pain relief.

STOPPING MEDICATIONS: Do not suddenly stop taking your medicine. Opioids must be stopped gradually. Call your pharmacist, nurse, or doctor before you stop taking your medicine.

REMEMBER!
- Keep count of your medicine.
- Do not mix medicines in the same container.
- Do not run out of medicine.
- In some states prescriptions for this medicine cannot be <u>re</u>filled or phoned in to your pharmacy. Check with your nurse, doctor, or pharmacist.
- Get a **new** prescription filled a few days before you will run out of medicine.
- **Call** your nurse or doctor if side effects occur or if pain changes or does not go away. Your medicine may need to be changed.
- Take unused, unneeded, or expired medicines out of their original containers and flush them down the toilet. Do not put them in the trash.

COMMENTS:

- <u>Warning</u>: Keep this medicine out of reach of children! A dose could be fatal to a child.
- <u>Be sure to keep this medicine in a safe place out of sight of others</u>. A locked box may be indicated to prevent someone else from taking this medicine.

Form IV-6 | Cont'd.

PATIENT MEDICATION INFORMATION

Hydromorphone (generic name)

BRAND NAMES: Dilaudid®, Hydromorphone Hydrochloride®

TYPE OF PAIN MEDICINE: Opioid (narcotic), short-acting. Sometimes called immediate-release.

DESCRIPTION: Hydromorphone is available in tablets and liquid. Common examples are listed below.

Tablets:
• Dilaudid 2 mg tablet, also available in 4 mg and 8 mg
• Hydromorphone Hydrochloride 2 mg tablet, also available in 4 mg and 8 mg

Liquid:
• Dilaudid 1 mg/mL Liquid

USES:
Relieves pain.
Sometimes used to control cough or shortness of breath.
Sometimes used for breakthrough pain (rescue doses) when other medicine is taken around the clock for persistent pain.

DOSAGE AND ADMINISTRATION:
• Take only as directed.
• These directions may change.
• For liquids, doses are prescribed in mL (milliliters) or mg (milligrams). Be careful not to confuse the two. They are not the same.
• When measuring liquid Dilaudid, do not use regular teaspoons or tablespoons since they are not accurate enough. Measure your dose with a dropper, medicine cup, or syringe. If one of these does not come with your medicine, ask the pharmacist for one.
• You should feel pain relief in 30 to 60 minutes.
• Usually taken every 2 to 4 hours.
• You may need to adjust your schedule. If so, call your nurse or doctor.
• There is no maximum dose or amount that your doctor may prescribe for you but the amount may be limited by state and federal laws, prescription plan rules, and pharmacy supply.
• May be taken alone or in addition to other pain medicines.
• May be taken with or without food.
• May be taken with other medicines.
• If you miss a dose of your medicine, take it as soon as possible. If it is almost time for the next dose, skip the missed dose. Do not take two doses at one time.
• Tell your nurse or doctor if you are pregnant, plan to become pregnant, or are breast-feeding.
• Tell your doctor, nurse, and pharmacist about all medicines you take.
• If you are having difficulty swallowing, talk with your nurse or doctor about the possibility of a suppository. Hydromorphone comes in Hydromorphone Hydrochloride 3 mg Rectal Suppository.

POSSIBLE SIDE EFFECTS:
• Constipation. Opioids block pain and block bowels. Constipation can be controlled with daily laxatives such as Senokot-S. Try to drink 8 large glasses of fluid a day. Increase your activity by walking or exercising. (For more helpful information, see Constipation Caused by Opioids form.)

Continued

Form IV-7 | Patient medication information: hydromorphone.

PATIENT MEDICATION INFORMATION—cont'd

Hydromorphone (generic name)

- Nausea and vomiting. Take your medicine with food to lessen this. If nausea and vomiting continue, call your nurse or doctor. May be controlled with medicines.
- Drowsiness. May occur when starting hydromorphone or increasing the dose. This usually goes away in about 2 to 3 days. Rest as needed.
- Confusion. This is less common than drowsiness. If this happens, call your nurse or doctor.

PRECAUTIONS:
- Be careful driving or using machinery such as lawn mowers, power tools, or saws. Do not do these things if you are drowsy.
- Be careful when drinking alcohol. Alcohol will increase drowsiness.
- Call your doctor or nurse if pain increases or if you do not get pain relief.

STOPPING MEDICATIONS: Do not suddenly stop taking your medicine. Opioids must be stopped gradually. Call your pharmacist, nurse, or doctor before you stop taking your medicine.

REMEMBER!
- Keep count of your medicine.
- Do not mix medicines in the same container.
- Do not run out of medicine.
- Prescriptions for this medicine cannot be refilled or phoned in to your pharmacy.
- Get a **new** prescription filled a few days before you will run out of medicine.
- **Call** your nurse or doctor if side effects occur or if pain changes or does not go away. Your medicine may need to be changed.
- Take unused, unneeded, or expired medicines out of their original containers and flush them down the toilet. Do not put them in the trash.

COMMENTS:

- Warning: Keep this medicine out of reach of children! A dose could be fatal to a child.
- Be sure to keep this medicine in a safe place out of sight of others. A locked box may be indicated to prevent someone else from taking this medicine.

Form IV-7 | Cont'd.

PATIENT MEDICATION INFORMATION

Methadone (generic name)

Safely Taking Methadone for Pain

Please read this handout carefully and share it with family members or caretakers.
It does not take the place of your health care provider's guidance or the methadone package insert.

Your health care provider has prescribed methadone to help control pain. Methadone (methuh-doan) is a strong pain reliever that has been used successfully for more than 60 years in millions of persons worldwide. It is a man-made, or synthetic, opioid (oh-pee-oyd) drug with actions similar to natural opioids like morphine or codeine that come from the opium poppy, except methadone is more potent.

Methadone is a very effective and economical medication. When used properly, it can help safely relieve pain even when other medications fail. However, since it is a long-lasting and powerful drug, its improper use or abuse can be harmful and even fatal (causing death).
Therefore, it is very important that you read, understand, and follow all of the safety instructions below.

Always take methadone exactly as directed.
- **Taking extra methadone or combining it with other drugs, alcohol, or over-the-counter products, unless approved by your health care provider, can be harmful or fatal.**
- Make sure the methadone prescriber knows of all health care products and drugs (prescribed or not) that you are using and your complete medical history.
- You must take only the prescribed amount of methadone and at the specified time intervals.
- If you were told to split methadone tablets for the proper dose, ask your health care provider or pharmacist how to do that accurately.
- Methadone builds up in the body over time, often taking a week or longer to achieve full effect. During that time, pain relief may be incomplete. However, unless told to do so by your health care provider, *never take extra methadone doses or other pain relievers,* as this could be harmful or fatal.
- If you forget to take your usual methadone dose on time, you can take it very soon thereafter. Otherwise, wait until it is time for the next dose and take only that; *do not* take extra methadone to make up for what was missed.
- To help avoid missing doses or taking extra ones, use a dosing chart or medication log to keep track of when you take each dose of methadone.
- If you are forgetful, have someone else give you each dose of methadone and keep a record of it.
- Do not take methadone with grapefruit or grapefruit juice. It can block the breakdown of methadone, causing a harmfully excessive amount to accumulate.
- Tell *all* of your healthcare providers that you are taking methadone. Unless they know of this, they might prescribe medications that alter methadone's effects. They should contact the methadone prescriber if there are questions.

Store methadone safely.
- Methadone *absolutely must be kept in a safe place* where others—children or adults—cannot gain access to it. A single tablet of methadone can be harmful, or even fatal, in an individual who is not used to the medication.
- Do not keep methadone on kitchen counters, in bathroom cabinets, or other obvious places. If necessary, store methadone in a locked box or cabinet and in an out of the way location.
- Remember, persons you may least suspect, family members or visitors, might look for drugs like methadone to use for illegal purposes.
- Never share your methadone with anyone else, since it could do them great harm.

Continued

Form IV-8 | Patient medication information: methadone.

As appears in Pasero, C., & McCaffery, M. (2011). *Pain assessment and pharmacologic management*, pp. 560-561, St. Louis, Mosby. From Leavitt, S. B. (2008). Methadone safety handout for patients. *Pain Treatment Topics.* Available at http://pain-topics.org/pdf/MethadoneHandout.pdf. Accessed Sept. 30, 2009.

PATIENT MEDICATION INFORMATION—cont'd

Methadone (generic name)

What are methadone side effects to watch for?

- Alert your family members or caretakers of ***important warning signs*** to watch for that may indicate you are reacting badly to methadone and are in distress. If you experience any of the following, they should call for emergency help:
  - Trouble staying awake.
  - Difficult or slow breathing.
  - Loud or unusual snoring at night and difficulty being awakened.
  - Fast heartbeat, unusual dizziness, or loss of consciousness (fainting).
- Methadone, like all other opioids, may cause constipation. Your health care provider or pharmacist can recommend approaches for preventing or treating this. Reducing the methadone dose will *not* help.
- Certain side effects, if they occur at all, usually become milder or go away with time, such as a lightheaded feeling, nausea, stomach upset, or mild drowsiness. Possible others may be more long-lasting, including: itching, dry mouth, flushing, or increased sweating. Contact your health care provider if any of these continue or worsen.
- Uncommon side effects include confusion, mood changes (depression or agitation), shaking, blurred vision, or difficulty urinating. If you experience any of these, tell your health care provider.
- Allergic reactions to methadone—including rash, hives, or swelling—are rare but require prompt medical attention.
- You should refrain from driving and other activities requiring balance or focused concentration until the effects of methadone are known, typically a week or longer.

Will you become dependent on or addicted to methadone?

- After awhile, methadone causes *physical dependence*. That is, if you suddenly stop the medication you may experience uncomfortable withdrawal symptoms, such as diarrhea, body aches, weakness, restlessness, anxiety, loss of appetite, and other ill feelings. These may take several days to develop.
- This is not the same as *addiction,* a disease involving craving for the drug, loss of control over taking it or compulsive use, and using it despite harm. Addiction to methadone in persons without a recent history of alcohol or drug problems is rare.
- If you ever want to stop taking methadone, do not do so on your own. Gradually reducing the methadone dose as directed by your health care provider will help prevent uncomfortable withdrawal reactions.

Form IV-8 | Cont'd.

PATIENT MEDICATION INFORMATION

Morphine Sulfate (generic name) short-acting

BRAND NAMES: Roxanol®, Morphine Sulfate®

TYPE OF PAIN MEDICINE: Opioid (narcotic), short-acting. Tablets are sometimes called immediate-release (IR).

DESCRIPTION: Morphine sulfate short-acting comes in pills and liquids. Common examples are listed below.

Tablets:
- Morphine Sulfate 15 mg tablet, also available in 30 mg.

Liquids:
- Morphine Sulfate 10 mg/5 ml Solution (10 mg per teaspoon), also available in 20 mg/5 mL (20 mg per teaspoon).
- Roxanol Concentrated 20 mg/ml Solution. 100 mg/5 ml = 100 mg/teaspoon.

USES:
Relieves pain.
Sometimes used to control cough or shortness of breath.
Often used for breakthrough pain (rescue doses) when other medicine is being taken around the clock for persistent pain.

DOSAGE AND ADMINISTRATION:
- Take only as directed.
- These directions may change.
- For liquids, doses are prescribed in mL (milliliters) or mg (milligrams). Be careful not to confuse the two. They are not the same.
- When measuring liquid morphine, do not use regular teaspoons or tablespoons since they are not accurate enough. Measure your dose with a dropper, medicine cup, or syringe. If one of these does not come with your medicine, ask the pharmacist for one.
- You should feel pain relief in 30 to 60 minutes.
- Usually taken every 3 to 4 hours.
- You may need to adjust your schedule. If so, call your nurse or doctor.
- There is no maximum dose or amount that your doctor may prescribe for you, but the amount may be limited by state and federal laws, prescription plan rules, and pharmacy supply.
- May be taken alone or in addition to other pain medicines.
- May be taken with or without food.
- May be taken with other medicines.
- If you miss a dose of your medicine, take it as soon as possible. If it is almost time for the next dose, skip the missed dose. Do not take two doses at one time.
- Tell your nurse or doctor if you are pregnant, plan to become pregnant, or are breast-feeding.
- Tell your doctor, nurse, and pharmacist about all medicines you take.
- If you are having difficulty swallowing, talk with your nurse or doctor about the possibility of suppositories. Morphine Sulfate Rectal Suppository is available in 5 mg, 10 mg, 20 mg, and 30 mg.

POSSIBLE SIDE EFFECTS:
- Constipation. Opioids block pain and block bowels. Constipation can be controlled with daily laxatives such as Senokot-S. Try to drink 8 large glasses of fluid a day. Increase your activity by walking or exercising. (For more helpful information, see Constipation Caused by Opioids form.)

Continued

Form IV-9 | Patient medication information: morphine sulfate, short-acting.

PATIENT MEDICATION INFORMATION—cont'd

Morphine Sulfate (generic name) short-acting

- Nausea and vomiting. Take your medicine with food to lessen this. If nausea and vomiting continue, call your nurse or doctor. May be controlled with medicines.
- Drowsiness. May occur when starting morphine or increasing the dose. This usually goes away in about 2 to 3 days. Rest as needed.
- Confusion. This is less common than drowsiness. If this happens, call your nurse or doctor.

PRECAUTIONS:
- Be careful driving or using machinery such as lawn mowers, power tools, or saws. Do not do these things if you are drowsy.
- Be careful when drinking alcohol. Alcohol will increase drowsiness.
- Call your doctor or nurse if pain increases or if you do not get pain relief.
- Protect liquid morphine from the light. Discard 90 days after opening.

STOPPING MEDICATIONS: Do not suddenly stop taking your medicine. Opioids must be stopped gradually. Call your pharmacist, nurse, or doctor before you stop taking your medicine.

REMEMBER!
- Keep count of your medicine.
- Do not mix medicines in the same container.
- Do not run out of medicine.
- Prescriptions for this medicine cannot be refilled or phoned in to your pharmacy.
- Get a **new** prescription filled a few days before you will run out of medicine.
- **Call** your nurse or doctor if side effects occur or if pain changes or does not go away. Your medicine may need to be changed.
- Take unused, unneeded, or expired medicines out of their original containers and flush them down the toilet. Do not put them in the trash.

COMMENTS:

- Warning: Keep this medicine out of reach of children! A dose could be fatal to a child.
- Be sure to keep this medicine in a safe place out of sight of others. A locked box may be indicated to prevent someone else from taking this medicine.

Form IV-9 | Cont'd.

PATIENT MEDICATION INFORMATION

Morphine Sulfate Modified-Release (generic name) every <u>12-hour dosing</u>

BRAND NAMES: MS Contin®, Morphine Sulfate Extended-Release®

TYPE OF PAIN MEDICINE: Opioid (narcotic). Sometimes called long-acting, extended-release, or controlled-release.

DESCRIPTION: Available in tablets.

<u>MS Contin</u> tablets are available in 15 mg, 30 mg, 60 mg, 100 mg, and 200 mg.
<u>Morphine Sulfate Extended-Release</u> tablets are available in 15 mg, 30 mg, 60 mg, 100 mg, and 200 mg.

USES:
Relieves pain.

DOSAGE AND ADMINISTRATION:
- <u>Take only as directed.</u>
- These directions may change.
- Usually taken every 12 hours, sometimes every 8 hours.
- Take at the same time every day.
- Do not chew, crush, or dissolve tablets. You may get too much medicine too fast, resulting in an overdose.
- Be sure to take your doses of modified-release morphine at the same time each day. With your first dose of MS Contin you should feel pain relief in about 2 to 3 hours. Then if you take your medicine on a regular schedule, pain relief should be about the same 24 hours a day. If pain returns before the next dose, call your doctor or nurse. Your dose or time between doses may need to be changed.
- There is no maximum dose or amount that your doctor may prescribe for you, but the amount may be limited by state and federal laws, prescription plan rules, and pharmacy supply.
- May be taken alone or in addition to other pain medicines.
- May be taken with or without food.
- May be taken with other medicines.
- <u>If you miss a dose</u> of your medicine, take it as soon as possible. If it has been longer than 2 to 3 hours since the missed dose, skip the missed dose. Call your nurse or doctor for directions. Do not take two doses at one time. If you have medicine for breakthrough pain (rescue doses) you may use this to treat your pain until it is time for your next dose of modified-release morphine.
- To avoid missing a dose of modified-release morphine, consider taking <u>one</u> dose with you when you leave home for several hours.
- If you are pregnant, planning to get pregnant, or breast-feeding, tell your nurse or doctor.
- You may see empty tablets in your stool. Do not worry. The medicine is in your body.

POSSIBLE SIDE EFFECTS:
- Constipation. Opioids block pain and block bowels. Constipation can be controlled with daily laxatives such as Senokot-S. Try to drink 8 large glasses of fluid a day. Increase your activity by walking or exercising. (For more helpful information, see Constipation Caused by Opioids form.)
- Nausea and vomiting. Take your medicine with food to lessen this. If nausea and vomiting continue, call your nurse or doctor. May be controlled with medicines.
- Drowsiness. May occur when starting morphine or increasing the dose. This usually goes away in about 2 to 3 days. Rest as needed.
- Confusion. This is less common than drowsiness. If this happens, call your nurse or doctor.

Continued

Form IV-10 | Patient medication information: morphine sulfate, modified-release, 12-hour dosing.

PATIENT MEDICATION INFORMATION—cont'd

Morphine Sulfate Modified-Release (generic name) every <u>12-hour dosing</u>

PRECAUTIONS:
- Be careful driving or using machinery such as lawn mowers, power tools, or saws. Do not do these things if you are drowsy.
- Be careful when drinking alcohol. Alcohol will increase drowsiness.
- Call your doctor or nurse if pain increases or if you do not get pain relief.

STOPPING MEDICATIONS: Do not suddenly stop taking your medicine. Opioids must be stopped gradually. Call your pharmacist, nurse, or doctor before you stop taking your medicine.

REMEMBER!
- Keep count of your medicine.
- Do not mix medicines in the same container.
- Do not run out of medicine.
- Prescriptions for this medicine cannot be <u>re</u>filled or phoned in to your pharmacy.
- Get a **new** prescription filled a few days before you will run out of medicine.
- <u>**Call**</u> your nurse or doctor if side effects occur or if pain changes or does not go away. Your medicine may need to be changed.
- Take unused, unneeded, or expired medicines out of their original containers and flush them down the toilet. Do not put them in the trash.
- Ask your <u>pharmacy not to substitute another brand</u> for the one you are taking. Although a different brand may have the same amount of morphine, it is distributed differently in the body. If a switch is necessary, call your nurse or doctor to inform them and ask about any differences you should know about.

COMMENTS:

- <u>Warning</u>: Keep this medicine out of reach of children! A dose could be fatal to a child.
- <u>Be sure to keep this medicine in a safe place out of sight of others</u>. A locked box may be indicated to prevent someone else from taking this medicine.

Form IV-10 | Cont'd.

PATIENT MEDICATION INFORMATION

Morphine Sulfate Modified-Release (generic name) every <u>24-hour dosing</u>

BRAND NAMES: Avinza®, Kadian®

TYPE OF PAIN MEDICINE: Opioid (narcotic). Sometimes called long-acting, extended-release, or controlled-release.

DESCRIPTION: Available in capsules.

<u>Avinza</u> Extended-Release Capsules are available in 30 mg, 60 mg, 90 mg, and 120 mg.
<u>Kadian</u> Extended-Release capsules are available in 10 mg, 20 mg, 30 mg, 50 mg, 60 mg, 80 mg, 100 mg, and 200 mg.

USES:
Relieves pain.

DOSAGE AND ADMINISTRATION:

- <u>Take only as directed.</u>
- These directions may change.
- Usually taken every 24 hours, sometimes every 12 hours. Take at the same time each day.
- You may need to adjust your schedule. If so, call your nurse or doctor.
- Do not chew, crush, or dissolve capsules. You may get too much medicine too fast.
- With your first dose of Avinza you should feel pain relief in about 30 to 45 minutes. With Kadian it takes longer to feel pain relief, up to a few hours. Then if you take your medicine on a regular schedule every 12 or 24 hours, pain relief should be about the same 24 hours a day. If pain returns before the next dose, call your doctor or nurse. Your dose or time between doses may need to be changed.
- There is no maximum dose or amount of Kadian that your doctor may prescribe for you. However, the maximum limit of Avinza is 1600 mg/day due to the possibility of kidney problems (from fumaric acid).
- May be taken alone or in addition to other pain medicines.
- May be taken with or without food.
- With AVINZA DO NOT TAKE ALCOHOL or any alcohol-containing medicines. Alcohol may cause the total dose to be released at once, resulting in an overdose. Alcohol may be consumed with Kadian but may make you drowsy.
- May be taken with other medicines.
- If you <u>miss a dose</u> of your medicine, take it as soon as possible based on the directions below:
  - If you are taking the medicine <u>every 24 hours</u> and you miss your dose for longer than 4 to 6 hours, skip the missed dose. Call your nurse or doctor for directions. If you have medicine for breakthrough pain (rescue doses) you may use these to treat your pain until it is time for your next dose of Avinza or Kadian.
  - If you are taking the medicine <u>every 12 hours</u> and you miss your dose for longer than 2 to 3 hours, skip the missed dose. Call your nurse or doctor for directions. Do not take two doses at one time. If you have medicine for breakthrough pain (rescue doses) you may use this to treat your pain until it is time for your next dose of Kadian or Avinza.
- If you are pregnant, planning to get pregnant, or breast-feeding, tell your nurse or doctor.
- There are two other ways to take these capsules.
  (1) If you have <u>difficulty swallowing</u> the capsules, try the following. Immediately before using, capsules may be opened and the contents sprinkled on a small amount of applesauce (at room temperature or cooler). Do not use foods other than applesauce. Swallow mixture right away without chewing or crushing the pellets. Be sure to eat all the applesauce so that you get all the medicine. Rinse your mouth and swallow to be sure you have gotten all the medicine.

Continued

Form IV-11 | Patient medication information: morphine sulfate, modified-release, 24-hour dosing.

PATIENT MEDICATION INFORMATION—cont'd

Morphine Sulfate Modified-Release (generic name) every 24-hour dosing

(2) If you have a gastrostomy tube, try the following. Capsules may be administered through a 16 French gastrostomy (stomach) tube (not a nasogastric tube which is inserted into the nose and down to the stomach). Flush the tube with 4 ounces of water. Sprinkle the capsule contents into 2 teaspoons to 1 ounce of water or apple juice in a container. Using a funnel and a swirling motion, pour water or apple juice mixed with pellets into the tube. Fill the container with about 2 teaspoons of water and pour into funnel. Repeat until no pellets remain in the container.

POSSIBLE SIDE EFFECTS:
• Constipation. Opioids block pain and block bowels. Constipation can be controlled with daily laxatives such as Senokot-S. Try to drink 8 large glasses of fluid a day. Increase your activity by walking or exercising. (For more helpful information, see Constipation Caused by Opioids form.)
• Nausea and vomiting. Take your medicine with food or milk to lessen this. If nausea and vomiting continue, call your nurse or doctor. May be controlled with medicines.
• Drowsiness. May occur when starting this medicine or increasing the dose. This usually goes away in about 2 to 3 days. Rest as needed.
• Confusion. This is less common than drowsiness. If this happens, call your nurse or doctor.

PRECAUTIONS:
• Be careful driving or using machinery such as lawn mowers, power tools, or saws. Do not do these things if you are drowsy.
• Be careful when drinking alcohol with Kadian. Alcohol will increase drowsiness.
• DO NOT USE ALCOHOL WITH AVINZA since it may result in an overdose. Check the contents of all liquid medicines to be sure they do not contain alcohol. Ask your pharmacist if you are not sure.
• Call your doctor or nurse if pain increases or if you do not get pain relief.

STOPPING MEDICATIONS: Do not suddenly stop taking your medicine. Opioids must be stopped gradually. Call your pharmacist, nurse, or doctor before you stop taking your medicine.

REMEMBER!
• Keep count of your medicine.
• Do not mix medicines in the same container.
• Do not run out of medicine.
• Prescriptions for this medicine cannot be refilled or phoned in to your pharmacy.
• Ask your pharmacy not to substitute another brand for the one you are taking. Although Avinza and Kadian have the same amount of morphine, it is distributed differently in the body.
• Get a **new** prescription filled a few days before you will run out of medicine.
• **Call** your nurse or doctor if side effects occur or if pain changes or does not go away. Your medicine may need to be changed.
• Take unused, unneeded, or expired medicines out of their original containers and flush them down the toilet. Do not put them in the trash.

COMMENTS:

• Warning: Keep this medicine out of reach of children! A dose could be fatal to a child.
• Be sure to keep this medicine in a safe place out of sight of others. A locked box may be indicated to prevent someone else from taking this medicine.

PATIENT MEDICATION INFORMATION

Oxycodone (generic name) short-acting

BRAND NAMES: Roxicodone®, OxyFast®, and generics

TYPE OF PAIN MEDICINE: Opioid (narcotic), short-acting. Sometimes called immediate-release.

DESCRIPTION: Oxycodone short-acting comes in pills and liquid. Common examples are listed below.

Tablets/capsules:
- Roxicodone tablets come in 5 mg, 15 mg, and 30 mg.
- Oxycodone capsules come in 5 mg.

Liquid:
- Roxicodone comes in 5 mg/5 mL (5 mg per teaspoon).
- Roxicodone comes in 20 mg/mL (NOTE: this is very concentrated).
- OxyFast comes in 20 mg/mL.

USES:
Relieves pain.
Often used for breakthrough pain (rescue doses) when other medicine is being taken around the clock for persistent pain.

DOSAGE AND ADMINISTRATION:
- Take only as directed.
- These directions may change.
- For liquids, doses are prescribed in mL (milliliters) or mg (milligrams). Be careful not to confuse the two. They are not the same.
- When measuring liquid oxycodone, do not use regular teaspoons or tablespoons since they are not accurate enough. Measure your dose with a dropper, medicine cup, or syringe. If one of these does not come with your medicine, ask the pharmacist for one.
- You should feel pain relief in 30 to 60 minutes.
- Usually taken every 3 to 4 hours.
- You may need to adjust your schedule. If so, call your nurse or doctor.
- There is no maximum dose or amount that your doctor may prescribe for you, but the amount may be limited by state and federal laws, prescription plan rules, and pharmacy supply.
- May be taken alone or in addition to other pain medicines.
- May be taken with or without food.
- May be taken with other medicines.
- If you miss a dose of your medicine, take it as soon as possible. If it is almost time for the next dose, skip the missed dose. Do not take two doses at one time.
- Tell your nurse or doctor if you are pregnant, plan to become pregnant, or are breast-feeding.
- Tell your doctor, nurse, and pharmacist about all medicines you take.

POSSIBLE SIDE EFFECTS:
- Constipation. Opioids block pain and block bowels. Constipation can be controlled with daily laxatives such as Senokot-S. Try to drink 8 large glasses of fluid a day. Increase your activity by walking or exercising. (For more helpful information, see Constipation Caused by Opioids form.)

Continued

Form IV-12 | Patient medication information: oxycodone, short-acting.

As appears in Pasero, C., & McCaffery, M. (2011). *Pain assessment and pharmacologic management*, pp. 568-569, St. Louis, Mosby. Modified from Fox Chase Cancer Center/Pain Management, Philadelphia, 2007. May be duplicated for use in clinical practice.

PATIENT MEDICATION INFORMATION—cont'd

Oxycodone (generic name) short-acting

- Nausea and vomiting. Take your medicine with food to lessen this. If nausea and vomiting continue, call your nurse or doctor. May be controlled with medicines.
- Drowsiness. May occur when starting oxycodone or increasing the dose. This usually goes away in about 2 to 3 days. Rest as needed.
- Confusion. This is less common than drowsiness. If this happens, call your nurse or doctor.

PRECAUTIONS:
- Be careful driving or using machinery such as lawn mowers, power tools, or saws. Do not do these things if you are drowsy.
- Be careful when drinking alcohol. Alcohol will increase drowsiness.
- Call your doctor or nurse if pain increases or if you do not get pain relief.

STOPPING MEDICATIONS: Do not suddenly stop taking your medicine. Opioids must be stopped gradually. Call your pharmacist, nurse, or doctor before you stop taking your medicine.

REMEMBER!
- Keep count of your medicine.
- Do not mix medicines in the same container.
- Do not run out of medicine.
- Prescriptions for this medicine cannot be <u>re</u>filled or phoned in to your pharmacy.
- Get a **<u>new</u>** prescription filled a few days before you will run out of medicine.
- **<u>Call</u>** your nurse or doctor if side effects occur or if pain changes or does not go away. Your medicine may need to be changed.
- Take unused, unneeded, or expired medicines out of their original containers and flush them down the toilet. Do not put them in the trash.

COMMENTS:

- <u>Warning</u>: Keep this medicine out of reach of children! A dose could be fatal to a child.
- <u>Be sure to keep this medicine in a safe place out of sight of others</u>. A locked box may be indicated to prevent someone else from taking this medicine.

Form IV-12 | Cont'd.

PATIENT MEDICATION INFORMATION

Oxycodone Modified-Release (generic name)

BRAND NAME: OxyContin® Extended-Release

TYPE OF PAIN MEDICINE: Opioid (narcotic). Sometimes called long-acting, extended-release, or controlled-release.

DESCRIPTION: OxyContin Extended-Release tablets available in 10 mg, 15 mg, 20 mg, 30 mg, 40 mg, 60 mg, and 80 mg.

USES:
Relieves pain.

DOSAGE AND ADMINISTRATION:
• <u>Take only as directed.</u>
• These directions may change.
• Usually taken every 12 hours, sometimes every 8 hours.
• Take at the same time every day.
• With your first dose you should feel pain relief within about an hour. Then if you take your medicine on a regular schedule, pain relief should be about the same 24 hours a day. If pain regularly returns before the next dose, discuss this with your doctor or nurse. Your dose or time between doses may need to be changed.
• Do not chew, crush, or dissolve tablets of OxyContin. You may get too much medicine too fast.
• There is no maximum dose or amount that your doctor may prescribe for you, but the amount may be limited by state and federal laws, prescription plan rules, and pharmacy supply.
• May be taken alone or in addition to other pain medicines.
• May be taken with or without food.
• May be taken with other medicines.
• If you are taking OxyContin every 12 hours and you <u>miss a dose</u> of your medicine, take it as soon as possible. If it has been longer than 2 to 3 hours since the missed dose, skip the missed dose. Call your nurse or doctor for directions. Do not take two doses at one time. If you have medicine for breakthrough pain (rescue doses) you may use this to treat your pain until it is time for your next dose of OxyContin.
• To avoid missing a dose of OxyContin, consider taking <u>one</u> dose with you when you leave home for several hours.
• If you are pregnant, planning to get pregnant, or breast-feeding, tell your nurse or doctor.
• You may see empty tablets in your stool. Do not worry. The medicine is in your body.

POSSIBLE SIDE EFFECTS:
• Constipation. Opioids block pain and block bowels. Constipation can be controlled with daily laxatives such as Senokot-S. Try to drink 8 large glasses of fluid a day. Increase your activity by walking or exercising. (For more helpful information, see Constipation Caused by Opioids form.)
• Nausea and vomiting. Take your medicine with food to lessen this. If nausea and vomiting continue, call your nurse or doctor. May be controlled with medicines.
• Drowsiness. May occur when starting OxyContin or increasing the dose. This usually goes away in about 2 to 3 days. Rest as needed.
• Confusion. This is less common than drowsiness. If this happens, call your nurse or doctor.

Continued

Form IV-13 | Patient medication information: oxycodone, modified-release.

PATIENT MEDICATION INFORMATION—cont'd

Oxycodone Modified-Release (generic name)

PRECAUTIONS:
- Be careful driving or using machinery such as lawn mowers, power tools, or saws. Do not do these things if you are drowsy.
- Be careful when drinking alcohol. Alcohol will increase drowsiness.
- Call your doctor or nurse if pain increases or if you do not get pain relief.

STOPPING MEDICATIONS: Do not suddenly stop taking your medicine. Opioids must be stopped gradually. Call your pharmacist, nurse, or doctor before you stop taking your medicine.

REMEMBER!
- Keep count of your medicine.
- Do not mix medicines in the same container.
- Do not run out of medicine.
- Prescriptions for this medicine cannot be <u>re</u>filled or phoned in to your pharmacy.
- Get a **new** prescription filled a few days before you will run out of medicine.
- **Call** your nurse or doctor if side effects occur or if pain changes or does not go away. Your medicine may need to be changed.
- Take unused, unneeded, or expired medicines out of their original containers and flush them down the toilet. Do not put them in the trash.

COMMENTS:

- <u>Warning</u>: Keep this medicine out of reach of children! A dose could be fatal to a child.
- <u>Be sure to keep this medicine in a safe place out of sight of others</u>. A locked box may be indicated to prevent someone else from taking this medicine.

Form IV-13 | Cont'd.

PATIENT MEDICATION INFORMATION

Oxycodone with Acetaminophen (generic name)

BRAND NAMES: Percocet®, Tylox®, Roxicet®

TYPE OF PAIN MEDICINE: Opioid (narcotic) and nonopioid

DESCRIPTION: Oxycodone plus acetaminophen comes in pill or liquid form. Acetaminophen is the same as Tylenol®. There are several brands and combinations of oxycodone and acetaminophen as well as generics. Common examples are listed below.

Tablets/caplets:

• Percocet 2.5/325 contains oxycodone 2.5 mg plus acetaminophen 325 mg.
• Percocet 5/325 contains oxycodone 5 mg plus acetaminophen 325 mg.
• Percocet 7.5/500 contains oxycodone 7.5 mg plus acetaminophen 500 mg.
• Tylox® 5/500 contains oxycodone 5 mg plus acetaminophen 500 mg.

Liquid:

• Roxicet®. One teaspoon contains oxycodone 5 mg plus acetaminophen 325 mg.

USES:
Relieves pain.

DOSAGE AND ADMINISTRATION:
• Take only as directed.
• These directions may change.
• You should feel pain relief in 30 to 60 minutes.
• Usually 1 to 2 tablets/caplets are taken every 3 to 4 hours. Take at the first sign of pain.
• The maximum number of tablets/caplets allowed in any 24-hour period is limited by the amount of acetaminophen. Do not take more than 4000 mg acetaminophen in 24 hours. For example, do not take more than 8 Tylox® 5/500 or 12 Percocet with acetaminophen 325 mg in 24 hours. Some patients should take less than 4000 mg; check with your nurse or doctor. Be aware that other medicines that you take such as certain cold medicines or sleep medicines may have acetaminophen in them.
• May be taken alone or in addition to other pain medicines.
• May be taken with or without food.
• May be taken with other medicines.
• Tell your nurse or doctor if you are pregnant, plan to become pregnant, or are breast-feeding.
• Tell your doctor, nurse, and pharmacist about all medicines you take.

POSSIBLE SIDE EFFECTS:
• Constipation. Opioids block pain and block bowels. Constipation can be controlled with daily laxatives such as Senokot-S. Try to drink 8 large glasses of fluid a day. Increase your activity by walking or exercising. (For more helpful information, see Constipation Caused by Opioids form.)
• Nausea and vomiting. Take your medicine with food to lessen this. If nausea and vomiting continue, call your nurse or doctor. May be controlled with medicines.
• Drowsiness. May occur when starting oxycodone plus acetaminophen or increasing the dose. This usually goes away in about 2 to 3 days. Rest as needed.
• Confusion. This is less common than drowsiness. If this happens, call your nurse or doctor.

Form IV-14 | Patient medication information: oxycodone with acetaminophen.

As appears in Pasero, C., & McCaffery, M. (2011). *Pain assessment and pharmacologic management*, pp. 572-573, St. Louis, Mosby. Modified from Fox Chase Cancer Center/Pain Management, Philadelphia, 2008. May be duplicated for use in clinical practice.

PATIENT MEDICATION INFORMATION—cont'd

Oxycodone with Acetaminophen (generic name)

PRECAUTIONS:
- Be careful driving or using machinery such as lawn mowers, power tools, or saws. Do not do these things if you are drowsy.
- Be careful when drinking alcohol. Alcohol will increase drowsiness. Your medicine contains acetaminophen, and drinking alcohol with acetaminophen may increase risk of liver damage.
- Call your doctor or nurse if pain increases or if you do not get pain relief.

STOPPING MEDICATIONS: Do not suddenly stop taking your medicine. Opioids must be stopped gradually. Call your pharmacist, nurse, or doctor before you stop taking your medicine.

REMEMBER!
- Keep count of your medicine.
- Do not mix medicines in the same container.
- Do not run out of medicine.
- Prescriptions for this medicine cannot be <u>re</u>filled or phoned in to your pharmacy.
- Get a **new** prescription filled a few days before you will run out of medicine.
- **Call** your nurse or doctor if side effects occur or if pain changes or does not go away. Your medicine may need to be changed.
- Take unused, unneeded, or expired medicines out of their original containers and flush them down the toilet. Do not put them in the trash.

COMMENTS:

- <u>Warning</u>: Keep this medicine out of reach of children! A dose could be fatal to a child.
- <u>Be sure to keep this medicine in a safe place out of sight of others</u>. A locked box may be indicated to prevent someone else from taking this medicine.

Form IV-14 | Cont'd.

PATIENT MEDICATION INFORMATION

Oxymorphone (generic name) short-acting

BRAND NAME: Opana®

TYPE OF PAIN MEDICINE: Opioid (narcotic), short-acting. Sometimes called immediate-release.

DESCRIPTION: Opana is available in tablets:
- Opana 5 mg tablet
- Opana 10 mg tablet

USES:

Relieves pain.

Sometimes used for breakthrough pain (rescue doses) when other medicine is taken around the clock for persistent pain.

DOSAGE AND ADMINISTRATION:
- <u>Take only as directed.</u>
- These directions may change.
- You should feel pain relief in 30 to 45 minutes.
- Usually taken every 4 to 6 hours.
- You may need to adjust your schedule. If so, call your nurse or doctor.
- There is no maximum dose or amount that your doctor may prescribe for you, but the amount may be limited by state and federal laws, prescription plan rules, and pharmacy supply.
- <u>May not be taken with food.</u> Opana should be taken on an empty stomach, 1 hour before eating or 2 hours after eating.
- <u>Do not use alcohol or alcohol-containing medicines</u> with Opana. Alcohol may increase the release of Opana and possibly cause an overdose.
- May be taken alone or in addition to other pain medicines, except those containing alcohol.
- May be taken with other medicines, except those containing alcohol.
- If you miss a dose of your medicine, take it as soon as possible. If it is almost time for the next dose, skip the missed dose. Do not take two doses at one time.
- Tell your nurse or doctor if you are pregnant, plan to become pregnant, or are breast-feeding.
- Tell your doctor, nurse, and pharmacist about all medicines you take, especially antipsychotics (phenothiazines such as Compazine) or amphetamines.
- If you are having difficulty swallowing, talk with your nurse or doctor about the possibility of a <u>suppository</u>. Oxymorphone is available as Numorphan 5 mg rectal suppository.

POSSIBLE SIDE EFFECTS:
- Constipation. Opioids block pain and block bowels. Constipation can be controlled with daily laxatives such as Senokot-S. Try to drink 8 large glasses of fluid a day. Increase your activity by walking or exercising. (For more helpful information, see Constipation Caused by Opioids form.)
- Nausea and vomiting. Call your nurse or doctor. May be controlled with medicines.
- Drowsiness. May occur when starting Opana or increasing the dose. This usually goes away in about 2 to 3 days. Rest as needed.
- Confusion. This is less common than drowsiness. If this happens, call your nurse or doctor.

Continued

Form IV-15 | Patient medication information: oxymorphone.

From Pasero, C., & McCaffery, M. *Pain assessment and pharmacologic management*, pp. 574-575, St. Louis, Mosby. © 2011, McCaffery M, Pasero C. May be duplicated for use in clinical practice.

PATIENT MEDICATION INFORMATION—cont'd

Oxymorphone (generic name) short-acting

PRECAUTIONS:
- Be careful driving or using machinery such as lawn mowers, power tools, or saws. Do not do these things if you are drowsy.
- Do not drink alcohol or alcohol-containing medicines when you are taking Opana. Alcohol may increase the release of Opana and possibly cause an overdose.
- Call your doctor or nurse if pain increases or if you do not get pain relief.

STOPPING MEDICATIONS: Do not suddenly stop taking your medicine. Opioids must be stopped gradually. Call your pharmacist, nurse, or doctor before you stop taking your medicine.

REMEMBER!
- Keep count of your medicine.
- Do not mix medicines in the same container.
- Do not run out of medicine.
- Prescriptions for this medicine cannot be <u>re</u>filled or phoned in to your pharmacy.
- Get a **new** prescription filled a few days before you will run out of medicine.
- **Call** your nurse or doctor if side effects occur or if pain changes or does not go away. Your medicine may need to be changed.
- Take unused, unneeded, or expired medicines out of their original containers and flush them down the toilet. Do not put them in the trash.

COMMENTS:

- <u>Warning</u>: Keep this medicine out of reach of children! A dose could be fatal to a child.
- <u>Be sure to keep this medicine in a safe place out of sight of others</u>. A locked box may be indicated to prevent someone else from taking this medicine.

Form IV-15 Cont'd.

PATIENT MEDICATION INFORMATION

Oxymorphone Modified-Release (generic name)

BRAND NAME: Opana® ER

TYPE OF PAIN MEDICINE: Opioid (narcotic), modified-release

DESCRIPTION: Sometimes called long-acting or extended-release. Available in tablets: Opana® ER comes in 5 mg, 7.5 mg, 10 mg, 15 mg, 20 mg, 30 mg, 40 mg,

USES:
Relieves pain.

DOSAGE AND ADMINISTRATION:
- <u>Take only as directed.</u>
- These directions may change.
- Usually taken every 12 hours.
- You may need to adjust your schedule. If so, call your nurse or doctor.
- With the first dose of Opana ER you may begin to feel some pain relief within 30 minutes to an hour. If you take your medicine on a regular schedule every 12 hours, pain relief should be about the same 24 hours a day. If pain returns before the next dose, call your doctor or nurse. Your dose or time between doses may need to be changed.
- Do not chew, crush, or dissolve tablets of Opana ER. You may get too much medicine too fast.
- There is no maximum dose or amount that your doctor may prescribe for you, but the amount may be limited by state and federal laws, prescription plan rules, and pharmacy supply.
- <u>May not be taken with food.</u> Opana ER should be taken on an empty stomach 1 hour before eating or 2 hours after eating.
- <u>Do not use alcohol or alcohol-containing medicines</u> with Opana ER. Alcohol may increase the release of Opana ER and possibly cause an overdose.
- May be taken alone or in addition to other pain medicines, except those containing alcohol.
- May be taken with other medicines, except those containing alcohol.
- <u>If you miss a dose</u> of your medicine, take it as soon as possible. If it has been longer than 2 to 3 hours since the missed dose, skip the missed dose and call your nurse or doctor for directions. Do not take two doses at one time. If you have medicine for breakthrough pain (rescue doses) you may use this to treat your pain until it is time for your next dose of Opana ER.
- Tell your nurse or doctor if you are pregnant, plan to become pregnant, or are breast-feeding.
- Tell your doctor, nurse, and pharmacist about all medicines you take, especially antipsychotics (phenothiazines such as Compazine) or amphetamines.
- If you are having difficulty swallowing, talk with your nurse or doctor about the possibility of a <u>suppository</u>. Oxymorphone is available as Numorphan 5 mg rectal suppository.

POSSIBLE SIDE EFFECTS:
- Constipation. Opioids block pain and block bowels. Constipation can be controlled with daily laxatives such as Senokot-S. Try to drink 8 large glasses of fluid a day. Increase your activity by walking or exercising. (For more helpful information, see Constipation Caused by Opioids form.)
- Nausea and vomiting. Call your nurse or doctor. May be controlled with medicines.
- Drowsiness. May occur when starting Opana ER or increasing the dose. This usually goes away in about 2 to 3 days. Rest as needed.

Continued

Form IV-16 | Patient medication information: oxymorphone, modified-release.

PATIENT MEDICATION INFORMATION—cont'd

Oxymorphone Modified-Release (generic name)

- Dryness of the mouth. Chewing sugarless gum or sucking hard candy, and drinking plenty of water may help.
- Dried eyes and blurred vision. If you wear contact lenses you may feel some discomfort. Lubricating drops may help. If this is severe or does not go away, call your nurse or doctor.
- Confusion. This is less common than drowsiness. If this happens, call your nurse or doctor.

PRECAUTIONS:
- Be careful driving or using machinery such as lawn mowers, power tools, or saws. Do not do these things if you are drowsy.
- Do not drink alcohol or alcohol-containing medicines when you are taking Opana ER. Alcohol may increase the release of Opana ER and possibly cause an overdose.
- Call your doctor or nurse if pain increases or if you do not get pain relief.

STOPPING MEDICATIONS: Do not suddenly stop taking your medicine. Opioids must be stopped gradually. Call your pharmacist, nurse, or doctor before you stop taking your medicine.

REMEMBER!
- Keep count of your medicine.
- Do not mix medicines in the same container.
- Do not run out of medicine.
- Prescriptions for this medicine cannot be <u>re</u>filled or phoned in to your pharmacy.
- Get a **new** prescription filled a few days before you will run out of medicine.
- <u>**Call**</u> your nurse or doctor if side effects occur or if pain changes or does not go away. Your medicine may need to be changed.
- Take unused, unneeded, or expired medicines out of their original containers and flush them down the toilet. Do not put them in the trash.

COMMENTS:

- <u>Warning</u>: Keep this medicine out of reach of children! A dose could be fatal to a child.
- <u>Be sure to keep this medicine in a safe place out of sight of others</u>. A locked box may be indicated to prevent someone else from taking this medicine.

Form IV-16 | Cont'd.

PATIENT MEDICATION INFORMATION

Propoxyphene Napsylate with Acetaminophen (generic name)

BRAND NAME: Darvocet®

TYPE OF PAIN MEDICINE: Opioid (narcotic) and nonopioid

DESCRIPTION: Darvocet is made up of 2 medicines: propoxyphene napsylate and acetaminophen. Acetaminophen is the same as Tylenol®.

Darvocet® comes In three strengths:
• Darvocet-N® 50—propoxyphene 50 mg + acetaminophen 325 mg
• Darvocet-N® 100—propoxyphene 100 mg + acetaminophen 650 mg
• Darvocet A-500®—propoxyphene 100 mg + acetaminophen 500 mg

USES:
Relieves mild to moderate pain.

DOSAGE AND ADMINISTRATION:
• <u>Take only as directed.</u>
• These directions may change.
• You should feel pain relief in 30 to 60 minutes.
• Usually taken every 4 hours. Take at the first sign of pain.
• Do not take more than 600 mg of propoxyphene in 24 hours.
• Do not take more than 4000 mg acetaminophen in 24 hours. Some patients should take less than 4000 mg; check with your nurse or doctor. Be aware that other medicines that you take such as certain cold medicines or sleep medicines may have acetaminophen in them.
• May be taken alone or in addition to other pain medicines.
• May be taken with or without food.
• May be taken with other medicines.
• One to two Darvocet-N® 50 may be taken every 4 hours, but only one Darvocet-N® 100 or one Darvocet A500® may be taken every 4 hours.
• Tell your nurse or doctor if you are pregnant, plan to become pregnant, or are breast-feeding.
• Tell your doctor, nurse, and pharmacist about all medicines you take.

POSSIBLE SIDE EFFECTS:
• Constipation. Opioids block pain and block bowels. Constipation can be controlled with daily laxatives such as Senokot-S®. Try to drink 8 large glasses of fluid a day. Increase your activity by walking or exercising. (For more helpful information, see Constipation Caused by Opioids form.)
• Nausea and vomiting. Take your medicine with food to lessen this. If nausea and vomiting continue, call your nurse or doctor. May be controlled with medicines.
• Drowsiness. May occur when starting Darvocet or increasing the dose. This usually goes away in about 2 to 3 days. Rest as needed.
• Confusion. This is less common than drowsiness. If this happens, call your nurse or doctor.

PRECAUTIONS:
• Be careful driving or using machinery such as lawn mowers, power tools, or saws. Do not do these things if you are drowsy.
• Be careful when drinking alcohol. Alcohol will increase drowsiness. Darvocet contains acetaminophen, and drinking alcohol with acetaminophen may increase risk of liver damage.

Continued

Form IV-17 │ Patient medication information: propoxyphene napsylate with acetaminophen.

PATIENT MEDICATION INFORMATION—cont'd

Propoxyphene Napsylate with Acetaminophen (generic name)

• Remember not to take more than 600 mg of propoxyphene napsylate or 4000 mg of acetaminophen in a 24-hour period.
• Call your doctor or nurse if pain increases or if you do not get pain relief.

STOPPING MEDICATIONS: Do not suddenly stop taking your medicine. Opioids must be stopped gradually. Call your pharmacist, nurse, or doctor before you stop taking your medicine.

REMEMBER!
• Keep count of your medicine.
• Do not mix medicines in the same container.
• Do not run out of medicine.
• In some states prescriptions for this medicine cannot be <u>re</u>filled or phoned in to your pharmacy. Check with your nurse or doctor.
• Get a **<u>new</u>** prescription filled a few days before you will run out of medicine.
• **<u>Call</u>** your nurse or doctor if side effects occur or if pain changes or does not go away. Your medicine may need to be changed.
• Take unused, unneeded, or expired medicines out of their original containers and flush them down the toilet. Do not put them in the trash.

COMMENTS:

• <u>Warning</u>: Keep this medicine out of reach of children! A dose could be fatal to a child.
• <u>Be sure to keep this medicine in a safe place out of sight of others</u>. A locked box may be indicated to prevent someone else from taking this medicine.

Form IV-17 | Cont'd.

References

Abd-El-Maeboud, K.H., Ghazy, A.A., Nadeem, A.A., et al. (2008). Effect of vaginal pH on the efficacy of vaginal misoprostol for induction of midtrimester abortion. *The Journal of Obstetrics and Gynaecology Research*, 34(1), 78–84.

Abnerthy, A. P., Currow, D. C., Frith, P., et al. (2003). Randomised, double blind, placebo controlled crossover trial of sustained release morphine for the management of refractory dyspnea. *BMJ (Clinical Research Ed.)*, 327(7414), 523–528.

Abou hammoud, H., Simon, N., Urien, S., et al. (2009). Intravenous morphine titration in immediate postoperative pain management: Population kinetic-pharmacodynamic and logistic regression analysis. *Pain*, 144(1–2), 139–146.

Acute Pain Management Guideline Panel. (1992). *Acute pain management: Operative or medical procedures and trauma.* AHCPR Pub. No. 92-0032. Agency for Health Care Policy and Research (AHCPR), Public Health Service, U.S. Department of Health and Human Services.

Adams, E. H., Chwiecko, P., Ace-Wagoner, Y., et al. (2006). A study of Avinza (morphine sulfate extended-release capsules) for chronic moderate-to-severe noncancer pain conducted under real-world treatment conditions – the ACCPT study. *Pain Practice*, 6(4), 254.

Adams, M., Pieniaszek, H. J., Jr., Gammaitoni, A. R., et al. (2005). Oxymorphone extended release does not affect CYP2C9 or CYP3A4 metabolic pathways. *Journal of Clinical Pharmacology*, 45(3), 337–345.

Agarwal, A., Gautam, S., Nath, S. S., et al. (2007). Comparison of the incidence and severity of cough induced by sufentanil and fentanyl: A prospective, randomised, double-blind study. *Anaesthesia*, 62(12), 1230–1232.

Agarwal, S., Polydefkis, M., Block, B., et al. (2007). Transdermal fentanyl reduces pain and improves functional activity in neuropathic pain states. *Pain Medicine*, 8(7), 554–562.

Agashe, G. S., Coakley, J., & Mannheimer, P. D. (2006). Forehead pulse oximetry: Headband use helps alleviate false low readings likely related to venous pulsation artifact. *Anesthesiology*, 105(6), 1111–1116.

Ahdieh, H., Ma, T., Babul, N., et al. (2004). Efficacy of oxymorphone extended release in postsurgical pain: A randomized clinical trial in knee arthroplasty. *Journal of Clinical Pharmacology*, 44(7), 767–776.

Alcoholics Anonymous (AA) World Services, Inc. (1984). *The A.A. Member – Medications and Other Drugs.* New York, NY: AA.

Alemdar, M., Pekdemir, M., & Selekler, H. M. (2007). Single-dose intravenous tramadol for acute migraine pain in adults: A single-blind, prospective, randomized, placebo-controlled clinical trial. *Clinical Therapeutics*, 29(7), 1441–1447.

Alford, D. P., Compton, P., & Samet, J. H. (2006). Acute pain management for patients receiving maintenance methadone or buprenorphine therapy. *Annals of Internal Medicine*, 144(2), 127–134.

Alkhazrajy, W. K., Macintyre, P. E., Upton, R. N., et al. (2007). An audit of the safety and effectiveness of an alfentanil:morphine mixture in the postanaesthesia care unit. *Acute Pain*, 9(1), 13–19.

Allan, L., Hays, H., Jensen, N. H., et al. (2001). Randomised crossover trial of transdermal fentanyl and sustained release oral morphine for treating chronic noncancer pain. *BMJ (Clinical Research Ed.)*, 322(7295), 1154–1158.

Allan, L., Richarz, U., Simpson, K., et al. (2005). Transdermal fentanyl versus sustained release oral morphine in strong-opioid naïve patients with chronic low back pain. *Spine*, 30(22), 2484–2490.

Allegri, M., Baldi, C., Pitino, E., et al. (2009). An accidental intravenous infusion of ropivacaine without any adverse effects. *Journal of Clinical Anesthesia*, 21(4), 312–313.

Allen, L.V., Stiles, M.L., & Tu, Y. H. (1990). Stability of fentanyl citrate in 0.9% sodium chloride solution in portable infusion pumps. *American Journal of Hospital Pharmacy*, 47(7), 1572–1573.

Allen, L. V., Stiles, M. L., & Wang, D. P. (1993). Stability of bupivacaine hydrochloride, epinephrine hydrochlorid, and fentanyl citrate in portable infusion-pump reservoirs. *American Journal of Hospital Pharmacy*, 50(4), 714–715.

Alpharma Pharmaceuticals. (2008). *Kadian prescribing information.* Elizabeth, NJ: Alpharma Pharmaceuticals. Available at http://www.kadian.com/pages/getfile.aspx?id=1C6197AB-8F83-43E7-B239-D4615293989B. Accessed April 17, 2008.

Alsahaf, M. H., & Stockwell, M. (2000). Respiratory failure due to the combined effects of transdermal fentanyl and epidural bupivacaine/diamorphine following radical nephrectomy. *Journal of Pain and Symptom Management*, 20(3), 210–213.

Alvarez, J. C., de Mazancourt, P., Chartier-Kastler, E., et al. (2004). Drug stability testing to support clinical feasibility investigations for intrathecal baclofen-clonidine admixture. *Journal of Pain and Symptom Management*, 28(3), 268–272.

Amabile, C. M., & Bowman, B. J. (2006). Overview of oral modified-release opioid products for the management of chronic pain. *The Annals of Pharmacotherapy*, 40(7/8), 1327–1335.

Amador, L. F., & Goodwin, J. S. (2005). Postoperative delirium in the older patient. *Journal of the American College of Surgeons*, 200(5), 767–773.

American Academy of Pain Medicine (AAPM), American Pain Society (APS), American Society of Addiction Medicine (ASAM). (2001). *Definitions related to the use of opioids for the treatment of pain.* Available at http://www.painmed.org/pdf/definition.pdf. Accessed July 28, 2009.

American Academy of Pediatrics (AAP). (2001). The transfer of drugs and other chemicals into human milk. *Pediatrics*, 108(3), 776–789. Available at http://aappolicy.aappublications.org/cgi/content/full/pediatrics%3b108/3/776. Accessed November 21, 2008.

American Association of Colleges of Nursing (AACN). (2009). *End of Life Nursing Education Consortium (ELNEC).* American Association of Colleges of Nursing (AACN). Available at http://www.aacn.nche.edu/ELNEC/factsheet.htm. Accessed September 1, 2009.

American Geriatrics Society (AGS). (2002). The management of persistent pain in older persons. *Journal of the American Geriatrics Society*, 50(1), S205–S224.

American Geriatrics Society (AGS). (2009). Panel on Pharmacological Management of Persistent Pain in the Older Persons. *Journal of the American Geriatrics Society*, 57(8), 1331–1346.

American Medical Association (AMA) Council on Ethical and Judicial Affairs. (1992). Decisions near the end of life. *JAMA: The Journal of the American Medical Association, 267*(16), 2229–2233.

American Nurses Association (ANA). (2003). *Pain management and control of distressing symptoms in dying patients.* Available at http://www.nursingworld.org/MainMenuCategories/HealthcareandPolicyIssues/ANAPositionStatements/EthicsandHumanRights.aspx. Accessed September 28, 2009.

American Pain Foundation. (2009). American Pain Foundation endorses opioid class REMS recommendations to FDA. Available at http://www.painfoundation.org/newsroom/position-statements/rems-recommendations.pdf. Accessed March 16, 2010.

American Pain Society (APS). (1987). *Principles of analgesic use in the treatment of acute pain and chronic cancer pain.* Washington DC: APS.

American Pain Society (APS). (2003). *Principles of analgesic use in the treatment of acute and cancer pain* (5th ed.). Glenview, IL: APS.

American Pharmacists Association. (2009). White paper on designing a risk evaluation and mitigation strategies (REMS) system to optimize the balance of patient access, medication safety, and impact on the health care system. *J Am Pharm Assoc, 49*(6), 729–743.

American Psychiatric Association. (2000). *Diagnostic and statistical manual of mental disorders* (4th ed. text revised). Washington DC: American Psychiatric Association.

American Society for Pain Management Nursing (ASPMN). (2004). *The use of "as needed" range orders for opioid analgesics in the management of acute pain: A consensus statement of the American Society for Pain Management Nursing and the American Pain Society.* Lenexa, KS: ASPMN.

American Society of Addiction Medicine (ASAM). (2001). *Definitions related to the use of opioids for the treatment of pain: Consensus Statement of the American Academy of Pain Medicine, the American Pain Society, and the American Society of Addiction Medicine.* Available at http://www.asam.org/DefinitionsRelatedtoUseofOpioidsforTreatmentofPain.html. Accessed March 22, 2009.

American Society of Anesthesiologists (ASA). (2004). Practice guidelines for acute pain management in the perioperative setting: An updated report. *Anesthesiology, 100*(6), 1573–1581.

American Society of Anesthesiologists (ASA). (2006). Practice guidelines for the perioperative management of patients with obstructive sleep apnea. *Anesthesiology, 104*(5), 1081–1093.

American Society of Anesthesiologists Task Force on Neuraxial Opioids. (2009). Practice guidelines for the prevention, detection, and management of respiratory depression associated with neuraxial opioid administration. *Anesthesiology, 110*(2), 218–230.

American Society of PeriAnesthesia Nurses (ASPAN). (2006). ASPAN's evidence-based clinical practice guideline for the prevention and/or management of PONV/PDNV. *J Perianesthesia Nursing, 21*(4), 230–250.

American Thoracic Society. (1999). Dyspnea. Mechanisms, assessment, and management: A consensus statement. *American Journal of Respiratory and Critical Care Medicine, 159*(1), 321–340.

Andersen, G., Christrup, L., & Sjøgren, P. (2003). Relationships among morphine metabolism, pain and side effects during long-term treatment: An update. *Journal of Pain and Symptom Management, 25*(1), 74–91.

Anderson, S. L., & Shreve, S. T. (2004). Continuous subcutaneous infusion of opiates at end-of-life. *The Annals of Pharmacotherapy, 38*(6), 1015–1023.

Andrieu, G., Roth, B., Ousmane, L., et al. (2009). The efficacy of intrathecal morphine with or without clonidine for postoperative analgesia after radical prostatectomy. *Anesthesia and Analgesia, 108*(6), 1954–1957.

Anghelescu, D. L., Burgoyne, L. L., Oakes, L. L., et al. (2005). The safety of patient-controlled analgesia by proxy in pediatric oncology patients. *Anesthesia and Analgesia, 101*(6), 1623–1627.

Angst, M. S., Chu, L. F., Tingle, M. S., et al. (2009). No evidence for the development of acute tolerance to analgesic, respiratory depessant and sedative opioid effects in humans. *Pain, 142*(1–2), 17–26.

Angst, M. S., & Clark, D. (2006). Opioid-induced hyperalgesia. *Anesthesiology, 104*(3), 570–587.

Angst, M. S., Koppert, W., Pahl, I., et al. (2003). Short-term infusion of the mu-opioid agonist remifentanil in humans causes hyperalgesia during withdrawal. *Pain, 106*(1–2), 49–57.

Angst, M. S., Ramaswamy, B., Riley, E. T., et al. (2000). Lumbar epidural morphine in humans and supraspinal analgesia to experimental heat pain. *Anesthesiology, 92*(2), 312–324.

Antonopolous, J., Bollinger, K., & Goshman, L. (1996). Guidelines for use of meperidine. *Drug Policy Perspect, 2*(3), 25–27.

Anwari, JS, & Iqbal, S. (2003). Antihistamines and potentiation of opioid induced sedation and respiratory depression. *Anaesthesia, 58*(5), 494–495.

Apfel, C. C., Korttila, K., Abdalla, M., et al. (2004). A factorial trial of six interventions for the prevention of postoperative nausea and vomiting. *The New England Journal of Medicine, 350*(24), 2441–2451.

Apfel, C. C., Kranke, P., Eberhart, L. H. J., et al. (2002). Comparison of predictive models for postoperative nausea and vomting. *British Journal of Anaesthesia, 88*(2), 234–240.

Apfel, C. C., Laara, E., Koivuranta, M., et al. (1999). A simplified risk score for predicting postoperative nausea and vomiting. *Anesthesiology, 91*(3), 693–700.

Apolone, G., Corli, O., Negri, E., et al. (2009). Effects of transdermal buprenorphine on patients-reported outcomes in cancer patients. *The Clinical Journal of Pain, 25*(8), 671–682.

Aqua, K., Gimbel, J. S., Singla, N., et al. (2007). Efficacy and tolerability of oxymorphone immediate release for acute postoperative pain after abdominal surgery: A randomized, double-blind, active- and placebo-controlled, parallel-group trial. *Clinical Therapeutics, 29*(6), 1000–1012.

Ardery, G., Herr, K., Hannon, B. J., et al. (2003). Lack of opioid administration in older hip fracture patients. *Geriatric Nursing (New York, N.Y.), 24*(6), 353–360.

Argoff, C. E. (2007). Tailoring chronic pain treatment to the patient: Long-acting, short-acting, and rapid-onset opioids. *Medscape Neurology Neurosurgery.* Available at http://www.medscape.com/viewarticle/554015. Accessed April 6, 2007.

Argoff, C. E. (2010). Clinical implications of opioid pharmacogenetics. *The Clinical Journal of Pain*, 26(Suppl. 1), S16–S20.

Argoff, C. E., Albrecht, P., Irving, G., et al. (2009). Multimodal analgesia for chronic pain: Rationale and future directions. *Pain Medicine (Malden, Mass.)*, 10(Suppl. 2), S53–S66.

Argoff, C. E., Backonja, M. M., Belgrade, M. J., et al. (2006). Consensus guidelines: Treatment and planning. *Mayo Clinic Proceedings*, 81(Suppl. 4), S12–S25.

Armstrong, P. J., Morton, C. P., & Nimmo, A. F. (1993). Pethidine has local anesthetic action on peripheral nerves in vivo. *Anaesthesia*, 48(5), 382–386.

Armstrong, S. C., Cozza, K. L., & Sandson, N. B. (2003). Six patterns of drug-drug interactions. *Psychosomatics*, 44(3), 255–258.

Armstrong, S. C., Wynn, G. H., & Sandson, N. B. (2009). Pharmacokinetic drug interactions of synthetic opiate analgesics. *Psychosomatics*, 50(2), 169–176.

Arpino, P. A., Klafatas, K., & Thompson, B. T. (2008). Feasibility of dexmedetomidine in facilitating extubation in the intensive care unit. *Journal of Clinical Pharmacy Therapeutics*, 33(1), 25–30.

Arsenjo, J. F., & Brecht, K. M. (2005). Opioids: Other routes for use in recovery room. *Current Drug Targets*, 6(7), 773–779.

Asao, T., Kuwano, H., Nakamura, J., et al. (2002). Gum chewing enhances early recovery from postoperative ileus after laparoscopic colectomy. *Journal of the American College of Surgeons*, 195(1), 30–32.

Ashburn, M. A., Caplan, R. A., Carr, D. B., et al. (2004). Practice guidelines for acute pain management in the perioperative setting. An updated report by the American Society of Anesthesiologists task force on acute pain management. *Anesthesiology*, 100(6), 1573–1581.

Ashburn, M. A., Fine, P. G., & Stanley, T. H. (1989). Oral transmucosal fentanyl citrate for the treatment of breakthrough cancer pain: A case report. *Anesthesiology*, 71(4), 615–617.

Ashburn, M. A., Love, G., & Pace, N. L. (1994). Respiratory-related critical events with intravenous patient-controlled analgesia. *The Clinical Journal of Pain*, 10(1), 52–56.

Ashburn, M. A., Ogden, L. L., Zhang, J., et al. (2003). The pharmacokinetics of transdermal fentanyl delivered with and without controlled heat. *The Journal of Pain*, 4(6), 291–297.

Aubrun, F., Bunge, D., Langeron, O., et al. (2003). Postoperative morphine consumption in the elderly patient. *Anesthesiology*, 99(1), 160–165.

Aubrun, F., Langeron, O., Quesnel, C., et al. (2003). Relationships between measurement of pain using visual analog score and morphine requirements during postoperative intravenous morphine titration. *Anesthesiology*, 98(6), 1415–1421.

Aubrun, F., & Marmion, F. (2007). The elderly patient and postoperative pain treatment. *Best Practice & Research Clinical Anaesthesiology*, 21(1), 109–127.

Aubrun, F., Monsel, S., Langeron, O., et al. (2001). Postoperative titration of intravenous morphine. *European Journal of Anaesthesiology*, 18(3), 159–165.

Aubrun, F., Monsel, S., Langeron, O., et al. (2002). Postoperative titration of intravenous morphine in the elderly patient. *Anesthesiology*, 96(1), 17–23.

Aubrun, F., & Riou, B. (2004). In reply to correspondence. *Anesthesiology*, 100(3), 745.

Aubrun, F., Salvi, N., Coriat, P., et al. (2005). Sex- and age-related differences in morphine requirements for postoperative pain relief. *Anesthesiology*, 105(1), 156–160.

Austin, K. L., Stapleton, J. V., & Mather, L. E. (1980a). Relationship between blood meperidine concentrations and analgesic response: A preliminary report. *Anesthesiology*, 53(6), 460–466.

Austin, K. L., Stapleton, J. V., & Mather, L. E. (1980b). Multiple intramuscular injections: A major source of variability in analgesic response to meperidine. *Pain*, 8, 47–62.

Ayonrinde, O. T., & Bridge, D. T. (2000). The rediscovery of methadone for cancer pain management. *The Medical Journal of Australia*, 173(10), 536–540.

Bach, S., Noreng, M. J., & Tjellden, N. U. (1988). Phantom pain in amputees during the first 12 months following limb amputation, after preoperative lumbar epidural blockade. *Pain*, 33(3), 297–301.

Badner, N. H., Doyle, J. A., Smith, M. H., et al. (1996). Effect of varying intravenous patient-controlled analgesia dose and lockout intervals while maintaining a constant hourly maximum dose. *Journal of Clinical Anesthesia*, 8(5), 382–385.

Bagri, A. S., Rico, A., & Ruiz, J. G. (2008). Evaluation and management of the elderly patient at risk for postoperative delirium. *Clinics in Geriatric Medicine*, 24(4), 667–686.

Bailie, G. R., & Johnson, C. A. (2002). Safety of propoxyphene in dialysis patients. *Seminars in Dialysis*, 15(5), 375.

Bainbridge, D., Martin, J. E., & Cheng, D. C. (2006). Patient-controlled versus nurse-controlled analgesia after cardiac surgery—a meta-analysis. *Canadian Journal of Anaesthesia*, 53(5), 492–499.

Baker, R. A., Zeller, R. A., Klein, R. I., et al. (2001). Burn wound itch control using H1 and H2 antagonists. *The Journal of Burn Care & Rehabilitation*, 22(4), 263–268.

Ballantyne, J. C. (2004). Does epidural analgesia improve surgical outcome? (Editorial). *British Journal of Anaesthesia*, 92(1), 4–6.

Ballantyne, J. C., & Carwood, C. (2005). Comparative efficacy of epidural, subarachnoid, and intracerebroventricular opioids in patients with pain due to cancer. *Cochrane Database of Systematic Reviews (Online)*, (1), CD005178.

Ballas, S. K., Viscusi, E. R., & Epstein, K. R. (2004). Management of acute chest wall sickle cell pain with nebulized morphine. *American Journal of Hematology*, 76(2), 190–191.

Baltali, S., Turkoz, A., Bozdogan, N., et al. (2009). The efficacy of intravenous patient-controlled remifentanil versus morphine anesthesia after coronary artery surgery. *Journal of Cardiothoracic and Vascular Anesthesia*, 23(2), 170–174.

Barkin, R. L., Barkin, S. J., & Barkin, D. S. (2006). Propoxyphene (dextropropoxyphene): A critical review of a weak opioid analgesic that should remain in antiquity. *American Journal of Therapeutics*, 13(6), 534–542.

Barkin, R. L., Lubenow, T. R., Bruehl, S., et al. (1996). Management of chronic pain. *Disease-A-Month*, 42(7), 389–454.

Barnhill, B. J., Holbert, M. D., Jackson, N. M., et al. (1996). Using pressure to decrease the pain of intramuscular injections. *Journal of Pain and Symptom Management*, 12(1), 52–58.

Bar-Oz, B., Bulkowstein, M., Benyamini, L., et al. (2003). Use of antibiotic and analgesic drugs during lactation. *Drug Safety: An International Journal of Medical Toxicology and Drug Experience*, 26(13), 925–935.

Basse, L., Billesbolle, P., & Kehlet, H. (2002). Early recovery after abdominal rectopexy with multimodal rehabilitation. *Diseases of the Colon and Rectum*, 45(2), 195–199.

Basse, L., Hjort Jakobsen, D., Billesbolle, P., et al. (2000). A clinical pathway to accelerate recovery after colonic surgery. *Annals of Surgery*, 232(1), 51–57.

Basse, L., Raskov, H. H., Hjort Jakobsen, D., et al. (2002). Accelerated postoperative recovery programme after colonic resection improves physical performance, pulmonary function, and body composition. *The British Journal of Surgery*, 89(4), 446–453.

Basse, L., Werner, M., & Kehlet, H. (2000). Is urinary drainage necessary during continuous epidural analgesia after colonic resection? *Regional Anesthesia and Pain Medicine*, 25(5), 498–501.

Bateman, D. N., & Eddleston, M. (2007). Clinical pharmacology: The basics. *The Foundation Years*, 3(6), 235–239.

Bates, J. J., Foss, J. F., & Murphy, D. B. (2004). Are peripheral opioid antagonists the solution to opioid side effects? *Anesthesia and Analgesia*, 98(1), 116–122.

Bauer, C., Hentz, J. G., Ducrocq, X., et al. (2007). Lung function after lobectomy: A randomized, double-blinded trial comparing thoracic epidural ropivacaine/sufentanil and intravenous morphine for patient-controlled analgesia. *Anesthesia and Analgesia*, 105(1), 238–244.

Beattie, W. S., Badner, N. H., & Choi, P. (2001). Epidural analgesia reduces postoperative myocardia infarction: A meta-analysis. *Anesthesia and Analgesia*, 93(4), 853–858.

Beaulé, P. E., Smith, M. I., & Nguyen, V. N. (2004). Meperidine-induced seizure after revision hip arthroplasty. *Journal of Arthroplasty*, 19(4), 516–519.

Beaver, W. T., & Frise, G. A. (1977). A comparison of the analgesic effect of oxymorphone by rectal suppository and intramuscular injection in patients with postoperative pain. *Journal of Clinical Pharmacology*, 17(5–6), 276–291.

Becker, G., & Blum, H. E. (2009). Novel opioid antagonists for opioid-induced bowel dysfunction and postoperative ileus. *Lancet*, 373(9670), 1198–1206.

Becker, G., Galandi, D., & Blum, H. E. (2007). Peripherally acting opioid antagonists in the treatment of opioid-related constipation: A systematic review. *Journal of Pain and Symptom Management*, 35(5), 547–565.

Bedder, M. D., Burchiel, K., & Larson, A. (1991). Cost analysis of two implantable narcotic delivery systems. *Journal of Pain and Symptom Management*, 6(3), 368–373.

Beers, M. H. (1997). Explicit criteria for determining potentially inappropriate medication use by the elderly. An update. *Archives of Internal Medicine*, 157(14), 1531–1536.

Beers, M. H., Ouslander, J. G., Rollingher, I., et al. (1991). Explicit criteria for determining inappropriate medication use in nursing home residents. *Archives of Internal Medicine*, 151(9), 1825–1832.

Beers, R., & Camporesi, E. (2004). Remifentanil update: Clinical science and utility. *CNS Drugs*, 18(15), 1085–1104.

Beilin, Y., Bernstein, H. H., Zucker-Pinchoff, B., et al. (1998). Subhypnotic doses of propofol do not relieve pruritus induced by intrathecal morphine after cesarean section. *Anesthesia and Analgesia*, 86(2), 310–313.

Beilin, Y., Bodian, C. A., Weiser, J., et al. (2005). Effect of labor epidural analgesia with and without fentanyl on infant breast-feeding. *Anesthesiology*, 103(6), 1211–1217.

Bell, J. G., Shaffer, L. E., & Schrickel-Feller, T. (2007). Randomized trial comparing 3 methods of postoperative analgesia in gynecology patients: Patient-controlled intravenous, scheduled intravenous, and scheduled subcutaneous. *American Journal of Obsetetrics and Gynecology*, 197(5), 472, e1–e7.

Beloeil, H., Corsia, G., Coriat, P., et al. (2002). Remifentanil compared with sufentanil during extra-corporeal shock wave lithotripsy with spontaneous ventilation: A double-blind, randomized study. *British Journal of Anaesthesia*, 89(4), 567–570.

Ben-David, B., Frankel, R., Arzumonov, T., et al. (2000). Minidose bupivacaine-fentanyl spinal anesthesia for surgical repair of hip fracture in the aged. *Anesthesiology*, 92(1), 6–10.

Bendiane, M. K., Bouhnik, A. D., Favre, R., et al. (2007). Morphine prescription in end-of-life care and euthanasia: French home nurses' opinions. *Journal of Opioid Management*, 3(1), 21–26.

Benítez-Rosario, M. A., Salinas-Martín, A., Aguirre-Jaime, A., et al. (2009). Morphine-methadone opioid rotation in cancer patients: Analysis of dose ratio predicting factors. *Journal of Pain and Symptom Management*, 37(6), 1061–1068.

Bennett, D., Burton, A.W., Fishman, S., et al. (2005a). Consensus panel recommendations for the assessment and management of breakthrough pain. Part I Assessment. *Pharmacology & Therapeutics*, 30(5): 296–301.

Bennett, D., Burton, A.W., Fishman, S., et al. (2005b). Consensus Panel Recommendations for the Assessment and Management of Breakthrough Pain. Part II Management. *Pharmacology & Therapeutics*, 30(6), 354–361.

Bennett, G., Burchiel, K., Buchser, E., et al. (2000). Clinical guidelines for intraspinal infusion: Report of an expert panel. *Journal of Pain and Symptom Management*, 20(2), S37–S43.

Bennett, G., Serafini, M., Burchiel, K., et al. (2000). Evidence-based review of the literature on intrathecal delivery of pain medication. *Journal of Pain and Symptom Management*, 20(2), S12–S36.

Bennett, J. A., Abrams, J. T., Van Riper, D. F., et al. (1997). Difficult or impossible ventilation after sufentanil-induced anesthesia is caused primarily by vocal cord closure. *Anesthesiology*, 87(5), 1070–1074.

Bercovitch, M., & Adunsky, A. (2004). Patterns of high-dose morphine use in a home-care hospice serve: Should we be afraid of it? *Cancer*, 101(6), 1473–1477.

Berde, C. B., Brennan, T. J., & Raja, S. N. (2003). Opioids: More to learn, improvements to be made. (Editorial). *Anesthesiology*, 98(6), 1309–1312.

Berdine, H. J., & Nesbit, S. A. (2006). Equianalgesic dosing of opioids. *Journal of Pain & Palliative Care Pharmacotherapy*, 20(4), 79–84.

Berghella, V., Lim, P. J., Hill, M. K., et al. (2003). Material methadone dose and neonatal withdrawal. *American Journal of Obstetrics and Gynecology*, 189(2), 312–317.

Berliner, M. N., Giesecke, T., & Bornhovd, K. D. (2007). Impact of transdermal fentanyl on quality of life in rheumatoid arthritis. *The Clinical Journal of Pain*, 23(6), 530–534.

Bernards, C. M. (2000). Rostral spread of epidural morphine. (Editorial). *Anesthesiology*, 92(2), 299–301.

Berntzen, D., & Gotestam, K. G. (1987). Effects of on-demand versus fixed-interval schedules in the treatment of chronic pain with analgesic compounds. *Journal of Consulting and Clinical Psychology, 55*(2), 213–217.

Beyea, S. C., & Nicoll, L. H. (1996). Back to basics: Administering IM injections the right way. *The American Journal of Nursing, 96*(1), 34–35.

Bhatnagar, S., Mishra, S., Srikanti, M., et al. (2008). Cancer pain management at a tertiary care cancer center in India—a retrospective analysis of 3238 patients. *Journal of Opioid Management, 46*(6), 361–368.

Bhimji, K. (2005). Opioid rotation from methadone: Fraught with difficulties. *Journal of Pain and Symptom Management, 29*(4), 334–335.

Bignami, E., Landoni, G., Biondi-Zoccai, G. G. L., et al. (2010). Epidural analgesia improves outcome in cardiac surgery: A meta-analysis of randomized controlled trials. *Journal of Cardiothoracic and Vascular Anesthesia*, in press. doi:10.1053/j.jvca.2009.09.015.

Bijur, P. E., Kenny, M. K., & Gallagher, E. J. (2005). Intravenous morphine at 0.1 mg/kg is not effective for controlling severe acute pain in the majority of patients. *Annals of Emergency Medicine, 46*(4), 362–367.

Bilsen, J., Norup, M., Deliens, L., et al. (2006). Drugs used to alleviate symptoms with life shortening as a possible side effect: End-of-life care in six European countries. *Journal of Pain and Symptom Management, 31*(2), 111–121.

BioDelivery Sciences International, Inc. (2009). Risk Evaluation and Mitigation Strategy (REMS): FOCUS™ Program for Onsolis™. Available at http://www. fda.gov/downloads/ Drugs/DrugSafety/PostmarketDrugSafetyInformationfor PatientsandProviders/UCM187537.pdf. Accessed March 16, 2010.

Birnbach, D. J., & Browne, I. M. (2005). Anesthesia for Obstetrics. In R. D. Miller (Ed.), *Miller's anesthesia* (6th ed., vol. 2, pp. 2307–2344). St. Louis: Churchill Livingstone.

Birnbaum, A., Esses, D., Bijur, P. E., et al. (2007). Randomized double-blind placebo-controlled trial of two intravenous morphine dosages (0.10 mg/kg and 0.15 mg/kg) in emergency department patients with moderate to severe acute pain. *Annals of Emergency Medicine, 49*(4), 445–453.

Blackburn, D., Somerville, Squire, J. (2002). Methadone: An alternative conversion regime. *Eur J Palliat Care, 9*(3), 92–96.

Blair, J. M., Hill, D. A., & Fee, J. P. H. (2001). Patient-controlled analgesia for labour using remifentanil: A feasibility study. *British Journal of Anaesthesia, 87*(3), 415–420.

Blaylock, V., Brinkman, M., Carver, S., et al. (2008). Comparison of finger and forehead oximetry sensors in postanesthesia care patients. *Journal of Perianesthesia Nursing, 23*(6), 379–386.

Blick, S. K., & Wagstaff, A. J. (2006). Fentanyl buccal tablet: In breakthrough pain in opioid-tolerant patients with cancer. *Drugs, 66*(18), 2387–2393.

Blum, D., Breithaupt, I., Hackett, S., et al. (2008). The safety of BEMA (BioErodible MucoAdhesive) fentanyl for breakthrough pain (BTP) in cancer patients. *Journal of Clinical Oncology, 26*(May 20 Suppl.) abstract 20486.

Blum, D., & Finn, A. (2008). Lack of adverse events affecting the mouth in three clinical trials of BEMA (BioErodible MucoAdhesive) fentanyl. *The Journal of Pain, 9*(4, Suppl. 1), P24.

Blumenthal, S., Min, K., Marquardt, M., et al. (2007). Postoperative intravenous morphine consumption, pain scores, and side effects with perioperative oral controlled-release oxycodone after lumbar discectomy. *Anesthesia and Analgesia, 105*(1), 233–237.

Blumstein, H. A., & Moore, D. (2003). Visual analog pain scores do not define desire for analgesia in paitents with acute pain. *Academic Emergency Medicine, 10*(3), 211–214.

Boitquin, L., Hecq, J. D., Evrard, J. M., et al. (2004). Long-term stability of sufentanil citrate with levobupivacaine hydrochloride in 0.9% sodium chloride infusion pvc bags at 4° C. *Journal of Pain and Symptom Management, 28*(1), 4–6.

Booth, J. V., Lindsay, D. R., Olufolabi, A. J., et al. (2000). Subarachnoid meperidine (pethidine) causes significant nausea and vomiting during labor. *Anesthesiology, 93*(2), 418–421.

Borgbjerg, F. M., Nielsen, K., & Franks, J. (1996). Experimental pain stimulates respiration and attenuates morphine-induced respiratory depression: A controlled study in human volunteers. *Pain, 64*(1), 123–128.

Borgeat, A., Ekatodramis, G., & Schenker, C. A. (2003). Postoperative nausea and vomiting in regional anesthesia. *Anesthesiology, 98*(2), 530–547.

Borgeat, A., Wilder-Smith, O., Saiah, M., et al. (1992). Subhypnotic doses of propofol relieves pruritus induced by epidural and intrathecal morphine. *Anesthesiology, 76*(4), 510–512.

Borland, M. L., Bergesio, R., Pascoe, E. M., et al. (2005). Intranasal fentanyl is an equivalent analgesic to oral morphine in paediatric burns patients for dressing changes: A randomised double blind crossover study. *Burns: Journal of the International Society for Burn Injuries, 31*(7), 831–837.

Bostrom, E., Hammarlund-Udenaes, M., & Simonsson, U. S. (2008). Blood-brain barrier transport helps to explain discrepancies in in vivo potency between oxycodone and morphine. *Anesthesiology, 108*(3), 495–505.

Bounes, V., Ducasse, J. L., Bona, A. M., et al. (2009). Nebulized morphine for analgesia in an emergency setting. *Journal of Opioid Management, 5*(1), 23–26.

Bourdeanu, L., Loseth, D. B., & Funk, M. (2005). Management of opioid-induced sedation in patients with cancer. *Clinical Journal of Oncology Nursing, 9*(6), 705–711.

Bowdle, T. A., Camporesi, E. M., Maysick, L., et al. (1996). A multi center evaluation of remifentanil for early postoperative analgesia. *Anesthesia and Analgesia, 83*(6), 1292–1297.

Bracco, D., & Hemmerling, T. M. (2008). Thoracic epidural analgesia in cardiac surgery: Impact on postoperative morbidity. *Techniques Reg Anesth Pain Manage, 12*(1), 32–40.

Bradshaw, A., & Price, L. (2007). Rectal suppository insertion: The reliability of the evidence as a basis for nursing practice. *Journal of Clinical Nursing, 16*(1), 98–103.

Brandman, J. F. (2005). Cancer patients, opioids, and driving. *Journal of Supportive Oncology, 3*(4), 317–320.

Brandsborg, B., Dueholm, M., Nikolajsen, L., et al. (2009). A prospective study of risk factors for pain persisting 4 months after hysterectomy. *The Clinical Journal of Pain, 25*(4), 263–268.

Breitbart, W., Chandler, S., Eagel, B., et al. (2000). An alternative algorithm for dosing transdermal fentanyl for cancer-related pain. *Oncology, 14*(5), 695–705. See discussion in same issue, pages 705, 709–710, 712, 717.

Brennan, M. J. (2009). Summary of short-term and long-term oxymorphone efficacy (pain) studies in low back pain, cancer pain, osteoarthritis, and neuropathic pain. *Pain Medicine (Malden, Mass.)*, 10(1 Suppl.), S11–S19.

Bridges, D., Thompson, S. W. N., & Rice, A. S. C. (2001). Mechanisms of neuropathic pain. *British Journal of Anaesthesia*, 87(1), 12–26.

Brimacombe, J., Archdeacon, J., Newell, S., et al. (1991). Two cases of naloxone-induced pulmonary oedema: The possible use of phentolamine in management. *Anesthesia Intens Care*, 19(4), 578–580.

Brodner, G., Van Aken, H., Hertle, L., et al. (2001). Multimodal perioperative management—combining thoracic epidural analgesia, forced mobilization, and oral nutrition—reduces hormonal and metabolic stress and improves convalescence after major urologic surgery. *Anesthesia and Analgesia*, 92(6), 1595–1600.

Brody, H., Campbell, M. L., Faber-Langendoen, K., et al. (1997). Withdrawing intensive life-sustaining treatment: Recommendations for compassionate clinical management. (Sounding Board). *The New England Journal of Medicine*, 336(9), 652–657.

Bromley, L. (2006). Pre-emptive analgesia and protective premedication. What is the difference? *Biomedicine & Pharmacotherapy*, 60(7), 336–340.

Brooks, K., Pasero, C., Hubbard, L., et al. (1995). The risk of infection associated with epidural analgesia. *Infection Contol and Hospital Epidemiology*, 16(12), 725–726.

Brown, D. L. (2005). Spinal, epidural, and caudal anesthesia. In R. D. Miller (Ed.), *Miller's anesthesia* (6th ed., vol. 2, pp. 1653–1683). Philadelphia: Elsevier.

Brown, D. R., Hofer, R. E., Patterson, D. E., et al. (2004). Intrathecal anesthesia and recovery from radical prostatectomy. *Anesthesiology*, 100(4), 926–934.

Brownridge, P., Cohen, S. E., & Ward, M. E. (1998). Neural blockade for obstetrics and gynecologic surgery. In M. J. Cousins, & P. O. Bridenbaugh (Eds.), *Neural blockade in clinical anesthesia and management of pain*. (3rd ed., pp. 557–604). Philadelphia: Lippincott-Raven.

Bruce, J., Drury, N., Poobalan, A. S., et al. (2003). The prevalence of chronic chest and leg pain following cardiac surgery: A historical cohort study. *Pain*, 104(1–2), 265–273.

Bruce, R. D., Altice, F. L., Gourevitch, M. N., et al. (2006). Pharmacokinetic drug interactions between opioid agonist therapy and antiretroviral medications: Implications and management for clinical practice. *Journal of Acquired Immune Deficiency Syndromes*, 41(5), 563–572.

Bruera, E., Brennels, C., Michaud, M., et al. (1987). Continuous SC infusion of narcotics using a portable disposable device in patients with advanced cancer. *Cancer Treatment Rep*, 71(6), 635–637.

Bruera, E., & Currow, D. (2009). Strategies for the palliation of dyspnea in cancer. *HIV/AIDS Cancer Pain Release*, 22(1–2), 1–5.

Bruera, E., Macmillan, K., Hanson, J., et al. (1989). The cognitive effects of the administration of narcotic analgesics in patients with cancer pain. *Pain*, 39(1), 13–16.

Bruera, E., Palmer, J. L., Bosnjak, S., et al. (2004). Methadone versus morphine as a first-line strong opioid for cancer pain: A randomized, double-blind study. *Journal of Clinical Oncology*, 22(1), 185–192.

Bruera, E., & Sweeney, C. (2002). Methadone use in cancer patients with pain: A review. *Journal of Palliative Medicine*, 5(1), 127–138.

Buck, M. L. (2002). Naloxone for reversal of opioid adverse effects. *Pediatric Pharmacology (New York, N. Y.)*, 8(8), 5–10. http://www.medscape.com/viewarticle/441915. Accessed February 8, 2007.

Buggy, D. J., Doherty, W. L., Hart, E. M., et al. (2002). Postoperative wound oxygen tension with epidural or intravenous analgesia. *Anesthesiology*, 97(4), 952–958.

Buntin-Mushock, C., Phillip, L., Moriyana, K., et al. (2005). Age-dependent opioid escalation in chronic pain patients. *Anesthesia and Analgesia*, 100(6), 1740–1745.

Burlacu, C. L., & Buggy, D. L. (2008). Update on local anesthetics: Focus on levobupivacaine. *Therap Clin Risk Manage*, 4(2), 381–392.

Burnham, R., McNeil, S., Hegedus, C., et al. (2006). Fibrous myopathy as a complication of repeated intramuscular injection for chronic headache. *Pain Research and Management*, 11(4), 249–252.

Burns, J. W., Hodsman, N. B. A., McLintock, T. T. C., et al. (1989). The influence of patient characteristics on the requirements for postoperative analgesia. *Anaesthesia*, 44(1), 2–6.

Burns, S. M., Cowan, C. M., Barclay, P. M., et al. (2001). Intrapartum epidural catheter migration: A comparative study of three dressing applications. *British Journal of Anaesthesia*, 86(4), 565–567.

Burton, A. W., Driver, L. C., Mendoza, T. R., et al. (2004). Oral transmucosal fentanyl citrate in the outpatient management of severe cancer pain crises: A retrospective case series. *The Clinical Journal of Pain*, 20(3), 195–197.

Busch, C. A., Shore, B. J., Bhandari, R., et al. (2006). Efficacy of periarticular multimodal drug injection in total knee Arthroplasty. *Journal of Bone and Joint Surgery*, 88a(5), 959–963.

Bussink, M., Gramke, H. F., van Kleef, M., et al. (2005). Bacterial meningitis ten days after spinal anesthesia. (Letter). *Regional Anesthesia and Pain Medicine*, 30(2), 210–211.

Butterworth, J., & Douglas-Akinwande, A. (2007). Lower extremity paralysis after thoracotomy or thoracic epidural: Image first, ask questions later. *Anesthesia and Analgesia*, 104(1), 201–203.

Buxton, I. L. O. (2006). Pharmacokinetics and pharmacodynamics. The dynamics of drug absorption, distribution, action, and elimination. In L. L. Brunton, J. S. Lazo, & K. L. Parker (Eds.), *Goodman, Gilman's the pharmacological basis of therapeutics*. (11th ed., pp. 1–39). New York: McGraw-Hill.

Buyse, I., Stockman, W., Columb, M., et al. (2007). Effect of sufentanil on minimum local analgesic concentrations of epidural bupivacaine, ropivacaine, and levobupivacaine in nullipara in early labour. *International Journal of Obstetric Anesthesia*, 16(1), 22–28.

Cai, Q., Huang, H., Sun, X., et al. (2008). Efficacy and safety of transdermal fentanyl for treatment of oral mucositis pain caused by chemotherapy. *Expert Opinion on Pharmacotherapy*, 9(18), 3137–3144.

Calderon, E., Pernia, A., De Antonio, P., et al. (2001). A comparison of two constant-dose continuous infusions of remifentanil for severe postoperative pain. *Anesthesia and Analgesia*, 92(3), 715–719.

Caldwell, J. R., Rapoport, R. J., Davis, J. C., et al. (2002). Efficacy and safety of a once-daily morphine formulation in chronic, moderate-to-severe osteoarthritis pain: Results from a randomized, placebo-controlled, double-blind trial and an open-label extension trial. *Journal of Pain and Symptom Management*, 23(4), 278–291.

Cameron, C. M., Scott, D. A., McDonald, W., et al. (2007). A review of neuraxial epidural morbidity. *Anesthesiology, 106*(5), 997–1002.

Candido, K. D., Franco, C. D., Khan, M. A., et al. (2001). Buprenorphine added to local anesthetic for brachial plexus block to provide postoperative analgesia in outpatients. *Regional Anesthesia and Pain Medicine, 26*(4), 352–356.

Candido, K. D., Winnie, A. P., Ghaleb, A. H., et al. (2002). Buprenorphine added to the local anesthetic for axillary brachial plexus block prolongs postoperative analgesia. *Regional Anesthesia and Pain Medicine, 27*(2), 162–167.

Candiotti, K. A., Kovac, A. L., Melson, T. I., et al. (2008). A randomized, double-blind study to evaluate the efficacy and safety of three different doses of palonosetron versus placebo for preventing postoperative nausea and vomiting. *Anesthesia and Analgesia, 107*(2), 445–451.

Caraceni, A., Martini, C., Zecca, E., et al. (2004). Working Group of an IASP Task Force on Cancer Pain. Breakthrough pain characteristics and syndromes in patients with cancer pain. An international survey. *Palliative Medicine, 18*(3), 177–183.

Carli, F., Mayo, N., Klubien, K., et al. (2002). Epidural analgesia enhances functional exercise capacity and health-related quality of life after colonic surgery. *Anesthesiology, 97*(3), 540–549.

Carli, F., Trudel, J. L., & Belliveau, P. (2005). The effect of intraoperative thoracic epidural anesthesia and postoperative analgesia on bowel function after colorectal surgery. *Diseases of the Colon and Rectum, 44*(8), 1083–1089.

Carlisle, J., & Stevenson, C. A. (2006). Drugs for preventing postoperative nausea and vomiting. *Cochrane Database of Systematic Reviews (Online), (3)* CD004125.

Carr, D. B., & Goudas, L. C., (2000). The Brietbart, et al article reviewed. *Oncology, 14*(5), 712, 717.

Carroll, I. R., Angst, M. S., & Clark, J. F. (2004). Management of perioperative pain in patients chronically consuming opioids. *Regional Anesthesia and Pain Med, 29*(6), 576–591.

Carvalho, B., Riley, E., Cohen, S. E., et al. (2005). Single-dose, sustained-release epidural morphine in the management of postoperative pain after elective cesarean delivery: Results of a multicenter randomized controlled study. *Anesthesia and Analgesia, 100*(4), 1150–1158.

Casarett, D. J., & Inouye, S. K. (2001). Diagnosis and management of delirium near the end of life. *Annals of Internal Medicine, 135*(1), 32–40.

Cashman, J. (2006). Patient-controlled analgesia. In G. Shorten, D. B. Carr, D. Harmon, M. M. Puig, & J. Browne (Eds.), *Postoperative pain management: An evidence-based guide to practice* (pp. 148–153). Philadelphia: Saunders.

Cashman, J. (2008). Routes of administration. In P. E. Macintyre, S. M. Walker, & D. J. Rowbotham (Eds.), *Acute pain*. (2nd ed., pp. 201–216). London, UK: Hodder Arnold.

Cashman, J. N., & Dolin, S. J. (2004). Respiratory and haemodynamic effects of acute postoperative pain management: Evidence from published data. *British Journal of Anaesthesia, 93*(2), 212–223.

Cassinelli, E. H., Dean, C. L., Garcia, R. M., et al. (2008). Ketorolac use for postoperative pain management following lumbar decompression surgery: A prospective, randomized, double-blinded, placebo-controlled trial. *Spine, 33*(12), 1313–1317.

Castillo, R. C., MacKenzie, E. J., Wegener, S. T., et al. (2006). Prevalence of chronic pain seven years following limb threatening lower extremity trauma. *Pain, 124*(3), 321–329.

Cata, J. P., Noguera, E. M., Parke, E., et al. (2008). Patient-controlled epidural analgesia (PCEA) for postoperative pain control after lumbar spine surgery. *Journal of Neurosurgical Anesthesiology, 20*(4), 256–260.

Centeno, C., & Vara, F. (2005). Intermittent subcutaneous methadone administration in the management of cancer pain. *Journal of Pain & Palliative Care Pharmacotherapy, 19*(2), 7–12.

Center for Drug Evaluation and Research (CDER). (2002). *Drug Information: Subutex (buprenorphine hydrochloride) and Suboxone tablets (buprenorphine hydrochloride and naloxone hydrochloride).* Available at http://www.fda.gov/cder/drug/infopage/subutex_suboxone/default.htm Accessed Feb 29, 2008.

Cepeda, M. S., Camargo, F., Zea, C., et al. (2006). Tramadol for osteoarthritis. *Cochrane Database of Systematic Reviews (Online), (3)* CD005522.

Cepeda, M. S., Camargo, F., Zea, C., et al. (2007). Tramadol for osteoarthritis: A systematic review and metaanalysis. *The Journal of Rheumatology, 34*(3), 543–555.

Cephalon. (2007). *Actiq prescribing information.* Frazer, PA: Cephalon Inc. Available at http://www.actiq.com/pdf/actiq_package_insert_4_5_07.pdf Accessed April 13, 2008.

Cephalon. (2008). *Fentora prescribing information.* Frazer, PA: Cephalon Inc. Available at http://www.fda.gov/cder/foi/label/2008/021947s006lbl.pdf Accessed April 13, 2008.

Chabbouh, T., Lentschener, C., Zuber, M., et al. (2005). Persistent cauda equine syndrome with no identifiable facilitating condition after uneventful single spinal administration of 0.5% hyperbaric bupivacaine. *Anesthesia and Analgesia, 101*(6), 1847–1848.

Chamberlin, B. H., Cross, K., Winston, J. L., et al. (2009). Methylnaltrexone treatment of opioid-induced constipation in patients with advanced illness. *Journal of Pain and Symptom Management, 38*(5), 683–690.

Chamberlin, K. W., Cottle, M., Neville, R., et al. (2007). Oral oxymorphone for pain management. *The Annals of Pharmacotherapy, 41*(7), 1144–1152.

Chan, J. D., Treece, P. D., Engelberg, R. A., et al. (2004). Narcotic and benzodiazepine use after withdrawal of life support. *Chest, 126*(1), 286–293.

Chandler, S. (1999). Nebulized opioids to treat dyspnea. *The American Journal of Hospice & Palliative Care, 16*(1), 418–422.

Chaney, M. A., Furry, P. A., Fluder, E. M., et al. (1997). Intrathecal morphine for coronary artery bypass grafting and early extubation. *Anesthesia and Analgesia, 84*(2), 241–248.

Chang, A., Emmel, D. W., Rossi, G. C., et al. (1998). Methadone analgesia in morphine-insensitive CXBK mice. *European Journal of Pharmacology, 351*(2), 189–191.

Chang, A. K., Bijur, P. E., Campbell, C. M., et al. (2009). Safety and efficacy of rapid titration using 1-mg doses of intravenous hydromorphone in emergency department patients with acute severe pain: The "1 +1" protocol. *Annals of Emergency Medicine, 54*(2), 221–225.

Chang, A. K., Bijur, P. E., Davitt, M., et al. (2009). Randomized clinical trial comparing a patient-driven titration protocol of intravenous hydromorphone with traditional physician-driven management of emergency department patients with acute severe pain. *Annals of Emergency Medicine*, (4), 561.e2–567.e2.

Chang, A. K., Bijur, P. E., Meyer, R. H., et al. (2006). Safety and efficacy of hydromorphone as an analgesic alternative to morphine in acute pain: A randomized clinical trial. *Annals of Emergency Medicine*, 48(2), 164–172.

Chang, A. K., Bijur, P. E., Napolitano, A., et al. (2009). Two milligrams IV hydromorphone is efficacious for treating pain but is associated with oxygen desaturation. *Journal of Opioid Management*, 5(2), 75–80.

Chang, K. Y., Dai, C. Y., Ger, L. P., et al. (2006). Determinants of patient-controlled epidural analgesia requirements. A prospective analysis of 1753 patients. *The Clinical Journal of Pain*, 22(9), 751–756.

Chao, J. (2005). Retrospective analysis of Kadian (morphine sulfate sustained-release capsules) in patients with chronic, nonmalignant pain. *Pain Medicine (Malden, Mass.)*, 6(3), 262–265.

Chapalain-Pargade, S., Laville, I., Paci, A., et al. (2006). Microbiological and physicochemical stability of fentanyl and sufentanil solutions for patient-controlled delivery systems. *Journal of Pain and Symptom Management*, 32(1), 90–97.

Chapman, S., Byas-Smith, M. G., & Reed, B. A. (2002). Effects of intermediate- and long-term use of opioids on cognition in patients with chronic pain. *The Clinical Journal of Pain*, 18, S83–S90.

Charlton, S. T., Davis, S. S., & Illum, L. (2007). Evaluation of bioadhesive polymers as delivery systems for nose to brain delivery: In vitro characterisation studies. *Journal of Controlled Release*, 118(2), 225–234.

Charoenkwan, K., Phillipson, G., & Vutyavanich, T. (2007). Early versus delayed oral fluids and food for reducing complications after major abdominal gynaecologic surgery. *Cochrane Database of Systematic Reviews (Online)*, (4) CD004508.

Charuluxananan, S., Kyokong, O., Somboonviboon, W., et al. (2003). Nalbuphine versus ondansetron for prevention of intrathecal morphine-induced pruritus after cesarean delivery. *Anesthesia and Analgesia*, 96(6), 1789–1793.

Charuluxananan, S., Somboonviboon, W., Kyokong, O., et al. (2000). Ondansetron for treatment of intrathecal morphine-induced pruritus after cesarean delivery. *Regional Anesthesia and Pain Medicine*, 25(5), 535–539.

Chelly, J. E., Greger, J., Gebhard, R., et al. (2001). Continuous femoral nerve blocks improve recovery and outcome of patients undergoing total knee arthroplasty. *The Journal of Arthroplasty*, 16(4), 436–445.

Chen, J., Hillman, K., Bellomo, R., et al. (2009). The impact of introducing medical emergency team system on the documentations of vital signs. *Resuscitation*, 80(1), 35–43.

Chen, P. P., Cheam, E. W., Ma, M., et al. (2001). Patient-controlled pethidine after major upper abdominal surgery: Comparison of the epidural and intravenous routes. *Anaesthesia*, 56(1), 1090–1115.

Chen, X., Qian, X., Fu, F., et al. (2009). Intrathecal sufentanil decreases the median effective dose (ED50) of intrathecal hyperbaric ropivacaine for caesarean delivery. *Acta Anaesthesiologica Scandinavica*, 10.1111/j.1399-6576.2009.02051.x.

Cheng, D. C. H., Newman, M. F., Duke, P., et al. (2001). The efficacy and resource utilization of remifentanil and fentanyl in fast-track coronary artery bypass graft surgery: A prospective randomized, double-blinded controlled, multi-center trial. *Anesthesia and Analgesia*, 92(5), 1094–1102.

Cherny, N., Ripamonti, C., Pereira, J., et al. (2001). Strategies to manage the adverse effects of oral morphine: An evidence-based report. *Journal of Clinical Oncology*, 19(9), 2542–2554.

Cherrier, M. M., Amory, J. K., Ersek, M., et al. (2009). Comparative cognitive and subjective side effects of immediate-release oxycodone in healthy middle-aged and older adults. *The Journal of Pain*, 10(10), 1038–1050.

Cheville, A., Chen, A., Oster, G., et al. (2001). A randomized trial of controlled-release oxycodone during inpatient rehabilitation following unilateral total knee arthroplasty. *Journal of Bone and Joint Surgery*, 83A(4), 572–576.

Chia, Y. Y., Kuo, M. C., Liu, K., et al. (2002). Does postoperative pain induce emesis? *The Clinical Journal of Pain*, 18(5), 317–323.

Chia, Y. Y., Wei, R. J., Chang, H. C., et al. (2009). Optimal duration of urinary catheterization after thoractomy in patients under postoperative patient-controlled epidural analgesia. *Acta Anaesthesiologica Taiwan*, 47(4), 173–179.

Choi, P., Bhandari, M., Scott, J., et al. (2003). Epidural analgesia for pain relief following hip or knee replacement. *Cochrane Database of Systematic Reviews (Online)*, (3) CD003071.

Choi, S. H., Koo, B. N., Nam, S. H., et al. (2008). Comparison of remifentanil and fentanyl for postoperative pain control after abdominal hysterectomy. *Yonsei Medical Journal*, 49(2), 204–210.

Chou, R., Fanciullo, G. J., Fine, P., et al. (2009). Opioid treatment guidelines: Clinical guidelines for the use of chronic opioid therapy in chronic noncancer pain. *The Journal of Pain*, 10(2), 113–130.

Chou, W. Y., Wang, C. H., Liu, C. C., et al. (2006). Human opioid receptor A118G polymorphism affects intravenous patient-controlled analgesia morphine consumption after total abdominal hysterectomy. *Anesthesiology*, 105(2), 334–337.

Christensen, K. S., Cohen, A. E., Mermelstein, F. H., et al. (2008). The analgesic efficacy and safety of a novel intranasal morphine formulation (morphine plus chitosan), immediate release oral morphine, intravenous morphine, and placebo in a postsurgical dental pain model. *Anesthesia and Analgesia*, 107(6), 2018–2024.

Christie, I. W., & McCabe, S. (2007). Major complications of epidural analgesia after surgery: Results of a six-year survey. *Anaesthesia*, 62(4), 334–341.

Chu, C. C., Shieh, J. P., Tzeng, J. I., et al. (2008). The prophylactic effect of haloperidol plus dexamethasone on postoperative nausea and vomiting in patients undergoing laparoscopically assisted vaginal hysterectomy. *Anesthesia and Analgesia*, 106(5), 1402–1406.

Chu, L. F., Angst, M. S., & Clark, D. (2008). Opioid-induced hperalgesia in humans: Molecular mechanisms and clinical considerations. *The Clinical Journal of Pain*, 24(6), 479–496.

Chu, L. F., Clark, K. J., & Angst, M. S. (2006). Opioid tolerance and hyperalgesia in chronic pain patients after one month of oral morphine therapy: A preliminary prospective study. *The Journal of Pain*, 7, 43–48.

Classen, A. M., Wimbish, G. H., & Kupiec, T. C. (2004). Stability of admixture containing morphine sulfate, bupivacaine hydrochloride, and clonidine hydrochloride in an implantable infusion system. *Journal of Pain and Symptom Management, 28*(6), 603–611.

Claxton, A. R., McGuire, G., Chung, F., et al. (1997). Evaluation of morphine versus fentanyl for postoperative analgesia after ambulatory surgical procedures. *Anesthesia and Analgesia, 84*(3), 509–514.

Clemens, K. E., & Klaschik, E. (2008a). Morphine in the management of dyspnoea in ALS. A pilot study. *European Journal of Neurology, 15*(5), 445–450.

Clemens, K. E., & Klaschik, E. (2008b). Effect of hydromorphone on ventilation in palliative care patients with dyspnea. *Supportive Care in Cancer, 16*(1), 93–99.

Clemens, K. E., Quednau, I., & Klaschik, E. (2008). Is there a higher risk of respiratory depression in opioid-naïve palliative care patients during symptomatic therapy of dyspnea with strong opioids? *Journal of Palliative Medicine, 11*(2), 204–216.

Clemens, K. E., Quednau, I., & Klaschik, E. (2009). Use of oxygen and opioids in the palliation of dyspnoea in hypoxic and non-hypoxic palliative care patients: A prospective study. *Supportive Care in Cancer, 17*(4), 367–377.

Coda, B. A. (2006). Opioids. In P. G Barash, B. F Cullen, & R. K Stoelting (Eds.), *Clinical anesthesia.* (5th ed.). Philadelphia: Lippincott, Williams, Wilkins.

Coddings, C., Levinsky, D., Hale, M., et al. (2008). *Analgesic efficacy and safety of controlled-release hydrocodone and acetaminophen tablets, dosed twice daily for moderate-to-severe mechanical chronic low back pain: A randomized, double-blind, placebo-controlled withdrawal trial.* Paper presented at American Pain Society Annual Meeting, Tampa, Florida, May 8–10.

Coelho, J. C. U., Runkel, N., Herfarth, C., et al. (1986). Effect of analgesic drugs on electromyographic activity of the gastrointestinal tract and sphincter of Oddi and on biliary pressure. *Annals of Surgery, 204*(1), 53–58.

Cohen, M. R., & Smetzer, J. (2005). Patient-controlled analgesia safety issues. *Journal of Pain & Palliative Care Pharmacotherapy, 19*(1), 45–50.

Cohen, R. S. (2009). Fentanyl transdermal analgesia during pregnancy and lactation. *Journal of Human Lactation, 25*(3), 359–361.

Collado, F., & Torres, L. M. (2008). Association of transdermal fentanyl and oral transmucosal fentanyl citrate in the treatment of opioid naïve patients with severe chronic noncancer pain. *Journal of Opioid Management, 4*(2), 111–115.

Coloma, M., White, P. F., Markowitz, S. D., et al. (2002). Dexamethasone in combination with dolasetron for prophylaxis in the ambulatory setting. *Anesthesiology, 96*(6), 1346–1350.

Coloma, M., White, P. F., Ogunnaike, B. O., et al. (2002). Comparison of acustimulation and ondansetron for the treatment of established postoperative nausea and vomiting. *Anesthesiology, 97*(6), 1387–1392.

Coluzzi, P. H., Schwartzberg, L., Conroy, J. D., et al. (2001). Breakthrough cancer pain: A randomized trial comparing oral transmucosal fentanyl citrate (OTFC) and morphine sulfate immediate release (MSIR). *Pain, 91*(1–2), 123–130.

Committee on the Safety of Medicines of the UK. (2006). Overdose risk prompts UK withdrawal of propoxyphene combination. *Journal of Pain & Palliative Care Pharmacotherapy, 20*(4), 49–50.

Compton, P. (1999). Substance abuse. In M. McCaffery, & C. Pasero (Eds.), *Pain: Clinical manual.* (2nd ed., pp. 429–466). St. Louis: Mosby.

Compton, P. (2008). The OIH paradox: Can opioids make pain worse? *Pain Treatment Topics.* Available at http://pain-topics.org/pdf/Compton-OIH-Paradox.pdf. Accessed Feb. 16, 2009.

Connelly, N. R., Parker, R. K., Rahimi, A., et al. (2000). Sumatriptan in patients with postdural puncture headache. *Headache, 40*(4), 316–319.

Connor, S. R., Horn, S. D., Smout, R. J., et al. (2005). The National Hospice Outcomes Project (NHOP): Development and implementation of a multi-site hospice outcomes study. *Journal of Pain and Symptom Management, 29*(3), 286–296.

Cook, D. J., & Rooke, G. A. (2003). Priorities in perioperative geriatrics. *Anesthesia and Analgesia, 96*(6), 1823–1836.

Correll, D. J., Viscusi, E. R., Grunwald, Z., et al. (2001). Epidural analgesia compared with intravenous morphine patient-controlled analgesia: Postoperative outcome measures after mastectomy with immediate TRAM flap breast reconstruction. *Regional Anesthesia and Pain Medicine, 26*(5), 444–449.

Cortinez, L. I., Munoz, H. R., De al Fuente, R., et al. (2005). Target-controlled infusión of remifentanil or fentanyl Turing extra-corporeal shock-wave lithotripsy. *European Journal of Anaesthsiology, 22*(1), 56–61.

Cousins, M. J. (2007). Advances in the long-term management of chronic pain: Recent evidence with OROS hydromorphone, a novel, once-daily, long-acting opioid analgesic. *Journal of Pain and Symptom Management, 33*(Suppl. 2), S1–S3.

Cousins, M. J., & Umedaly, H. S. (1996). Postoperative pain management in the neurosurgical patient. *International Anesthesiology Clinics, 34*(4), 179–193.

Cousins, M. J., & Veering, B. T. (1998). Epidural neural blockade. In M. J. Cousins, & P. O. Bridenbaugh (Eds.), *Neural blockade in clinical anesthesia and management of pain* (pp. 243–321). Philadelphia: Lippincott-Raven Publishers.

Covino, B. G., & Wildsmith, J. A. W. (1998). Clinical pharmacology of local anesthetic agents. In M. J. Cousins, & P. O. Bridenbaugh (Eds.), *Neural blockade in clinical anesthesia and management of pain* (pp. 97–128). Philadelphia: Lippincott.

Coyle, N. (1996). Cancer patients and subcutaneous infusions. *The American Journal of Nursing, 96*(3), 61.

Coyle, N., Adelhardt, J., Foley, K. M., et al. (1990). Character of terminal illness in the advanced cancer patient: Pain and other symptoms during the last four weeks of life. *Journal of Pain and Symptom Management, 5*(2), 83–93.

Coyle, N., Cherny, N., & Portenoy, R. K. (1995). Pharmacologic management of cancer pain. In D. McGuire, C. H. Yarbro, & B. R Ferrell (Eds.), *Cancer pain management.* (2nd ed., pp. 89–130). Boston: Jones, Bartlett Publishers.

Coyle, N., Mauskop, A., Maggard, J., et al. (1986). Continuous subcutaneous infusions of opiates in cancer patients with pain. *Oncology Nursing Forum, 13*(4), 53–57.

Coyle, N., & Portenoy, R. K. (1996). Pharmacologic management of cancer pain. In *Cancer Nursing.* (2nd ed., pp. 1035–1055). Philadelphia: WB Saunders.

Coyne, P. J., Paice, J. A., Ferrell, B. R., et al. (2007). Oncology End-of-Life Nursing Education Consortium training program: Improving palliative care in cancer. *Oncology Nursing Forum, 34*(4), 801–807.

Coyne, P. J., Viswanathan, R., & Smith, T. J. (2002). Nebulized fentanyl citrate improves patients' perception of breathing, respiratory rate, and oxygen saturation in dyspnea. *Journal of Pain and Symptom Management, 23*(2), 157–160.

Cretikos, M. A., Bellomo, R., Hillman, K., et al. (2008). Respiratory rate: The neglected vital sign. *MJA, 188*(11), 657–659.

Cruciani, R. A. (2008). Methadone: To ECG or not to ECG... That is still the question. *Journal of Pain and Symptom Management, 36*(5), 545–552.

Currow, D. C., Plummer, J. L., Cooney, N. J., et al. (2007). A randomized, double-blind, multi-site, crossover, placebo-controlled equivalence study of morning versus evening once-daily sustained-release morphine sulfate in people with pain from advanced cancer. *Journal of Pain and Symptom Management, 34*(1), 17–23.

Curry, C. E., & Butler, D. M. (2006). Constipation. In R. R. Berardi, A. L. Kroon, & J. H. McDermott, et al: *Handbook of nonprescription drugs. An interactive approach to self care*, ed 15, Washington DC, American Pharmacists Association.

Cywinski, J. B., Parker, B. M., Xu, M., et al. (2004). A comparison of postoperative pain control in patients after right lobe donor hepatectomy and major hepatic resection for tumor. *Anesthesia and Analgesia, 99*(6), 1747–1752.

Czarnecki, M. L., Ferrise, A. S., Jastrowski Mano, K. E., et al. (2008). Parent/nurse-controlled analgesia for children with developmental delay. *The Clinical Journal of Pain, 24*(9), 817–824.

Dabu-Bondoc, S., Franco, S. A., & Sinatra, R. S. (2009). Neuraxial analgesia with hydromorphone, morphine, and fentanyl: Dosing and safety guidelines. In R. S Sinatra, O. A de Leon-Casasola, B. Ginsberg, & E. R Viscusi (Eds.), *Acute pain management* (pp. 230–244). Cambridge, New York: Cambridge University Press.

Daeninck, P. J., & Bruera, E. (1999). Reduction in constipation and laxative requirements following opioid rotation to methadone: A report of four cases. *Journal of Pain and Symptom Management, 18*(4), 303–309.

Dahaba, A. A., Grabner, T., Rehak, P. H., et al. (2004). Remifentanil versus morphine analgesia and sedation for mechanically ventilated critically ill patients. *Anesthesiology, 101*(3), 640–646.

Dahan, A., Aarts, L., & Smith, T. W. (2010). Incidence, reversal, and prevention of opioid-induced respiratory depression. *Anesthesiology, 112*(1), 226–238.

Dahan, A., van Dorp, E., Smith, T., et al. (2008). Morphine-6-glucuronide (M6G) for postoperative pain relief. *European Journal of Pain (London, England), 12*(4), 403–411.

Dahan, A., Yassen, A., Bijl, H., et al. (2005). Comparison of the respiratory effects of intravenous buprenorphine and fentanyl in humans and rats. *British Journal of Anaesthesia, 94*(6), 325–334.

Dahan, A., Yassen, A., Romberg, R., et al. (2006). Buprenorphine induces ceiling in respiratory depression but no in analgesia. *British Journal of Anaesthesia, 96*(5), 627–632.

Dahl, J. B., & Moiniche, S. (2004). Pre-emptive analgesia. *British Medical Bulletin, 71*(1), 13–27.

Dahmani, S., Dupont, H., Mantz, J., et al. (2001). Predictive factors of early morphine requirements in the post-anaesthesia care unit (PACU). *British Journal of Anaesthesia, 87*(3), 385–389.

Dal, D., Canbak, M., Cagler, M., et al. (2003). A background infusion of morphine does not enhance postoperative analgesia after cardiac surgery. *Canadian Journal of Anesthesia, 50*(3), 476–479.

Dale, O., Hjortkjær, R., & Kharasch, E. D. (2002). Nasal administration of opioids for pain management in adults. *Acta Anaesthesiologica Scandinavica, 46*(7), 759–770.

Dale, O., Hoffer, C., Sheffels, P., et al. (2002). Disposition of nasal, intravenous, and oral methadone in healthy volunteers. *Clinical Pharmacology and Therapeutics, 72*(5), 536–545.

Dale, O., Piribauer, M., Kaasa, S., et al. (2009). A double-blind, randomized, crossover comparison between single-dose and double-dose immediate-release oral morphine at bedtime in cancer patients. *Journal of Pain and Symptom Management, 37*(1), 68–76.

Dale, O., Sheffels, P., & Kharasch, E. D. (2004). Bioavailabilities of rectal and oral methadone in healthy subjects. *British Journal of Clinical Pharmacology, 58*(2), 156–162.

Daniels, S., Casson, E., Stegmann, J. U., et al. (2009). A randomized, double-blind, placebo-controlled phase 3 study of the relative efficacy and tolerability of tapentadol IR and oxycodone IR for acute pain. *Current Medical Research and Opinion, 25*(6), 1551–1556.

Darwish, M., Kirby, M., Jiang, J. G., et al. (2008). Bioequivalence following buccal and sublingual placement of fentanyl buccal tablet 400 microg in healthy subjects. *Clinical Drug Investigation, 28*(1), 1–7.

Darwish, M., Kirby, M., Robertson, P., Jr., et al. (2007). Absolute and relative bioavailability of fentanyl buccal tablet and oral transmucosal fentanyl citrate. *Journal of Clinical Pharmacology, 47*(3), 343–350.

Davies, A. N., Vriens, J., Kennett, A., et al. (2008). An observational study of oncology patients' utilization of breakthrough pain medication. *Journal of Pain and Symptom Management, 35*(4), 406–411.

Davis, G. A., Rudy, A. C., Archer, S. M., et al. (2004). Bioavailability and pharmacokinetics of intranasal hydromorphone in patients experiencing vasomotor rhinitis. *Clinical Drug Investigation, 24*(11), 633–639.

Davis, G. A., Rudy, A. I. A., Archer, S. M., et al. (2005). Bioavailability of intranasal butorphanol administered from a single-dose sprayer. *American Journal of Health-System Pharmacy: AJHP, 62*(1), 48–53.

Davis, J. J., Johnson, K. B., Egan, T. D., et al. (2003). Preoperative fentanyl infusion with pharmacokinetic simulation for anesthetic and perioperative management of an opioid-tolerant patient. *Anesthesia and Analgesia, 97*(6), 1661–1662.

Davis, K. M., Esposito, M. A., & Meyer, B. A. (2006). Oral analgesia compared with intravenous patient-controlled analgesia for pain after cesarean delivery: A randomized controlled trial. *American Journal of Obstetrics and Gynecology, 194*(4), 967–971.

Davis, M. P. (2004). Acute pain in advanced cancer: An opioid dosing strategy and illustration. *The American Journal of Hospice & Palliative Care, 21*(1), 47–140.

Davis, M. P. (2005). Buprenorphine in cancer pain. *Supportive Care in Cancer, 13*(11), 878–887.

Davis, M. P., Varga, J., Dickerson, D., et al. (2003). Normal-release and controlled-release oxycodone: Pharmacokinetics, pharmacodynamics, and controversy. *Supportive Care in Cancer, 11*(2), 84–92.

Davis, M. P., & Walsh, D. (2001). Methadone for relief of cancer pain: A review of pharmacokinetics, pharmacodynamics, drug interactions and protocols of administration. *Supportive Care in Cancer*, 9(2), 73–83.

Davis, M. P., Walsh, D., LeGrand, S. B., et al. (2002). Symptom control in cancer patients: The clinical pharmacology and therapeutic role of suppositories and rectal suspensions. *Supportive Care in Cancer*, 10(2), 117–138.

Dawn, A. G., & Yosipovitch, G. (2006). Butorphanol for treatment of intractable pruritus. *Journal of the American Academy of Dermatology*, 54(3), 527–531.

Dawson, P., Rosenfeld, J. V., Murphy, M. A., et al. (1991). Epidural abscess associated with postoperative epidural analgesia. *Anaesthesia and Intensive Care*, 19(4), 569–572.

Dean, M. (2004). Opioids in renal failure and dialysis patients. *Journal of Pain and Symptom Management*, 28(5), 497–504.

De Beer Jde, V., Winemaker, M. J., Donnelly, G. A. E., et al. (2005). Efficacy and safety of controlled-release oxycodone and standard therapies for postoperative pain after knee or hip replacement. *Canadian Journal of Surgery*, 48(4), 277–283.

De Cicco, M., Matovic, M., Castellani, G. T., et al. (1995). Time-dependent efficacy of bacterial filters and infection risk in long-term epidural catheterization. *Anesthesiology*, 82(3), 765–771.

De Cosmo, G., Congedo, E., Lai, C., et al. (2008). Ropivacaine vs. levobupivacaine combined with sufentanil for epidural analgesia after lung surgery. *European Journal of Anaesethesiology*, 25(12), 1020–1025.

Deer, T., Krames, E. S., Hassenbusch, S. J., et al. (2007). Polyanalgesic consensus conference: Recommendations for the management of pain by intrathecal (intraspinal) drug delivery; report of an interdisciplinary expert panel. *Neuromodulation*, 10(4), 300–328.

De Kock, M., Lavand'homme, P., & Waterloos, H. (2005). The short-lasting analgesia and long-term antihyperalgesic effect of intrathecal clonidine in patients undergoing colonic surgery. *Anesthesia and Analgesia*, 101(2), 566–572.

de Leon-Casasola, O. A. (2008). Current developments in opioid therapy for management of cancer pain. *The Clinical Journal of Pain*, 24(4), S3–S7.

Delvecchio, L., Bettinelli, S., Klersy, C., et al. (2008). Comparing the efficacy and safety of continuous epidural analgesia in abdominal and urological surgery between two opioids with different kinetic properties: Morphine and sufentanyl. *Minerva Anestesiologica*, 74(3), 69–76.

Demeure, M. J., & Fain, M. J. (2006). The elderly surgical patient and postoperative delirium. *Journal of the American College of Surgeons*, 203(5), 752–757.

Dempsey, S. J., Davidson, J., Cahill, D., et al. (2008). *Selection of a sedation assessment scale for clinical practice: Interrater reliability, ease of use, and applicability testing of the Richmond-Agitation-Sedation and Pasero Opioid-induced Sedation Scale.* Poster presentation, National Association of Orthopedic Nurses Congress, Tampa, FL, May 6–10.

De Pinto, M., Dunbar, P. J., & Edwards, W. T. (2006). Pain management. *Anesthesiology Clin N Am*, 24(1), 19–37.

Dershwitz, M., Landow, L., & Joshi-Ryzewicz, W. (2003). Anesthesia for bedside procedures. In R. S. Irwin, & J. M. Rippe (Eds.), *Irwin, Rippe's intensive care medicine.* Philadelphia: Lippincott Williams, Wilkins.

Devulder, J., Jacobs, A., Richarz, U., et al. (2009). Impact of opioid rescue medication for breakthrough pain on the efficacy and tolerability of long-acting opioids in patients with chronic non-malignant pain. *British Journal of Anaesthesia*, 103(4), 576–585.

Dewachter, P., Lefebvre, D., Kalaboka, S., et al. (2009). An anaphylactic reaction to transdermal delivered fentanyl. *Acta Anaesthesiologica Scandinavica*, 53(8), 1092–1093.

Dillon, A. E., Wagner, C. L., Wiest, D., et al. (1997). Drug therapy in the nursing mother. *Obstetrics and Gynecology Clinics of North America*, 24(3), 675–696.

Dix, P., Sandhar, B., Murdoch, J., et al. (2004). Pain on medical wards in a district general hospital. *British Journal of Anaesthesia*, 92(2), 235–237.

D'Onofrio, P., Novelli, A. M. M., Mecacci, F., et al. (2009). The efficacy and safety of continuous intravenous administration of remifentanil for birth pain relief: An open study of 205 parturients. *Anesthesia and Analgesia*, 109(6), 1922–1924.

Dole, V., & Nyswander, M. E. (1965). A medical treatment for diacetylmorphine (heroin) addiction. *J Am Med Assoc*, 193, 646–650.

Dolin, S. J., & Cashman, J. N. (2005). Tolerability of acute postoperative pain management: Nausea, vomiting, sedation, pruritus, and urinary retention. Evidence from published data. *British Journal of Anaesthesia*, 95(5), 584–591.

Donnelly, S., Davis, M. P., Walsh, D., et al. (2002). Morphine in cancer pain management: A practical guide. *Supportive Care in Cancer*, 10(1), 13–35.

Donner, B., Zenz, M., Tryba, M., et al. (1996). Direct conversion from oral morphine to transdermal fentanyl: A multicenter study in patients with cancer pain. *Pain*, 64(3), 527–534.

Donshik, P. C., Pearlman, D., Pinnas, J., et al. (2000). Efficacy and safety of ketorolac tromethamine 0.5% and levocabastin 0.05%: A multicenter comparison in patients with seasonal allergic conjunctivitis. *Advances in Therapy*, 17(2), 94–102.

Dorr, L. D., Raya, J., Long, W. T., et al. (2008). Multimodal analgesia without parenteral narcotics for total knee arthroscopy. *The Journal of Arthroplasty*, 23(4), 502–508.

Dosa, D. M., Dore, D. D., Mor, V., et al. (2009). Frequency of long-acting opioid analgesic initiation in opioid-naive nursing home residents. *Journal of Pain and Symptom Management*, 38(4), 515–521.

Doss, N. W., Ipe, J., Crimi, T., et al. (2001). Continuous thoracic epidural anesthesia with 0.2% ropivacaine versus general anesthesia for perioperative management of modified radical mastectomy. *Anesthesia and Analgesia*, 92(6), 1552–1557.

Douma, M. R., Verwey, R. A., Kam-Endtz, C. E., et al. (2010). Obstetric analgesia: A comparison of patient-controlled meperidine, remifentanil, and fentanyl in labour. *British Journal of Anaesthesia*, 104(2), 209–215.

Doverty, M., White, J. M., Somogyi, A. A., et al. (2001). Hyperalgesic responses in methadone maintenance patients. *Pain*, 90(1–2), 91–96.

Downing, G. M., Kuziemsky, C., Lesperance, M., et al. (2007). Development and reliability testing of the Victoria Bowel Performance Scale (BPS). *Journal of Pain and Symptom Management*, 34(5), 513–522.

Drug Enforcement Administration. (2008). *Drugs and chemicals of concern.* Available at http://www.deadiversion.usdoj.gov/drugs_concern/tramadol.htm. Accessed June 30, 2009.

Drug Topics (2008). *Top 200 drugs.* Available at http://drug-topics.modernmedicine.com/drugtopics/data/articlestandard/drugtopics/222009/599844/article.pdf. Accessed 9 June 2008.

Duggleby, W., & Lander, J. (1994). Cognitive status and postoperative pain: older adults. *Journal of Pain and Symptom Management, 9*(1), 19–27.

Dunbar, P. J., Chapman, C. R., Buckley, F. P., et al. (1996). Clinical analgesic equivalence for morphine and hydromorphone with prolonged PCA. *Pain, 68*(2–3), 265–270.

Duncan, A. (2002). The use of fentanyl and alfentanil sprays for episodic pain. *Palliative Medicine, 16*(6), 550.

Dunteman, E., Karanikolas, M., & Filos, K. S. (1996). Transnasal butorphanol for the treatment of opioid-induced pruritus unresponsive to antihistamines. *Journal of Pain and Symptom Management, 12*(4), 255–260.

DuPen, A., Shen, D., & Ersek, M. (2007). Mechanisms of opioid-induced tolerance and hyperalgesia. *Pain Management Nursing, 8*(3), 113–121.

DuPen, S., DuPen, A., & Hillyer, J. (2006). Intrathecal hydromorphone for intractable nonmalignant pain: A retrospective study. *Pain Medicine (Malden Mass.), 7*(1), 10–15.

DuPen, S. L., & DuPen, A. R. (1998). Spinal analgesia. In M. A. Ashburn, & L. J. Rice (Eds.), *The management of pain* (pp. 171–186). New York: Churchill Livingstone.

Dworkin, R. H., Barbano, R. L., Tyring, S. K., et al. (2009). A randomized, placebo-controlled trial of oxycodone and of gabapentin for acute pain in herpes zoster. *Pain, 142*(3), 209–217.

Dworkin, R. H., O'Connor, A. B., Backonja, M., et al. (2007). Pharmacologic management of neuropathic pain: Evidence-based recommendations. *Pain, 132*(3), 237–251.

Eberhart, L. H., Mauch, M., Morin, A. M., et al. (2002). Impact of a multimodal anti-emetic prophylaxis on patient satisfaction in high-risk patients for postoperative nausea and vomting. *Anaesthesia, 57*(10), 1022–1027.

Ebner, N., Rohrmeister, K., Winklbaur, B., et al. (2007). Management of neonatal abstinence syndrome in neonates born to opioid maintained women. *Drug and Alcohol Dependence, 87*(2–3), 131–138.

Edmonds, P., Higginson, I., Altmann, D., et al. (2000). Is the presence of dyspnea a risk factor for morbidity in cancer patients? *Journal of Pain and Symptom Management, 19*(1), 15–22.

Edwards, J. E., McQuay, H. J., & Moore, R. A. (2004). Single dose oral dihydrocodeine for acute postoperative pain. *Cochrane Database of Systematic Reviews (Online),* (4) D002760.

Edwards, S. M., & Murdin, L. (2001). Respiratory rate – an under-documented clinical assessment. *Clinical Medicine (London, England), 1*(1), 85.

Egan, T. D., Huizinga, B., Gupta, S. K., et al. (1998). Remifentanil pharmcokinetics in obese versus lean patients. *Anesthesiology, 89*(3), 562–573.

Egan, T. D., Kern, S. E., Muir, K. T., et al. (2004). Remifentanil by bolus injection: A safety pharmacokinetic, pharmacodynamic, and age effect investigation in human volunteers. *British Journal of Anaesthesia, 92*(3), 335–343.

Egan, T. D., Sharma, A., Ashburn, M. A., et al. (2000). Multiple dose pharmacokinetics of oral transmucosal fentanyl citrate in healthy volunteers. *Anesthesiology, 92*(3), 665–673.

Egbert, A. M., Parks, L. H., Short, L. M., et al. (1990). Randomized trial postoperative patient-controlled analgesia vs. Intramuscular narcotics in frail elderly men. *Archives of Internal Medicine, 150,* 1897–1903.

Einarson, A., Bozzo, P., & Taguchi, N. (2009). Use of fentanyl patch throughout pregnancy. (Letter). *Journal of Obstet Gynecol Can, 31*(1), 20.

Eisenberg, E., Berkey, C. S., Carr, D. B., et al. (1994). Efficacy and safety of nonsteroidal antiinflammatory drugs for cancer pain: A meta-analysis. *Journal of Clinical Oncology, 12*(12), 2756–2765.

Eisenberg, E., Marinangeli, F., Birkhahn, J., et al. (2005). Time to modify the WHO analgesic ladder? *Pain. Clinical Updates. IASP, 13*(5), 1–4.

Eisenberg, E., McNicol, E. D., & Carr, D. B. (2006). Efficacy of mu-opioid agonists in the treatment of evoked neuropathic pain: Systematic review of randomized controlled trials. *European Journal of Pain (London, England), 10*(8), 667–676.

Eisenkraft, J. B. (2006). Forehead pulse oximetry. Friend and foe. (Editorial). *Anesthesiology, 105*(6), 1075–1077.

Elia, N., Culebras, X., Mazza, C., et al. (2008). Clonidine as an adjuvant to intrathecal local anesthetics for surgery: Systematic review of randomized trials. *Regional Anesthesia and Pain Medicine, 33*(2), 159–167.

Eliot, L., Geiser, R., & Loewen, G. (2001). Steady-state pharmacokinetic comparison of a new, once-daily, extended-release morphine formulation (Morphelan) and OxyContin twice daily. *Journal of Oncology Pharmacy Practice, 7*(1), 1–8.

Elliott, P., O'Hare, R., Bill, K. M., et al. (2000). Severe cardiovascular depression with remifentanil. *Anesthesia and Analgesia, 91*(1), 58–61.

Ely, E. W., Truman, B., Shintani, A., et al. (2003). Monitoring sedation status over time in ICU patients. *JAMA: The Journal of the American Medical Association, 289*(22), 2983–2991.

Endo (2006). *Opana prescribing information.* Chadds Ford, PA: Endo Pharmaceuticals. Available at http://www.endo.com/pdf/Opana_IR_PI.pdf. Accessed April 17, 2008.

Engoren, M., Luther, G., & Fenn-Buderer, N. (2001). A comparison of fentanyl, sufentanil, and remifentanil for fast-track cardiac anesthesia. *Anesthesia and Analgesia, 93*(4), 859–864.

Ernst, A. A., Weiss, S. J., Park, S., et al. (2000). Prochlorperazine versus promethazine for uncomplicated nausea and vomiting in the emergency department: A randomized, double-blind clinical trial. *Annals of Emergency Medicine, 36*(2), 89–94.

Erstad, B. L., Puntillo, K., Gilbert, H. C., et al. (2009). Pain management principles in the critically ill. *Chest, 135*(4), 1075–1086.

Estfan, B., Mahmoud, F., Shaheen, P., et al. (2007). Respiratory function during parenteral opioid titration for cancer pain. *Palliative Medicine, 21*(1), 81–86.

Etches, R. C. (1994). Respiratory depression associated with patient-controlled analgesia: A review of eight cases. *Canadian Journal of Anaesthesia, 41,* 125–132.

Etches, R. C., Gammer, T.-L., & Cornish, R. (1996). Patient-controlled epidural analgesia after thoracotomy: A comparison of meperidine with and without bupivacaine. *Anesthesia and Analgesia, 83*(1), 81–86.

Ethuin, F., Boudaoud, S., Leblanc, I., et al. (2003). Pharmacokinetics of long-term sufentanil infusion for sedation in ICU patients. *Intensive Care Medicine, 29*(11), 1916–1920.

Etropolski, M., Rauschkolb-Loffler, C., Shapiro, D., et al. (2009). A randomized, double-blind, placebo- and active-controlled phase III study of tapentadol ER for chronic low back pain: Analysis of efficacy endpoint sensitivity. (Abstract). *The Journal of Pain: Official Journal of the American Pain Society, 10*(Suppl. 4), S51.

Evans, T. N., & Park, G. R. (1997). Remifentanil in the critically ill. *Anaesthesia, 52*(8), 797–811.

Evron, S., Glezerman, M., Sadan, O., et al. (2005). Remifentanil: A novel systemic analgesic for labor pain. *Anesthesia and Analgesia, 100*(1), 233–238.

Evron, S., Sessler, D., Sadan, O., et al. (2004). Identification of the epidural space: Loss of resistance with air, lidocaine, or the combination of air and lidocaine. *Anesthesia and Analgesia, 99*(1), 245–250.

Ewalenko, P., Janny, S., Dejonckheere, M., et al. (1996). Antiemetic effect of subhypnotic doses of propofol after thyroidectomy. *British Journal of Anaesthesia, 77*(4), 463–467.

Ezri, T., Lurie, S., Stein, A., et al. (2002). Postoperative nausea and vomiting: Comparison of the effect of postoperative meperidine or morphine in gynecologic surgery patients. *Journal of Clinical Anesthesia, 14*(4), 262–266.

Fairlie, F. M., Marshall, L., Walker, J. J., et al. (1999). Intramuscular opioids for maternal pain relief in labor: A randomized controlled trial comparing pethidine with diamorphine. *Britsh Journal of Obstetrics and Gynaecology Research, 106*(11), 1181–1187.

Fajemirokun-Odudeyi, O., Sinha, C., Tutty, S., et al. (2006). Pregnancy outcome in women who use opiates. *European Journal of Obstetrics Gynecology and Reproductive Biology, 126*(2), 170–175.

Fakuda, K. (2005). Intravenous opioid anesthetics. In R. D. Miller (Ed.), *Miller's anesthesia* (6th ed., vol. 1, pp. 379–437). Philadelphia: Elsevier.

Farragher, R. A., & Laffey, J. G. (2006). Postoperative pain management after cesarean section. In G. Shorten, D. B. Carr, D. Harmon, M. M. Puig, & J. Browne (Eds.), *Postoperative pain management: An evidence-based guide to practice* (pp. 225–238). Philadelphia: Saunders.

Ferrell, B. R., & Griffith, H. (1994). Cost issues related to pain management: Report from the cancer pain panel of the Agency for Health Care Policy and Research. *Journal of Pain and Symptom Management, 9*(4), 221–234.

Ferrell, B. R., Virani, R., Paice, J. A., et al. (2009). Evaluation of palliative care nursing education seminars. *European Journal of Oncology Nursing,* doi: 10.1016/j.ejon.2009.08.004.

Fick, D. M., Cooper, J. W., Wade, W. E., et al. (2003). Updating the Beers criteria for potentially inappropriate medication use in older adults: Results of a US consensus panel of experts. *Archives of Internal Medicine, 163*(22), 2716–2724.

Filitz, J., Ihmsen, H., Gunther, W., et al. (2008). Supra-additive effects of tramadol and acetaminophen in a human pain model. *Pain, 136*(3), 262–270.

Fillingim, R. B. (2005). Individual differences in pain responses. *Current Rheumatology Reports, 7*(5), 342–347.

Fine, P. G., Mahajan, G., & McPherson, M. L. (2009). Long-acting opioids and short-acting opioids: Appropriate use in chronic pain management. *Pain Medicine (Malden, Mass.), 10*(Suppl 2), S79–S88.

Fine, P. G., & Portenoy, R. K. (2007). *A clinical guide to opioid analgesia.* New York: Vendome Group, LLC.

Fine, P. G., Portenoy, R. K., & Ad Hoc Expert Panel on Evidence Review and Guidelines for Opioid Rotation. (2009). Establishing "Best practices" for opioid rotation: Conclusions of an expert panel. *Journal of Pain and Symptom Management, 38*(3), 418–425.

Finn, J., Wright, J., Fong, J., et al. (2004). A randomised cross-over trial of patient controlled intranasal fentanyl and oral morphine for procedural wound care in adult patients with burns. *Burns: Journal of the International Society for Burn Injuries, 30*(3), 262–268.

Finnerup, N. B., Otto, M., McQuay, H. J., et al. (2005). Algorithm for neuropathic pain treatment: An evidence-based proposal. *Pain, 118*(3), 289–305.

Finucane, B. T., Ganapathy, S., Carli, F., et al. (2001). Prolonged epidural infusions of ropivacaine (2 mg/mL) after colonic surgery: The impact of adding fentanyl. *Anesthesia and Analgesia, 92*(5), 1276–1285.

Fishbain, D. A. (2009). Oxymorphone status. *Pain Medicine (Malden, Mass.), 10*(Suppl. 1), S1–S2.

Fishbain, D. A., Cole, B., Lewis, J., et al. (2008). What percentage of chronic nonmalignant pain patients exposed to chronic opioid analgesic therapy develop abuse/addiction and/or aberrant drug-related behaviors? A structured evidence-based review. *Pain Medicine (Malden, Mass.), 9*(4), 444–459.

Fishbain, D. A., Cutler, R. B., Rosomoff, H. L., et al. (2002). Can patients taking opioids drive safely? A structured evidence-based review. *Journal Pain Palliative Care Pharmacotherapy, 16*(1), 9–28.

Fishbain, D. A., Cutler, R. B., Rosomoff, H. L., et al. (2003). Are opioid-dependent/tolerant patients impaired in driving-related skills? A structured evidence-based review. *Journal of Pain and Symptom Management, 25*(6), 559–577.

Fishbain, D. A., Lewis, J. E., Cole, B., et al. (2007). Medicolegal rounds: Medicolegal issues and alleged breaches of standards of medical care in a patient motor vehicle accident allegedly related to chronic opioid analgesic therapy. *Journal of Opioid Management, 3*(1), 16–20.

Fisher, K., Stiles, C., & Hagen, N. A. (2004). Characterization of the early pharmacodynamic profile of oral methadone for cancer-related breakthrough pain: A pilot study. *Journal of Pain and Symptom Management, 28*(6), 619–625.

Fisher, K., Stiles, C., Heim, B., et al. (2006). Can fentanyl be systemically absorbed when administered vaginally? A feasibility study. *Journal of Palliative care, 22*(1), 54–56.

Fishman, S. M., Bandman, T. B., Edwards, A., et al. (1999). The opioid contract in the management of chronic pain. *Journal of Pain and Symptom Management, 18*(1), 27–37.

Fishman, S. M., & Webster, L. R. (2009). Unintended harm from opioid prescribing guidelines. *Pain Medicine (Malden, Mass.), 10*(2), 285–286.

Fitzgibbon, D., Morgan, D., Dockter, D., et al. (2003). Initial pharmacokinetic, safety and efficacy evaluation of nasal morphine gluconate for breakthrough pain in cancer patients. *Pain, 106*(3), 309–315.

Fleming, A., Noonan, P., Wheeler, A., et al. (2008). Abuse-deterrent properties and pharmacokinetics of a novel sustained release formulation of oxycodone for the treatment of moderate to severe pain. *The Journal of Pain, 9*(4, Suppl. 1), P46.

Flemming, K. (2010). The use of morphine to treat cancer-related pain: A synthesis of quantitative and qualitative research. *Journal of Pain and Symptom Management*, 39(1), 139–154.

Flisberg, P., Rudin, A., Linner, R., et al. (2003). Pain relief and safety after major surgery. A prospective study of epidural and intravenous analgesia in 2696 patients. *Acta Anaesthesiologica Scandinavica*, 47(4), 457–465.

Foley, K. M. (1993). Opioids. *Neurologic Clinics*, 11(3), 503–522.

Foley, K. M. (1995). Misconceptions and controversies regarding the use of opioids in cancer pain. *Anti-Cancer Drugs*, 6(Suppl 3), 4–13.

Foley, K. M. (2004). Acute and chronic cancer pain syndromes. In D. Doyle, G. Hanks, N. I. Cherny, & K. Calman (Eds.), *Oxford textbook of palliative medicine*. (3rd ed., pp. 298–316). New York: Oxford Press.

Foley, K. M., & Houde, R. W. (1998). Methadone in cancer pain management: Individualize dose and titrate to effect. *Journal of Clinical Oncology*, 16(10), 3213–3215.

Follett, K. A., Boortz-Marx, R. L., Drake, J. M., et al. (2004). Prevention and management of intrathecal drug delivery and spinal cord stimulation system infections. *Anesthesiology*, 100(6), 1582–1594.

Fong, C. C., & Kwan, A. (2005). Patient-controlled sedation using remifentanil for third molar extraction. *Anaesthesia and Intensive Care*, 33(1), 73–77.

Fong, H. K., Sands, L. P., & Leung, J. M. (2006). The role of postoperative analgesia in delirium and cognitive decline in elderly patients: A systematic review. *Anesthesia and Analgesia*, 102(4), 1255–1266.

Forster, J. G., & Rosenberg, P. H. (2004). Small dose of clonidine mixed with low-dose ropivacaine and fentanyl for epidural analgesia after total knee arthroplasty. *British Journal of Anaesthesia*, 93(5), 670–677.

Foss, N. B., Kristensen, M. T., Kristensen, B. B., et al. (2005). Effect of postoperative epidural analgesia on rehabilitation and pain after hip fracture surgery. *Anesthesiology*, 102(6), 1197–1204.

Foster, A., Mobley, E., & Wang, Z. (2007). Complicated pain management in a CYP450 2D6 poor metabolizer. *Pain Practice*, 7(4), 352–356.

Fournier, R., Weber, A., & Gamulin, Z. (2005). Intrathecal sufentanil is more potent than intravenous for postoperative analgesia after total hip replacement. *Regional Anesthesia and Pain Medicine*, 30(3), 249–254.

Fragen, R. J., Vilich, F., Spies, S. M., et al. (1999). The effect of remifentanil on biliary tract drainage into the duodenum. *Anesthesia and Analgesia*, 89(6), 1561–1564.

Fredheim, O. M., Moksnes, K., & Borchgrevink, P. C., et al. (2008). Clinical pharmacology of methadone for pain. *Acta Anaesthesiologica Scandinavica*, 52(7), 879–889.

Freye, E. (2008). *Opioids in medicine*. The Netherlands: Springer.

Frolich, M., Giannotti, A., & Modell, J. H. (2001). Opioid overdose in a patient using a fentanyl patch during treatment with a warming blanket. *Anesthesia and Analgesia*, 93(3), 647–648.

Fromm, M. F., Eckhardt, K., Li, S., et al. (1997). Loss of analgesic effect of morphine due to coadministration of rifampin. *Pain*, 72(1, 2), 261–267.

Fujii, Y., Saitoh, Y., Tanaka, H., et al. (1999). Granisetron/dexamethasone combination for reducing nausea and vomiting during and after spinal anesthesia for cesarean section. *Anesthesia and Analgesia*, 88(6), 1346–1350.

Fukuda, K. (2005). Intravenous opioid anesthetics. (2005). In R. D. Miller (Ed.), *Miller's anesthesia*. (6th ed., pp. 379–437). St. Louis: Churchill Livingstone.

Furlan, A., Lakha, S. F., Yegneswaran, B., et al. (2007). A systematic review of the effects of opioids on driving and working performances. *Pain Research & Management*, 12, 126–127. Poster presented at Canadian Pain Society Conference, May, 2007, Ottawa, Ontario.

Furlan, A. D., Sandoval, J. A., Mailis-Gagnon, A., et al. (2006). Opioids for chronic noncancer pain: A meta-analysis of effectiveness and side effects. *Canadian Medical Association Journal*, 174(11), 1589–1594.

Gabrail, N. Y., Dvergsten, C., & Ahdieh, H. (2004). Establishing the dosage equivalency of oxymorphone extended release and oxycodone controlled release in patients with cancer pain: A randomized controlled study. *Current Medical Research and Opinion*, 20(6), 911–918.

Gaertner, J., Radbruch, T., Giesecke, H., et al. (2006). Assessing cognition and psychomotor function under long-term treatment with controlled release oxycodone in non-cancer patients. *Acta Anesthesiologica Scandinavica*, 50(6), 664–672.

Gagliese, L., Gauthier, L. R., Macpherson, A. K., et al. (2008). Correlates of postoperative pain and intravenous patient-controlled analgesia use in younger and older surgical patients. *Pain Medicine (Malden, Mass.)*, 9(3), 299–314.

Gagliese, L., Jackson, M., Ritvo, P., et al. (2000). Age is not an impediment to effective use of patient-controlled analgesia by surgical patients. *Anesthesiology*, 93(3), 601–610.

Gagnon, P., Allard, P., Masse, B., et al. (2000). Delirium in terminal cancer: A prospective study using daily screening, early diagnosis, and continuous monitoring. *Journal of Pain and Symptom Management*, 19(6), 412–426.

Gallagher, P. F., Barry, P. J., Ryan, C., et al. (2008). Inappropriate prescribing in an acutely ill population of elderly patients as determined by Beers' Criteria. *Age and Ageing*, 37(1), 96–101.

Gallagher, R. E., Arndt, D. R., & Hunt, K. L. (2005). Analgesic effects of topical methadone: A report of four cases. *The Clinical Journal of Pain*, 21(2), 190–192.

Gallagher, R. M., Welz-Bosna, M., & Gammaitoni, A. (2007). Assessment of dosing frequency of sustained-release opioid preparations in patients with chronic nonmalignant pain. *Pain Medicine (Malden, Mass.)*, 8(1), 71–74.

Gallagher, S. F., Haines, K. L., Osterlund, L. G., et al. (2010). Postoperative hypoxemia: Common, undetected, and unsuspected after bariatric surgery. *The Journal of Surgical Research*, doi:10.1016/j.jss.2009.09.003.

Galski, T., Williams, J. B., & Ehle, H. T. (2000). Effects of opioids on driving ability. *Journal of Pain and Symptom Management*, 19(3), 200–208.

Gambling, D., Hughes, T., Martin, G., et al. (2005). A comparison of DepoDur, a novel, single-dose extended-release epidural morphine with conventional, preservative-free epidural morphine for pain relief after lower abdominal surgery. *Anesthesia and Analgesia*, 100(4), 1065–1074.

Gan, T. J. (2002). Postoperative nausea and vomiting—can it be eliminated? *JAMA: The Journal of the American Medical Association*, 287(10), 1233–1236.

Gan, T. J. (2006). Risk factors for postoperative nausea and vomiting. *Anesthesia and Analgesia*, 102(6), 1884–1898.

Gan, T. J., Coop, A., Philip, B. K., et al. (2005). A randomized, double-blind study of granisetron plus dexamethasone versus ondansetron plus dexamethasone to prevent postoperative nausea and vomiting in patients undergoing abdominal hysterectomy. *Anesthesia and Analgesia, 101*(5), 1323–1329.

Gan, T. J., Franiak, R., & Reeves, J. (2002). Ondansetron orally disintegrating tablet versus placebo for the prevention of postdischarge nausea and vomiting after ambulatory surgery. *Anesthesia and Analgesia, 94*(5), 1199–1200.

Gan, T. J., Jiao, K. R., Zenn, M., et al. (2004). A randomized controlled comparison of electro-acupoint stimulation or ondannsetron versus placebo for the prevention of postoperative nausea and vomiting. *Anesthesia and Analgesia, 99*(4), 1070–1075.

Gan, T. J., Meyer, T., Apfel, C. C., et al. (2003). Consensus guidelines for managing postoperative nausea and vomiting. *Anesthesia and Analgesia, 97*(1), 62–71.

Gan, T. J., Meyer, T., Apfel, C. C., et al. (2007). Society for Ambulatory Anesthesia guidelines for the management of postoperative nausea and vomiting. *Anesthesia and Analgesia, 105*(6), 1615–1628.

Gan, T. J., Sinha, A. C., Kovac, A. L., et al. (2009). A randomized, double-blind, multicenter trial comparing transdermal scopolamine plus ondansetron to ondansetron alone for the prevention of postoperative nausea and vomiting in the outpatient setting. *Anesthesia and Analgesia, 108*(5), 1498–1504.

Gan, T.J., Sloan, F., de L Dear, G., et al. (2001). How much are patients willing to pay to avoid postoperative nausea and vomiting? *Anesthesia and Analgesia, 92*(2), 393–400.

Gan, T. J., White, P. F., Scuderi, P. E., et al. (2002). FDA "Black Box" warning regarding use of droperidol for postoperative nause and vomiting: Is it justified? (Letter). *Anesthesiology, 97*(1), 287.

Ganesh, A., & Maxwell, L. G. (2007). Pathophysiology and management of opioid-induced pruritus. *Drugs, 67*(6), 2323–2333.

Gannon, R. H. (2007). Current strategies for preventing or ameliorating postoperative ileus: A multimodal approach. *American Journal of Health-System Pharmacy: AJHP, 64*(20 Suppl. 13), S8–S12.

Gardner-Nix, J. (1996). Oral methadone for managing chronic nonmalignant pain. *Journal of Pain and Symptom Management, 11*(5), 321–328.

Gardner-Nix, J. (2001a). Oral transmucosal fentanyl and sufentanil for incident pain. (Letter). *Journal of Pain and Symptom Management, 22*(2), 627–629.

Gardner-Nix, J. (2001b). Caregiver toxicity from transdermal fentanyl. (Letter). *Journal of Pain and Symptom Management, 21*(6), 447–448.

Gardner-Nix, J., & Mercadante, S. (2010). The role of OROS hydromorphone in the management of cancer pain. *Pain Practice, 10*(1), 72–77.

Gasche, Y., Daali, Y., Fathi, M., et al. (2004). Codeine intoxication associated with ultrarapid CYP2D6 metabolism. *The New England Journal of Medicine, 351*(27), 2827–2831.

Gaskell, H., Derry, S., Moore, R. A., et al. (2009). Single dose oral oxycodone and oxycodone plus paracetamol (acetaminophen) for acute postoperative pain in adults. *Cochrane Database of Systematic Reviews (Online),* (3), CD002763.

Gasse, C., Derby, L., Vasilakis-Scaramozza, C., et al. (2000). Incidence of first-time idiopathic seizures in users of tramadol. *Pharmacotherapy, 20*(6), 629–634.

Gautier, P. E., Debry, F., Fanard, L., et al. (1997). Ambulatory combined spinal-epidural analgesia for labor: Influence of epinephrine on bupivacaine-sufentanil combination. *Regional Anesthesia, 22*(2), 143–149.

Gharagozlou, P., Hashemi, E., DeLorey, T. M., et al. (2006). Pharmacological profiles of opioid ligands at kappa opioid receptors. *BMC Pharmacology, 6,* 3.

Ghori, M. K., Zhang, Y. F., & Sinatra, R. S. (2009). Pathophysiology of acute pain. In R. S Sinatra, O. A de Leon-Casasola, B. Ginsberg, & E. R Viscusi (Eds.), *Acute pain management* (pp. 21–32). Cambridge, New York: Cambridge University Press.

Gianino, J. M., York, M. M., & Paice, J. A. (1996). *Intrathecal drug therapy for spasticity and pain.* New York: Springer.

Gibbison, B., & Spencer, R. (2009). Post-operative nausea and vomiting. *Anaesthesia and Intensive Care Medicine, 10*(12), 583–585.

Gilron, I. (2008). Analgesia controlled with patience: Towards a better understanding of analgesic self-administration behaviour. *Canadian Journal of Anesthesia, 55*(2), 75–81.

Gilron, I., Bailey, J. M., Tu, D., et al. (2005). Morphine, gabapentin, or their combination for neuropathic pain. *The New England Journal of Medicine, 352*(13), 1324–1334.

Gimbel, J. S., & Ahdieh, H. (2004). The efficacy and safety of oral immediate-release oxymorphone for postsurgical pain. *Anesthesia and Analgesia, 99*(5), 1472–1477.

Gimbel, J.S, Richards, P., & Portenoy, R. K. (2003). Controlled-release oxycodone for pain in diabetic neuropathy. A randomized controlled trial. *Neurology, 60*(6), 927–934.

Gimbel, J. S., Walker, D., Ma, T., et al. (2005). Efficacy and safety of oxymorphone immediate release for the treatment of mild to moderate pain after ambulatory orthopedic surgery: Results of a randomized, double-blind, placebo-controlled trial. *Archives of Physical Medicine and Rehabilitation, 86*(12), 2284–2289.

Ginsberg, B., Cohen, N. A., Ossey, K. D., et al. (1989). The use of PCA to assess the influence of demographic factors on analgesic requirements. *Anesthesiology, 71,* A688 (abstract).

Ginsberg, B., Sinatra, R. S., Adler, L. J., et al. (2003). Conversion to oral controlled-release oxycodone from intravenous opioid analgesic in the postoperative setting. *Pain Medicine (Malden, Mass.), 4*(1), 31–38.

Glare, P., Walsh, D., & Sheehan, D. (2006). The adverse effects of morphine: A prospective survey of common symptoms during repeated dosing for chronic pain. *The American Journal of Hospice & Palliative Care, 23*(3), 229–235.

GlaxoSmithKline. (2009). *Entereg prescribing information.* Research Triangle Park, NC: GlaxoSmithKline.

Goldberg, M., Vatashsky, E., Haskel, Y., et al. (1987). The effect of meperidine on the guinea pig extrahepatic biliary tract. *Anesthesia and Analgesia, 66*(12), 1282–1286.

Gold Standard Clinical Pharmacology. (2009). *Relistor monograph.* Available at http://clinicalpharmacology.com/Forms/Monograph/monograph.aspx?cpnum=3386&sec=monindi. Accessed August 19, 2009.

Golembiewski, J. A. (2003). Morphine and hydromorphone for postoperative analgesia: Focus on safety. *Journal of Perianesthesia Nursing, 18*(2), 120–122.

Golembiewski, J. A., Chernin, E., & Chopra, T. (2005). Prevention and treatment of postoperative nausea and vomiting. *American Journal of Health-System Pharmacy, 62*(5), 1247–1262.

Golf, M., Robson, M., Pollak, R., et al. (2008). *Safety and efficacy of 12-hour controlled-release hydrocodone/acetaminophen for acute pain following bunionectomy: A phase 3, randomized, multi-center, double-blind study.* Paper presented at *American Academy of Pain Medicine Annual Meeting*, Orlando, Florida, February 12–16.

Goll, V., Akca, O., Grief, R., et al. (2001). Ondansetron is no more effective than supplemental intraoperative oxygen for prevention of postoperative nausea and vomiting. *Anesthesia and Analgesia, 92*(1), 112–117.

Goodfriend, B. (1987). Slap down injection discomfort. *Consultant, 27*, 154.

Goodheart, C. R., & Leavitt, S. B. (2006). Managing opioid-induced constipation in ambulatory-care patients. *Pain Treatment Topics.* Available at http://pain-topics.org/pdf/Managing_Opioid-Induced_Constipation.pdf#search="constipation". Accessed July 28, 2007.

Goodman, M., Low, J., & Wilkinson, S. (2005). Constipation management in palliative care: A survey of practices in the United Kingdom. *Journal of Pain and Symptom Management, 29*(3), 238–244.

Goodwin, K., Kim, N. H., & Zuniga, R. (2001). Stability of a baclofen and clonidine hydrochloride admixture for intrathecal administration. *Hospital pharmacy, 36*(9), 950–954.

Gordon, A. F., Levine, J. D., Dubois, M. Y., et al. (2007). Open-label exploration of an intravenous nalbuphine and naloxone mixture as an analgesic agent following gynecologic surgery. *Pain Medicine (Malden, Mass.), 8*(6), 525–530.

Gordon, D. (1995). Hydroxyzine doesn't "help" opioids. *The American Journal of Nursing, 95*(8), 20.

Gordon, D. B. (2006). Oral transmucosal fentanyl citrate for cancer breakthrough pain: A review. *Oncology Nursing Forum, 33*(2), 257–264.

Gordon, D. B. (2008). Continuous infusion subcutaneous morphine. Personal email communication on September, 20, 2008.

Gordon, D. B., Dahl, J., Phillips, P., et al. (2004). The use of "as needed" range orders for opioid analgesics in the management of acute pain: A consensus statement from the American Society for Pain Management Nursing and the American Pain Society. *Pain Management Nursing, 5*(2), 53–58.

Gordon, D. B., Jones, H. D., Goshman, L. M., et al. (2000). A quality improvement approach to reducing use of meperidine. *Joint Commission Journal on Quality and Improvement, 26*(12), 686–699.

Gordon, D. B., Pellino, T. A., Higgins, G. A., et al. (2008). Nurses' opinions on appropriate administration of PRN range opioid analgesic orders for acute pain. *Pain Management Nursing, 9*(3), 131–140.

Gordon, N. B. (1973). The functional status of the methadone maintained person. In L. R. S. Simmons, & M. B. Gold (Eds.), *Discrimination and the addict* (pp. 101–121). Beverly Hills: Sage Publications.

Gottschalk, A. (2009). Craniotomy pain: Trying to do better. *Anesthesia and Analgesia, 109*(5), 1379–1381.

Gottschalk, A., Freitag, M., Burmeister, M.A, et al. (2002). Patient-controlled thoracic epidural infusion with ropivacaine 0.375% provides comparable pain relief as bupivacaine 0.125% plus sufentanil after major abdominal gynecologic tumor surgery. *Regional Anesthesia and Pain Medicine, 27*(4), 367–373.

Gould, E. M., Jensen, M. P., Victor, T. W., et al. (2009). The pain quality response profile of oxymorphone extended release in the treatment of low back pain. *The Clinical Journal of Pain, 25*(2), 116–122.

Gourevitch, M. N. (2009). First, do no harm . . . reduction? *Annals of Internal Medicine, 150*(6), 417–418.

Gourevitch, M. N., & Friedland, G. H. (2000). Interactions between methadone and medications used to treat HIV infection: A review. *The Mount Sinai Journal of Medicine New York, 67*(5–6), 429–436.

Graf, C., & Puntillo, K. (2003). Pain in the older adult in the intensive care unit. *Critical Care Clinics, 19*, 749–770.

Gralow, I. (2002). Cancer pain: An update of pharmacological approaches in pain therapy. *Current Opinion in Anaesthesiology, 15*(5), 555–561.

Grape, S., & Schug, S. A. (2008). Epidural and spinal analgesia. In P. E Macintyre, S. M Walker, & D. J. Rowbotham (Eds.), *Clinical pain management. Acute pain* (pp. 255–270). London: Hodder Arnold.

Grape, S., & Tramer, M. R. (2007). Do we need preemptive analgesia for the treatment of postoperative pain? *Best Practice & Research Clinical Anaesthesiology, 21*(1), 51–63.

Grass, J. A. (2005). Patient-controlled analgesia. *Anesthesia and Analgesia, 101*(Suppl. 1), S44–S61.

Grauer, P. A., Bass, J., Wenzel, E., et al. (1992). A feasibility study of the rectal and vaginal administration of sustained release morphine sulfate tablets for the treatment of cancer-related pain. *Proc Am Soc Clin Oncol, 11*, 1392.

Grover, V. K., Mathew, P. J., & Hegde, H. (2009). Efficacy of orally disintegrating ondansetron in preventing postoperative nausea and vomiting after laparoscopic cholecystectomy: A randomised, double-blind placebo controlled study. *Anaesthesia, 64*(6), 595–600.

Gruber, E. M., Tschernko, E. M., Kritzinger, M., et al. (2001). The effects of thoracic epidural analgesia with bupivacaine 0.25% on ventilatory mechanics in patients with severe chronic obstructive pulmonary disease. *Anesthesia and Analgesia, 92*(4), 1015–1019.

Guay, D. R. (2007). Use of oral oxymorphone in the elderly. *The Consultant Pharmacist: The Journal of the American Society of Consultant Pharmacists, 22*(5), 417–430.

Guignard, B., Bossard, A. E., Cost, C., et al. (2000). Acute opioid tolerance. Intraoperative remifentanil increases postoperative pain and morphine requirement. *Anesthesiology, 93*(2), 409–417.

Guler, T., Unlugenc, H., Gundogan, Z., et al. (2004). A background infusion of morphine enhances patient-controlled analgesia after cardiac surgery. *Canadian Journal of Anesthesia, 51*(7), 718–722.

Gunion, M. W., Marchionne, A. M., & Anderson, C. T. M. (2004). Use of the mixed agonist antagonist nalbuphine in opioid based analgesia. *Acute Pain, 6*(1), 29–39.

Gupta, A., Fant, F., Axelsson, K., et al. (2006). Postoperative analgesia after radical retropublic prostatectomy. *Anesthesiology, 105*(4), 784–793.

Gupta, S., & Sathyan, G. (2007). Providing constant analgesia with OROS hydromorphone. *Journal of Pain and Symptom Management, 33*(2S), S19–S24.

Gurkan, Y., & Toker, K. (2002). Prophylactic ondansetron reduces the incidence of intrathecal fentanyl-induced pruritus. *Anesthesia and Analgesia, 96*(6), 1763–1766.

Gutstein, H. B., & Akil, H. (2006). Opioid analgesics. In L. L. Brunton, J. S. Lazo, & K. L. Parker (Eds.), *Goodman, Gilman's the pharmacological basis of therapeutics.* (11th ed., pp. 547–590). New York: McGraw-Hill.

Habib, A. S., Breen, T. W., & Gan, T. J. (2005). Promethazine adverse events after implementation of a medication shortage interchange. (Letter). *The Annals of Pharmacotherapy, 39*(7–8), 1370.

Habib, A. S., El-Moalem, H. E., & Gan, T. J. (2004). The efficacy of the 5-HT3 receptor antagonists combined with droperidol for PONV prophylaxis is similar to their combination with dexamethasone: A meta-analysis of randomized controlled trials. *Canadian Journal of Anesthesia, 51*(4), 311–319.

Habib, A. S., & Gan, T. J. (2003). Food and Drug Administration Black Box Warning on the perioperative use of droperidol: A review of the cases. *Anesthesia and Analgesia, 96*(5), 1377–1379.

Habib, A. S., & Gan, T. J. (2004). Evidence-based management of postoperative nausea and vomiting: A review. *Canadian Journal of Anesthesia, 51*(4), 326–341.

Habib, A. S., & Gan, T. J. (2010). CON: Postoperative nausea and vomiting database research: Limitations and opportunities. (Editorial). *Anesthesia and Analgesia, 110*(2), 412–414.

Habib, A. S., Reuveni, J., Taguchi, A., et al. (2007). A comparison of ondansetron with promethazine for treating postoperative nausea and vomiting in patients who received prophylaxis with ondansetron: A retrospective database analysis. *Anesthesia and Analgesia, 104*(3), 548–551.

Habib, A. S., White, W. D., Eubanks, S., et al. (2004). A randomized comparison of a multimodal management strategy versus combination antiemetics for the prevention of postoperative nausea and vomiting. *Anesthesia and Analgesia, 99*(1), 77–81.

Hadi, I., da Silva, O., Natale, R., et al. (2006). Opioids in the parturient with chronic nonmalignant pain: A retrospective review. *Journal of Opioid Management, 2*(1), 31–34.

Hagen, N. A., & Babul, N. (1997). Comparative clinical efficacy and safety of a novel controlled-release oxycodone formulation and controlled-release hydromorphone in the treatment of cancer pain. *Cancer, 79*, 1428–1437.

Hagen, N. A., Fisher, K., & Stiles, C. (2007). Sublingual methadone for the management of cancer-related breakthrough pain: A pilot study. *Journal of Palliative Medicine, 10*(2), 331–337.

Hagen, N. A., & Swanson, R. (1997). Strychnine-like multifocal myoclonus and seizures in extremely high-dose opioid administration: Treatment strategies. *Journal of Pain and Symptom Management, 14*(1), 51–58.

Hair, P. I., Keating, G. M., & McKeage, K. (2008). Transdermal matrix fentanyl membrane patch (matrifen): In severe cancer-related chronic pain. *Drugs, 68*(14), 2001–2009.

Hale, M. E., Ahdieh, H., Ma, T., et al. (2007). Efficacy and safety of OPANA ER (oxymorphone extended release) for relief of moderate to severe chronic low back pain in opioid-experienced patients: A 12-week, randomized, double-blind, placebo-controlled study. *The Journal of Pain, 8*(2), 175–184.

Hale, M. E., Dvergsten, C., & Gimbel, J. (2005). Efficacy and safety of oxymorphone extended-release in chronic low back pain: Results of a randomized, double-blind, placebo- and active-controlled study. *The Journal of Pain, 6*(1), 21–28.

Hale, M., Tudor, I. C., Khanna, S., et al. (2007). Efficacy and tolerability of once-daily OROS hydromorphone and twice-daily extended-release oxycodone in patients with chronic, moderate to severe osteoarthritis pain: Results of a 6-week, randomized, open-label, noninferiority analysis. *Clinical Therapeutics, 29*(5), 874–888.

Hale, M., Upmalis, D., Okamoto, A., et al. (2009). Tolerability of tapentadol immediate release in patients with lower back pain or osteoarthritis of the hip or knee over 90 days: A randomized, double-blind study. *Current Medical Research and Opinion, 25*(5), 1095–1104.

Halker, R. B., Demaerschalk, B. M., Wellik, K. E., et al. (2007). Caffeine for the prevention and treatment of postdural puncture headache: Debunking the myth. *The Neurologist, 13*(5), 323–327.

Han, P. K. J., Arnold, R., & Bond, G. (2002). Myoclonus secondary to withdrawal from transdermal fentanyl: Case report and literature review. *Journal of Pain and Symptom Management, 23*(1), 66–72.

Hanks, G., Cherny, N. I., & Fallon, M. (2004). Opioid analgesic therapy. In D. Doyle, G. Hanks, N. I. Cherny, & K. Calman (Eds.), *Oxford textbook of palliative medicine.* (3rd ed., pp. 316–341). New York: Oxford Press.

Hanks, G. W., De Conno, F., Cherny, N., et al. (2001). Morphine and alternative opioids in cancer pain: The EAPC recommendations. *British Journal of Cancer, 84*(5), 587–593.

Hanks, G. W., & Reid, C. (2005). Contribution to variability in response to opioids. *Supportive Care in Cancer, 13*(3), 145–152.

Hanley, M. A., Jensen, M. P., Smith, D. G., et al. (2007). Preamputation pain and acute pain predict chronic pain after lower extremity amputation. *The Journal of Pain, 8*(2), 102–109.

Hanna, M. H., Elliott, K. M., & Fung, M. (2005). Randomized, double-blind study of the analgesic efficacy of morphine-6-glucuronide versus morphine sulfate for postoperative pain in major surgery. *Anesthesiology, 102*(4), 815–821.

Hanna, M., O'Brien, C., & Wilson, M. C. (2008). Prolonged-release oxycodone enhances the effects of existing gabapentin therapy in painful diabetic neuropathy patients. *European Journal of Pain (London, England), 12*(6), 804–813.

Hanna, M., Thipphawong, J., 118 Study Group. (2008). A randomized, double-blind comparison of OROS hydromorphone and controlled-release for the control of chronic cancer pain. *BMC Palliative Care, 7*(1), 17.

Hans, G. (2007). Buprenorphine—a review of its role in neuropathic pain. *Journal Opioid Management, 2*(4), 195–206.

Hansen, L. A., Noyes, M. A., & Lehman, M. E. (1991). Evaluation of patient-controlled analgesia (PCA) versus PCA plus continuous infusion in postoperative cancer patients. *Journal of Pain and Symptom Management, 6*(1), 4–14.

Harnett, M. J. P., O'Rourke, N., Walsh, M., et al. (2007). Transdermal scopolamine for prevention of intrathecal morphine-induced nausea and vomiting after cesarean delivery. *Anesthesia and Analgesia, 105*(3), 764–769.

Harris, J. D. (2008). Management of expected and unexpected opioid-related side effects. *The Clinical Journal of Pain*, 24(4, Suppl. 10), S8–S13.

Harris, J. D., & Kotob, F. (2006). In de Leon-Casasola (Eds.), *Cancer pain. Pharmacological, interventional and palliative care approaches* (pp. 207–234). Philadelphia: Saunders.

Hartrick, C. T., & Hartrick, K. A. (2008). Extended-release epidural morphine (DepoDur): Review and safety analysis. *Expert Review of Neurotherapeutics*, 8(11), 1641–1648.

Hartrick, C., Van Hove, I., Stegmann, J. U., et al. (2009). Efficacy and tolerability of tapentadol immediate release and oxycodone HCL immediate release in patients awaiting primary joint replacement surgery for end-stage joint disease: A 10-day, phase III, randomized, double-blind, active- and placebo-controlled study. *Clinical Therapeutics*, 31(2), 260–271.

Hartrick, C. T., Martin, G., Kantor, G., et al. (2006). Evaluation of a single-dose extended-release epidural morphine formulation for pain after knee arthroplasty. *Journal of Bone and Joint Surgery*, 88A(11), 271–281.

Hartsell, T., Long, D., & Kirsch, J. R. (2005). The efficacy of postoperative ondansetron (Zofran®) orally disintegrating tablets for preventing nausea and vomiting after acoustic neuroma surgery. *Anesthesia and Analgesia*, 101(5), 1492–1496.

Hassenbusch, S. J., Portenoy, R. K., Cousins, M., et al. (2004). Polyanalgesic consensus conference 2003: An update on the management of pain by intraspinal drug delivery—report of an expert panel. *Journal of Pain and Symptom Management*, 27(6), 540–563.

Hawton, K., Bergen, H., Simkin, S., et al. (2009). Effect of withdrawal of co-proxamol on prescribing and deaths from drug poisoning in England and Wales: Time series analysis. *BMJ (Clinical Research Ed.)*, 338, b2270.

Hebl, J. R. (2006). The importance and implications of aseptic techniques during regional anesthesia. *Regional Anesthesia and Pain Medicine*, 31(4), 311–323.

Heid, F., Piepho, T., Stengel, S., et al. (2009). Premature termination of epidural analgesia—a prospective analysis to improve quality. *Acute Pain*, 11(3–4), 75–81.

Heinomen, O. P., Slone, S., & Shapiro, S. (1977). *Birth defects and drugs in pregnancy*. Littleton, MA: Publishing Science Group.

Heiskanen, T., Matzke, S., Haakana, S., et al. (2009). Transdermal fentanyl in cachectic cancer patients. *Pain*, 144(1–2), 218–222.

Heit, H. A., & Gourlay, D. L. (2008). Buprenorphine: New tricks with an old molecule for pain management. *The Clinical Journal of Pain*, 24(2), 93–97.

Heitz, J. W., & Viscusi, E. R. (2009). In R. S. Sinatra, O. A. de Leon-Casasola, B. Ginsberg, & E.R Viscusi (Eds.), *Acute pain management* (pp. 323–331). Cambridge, New York: Cambridge University Press.

Helm, J. F., Venu, R. P., Geenen, J. E., et al. (1988). Effects of morphine on the human sphincter of Oddi. *Gut*, 29(10), 1402–1407.

Hemmelgarn, B., Suissa, S., Huang, A., et al. (1997). Benzodiazepine use and the risk of motor vehicle crash in the elderly. *J Am Med Assoc*, 278, 27–31.

Hemstapat, K., Monteith, G. R., Smith, D., et al. (2003). Morphine-3 glucuronide's neuro-excitatory effects are mediated via indirect activation of N-methyl-D-aspartic acid receptors: Mechanistic studies in embryonic cultured hippocampal neurones. *Anesthesia and Analgesia*, 97(2), 494–505.

Hendler, N., Cimini, C., & Long, D. (1980). A comparison of cognitive impairment due to benzodiazepines and to narcotics. *The American Journal of Psychiatry*, 137(7), 828–830.

Henry, A., Tetzlaff, J. E., & Steckner, K. (2002). Ondansetron is effective in treatment of pruritus after intrathecal fentanyl. (Letter). *Regional Anesthesia and Pain Medicine*, 27(5), 538–539.

Herrick, I. A., Ganapathy, S., Komar, W., et al. (1996). Postoperative cognitive impairment in the elderly. *Anaesthesia*, 51, 356–360.

Hersh, E. V., Pinto, A., & Moore, P. A. (2007). Adverse drug interactions involving common prescription and over-the-counter analgesic agents. *Clinical Therapeutics*, 29(Suppl.), 2477–2497.

Hess, P., & Aleshi, P. (2008). Pain in pregnancy, childbirth, and the puerperium. In P. E. Macintyre, S. M. Walker, & D. J. Rowbotham (Eds.), *Acute pain*. (2nd ed., pp. 460–476). London, UK: Hodder Arnold.

Hewitt, D. J. (2000). The Brietbart, et al article reviewed. *Oncology*, 14(5), 705–710.

Hewitt, D. J., Todd, K. H., Xiang, J., et al. (2007). Tramadol/acetaminophen or hydrocodone/acetaminophen for the treatment of ankle sprain: A randomized, placebo-controlled trial. *Annals of Emergency Medicine*, 49(4), 468–480.

Hicks, R. W., Heath, M., Sikirica, V., et al. (2008). Medication errors involving patient-controlled analgesia. *Joint Commission Journal on Quality and Patient Safety/Joint Commission Resources*, 34(12), 734–742.

Hildebrand, K. R., Elsberry, D. E., & Anderson, V. C. (2001a). Stability and compatibility of hydromorphone hydrochloride in an implantable infusion system. *Journal of Pain and Symptom Management*, 22(6), 1042–1047.

Hildebrand, K. R., Elsberry, D. D., & Deer, T. R. (2001b). Stability, compatibility, and safety of intrathecal bupivacaine administered chronically via an implantable delivery system. *The Clinical Journal of Pain*, 17(3), 238–244.

Hildebrand, K. R., Elsberry, D. D., & Hassenbusch, S. J. (2003). Stability and compatibility of morphine—clonidine admixtures in an implantable infusion system. *Journal of Pain and Symptom Management*, 25(5), 464–471.

Hillman, H., & Jarman, D. (1986). Freezing skin. *Nursing times*, 82, 40–41.

Hinrichs, M., & Huseboe, J. (2001). Research-based protocol: Management of constipation. *Journal of Gerontology Nursing*, 27(2), 17–28.

Ho, K. T., & Gan, T. J. (2009). Opioid-related adverse effects and treatment options. In R. S Sinatra, O. A. de Leon-Casasola, B. Ginsberg, & E. R Viscusi (Eds.), *Acute pain management* (pp. 406–415). Cambridge: New York, Cambridge University Press.

Ho, T., Vrabec, J. T., & Burton, A. W. (2007). Hydrocodone use and sensorineural hearing loss. *Pain Physician*, 10(3), 467–472.

Hodgson, P. S., & Liu, S. S. (2001). A comparison of ropivacaine with fentanyl to bupivacaine with fentanyl for postoperative patient-controlled epidural analgesia. *Anesthesia and Analgesia*, 92(4), 1024–1028.

Hodgson, P. S., Neal, J. M., Pollock, J. E., et al. (1999). The neurotoxicity of drugs given intrathecally (spinal). *Anesthesia and Analgesia*, 88(4), 798–809.

Hogan, J. (2006). Why don't nurses monitor the respiratory rate of patients? *British Journal of Nursing (Mark Allen Publishing)*, 15(9), 489–492.

Hoke, J. F., Shlugman, D., Dershwitz, M., et al. (1997). Pharmacokinetics and pharmacodynamics of remifentanil in persons with renal failure compared with healthy volunteers. *Anesthesiology*, 87, 533–541.

Holmfred, A., Vikersfors, T., Berggren, L., et al. (2006). Intrathecal catheters with subcutaneous port systems in patients with severe cancer-related pain managed out of hospital: The risk of infection. *Journal of Pain and Symptom Management*, 31(6), 568–572.

Holmquist, G. (2009). Opioid metabolism and effects of cytochrome P450. *Pain Medicine (Malden, Mass.)*, 10(Suppl. 1), S20–S29.

Holt, D. V., Viscusi, E. R., & Wordell, C. J. (2007). Extended-duration agents for perioperative pain management. *Current pain and Headache Reports*, 11(1), 33–37.

Holte, K., Kehlet (2002). Postoperative ileus: Progress towards effective management. *Drugs*, 62(18), 2603–2615.

Hong, D., Flood, P., & Diaz, G. (2008). The side effects of morphine and hydromorphone patient-controlled analgesia. *Anesthesia and Analgesia*, 107(4), 1384–1389.

Horlocker, T. T., & Wedel, D. J. (2006). Regional anesthesia in the immunocompromised patient. *Regional Anesthesia and Pain Medicine*, 31(4), 334–345.

Huang, P., Kehner, G. B, Cowan, A., et al. (2001). Comparison of pharmacological activities of buprenorphine and norbuprenorphine: Norbuprenorphine is a potent opioid agonist. *Journal of Pharmacology and Experimental Therapeutics*, 297(2), 688–695.

Huang, Y. S., Lin, L. C., Huh, B. K., et al. (2007). Epidural clonidine for postoperative pain after total knee arthroplasty: A dose-response study. *Anesthesia and Analgesia*, 104(5), 1230–1235.

Huang, Y. M., Wang, C. M., Wang, C. T., et al. (2008). Perioperative celebrex administration for pain management after total knee arthroplasty—A randomized, controlled study. *BMC Musculoskeletal Disorders*, 9, 77.

Hubbard, G. P., & Wolfe, K. R. (2003). Meperidine misuse in a patient with sphincter of Oddi dysfunction. *The Annals of Pharmacotherapy*, 37(4), 534–537.

Hudcova, J., McNicol, E. D., Quah, C. S., et al. (2006). Patient controlled opioid analgesia versus conventional opioid analgesia for postoperative pain. *Cochrane Database of Systematic Reviews (Online)*, (4), CD003348.

Hudziak, B. (1983). Contralateral ice massage during bone marrow aspiration. *PRN Forum*, 2, 5.

Hum, A., Fainsinger, R. L., & Bielech, M. (2007). Subcutaneous methadone—An issue revisited. *Journal of Pain and Symptom Management*, 34(6), 573–575.

Hunt, R., Fazekas, B., Thorne, D., et al. (1999). A comparison of subcutaneous morphine and fentanyl in hospice cancer patients. *Journal of Pain and Symptom Management*, 18, 111–119.

Hutchison, R. W., Chon, E. H., Tucker, W. F., et al. (2006). A comparison of a fentanyl, hydromorphone, and morphine patient-controlled intravenous delivery for acute postoperative analgesia: A multicenter study of opioid-induced adverse effects. *The American Journal of Nursing*, 41(7), 659–663.

Iatrou, C. A., Dragoumanis, C. K., Vogiatzaki, T. D., et al. (2005). Prophylactic intravenous ondansetron and dolasetron in intrathecal morphine-induced pruritus: A randomized, double-blinded, placebo-controlled study. *Anesthesia and Analgesia*, 101(5), 1516–1520.

Iijima, T., Ishiyama, T., Kashimoto, S., et al. (2007). A comparison of three different concentrations if ropivacaine with fentanyl for patient-controlled analgesia. *Anesthesia and Analgesia*, 105(2), 507–511.

Indelicato, R. A., & Portenoy, R. K. (2002). Opioid rotation in the management of refractory cancer pain. *Journal of Clinical Oncology*, 20(1), 348–352.

Inouye, S. M., van Dyck, C., Alessi, C., et al. (1990). Clarifying confusion: The confusion assessment method. *Annals of Internal Medicine*, 113(12), 941–948.

Institute for Safe Medication Practices (ISMP). (2003a). Safety issues with patient-controlled analgesia. Part I. *ISMP Medication Safety Alert!*, 8(14), 1–3. http://www.ismp.org/Newsletters/acutecare/articles/20030710.asp. Accessed July 30, 2003.

Institute for Safe Medication Practices (ISMP). (2003b). Safety issues with patient-controlled analgesia. Part II. *ISMP Medication Safety Alert!*, 8(15), 1–3. Available at http://www.ismp.org/Newsletters/acutecare/articles/20030724.asp. Accessed July 30, 2003.

Institute for Safe Medication Practices (ISMP). (2003c). How fast is too fast for IV push medications? *ISMP Medication Safety Alert!*, 8(11), 1–2. Available at http://www.ismp.org/Newsletters/acutecare/articles/20030515.asp. Accessed May 6, 2005.

Institute for Safe Medication Practices (ISMP). (2004a). An omnipresent risk of morphine hydromorphone mix-ups. *ISMP Medication Safety Alert!*, 8(15), 1–3. Available at http://www.ismp.org/Newsletters/acutecare/articles/20040701.asp. Accessed April 4, 2008.

Insititue for Safe Medication Practices (ISMP). (2004b). Misprogram a PCA pump? It's easy! *ISMP Medication Safety Alert!*, 9(15), 1–2.

Institute for Safe Medication Practices (ISMP). (2004c). The five rights cannot stand alone. *Nurse-Advise ERR*, 2(11), 1. Available at http://www.ismp.org/Newsletters/nursing/Issues/NurseAdviseERR200411.pdf. Accessed September 4, 2009.

Institute for Safe Medication Practices (ISMP). (2006a). Action needed to prevent serious tissue injury with IV promethazine. *ISMP Medication Safety Alert!*, 4(6), 1–2.

Institute for Safe Medication Practices (ISMP). (2006b). Promethazine survey spurs renewed efforts to prevent tissue injury. *ISMP Medication Safety Alert!*, 4(6), 1–2.

Institute for Safe Medication Practices (ISMP). (2007). Reducing patient harm from opiates. *ISMP Medication Safety Alert! Acute Care Edition*. Available at http://www.ismp.org/Newsletters/acutecare/articles/20070222.asp.

Institute for Safe Medication Practices (ISMP). (2008). Keeping patients safe from iatrogenic methadone overdoses. *ISMP Medication Safety Alert: Acute Care Edition*. Available at http://www.ismp.org/newsletters/acutecare/articles/20080214.asp. Accessed July 31, 2009.

Institute for Safe Medication Practices (ISMP). (2009). Various release formulations of oral opioids confusion. *ISMP Medication Safety Alert! Nurse Advise-ERR*, 7(3), 1–3.

Insititue for Safe Medication Practices (ISMP). (2010). Intrathecal injection warrants mask worn by clinicians during procedure. *ISMP Medication Safety Alert! Nurse Advise-ERR*, 8(1), 1–2.

Inturrisi, C. E. (2002). Clinical pharmacology of opioids for pain. *The Clinical Journal of Pain*, 18(S3), S3–S13.

Inturrisi, C. E. (2009). Speaking for you: APS Develops and Promulgates REMS Position. *APS Bulletin, 19*(3). Available at http://www.ampainsoc.org/pub/bulletin/fall09/pres.htm. Accessed March 16, 2010.

Iocolano, C. F. (2000). Perioperative pain management in the chemically dependent patient. *Journal of Perianesthesia Nursing, 155*(5), 329–347.

Ionescu, D., Badescu, C., & Acalovschi, I. (2007). Nicotine patch for the prevention of postoperative nausea and vomiting. *Clinical Drug Investigation, 27*(8), 559–564.

Ishiyama, T., Iijima, T., Sugawara, T., et al. (2007). The use of patient-controlled epidural fentanyl in elderly patients. *Anaesthesia, 62*(2), 1246–1250.

Isono, S., Tanaka, A., & Nishino, T. (2002). Lateral position decreases collapsibility of the passive pharynx in patients with obstructive sleep apnea. *Anesthesiology, 97*(4), 771–773.

Jackson, K., Ashby, M., & Keech, J. (2002). Pilot dose finding study of intranasal sufentanil for breakthrough and incident cancer-associated pain. *Journal of Pain and Symptom Management, 23*(6), 450–452.

Jacobi, J., Fraser, G., Coursin, D., et al. (2002). Clinical practice guidelines for the sustained use of sedatives and analgesics in the critically ill adult. *Critical Care Medicine, 30*(1), 119–141.

Jacobsen, R., Sjogren, P., Moldrup, C., et al. (2007). Physician-related barriers to cancer pain management with opioid analgesics: A systematic review. *Journal of Opioid Manage, 5*(4), 207–214.

Jacox, A., Carr, D. B., Payne, R., et al. (1994). *Management of cancer. Clinical practice guideline.* No. 9 AHCPR publication No.94-0592. Rockville, MD: Agency for Health Care Policy and Research, U.S. Department of Health and Human Services, Public Health Service.

Jamison, R. N., Schein, J. R., Vallow, S., et al. (2003). Neuropsychological effects of long-term opioid use in chronic pain patients. *Journal of Pain and Symptom Management, 26*(4), 913–921.

Janssen. (2008). *Duragesic® (fentanyl transdermal CII system) prescribing information.* Titusville, NJ: Janssen, Division of Ortho-McNeil-Janssen Pharmaceuticals, Inc.

Jenkins, H. H., Spencer, E. D., Weissgerber, A. J., et al. (2009). Correlating an 11-point verbal nscale to a 4-point verbal rating scale in the measurement of pruritus. *Journal of Perianesthesia Nursing, 24*(3), 152–155.

Jennings, A. L., Davies, A. N., Higgins, J. P. T., et al. (2001). Opioids for palliation of breathlessness in terminal illness. *Cochrane Database of Systematic Reviews,* (3) CD002066. DOI:10.1002/14651858.CD002066.

Johnson, F., Sun, S., Stauffer, J., et al. (2007). Morphine release profile in a formulation containing polymer-coated extended-release morphine sulfate plus sequestered naltrexone. *The Journal of Pain, 8*(4), S40.

Johnson, F., Wagner, G., Sun, S., et al. (2008). Effect of concomitant ingestion of alcohol on the in vivo pharmacokinetics of Kadian (morphine sulfate extended-release) capsules. *The Journal of Pain, 9*(4), 330–336.

Johnson, K. B., Swenson, J. D., Egan, T. D., et al. (2002). Midazolam and remifentanil by bolus injection for intensely stimulating procedures of brief duration: Experience with awake laryngoscopy. *Anesthesia and Analgesia, 94*(5), 1241–1243.

Johnson, R. E., Fudala, P. J., & Payne, R. (2005). Buprenorphine: Considerations for pain management. *Journal of Pain and Symptom Management, 29*(3), 297–326.

Johnson, R. E., Strain, E. C., & Amass, L. (2003). Buprenorphine: How to use it right. *Drug and Alcohol Dependence, 70*(Suppl. 2), S59–S77.

Johnson, S. J. (2007). Opioid safety in patients with renal or hepatic dysfunction. *Pain Treatment Topics.* www.pain-topics.org. Accessed February 2, 2009.

Joint Commission, The (TJC). (2004). *Sentinel event alert: Patient-controlled analgesia by proxy.* http://www.jointcommission.org/SentinelEvents/SentinelEventAlert/sea_33.htm. Accessed January 9, 2005.

Jokela, R. M., Cakmakkaya, O. S., Danzeisen, O., et al. (2009). Ondansetron has similar clinical efficacy against both nausea and vomiting. *Anaesthesia, 64*(2), 147–151.

Joly, V., Richebe, P., Guignard, B., et al. (2005). Remifentanil-induced postoperative hyperalgesia preventions with small dose ketamine. *Anesthesiology, 103*(1), 147–155.

Jones, H. E., O'Grady, K., Johnson, R., et al. (2009). Management of acute postpartum pain in patients maintained on methadone or buprenorphine during pregnancy. *The American Journal of Drug and Alcohol Abuse, 35*(3), 151–156.

Jones, J. B., Johnson, F., Wagner, G., et al. (2008). Evaluation of abuse potential of ALO-01, an extended-release morphine sulfate plus sequestered naltrexone formulation, among recreational opioid users. *The Journal of Pain, 9*(4, Suppl. 1), P34.

Jones, L. (1987). Patient-controlled oral analgesia. *Orthopaedic Nursing/National Association of Orthopaedic Nurses, 6*(1), 38–41.

Joo, H. S., Perks, W. J., Kataoka, M. T., et al. (2001). A comparison of patient-controlled sedation using either remifentanil or remifentanil-propofol for shock wave lithotripsy. *Anesthesia and Analgesia, 93*(5), 1227–1232.

Jorgensen, H., Fomsgaard, J. S., Dirks, J., et al. (2000). Effect of continuous epidural 0.2% ropivacaine vs 0.2% bupivacaine on postoperative pain, motor block and gastrointestinal function after abdominal hysterectomy. *British Journal of Anaesthesia, 84*(2), 144–150.

Jorgensen, H., Wetterslev, J., Moiniche, S., et al. (2001). Epidural local anaesthetics versus opioid-based analgesic regimens for postoperative gastrointestinal paralysis, PONV and pain after abdominal surgery. *Cochrane Database of Systematic Reviews (Online),* (4) CD001893.

Joyce, M., McSweeney, M., Carrieri-Kohlman, V. L., et al. (2004). The use of nebulized opioids in the management of dyspnea: Evidence synthesis. *Oncology Nursing Forum, 31*(3), 551–559.

Juan, G., Ramon, M., Valia, J. C., et al. (2005). Palliative treatment of dyspnea with epidural methadone in advanced emphysema. *Chest, 128*(5), 3322–3328.

Kabon, B., Fleischmann, E., Treschan, T., et al. (2003). Thoracic epidural anesthesia increases tissue oxygenation during major abdominal surgery. *Anesthesia and Analgesia, 97*(6), 1812–1817.

Kaestli, L. Z., Wasilewski-Rasca, A. F., Bonnabry, P., et al. (2008). Use of transdermal drug formulations in the elderly. *Drugs and Aging, 25*(4), 269–280.

Kahl, L., Parvizi, J., Viscusi, E. R., et al. (2010). Lessons learned with extended-release epidural morphine after total hip arthroplasty. *Clinical Orthopaedics and Related Research,* in press. 10.1007/s11999-009-1181-3.

Kaiko, R. F., Foley, K. M., Grabinski, P. Y., et al. (1983). Central nervous system excitatory effects of meperidine in cancer patients. *Annals of Neurology, 13*, 180–185.

Kalso, E. (2005). Oxycodone. *Journal of Pain and Symptom Management, 29*(Suppl 5), S47–S56.

Kalso, E. (2007). How different is oxycodone from morphine? *Pain, 132*(3), 227–228.

Kalso, E., Simpson, K. H., Slappendel, R., et al. (2007). Predicting long-term response to strong opioids in patients with low back pain: Findings from a randomized, controlled trial of transdermal fentanyl and morphine. *BMC Medicine, 5,* 39.

Kamal-Bahl, S. J., Stuart, B. C., & Beers, M. H. (2006). Propoxyphene use and risk for hip fractures in older adults. *The American Journal of Geriatric Pharmacotherapy, 4*(3), 219–226.

Kampe, S., Warm, M., Kaufmann, J., et al. (2004). Clinical efficacy of controlled-release oxycodone 20 mg administered on a 12-h dosing schedule on the management of postoperative pain after breast surgery for cancer. *Curr Res Opin, 20*(2), 199–202.

Kanazi, G. E., Aouad, M. T., Jabbour-Khoury, S. L., et al. (2006). Effect of low-dose dexmedetomidine or clinidine on the characterstics of bupivacaine spinal block. *Acta Anaesthesiologica Scandinavica, 50*(2), 222–227.

Kaplan, R., Slywka, J., Slagle, S., et al. (2000). A titrated morphine analgesic regimen comparing substance users and nonusers with AIDS-related pain. *Journal of Pain and Symptom Management, 19*(4), 265–273.

Kastanias, P., Snaith, K. E., & Robinson, S. (2006). Patient-controlled oral analgesia: A low-tech solution in a high-tech world. *Pain Management Nursing, 7*(3), 126–132.

Katz, J. (1997). Pain begets pain. Predictors of long-term phantom limb pain and post-thoracotomy pain. *Pain Forum, 6*(2), 140–144.

Katz, J., Buis, T., & Cohen, L. (2008). Locked out and still knocking: Predictors of excessive demands for postoperative intravenous patient-controlled analgesia. *Canadian Journal of Anesthesia, 55*(2), 88–99.

Katz, N., & Mazer, N. A. (2009). The impact of opioids on the endocrine system. *The Clinical Journal of Pain, 25*(2), 170–175.

Katz, N., Rauck, R., Ahdieh, H., et al. (2007). A 12-week, randomized, placebo-controlled trial assessing the safety and efficacy of oxymorphone extended release for opioid-naive patients with chronic low back pain. *Current Medical Research and Opinion, 23*(1), 117–128.

Katz, N., Sun, S., Fox, L., et al. (2008). Efficacy and safety evaluation of an extended-release morphine sulfate formulation with sequestered naltrexone for the treatment of osteoarthritis. *The Journal of Pain, 9*(4, Suppl. 1), P41.

Katz, N., Sun, S., Johnson, F., et al. (2009). ALO-01 (morphine sulfate and naltrexone hydrochloride) extended-release capsules in the treatment of chronic pain of osteoarthritis of the hip or knee: Pharmacokinetics, efficacy, and safety. *The Journal of Pain,* doi: 10.1016/j.jpain.2009.07.017.

Katz, N. P., Adams, E. H., Chilcoat, H., et al. (2007). Challenges in the development of prescription opioid abuse-detrrent formulation. *The Clinical Journal of Pain, 23*(8), 648–660.

Kaya, M., Sariyildiz, O., Karakus, D., et al. (2003). Tramadol versus meperidine in the treatment of shivering during spinal anaesthesia. *European Journal of Anaesthesiology, 20*(4), 332–333.

Kaya, T., Buyukkocak, U., Basar, H., et al. (2008). Comparison of epidural ropivacaine 0.2% and ropivacaine 0.2% in combination with sufentanil 0.75 microg mL-1 for postcaesarean analgesia. *Agri: The Journal of the Turkish Society of Algology, 20*(4), 30–37.

Kazemi-Kjellberg, F., Henzi, I., & Tramer, M. R. (2001). Treatment of established postoperative nausea and vomiting: A quantitative systematic review. *BMC Anesthesiology, 1*(1), 2.

Kedlaya, D., Reynolds, L., & Waldman, S. (2002). Epidural and intrathecal analgesia for cancer pain. *Best Practice & Research. Clinical Anaesthesiology, 16*(4), 651–665.

Keen, M. F. (1986). Comparison of intramuscular injection techniques to reduce site discomfort and lesions. *Nursing Research, 35,* 207–210.

Kehlet, H. (2005). Preventive measures to minimize or avoid postoperative ileus. *Sem Colon Rec Surg, 16*(4), 203–206.

Kehlet, H., & Dahl, J. (2002). Epidural analgesia and postoperative outcome? *Anesthesiology, 97*(4), 1025–1026.

Kehlet, H., & Holte, K. (2001). Review of postoperative ileus. *American Journal of Surgery, 182*(Suppl. 5A), 3S–10S.

Kehlet, H., Jensen, T. S., & Woolf, C. J. (2006). Persistent postsurgical pain: Risk factors and prevention. *Lancet, 367*(9522), 1618–1625.

Kehlet, H., & Wilmore, D. W. (2008). Evidence-based surgical care and the evolution of fast-track surgery. *Annals of Surgery, 248*(2), 189–198.

Keita, H., Diouf, E., Tubach, F., et al. (2005). Predictive factors of early postoperative urinary retention in the postanesthesia care unit. *Anesthesia and Analgesia, 101*(2), 592–596.

Keita, H., Tubach, F., Maalouli, J., et al. (2008). Age-adapted morphine titration produces equivalent analgesia and adverse effects in younger and older patients. *European Journal of Anaesthesiology, 25*(5), 352–356.

Kelly, D. J., Ahmad, M., & Brull, S. J. (2001). Preemptive analgesia II: Recent advances and current trends. *Canadian Journal of Anesthesia, 48*(11), 1091–1101.

Kent, C. D., Kaufman, B. S., & Lowry, J. (2005). Dexmedetomidine facilitates the withdrawal of ventilatory support in palliative care. *Anesthesiology, 103*(2), 439–441.

Kerger, K. H., Mascha, E., Steinbrecher, B., et al. (2009). Routine use of nasogastric tubes does not reduce postoperative nausea and vomiting. *Anesthesia and Analgesia, 109*(3), 769–773.

Kerr, D., Kelly, A. M., Dietze, P., et al. (2009). Randomized controlled trial comparing the effectiveness and safety of intranasal and intramuscular naloxone for the treatment of heroin overdose. *Addiction (Abingdon, England), 104*(12), 2067–2074.

Kerr, I. G., Sone, M., DeAngelis, C., et al. (1988). Continuous narcotic infusion with patient-controlled analgesia for chronic cancer pain in outpatients. *Annals of Internal Medicine, 108*(4), 554–557.

Kessler, P., Neidhart, G., Bremerich, D. H., et al. (2002). High thoracic epidural anesthesia for coronary artery bypass grafting using two different surgical approaches in conscious patients. *Anesthesia and Analgesia, 95*(4), 791–797.

Kharasch, E. D., Hoffer, C., & Whittington, D. (2004). Influence of age on the pharmacokinetics and pharmacodynamics of oral transmucosal fentanyl citrate. *Anesthesiology, 101*(3), 738–743.

Kim, S. Y., Kim, E. M., Nam, K. H., et al. (2008). Postoperative intravenous patient-controlled analgesia in thyroid surgery: Comparison of fentanyl and ondansetron regimens with and without the nonsteroidal anti-inflammatory drug ketorolac. *Thyroid, 18*(12), 1285–1290.

King Pharmaceuticals. (2008a). *Avinza prescribing information.* Bristol, TN: King Pharmaceuticals. Available at http://www.

kingpharm.com/kingpharm/uploads/pdf_inserts/AVINZA_ PI.pdf. Accessed April 17, 2008.

King Pharmaceuticals. (2008b). *King provides additional information on the REMOXY® NDA resubmission plan.* Bristol, TN: King Pharmaceuticals. Available at http://www. kingpharm.com/Investors/News_Details.cfm?news_item_ id=522. Accessed July 16, 2009.

King Pharmaceuticals. (2009). *Embeda prescribing information.* Bristol, TN: King Pharmaceuticals. http://www.embeda.com/. Accessed August 16, 2009.

Kivitz, A., Ma, C., Ahdieh, H., et al. (2006). A 2-week multicenter, randomized, double blind, placebo-controlled dose ranging, phase III trial comparing the efficacy of oxymorphone extended release and placebo in adults with pain associated with osteoarthritis of the hip or knee. *Clinical Therapeutics, 3*(28), 352–364.

Kizilkaya, M., Yildirim, O. S., Dogan, N., et al. (2004). Analgesic effects of intraarticular sufentanil and sufentanil plus methylprednisolone after arthroscopic knee surgery. *Anesthesia and Analgesia, 98*(4), 1062–1965.

Kleinert, R., Lange, C., Steup, A., et al. (2008). Single dose analgesic efficacy of tapentadol in postsurgical dental pain: The results of a randomized, double-blind, placebo-controlled study. *Anesthesia and Analgesia, 107*(6), 2048–2055.

Klepstad, P., Kaasa, S., Jystad, A., et al. (2003). Immediate- or sustained-release morphine for dose finding during start of morphine to cancer patients: A randomized, double-blind trial. *Pain, 101*(1–2), 193–198.

Klepstad, P., Kaasa, S., Skauge, M., et al. (2000). Pain intensity and side effects during titration of morphine to cancer patients using a fixed schedule dose escalation. *Acta Anaesthesiologica Scandinavica, 44*(6), 656–664.

Kneip, C., Terlinden, R., Beier, H., et al. (2008). Investigations into the drug-drug interaction potential of tapentadol in human liver microsomes and fresh human hepatocytes. *Drug Metab Lett, 2*(1), 67–75.

Knotkova, H., Fine, P. G., & Portenoy, R. K. (2009). Opioid rotation: The science and limitations of the equianalgesic dose table. *Journal of Pain and Symptom Management, 38*(3), 426–439.

Ko, W. M., & Ferrante, F. M. (2006). New onset lumbar radicular pain after implantation of an intrathecal drug delivery system: Imaging catheter migration. *Regional Anesthesia and Pain Medicine, 31*(4), 363–367.

Kolesnikov, Y. A., Wilson, R. S., & Pasternak, G. W. (2003). The synergistic analgesic interactions between hydrocodone and ibuprofen. *Anesthesia and Analgesia, 97*(6), 1721–1723.

Koo, H. C., Moon, J. H., Choi, H. J., et al. (2009). Effect of transdermal fentanyl patch on sphincter of Oddi—For application of pain management in pancreatitis. (Abstract). *Gastrointestinal Endoscopy, 69*(5), AB270.

Kopka, A., Wallace, E., Reilly, G., et al. (2007). Observational study of perioperative Ptc$_{cO2}$ and SpO2 in non-ventilated patients receiving epidural infusion or patient-controlled analgesia using a single earlobe monitor (TOSCA). *British Journal of Anaesthesia, 99*(4), 567–571.

Kornick, C. A., Santiago-Palma, J., Moryl, N., et al. (2003). Benefit-risk assessment of transdermal fentanyl for treatment of chronic pain. *Drug safety: an International Journal of Medical Toxicology and Drug Experience, 26*(13), 951–973.

Kornick, C. A., Santiago-Palma, J., Schulman, G., et al. (2003). A safe and effective method for converting patients from

transdermal to intravenous fentanyl for treatment of acute cancer-related pain. *Cancer, 97*(12), 3121–3124.

Kornitzer, B. S., Manace, L. C., Fischberg, D. J., et al. (2006). Prevalence of meperidine use in older surgical patients. *Archives of Surgery, 141*(8), 76–81.

Kothari, S. N., Boyd, W. C., Bottcher, M. L., et al. (2000). Antiemetic efficacy of prophylactic dimenhydrinate (Dramamine) vs ondansetron (Zofran). *Surgical Endoscopy, 14*(10), 926–929.

Kraft, M. D. (2007). Emerging pharmacologic options for treating postoperative ileus. *American Journal of Health-System Pharmacy, 64*(20), S13–S20.

Kranke, P., Eberhart, L. H., Roewer, N., et al. (2004). Single-dose parenteral pharmacological interventions for prevention of postoperative shivering: A quantitative systematic review of randomized controlled trials. *Anesthesia and Analgesia, 99*(3), 718–727.

Kranke, P., Morin, A. M., Roewer, N., et al. (2002). The efficacy and safety of transdermal scopolamine for the prevention of postoperative nausea and vomiting: A quantitative systematic review. *Anesthesia and Analgesia, 95*(1), 133–143.

Krantz, M. J., Martin, J., Stimmel, B., et al. (2009). QTc interval screening in methadone treatment. *Annals of Internal Medicine, 150*(6), 387–395.

Krenzischek, D., & Wilson, L. (2003). Introduction to the ASPAN pain and comfort clinical practice guideline. *Journal of Perianesthesia Nursing, 18*(4), 228–231.

Kress, H. G., Von der Laage, D., Hoerauf, K. H., et al. (2008). A randomized, open, parallel group, multicenter trial to investigate analgesic efficacy and safety of the new transdermal fentanyl patch compared to standard opioid treatment in cancer pain. *Journal of Pain and Symptom Management, 36*(3), 268–279.

Kshatri, A. M., & Foster, P. A. (1997). Adrenocorticotropic hormone infusion as a novel treatment for postdural puncture headache. *Regional Anesthesia, 22*(5), 432–434.

Kumar, K., Bodani, V., Bishop, S., et al. (2009). Use of intrathecal bupivacaine in refractory chronic nonmalignant pain. *Pain Medicine (Malden, Mass.), 10*(5), 819–828.

Kumar, M. G., & Lin, S. (2007). Hydromorphone in the management of cancer-related pain: An update on routes of administration and dosage forms. *Journal of Pharmacy & Pharmaceutical Sciences, 10*(4), 504–518.

Kunz, K. (1994). Opioid cost factors. *Cancer Pain Update,* Fall, 3.

Kurella, M., Bennett, W. M., & Chertow, G. M. (2003). Analgesia in patients with ESRD: A review of available evidence. *American Journal of Kidney Diseases, 42*(2), 217–228.

Ladak, S. S. J., Katznelson, R., Muscat, M., et al. (2009). Incidence of urinary retention in patients with thoracic patient-controlled epidural analgesia (TPCEA) undergoing thoractomy. *Pain Management Nursing, 10*(2), 94–98.

Lagan, G., & McLure, H. A. (2004). Review of local anaesthetic agents. *Curr Anaesth Crit Care, 15*(4–5), 247–254.

Lahtinen, P., Kokki, H., & Hynynen, M. (2008). Remifentanil infusion does not induce opioid tolerance after cardiac surgery. *Journal of Cardiothoracic and Vascular Anesthesia, 22*(2), 225–229.

Lalley, P. M. (2005). D1-dopamine receptor agonists prevent and reverse opiate depression of breathing but not antinociception in the cat. *American Journal of Physiology. Regulatory, Integrative and Comparative Physiology, 289*(1), R45–R51.

Lalovic, B., Kharasch, E., Hoffer, C., et al. (2006). Pharmacokinetics and pharmacodynamics of oral oxycodone in healthy human subjects: Role of circulating active metabolites. *Clinical Pharmacology and Therapeutics, 79*(5), 461–479.

Lamb, E. (2008). Top 200 prescription drugs of 2007. *Pharmacy Times, 74*(5), 20–23. Available at http://www.pharmacytimes.com/issues/articles/2008-05_003.asp. Accessed June 9, 2008.

Landau, R. (2006). One size does not fit all. (Editorial). *Anesthesiology, 105*(2), 235–237.

Langevin, P. B. (2000). How should we handle epidural solutions: One view. (Editorial). *Regional Anesthesia and Pain Medicine, 25*(4), 343–346.

Langevin, P. B., Gravenstein, N., Langevin, S. O., et al. (1996). Epidural catheter reconnection. Safe and unsafe practice. *Anesthesiology, 85*(4), 883–888.

Langford, R., McKenna, F., Ratcliffe, S., et al. (2006). Transdermal fentanyl for improvement of pain and functioning in osteoarthritis: A randomized, placebo-controlled trial. *Arthritis and Rheumatism, 54*(6), 1829–1837.

Larijani, G. E., & Goldberg, M. E. (2004). Analgesic evaluation in postoperative patients. (Letter). *Anesthesiology, 100*(3), 744–745.

Larijani, G. E., Goldberg, M. E., Gratz, I., et al. (2004). Analgesic and hemodynamic effects of a single 7.5 mg intravenous dose of morphine in patients with moderate-to-severe postoperative pain. *Pharmacotherapy, 24*(12), 1675–1680.

Latta, K. S., Ginsberg, B., & Barkin, R. L. (2002). Meperidine: A critical review. *American Journal of Therapeutics, 9*(1), 53–68.

Lattermann, R., Wykes, L., Eberhart, L., et al. (2007). A randomized controlled trial of the anticatabolic effect of epidural analgesia and hypocaloric glucose. *Regional Anesthesia and Pain Medicine, 32*(3), 227–232.

Launay-Vacher, V., Karie, S., Fau, J. B., et al. (2005). Treatment of pain in patients with renal insufficiency: The World Health Organization three-step ladder adapted. *The Journal of Pain, 6*(3), 137–148.

Lauretti, G. R., Oliveira, G. M., & Pereira, N. L. (2003). Comparison of sustained-release morphine with sustained-release oxycodone in advanced cancer patients. *British Journal of Cancer, 89*(11), 2027–2030.

Lavelle, W., Lavelle, E. D., & Lavelle, L. (2007). Intra-articular injections. *The Medical Clinics of North America, 91*(2), 241–250.

Laverty, D. (2007). Treating cancer-related breakthrough pain: The oral transmucosal route. *International Journal of Palliative Nursing, 13*(7), 326–331.

Lawlor, P., Turner, K., Hanson, J., et al. (1997). Dose ratio between morphine and hydromorphone in patients with cancer pain: A retrospective study. *Pain, 72*(1–2), 79–85.

Lawlor, P. G., Turner, K. S., Hanson, J., et al. (1998). Dose ratio between morphine and methadone in patients with cancer pain: A retrospective study. *Cancer, 82*(6), 1167–1173.

Leavitt, S. B. (2005). *Methadone-drug interactions.* (3rd ed.). Addiction Treatment Forum. Available at http://www.atforum.com/SiteRoot/pages/addiction_resources/Drug_Interactions.pdf. Accessed June 8, 2008.

Leavitt, S. B. (2006). Methadone-drug interactions. *Pain Treatment Topics.* Available at http://pain-topics.org/pdf/Methadone-Drug_Intx_2006.pdf. Accessed July 31, 2009.

Leavitt, S. B. (2008). Methadone safety handout for patients. *Pain Treatment Topics.* Available at http://pain-topics.org/pdf/MethadoneHandout.pdf. Accessed July 31, 2009.

Leavitt, S. B. (2009). Misguided pain guidelines? When strong claims follow from weak evidence. *Pain Treatment Topics e-Briefing, 4*(1), 1–8.

LeBon, B., Zeppetella, G., Higginson, I. J., et al. (2009). Effectiveness of topical administration of opioids in palliative care: A systematic review. *Journal of Pain and Symptom Management, 37*(5), 913–917.

Lee, A., & Done, M. L. (1999). The use of nonpharmacologic techniques to prevent postoperative nausea and vomiting: A meta-analysis. *Anesthesia and Analgesia, 88*(6), 1362–1369.

Lee, A., & Fan, L. T. Y. (2009). Stimulation of the wrist acupuncture point P6 for preventing postoperative nausea and vomiting. *Cochrane Database of Systematic Reviews (Online)*, (2) CD003281.

Lee, E. Y., Lee, E. B., Park, B. J., et al. (2006). Tramadol 37.5-mg/acetaminophen 325-mg combination tablets added to regular therapy for rheumatoid arthritis pain: A 1-week, randomized, double-blind, placebo-controlled trial. *Clinical Therapeutics, 28*(12), 2052–2060.

Lee, F., & Cundiff, D. (1998). Meperidine vs morphine in pancreatitis and cholecystitis. (Letter). *Archives of Internal Medicine, 158*(21), 2399.

Lehmann, K. A. (2005). Recent developments in patient-controlled analgesia. *Journal of Pain and Symptom Management, 29*(Suppl. 5), S72–S89.

Lehne, R. A. (2004). *Pharmacology for Nursing Care* (5th ed.). St. Louis: Saunders.

Lehr, V. T., & BeVier, P. (2003). Patient-controlled analgesia for the pediatric patient. *Orthopaedic Nursing/National Association of Orthopaedic Nurses, 22*(4), 298–304.

Lemberg, K. K., Siiskonen, A. O., Kontinen, V. K., et al. (2008). Pharmacological characterization of noroxymorphone as a new opioid for spinal analgesia. *Anesthesia and Analgesia, 106*(2), 463–470.

Lennernas, B., Hedner, T., Holmberg, M., et al. (2005). Pharmacokinetics and tolerability of different doses of fentanyl following sublingual administration of a rapidly dissolving tablet to cancer patients: A new approach to treatment of incident pain. *British Journal of Clinical Pharmacology, 59*(2), 249–253.

Lentschener, C., Tostivint, P., White, P. F., et al. (2007). Opioid-induced sedation in the postanesthesia care unit does not insure adequate pain relief: A case-control study. *Anesthesia and Analgesia, 105*(4), 1143–1147.

Lenz, H., Sandvik, L., Qvigstad, E., et al. (2009). A comparison of intravenous oxycodone and intravenous morphine in patient-controlled postoperative analgesia after laparoscopic hysterectomy. *Anesthesia and Analgesia, 109*(4), 1279–1283.

Leone, M., Albanese, J., Viviand, X., et al. (2004). The effects of remifentanil on endotracheal suction-induced increases in intracranial pressure in head-injured patients. *Anesthesia and Analgesia, 99*(4), 1193–1198.

Leppert, W. (2009). The role of methadone in cancer pain treatment—A review. *International Journal of Clinical Practice, 63*(7), 1095–1109.

Leppert, W., & Łuczak, J. (2005). The role of tramadol in cancer pain treatment—A review. *Supportive Care in Cancer, 13*(1), 5–17.

Leslie, J. B. (2005). Alvimopan for the management of postoperative ileus. *The Annals of Pharmacotherapy, 39*(9), 1502–1510.

Levy, M. H. (1989). Integration of pain management into comprehensive cancer care. *Cancer, 63*(11 suppl), 2328–2335.

Levy, M. H. (1993). Medical management of cancer pain. In C. Warfield (Ed.), *Principles and practice of pain management* (pp. 235–250). New York: McGraw-Hill.

Lew, E., Yeo, S. W., & Thomas, E. (2004). Combined spinal-epidural anesthesia using epidural volume extension leads to faster motor recovery after elective cesarean delivery: A prospective, randomized, double-blind study. *Anesthesia and Analgesia*, 98(3), 810–814.

Li Wan Po, A., & Zhang, W. Y. (1997). Systematic overview of co-proxamol to assess analgesic effects of addition of dextropropoxyphene to paracetamol. *BMJ (Clinical Research Ed.)*, 315(7122), 1565–1571.

Likar, R., Vadlau, E. M., Breschan, C., et al. (2008). Comparable analgesic efficacy of transdermal buprenorphine in patients over and under 65 years of age. *The Clinical Journal of Pain*, 25(6), 536–543.

Likar, R., Wittels, M., Molnar, M., et al. (2006). Pharmacokinetic and pharmacodynamic properties of tramadol IR and SR in elderly patients: A prospective, age-group-controlled study. *Clinical Therapeutics*, 28(12), 2022–2039.

Lilker, S., Rofaeel, A., Balki, M., et al. (2009). Comparison of fentanyl and sufentanil as adjuncts to bupivacaine for labor epidural analgesia. *Journal of Clinical Anesthesia*, 21(2), 108–112.

Lim, S., Prasad, M., Samuels, P., et al. (2009). High-dose methadone in pregnant women and its effect on duration of neonatal abstinence syndrome. *American Journal of Obstetrics and Gynecology*, 200(1), 70.e1–70.e5.

Lim, Y., Wilson, S., & Katz, S. (2006). A comparison of patient-controlled epidural pethidine vs. nurse-administered epidural pethidine for analgesia after caesarean section. *Journal of Opioid Management*, 2(2), 99–104.

Litman, R. S. (2000). Conscious sedation with remifentanil during painful medical procedures. *Journal of Pain and Symptom Management*, 19(6), 468–471.

Little, B. B., Snell, L. M., Van Beveren, T. T., et al. (2003). Treatment of substance abuse during pregnancy and infant outcome. *American Journal of Perinatology*, 20(5), 255–262.

Liu, G. G., & Christensen, D. B. (2002). The continuing challenge of inappropriate prescribing in the elderly: An update of the evidence. *Journal of the American Pharmaceutical Association*, 42(6), 847–857.

Liu, L. L., & Gropper, M. A. (2003). Postoperative analgesia and sedation in the adult intensive care unit: A guide to drug selection. *Drugs*, 63(8), 755–767.

Liu, M., & Wittbrodt, E. (2002). Low-dose oral naloxoen reverses opioid-induced constipation and analgesia. *Journal of Pain and Symptom Management*, 23(1), 48–53.

Liu, S. S., Carpenter, R. L., Mulroy, M. F., et al. (1995). Intravenous versus epidural administration of hydromorphone. *Anesthesiology*, 82(3), 682–688.

Liu, S. S., Moore, J. M., Luo, A. M., et al. (1999). Comparison of three solutions of ropivacaine/fentanyl for postoperative patient-controlled epidural analgesia. *Anesthesiology*, 90(3), 727–733.

Liu, S. S., & Wu, C. L. (2007a). The effect of analgesic technique on postoperative patient-reported outcomes including analgesia: A systematic review. *Anesthesia and Analgesia*, 105(3), 789–808.

Liu, S. S., & Wu, C. L. (2007b). Effect of postoperative analgesia on major postoperative complications: A systematic update of the evidence. *Anesthesia and Analgesia*, 104(3), 689–702.

Locniskar, A., Greenblatt, D. J., & Zinny, M. A. (1986). Pharmacokinetics of dezocine, a new analgesic: Effect of dose and route of administration. *European Journal of Clinical Pharmacology*, 30(1), 121–123.

Locsin, R. G. (1985). Pinch-grasp technique. *PRN Forum*, 4, 4–5.

Lorenz, J., Beck, H., & Bromm, B. (1997). Cognitive performance, mood and experimental pain before and during morphine-induced analgesia in patients with chronic nonmalignant pain. *Pain*, 73(3), 369–375.

Lotsch, J. (2005). Opioid metabolites. *Journal of Pain and Symptom Management*, 29(Suppl. 5), S10–S24.

Lotsch, J., Dudziak, R., Freynhagen, R., et al. (2006). Fatal respiratory depression after multiple morphine injections. *Clin Pharmacokinet*, 45(11), 1051–1060.

Lovovschi, V., Aubrun, F., Bonnet, P., et al. (2008). Intravenous morphine titration to treat severe pain in the ED. *The American Journal of Emergency Medicine*, 26(4), 676–682.

Lucas, C. E., Vlahos, A. L., & Ledgerwood, A. M. (2007). Kindness kills: The negative impact of pain as the fifth vital sign. *Journal of the American College of Surgeons*, 205(1), 101–107.

Lugo, R. A., & Kern, S. E. (2004). The pharmacokinetics of oxycodone. *Journal of Pain & Palliative Care Pharmacotherapy*, 18(4), 17–30.

Lugo, R. A., Satterfield, K. L., & Kern, S. E. (2005). Pharmacokinetics of methadone. *Journal of Pain & Palliative Care Pharmacotherapy*, 19(4), 13–24.

Lynch, M. E. (2005). A review of the use of methadone for the treatment of chronic noncancer pain. *Pain Research & Management*, 10(3), 133–144.

Lynn, J., Teno, J. M., & Phillips, R. S. (1997). Perceptions by family members of the dying experience of older and seriously ill patients. *Annals of Internal Medicine*, 126(2), 97–106.

Ma, K., Jiang, W., Zhou, Q., et al. (2008). The efficacy of oxycodone for management of acute pain episodes in chronic neck pain patients. *International Journal of Clinical Practice*, 62(2), 241–247.

Maalouf, D. B., & Liu, S. S. (2009). Clinical application of epidural analgesia. In R. S. Sinatra, O. A. de Leon-Casasola, B. Ginsberg, & E. R. Viscusi (Eds.), *Acute pain management* (pp. 221–229). Cambridge, New York: Cambridge University Press.

Macario, A. (2005). Systematic literature review of the economics of intravenous patient-controlled analgesia. *P, T*, 30(7), 392–399.

Machelska, H. (2007). Targeting of opioid-producing leukocytes for pain control. *Neuropeptides*, 41(6), 355–363.

MacIntyre, P. A., Margetts, L., Larsen, D., et al. (2007). Oral transmucosal fentanyl citrate versus placebo for painful dressing changes: A crossover trial. *Journal of Wound Care*, 16(3), 118–121.

Macintyre, P. E., & Coldrey, J. (2008). Patient-controlled analgesia. In P. E. Macintyre, S. M. Walker, & D. J. Rowbotham (Eds.), *Acute pain*. (2nd ed., pp. 217–235). London: UK, Hodder Arnold.

Macintyre, P. E., & Coldrey, J. (2009). Intravenous patient-controlled analgesia. In: R. S. Sinatra, O. A. de Leon-Casasola, B. Ginsberg, & E. R. Viscusi (Eds.), *Acute pain management* (pp. 204–220). Cambridge, New York: Cambridge University Press.

Madacsy, L., Bertalan, V., Szepes, A., et al. (2003). Effect of nalbuphine on the motility of the sphincter of Oddi in patients with suspected sphincter of Oddi dysfunction. *Gastrointestinal Endoscopy*, 57(3), 319–323.

Maddux, J. F., Williams, T. R., & Ziegler, J. A. (1977). Driving records before and during methadone maintenance. *The American Journal of Drug and Alcohol Abuse*, 4(1), 91–100.

Maier, C., Hildebrandt, J., Klinger, R., et al. (2002). Morphine responsiveness, efficacy and tolerability in patients with chronic non-tumor associated pain – results of a double-blind placebo-controlled trial (MONTAS). *Pain*, 97(3), 223–233.

Makin, M. K. (2000). Subcutaneous methadone in terminally-ill patients. *Journal of Pain and Symptom Management*, 19(4), 237–238.

Malkin, J. D., Ackerman, S. J., Schein, J. R., et al. (2001). Outcomes associated with fentanyl transdermal system and oxycodone controlled-release in a California Medicaid population. *Pain Medicine (Malden, Mass.)*, 2(3), 246–247.

Malloy, P., Paice, J., Virani, R., et al. (2008). End-of-Life Nursing Education Consortium: 5 years of educating graduate nursing faculty in excellent palliative care. *Journal of Professional Nursing*, 24(6), 352–357.

Maloney, C. M., Kesner, R. K., Klein, G., et al. (1989). The rectal administration of MS Contin: Clinical implications of use in end stage cancer. *The American Journal of Hospice Care*, 6(4), 34–35.

Maltoni, M., Pittureri, C., Scarpi, E., et al. (2009). Palliative sedation does not hasten death: Results from a prospective multicenter study. *Annals of Oncology*, 20(7), 1163–1169.

Maltoni, M., Scarpi, E., Modonesi, C., et al. (2005). A validation study of the WHO analgesic ladder: A two-step vs three-step strategy. *Supportive Care in Cancer*, 13(11), 888–894.

Manfredi, P. L., & Houde, R. W. (2003). Prescribing methadone, a unique analgesic. *The Journal of Supportive Oncology*, 1(3), 216–220.

Manfredi, P. L., Ribeiro, S., & Chandler, S. W. (1996). Inappropriate use of naloxone in cancer patients with pain. *Journal of Pain and Symptom Management*, 11(2), 131–134.

Mann, C., Pouzeratte, Y., Boccara, G., et al. (2000). Comparison of intravenous or epidural patient-controlled analgesia in the elderly after major abdominal surgery. *Anesthesiology*, 92(2), 433–441.

Mannino, R., Coyne, P., Swainey, C., et al. (2006). Methadone for cancer-related neuropathic pain: A review of the literature. *Journal of Opioid Management*, 2(5), 269–276.

Manworren, R. C. B. (2006). A call to action to protect range orders. *The American Journal of Nursing*, 106(7), 30–33.

Marcantonio, E. R., Juarez, G., Goldman, L., et al. (1994). The relationship of postoperative delirium with psychoactive medications. *JAMA: The Journal of the American Medical Association*, 272(19), 1518–1522.

Marcou, T. A., Marque, S., Mazoit, J. X., et al. (2005). The median effective dose of tramadol and morphine for postoperative patients: A study of interactions. *Anesthesia and Analgesia*, 100(2), 469–474.

Marier, J. F., Lor, M., Morin, J., et al. (2006). Comparative bioequivalence study between a novel natrix transdermal delivery system of fentanyl and a commercially available reservoir formulation. *British Journal of Clinical Pharmacology*, 63(1), 121–124.

Marier, J. F., Lor, M., Potvin, D., et al. (2006). Pharmacokinetics, tolerability, and performance of a novel matrix transdermal delivery system of fentanyl relative to the commercially

available reservoir formulation in healthy subjects. *Journal of Clinical Pharmacology*, 46(6), 642–653.

Marinangeli, F., Ciccozzi, A., Aloisio, L., et al. (2007). Improved cancer pain treatment using combined fentanyl-TTS and tramadol. *Pain Practice*, 7(4), 307–312.

Marinangeli, F., Ciccozzi, A., Leonardis, M., et al. (2004). Use of strong opioids in advanced cancer pain: A randomized trial. *Journal of Pain and Symptom Management*, 27(5), 409–416.

Marquardt, K. A., Alsop, J. A., & Albertson, T. E. (2005). Tramadol exposures reported to statewide poison control system. *The Annals of Pharmacotherapy*, 39(6), 1039–1044.

Marret, E., Kurdi, O., Zufferey, P., et al. (2005). Effects of nonsteroidal antiinflammatory drugs on patient-controlled analgesia morphine side effects. *Anesthesiology*, 102(6), 1249–1260.

Martinez, J. B., Moos, D. D., & Dahlen, L. L. (2006). Droperidol's effect on QT interval. *Journal of Perianesthesia Nursing*, 21(1), 82–87.

Mathew, P., & Storey, P. (1999). Subcutaneous methadone in terminally ill patients: Manageable local toxicity. *Journal of Pain and Symptom Management*, 18(1), 49–52.

Mathieu, N., Cnudde, N., Engelman, E., et al. (2006). Intranasal sufentanil is effective for postoperative analgesia in adults. *Canadian Journal of Anesthesia*, 53(1), 60–66.

Matot, I., Drenger, B., Weissman, C., et al. (2004). Epidural clonidine, bupivacaine and methadone as the sole agent after thoractomy for lung resection. *Anaesthesia*, 59(9), 861–866.

Matot, I., Scheinin, O., Eid, A., et al. (2002). Epidural anesthesia and analgesia in liver resection. *Anesthesia and Analgesia*, 95(5), 1179–1181.

Matsumoto, A. K., Babul, N., & Ahdieh, H. (2005). Oxymorphone extended-release tablets relieve moderate to severe pain and improve physical function in osteoarthritis: Results of a randomized, double-blind, placebo- and active-controlled phase III trial. *Pain Medicine (Malden, Mass.)*, 6(5), 357–366.

May, J. A., White, H. C., Leonard-White, A., et al. (2001). The patient recovering from alcohol or drug addiction: Special issues for the anesthesiologist. *Anesthesia and Analgesia*, 92(6), 1601–1608.

Mayer, J., Boldt, J., Schellhaafs, A., et al. (2007). Bispectral index-guided general anesthesia in combination with thoracic epidural analgesia reduces recovery time in fast-track colon surgery. *Anesthesia and Analgesia*, 104(5), 1145–1149.

Mazzocato, C., Buclin, T., & Rapin, C. H. (1999). The effects of morphine on dyspnea and ventilatory function in elderly patients with advanced cancer: A randomized double-blind controlled trial. *Annals of Oncology*, 10(12), 1511–1514.

McBride, J., Knight, D., Piper, J., et al. (2005). Long-term effect of introducing an early warning score on respiratory rate charting on general wards. *Resuscitation*, 65(1), 41–44.

McCaffery, M., Herr, K., & Pasero, C. Assessment: Basic problems, misconceptions, and practical tools. In C. Pasero, & M. McCaffery (Eds.), *Pain: Assessment and pharmacologic management* (in press). St. Louis: Mosby.

McCaffery, M., & Lochman, C. (1996). Controlled release morphine products. *The American Journal of Nursing*, 96(4), 65.

McCaffery, M., Martin, L., & Ferrell, B. R. (1992). Analgesic administration via rectum or stoma. *Journal of ET Nursing*, 19(4), 114–121.

McCaffery, M., & Vourakis, C. (1992). Assessment and relief of pain in chemically dependent patients. *Orthopaedic Nursing/National Association of Orthopaedic Nurses,* *11*(2), 13–27.

McCartney, C. J. L., & Niazi, A. (2006). Use of opioid analgesics in the perioperative period. In G. Shorten, D. B. Carr, D. Harmon, M. M. Puig, & J. Browne (Eds.), *Postoperative pain management: An evidence-based guide to practice* (pp. 137–147). Philadelphia: Saunders.

McClean, R. (2005). Standard IV morphine dose given in the ER may be ineffective. *Pain Medicine News, 3*(10), 5.

McClellan, K., & Scott, L. J. (2003). Tramadol/paracetamol. *Drugs, 63*(11), 1079–1086.

McGee, J. L., & Alexander, M. R. (1979). Phenothiazine analgesia: Fact or fantasy? *American Journal of Hospital Pharmacy, 36*(5), 633–640.

McIlwain, H., & Ahdieh, H. (2005). Safety, tolerability, and effectiveness of oxymorphone extended release for moderate to severe osteoarthritis pain. A one year study. *American Journal of Therapeutics, 12*(2), 105–112.

Mcintyre, P. E., & Upton, R. (2008). Acute pain management in the elderly patient. In P. E. Macintyre, S. M. Walker, & D. J. Rowbotham (Eds.), *Acute pain.* (2nd ed., pp. 504–525). London: UK, Hodder Arnold.

McMillan, S. C., & Williams, F. A. (1989). Validity and reliability of the Constipation Assessment Scale. *Cancer Nursing, 12*(3), 183–188.

McNicol, E., Boyce, D. B., Schumann, R., et al. (2008). Efficacy and safety of mu-opioid antagonists in the treatment of opioid-induced bowel dysfunction: Systematic review and meta-analysis of randomized controlled trials. *Pain Medicine (Malden, Mass.), 9*(6), 634–659.

McNulty, J. P. (2007). Can levorphanol be used like methadone for intractable refractory pain? *Journal of Palliative Medicine, 10,* 293–296.

Medical News Today. (2008). *TheraQuest's IND for abuse deterrent strong opioid (TQ-1015) accepted by FDA.* http://www.medicalnewstoday.com/articles/129330.php. Accessed September 10, 2009.

Medina, H. J., Gavin, E. M., Dirckx, M., et al. (2005). Remifentanil as a single drug for extracorporeal shock wave lithotripsy: A comparison of infusion doses in terms of analgesic potency and side effects. *Anesthesia and Analgesia, 101*(2), 365–370.

Meek, T. (2004). Epidural anaesthesia and analgesia in major surgery. *Curr Anaesth Crit Care, 15*(4–5), 239–246.

Mehta, V., & Langford, R. M. (2006). Acute pain management for opioid dependent patients. *Anaesthesia, 61,* 269–276.

Meissner, W., Leyendecker, P., Mueller-Lissner, S., et al. (2009). A randomised controlled trial with prolonged-release oral oxycodone and naloxone to prevent and reverse opioid-induced constipation. *European Journal of Pain (London, England), 13*(9), 56–64.

Meldrum, M. (2005). The ladder and the clock: Cancer pain and public policy at the end of the twentieth century. *Journal of Pain and Symptom Management, 29*(1), 41–54.

Melzack, R., Abbott, F. V., Zackon, W., et al. (1987). Pain on a surgical ward: A survey of duration and intensity of pain and the effectiveness of medication. *Pain, 29*(1), 67–72.

Mendola, C., Ferrante, D., Oldani, E., et al. (2009). Thoracic epidural analgesia in post-thoracotomy patients: Comparison of three different concentrations of levobupivacaine and sufentanil. *British Journal of Anaesthesia, 102*(3), 418–423.

Menefee, L. A., Frank, E. D., Crerand, C., et al. (2004). The effects of transdermal fentanyl on driving, cognitive performance, and balance in patients with chronic nonmalignant pain conditions. *Pain Medicine (Malden, Mass.), 5*(1), 42–49.

Menefee, L. A., Katz, N. P., & Zacharoff, K. L. (2007). *PainEDU.org Manual.* (3rd ed.). Newton, MA: Inflexxion.

Menigaux, C., Guignard, B., Fletcher, D., et al. (2001). More epidural than intravenous sufentanil is required to provide comparable postoperative pain relief. *Anesthesia and Analgesia, 93*(2), 472–476.

Mercadante, S. (1995). Dantrolene treatment of opioid-induced myoclonus. *Anesthesia and Analgesia, 81*(6), 1307–1308.

Mercadante, S. (2006a). Breakthrough (episodic) vs. baseline pain in cancer. *Cancer Pain Release, 17*(4), 1–3.

Mercadante, S. (2006b). Breakthrough pain in cancer patients. *Pain Clinical Updates. IASP, 14*(1), 1–4.

Mercadante, S., & Arcuri, E. (2007). Pharmacological management of cancer pain in the elderly. *Drugs and Aging, 24*(9), 761–776.

Mercadante, S., Arcuri, E., Ferrera, P., et al. (2005). Alternative treatments of breakthrough pain in patients receiving spinal analgesics for cancer pain. *Journal of Pain and Symptom Management, 30*(5), 485–491.

Mercadante, S., Arcuri, E., Fusco, F., et al. (2005). Randomized double-blind, double-dummy crossover clinical trial of oral tramadol versus rectal tramadol administration in opioid-naive cancer patients with pain. *Supportive Care in Cancer, 13*(9), 702–707.

Mercadante, S., & Bruera, E. (2006). Opioid switching: A systematic and critical review. *Cancer Treatment Reviews, 32*(4), 304–315.

Mercadante, S., Casuccio, A., & Calderone, L. (1999). Rapid switching from morphine to methadone in cancer patients with poor response to morphine. *Journal of Clinical Oncology, 17*(10), 3307–3312.

Mercadante, S., Casuccio, A., Fulfaro, F., et al. (2001). Switching from morphine to methadone to improve analgesia and tolerability in cancer patients: A prospective study. *Journal of Clinical Oncology, 19*(11), 2898–3904.

Mercadante, S., Costanzo, B. V., Fusco, F., et al. (2009). Breakthrough pain in advanced cancer patients followed at home: A longitudinal study. *Journal of Pain and Symptom Management, 38*(4), 554–560.

Mercadante, S., Ferrera, P., Villari, P., et al. (2006). Opioid escalation in patients with cancer pain: The effect of age. *Journal of Pain and Symptom Management, 32*(5), 413–419.

Mercadante, S., Ferrera, P., Villari, P., et al. (2009). Frequency, indications, outcomes, and predictive factors of opioid switching in an acute palliative care unit. *Journal of Pain and Symptom Management, 37*(4), 632–641.

Mercadante, S., Intravaia, G., Villari, P., et al. (2008). Intravenous morphine for breakthrough (episodic-) pain in an acute palliative care unit: A confirmatory study. *Journal of Pain and Symptom Management, 35*(3), 307–313.

Mercadante, S., Porzio, G., Ferrera, P., et al. (2006). Low morphine doses in opioid-naïve cancer patients with pain. *Journal of Pain and Symptom Management, 31*(3), 242–247.

Mercadante, S., Porzio, G., Ferrera, P., et al. (2008). Sustained-release oral morphine versus transdermal fentanyl and oral methadone in cancer pain management. *European Journal of Pain (London, England), 12*(8), 1040–1046.

Mercadante, S., Radbruch, L., Caraceni, A., et al. (2002). Episodic (breakthrough) pain. *Cancer, 94*(3), 832–839.

Mercadante, S., & Villari, P. (2001). Clinical problems with transdermal titration from 25 mcg to 50 mcg/hr. (Letter). *Journal of Pain and Symptom Management, 21*(6), 448–449.

Mercadante, S., Villari, P., Ferrera, P., et al. (2002). Rapid titration with intravenous morphine for severe cancer pain and immediate oral conversion. *Cancer, 95*(1), 203–208.

Mercadante, S., Villari, P., Ferrera, P., et al. (2004). Optimization of opioid therapy for preventing incident pain associated with bone metastases. *Journal of Pain and Symptom Management, 28*(5), 505–510.

Mercadante, S., Villari, P., Ferrera, P., et al. (2007). Transmucosal fentanyl vs intravenous morphine in doses proportional to basal opioid regimen for episodic-breakthrough pain. *British Journal of Cancer, 6*(12), 1828–1833.

Miaskowski, C. (2005). Patient-controlled modalities for acute postoperative pain management. *Journal of Perianesthesia Nursing, 20*(4), 255–267.

Miaskowski, C. (2009). A review of the incidence, causes, consequences, and management of gastrointestinal effects associated with postoperative opioid administration. *Journal of Perianesthesia Nursing, 24*(4), 222–228.

Miaskowski, C., Cleary, J., Burney, R., et al. (2005). *Guideline for the management of cancer pain in adults and children IL.* Glenview: American Pain Society.

Miaskowski, C., Dodd, M. J., West, C., et al. (2001). Lack of adherence with the analgesic regimen: A significant barrier to effective cancer pain management. *Journal of Clinical Oncology, 19*(23), 4275–4279.

Miaskowski, C., Mack, K. A., Dodd, M. J., et al. (2002). Oncology outpatients with pain from bone metastasis require more than around-the-clock dosing of analgesics to achieve adequate pain control. *The Journal of Pain, 3*(1), 12–20.

Mikkelsen, L. P., Butler, J., Huerta, D., et al. (2000). A pharmacokinetic and tolerability evaluation of two continuous subcutaneous infusions systems compared to an oral controlled-release morphine. *Journal of Pain and Symptom Management, 19*(5), 348–356.

Mildh, L. H., Scheinin, H., & Kirvelä, O. A. (2001). The concentration-effect relationship of the respiratory depressant effects of alfentanil and fentanyl. *Anesthesia and Analgesia, 93*(4), 939–946.

Miller, M. G., McCarthy, N., O'Boyle, C. A., et al. (1999). Continuous subcutaneous infusion of morphine vs. hydromorphone: A controlled trial. *Journal of Pain and Symptom Management, 18*(1), 9–16.

Miller, P. L., & Ernst, A. A. (2004). Sex differences in analgesia: A randomized trial of mu versus kappa opioid agonists. *Southern Medical Journal, 97*(1), 35–41.

Milligan, K., Lanteri-Minet, M., Borchert, K., et al. (2001). Evaluation of long-term efficacy and safety of transdermal fentanyl in the treatment of chronic noncancer pain. *The Journal of Pain, 2*(4), 197–204.

Minozzi, S., Amato, L., Vecchi, S., et al. (2008). Maintenance agonist treatments for opiate dependent pregnant women. *Cochrane Database of Systematic Reviews (Online), (2),* CD006318.

Mishra, S., Bhatnagar, S., Gupta, D., et al. (2008). Incidence and management of phantom limb pain according to World Health Organization analgesic ladder in amputees of malignant origin. *The American Journal of Hospice & Palliative Care, 24*(6), 455–462.

Mitchell, A., van Zanten, S. V., Inglis, K., et al. (2008). A randomized controlled trial comparing acetaminophen plus ibuprofen versus acetaminophen plus codeine plus caffeine after outpatient general surgery. *Journal of the American College of Surgeons, 206*(3), 472–479.

Mitra, S. (2008). Opioid-induced hyperalgesia: Pathophysiology and clinical implications. *Journal of Opioid Management, 4*(3), 123–130.

Mitra, S., & Sinatra, R. S. (2004). Perioperatiave management of acute pain in the opioid dependent patient. *Anesthesiology, 101*(1), 212–227.

Mohta, M., Kumari, N., Tyagi, A., et al. (2009). Tramadol for prevention of postanaesthestic shivering: A randomised double-blind comparison with pethidine. *Anaesthesia, 64*(2), 141–146.

Moinche, S., Kehlet, H., & Dahl, J. B. (2002). A qualitative and quantitative systematic review of preemptive analgesia for postoperative pain relief. *Anesthesiology, 96*(3), 725–741.

Monitto, C. L., Greenberg, R. S., Kost-Byerly, S., et al. (2000). The safety and efficacy of parent-/nurse-controlled analgesia in patients less than six years of age. *Anesthesia and Analgesia, 91*(3), 573–579.

Monk, T. G., Parker, R. K., & White, P. F. (1990). Use of PCA in geriatric patients: Effect of aging on the postoperative analgesic requirement. *Anesthesia and Analgesia, 70,* S272.

Monsivals, D., & McNeill, J. (2007). Multicultural influences on pain medication attitudes and beliefs in patients with nonmalignant chronic pain syndromes. *Pain Management Nursing, 8*(2), 64–71.

Moore, B. A., Kalff, J. C., & Bauer, A. J. (2005). Molecular and cellular inflammatory mechanisms in the development of postoperative ileus. *Sem Colon Rec Surg, 16*(4), 184–187.

Morita, T., Takigawa, C., Onishi, H., et al. (2005). Opioid rotation from morphine to fentanyl in delirious cancer patients: An open-label trial. *Journal of Pain and Symptom Management, 30*(1), 96–103.

Morita, T., Tei, Y., Tsunoda, J., et al. (2002). Increased plasma morphine metabolites in terminally ill cancer patients with delirium: An intra-individual comparison. *Journal of Pain and Symptom Management, 23*(2), 107–113.

Morita, T., Tsunoda, J., Inoue, S., et al. (2001). Effects of high dose opioids and sedatives on survival in terminally ill cancer patients. *Journal of Pain and Symptom Management, 21*(4), 282–289.

Morley, J. S., & Makin, M. K. (1997). Comments on Ripamonti, et al. *Pain, 73*(1), 114.

Moryl, N., Coyle, N., & Foley, K. M. (2008). Managing an acute pain crisis in a patient with advanced cancer: "This is as much of a crisis as a code". *JAMA: The Journal of the American Medical Association, 299*(12), 1457–1467.

Moser, J. D., Caldwell, J. B., & Rhule, F. J. (2006). No more than necessary: Safety and efficacy of low-dose promethazine. *The Annals of Pharmacotherapy, 40*(1), 45–48.

Moss, D. D., & Hansen, D. J. (2008). Metoclopramide and extrapyramidal symptoms: A case report. *Journal of Perianesthesia Nursing, 23*(5), 292–299.

Mouallem, M., Schwartz, E., & Farfel, Z. (2000). Prolonged oral morphine therapy for severe angina pectoris. *Journal of Pain and Symptom Management, 19*(5), 393–397.

Moulin, D. E., Clark, A. J., Gilron, I., et al. (2007). Pharmacological management of chronic neuropathic pain—consensus statement and guidelines from the Canadian Pain Society. *Pain Research & Management, 12*(1), 13–21.

Moulin, D. E., Johnson, N. G., Murray-Parsons, N., et al. (1992). Subcutaneous narcotic infusions for cancer pain: Treatment outcome and guidelines for use. *Canadian Medical Association Journal, 146*(6), 891–897.

Mousa, S. A. (2003). Morphological correlates of immune-mediated peripheral opioid analgesia. *Advances in Experimental Medicine and Biology, 521,* 77–87.

Muellejans, B., Lopez, A., Cross, M. H., et al. (2004). Remifentanil versus fentanyl for analgesia based sedation to provide patient comfort in the intensive care unit: A randomized double-blind controlled trial [ISRCTN43755713]. *Critical Care (London, England), 8*(1), R1–R11.

Mularski, R. A., Puntillo, K., Varkey, B., et al. (2009). Pain management within the palliative care and end-of-life care experience in the ICU. *Chest, 135*(5), 1360–1369.

Muller, S., Zalunardo, M. P., Hubner, M., et al. (2009). A fast-track program reduces complicaitons and length of hospital stay after open colonic surgery. *Gastroenterology, 136*(3), 842–847.

Mullins, C. R., & Wild, T. L. (2003). Pain management in a long-term care facility: Compliance with JCAHO standards. *Journal of Pain & Palliative Care Pharmacotherapy, 17*(2), 63–70.

Murphy, D. (2006). Applied clinical pharmacology of opioids. In G. Shorten, D. B. Carr, D. Harmon, M. M. Puig, & J. Browne (Eds.), *Postoperative pain management: An evidence-based guide to practice* (pp. 127–136). Philadelphia: Saunders.

Murphy, G. S., Szokol, J. W., Marymont, J. H., et al. (2007). The effects of morphine and fentanyl on the inflammatory response to cardiopulmonary bypass in patients undergoing elective coronary artery bypass graft surgery. *Anesthesia and Analgesia, 104*(6), 1334–1342.

Murray, A., & Hagen, N. A. (2005). Hydromorphone. *Journal of Pain and Symptom Management, 29*(Suppl. 5), S57–S66.

Murtagh, F. E., Chai, M. O., Donohoe, P., et al. (2007). The use of opioid analgesia in end-stage renal disease patients managed without dialysis: Recommendations for practice. *Journal of Pain & Palliative Care Pharmacotherapy, 21*(2), 5–16.

Myles, P. S. (2004). The pain visual analog scale: Linear or nonlinear? (Letter). *Anesthesiology, 100*(3), 744.

Mystakidou, K., Katsouda, E., Parpa, E., et al. (2005). Oral transmucosal fentanyl citrate for the treatment of breakthrough pain in cancer patients: An overview of its pharmacological and clinical characteristics. *The American Journal of Hospice & Palliative Care, 22*(3), 228–232.

Mystakidou, K., Parpa, E., Tsilika, E., et al. (2003). Long-term management of noncancer pain with transdermal therapeutic system-fentanyl. *The Journal of Pain, 4*(6), 298–306.

Mystakidou, K., Parpa, E., Tsilika, E., et al. (2004). Pain management of cancer patients with transdermal fentanyl: A study of 1828 step I, II, III transfers. *The Journal of Pain, 5*(2), 119–132.

Mystakidou, K., Tsilika, E., Parpa, E., et al. (2003). Long-term cancer pain management in morphine pre-treated and opioid naïve patients with transdermal fentanyl. *International Journal of Cancer, 107*(3), 486–492.

Mythen, M. G. (2005). Postoperative gastrointestinal tract dysfunction. *Anesthesia and Analgesia, 100*(1), 196–204.

Nafiu, O. O., & Bullough, A. S. (2007). Pneumocephalus and headache after epidural analgesia: Should we really be using air? (Letter). *Anesthesia and Analgesia, 105*(4), 1172–1173.

National Comprehensive Cancer Network (NCCN). (2008). *NCCN Clinical Practice Guidelines in Oncology: Adult Cancer Pain.* http://www.nccn.org/professionals/physician_gls/PDF/pain.pdf. Accessed May 1, 2008.

Nauta, M., Landsmeer, M. L. A., & Koren, G. (2009). Codeine-acetaminophen versus nonsteroidal anti-inflammatory drugs in the treatment of post-abdominal surgery pain: A systematic review of randomized trials. *American Journal of Surgery, 198*(2), 256–261.

Neal, J. M. (2008). Anatomy and physiology of spinal cord injury associated with regional anesthesia and pain medicine. *Regional Anesthesia and Pain Medicine, 33*(5), 423–434.

Neary, P., & Delaney, C. P. (2005). Alvimopan. *Expert Opinion on Investigational Drugs, 14*(4), 479–488.

Negro, S., Martin, A., Azuara, M. L., et al. (2005). Stability of tramadol and haloperidol for continuous subcutaneous infusion at home. *Journal of Pain and Symptom Management, 30*(2), 192–199.

Nelson, J. E., Meier, D. E., Oei, E. J., et al. (2001). Self-reported symptom experiences of critically ill cancer patients receiving intensive care. *Critical Care Medicine, 29*(2), 277–282.

Nelson, R., Tse, B., & Edwards, S. (2005). Systematic review of prophylactic nasogastric decompression after abdominal operations. *The British Journal of Surgery, 92*(6), 673–680.

Nemergut, E. C., Durieux, M. E., Missaghi, N. B., et al. (2007). Pain management after craniotomy. *Best Practice & Research Clinical Anaesthesiology, 21*(4), 557–573.

Neruda, B. (2008). The search for the originator of the hanging drop technique. *Regional Anesthesia and Pain Medicine, 33*(3), 276–277.

New Hampshire Hospice and Palliative Care Organization. *Opioid use guidelines.* Available at http://www.nhhpco.org/opioid.htm. Accessed July 30, 2009.

Newshan, G., & Lefkowitz, M. (2001). Transdermal fentanyl for chronic pain in AIDS: A pilot study. *Journal of Pain and Symptom Management, 21*(1), 69–77.

Newton, P. J., Davidson, P. M., Macdonald, P., et al. (2008). Nebulized furosemide in the management of dyspnea: Does the evidence support its use? *Journal of Pain and Symptom Management, 36*(4), 424–441.

Nichols, R. (2003). Pain management in patients with addictive disease. *The American Journal of Nursing, 103*(3), 87–90.

Nicholson, B., & Passik, S. D. (2007). Management of chronic noncancer pain in the primary care setting. *Southern Medical Journal, 100*(10), 1028–1036.

Nicholson, B., Ross, E., Weil, A., et al. (2006). Treatment of chronic moderate-to-severe non-malignant pain with polymer-coated extended-release morphine sulfate capsules. *Current Medical Research and Opinion, 22*(3), 539–550.

Nielsen, C. K., Ross, F. B., Lotfipour, S., et al. (2007). Oxycodone and morphine have distinctly different pharmacological profiles: Radioligand binding and behavioural studies in two rat models of neuropathic pain. *Pain, 132*(3), 289–300.

Nielsen, C. S., Stubhaug, A., Price, D. D., et al. (2008). Individual differences in pain sensitivity: Genetic and environmental contributions. *Pain, 136*(1), 21–29.

Nieminen, T. H., Hagelberg, N. M., Saari, T. I., et al. (2009). Rifampin greatly reduces the plasma concentrations of intravenous and oral oxycodone. *Anesthesiology, 110*(6), 1371–1378.

Nightingale, J. J., Knight, M. V., Higgins, B., et al. (2007). Randomized, double-blind comparison of patient-controlled epidural infusion vs nurse-administered epidural infusion for postoperative analgesia in patients undergoing colonic resection. *British Journal of Anaesthesia, 98*(3), 380–384.

Nikolajsen, L., Ilkjaer, S., Kroner, K., et al. (1997). The influence of preamputation pain on postamputation stump and phantom pain. *Pain, 72*(3), 393–405.

Nisbet, A. T., & Mooney-Cotter, F. (2008). *Post opioid induced sedation scales. Validity, reliability, accuracy, and performance in adult non-critical care settings.* Poster presentation, American Society for Pain Management Nursing National Meeting, Tucson, AZ, September 4–6.

Nisbet, A. T., & Mooney-Cotter, F. (2009). Selected scales for reporting opioid-induced sedation. *Pain Management Nursing, 10*(3), 154–164.

Nishimori, M., Ballantyne, J. C., & Low, J. H. (2006). Epidural pain relief versus systemic opioid-based pain relief for abdominal aortic surgery. *Cochrane Database of Systematic Reviews (Online),* (3), CD005059.

Nitescu, P., Hultman, E., Appelgren, L., et al. (1992). Bacteriology, drug stability and exchange of percutaneous delivery systems and antibacterial filters in long-term intrathecal infusion of opioid drugs and bupivacaine in "refractory" pain. *The Clinical Journal of Pain, 8*(4), 324–337.

Noble, F., & Roques, B. P. (2007). Protection of endogenous enkephalin catabolism as a natural approach to novel analgesic and antidepressant drugs. *Expert Opinion on Therapeutic Targets, 11*(2), 145–159.

Noble, M., Tregear, S. T., Treadwell, J. R., et al. (2008). Long-term opioid therapy for chronic noncancer pain: A systematic review and meta-analysis of efficacy and safety. *Journal of Pain and Symptom Management, 35*(2), 214–228.

Norman, P. H., Daley, M. D., & Lindsey, R. W. (2001). Preemptive analgesic effects of ketorolac in ankle fracture surgery. *Anesthesiology, 94*(4), 599–603.

North, J., Kapoor, R., Bull, J., et al. (2008). Rapid and effective control of breakthrough pain (BTP) and tolerability in cancer patients treated with BEMA (BioErodible MucoAdhesive) fentanyl. *The Journal of Pain, 9*(4, Suppl. 1), P23.

Nugent, M., Davis, C., Brooks, D., et al. (2001). Long-term observations of patients receiving transdermal fentanyl after a randomized trial. *Journal of Pain and Symptom Management, 21*(5), 385–391.

Nunez, S., Lee, J. S., Zhang, Y., et al. (2007). Role of peripheral mu-opioid receptors in inflammatory orofacial muscle pain. *Neuroscience, 146*(3), 1346–1354.

Nunley, C., Wakim, J., & Guinn, C. (2008). The effects of stimulation of acupressure point p6 on postoperative nausea and vomiting: A review of the literature. *Journal of Perianesthesia Nursing, 23*(4), 247–261.

Odom-Forren, J., & Watson, D. (2005). *Practical guide to moderate sedation/analgesia.* St. Louis: Mosby.

Office of Drug Control Policy (ODCP). (2007). *Proper disposal of prescription drugs.* http://www.whitehousedrugpolicy.gov/news/press07/022007.html. Accessed April 12, 2008.

Okamoto, Y., Tsuneto, S., Matsuda, Y., et al. (2007). A retrospective chart review of the antiemetic effectiveness of risperidone in refractory opioid-induced nausea and vomiting in advanced cancer patients. *Journal of Pain and Symptom Management, 34*(2), 217–222.

Okon, T. R., & George, M. L. (2008). Fentanyl-induced neurotoxicity and paradoxic pain. *Journal of Pain and Symptom Management, 35*(3), 327–333.

Olson, D. W., Lynn, M., Thoyre, S. M., et al. (2007). The limited reliability of the Ramsay Scale. *Neurocritical Care, 7*(3), 227–231.

O'Malley-Dafner, L., & Davies, P. (2000). Naloxone-induced pulmonary edema. *The American Journal of Nursing, 100*(11), 24AA–24JJ.

Ong, C. K. S., Lirk, P., Seymour, R. A., et al. (2005). The efficacy of preemptive analgesia for acute postoperative pain management: A meta-analysis. *Anesthesia and Analgesia, 100*(3), 757–773.

Osborn, D. A., Jeffery, HE., & Cole, M. J. (2005a). Opiate treatment for opiate withdrawal in newborn infants. *Cochrane Database of Systematic Reviews (Online),* (3), CD002059.

Osborn, D. A., Jeffery, H. E., & Cole, M. J. (2005b). Sedatives for opiate withdrawal in newborn infants. *Cochrane Database of Systematic Reviews (Online),* (3), CD002053.

Ostrop, N. J., Lamb, J., & Reid, G. (1998). Intravaginal morphine: An alternative route of administration. *Pharmacotherapy, 18*(4), 863–865.

Overdyk, F., & Ahmed, Q. (2009). Postoperative monitoring of obese patients with obstructive sleep apnea. (Letter). *Anesthesia and Analgesia, 108*(3), 1044–1045.

Overdyk, F., Carter, R., & Maddox, R. R. (2006). New JCAHO pain standard bigger threat to patient safety than envisioned. (Letter). *Anesthesie Analgesie, 102,* 1596.

Overdyk, F., Carter, R., Maddox, R. R., et al. (2007). Continuous oximetry/capnography monitoring reveals frequent desaturation and bradypnea during patient-controlled analgesia. *Anesthesia and Analgesia, 105*(2), 412–418.

Owen, H., Plummer, J. L., Armstrong, I., et al. (1989). Variables of patient-controlled analgesia. 1: Bolus size. *Anaesthesia, 44*(1), 7–10.

Paech, M. J., Moore, J. S., & Evans, S. F. (1994). Meperidine for patient-controlled analgesia after cesarean section. *Anesthesiology, 80*(6), 1268–1276.

Paech, M. J., Pavy, T. J. G., Orlikowski, C. E. P., et al. (2000). Postoperative intraspinal opioid analgesia after caesarean section; a randomised comparison of subarachnoid morphine and epidural pethidine. *International Journal of Obstetric Anesthesia, 9*(4), 238–245.

Paech, M. J., Rucklidge, M. W. M., Lain, J., et al. (2007). Ondansetron and dexamethasone dose combinations for prophylaxis against postoperative nausea and vomiting. *Anesthesia and Analgesia, 104*(4), 808–814.

Page, G. (2005). Immunologic effects of opioids in the presence or absence of pain. *Journal of Pain and Symptom Management, 29*(5S), S25–W31.

Paice, J. A. (2008). Pharmacokinetics, pharmacodynamics, and pharmacogenomics of opioids. *Pain Management Nursing, 8*(3, Suppl. 1), S2–S5.

Paice, J. A., Noskin, G. A., Vanagunas, A., et al. (2005). Efficacy and safety of scheduled dosing of opioid analgesics: A quality improvement study. *The Journal of Pain, 6*(10), 639–643.

Paice, J. A., Von Roenn, J. H., Hudgins, J. C., et al. (2008). Morphine bioavailability from a topical gel formulation in volunteers. *Journal of Pain and Symptom Management, 35*(3), 314–320.

Paice, J. A., & Williams, A. R. (1995). Intraspinal drugs for pain. In D. McGuire, C. H. Yarbro, & B. R. Ferrell (Eds.), *Cancer pain management.* (2nd ed., pp. 131–158). Boston: Jones, Bartlett Publishers.

Paiste, J., Bjerke, R. J., Williams, J. P., et al. (2001). Minimally invasive direct coronary artery bypass surgery under high thoracic epidural. *Anesthesia and Analgesia, 93*(6), 1486–1488.

Palacioz, K. (2001). Inappropriate meperidine use. *Pharm Letters, 17,* document 171117-8.

Palangio, M., Northfelt, D. W., Portenoy, R. K., et al. (2002). Dose conversion and titration with a novel, once-daily, OROS technology, extended-release hydromorphone formulation in the treatment of chronic malignant or nonmalignant pain. *Journal of Pain and Symptom Management, 23*(5), 355–368.

Palm, S., Lehzen, S., Mignat, C., et al. (1998). Does prolonged oral treatment with sustained-release morphine tablets influence immune function? *Anesthesia and Analgesia, 86,* 166–172.

Palmer, S. N., Giesecke, N. M., Body, S. C., et al. (2005). Pharmacogenetics of anesthetic and analgesic agents. *Anesthesiology, 102*(3), 663–671.

Pan, H., Zhang, Z., Zhang, Y., et al. (2007). Efficacy and tolerability of oxycodone hydrochloride controlled-release tablets in moderate to severe cancer pain. *Clinical Drug Investigation, 27*(4), 259–267.

Pan, P. H., Lee, S. C., & Harris, L. C. (2008). Antiemetic prophylaxis for postdischarge nausea and vomiting and impact on functional quality of living during recovery in patients with high emetic risks: A prospective randomized, double-blind comparison of two prophylactic antiemetic regimens. *Anesthesia and Analgesia, 107*(2), 429–438.

Pandey, C. K., Raza, M., Ranjan, R., et al. (2005). Intravenous lidocaine 0.5 mg.kg-1 effectively suppresses fentanyl-induced cough. *Canadian Journal of Anesthesia, 52*(2), 172–175.

Panjabi, S. S., Panjabi, R. S., Shepherd, M. D., et al. (2008). Extended-release, once-daily morphine (Avinza) for the treatment of chronic nonmalignant pain: Effect on pain, depressive symptoms, and cognition. *Pain Medicine (Malden, Mass.), 9*(8), 985–993.

Pantanwala, A. E., Jarzyna, D. L., Miller, M. D., et al. (2008). Comparison of opioid requirements and analgesic response in opioid-tolerant versus opioid-naïve patients after total knee arthroplasty. *Pharmacotherapy, 28*(12), 1453–1460.

Paqueron, X., Lumbroso, A., Mergoni, P., et al. (2002). Is morphine-induced sedation synonymous with analgesia during intravenous morphine titration? *British Journal of Anaesthesia, 89*(5), 687–701.

Park, W. Y., Thompson, J. S., Lee, K. K., et al. (2001). Effect of epidural anesthesia and analgesia on perioperative outcome. *Annals of Surgery, 234*(4), 560–569.

Parker, R. K., Holtmann, B., & White, P. F. (1991). Patient-controlled analgesia: Does a concurrent opioid infusion improve pain management after surgery? *JAMA: The Journal of the American Medical Association, 266*(14), 1947–1952.

Parker, R. K., Holtmann, B., & White, P. F. (1997). Patient-controlled epidural analgesia: Interactions between nalbuphine and hydromorphone. *Anesthesia and Analgesia, 84*(4), 757–763.

Parker, R. K., Sawaki, Y., & White, P. F. (1992). Epidural patient-controlled analgesia: influence of bupivacaine and hydromorphone basal infusion on pain control after cesarean section. *Anesthesia and Analgesia, 75*(5), 740–746.

Parker, R. K., & White, P. F. (1992). Epidural patient-controlled analgesia: an alternative to intravenous patient-controlled analgesia for pain relief after cesarean section. *Anesthesia and Analgesia, 75*(2), 245–251.

Parpaglioni, R., Baldassini, B., Barbati, G., et al. (2009). Adding sufentanil to levobupivacaine or ropivacaine intrathecal anaesthesia affects the minimum local anesthetic dose required. *Acta Anaesthesiologica Scandinavica, 53*(9), 1214–1220.

Parramon, F., Garcia, C. H., Gambus, P., et al. (2003). Postoperative patient-controlled analgesia is more effective with epidural methadone than with intravenous methadone in thoracic surgery. *Revista Espanola de Anesthesiologia Reanimacion, 50*(7), 326–331.

Parris-Piper, T. (2008). Post caesarean delivery pain management: Do not dismiss pethidine. *International Journal of Obstetric Anesthesia, 17*(1), 95–96.

Pasero, C. (2003). Multimodal analgesia in the PACU. *Journal of Perianesthesia Nursing, 18*(4), 265–268.

Pasero, C. (2005). Fentanyl for acute pain management. *Journal of Perianesthesia Nursing, 20*(4), 279–284.

Pasero, C. (2007). Procedure-specific pain management: PROSPECT. *Journal of Perianesthesia Nursing, 22*(5), 335–340.

Pasero, C. (2009a). Challenges in pain assessment. *Journal of Perianesthesia Nursing, 24*(1), 50–54.

Pasero, C. (2009b). Assessment of sedation during opioid administration for pain management. *Journal of Perianesthesia Nursing, 24*(3), 186–190.

Pasero, C., & Belden, J. (2006). Evidence-based perioperative care: Accelerated postoperative recovery programs. *Journal of Perianesthesia Nursing, 21*(3), 168–177.

Pasero, C., Eksterowicz, N., Primeau, M., et al. (2007). Registered nurse management and monitoring of analgesia by catheter techniques. *Pain Management Nursing, 8*(2), 48–54.

Pasero, C., Manworren, R. C. B., & McCaffery, M. (2007). IV Opioid range orders for acute pain management. *The American Journal of Nursing, 107*(2), 52–59.

Pasero, C., & McCaffery, M. (1993). Unconventional PCA: Making it work for your patient. *The American Journal of Nursing, 93*(9), 38–41.

Pasero, C., & McCaffery, M. (2001). Multimodal balanced analgesia in the critically ill. *Critical Care Nursing Clinics of North America, 13*(2), 195–206.

Pasero, C., & McCaffery, M. (2002). Monitoring sedation. *The American Journal of Nursing, 102*(2), 67–69.

Pasero, C., & McCaffery, M. (2003). Accountability for pain relief: Use of comfort-function goals. *Journal of Perianesthesia Nursing, 18*(1), 50–52.

Pasero, C., & McCaffery, M. (2004). Safe use of a continuous infusion with IV PCA. *Journal of Perianesthesia Nursing, 19*(1), 42–45.

Pasero, C., & McCaffery, M. (2005a). Authorized and unauthorized use of PCA pumps. *The American Journal of Nursing, 105*(7), 30–33.

Pasero, C., & McCaffery, M. (2005b). Extended-release epidural morphine (Depodur™). *Journal of Perianesthesia Nursing, 20*(5), 345–350.

Pasero, C., & McCaffery, M. (2007). Orthopaedic postoperative pain management. *Journal of Perianesthesia Nursing, 22*(3), 160–173.

Pasero, C., Portenoy, R. K., & McCaffery, M. (1999). Opioid analgesics. In M. McCaffery, & C. Pasero (Eds.), *Pain: Clinical manual.* (2nd ed., pp. 161–299). St. Louis: Mosby.

Passik, S. D., & Kirsh, K. L. (2004). Opioid therapy in patients with a history of substance abuse. *CNS drugs, 18*(1), 13–25.

Pasternak, G. W. (2001). Incomplete cross tolerance and multiple mu opioid peptide receptors. *Trends in Pharmacological Sciences*, 22(2), 67–70.

Pasternak, G. W. (2005). Molecular biology of opioid analgesia. *Journal of Pain and Symptom Management*, 29(5S), S2–S9.

Pasternak, G. W. (2010). Molecular insights into μ opioid pharmacology from the clinic to the bench. *The Clinical Journal of Pain*, 26(Suppl. 1), S3–S9.

Patanwala, A. E., Jarzyna, D. L., Miller, M. D., et al. (2008). Comparison of opioid requirements and analgesic response in opioid-tolerant versus opioid-naïve patients after total knee arthroplasty. *Pharmacotherapy*, 28(12), 1453–1460.

Patt, R. B. (1998). Co-proxamol/Propoxyphene: It is the wise doctor who listens to their patients. *BMJ (Clinical Research Ed.)*. Rapid Response 29 Sep. http://phstwlp1.partners.org:2352/cgi/eletters/315/7122/1565#880. Accessed March 9, 2008.

Pavis, H., Wilcock, A., Edgecombe, J., et al. (2002). Pilot study of nasal morphine-chitosan for the relief of breakthrough pain in patients with cancer. *Journal of Pain and Symptom Management*, 24(6), 598–602.

Payne, R. (2007). Recognition and diagnosis of breakthrough pain. *Pain Medicine (Malden, Mass.)*, 8(Suppl. 1), S3–S7.

Payne, R., Mathias, S. D., Pasta, D. J., et al. (1998). Quality of life and cancer pain: Satisfaction and side effects with transdermal fentanyl versus oral morphine. *Journal of Clinical Oncology*, 16(4), 1588–1593.

Pearl, M. L., McCauley, D. L., Thompson, J., et al. (2002). A randomized controlled trial of early oral analgesia in gynecologic oncology patients undergoing intra-abdominal surgery. *Obstetrics Gynecology*, 99(5), 704–708.

Peck, M., & Down, J. (2009). Use of sedatives in the critically ill. *Anaesth Intens Care Med*, 11(1), 12–15.

Pedersen, T., Moller, A. M., & Pederson, B. D. (2003). Pulse oximetry for perioperative monitoring: Systematic review of randomized, controlled trials. *Anesthesia and Analgesia*, 97(2), 426–431.

Peng, P., Tumber, P., Stafford, M., et al. (2008). Experience of methadone therapy in 100 consecutive chronic pain patients in a multidisciplinary pain center. *Pain Medicine (Malden, Mass.)*, 9(7), 786–794.

Peng, P. W., Tumber, P. S., & Gourlay, D. (2005). Review article: Perioperative pain management of patients on methadone therapy. *Canadian Journal of Anaesthesia*, 52(5), 513–523.

Peng, Y. R., Sun, W. Z., & Mok, M. S. (2005). Mini-dose titration of the transdermal fentanyl patch—A novel approach by adjusting the area of absorption. *Journal of Pain and Symptom Management*, 30(1), 7–8.

Penniston, J. H., & Gould, E. (2009). Oxymorphone extended release for the treatment of chronic low back pain: A retrospective pooled analysis of enriched-enrollment clinical trial data stratified according to age, sex, and prior opioid use. *Clinical Therapeutics*, 31(2), 347–359.

Pereira, J., Lawlor, P., Vigano, A., et al. (2001). Equianalgesic dose ratios for opioids. A critical review and proposals for long-term dosing. *Journal of Pain and Symptom Management*, 22(2), 672–687.

Perkins, F. M., & Kehlet, H. (2000). Chronic pain as an outcome of surgery. *Anesthesiology*, 93(4), 1123–1133.

Perri, M., 3rd, Menon, A. M., Deshpande, A. D., et al. (2005). Adverse outcomes associated with inappropriate drug use in nursing homes. *The Annals of Pharmacotherapy*, 39(3), 405–411.

Persec, J., Persec, Z., Bukovic, D., et al. (2007). Effects of clonidine preemptive analgesia on acute postoperative pain in abdominal surgery. *Collegium Antropologicum*, 31(4), 1071–1075.

Phillips, T. W., Broussard, D. M., Sumrall, W. D., et al. (2007). Intraoperative oxygen administration does not reduce the incidence or severity of nausea or vomiting associated with neuraxial anesthesia for cesarean delivery. *Anesthesia and Analgesia*, 105(4), 1113–1117.

Picker, M. J. (1997). Discriminative stimulus effects of the mixed-opioid agonist/antagonist dezocine: Cross-substitution by mu and delta opioid agonists. *Journal of Pharmacology Experimental Therapeutics*, 283(3), 1009–1017.

Pirat, A., Tuncay, S. F., Torgay, A., et al. (2005). Ondansetron, orally disintegrating tablets versus intravenous injection for prevention of intrathecal morphine-induced nausea, vomiting and pruritus in young males. *Anesthesia and Analgesia*, 101(5), 1330–1336.

Pitsiu, M., Wilmer, A., Bodenham, A., et al. (2004). Pharmacokinetics of remifentanil and its major metabolite, remifentanil acid, in ICU patients with renal impairment. *British Journal of Anaesthesia*, 92(4), 493–503.

Pittelkow, M. R., & Loprinzi, C. L. (2004). Pruritus and sweating in palliative medicine. In D. Doyle, G. Hanks, N. I. Cherny, & K. Calman (Eds.), *Oxford textbook of palliative medicine*. (3rd ed., pp. 573–587). New York: Oxford Press.

Platt, A., Eckman, J. R., Beasley, J. A., et al. (2002). Treating sickle cell pain: An update from the Georgia Comprehensive Sickle Cell Center. *The Journal of Emergency Medicine*, 28(4), 297–303.

Pleuvry, B. J. (2009). Physiology and pharmacology of nausea and vomiting. *Anaesth Intens Care Med*, 10(12), 587–601.

Plonk, W. M. (2005). Simplified methadone conversion. *Journal of Palliative Medicine*, 8(3), 478–479.

Poobalan, A. S., Bruce, J., King, P. M., et al. (2001). Chronic pain and quality of life following open inguinal hernia repair. *The British Journal of Surgery*, 88(8), 1122–1126.

Poobalan, A. S., Bruce, J., Smith, W. C., et al. (2003). A review of chronic pain after inguinal herniorrhaphy. *The Clinical Journal of Pain*, 19(1), 48–54.

Portenoy, R. K. (1996). Opioid analgesics. In R. K. Portenoy, & R. M. Kanner (Eds.), *Pain management: Theory and practice* (pp. 249–276). Philadelphia: FA Davis.

Portenoy, R. K. (2005). Prevalence and characteristics of breakthrough pain in opioid-treated patients with chronic noncancer pain. *The Journal of Pain*, 7(8), 583–591.

Portenoy, R. K., Bennett, D. S., Rauck, R., et al. (2006). Prevalence and characteristics of breakthrough pain in opioid-treated patients with chronic noncancer pain. *The Journal of Pain*, 7(8), 583–591.

Portenoy, R. K., Farrar, J. T., Backonja, M. M., et al. (2007). Long-term use of controlled-release oxycodone for noncancer pain: Results of a 3-year registry study. *The Clinical Journal of Pain*, 23(4), 287–299.

Portenoy, R. K., & Foley, K. M. (1986). Chronic use of opioid analgesics in non-malignant pain: Report of 38 cases. *Pain*, 15(2), 171–186.

Portenoy, R. K., Forbes, K., Lussier, D., et al. (2004). Difficult pain problems: An integrated approach. In D. Doyle, G. Hanks, N. I. Cherny, & K. Calman (Eds.), *Oxford textbook of palliative medicine*. (3rd ed., pp. 438–458). New York: Oxford Press.

Portenoy, R. K., & Hagen, N. A. (1990). Breakthrough pain: Definition, prevalence and characteristics. *Pain, 41*(3), 273–281.

Portenoy, R. K., Maldonado, M., Fitzmartin, R., et al. (1989). Oral controlled-release morphine sulfate. Analgesic efficacy and side effects of a 100 mg tablet in cancer pain patients. *Cancer, 63*(Suppl. 11), 2284–2288.

Portenoy, R. K., Sciberras, A., Eliot, L., et al. (2002). Steady-state pharmacokinetic comparison of a new, extended-release, once-daily morphine formulation, Avinza, and a twice-daily controlled-release morphine formulation in patients with chronic moderate-to-severe pain. *Journal of Pain and Symptom Management, 23*(4), 292–300.

Portenoy, R. K., Sibirceva, U., Smout, R., et al. (2006). Opioid use and survival at the end of life: A survey of a hospice population. *Journal of Pain and Symptom Management, 32*(6), 532–540.

Portenoy, R. K., Taylor, D., Messina, J., et al. (2006). A randomized, placebo-controlled study of fentanyl buccal tablet for breakthrough pain in opioid-treated patients with cancer. *The Clinical Journal of Pain, 22*(9), 805–811.

Portenoy, R. K., Thomas, J., Moehl Boatwright, M. L., et al. (2008). Subcutaneous methylnaltrexone for the treatment of opioid-induced constipation in patients with advanced illness: A double-blind, randomized, parallel group, dose-ranging study. *Journal of Pain and Symptom Management, 35*(5), 458–468.

Pouzeratte, Y., Delay, J. M., Brunat, G., et al. (2001). Patient-controlled epidural analgesia after abdominal surgery: Ropivacaine versus bupivacaine. *Anesthesia and Analgesia, 93*(6), 1587–1592.

Prager, J., & Rauck, R. (2004). *Oxymorphone extended release for moderate to severe neuropathic pain: An open label, long-term study of safety and effectiveness.* Paper presented at The Second Joint Scientific Meeting of the APS and the Canadian Pain Society, Vancouver, BC Canada; May 6–9.

Prakash, S., Fatima, T., & Pawar, M. (2004). Patient-controlled analgesia with fentanyl for burn dressing changes. *Anesthesia and Analgesia, 99*(2), 552–555.

Prettyman, J. (2005). Subcutaneous or intramuscular? Contronting a parenteral administration dilemma. *Medsurg Nursing, 14*(2), 93–98.

Pricara, (2008). *Nucynta package insert. Pricara, Division of Ortho McNeil Pharmaceuticals.* Available at http://www.nucynta.com/nucynta/assets/Nucynta-PI.pdf. Accessed July 1, 2009.

Priestley, M. C., Cope, L., Halliwell, R., et al. (2002). Thoracic epidural anesthesia for cardiac surgery: The effects on tracheal intubation time and length of hospital stay. *Anesthesia and Analgesia, 94*(2), 275–282.

Prieto-Alvarez, P., Tello-Galindo, I., Cuenca-Pena, J., et al. (2002). Continuous epidural infusion of racemic methadone results in effective postoperative analgesia and low plasma concentrations. *Canadian Journal of Anesthesia, 49*(1), 25–31.

Prime Therapeutics. (2007). *Study finds 90 percent of Actiq "lollipop" prescriptions are off-label.* http://www.primetherapeutics.com/pdf/Actiq.pdf. Accessed April 13, 2007.

Prommer, E. (2005). Tramadol: Does it have a role in cancer pain management? *Journal of Opioid Management, 1*(3), 131–138.

Prommer, E. (2006a). Rotating methadone to other opioids: A lesson in the mechanisms of opioid tolerance and opioid-induced pain. *Journal of Palliative Medicine, 9*(2), 488–493.

Prommer, E. (2006b). Oxymorphone: A review. *Supportive Care in Cancer, 14*(2), 109–115.

Prommer, E. (2007a). Levorphanol: The forgotten opioid. *Supportive Care in Cancer, 15,* 259–264.

Prommer, E. (2007b). Levorphanol revisited. *Journal of Palliative Medicine, 10*(6), 1228–1230.

Puntillo, K., Pasero, C., Li, D., et al. (2009). Evaluation of pain in the ICU patients. *Chest, 135*(4), 1069–1074.

Puntillo, K. A., White, C., Morris, A. B., et al. (2001). Patient's perceptions and responses to procedural pain: Results from Thunder Project II. *American Journal of Critical Care, 10*(4), 238–251.

Purdue Pharma, L. P. (2007). *OxyContin prescribing information.* Stamford, CT: Purdue Pharma LP. Available at http://www.purduepharma.com/PI/Prescription/Oxycontin.pdf. Accessed Apr 18, 2008.

Purhonen, S., Turunen, M., Ruohoaho, U. M., et al. (2003). Supplemental oxygen dose not reduce the incidence of postoperative nausea and vomiting after ambulatory gynecologic laparoscopy. *Anesthesia and Analgesia, 96*(1), 91–96.

Purkayastha, S., Tilney, H. S., Darzi, A. W., et al. (2008). Meta-analysis of randomized studies evaluating chewing gum to enhance postoperative recovery following colectomy. *Archives of Surgery, 143*(8), 788–793.

Qaseem, A., Snow, V., Shekelle, P., et al. (2008). Evidence-based interventions to improve the palliative care of pain, dyspnea, and depression at the end of life: A clinical practice guideline from the American College of Physicians. *Annals of Internal Medicine, 148*(2), 141–146.

Quigley, C. (2002). Hydromorphone for acute and chronic pain. *Cochrane Database of Systematic Reviews (Online),* (1), CD003447.

Quigley, C. (2004). Opioid switching to improve pain relief and drug tolerability. *Cochrane Database of Systematic Reviews (Online),* (3), CD004847.

Quigley, C., & Wiffen, P. (2003). A systematic review of hydromorphone in acute and chronic pain. *Journal of Pain and Symptom Management, 5*(2), 169–178.

Quinlan-Colwell, A., Ballato, S., & Holmes, W. (2009). *Exploring the correlation among reports of pain, analgesia and the instance of falling.* Poster Presentation at *Connecting the Dots – Geriatric Nursing, Education and Clinical Simulation International Conference,* April 2–3, Durham, North Carolina.

Radnay, P. A., Brodman, E., Mankikar, D., et al. (1980). The effect of equianalgesic doses of fentanyl, morphine, meperidine, and pentazocine on common bile duct pressure. *Anaesthetist, 29,* 26–29.

Radnay, P. A., Duncalf, D., Novakovic, M., et al. (1984). Common bile duct pressure changes after fentanyl, morphine, meperidine, butorphanol, and naloxone. *Anesthesia and Analgesia, 63*(4), 441–444.

Raffa, R. B., & Stone, D. J. (2008). Unexceptional seizure potential of tramadol or its enantiomers or metabolites in mice. *The Journal of Pharmacology and Experimental Therapeutics, 325*(2), 500–506.

Raja, S. N., Haythornthwaite, J. A., Pappagallo, M., et al. (2002). Opioids versus antidepressants in postherpetic neuralgia. A randomized, placebo-controlled trial. *Neurology, 59*(7), 1015–1021.

Ramsay, M., Savege, T., Simpson, B., et al. (1974). Controlled sedation with akphaxolone-alphadolone. *BMJ (Clinical*

Research Ed.), 2(5920), 656–659. Ramsay Scale available at http://5jsnacc.umin.ac.jp/How%20to%20use%20the%20 Ramsay%20Score%20to%20assess%20the%20level%20 of%20ICU%20Sedation.htm. Accessed August 28, 2009.

Raphael, J. H., Southall, J. L., Gnanadurai, T. V., et al. (2002). Long-term experience with implanted intrathecal drug administration systems for failed back syndrome and chronic mechanical low back pain. *BMC Musculoskeletal Disorders, 3*, 17.

Rapoport, A. M., Bigal, M. E., Tepper, S. J., et al. (2004). Intranasal medications for the treatment of migraine and cluster headache. *CNS Drugs, 18*(10), 671–685.

Rapp, S. E., Egan, K. J., Ross, B. K., et al. (1996). A multi-dimensional comparison of morphine and hydromorphone patient-controlled analgesia. *Anesthesia and Analgesia, 82*(5), 1043–1048.

Rathmell, J. P., Lake, T., & Ramundo, M. B. (2006). Infectious risk of chronic pain treatments: Injection therapy, surgical implants, and intradiscal techniques. *Regional Anesthesia and Pain Medicine, 31*(4), 346–352.

Rathmell, J. P., Viscomi, C. M., & Ashburn, M. A. (1997). Management of nonobstetric pain during pregnancy and lactation. *Anesthesia and Analgesia, 85*(5), 1074–1087.

Rauck, R. L., Bookbinder, S. A., Bunker, T. R., et al. (2006). The ACTION study: A randomized, open-label, multicenter trial comparing once-a-day extended-release morphine sulfate capsules (Avinza) to twice-a-day controlled-release oxycodone hydrochloride tablets (OxyContin) for the treatment of chronic, moderate to severe low back pain. *Journal of Opioid Management, 2*(3), 155–166.

Rauck, R. L., Bookbinder, S. A., Bunker, T. R., et al. (2007). A randomized, open-label, multicenter trial comparing once-a-day Avinza (morphine extended-release capsules) versus twice-a-day OxyContin (oxycodone hydrochloride controlled-release tablets for the treatment of chronic, moderate to severe low back pain: Improved physical functioning in the ACTION trial. *Journal of Opioid Management, 3*(1), 35–43.

Rauck, R., Ma, T., Kerwin, R., et al. (2008). Titration with oxymorphone extended release to achieve effective long-term pain relief and improve tolerability in opioid-naive patients with moderate to severe pain. *Pain Medicine (Malden, Mass.), 9*(7), 777–785.

Ray, W. A., Fought, R. L., & Decker, M. D. (1992). Psychoactive drugs and the risk of injurious motor vehicle crashes in elderly drivers. *American Journal of Epidemiology, 136*(7), 33–47.

Rayburn, W. F., Smith, C. V., & Woods, M. P. (1989). Continuous and demand narcotic dosing for patient-controlled analgesia after cesarean section. *Anesthesiology Review, 17*(5), 58–62.

Raymo, L.L, Camejo, M., & Fudin, J. (2007). Eradicating analgesic use of meperidine in a hospital. *American Journal of Health-System Pharmacy: AJHP, 64*(11), 1148, 1150–1152.

Redelmeier, D. (2007). New thinking about postoperative delirium. *Canadian Medical Association Journal, 177*(4), 424.

Rees, D. C., Olujohungbe, A. D., Parker, N. E., et al. (2003). Guideline for the management of the acute painful crisis in sickle cell disease. *British Journal of Haematology, 120*(5), 744–752.

Reich, D. L., Timcenko, A., Bodian, C. A., et al. (1996). Predictors of pulse oximetry data failure. *Anesthesiology, 84*(4), 859–864.

Reid, C. M., Martin, R. M., Sterne, J. A., et al. (2006). Oxycodone for cancer-related pain: Meta-analysis of randomized controlled trials. *Archives of Internal Medicine, 166*(8), 837–843.

Reisfield, G. M., & Wilson, G. R. (2007). Rational use of sublingual opioids in palliative medicine. *Journal of Palliative Medicine, 10*(2), 465–475.

Reuben, D. B., & Mor, V. (1986). Dyspnea in terminally ill cancer patients. *Chest, 89*(2), 234–236.

Reynvoet, M. E. J., Cosaert, P.A.J.M., Desmet, M. F. R., et al. (1997). Epidural dextran 40 patch for postdural puncture headache. *Anaesthesia, 52*(9), 886–888.

Ribeiro, M. D. C., Joel, S. P., & Zeppetella, G. (2004). The bioavailability of morphine applied topically to cutaneous ulcers. *Journal of Pain and Symptom Management, 27*(5), 434–439.

Ricard-Hibon, A., Belpomme, V., Chollet, C., et al. (2008). Compliance with a morphine protocol and effect on pain relief in out-of-hospital patients. *The Journal of Emergency Medicine, 34*(3), 305–310.

Rickard, C., O'Meara, P., McGrail, M., et al. (2007). A randomized controlled trial of intranasal fentanyl vs intravenous morphine for analgesia in the prehospital setting. *The American Journal of Emergency Medicine, 25*(8), 911–917.

Ridley, S. (2005). The recognition and early management of critical illness. *Annals of the Royal College of Surgeons of England, 87*(5), 315–322.

Riley, J., Eisenberg, E., Müller-Schwefe, G., et al. (2008). Oxycodone: A review of its use in the management of pain. *Current Medical Research and Opinion, 24*(1), 175–192.

Riley, J., Ross, J. R., Rutter, D., et al. (2006). No pain relief from morphine? Individual variation in sensitivity to morphine and the need to switch to an alternative opioid in cancer patients. *Supportive Care in Cancer, 14*(1), 56–64.

Riordan, S. W., Beam, K., & Okabe-Yamamura, T. (2004). Introducing patient-controlled oral analgesia. *Nursing, 34*(9), 20.

Ripamonti, C. I., & Bandieri, E. (2009). Pain therapy. *Critical Reviews in Oncology/Hematology, 70*(2), 145–159.

Ripamonti, C. I., Campa, T., Fagnoni, E., et al. (2009). Normal-release oral morphine startign dose in cancer patients with pain. *The Clinical Journal of Pain, 25*(5), 386–390.

Ripamonti, C. I., Groff, L., Brunelli, C., et al. (1998). Switching from morphine to oral methadone in treating cancer pain: What is the equianalgesic dose ratio? *Journal of Clinical Oncology, 16*(10), 3216–3221.

Rittner, H. L., & Brack, A. (2007). Leukocytes as mediators of pain and analgesics. *Current Rheumatology Reports, 9*(6), 503–510.

Rivara, F. P., MacKenzie, E. J., Jurkovich, G. J., et al. (2008). Prevalence of pain in patients 1 year after major trauma. *Archives of Surgery, 143*(3), 282–287.

Roberts, G. (2004). A review of the efficacy and safety of opioid analgesics. *Nursing in Critical Care, 9*(6), 277–283.

Robertson, T. M., Hendey, G. W., Stroh, G., et al. (2009). Intranasal naloxone is a viable alternative to intravenous naloxone for prehospital narcotic overdose. *Prehospital Emergency Care, 13*(4), 512–515.

Robinson, J. M., Wilkie, D. J., & Campbell, B. (1995). Sublingual and oral morphine administration. *The Nursing Clinics of North America, 30*(4), 725–743.

Rocker, G. M., Heyland, D. K., Cook, D., et al. (2004). Most critically ill patients are perceived to die in comfort during withdrawal of life support: A Canadian multicentre study. *Canadian Journal of Anesthesia, 51*(6), 623–630.

Rockford, M. A., & DeRuyter, M. L. (2009). Perioperative epidural analgesia. In H. S. Smith (Ed.), *Current therapy in pain* (pp. 78–84). Philadelphia: Saunders.

Rodgers, A., Walker, N., Schug, S., et al. (2008). Reduction of postoperative mortality and morbidity with epidural or spinal anaesthesia: Results from overview of randomised trials. *BMJ (Clinical Research Ed.), 321*(7275), 1493.

Rodriguez, R. F., Bravo, L. E., Castro, F., et al. (2007). Incidence of weak opioids adverse events in the management of cancer pain: A double-blind comparative trial. *Journal of Palliative Medicine, 10*(1), 56–60.

Rodriguez, R. F., Castillo, J. M., Del Pilar Castillo, M., et al. (2007). Codeine/acetaminophen and hydrocodone/acetaminophen combination tablets for the management of chronic cancer pain in adults: A 23-day, prospective, double-blind, randomized, parallel-group study. *Clinical Therapeutics, 29*(4), 581–587.

Rohm, K. D., & Boldt, J. (2006). Persisting neurological symptoms after uncomplicated intrathecal bupivacaine. (Letter). *Anesthesia and Analgesia, 103*(4), 1047.

Rosati, J., Gallagher, M., Shook, B., et al. (2007). Evaluation of an oral patient-controlled analgesia device for pain management in oncology inpatients. *The Journal of Supportive Oncology, 5*(9), 443–448.

Roscoe, J. A., Bushunow, P., Jean-Pierre, P., et al. (2009). Acupressure bands are effective in reducing radiation therapy-related nausea. *Journal of Pain and Symptom Management, 38*(3), 381–389.

Rosen, D., & DeGaetano, N. P. (2006). Perioperative management of opioid-tolerance chronic pain patients. *Journal of Opioid Management, 2*(6), 353–363.

Rosenthal, M., Moore, P., Groves, E., et al. (2007). Sleep improves when patients with chronic OA pain are managed with morning dosing of once a day extended-release morphine sulfate (AVINZA): Findings from a pilot study. *Journal of Opioid Management, 3*(3), 145–154.

Rosielle, D. A. (2007). *Fast fact and concept #166: Once-daily oral morphine formulations.* Available at http://www.eperc.mcw.edu/fastFact/ff_166.htm. Accessed July 3, 2009.

Rosow, C. E., Gomery, P., Chen, T. Y., et al. (2007). Reversal of opioid-induced bladder dysfunction by intravenous naloxone and methylnaltrexone. *Clinical Pharmacology and Therapeutics, 82*(1), 48–53.

Ross, F. B., Wallis, S. C., & Smith, M. T. (2000). Co-administration of sub-antinociceptive doses of oxycodone and morphine produces marked antinociceptive synergy with reduced CNS side-effects in rats. *Pain, 84*(2–3), 421–428.

Ross, J. R., & Quigley, C. (2003). Transdermal fentanyl: Informed prescribing is essential. *European Journal of Pain (London, England), 7*(5), 481–483.

Roth, C. S., & Burgess, D. J. (2008). Changing residents' beliefs and concerns about treating chronic noncancer pain with opioids: Evaluation of a pilot workshop. *Pain Medicine (Malden, Mass.), 9*(7), 890–902.

Roth, S. H., Fleischmann, R. M., Burch, F. X., et al. (2000). Around-the-clock controlled-release oxycodone therapy for osteoarthritis-related pain. *Archives of Internal Medicine, 160*(6), 853–860.

Rothwell, M., Pearson, D., Wright, K., et al. (2009). Bacterial contamination of PCA and epidural infusion devices. *Anaesthesia, 64*(7), 751–753.

Rowbotham, M. C., Twilling, L., Davies, P. S., et al. (2003). Oral opioid therapy for chronic peripheral and central neuropathic pain. *The New England Journal of Medicine, 348*(13), 1223–1232.

Royse, C. F., Royse, A. G., Soeding, P. F., et al. (2000). Towards pain free cardiac surgery—High thoracic epidural analgesia. *Acute Pain, 3*(4), 7–14.

Royse, C. F., Soeding, P. F., & Royse, A. G. (2007). High thoracic epidural analgesia for cardiac surgery: An audit of 874 cases. *Anaesthesia and Intensive Care, 35*(3), 374–377.

Rozans, M., Dreisbach, A., Lertora, J. J. L., et al. (2002). Palliative uses of methylphenidate in patients with cancer: A review. *Journal of Clinical Oncology, 20*(1), 335–339.

Rozen, D., & DeGaetano, N. P. (2006). Perioperative management of opioid-tolerant chronic pain patients. *Journal of Opioid Management, 2*(6), 353–363.

Rudich, Z., Peng, P., Dunn, E., et al. (2004). Stability of clonidine in clonidine-hydromorphone mixture from implanted intrathecal infusion pumps in chronic pain patients. *Journal of Pain and Symptom Management, 28*(6), 599–602.

Rudin, A., Lundberg, J. F., Hammarlund-Udenaes, M., et al. (2007). Morphine metabolism after major liver surgery. *Anesthesia and Analgesia, 104*(6), 1409–1414.

Rudy, A. C., Coda, B. A., Archer, S. M., et al. (2004). A multiple-dose phase I study of intranasal hydromorphone hydrochloride in healthy volunteers. *Anesthesia and Analgesia, 99*(5), 1379–1386.

Ruiz, J. R., Kee, S. S., Frenzel, J. C., et al. (2010). The effect of an anatomically classified procedure on antiemetic administration in the postanesthesia care unit. *Anesthesia and Analgesia, 110*(2), 403–409.

Rusch, D., Arndt, C., Martin, H., et al. (2007). The addition of dexamethasone to dolasetron or haloperidol for treatment of established postoperative nausea and vomiting. *Anaesthesia, 62*(8), 810–817.

Russell, A. W., Owen, H., Ilsley, A. H., et al. (1996). Background infusion with patient-controlled analgesia: Effect on postoperative oxyhaemoglobin saturation and pain control. *Anaesthesia and Intensive Care, 21*(2), 174–179.

Saarialho-Kere, U., Julkunen, H., Mattila, M. J., et al. (1988). Psychomotor performance of patients with rheumatoid arthritis: Cross-over comparison of dextropropoxyphene, dextropropoxyphen plus amitriptyline, indomethacin, and placebo. *Pharmacology & Toxicology, 63*(4), 286–292.

Sabatowski, R., Schwalen, S., Rettig, K., et al. (2003). Driving ability under long-term treatment with transdermal fentanyl. *Journal of Pain and Symptom Management, 25*(1), 38–47.

Saclarides, T. J. (2006). Current choices—good or bad—for the proactive management of postoperative ileus: A surgeon's view. *Journal of Perianesthesia Nursing, 21*(Suppl. 2A), S7–S15.

Sah, N., Ramesh, V., Kaul, B., et al. (2009). Transdermal scopolamine patch in addition to ondansetron for postoperative nausea and vomiting prophylaxis in patients undergoing ambulatory cosmetic surgery. *Journal of Clinical Anesthesia, 21*(4), 249–252.

Sakai, T., Fukano, T., & Sumikawa, K. (2001). IV butorphanol reduces analgesia but not pruritus or nausea associated with intrathecal morphine. *Canadian Journal of Anesthesia, 48*(8), 831–832.

Sakuramoto, C., Kanai, I., Matoba, M., et al. (1996). Treatment of postoperative pain with thoracic epidural morphine in oral malignant tumor patients. *The Clinical Journal of Pain*, 12(2), 142–144.

Salisbury, E. M., Game, D. S., Al-Shakarchi, I., et al. (2009). Changing practice to improve pain control for renal patients. *Postgraduate Medical Journal*, 85(1), 30–33.

Salmon, P., & Hall, G. M. (2001). PCA: Patient-controlled analgesia or politically correct analgesia? (Editorial). *British Journal of Anaesthesia*, 87(6), 815–818.

Salzman, R. T., Roberts, M. S., & Wild, J. (1999). Can a controlled-release oral dose form of oxycodone be used as readily as an immediate-release form for the purpose of titrating to stable pain control? *Journal of Pain and Symptom Management*, 18(4), 271–279.

Sanchez-Ledesma, M. J., Lopez-Olaondo, L., Pueyo, F. J., et al. (2002). A comparison of three antiemetic combinations for prevention of postoperative nausea and vomiting. *Anesthesia and Analgesia*, 95(6), 1590–1595.

Sanchez del Aguila, M. J., Jones, M. F., & Vohra, A. (2003). Premixed solutions of diamorphine in ropivacaine for epidural anaesthesia: A study on their long-term stability. *British Journal of Anaesthesia*, 90(2), 179–182.

Sarbu, A., Radulescu, F., Robertson, S., et al. (2007). 425: Onset of analgesic effect and plasma levels of a controlled release tramadol (tramadol contramid® once-a-day) 200 mg in patients with acute low back pain. *Regional Anesthesia and Pain Medicine*, 32(5 Supp. 1), 163.

Sarhill, N., Davis, M. P., Walsh, D., et al. (2001). Methadone-induced myoclonus in advanced cancer. *The American Journal of Hospice & Palliative Care*, 18(1), 51–53.

Sarhill, N., Walsh, D., & Nelson, K. A. (2001). Hydromorphone: Pharmacology and clinical applications in cancer patients. *Supportive Care in Cancer*, 9(2), 84–96.

Sasson, M., & Shvartzman, P. (2006). Fentanyl patch sufficient analgesia for only one day. (Letter). *Journal of Pain and Symptom Management*, 31(5), 389–390.

Sathyan, G., Sivakumar, K., Thipphawong, J., et al. (2008). Pharmacokinetic profile of 24-hour controlled-release OROS formulation of hydromorphone in the presence of alcohol. *Current Medical Research and Opinion*, 24(1), 297–305.

Sathyan, G., Xu, E., Thipphawong, J., et al. (2007a). Pharmacokinetic investigation of dose proportionality with a 24-hour controlled-release formulation of hydromorphone. *BMC Clinical Pharmacology*, 7, 3.

Sathyan, G., Xu, E., Thipphawong, J., et al. (2007b). Pharmacokinetic profile of a 24-hour controlled-release OROS formulation of hydromorphone in the presence and absence of food. *BMC Clinical Pharmacology*, 7, 2.

Saunders, T. A., & Glass, P. S. A. (2002). A trial of labor for remifentanil (editorial). *Anesthesia and Analgesia*, 94(4), 771–773.

Savage, S. R. (2002). Assessment for addiction in pain-treatment settings. *The Clinical Journal of Pain*, 18, S28–S38.

Savage, S. R., & Schofferman, J. (1995). Pharmacological therapies of pain in drug and alcohol addictions. In N. Miller, & M. Gold (Eds.), *Pharmacological therapies for drug and alcohol addictions* (pp. 373–409). New York: Dekker.

Sawynok, J. (2003). Topically and peripherally acting analgesics. *Pharmacological Reviews*, 55(1), 1–20.

Schenk, M. R., Putzier, M., Kugler, B., et al. (2006). Postoperative analgesia after major spine surgery: Patient-controlled epidural analgesia versus patient-controlled intravenous analgesia. *Anesthesia and Analgesia*, 103(5), 1311–1317.

Schmid, R., Koren, G., Klein, J., et al. (2002). The stability of a ketamine-morphine solution. *Anesthesia and Analgesia*, 94(4), 898–900.

Schmittner, J., & Krantz, M. J. (2006). High-dose methadone and QTc prolongation: Strategies to optimize safety. *Journal of Opioid Management*, 2(1), 49–55.

Schricker, T., Meterissian, S., Wykes, L., et al. (2004). Postoperative protein sparing with epidural analgesia and hypocaloric dextrose. *Annals of Surgery*, 240(5), 916–921.

Schug, S. A. (2006). The role of COX-2 inhibitors in the treatment of postoperative pain. *Journal of Cardiovascular Pharmacology*, 47(Suppl. 1), S82–S86.

Schug, S. A., & Manopas, A. (2007). Update on the role of non-opioids for postoperative pain treatment. *Best Practice & Research. Clinical Anaesthesiology*, 21(1), 15–30.

Schug, S. A., Saunders, D., Kurowski, I., et al. (2006). Neuraxial drug administration: A review of treatment options for anaesthesia and analgesia. *CNS Drugs*, 20(11), 917–933.

Schultz, T. K. (Eds.), *Principles of addiction medicine* (2nd ed., pp. 919–944). Chevy Chase, MD: American Society of Addiction Medicine, Inc.

Schumacher, K. L., West, C., Dodd, M., et al. (2002). Pain management autobiographies and reluctance to use opioids for cancer pain management. *Cancer Nursing*, 25(2), 125–133.

Schuster, R., Grewal, N., Greaney, G. C., et al. (2006). Gum chewing reduces ileus after elective open sigmoid colectomy. *Archives of Surgery*, 141(2), 174–176.

Schuurmans, J. M., Shortridge-Baggett, L. M., & Duursma, S. A. (2003). The Delirium Observation Screening Scale: A screening instrument for delirium. *Research and Theory for Nursing Practice*, 17(1), 31–50.

Schuurmans, M. J., Deschamps, P. I., Markham, S. W., et al. (2003). The measurement of delirium: A review of scales. *Research and Theory for Nursing Practice*, 17(3), 207–224.

Schwartz, A. E., Matteo, R. S., Ornstein, E., et al. (1991). Pharmacokinetics of sufentanil in obese patients. *Anesthesia and Analgesia*, 73(6), 790–793.

Schwarzkopf, K. R. G., Hoff, H., Hartmann, M., et al. (2001). A comparison between meperidine, clonidine and urapidil in the treatment of postanesthetic shivering. *Anesthesia and Analgesia*, 92(1), 257–260.

Schwenk, W., Haase, O., Neudecker, J. J., et al. (2005). Short term benefits for laparoscopic colorectal resection. *Cochrane Database of Systematic Reviews (Online)*, (3), CD003145.

Scott, D. G. (2005). In the days of patients' choice, why is the patient being ignored? *Lancet*, 366(9482), 287–288.

Scott, L. J., & Perry, C. M. (2000). Tramadol: A review of its use in perioperative pain. *Drugs*, 60(1), 139–176.

Scuderi, P. E. (2010). PRO: Anatomical classification of surgical procedures improves our understanding of the mechanisms of postoperative nausea and vomiting. (Editorial). *Anesthesia and Analgesia*, 110(2), 410–411.

Scuderi, P. E., James, R. L., Harris, L., et al. (2000). Multimodal antiemetic management prevents early postoperative vomiting after outpatient laparoscopy. *Anesthesia and Analgesia*, 91(6), 1408–1414.

Seifert, C. F., & Kennedy, S. (2004). Meperidine is alive and well in the new millennium: Evaluation of meperidine usage patterns and frequency of adverse drug reactions. *Pharmacotherapy*, 24(6), 776–783.

Sekine, R., Obens, E.A.M.T., Coyle, N., et al. (2007). The successful use of parenteral methadone in a patient with a prolonged QTc interval. *Journal of Pain and Symptom Management, 34*(5), 566–569.

Semple, T. J., Macintyre, P. E., & Hooper, M. (1993). Parenteral codeine. *Anaesthesia, 48*(6), 539–540.

Servin, F. S., & Billard, V. (2008). Remifentanil and other opioids. *Handbook of Experimental Pharmacology*, (182), 283–311.

Sessler, C. N., Gosnell, M. S., Grap, M. J., et al. (2002). The Richmond Agitation-Sedation Scale. Validity and reliability in adult intensive care unit patients. *American Journal of Respiratory and Critical Care Medicine, 166*(10), 1338–1344.

Sevarino, F. B., Pizarro, C. W., & Sinatra, R. (2000). Sterility of epidural solutions—Recommendations for cost-effective use. *Regional Anesthesia and Pain Medicine, 25*(4), 368–371.

Shaheen, P. E., Walsh, D., Lasheen, W., et al. (2009). Opioid equianalgesic tables: Are they all equally dangerous? *Journal of Pain and Symptom Management, 38*(3), 409–417.

Shaiova, L., Berger, A., Blinderman, C. D., et al. (2008). Consensus guideline on parenteral methadone use in pain and palliative care. *Palliative & Supportive Care, 6*(2), 165–176.

Shaiova, L., & Wallenstein, D. (2004). Outpatient management of sickle cell pain with chronic opioid pharmacotherapy. *Journal of the National Medical Association, 96*(7), 984–986.

Shane, R. (2009). Risk evaluation and mitigation strategies: Impact on patients, health care providers, and health systems. *Am J Health Syst Pharm, 66*(24 Suppl 7), S6–S12.

Sharke, C., Geisslinger, G., & Lotsch, J. (2005). Is morphine-3-glucuronide of therapeutic relevance? *Pain, 116*(3), 177–180.

Sharma, P. T., Sieber, F. E., Zakriya, K. J., et al. (2005). Recovery room delirium predicts postoperative delirium after hip-fracture repair. *Anesthesia and Analgesia, 101*(4), 1215–1220.

Sheen, M. J., Ho, S. T., Lee, C. H., et al. (2008). Preoperative gabapentin prevents intrathecal morphine-induced pruritus after orthopedic surgery. *Anesthesia and Analgesia, 106*(6), 1868–1872.

Shelley, K., & Paech, M. J. (2008). The clinical applications of intranasal opioids. *Current Drug Delivery, 5*(1), 55–58.

Sherman, B., Enu, I., & Sinatra, R. S. (2009). Patient-controlled analgesia devices and analgesic infusion pumps. In R. S. Sinatra, O. A. de Leon-Casasola, & B. Ginsberg, et al. (Eds.), *Acute pain management*. Cambridge, NY: Cambridge University Press.

Sheth, H. S., Verrico, M. M., Skledar, S. J., et al. (2005). Promethazine adverse events after implementation of a medication shortage interchange. *The Annals of Pharmacotherapy, 39*(2), 255–261.

Shibutani, K., Inchiosa, M. A., Jr., Sawada, K., et al. (2004). Accuracy of pharmacokinetic models for predicting plasma fentanyl concentrations in lean and obese surgical patients: Derivation of dosing weight ("pharmacokinetic mass"). *Anesthesiology, 101*(3), 603–613.

Shibutani, K., Inchiosa, M. A., Jr., Sawada, K., et al. (2005). Pharmacokinetic mass of fentanyl for postoperative analgesia in lean and obese patients. *British Journal of Anaesthesia, 95*(3), 377–383.

Shirk, M. B., Donahue, K. R., & Shirvani, J. (2006). Unlabeled uses of nebulized medications. *American Journal of Health-System Pharmacy: AJHP, 63*(18), 1704–1716.

Siddiqi, N., Holt, R., Britton, A. M., et al. (2007). Interventions for preventing delirium in hospitalised patients. *Cochrane Database of Systematic Reviews (Online)*, (2), CD005563.

Sidebotham, D., Dijkhuizen, M. R. J., & Schug, S. A. (1997). The safety and utilization of patient-controlled analgesia. *Journal of Pain and Symptom Management, 14*(4), 202–209.

Silvasti, M., & Pitkanen, M. (2001). Patient-controlled epidural analgesia versus continuous epidural analgesia after total knee arthroplasty. *Acta Anaesthesiologica Scandinavica, 45*(4), 471–476.

Simonnet, G. (2009). Acute tolerance to opioids: Methodological, theoretical and clinical implications. *Pain, 142*(1–2), 3–4.

Simopoulos, T. T., Smith, H. S., Peeters-Asdourian, C., et al. (2002). Use of meperidine in patient-controlled analgesia and the development of a normeperidine toxic reaction. *Archives of Surgery, 137*(1), 84–88.

Simpson, K. H., & Jones, I. (2008). Intrathecal drug delivery for the management of cancer and noncancer pain. *Journal of Opioid Management, 4*(5), 293–304.

Simpson, R. S., Macintyre, P. E., Shaw, D., et al. (2000). Epidural catheter tip cultures: Results of a 4-year audit and implications for clinical practice. *Regional Anesthesia and Pain Medicine, 25*(4), 360–367.

Sinatra, R. S. (2006). Peripherally acting mu-opioid-receptor antagonists and the connection between postoperative ileus and pain management: The anesthesiologists's view and beyond. *Journal of Perianesthesia Nursing, 21*(Suppl. 2A), S16–S23.

Sinatra, R. S. (2009). Oral and parenteral opioid analgesics for acute pain management. In R. S. Sinatra, O. A. de Leon-Casasola, B. Ginsberg, & E. R. Viscusi (Eds.), *Acute pain management* (pp. 188–203). Cambridge, New York: Cambridge University Press.

Singh, H., Bossard, R. F., White, P. F., et al. (1997). Effects of ketorolac versus bupivacaine coadministration during patient-controlled hydromorphone epidural analgesia after thoractotomy procedures. *Anesthesia and Analgesia, 84*(3), 564–569.

Singh, S., Sleeper, R. B., & Seifert, C. F. (2007). Propoxyphene prescribing among populations older and younger than age 65 in a tertiary care hospital. *The Consultant Pharmacist: The Journal of the American Society of Consultant Pharmacists, 22*(2), 141–148.

Singla, N., Pong, A., Newman, K., et al. (2005). Combination oxycodone 5mg/ibuprofen 400 mg for the treatment of pain after abdominal or pelvic surgery in women: A randomized, double-blind, placebo- and active-controlled parallel-group study. *Clinical Therapeutics, 27*(1), 45–57.

Sittl, R., Likar, R., & Nautrup, B. P. (2005). Equipotent doses of transdermal fentanyl and transdermal buprenorphine in patients with cancer and noncancer pain: Results of a retrospective cohort study. *Clinical Therapeutics, 27*(2), 225–237.

Skaer, T. L. (2004). Practice guidelines for transdermal opioids in malignant pain. *Drugs, 64*(23), 2629–2638.

Skaer, T. L. (2006). Transdermal opioids for cancer pain. *Health and Quality of Life Outcomes, 31*(4), 24.

Slatkin, N., Hill, W., Finn, A. (2008). The safety of BEMA (BioErodible MucoAdhesive) fentanyl use for breakthrough pain (BTP) in cancer patients. *The Journal of Pain, 9*(4 Suppl. 1), P23.

Slatkin, N., Rhiner, M., & Bolton, T. M. (2001). Donepezil in the treatment of opioid-induced sedation: Report of six cases. *Journal of Pain and Symptom Management, 21*(5), 425–438.

Slatkin, N., Tormo, V., & Ahdieh, H. (2004). *Neuropathic pain treated with oxymorphone.* Paper presented at Neuropathic Pain: Changing Paradigms in Diagnosis and Treatment. An International Congress of NeuPSIG, Madrid, Spain, May 13–16.

Slatkin, N. E., Xie, F., Messina, J., et al. (2007). Fentanyl buccal tablet for relief of breakthrough pain in opioid-tolerant patients with cancer-related chronic pain. *The Journal of Supportive Oncology, 5*(7), 327–334.

Slinger, P., Shennib, H., & Wilson, S. (1995). Postthoracotomy pulmonary function: A comparison of epidural versus intravenous meperidine infusions. *Journal of Cardiothoracic and Vascular Anesthesia, 9*(2), 128–134.

Sloan, P. A., & Barkin, R. L. (2008). Oxymorphone and oxymorphone extended release: A pharmacotherapeutic review. *Journal of Opioid Management, 4*(3), 131–144.

Sloan, P., & Harmann, S. (2006). Ultra-low-dose opioid antagonists to enhance opioid analgesia. *Journal of Opioid Management, 2*(5), 295–304.

Sloan, P., Slatkin, N., & Ahdieh, H. (2005). Effectiveness and safety of oral extended-release oxymorphone for the treatment of cancer pain: A pilot study. *Supportive Care in Cancer, 13*(1), 57–65.

Smith, H. S. (2009). Clinical pharmacology of oxymorphone. *Pain Medicine (Malden, Mass.), 10*(Suppl. 1), S3–S10.

Smith, M. T. (2000). Neuroexcitatory effects of morphine and hydromorphone: Evidence implicating the 3-glucuronide metabolites. *Clinical and Experimental Pharmacology & Physiology, 27*(7), 524–528.

Smith, M. T., & South, S. M. (2001). The role of morphine-6-glucuronide (M6G) in pain control. *Pain Rev, 8*(2), 171–191.

Smith, T. W., Binning, A. R., & Dahan, A. (2009). Efficacy and safety of morphine-6-glucuronide (M6G) for postoperative pain relief: A randomized, double-blind study. *European Journal of Pain (London, England), 13*(2), 293–299.

Smith, W. C. S., Bourne, D., Squair, J., et al. (1999). A retrospective cohort study of post mastectomy pain syndrome. *Pain, 83*(1), 91–95.

Smythe, M. A., Zak, M. B., & O'Donnell, M. P. (1996). Patient-controlled analgesia versus patient-controlled analgesia plus continuous infusion after hip replacement surgery. *The Annals of Pharmacotherapy, 30*(3), 224–227.

Soares, L. G. (2005). Methadone for cancer pain: What have we learned from clinical studies? *The American Journal of Hospice & Palliative Care, 22*(3), 223–227.

Soares, L., Martins, M., & Uchoa, R. (2003). Intravenous fentanyl for cancer pain: A "fast titration" protocol for the emergency room. *Journal of Pain and Symptom Management, 26*(3), 876–881.

Soltesz, S., Biedler, A., Silomon, M., et al. (2001). Recovery after remifentanil and sufentanil for analgesia and sedation of mechanically ventilated patients after trauma or major surgery. *British Journal of Anaesthesia, 86*(6), 763–768.

Somogyi, A. A., Barratt, D. T., & Coller, J. K. (2007). Pharmacogenetics of opioids. *Clinical Pharmacology and Therapeutics, 81*(3), 429–444.

South, S. M., & Smith, M. T. (2001). Analgesic tolerance to opioids. *Pain. Clinical Updates. IASP, 9*(5), 1–9.

Spiegel, B. (2001). Meperidine or morphine in acute pancreatitis? (Letter). *American Family Physician, 64*(2), 219.

Staats, P. S., Markowitz, J., & Schein, J. (2004). Incidence of constipation associated with long-acting opioid therapy: A comparative study. *Southern Medical Journal, 97*(2), 129–134.

Stamenkovic, D. M., Geric, V., Slavkovic, Z., et al. (2008). Combined spinal-epidural analgesia vs. intermittent bolus epidural analgesia for pain relief after major abdominal surgery. A prospective, randomised, double blind clinical trial. *Intrnational Journal of Clinical Practice, 62*(2), 255–262.

Stanik-Hutt, J. A., Soeken, K. L., Belcher, A. E., et al. (2001). Pain experiences of traumatically injured patients in a critical care setting. *American Journal of Critical Care, 10*(4), 252–259.

Stemp, L. I., & Ramsay, M. (2005). Oxygen may mask hypoventilation—patient breathing must be ensured. (Letter). *APSF Newsletter, 20*, (Winter), 80.

Stevens, B. (1999). Pain in infants. In M. McCaffery, & C. Pasero (Eds.), *Pain: Clinical manual* (2nd ed., pp. 626–673). St. Louis: Mosby.

Stevens, R. A., & Ghazi, S. M (2000). *Routes of opioid analgesic therapy in the management of cancer pain.* Available at www.medscape.com/viewarticle/408974. Accessed 1/9/09.

Stiller, C. O., Lundblad, H., Weidenhielm, L., et al. (2007). The addition of tramadol to morphine via patient-controlled analgesia does not lead to better post-operative pain relief after total knee arthroplasty. *Acta Anaesthesiologica Scandinavica, 51*(3), 322–330.

Stoker, D. G., Reber, K. R., Waltzman, L. S., et al. (2008). Analgesic efficacy and safety of morphine-chitosan nasal solution in patients with moderate to severe pain following orthopedic surgery. *Pain Medicine (Malden, Mass.), 9*(1), 3–12.

St. Onge, S., Fugere, F., & Girard, M. (1997). Bupivacaine decreases epidural meperidine requirements after abdominal surgery. *Canadian Journal of Anesthesia, 44*(4), 360–366.

Strassels, S. A., McNicol, E., & Suleman, R. (2008). Pharmacotherapy of pain in older adults. *Clinics in Geriatric Medicine, 24*(2), 275–298.

Strichartz, G. R. (1998). Neural phyisology and local anesthetic action. In M. J. Cousins, & P. O. Bridenbaugh (Eds.), *Neural blockade in clinical anesthesia and management of pain* (pp. 35–54). Philadelphia: Lippincott.

Strichartz, G. R., & Berde, C. B. (2005). Local anesthetics. In Miller, R. D. (Ed.), *Miller's anesthesia.* (6th ed., vol. 2, pp. 573–603). St. Louis: Elsevier.

Striebel, H. W., Scheitza, W., Philippi, W., et al. (1998). Quantifying oral analgesic consumption using a novel method and comparison with patient-controlled intravenous analgesic consumption. *Anesthesia and Analgesia, 86*(5), 1051–1053.

Strong, W. E. (1991). Epidural abscess associated with epidural catheterization: A rare event? Report of two cases with markedly delayed presentation. (Letter). *Anesthesiology, 74*(5), 942–946.

Sudheer, P. S., Logan, C., Terblanche, B., et al. (2007). Comparison of the analgesic efficacy and respiratory effects of morphine, tramadol and codeine after craniotomy. *Anaesthesia, 62*(6), 555–560.

Sudlow, C. L. M., & Warlow, C. C. (2001). Epidural blood patching for preventing and treating post-dural puncture headache. *Cochrane Database of Systematic Reviews (Online), (2),* CD001791.

Sumida, S., Lesley, M. R., Hanna, M. N., et al. (2009). Meta-analysis of the effect of extended-release epidural morphine versus intravenous patient-controlled analgesia on respiratory depression. *Journal of Opioid Management, 5*(5), 301–312.

Sun, T., Sacan, O., White, P. F., et al. (2008). Perioperative versus postoperative celecoxib on patient outcomes after major plastic surgery procedures. *Anesthesia and Analgesia, 106*(3), 950–958.

SUPPORT Principle Investigators. (1995). A controlled trial to improve care for seriously ill hospitalized patients. *JAMA: The Journal of the American Medical Association, 274*(20), 1591–1598.

Susce, M. T., Murray-Carmichael, E., & de Leon, J. (2006). Response to hydrocodone, codeine and oxycodone in a CYP2D6 poor metabolizer. *Progress in Neuro-Psychopharmacology & Biological Psychiatry, 30*(7), 1356–1358.

Sutters, K. A., Miaskowski, C., Holdridge-Zeuner, D., et al. (2004). A randomized clinical trial of the effectiveness of a scheduled oral analgesic dosing regimen for the management of postoperative pain in children following tonsillectomy. *Pain, 110*(1–2), 49–55.

Sutters, K. A., Miaskowski, C., Holdridge-Zeuner, D., et al. (2005). Time-contingent dosing of an opioid analgesic after tonsillectomy does not increase moderate-to-severe side effects in children. *Pain Management Nursing, 6*(2), 49–57.

Swarm, R. A., Karanikolas, M., & Cousins, M. J. (2004). In D. Doyle, G. Hanks, N. I. Cherny, & K. Calman (Eds.), *Oxford textbook of palliative medicine.* (3rd ed., pp. 378–396). New York: Oxford Press.

Sykes, N., & Thorns, A. (2003a). Sedative use in the last week of life and the implications for end-of-life decision making. *Archives of Internal Medicine, 163*(93), 341–344.

Sykes, N., & Thorns, A. (2003b). The use of opioids and sedatives at end of life. *The Lancet Oncology, 4*(5), 312–318.

Szarvas, S., Chellapuri, R. S., Harmon, D. C., et al. (2003). A comparison of dexamethasone, ondansetron, and dexamethasone plus ondansetron as prophylactic antiemetic and antipruritic therapy in patients receiving intrathecal morphine for major orthopedic surgery. *Anesthesia and Analgesia, 97*(1), 259–263.

Taillefer, M. C., Carrier, M., Belisle, S., et al. (2006). Prevalence, characteristics, and predictors of chronic nonanginal postoperative pain after a cardiac operation: A cross-sectional study. *The Journal of Thoracic and Cardiovascular Surgery, 1131*(6), 1274–1280.

Tang, R., Evans, H., Chaput, A., et al. (2009). Multimodal analgesia for hip arthroplasty. *Orthopedic Clinics of North America, 40*(3), 377–387.

Tarcatu, D., Tamasdan, C., Moryl, N., et al. (2007). Are we still scratching the surface? A case of intractable pruritus following systemic opioid analgesia. *Journal of Opioid Management, 3*(3), 167–170.

Tassinari, D., Sartori, S., Tamburini, E., et al. (2008). Adverse effects of transdermal opiates treating moderate-severe cancer pain in comparison to long-acting morphine: A meta-analysis and systematic review of the literature. *Journal of Palliative Medicine, 11*(3), 492–501.

Taylor, D. R. (2005). The pharmacology of fentanyl and its impact on the management of pain. *Medscape Neurology Neurosurgery, 7*(2). http://www.medscape.com/viewarticle/518441. Accessed December 21, 2005.

Taylor, D. R. (2007). Fentanyl buccal tablet: Rapid relief from breakthrough pain. *Expert Opinion on Pharmacotherapy, 8*(17), 3043–3051.

Taylor, D. R., Webster, L. R., Chun, S. Y., et al. (2007). Impact of breakthrough pain on quality of life in patients with chronic, noncancer pain: Patient perceptions and effect of treatment with oral transmucosal fentanyl citrate (OTFC, Actiq). *Pain Medicine (Malden, Mass.), 8*(3), 281–288.

Taylor, S., Kirton, O. C., Staff, I., et al. (2005). Postoperative day one: A high risk period for respiratory events. *American Journal of Surgery, 190*(5), 752–756.

Taylor, S., Voytovich, A. E., & Kozol, R. A. (2003). Has the pendulum swung too far in postoperative pain control? *American Journal of Surgery, 186*(5), 472–475.

Tennant, F., & Hermann, L. (2002). Self-treatment with oral transmucosal fentanyl citrate to prevent emergency room visits for pain crises: Patient self-reports of efficacy and utility. *Journal of Pain & Palliative Care Pharmacotherapy, 16*(3), 37–44.

Teno, J. M., Clarridge, B. R., Casey, V., et al. (2004). Family perspectives on end-of-life care at the last place of care. *JAMA: The Journal of the American Medical Association, 291*(1), 88–93.

Teoh, W. H., Thomas, E., & Tan, H. M. (2006). Ultra-low dose combined spinal-epidural anesthesia with intrathecal bupivacaine 3.75,g fpr cesarean delivery. *International Journal of Obstetric Anesthesia, 15*(4), 273–278.

Terlinden, R., Ossig, J., Fliegert, F., et al. (2007). Absorption, metabolism, and excretion of 14C-labeled tapentadol HCL in healthy male subjects. *European Journal of Drug Metabolism and Pharmacokinetics, 32*(2), 163–169.

Thakore, B., D'Mello, J., Saksena, S., et al. (2009). Comparison of fentanyl and butorphanol for postoperative pain relief with intravenous patient controlled analgesia. *Acute Pain, 11*(3–4), 93–99.

Thipphawong, J. B., Babul, N., Morishige, R. J., et al. (2003). Analgesic efficacy of inhaled morphine in patients after bunionectomy surgery. *Anesthesiology, 99*(3), 693–700.

Thomas, J. (2008). Opioid-induced bowel dysfunction. *Journal of Pain and Symptom Management, 35*(1), 103–113.

Thomas, J., Karver, S., Cooney, G. A., et al. (2008). Methylnaltrexone for opioid-induced constipation in advanced illness. *The New England Journal of Medicine, 358*(22), 2332–2343.

Thomas, Z., & Bruera, E. (1995). Use of methadone in a highly tolerant patient receiving parenteral hydromorphone. *Journal of Pain and Symptom Management, 10*(4), 315–317.

Thompson, D. R. (2001). Narcotic analgesic effects on the sphincter of Oddi: A review of the data and therapeutic implications in treating pancreatitis. *The American Journal of Gastroenterology, 96*(4), 1266–1272.

Thorns, A., & Sykes, N. (2000). Opioid use in last week of life and implications for end-of-life decision making. (Research Letter). *Lancet, 356*(9227), 398–399.

Thune, A., Baker, R. A., Saccone, G. T. P., et al. (1990). Differing effects of pethidine and morphine on human sphincter of Oddi motility. *The British Journal of Surgery, 77*(9), 992–995.

Thwaites, D., McCann, S., & Broderick, P. (2004). Hydromorphone neuroexcitation. *Journal of Palliative Medicine, 7*(4), 545–550.

Timmers, J., Kalisvaart, K., Schuurmans, M., et al. (2004). A review of delirium scales. *Tijdschrift Voor Gerontologie en Geriatrie, 35*(1), 5–14.

Titler, M. G., Herr, K., Schilling, M. L., et al. (2003). Acute pain treatment for older adults hospitalized with hip fracture: Current nursing practices and perceived barriers. *Applied Nursing Research: ANR, 16*(4), 211–217.

Todd, J., Rees, E., Gwilliam, B., et al. (2002). An assessment of the efficacy and tolerability of a 'double dose' of normal-release morphine sulphate at bed-time. *Palliative Medicine, 16*(6), 507–512.

Toombs, J. D. (2008). Oral methadone dosing for chronic pain: A practitioner's guide. *Pain Treatment Topics.* Available at http://pain-topics.org/pdf/OralMethadoneDosing.pdf. Accessed July 31, 2009.

Trafton, J. A., & Ramani, A. (2009). Methadone: A new old drug with promises and pitfalls. *Current Pain and Headache Reports, 13*(1), 24–30.

Traynor, K. (2009). *Close vote by FDA advisers favors propoxyphene withdrawal.* http://www.ashp.org/import/news/HealthSystemPharmacyNews/newsarticle.aspx?id=3037. Accessed June 22, 2009.

Treece, P. D., Engelberg, R. A., Crowley, L., et al. (2004). Evaluation of a standardized order form for the withdrawal of life support in the intensive care unit. *Critical Care Medicine, 32*(5), 1141–1148.

Trissel, A. L., & Pham, L. (2002). Physical and chemical stability of low and high concentrations of morphine sulfate and bupivacaine hydrochloride packaged in plastic syringes. *Int J Pharm Compounding, 6*(1), 70–73.

Trissel, A. L., Xu, Q. A., & Pham, L. (2002). Physical and chemical stability of low and high concentrations of morphine sulfate with clonidine hydrochloride packaged in plastic syringes. *Int J Pharm Compounding, 6*(1), 66–69.

Troster, A., Sittl, R., Singler, B., et al. (2006). Modulation of remifentanil-induced analgesia and postinfusion hyperalgesia by paracoxib in humans. *Anesthesiology, 105,* 1016–1023.

Tsui, S. L., Irwin, M. G., Wong, C. M., et al. (1997). An audit of the safety of an acute pain service. *Anaesthesia, 52*(11), 1042–1071.

Tu, Y. H., Stiles, L., & Allen, L. V. (1990). Stability of fentanyl citrate and bupivacaine hydrochloride in portable pump reservoirs. *American Journal of Hospital Pharmacy, 47*(9), 2037–2039.

Tuca, A., Roca, R., Sala, C., et al. (2009). Efficacy of granisetron in the antiemetic control of nonsurgical intestinal obstruction in advanced cancer: A phase II clinical trial. *Journal of Pain and Symptom Management, 37*(2), 259–270.

Turnbull, D. K., & Shepherd, D. B. (2003). Post-dural puncture headache: Pathogenesis, prevention and treatment. *British Journal of Anaesthesia, 91*(5), 718–729.

Turner, J. A., Sears, J. M., & Loeser, J. D. (2007). Programmable intrathecal opioid delivery systems for chronic noncancer pain: A systematic review of effectiveness and complications. *The Clinical Journal of Pain, 23*(2), 180–195.

Tveita, T., Thoner, J., Klepstad, P., et al. (2008). A controlled comparison between single doses of intravenous and intramuscular morphine with respect to analgesic effects and patient safety. *Acta Anaesthesiologica Scandinavica, 52*(7), 920–925.

Twycross, R., & Wilcock, A. (Eds.). (2007). *Hospice and palliative care formulary USA.* Nottingham, UK: Palliativedrugs.com.

Tzschentke, T. M., De Vry, J., Terlinden, R., et al. (2006). Tapentadol hydrochloride. *Drugs of the Future, 31*(12), 1053–1061.

Ungar, J. R., Brandes, D., Reinoehi, B. M., et al. (1999). Pain management. In G. R. Schwartz (Ed.), *Principles and practice of emergency medicine* (4th ed.). Baltimore, MD: Williams, Wilkins.

United States Food and Drug Administration (FDA). (2005). *Safety warnings regarding use of fentanyl transdermal (skin) patches. FDA Public Health Advisory.* Available at http://www.fda.gov/CDER/DRUG/advisory/fentanyl.htm. Accessed April 12, 2008.

United States Food and Drug Administration (FDA). (2006). *FDA Alert: Death, narcotic overdose, and serious cardiac arrhythmias.* Available at http://www.fda.gov/downloads/Drugs/DrugSafety/PostmarketDrugSafetyInformationforPatientsandProviders/UCM142839.pdf. Accessed July 31 2009.

United States Food and Drug Administration (FDA). (2007a). *Use of codeine by some breastfeeding mothers may lead to life-threatening side effects in nursing babies. FDA Public Health Advisory.* Available at http://www.fda.gov/CDER/Drug/advisory/codeine.htm. Accessed January 9, 2008.

United States Food and Drug Administration (FDA). (2007b). *FDA warns of potential serious side effects with breakthrough cancer pain drug.* Available at http://www.fda.gov/bbs/topics/NEWS/2007/NEW01711.html. Accessed April 13, 2007.

United States Food and Drug Administration (FDA). (2007c). *Important information for the safe use of fentanyl transdermal system (patch). FDA Public Health Advisory.* Available at http://www.fda.gov/CDER/DRUG/advisory/fentanyl_2007.htm. Accessed Apil 12, 2008.

United States Food and Drug Administration (FDA). (2009a). *Questions and answers about Onsolis (fentanyl buccal soluble film).* Available at http://www.fda.gov/Drugs/DrugSafety/PostmarketDrugSafetyInformationforPatientsandProviders/ucm172039.htm. Accessed July 18, 2009.

United States Food and Drug Administration (FDA). (2009b). *Acetaminophen information.* Available at http://www.fda.gov/Drugs/DrugSafety/InformationbyDrugClass/ucm165107.htm. http://www.fda.gov/ForConsumers/ConsumerUpdates/ucm168830.htm. Accessed August 30, 2009.

United States Food and Drug Administration (FDA). (2009c). *Promethazine hydrochloride injection.* Available at http://www.fda.gov/Safety/MedWatch/SafetyInformation/SafetyAlertsforHumanMedicalProducts/ucm182500.htm. Accessed September 20, 2009.

United States Food and Drug Administration. (2009d). Guidance for industry: Format and content of proposed Risk Evaluation and Mitigation Strategies (REMS), REMS assessments, and proposed REMS modifications. Available at http://www.fda.gov/downloads/Drugs/GuidanceComplianceRegulatoryIlnformation/Guidances/UCM184128.pdf. Accessed March 14, 2010.

United States Food and Drug Administration. (2010). Approved Risk Evaluation and Mitigation Strategies (REMS). Available at http: //www. fda. gov/Drugs/DrugSafety/PostmarketDrugSafetyInformationforPatientsandProviders/ucm111350.htm. Accessed March 16, 2010.

United States Pharmacopeia. (2004). Patient-controlled analgesia pumps. *USP Quality Review, 81,* 1–3.

University of Arizona Center for Education and Research on Therapeutics. *Drugs with risk of torsade de pointes.* Available at http://www.azcert.org/medical-pros/drug-lists/bycategory.cfm Accessed July 30, (2009).

Upton, R. N. (2007). Cerebral uptake of drugs in humans. *Clinical and Experimental Pharmacology & Physiology, 4*(8), 695–701.

Urch, C. E., Carr, S., & Minton, O. (2004). A retrospective review of the use of alfentanil in a hospital palliative care setting. *Palliative Medicine, 18*(6), 516–519.

Vachharajani, N. N., Shyu, W. C., Garnett, W. R., et al. (1996). The absolute bioavailability and pharmacokinetics of butorphanol nasal spray in patients with hepatic impairment. *Clinical Pharmacology and Therapeutics*, 60(3), 283–294.

Vadalouca, A., Moka, E., Argyra, E., et al. (2008). Opioid rotation in patients with cancer: A review of the current literature. *Journal of Opioid Management*, 4(4), 213–250.

Vadalouca, A. N., Mavromati, P. D., Goudas, L. C., et al. (2000). Haemodynamic, endocrine and nociceptive response to gynaecological procedures under epidural local anaesthesia during continuous epidural infusion or bolus epidural fentanyl dosing. *Acute Pain*, 3(3), 1–6.

Vadivelu, N., & Hines, R. L. (2007). Buprenorphine: A unique opioid with broad clinical applications. *Journal of Opioid Managementment*, 3(1), 49–58.

Vallerand, A., & Nowak, L. A. (2009). Chronic opioid therapy for nonmalignant pain: The patient's perspective. Part I—life before and after opioid therapy. *Pain Management Nursing*, 10(3), 165–172.

van den Bosch, J. E., Kalkman, C. J., Vergouwe, Y., et al. (2005). Assessing the applicability of scoring systems for predicting postoperative nausea and vomiting. *Anaesthesia*, 60(4), 323–331.

Varadarajan, J. L., & Weisman, S. J. (2009). Acute pain management in sickle cell disease patients. In R. S. Sinatra, O. A. de Leon-Casasola, B. Ginsberg, & E. R. Viscusi (Eds.), *Acute pain management* (pp. 550–563). Cambridge, New York: Cambridge University Press.

Vascello, L., & McQuillan, R. J. (2006). Opioid analgesics and routes of administration. In O. A. de Leon-Casasola (Eds.), *Cancer pain. Pharmacological, interventional and palliative care approaches* (pp. 171–193). Philadelphia: Saunders.

Vasisht, N., Stark, J., & Finn, A. (2008). Dose linearity and absolute bioavailability of BEMA (BioErodible MucoAdhesive) fentanyl in healthy volunteers. *The Journal of Pain*, 9(4, Suppl. 1), P23.

Vaughn, C. W., & Connor, M. (2003). In search of a role for the morphine metabolite morphine-3-glucuronide. (Editorial). *Anesthesia and Analgesia*, 97(2), 3111–3112.

Vaurio, L. E., Sands, L. P., Wang, Y., et al. (2006). Postoperative delirium: The importance of pain and pain management. *Anesthesia and Analgesia*, 102(4), 1267–1273.

Vermiere, A., & Remon, J. P. (1999). Stability and compatibility of morphine. *International journal of pharmaceutics*, 187(1), 17–51.

Vevs, A., Backonja, M., & Malik, R. A. (2008). Painful diabetic neuropathy: Epidemiology, natural history, early diagnosis, and treatment options. *Pain Medicine (Malden, Mass.)*, 9(6), 660–674.

Vieira, Z. E., Zsigmond, E. K., Duarte, B., et al. (1993). Double-blind comparison of butorphanol and nalbuphine on the common bile duct by ultrasonography in man. *International Journal of Clinical Pharmacology and Therapeutics*, 31(11), 564–567.

Vieira, Z. E., Zsigmond, E. K., Duarte, B., et al. (1994). Evaluation of fentanyl and sufentanil on the diameter of the common bile duct by ultrasonography in man: A double-blind, placebo-controlled study. *International Journal of Clinical Pharmacology and Therapeutics*, 32(6), 274–277.

Vielvoye-Kerkmeer, A. P. E., Mattern, C., & Uitendaal, M. P. (2000). Transdermal fentanyl in opioid-naïve cancer pain patients: An open trial using transdermal fentanyl for the treatment of chronic cancer pain in opioid-naïve patients and a group using codeine. *Journal of Pain and Symptom Management*, 19(3), 185–192.

Vila, H., Smith, R. A., Augustyniak, M. J., et al. (2005). The efficacy and safety of pain management before and after implementation of hospital-wide pain management standards: Is patient safety compromised by treatment based solely on numerical pain ratings. *Anesthesia and Analgesia*, 101(2), 474–480.

Villesen, H. H., Banning, A. M., Petersen, R. H., et al. (2007). Pharmacokinetics of morphine and oxycodone following intravenous administration in elderly patients. *Ther Clin Risk Manag*, 3(5), 961–967.

Vilming, S. T., Kloster, R., & Sandvik, L. (2005). When should an epidural blood patch be performed in postlumbar puncture headache? A theoretical approach based on a coher of 79 patients. *Cephalagia: An International Journal of Headache*, 25(7), 523–527.

Virani, R., Malloy, P., Ferrell, B. R., et al. (2008). Statewide efforts in promoting palliative care. *Journal of Palliative Medicine*, 11(7), 991–996.

Viscomi, C. M., & Rathmell, J. P. (1998). Pain management issues in the pregnant patient. In M. A. Ashburn, & L. J. Rice (Eds.), *The management of pain* (pp. 363–381). New York: Churchill Livingstone.

Viscusi, E. R., Gan, T. J., Leslie, J. B., et al. (2009). Peripherally acting mu-opioid receptor antagonists and postoperative ileus: Mechanisms of action and clinical applicability. *Anesthesia and Analgesia*, 1108(6), 1811–1822.

Viscusi, E. R., Goldstein, S., Witkowski, T., et al. (2006). Alvimopan, a peripherally acting mu-opioid receptor antagonist compared with placebo in postoperative ileus after major abdominal surgery: Results of a randomized, double-blind, controlled study. *Surgical Endoscopy*, 20(1), 64–70.

Viscusi, E. R., Kopacz, D., Hartrick, C. T., et al. (2006). Single-dose extended-release epidural morphine for pain following hip arthroplasty. *American Journal of Therapeutics*, 13(5), 423–431.

Viscusi, E. R., Martin, G., Hartrick, C. T., et al. (2005). Forty-eight hours of postoperative pain relief after total hip arhtroplasty with a novel, extended-release epidural morphine formulation. *Anesthesiology*, 102(5), 1014–1022.

Voepel-Lewis, T., Marinkovic, A., Kostrzewa, A., et al. (2008). The prevalence of and risk factors for adverse events in children receiving patient-controlled analgesia by proxy or patient-controlled analgesia after surgery. *Anesthesia and Analgesia*, 107(1), 70–75.

Volmanen, P., Akural, E. I., Raudaskoski, T., et al. (2002). Remifentanil in obstetric analgesia: A dose-finding study. *Anesthesia and Analgesia*, 94(4), 913–917.

Voronov, P., Przybylo, H. J., & Jagannathan, N. (2007). Apnea in a child after oral codeine: A genetic variant—An ultra-rapid metabolizer. *Pediatric Anesthesia*, 17(7), 684–687.

Vorsanger, G., Xiang, J., Jordan, D., et al. (2007). Post hoc analysis of a randomized, double-blind, placebo-controlled efficacy and tolerability study of tramadol extended release for the treatment of osteoarthritis pain in geriatric patients. *Clinical Therapeutics*, 29(Suppl.), 2520–2535.

Vranken, J. H., van Kan, H. J. M., & van der Vegt, M. H. (2006). Stability and compatibility of a meperidine-clonidine mixture in portable pump reservoirs for the management of cancer pain syndromes. (Letter). *Journal of Pain and Symptom Management*, 32(4), 297–299.

Walder, B., Schafer, M., Henzi, I., et al. (2001). Efficacy and safety of patient-controlled opioid analgesia for acute postoperative pain: A quantitative systematic review. *Acta Anaesthesiologica Scandinavica, 45*(7), 795–804.

Waldman, S. D. (1991). Epidural abscess associated with epidural catheterization. *Anesthesiology (Letter), 75*(4), 708–709.

Walker, P. W., Palla, S., Pei, B. L., et al. (2008). Switching from methadone to a different opioid: What is the equianalgesic dose ratio? *Journal of Clinical Oncology, 11*(8), 1103–1108.

Walker, S. E., Law, S., & DeAngelis, C. (2001). Stability and compatibility of hydromorphone and ketamine in normal saline. *The Canadian Journal of Hospital Pharmacy, 54*(2), 193–201.

Wallace, M., Moulin, D. E., Rauck, R. L., et al. (2009). Long-term safety, tolerability, and efficacy of OROS hydromorphone in patients with chronic pain. *Journal of Opioid Management, 5*(2), 97–105.

Wallace, M., Rauck, R. L., Moulin, D., et al. (2007). Once-daily OROS hydromorphone for the management of chronic nonmalignant pain: A dose-conversion and titration study. *International Journal of Clinical Practice, 61*(10), 1671–1676.

Wallace, M. S., & Thipphawong, J. (2007). Clinical trial results with OROS hydromorphone. *Journal of Pain and Symptom Management, 33*(Suppl. 2), S25–S32.

Wallenborn, J., Gelbrich, G., Bulst, D., et al. (2006). Prevention of postoperative nausea and vomiting by metoclopramide combined with dexamethasone: Randomised double blind multicentre trial. *BMJ (Clinical Research Ed.), 333*(7563), 324–327.

Walsh, D., & Tropiano, P. S. (2002). Long-term rectal administration of high-dose sustained-release morphine tablets. *Supportive Care in Cancer, 10*(8), 653–655.

Wang, J., Pennefather, S., & Russell, G. (1998). Low-dose naloxone in the treatment of urinary retention during extradural fentanyl causes excessive reversal of analgesia. (Letter). *British Journal of Anaesthesia, 80*(4), 565–566.

Wang, J. J., Ho, S. T., Uen, Y. H., et al. (2002). Small-dose dexamethasone reduces nausea and vomiting after laparoscopic cholecystectomy: A comparison of tropisetron with saline. *Anesthesia and Analgesia, 95*(1), 229–232.

Wang, J. K., Nauss, L. A., & Thomas, J. E. (1979). Pain relief by intrathecally applied morphine in man. *Anesthesiology, 50*, 149–150.

Warren, D. E. (1996). Practical use of rectal medications in palliative care. *Journal of Pain and Symptom Management, 11*(6), 378–387.

Washington State Agency Medical Directors' Group (AMDG). (2007). *Interagency guideline on opioid treatment.* Olympia, WA: Washington State Department of Labor and Industries. Summary available at www.guidelines.gov/summary/summary.aspx?doc_id=12243. Accessed July 28, 2009.

Watanabe, S., Belzile, M., Kuehn, N., et al. (1996). Capsules and suppositories of methadone for patients on high-dose opioids for cancer pain: Clinical and economic considerations. *Cancer Treatment Reviews, 22*, 131–136.

Watcha, M. F. (2000). The cost-effective management of postoperative nausea and vomiting. (Editorial). *Anesthesiology, 92*(4), 931–933.

Watcha, M. F., & White, P. F. (1995). Post-operative nausea and vomiting: Do they matter? *European Journal of Anaesthesiology, 12*(Suppl. 10), 18–23.

Watson, C. P. N., Moulin, D., Watt-Watson, J., et al. (2003). Controlled-release oxycodone relieves neuropathic pain: A randomized controlled trial in painful diabetic neuropathy. *Pain, 105*(1–2), 71–78.

Watson, D. G., Lin, M., Morton, A., et al. (2005). Compatibility and stability of dexamethasone sodium phosphate and ketamine hydrochloride subcutaneous infusions in polypropylene syringes. *Journal of Pain and Symptom Management, 30*(1), 80–86.

Waxler, B., Dadabhoy, Z. P., Stojiljkovic, L., et al. (2005). Primer of postoperative pruritus for anesthesiologists. *Anesthesiology, 103*(1), 168–178.

Webb, A., & Leong, S. (2005). The combination of tramadol and morphine may be recommended for postoperative analgesia. *Anesthesia and Analgesia, 101*(6), 1884–1885.

Webster, L. R. (2008). Maximizing safety with methadone and other opioids. *Practical Pain Management, 8*(3), 51–55. Also available at http://pain-topics.org/pdf/Webster-MaximizingOpioidSafety.pdf. Accessed June 25, 2008.

Webster, L. R., Choi, Y., Desai, H., et al. (2008). Sleep-disordered breathing and chronic opioid therapy. *Pain Medicine (Malden, Mass.), 9*(4), 425–432.

Webster, L. R., & Dove, B. (2007). *Avoiding opioid abuse while managing pain.* North Branch, MN: Sunrise River Press.

Wedam, E. F., Bigelow, G. E., Johnson, R. E., et al. (2007). QT-interval effects of methadone, levomethadyl, and buprenorphine in a randomized trial. *Archives of Internal Medicine, 167*(22), 2469–2475.

Wedel, D. J., & Horlocker, T. T. (2006). Regional anesthesia in the febrile or infected patient. *Regional Anesthesia and Pain Medicine, 31*(4), 324–333.

Weil, A. J., Nicholson, B., & Sasaki, J. (2009). Factors affecting dosing regimens of morphine sulfate extended-release (Kadian) capsules. *Journal of Opioid Management, 5*(1), 39–45.

Weiler, J. M., Bloomfield, J. R., Woodworth, G. G., et al. (2000). Effects of fexofenadine, diphenhydramine, and alcohol on driving performance: A randomized, placebo-controlled trial in the Iowa Driving Simulator. *Annals of Internal Medicine, 132*, 354–363.

Weinberg, D. S., Inturrisi, C. E., Reidenberg, B., et al. (1988). Sublingual absorption of selected opioid analgesics. *Clinical Pharmacology and Therapeutics, 44*, 335–342.

Weinstein, S. M. (1994). In patients with chronic pain, what is the suggested maximum dose of sustained-release morphine? *Primary Care Cancer, 14*(1), 15.

Weissman, D.E, & Haddox, J. D. (1989). Opioid pseudoaddiction—an iatrogenic syndrome. *Pain, 36*(3), 363–366.

Wellington, J., & Chia, Y. Y. (2009). Patient variables influencing acute pain management. In R. S. Sinatra, O. A. de Leon-Casasola, B. Ginsberg, & E. R. Viscusi (Eds.), *Acute pain management* (pp. 33–40). Cambridge, New York: Cambridge University Press.

Werawatganon, T., & Charuluxananan, S. (2005). Patient controlled intravenous opioid analgesia versus continuous epidural analgesia for pain after intra-abdominal surgery. *Cochrane Database of Systematic Reviews (Online),* (1) CD004088.

Wermeling, D. P., Clinch, T., Rudy, A. C., et al. (2009). A multicenter, open-label, exploratory dose-ranging trial of intranasal hydromorphone for managing acute pain from traumatic injury. *Acute Pain, 11*(3), 151–152.

Wermeling, D. P., Grant, G. M., Lee, A., et al. (2005). Analgesic effects of intranasal butorphanol tartrate administered via a unit-dose device in the dental impaction pain model: A randomized, double-blind, placebo-controlled, parallel-group study. *Clinical Therapeutics, 27*(4), 430–440.

Weschules, D. J., & Bain, K. T. (2008). A systematic review of opioid conversion ratios used with methadone for the treatment of pain. *Pain Medicine (Malden, Mass.), 9*(5), 595–612.

Weschules, D. J., Bain, K. T., & Richeimer, S. (2008). Actual and potential drug interactions associated with methadone. *Pain Medicine (Malden, Mass.)*, 9(3), 315–344.

Westin, U. E., Boström, E., Gråsjö, J., et al. (2006). Direct nose-to-brain transfer of morphine after nasal administration to rats. *Pharmaceutical Research*, 23(3), 565–572.

Wheatley, R. G., Shepherd, D., Jackson, I. J., et al. (1992). Hypoxaemia and pain relief after upper abdominal surgery: Comparison of IM and patient-controlled analgesia. *British Journal of Anaesthesia*, 69(6), 558–661.

Wheatley, R. G., Schug, S. A., & Watson, D. (2001). Safety and efficacy of postoperative epidural analgesia. *British Journal of Anaesthesia*, 87(1), 47–61.

Wheeler, M., Oderda, G. M., Ashburn, M. A., et al. (2002). Adverse events associated with postoperative opioid analgesia: A systematic review. *The Journal of Pain*, 3(3), 159–180.

White, C., Hardy, J., Boyd, A., et al. (2008). Subcutaneous sufentanil for palliative care patients in a hospital setting. *Palliative Medicine*, 22(1), 89–90.

White, P. F. (2002). Droperidol: A cost-effective antiemetic for over thirty years. (Editorial). *Anesthesia and analgesia*, 95(4), 789–790.

White, P. F. (2005). The changing role of non-opioid analgesic techniques in the management of postoperative pain. *Anesthesia and Analgesia*, 105(Suppl. 5), S5–S22.

White, P. F., & Freire, A. R. (2005). Ambulatory (outpatient) anesthesia. In Miller, R. D. (Ed.), *Miller's anesthesia* (6th ed.,Vol. 2. pp. 2589–2635). St. Louis: Elsevier.

White, P. F., Hamza, M. A., Recart, A., et al. (2005). Optimal timing of acustimulation for antiemetic prophylaxis as an adjunct to ondansetron in patients undergoing plastic surgery. *Anesthesia and Analgesia*, 100(2), 367–372.

White, P. F., Issioui, T., Hu, J., et al. (2002). Comparative efficacy of acustimulation (ReliefBand®) versus ondansetron in combination with droperidol for preventing nausea and vomiting. *Anesthesiology*, 97(5), 1075–1081.

White, P. F., O'Hara, J. F., Roberson, C. R., et al. (2008). The impact of current antiemetic practices on patient outcomes: A prospective study on high-risk patients. *Anesthesia and Analgesia*, 107(2), 452–458.

White, P. F., Sacan, O., Nuangchamnog, N., et al. (2008). The relationship between patient risk factors and early versus late postoperative emetic symptoms. *Anesthesia and Analgesia*, 107(2), 459–463.

White, P. F., Song, D., Abrao, J., et al. (2005). Effect of low-dose droperidol on the QT interval during and after general anesthesia. *Anesthesiology*, 102(6), 1101–1105.

White, P. F., Tang, J., Song, D., et al. (2007). Transdermal scopolamine: An alternative to ondansetron and droperidol for the prevention of postoperative and postdischarge emetic symptoms. *Anesthesia and Analgesia*, 104(1), 92–96.

Wiffen, P. J., & McQuay, H. J. (2007). Oral morphine for cancer pain. *Cochrane Database of Systematic Reviews (Online)*, (4), CD003868.

Wilbeck, J., Schorn, M. N., & Daley, L. (2008). Pharmacologic management of acute pain in breastfeeding women. *Journal of Emergency Nursing: JEN*, 34(4), 340–344.

Wilhelm, S. M., Dehoorne-Smith, M. L., & Kale-Pradhan, P. B. (2007). Prevention of postoperative nausea and vomiting. *The Annals of Pharmacotherapy*, 41(1), 68–78.

Wilhelm, W., Schlaich, N., Harrer, J., et al. (2001). Recovery and neurological examination after remifentanil—desflurane or fentanyl-desflurane anaesthesia for carotid artery surgery. *British Journal of Anaesthesia*, 86(1), 44–49.

Williams, M. A. (1991). Delirium/acute confusional states: Evaluation devices in nursing. *International Psychogeriatrics/IPA*, 3(2), 301–308.

Williams-Russo, P., Urquhart, B. L., Sharrock, N. E., et al. (1992). Post-operative delirium predictors and prognosis in elderly orthopedic patients. *Journal of the American Geriatrics Society*, 40(8), 759–767.

Wilmore, D. W., & Kehlet, H. (2001). Management of patients in fast track surgery. *BMJ (Clinical Research Ed.)*, 322(7284), 473–476.

Wilmore, D. W., & Kehlet, H. (2008). Evidence-based surgical care and the evolution of fast-track surgery. *Annals of Surgery*, 248(2), 189–198.

Wilson, A. (2009). Regional analgesia and orthopaedic surgery. *Orthopaed Trauma*, 23(6), 441–449.

Wilson, J. M., Cohen, R. I., Kezer, E. A., et al. (1995). Single and multiple-dose pharmacokinetics of dezocine in patients with acute and chronic pain. *Journal of Clinical Pharmacology*, 35(4), 395–403.

Wilson, M. J. A., MacArthur, C., Cooper, G. M., et al. (2010). Epidural analgesia and breastfeeding: A randomised controlled trial of epidural techniques with and without fentanyl and a non-epidural comparison group. *Anaesthesia*, 65(2), 145–153.

Wilson, W. C., Smedira, N. G., Fink, C., et al. (1992). Ordering and administration of sedatives and analgesics during the withholding and withdrawal of life support from critically ill patients. *JAMA: The Journal of the American Medical Association*, 267(1), 949–953.

Wirz, S., Wartenberg, H. C., Elsen, C., et al. (2006). Managing cancer pain and symptoms of outpatient rotation to sustained-release hydromorphone. A prospective clinical trial. *The Clinical Journal of Pain*, 22(9), 770–775.

Wirz, S., Whittmann, M., Schenk, M., et al. (2009). Gastrointestinal symptoms under opioid therapy: A prospective comparison of oral sustained-release hydromorphone, transdermal fentanyl, and tranderaml buprenorphine. *European Journal of Pain (London, England)*, 13(7), 737–743.

Wisner, A., Dufour, E., Messaoudi, M., et al. (2006). Human opiorphin, a natural antinociceptive modulator of opioid-dependent pathways. *Proceedings of the National Academy of Sciences of the United States of America*, 103(47), 17979–17984.

Wittels, B., Glosten, B., & Faure, E. A. M. (1997). Postcesarean analgesia with both epidural morphine and intravenous patient-controlled analgesia: Neurobehavioral outcomes among nursing neonates. *Anesthesia and Analgesia*, 85(3), 600–606.

Wittwer, E., & Kern, S. E. (2006). Role of morphine's metabolites in analgesia: Concepts and controversies. *The AAPS Journal*, 8(2), E348–E352.

Wolfe, T. (2007). Intranasal fentanyl for acute pain: Techniques to enhance efficacy. *Annals of Emergency Medicine*, 49(5), 721–722.

Wood, G. J., Shega, J. W., Lynch, B., et al. (2007). Management of intractable nausea and vomiting in patients at the end of life. *JAMA: The Journal of the American Medical Association*, 298(10), 1196–1207.

Wood, J. D. (2005). Opioids, the enteric nervous system, and postoperative ileus. *Sem Colon Rec Surg*, 16(4), 188–196.

Woodall, H. E., Chiu, A., & Weissman, D. E. (2008). Opioid allergic reactions #175. *Journal of Palliative Medicine*, 11(10), 1340–1341.

Woolf, C. J. (1983). Evidence for a central component of post-injury pain hypersensitivity. *Nature, 306*(5944), 686–688.

Woolf, C. J., & Chong, M. S. (1993). Preemptive analgesia: Treating postoperative pain by preventing the establishment of central sensitization. *Anesthesia and Analgesia, 77*(2), 362–379.

World Health Organization (WHO). (1986). *Cancer pain relief.* Geneva: WHO.

World Health Organization (WHO). (1996). *Cancer Pain Relief.* (2nd ed.). Available at http://www.painpolicy.wisc.edu/publicat/cprguid.htm#WHO. Accessed May 15, 2008.

Wright, A. W., Mather, L. E., & Smith, M. T. (2001). Hydromorphone-3-glucuronide: A more potent neuro-excitant than its structural analogue, morphine-3-glucuronide. *Life Sciences, 69*(4), 409–420.

Wu, C. L. (2005). Acute postoperative pain. In R. D. Miller (Ed.), *Miller's anesthesia.* (6th ed. Vol. 2. pp. 2729–2762). Philadelphia: Elsevier.

Wuhrman, E., Cooney, M. F., Dunwoody, C. J., et al. (2007). Authorized and unauthorized ("PCA by proxy") dosing of analgesic infusion pumps: Position statement with clinical practice recommendations. *Pain Management Nursing, 8*(1), 4–11. Available at http://www.aspmn.org/Organization/documents/PMNVersionPCA.pdf. Accessed January 14, 2008.

Wulf, H., Gleim, M., & Mignat, C. (1994). The stability of mixtures of morphine hydrochloride, bupivacaine hydrochloride, and clonidine hydrochloride in portable pump reservoirs for the management of chronic pain syndromes. *Journal of Pain and Symptom Management, 9*(5), 308–311.

Wyeth Pharmaceuticals, Inc. (2009). *Relistor prescribing information.* Philadelphia, PA: Wyeth Pharmaceuticals, Inc.

Xanodyne Pharmaceuticals. (2008). *Oramorph SR prescribing information.* Newport, KY: Xanodyne Pharmaceuticals.

Yaksh, T. L., & Harty, G. J. (1988). Pharmacology of the allodynia in rats evoked by high dose intrathecal morphine. *The Journal of Pharmacology and Experimental Therapeutics, 244,* 501–507.

Yeh, H. M., Chen, L. K., Lin, C. J., et al. (2000). Prophylactic intravenous ondansetron reduces the incidence of intrathecal morphine-induced pruritus in patients undergoing cesarean delivery. *Anesthesia and Analgesia, 91*(1), 172–175.

Young-McCaughan, S., & Miaskowski, C. (2001). Definition of and mechanism for opioid-induced sedation. *Pain Management Nursing, 2*(3), 84–97.

Yu, S. C., Ngan Kee, W. D., & Kwan, A. S. K. (2002). Addition of meperidine to bupivacaine for spinal anaesthesia for caesarean section. *British Journal of Anaesthesia, 88*(3), 379–383.

Yuan, C. S. (Ed.). (2005). *Handbook of opioid bowel dysfunction.* New York: Haworth Medical Press.

Yuan, C. S., Foss, J. F., O'Connor, M., et al. (1998). Efficacy of orally administered methylnaltrexone in decreasing subjective effects after intravenous morphine. *Drug and Alcohol Dependence, 52*(2), 161–165.

Yuan, C. S., Foss, J. F., O'Connor, M., et al. (2000). Methylnaltrexone for reversal of constipation due to chronic methadone use. *The New England Journal of Medicine, 283*(3), 367–372.

Yuan, H. B., Zuo, Z., Yu, K. W., et al. (2008). Bacterial colonization of epidural catheters used for short-term postoperative analgesia. *Anesthesiology, 108*(1), 130–137.

Zacny, J. P. (1996). Should people taking opioids for medical reasons be allowed to work and drive? *Addiction (Abingdon, England), 91*(11), 1581–1584.

Zajaczkowska, R., Wlodzimierz, W., Wordliczek, J., et al. (2004). Peripheral opioid analgesia in laparoscopic cholecystectomy. *Regional Anesthesia and Pain Medicine, 29*(5), 424–429.

Zakriya, K. J., Christmas, C., Wenz, J. F., et al. (2002). Preoperative factors associated with postoperative change in confusion assessment method score in hip fracture patients. *Anesthesia and Analgesia, 94*(6), 1628–1632.

Zangrillo, A., Bignami, E., Biondi-Zoccai, G. G. L., et al. (2009). Spinal analgesia in cardiac surgery: A meta-analysis of randomized controlled trials. *Journal of Cardiothoracic and Vascular Anesthesia, 23*(6), 813–821.

Zaslansky, R., Eisenberg, E., Peskin, B., et al. (2006). Early administration of oral morphine to orthopedic patients after surgery. *Journal Opioid Management, 2*(2), 88–92.

Zech, D. F. J., Grond, S. U. A., Lynch, J., et al. (1995). Validation of World Health Organization Guidelines for cancer pain relief: A 10-year prospective study. *Pain, 63*(1), 65–76.

Zeppetella, G. (2000a). An assessment of the safety, efficacy, and acceptability of intranasal fentanyl citrate in the management of cancer-related breakthrough pain: A pilot study. *Journal of Pain and Symptom Management, 20*(4), 253–258.

Zeppetella, G. (2000b). Nebulized and intranasal fentanyl in the management of cancer-related breakthrough pain. *Palliative Medicine, 14*(1), 57–58.

Zeppetella, G. (2008). Opioids for cancer breakthrough pain: A pilot study reporting patient assessment of time to meaningful pain relief. *Journal of Pain and Symptom Management, 35*(5), 563–567.

Zeppetella, G., Porzio, G., & Aielli, F. (2007). Opioids applied topically to painful cutaneous malignant ulcers in a palliative care setting. *Journal of Opioid Management, 3*(3), 161–166.

Zeppetella, G., & Ribeiro, M. D. C. (2006). Opioids for the management of breakthrough (episodic) pain in cancer patients. *Cochrane Database of Systematic Reviews (Online),* (1), CD004311.

Zhan, C., Sangl, J., Bierman, A. S., et al. (2001). Potentially inappropriate medication use in the community-dwelling elderly: Findings from the 1996 Medical Expenditure Panel Survey. *JAMA: The Journal of the American Medical Association, 286*(22), 2823–2829.

Zhang, H., Zhang, J., & Streisand, J. B. (2002). Oral mucosal drug delivery: Clinical pharmacokinetics and therapeutic applications. *Clinical Pharmacokinetics, 41*(9), 661–680.

Zhao, S. Z., Chung, F., Hanna, D. B., et al. (2004). Dose-response relationship between opioid use and adverse effects after ambulatory surgery. *Journal of Pain and Symptom Management, 28*(1), 35–46.

Zhou, S., Chan, E., Pan, S. Q., et al. (2004). Pharmacokinetic interactions of drugs with St John's wort. *Journal of Psychopharmacology (Oxford, England), 18*(2), 262–276.

Zimmermann, C., Seccareccia, D., Booth, C. M., et al. (2005). Rotation to methadone after opioid dose escalation: How should individualization of dosing occur? *Journal of Pain & Palliative Care Pharmacotherapy, 19*(2), 25–31.

Zsigmond, E. K., Vieira, Z. E., Duarte, B., et al. (1993). Double-blind placebo-controlled ultrasonographic confirmation of constriction of the common bile duct by morphine. *International Journal of Clinical Pharmacology, Therapy, and Toxicology, 31*(10), 506–509.

Adjuvant Analgesics

Chris Pasero, Rosemary C. Polomano,
Russell K. Portenoy, and Margo McCaffery

Terminology

Acetaminophen Other generic names include *paracetamol* and *acetylparaaminophenol (APAP)*. Also referred to as "aspirin-free" drugs.

Addiction A chronic neurologic and biologic disease. As defined by pain specialists, it is characterized by behaviors that include one or more of the following: impaired control over drug use, compulsive use, continued use despite harm, and craving. Continued craving for an opioid and the need to use the opioid for effects other than pain relief. Physical dependence and tolerance are not the same as addiction.

Adjuvant analgesic A drug that has a primary indication other than pain (e.g., anticonvulsant, antidepressant, sodium channel blocker, or muscle relaxant) but is analgesic for some painful conditions.

Allodynia Pain due to a stimulus that does not normally provoke pain, such as touch. Typically experienced in the skin around areas affected by nerve injury; commonly seen with many neuropathic pain syndromes.

Analgesic ceiling A dose beyond which further increases in dose do not provide additional analgesia.

Bioavailability The extent to which a dose of a drug reaches its site of action.

Breakthrough dose (BTD) Also referred to as *supplemental dose* or *rescue dose*; the dose of analgesic taken to treat breakthrough pain.

Breakthrough pain (BTP) A transitory increase in pain that occurs on a background of otherwise controlled persistent pain.

Ceiling effect A dose above which further dose increments produce no change in effect.

Comfort-function goal The pain rating identified by the individual patient above which the patient experiences interference with function and quality of life, that is, activities that the patient needs or wishes to perform.

Controlled release See modified release.

Crescendo pain A period of rapid pain escalation often associated with increasing distress and functional impairment.

Distribution half-life The time it takes a drug to move from the blood and plasma to other tissues. Distribution half-life differs from half-life (terminal) (see **half-life**).

Dysesthesia An unpleasant abnormal sensation (whether spontaneous or evoked) that is usually associated with neuropathic pain and described as "pins and needles" (e.g., a limb "falling asleep," burning, electrical shock–like, tingling) and may be intermittent or continuous and experienced in an area of sensory loss. A dysesthesia is always unpleasant, whereas a paresthesia is not unpleasant. It may be difficult to differentiate dysesthesias from paresthesias.

Efficacy The extent to which a drug or another treatment "works" and can produce the effect in question—analgesia in this context. To determine whether or not this is the case, the treatment must be compared to another, typically a placebo, but sometimes an active comparator. *Maximal efficacy* refers to the maximum effect that can be produced by a drug, and *comparative efficacy* refers to the relative effects of two or more treatments compared at comparable treatment intensities.

Extended release See modified release.

Half-life The time it takes for the plasma concentration (amount of drug in the body) to be reduced by 50%. After starting a drug, or increasing its dose, four to five half-lives are required to approach a steady-state level in the blood, irrespective of the dose, dosing interval, or route of administration; after four to five half-lives, a drug that has been discontinued generally is considered to be mostly eliminated from the body.

Hydrophilic Readily absorbed in aqueous solution.

Hyperalgesia Increased pain response to noxious stimuli.

Intractable In reference to pain that is unresponsive to all other recommended therapeutic options (e.g., first-line and second-line analgesics).

Intraspinal "Within the spine"; term referring to the spaces or potential spaces surrounding the spinal cord into which medications can be administered. Most often, the term is used when referring to the epidural and intrathecal routes of administration. Sometimes used interchangeably with the term *neuraxial.*

Lipophilic Readily absorbed in fatty tissues.

Medically ill patients Patients with existing debilitating pathologic condition/illness that may be progressive or stable, as opposed to those who have only the symptom of pain and are otherwise healthy.

Metabolite The product of biochemical reactions during drug metabolism.

Modified release Analgesics that are formulated to release over a prolonged period of time; often used interchangeably with the terms *extended release, sustained release,* and *controlled release.* The term *modified release* will be used in this book to describe these drugs.

Narcotic See **opioid.** Obsolete term for *opioid,* in part because the government and media use the term loosely to refer to a variety of substances of potential abuse. Legally, controlled substances classified as narcotics include opioids, cocaine, and various other substances.

Neuralgia Pain in the distribution of a nerve (e.g., sciatica, trigeminal neuralgia). Often felt as an electrical shock–like pain.

Neuropathic pain Pain that is sustained by injury or dysfunction of the peripheral or central nervous system.

NMDA N-methyl-D-aspartate. In this book, the term is used in conjunction with drugs that are NMDA receptor antagonists or blockers, such as ketamine or dextromethorphan.

Nociceptive pain Pain that is sustained by ongoing activation of the sensory system that subserves the perception of noxious stimuli; implies the existence of damage to somatic or visceral tissues sufficient to activate the nociceptive system.

Nociceptor A primary afferent nerve that has the ability to respond to a noxious stimulus or to a stimulus that would be noxious if prolonged.

Nonopioid Used instead of *nonnarcotic.* Refers to acetaminophen and nonsteroidal antiinflammatory drugs (NSAIDs).

NSAID An acronym for *nonsteroidal antiinflammatory drug.* (Pronounced "in said.") Also referred to as *aspirin-like* drugs.

Opioid This term is preferred to **narcotic.** Opioid refers to codeine, morphine, and other natural, semisynthetic, and synthetic drugs that relieve pain by binding to multiple types of opioid receptors.

Opioid dose-sparing effect The dose of opioid may be lowered when another analgesic, such as a nonopioid, is added.

Opioid-induced hyperalgesia (OIH) A phenomenon clearly demonstrated in experimental models, but of uncertain significance in humans, by which exposure to the opioid induces increased sensitivity, or a lowered threshold, to the neural activity subserving pain perception; it is the "flip side" of analgesic tolerance, which is defined by the loss of analgesic activity due to exposure to the drug.

Opioid-naïve An opioid-naïve person has not recently taken enough opioid on a regular enough basis to become tolerant to the effects of an opioid.

Opioid-tolerant An opioid-tolerant person has taken opioids long enough at doses high enough to develop tolerance to many of the effects of an opioid, including analgesia and sedation, but there is no time frame for developing tolerance.

Paresthesia An abnormal sensation, whether spontaneous or evoked, manifested by sensations of numbness, prickling, tingling, and heightened sensitivity that is typically not unpleasant.

Paroxysmal Sudden periodic attack or recurrence.

Physical dependence Potential for withdrawal symptoms if the opioid is abruptly stopped or an antagonist is administered; not the same as **addiction.**

Potency The dose required to produce a specified effect; relative potency is the ratio of the doses of two or more analgesics required to produce the same analgesic effect.

Preemptive analgesia Preinjury pain treatments (e.g., preoperative epidural analgesia and preincision local anesthetic infiltration) to prevent the establishment of peripheral and central sensitization of pain.

Primary afferent neuron See nociceptor.

Prodrug An inactive precursor of a drug, converted into its active form in the body by normal metabolic processes.

Protective analgesia An aggressive, sustained multimodal intervention administered perioperatively (e.g., local anesthetic block, acetaminophen, NSAID, and anticonvulsant initiated preoperatively and continued throughout the intraoperative and postoperative periods) and directed toward prevention of pathologic pain (e.g., persistent neuropathic postsurgical pain syndromes).

Refractory Nonresponsive or resistant to therapeutic interventions such as first-line or second-line analgesics.

Rescue dose Also referred to as *supplemental dose* or *breakthrough dose.* Administered on a PRN basis (as needed) in combination with the regularly scheduled analgesic to relieve pain that exceeds, or breaks through, the ongoing pain.

Sustained release See modified release.

Systemic drug treatment; systemic administration Administration of a drug by a given route that allows absorption into the systemic circulation. Routes include oral, parenteral (IV, IM, SC), rectal, vaginal, topical application, transdermal, intranasal, and transmucosal. By contrast, the spinal route of administration deposits the drug directly into the central nervous system, minimizing the amount of drug that reaches the systemic circulation.

Titration Adjusting the amount (e.g., adjusting the dose of opioid).

Tolerance A process characterized by decreasing effects of a drug at its previous dose, or the need for a higher dose of drug to maintain an effect; not the same as **addiction.**

Up-regulation An increase in a cellular component (e.g., an increase in the number of receptors) that makes the cells more sensitive to a particular drug or other agent.

Terms Related to Research

Anecdotal evidence Evidence derived from clinical observations, clinical experience, or published case reports.

Case reports Published reports of one or more patient cases describing patient experiences, circumstances, or situations that infer specific outcomes that are not based on any scientific method of study.

Case-control study A retrospective observational study used most often to evaluate risk factors that may help explain the appearance or presentation of a disease or condition. Subjects with a known disease or condition are matched with similar individuals who do not possess it. Various potential risk factors, such as age or sex, or lifestyle factors, are then statistically evaluated to determine their levels of association with the disease or condition.

Cohort study A retrospective or prospective study in which a group of subjects who have a specific condition or receive a particular treatment are evaluated over time for a defined period. Data may be compared with another group of subjects who do not have the same condition or receive the same treatment, or subgroups within the cohort may be compared.

Controlled studies/trials Research studies that exert some or total control over the various treatment effects by using a comparison group (placebo group or comparator treatment group) and may use a single- or double-blind design, or a random assignment of subjects.

Double-blind study Neither the investigator nor the subject know the critical aspects of the study (e.g., in a placebo-controlled trial, neither the person administering the intervention nor the subject receiving the intervention know if the intervention is experimental or placebo); used to reduce investigator and subject bias.

Meta-analysis Data analysis in which the results of several studies that address related research are combined and analyzed to arrive at one overall measurement of treatment effect.

Number needed to treat (NNT) A parameter that is often used in reporting the results of epidemiologic studies, clinical trials, systematic reviews, and meta-analyses. It is an estimate of how many people would need to receive an intervention to prevent one undesirable outcome or how many people need to receive a treatment in order that one derives a well-defined benefit (e.g., a 50% reduction in pain). NNT is calculated by using a formula that involves a known risk reduction or benefit analysis. Investigators typically determine and define the outcome that is used to compute the NNT for their study.

Open-label Both the investigators and the subjects know what treatment subjects are receiving. An investigator studies the response to an analgesic in a sample of patients and follows them through the treatment phase, observing and recording the effects. A disadvantage of this study design is potential bias for patient selection, observations, and conclusions.

Placebo-controlled trial A study that compares a treatment to a placebo, which is a treatment with no known therapeutic value. The placebo typically resembles the active intervention and is used as the control to determine the active intervention's efficacy.

Randomized controlled trial (RCT) A study in which subjects are randomly assigned (by chance alone) to receive the various interventions in a study. Randomization increases the likelihood that factors that could influence the effects produced by a treatment are distributed evenly across treatment groups, thereby limiting the risk of bias.

Relative risk (RR) A measure of the risk of a certain event happening in one group compared with the risk of the same event happening in another group. For example, in cancer research, relative risk is used in prospective (forward-looking) studies, such as cohort studies and clinical trials. A relative risk of 1 means there is no difference between groups in terms of their risk of cancer, based on whether or not they were exposed to a certain substance or factor, or how they responded to two treatments being compared. A relative risk greater than 1 or less than 1 means that being exposed to a certain substance or factor either increases (relative risk greater than 1) or decreases (relative risk less than 1) the risk of cancer, or that the treatments being compared do not have the same effects (e.g., a relative risk of 2 would mean that those exposed to a certain substance or factor have twice the risk of cancer compared with those who are not exposed to a certain substance or factor). Relative risk is also often called *relative ratio*.

Sequential trials One drug is tried and if the results are unfavorable, it is discontinued and another drug is tried. A trial-and-error approach in which one drug after another is tried until the desired effects occur.

Single-blind study The investigators know to what treatment conditions subjects are assigned, but subjects are "blinded" (not aware) of what they are receiving.

The term *adjuvant analgesic* describes any drug that has a primary indication other than for pain but is analgesic for some painful conditions. This term, while widely accepted, is actually now a misnomer. Some adjuvant analgesics are indicated for specific types of pain, and, in this context, are not "adjuvant" to some other primary therapy. The adjuvant analgesics, therefore, are better considered nontraditional pain relievers that can be used both as "add-on" therapy to an opioid regimen or as distinct primary therapy for specific painful disorders.

More generally, adjuvant analgesics may be distinguished from "adjuvant therapy," which also has a different meaning in some contexts. For example, in the palliative care literature, adjuvant therapies comprise both analgesics (which may be combined with nonopioid analgesics, such as the NSAIDs, into a grouping called *coanalgesics*) and drugs used to counteract the adverse effects of analgesics. In this literature, emphasis is given to the treatment of pain using combination therapy consisting of opioids combined with coanalgesics and other drugs to manage opioid adverse effects; the adjuvant analgesics (e.g., antidepressants, anticonvulsants, corticosteroids, or bisphosphonates) are used to enhance opioid pain relief, treat pain less responsive or refractory to opioids, or reduce the doses of opioids to limit adverse effects (Ferrell, Levy, Paice, 2008; Klepstad, Kaasa, Cherny, et al., 2005; Lussier, Portenoy, 2004).

Clinical experience with most of the adjuvant analgesics initially evolved from the treatment of persistent neuropathic pain (see Section I); however, the role of adjuvant analgesics has expanded to include other types of persistent (chronic) pain syndromes as well as acute pain from surgery, trauma, or burns. For persistent pain unrelated to cancer or other progressive diseases, adjuvant analgesics are often used alone—not as an adjuvant to any other pharmacologic therapy. Some adjuvant analgesics are potentially useful for a variety of painful disorders (they may be considered multipurpose analgesics), and others are used for specific pain disorders because the literature is limited or they exert an action that targets a particular pain mechanism (Portenoy, 2000). The practice of administering adjuvant agents as primary analgesics has gained widespread acceptance in the treatment of some types of persistent noncancer pain, such as fibromyalgia, painful diabetic neuropathy, and postherpetic neuralgia.

Considerable research is underway to examine the role of adjuvant analgesics and to determine their benefits in the armamentarium of therapeutics for the treatment of pain. This section focuses on the knowledge, clinical experience, research, and evidence that are available to support the use of adjuvant analgesics in a wide range of painful conditions. Although there are still significant gaps in the evidence supporting the role of these drugs as analgesics, significant progress has been made in drug development and testing, in establishing indications for new and existing adjuvant analgesics, and in positioning these therapies through a growing clinical experience.

Various research terms are applied to discussions of investigations on adjuvant therapies, and these are defined in the glossary of terms appearing in the beginning of this section (Terminology). See also Table 3-4 (p. 130) for more research definitions. These definitions help to enhance the understanding of published studies and reports pertaining to adjuvant therapy and enable clinicians to evaluate the relative strength of evidence currently available. For example, clinical observations of astute clinicians, often referred to as *anecdotal evidence*, and guidelines derived largely from observational studies, anecdotal reports, and expert consensus can make valuable contributions to practice when research is inconclusive. Evidence-based guidelines developed from the data generated by randomized, placebo-controlled, double-blind studies, and especially from the systematic reviews or meta-analyses that may be done if the number of studies is sufficient, usually are more convincing and provide considerably stronger evidence to guide treatment decisions.

Adjuvant analgesics compose an extraordinarily diverse group of drug classes. A generally useful, broad classification distinguishes those that may be considered nonspecific, multipurpose analgesics from those that have more specific indications for selected types of pain (pp. 627-628). The availability of these drugs helps promote the concept of multimodal analgesia and effective symptom management. Growing research has dispelled common misconceptions about these drugs (table on pp. 627-628). Major classes of adjuvant analgesics, along with examples, are listed in the Adjuvant Analgesics table (pp. 628-630). The appropriate use of any of the analgesics discussed in this book requires an understanding of the underlying mechanisms of pain and analgesics. The reader is referred to Section I for a detailed discussion of the underlying mechanisms of nociceptive (physiologic) pain and the pathophysiology of neuropathic pain.

Selected Adjuvant Analgesics

Role of adjuvants in analgesic therapy: Adjuvants may be used in addition to other analgesics or alone as distinct primary therapy for certain painful conditions. Most experience with adjuvant analgesics has been in the treatment of persistent (chronic) pain, but use of adjuvants is now expanding to include treatment of acute pain.

TWO CLASSES:

1. Multipurpose adjuvant analgesics useful for persistent pain and symptom management, and in some cases acute pain. Examples of drug classes are as follows:
   a. Antidepressants
   b. Corticosteroids
   c. Alpha$_2$-adrenergic agonists
   d. Cannabinoids
   e. Topical analgesics
2. Adjuvant analgesics for specific types of pain. Examples of pain conditions and recommended adjuvant analgesic classes/drugs are as follows:
   a. Persistent neuropathic pain (e.g., anticonvulsants, antidepressants, sodium channel blockers, cannabinoids, topical analgesics)
   b. Persistent bone pain such as bony metastasis or osteoporosis (e.g., bisphosphonates, calcitonin, radiopharmaceuticals)
   c. Malignant bowel obstruction (e.g., anticholinergics, corticosteroids, octreotide)
   d. Musculoskeletal pain (e.g., muscle relaxants, benzodiazepines)
   e. Procedural pain (e.g., propofol, dexmedetomidine, ketamine, local anesthetic)
   f. Goal-directed sedation in the critically ill (propofol, fospropofol, local anesthetic)
   g. Postoperative pain, other types of acute inflammatory pain, prevention of persistent neuropathic postsurgical pain (e.g., anticonvulsants, clonidine, ketamine, sodium channel blockers)

From Pasero, C., & McCaffery, M. *Pain assessment and pharmacologic management*, p. 627, St. Louis, Mosby. © 2011, Pasero C, McCaffery M. May be duplicated for use in clinical practice.

Common Misconceptions about Adjuvant Analgesics

Misconception	Correction
Adjuvant analgesics are as reliable in providing pain relief as opioid and nonopioid analgesics.	Fewer patients respond adequately to adjuvant analgesics than to opioids and nonopioids. Furthermore, many adjuvant analgesics tend to have a much slower onset of analgesia and more adverse effects.
Adjuvants are only effective for neuropathic pain.	Some adjuvant analgesics such as antidepressants, corticosteroids, alpha$_2$-adrenergic agonists (e.g., clonidine), and cannabinoids are multipurpose analgesics that may be useful for both neuropathic and nociceptive (somatic and visceral) pain.
Adjuvant analgesics are appropriate only for persistent (chronic), not acute, pain.	There is growing evidence to support the role of adjuvant analgesics (e.g., anticonvulsants, sodium channel blockers, ketamine) in the treatment of both acute and persistent pain.
Use of adjuvant analgesics is no more time-consuming than use of other analgesic groups.	Drug selection and dose titration of adjuvants are usually more challenging and "labor intensive" than administration of opioid and nonopioid analgesics.
Pain relief from antidepressants depends on their ability to relieve depression in the patient with pain.	The analgesic effects of antidepressants are independent of their antidepressant activity. Patients who are depressed and those who are not depressed with pain report analgesia. Furthermore, the analgesic dose is often lower than that required to treat depression, and the onset of analgesia typically occurs much sooner, usually within 1 week.

Continued

Common Misconceptions about Adjuvant Analgesics—cont'd

Misconception	Correction
Antidepressants are more appropriate analgesics for burning neuropathic pain than for stabbing and lancinating (knifelike) neuropathic pain.	Research shows that antidepressants may be effective for both lancinating (knifelike) and continuous neuropathic pain.
Anticonvulsants are only used for persistent neuropathic pain.	Anticonvulsants now have a role in the treatment of acute pain, such as postoperative pain and prevention of persistent neuropathic postsurgical pain, as well as persistent mixed pain syndromes, such as fibromyalgia and some back pain.
Topical analgesics relieve only superficial pain.	Topical analgesics, such as lidocaine patch 5% and capsaicin, have been shown to be effective in relieving a variety of types of pain including some types of neuropathic pain.
Sedation alone is sufficient for painful procedures.	The low doses of sedative agents used for procedural sedation do not produce sufficient pain relief or entirely eliminate the memory of pain during the procedure. Sedation protocols for procedures thought to be painful should include the provision of analgesia regardless of the amnestic qualities of the sedative agent.
Drugs marketed as muscle relaxants, such as methocarbamol (Robaxin), relieve muscle pain by relaxing the muscle.	Well-controlled research is lacking to demonstrate that "muscle relaxants" relax skeletal muscle in humans. Although these drugs can relieve musculoskeletal pain, this may not be due to relaxation of skeletal muscle.

From Pasero, C., & McCaffery, M. *Pain assessment and pharmacologic management*, pp. 627-628, St. Louis, Mosby. © 2011, Pasero C, McCaffery M. May be duplicated for use in clinical practice.

Adjuvant Analgesics: Major Classes and Examples of Drugs

Pharmacologic Class/Generic Drug Names	Brand Name
Alpha$_2$-Adrenergic Agonists	
Clonidine	Catapres, Catapres TTS, Duraclon
Dexmedetomidine	Precedex
Tizanidine	Zanaflex
Anticonvulsants	
Carbamazepine	Tegretol
Clonazepam	Klonopin
Divalproex sodium	Depakote Sprinkle, Depakote DR, ER
Gabapentin	Neurontin
Lacosamide	Vimpat
Lamotrigine	Lamictal
Oxcarbazepine	Trileptal
Phenytoin	Dilantin
Pregabalin	Lyrica
Tiagabine	Gabitril
Topiramate	Topamax

Continued

Adjuvant Analgesics: Major Classes and Examples of Drugs—cont'd

Pharmacologic Class/Generic Drug Names	Brand Name
Valproic acid	Depacon (IV), Depakene (PO), Stavzor DR (PO), Valproate Sodium (IV) (valproates include divalproex sodium and valproic acid)
Zonisamide	Zonegran
Antidepressants	
Amitriptyline	Elavil
Bupropion	Aplenzin, Budeprion, Wellbutrin
Clomipramine	Anafranil
Desipramine	Norpramin
Doxepin	Sinequan
Duloxetine	Cymbalta
Fluoxetine	Prozac
Imipramine	Tofranil
Maprotiline	Ludiomil
Milnacipran	Savella
Mirtazapine	Remeron
Nefazodone	Serzone
Nortriptyline	Aventyl, Pamelor
Paroxetine	Paxil
Sertraline	Zoloft
Trazodone	Desyrel
Venlafaxine	Effexor
Cannabinoids	
Cannabis derivative	Sativex
Dronabinol	Marinol
Corticosteroids	
Dexamethasone	Baycadron, Decadron, Dexamethasone Intensol
Methylprednisolone	Depo-Medrol, Medrol, Solu-Medrol
Prednisone	Sterapred, Sterapred DS, Prednisone Intensol
Gamma Aminobutyric Acid (GABA) Agonists	
Baclofen	Lioresal
Fospropofol	Lusedra
Propofol	Diprivan
Sodium Channel Blockers	
Flecainide	Tambocor
Lidocaine (IV)	Lidocaine
Lidocaine patch 5%	Lidoderm

Continued

Adjuvant Analgesics: Major Classes and Examples of Drugs—cont'd

Pharmacologic Class/Generic Drug Names	Brand Name
Mexiletine	Mexitil
Tocainide	Tonocard
***N*-methyl-D-Aspartate (NMDA) Receptor Antagonists**	
Dextromethorphan	Delsym, Robafin Cough, Robitussin CoughGels
Ketamine	Ketalar
Neuroleptics	
Haloperidol	Haldol
Olanzapine	Zyprexa, Zydis
Pimozide	Orap
Psychostimulants	
Dextroamphetamine	Dexedrine
Methylphenidate	Concerta, Daytrana, Metadate, Methylin, Ritalin
Modafinil	Provigil
Skeletal "Muscle Relaxants"	
Carisoprodol	Soma
Chlorzoxazone	Parafon Forte DSC
Cyclobenzaprine	Flexeril
Methocarbamol	Robaxin
Orphenadrine	Norflex
Topical Agents	
Antidepressants (amitriptyline; doxepin) (compounded)	Elavil; Sinequan
Anticonvulsants (clonazepam) (compounded)	Klonopin
Capsaicin	Arthritis Formula Capiscum; Capzasin; Trixaicin; Zostrix; others
Clonidine	Catapres TTS
Ketamine (compounded)	Ketalar
Local anesthetics	EMLA; Lidoderm, L.M.X.4; Synera

Chapter 21 General Considerations in the Use of Adjuvant Analgesics

THE use of adjuvant analgesics in the management of pain is a "labor intensive" endeavor that includes careful patient selection, evaluating and selecting the best agent and dosing regimen, assessing response to treatment, and adjusting therapy to achieve the greatest benefit. All these activities are predicated on a systematic assessment of the patient, both initially and throughout the course of therapy. Over time, changes in pain, adverse effects, or any concerns regarding quality of life may lead to modifications in therapeutic approaches to managing pain.

Few studies actually capture the frequency with which adjuvant therapy is used. In one study on the use of treatment modalities, 723 community residents with moderate to severe pain were surveyed about their use of analgesics (Vallerand, Fouladbakhsh, Templin, 2005). Approximately 75% reported taking nonopioids, 15% reported taking opioids, and 11.6% reported taking adjuvant analgesics. Of concern, fully 28% were taking drugs for pain but had not informed their primary care providers. This finding underscores the importance of patient education about the need for communication with the health care provider who prescribes their analgesics. The safe prescription of the adjuvant analgesics depends on accurate information about all the drugs taken by the patient (see the discussion of patient education at the end of Section V).

Drug Selection

The selection of a specific adjuvant analgesic is usually based on the nature and characteristics of pain and the presence of other symptoms and co-morbidities. For example, an early trial of an analgesic antidepressant is justified by the existence of a co-morbid depression, which would be considered a separate target for this therapy.

Drug selection also may be influenced by the results of specific studies and accumulated clinical experience. For example, there are both controlled trials and several decades of experience suggesting the efficacy of carbamazepine in trigeminal neuralgia, and patients with this disorder often are offered a trial of this drug first. Similarly, patients with fibromyalgia usually are considered for a trial of the drugs that have been studied and are now approved for this condition, such as pregabalin and duloxetine.

In most circumstances, both the existing data and experience are insufficient to narrow the choice of drug substantially. Many options exist, and drug selection is based on guidelines or other factors; if one drug fails to provide adequate pain relief, others may be tried. In short, most of the therapeutic process involving the adjuvant analgesics follows an "informed trial-and-error" strategy in which drugs are offered in sequential trials based on the current evidence base, clinical experience, and other factors, such as age, co-existing medical conditions, prior response to a particular drug, issues with convenience and adherence to therapy, cost and availability of agents, and access to care and follow-up treatment. Decisions should be thoughtfully determined by an examination of the potential benefits and risks associated with therapy (Gatchel, Okifuji, 2006).

Cost comparison research is largely lacking, and the complex issue of cost-effectiveness usually ends with a decision influenced by the need for out-of-pocket expenses (a so-called *cost-minimization strategy*). A more sophisticated analysis involves assessment of pain intensity and distress, drug options, dosing regimen, likelihood of adherence, ancillary costs (e.g., other medications needed to control the adverse effects of the analgesics), and third-party payer influence (Gore, Sadosky, Tai, et al., 2007; O'Connor, Noyes, Holloway, 2007; Tarride, Gordon, Vera-Llonch, et al., 2006). The limited information about these factors at the start of therapy typically results in a prediction about overall costs that is highly tentative. An excellent cost analysis of the effect of pregabalin in the treatment of radiculopathy in the primary care setting found that pregablin alone or as an add-on therapy at doses within the recommended range significantly reduced pain, which translated into meaningful reductions in the use of both health care and non–health care resources (Saldana, Navarro, Perez, et al., 2010). The increases in drug cost were offset by a significant decrease in the costs associated with other components of health care, such as complementary tests, medical visits, and nondrug therapies.

Patient preference also is critical to consider in drug selection. Patients may express preferences that are idiosyncratic (e.g., knowledge of a family member who experienced benefit or adverse effects from a drug) or informed by factors that may influence their ability to tolerate a drug or adhere to therapy. Collaborative decision making around the use of therapeutic options for pain relief increases the likelihood that the patient will be adherent with the treatment plan (Manias, Williams, 2008).

Dosing

The adjuvant analgesics are heterogeneous, and dosing regimens vary. A few of the drugs are available as parenteral formulations, which can be used in monitored environments and administered at full doses promptly (e.g., a relatively large, intravenous [IV] loading dose of a corticosteroid, lidocaine, or valproate in the management of severe neuropathic pain).

In the more common scenario of oral drug administration in the ambulatory setting, low initial doses and gradual dose escalation may avoid early adverse effects or allow tolerance or adjustment to the adverse effects. In medically ill patients, this precaution is especially appropriate when adjuvant analgesics are initiated. When low doses and gradual titration to therapeutic effects are employed, it is easier to optimize therapy and balance pain relief with adverse effects. In some cases, patients must be forewarned that onset of analgesia with adjuvant drugs is likely to be delayed. Otherwise, patients may become discouraged and stop taking the drug.

Variability in Response

There is considerable variability among individuals in their response to adjuvant analgesics, including agents within the same class. While specific patient characteristics (e.g., advanced age, co-existing organ dysfunction or failure, and inherent differences in the ways patients metabolize and respond to drugs) may increase the likelihood of some common adverse effects, it is nonetheless true that neither beneficial nor unfavorable effects from any specific medication can be reliably predicted. The potential utility of adjuvant analgesics may only be established through repeated trial and error, allowing sufficient time to determine whether an adjuvant agent is likely to reduce pain.

The existence of significant intraindividual variation in the response to the large group of adjuvant analgesics must be explained to patients. If a treatment regimen is not successful, it is also critical that patients are aware of other options that can be tried. Frustration with the delay in finding an effective drug and the time required with each drug to explore the dose range should be acknowledged, but patients also should be encouraged to hold on to hope that a useful therapy will be found.

Patient Co-Morbidities

As noted, a medical or psychiatric co-morbidity may be an independent target for therapy, and as such, help guide the decision to try one type of adjuvant analgesic over another. Co-morbidities also must be recognized as potential impediments to the safe use of these drugs. For example, patients with pulmonary disease may be susceptible to the sedating effects of drugs and be placed at increased risk for respiratory problems or respiratory depression with the addition of sedating adjuvant analgesics. Debilitated patients are more prone to adverse effects such as sedation or confusion that may lead to falls or further functional decline. Renal and hepatic dysfunction can interfere with drug metabolism and excretion. Older adults may already have complex medication regimens for the management of other health problems. Therefore, it is important to identify potential drug-drug interactions that could alter risk assessment.

Adjuvant Analgesics During Pregnancy and Breast-Feeding

Teratogenic effects have been reported with some of the adjuvant analgesics, but little data exist to fully assess safety. Many have warnings against their use during pregnancy or recommendations for careful consideration of risk versus benefit (Lacy, Armstrong, Goldman, et al., 2008). For example, although the risk/benefit ratio is not defined for steroid use during the second and third trimesters of pregnancy, they should be avoided during the first trimester because they are associated with teratogenic effects (Hess, Aleshi, 2008).

Anticonvulsants (e.g., carbamazepine and valproic acid) have been studied during pregnancy primarily in women with epilepsy. There is twice the risk of congenital defects, such as cleft palate and congenital heart disease, in offspring of women who take them during pregnancy compared with the general population (Viscomi, Rathmell, 1998). Phenytoin should be avoided, as use is associated with a 7% increased risk of fetal hydantoin syndrome (microencephaly, mental deficiency, and craniofacial abnormalities). Tricyclic antidepressants (TCAs) are generally not recommended during pregnancy, but their benefit may outweigh the risk in some patients (Viscomi, Rathmell, 1998). First-trimester exposure to benzodiazepines (e.g., diazepam) may also carry an elevated risk of fetal congenital malformation, although this is poorly studied (Viscomi, Rathmell, 1998). Maternal benzodiazepine use can cause sedation and poor feeding in nursing infants so should be avoided.

Local anesthetics are generally considered safe, but due to progesterone-induced sensitivity to local anesthetics, dose is often reduced (Hess, Aleshi, 2008). All local anesthetic drugs cross the placenta, and the factors that influence maternal toxicity will influence fetal toxicity. Maternal administration of lidocaine and mepivacaine has been implicated in reduction of muscle tone in the neonate, but this appears to be less of a problem with bupivacaine because it binds to maternal plasma proteins better (Woods, DiFazio, 1995). Local anesthetics are considered safe during breast-feeding. Clonidine also is thought to produce minimal effects on infants during pregnancy and breast-feeding (Viscomi, Rathmell, 1998).

Women are advised to discuss the need to discontinue or avoid some of the adjuvant analgesics prior to becoming pregnant or breast-feeding whenever possible. Alternate methods for managing pain may be warranted in patients with underlying persistent pain and can be implemented in advance (e.g., opioid administration for some types of neuropathic pain; see Section IV). Clearly, more research is needed regarding the safe use of adjuvant analgesics during pregnancy and breast-feeding.

Multimodal Therapy

Broad acceptance of a role in pain management for the adjuvant analgesic drugs is premised on the growing importance of multimodal treatment for persistent (chronic) pain. As discussed in Section I, multimodal therapy is a relatively new concept, first proposed in the early 1990s and applied primarily to the treatment of acute pain and prevention of persistent postsurgical pain (Buvanendran, Kroin, 2009; Buvanendran, Kroin, Della Valle, et al., 2010; Gartner, Kroman, Callesen, et al., 2008; Kehlet, Jensen, Woolf, 2006; Milch, 2005; Pasero,

2003a; Polomano, Rathmell, Krenzischek, et al., 2008; Tang, Evans, Chaput, et al., 2009). Multimodal therapy involves the use of two or more classes of analgesics to target different pain mechanisms in the peripheral or central nervous system (see Section I). It relies on the thoughtful and rational combination of analgesics to maximize pain relief and prevent analgesic gaps that may lead to worsening pain or unnecessary bouts of uncontrolled pain (Carr, Reines, Schaffer, et al., 2005).

A multimodal approach may allow lower doses of each of the drugs in the treatment plan, and lower doses have the potential to produce fewer adverse effects (Ashburn, Caplan, Carr, et al., 2004; Brodner, Van Aken, Hertle, et al., 2001). Further, multimodal analgesia can result in comparable or greater pain relief than can be achieved with any single analgesic (Busch, Shore, Bhandari, et al., 2006; Butterfield, Schwarz, Ries, et al., 2001; Cassinelli, Dean, Garcia, et al., 2008; Huang, Wang, Wang, et al., 2008; White, 2005). In the setting of postoperative pain, the use of combination therapy to prevent both inflammatory and neuropathic pain is likely to yield the best immediate results and also offers the promise of reducing the incidence of prolonged or persistent postsurgical pain (Kehlet, Jensen, Woolf, 2006).

The multimodal strategy also has a role in the management of persistent pain. This is true in all of the various practice settings, including the emergency department (Baker, 2005), outpatient treatment sites (Gatchel, Okifuji, 2006), and settings providing specialist palliative care (Soares, Chan, 2007). The complex nature of the many persistent pain conditions indicates the need for appropriate combinations of analgesics to target different underlying mechanisms (Argoff, Albrecht, Irving, et al., 2009).

Multimodal therapy also is a useful strategy for addressing the common problem of symptom distress related to symptoms other than pain. Patients with acute or persistent pain often experience additional symptoms, which as noted, may influence the decision to try one of the adjuvant analgesics over another. More broadly, the experience of multiple symptoms also may guide the use of multiple drugs, some of which are targeted to distressing conditions, such as insomnia, that accompany pain and may be a factor in worsening it (Gan, Meyer, Apfel, et al., 2003; 2007; Gartner, Kroman, Callesen, et al., 2008).

Polypharmacy

The term *polypharmacy* carries a negative connotation, in contrast to multimodal therapy or combination therapy. Whereas multimodal therapy is based on rational combinations of analgesics with differing underlying mechanisms to achieve the most benefit in pain control, polypharmacy suggests the use of drug combinations that are irrational and less effective or safe than a regimen that has fewer or different agents.

Polypharmacy is most likely to occur in populations and settings in which rational multimodal therapy is appropriate and encouraged. For example, in the palliative care setting, adjuvant analgesics are typically administered to patients who are already receiving multiple drugs. Although complex regimens are widely regarded as appropriate in the care of terminally ill patients, the potential for additive or unpredictable adverse effects must be anticipated whenever an adjuvant is added to an existing drug regimen.

Polypharmacy is often a problem in older adults who may have complex medical conditions, are more susceptible to adverse effects of medications and combinations of drugs, and may be less adherent to complex medication schedules (American Geriatrics Society, 2002; Ruoff, 2002). A longitudinal cohort study of 2737 adults age 65 years and older found an association between cognitive decline and the combined use of medications that act on the central nervous system (CNS), especially when taken in high doses (Wright, Roumani, Boudreau, et al., 2009). The researchers emphasized the importance of careful drug selection and using the lowest effective doses, especially when treating the co-morbidities of pain and psychiatric conditions in older adults. These principles apply to all patients with pain.

Many of the adjuvant analgesics are metabolized in the liver by the cytochrome P450 system of isoenzymes (Virani, Mailis, Shapiro, et al., 1997) (see Chapter 11 for more on this). This also raises concern about the potential for drug-drug interactions. Patients may take drugs that either induce or block specific isoenzymes. An enzyme that is induced can metabolize substrates faster or more completely, leading to plasma drug concentrations less than would be expected at a specific dose. Conversely, an enzyme that is blocked could slow metabolism and lead to higher than anticipated concentrations of newly added drugs.

There are many examples of potentially problematic interactions. Some chemotherapeutic agents (Novy, Stupp, Rossetti, 2009; Yap, Chui, Chan, 2008) and oral antidiabetic agents (Schiltmeyer, Kropeit, Cawello, et al., 2006) may interfere with some analgesics. Concurrent administration of antidepressants that are substrates for the CYP2D6 enzyme (e.g., serotonin norepinephrine reuptake inhibitors [SNRIs] and TCAs) can increase tricyclic levels and lead to seizure activity (Lamoure, 2007). Clinicians who care for individuals with pain must become familiar with each drug's metabolism and the way the various drugs interact with the cytochrome P450 enzymes to provide safe and effective therapy. Patients must be told to report adverse effects promptly, and in some cases serum drug concentrations should be closely monitored to prevent toxicity, such as in patients who take multiple other medications.

Polypharmacy may lead to negative effects that are more subtle than potentially dangerous plasma levels of a drug. When a patient is receiving opioid and nonopioid analgesics, for example, the decision to initiate or continue an adjuvant analgesic must be based on careful assessment of patient outcomes and a clear understanding of the goals of therapy. If adjuvant medications yield demonstrable benefits without adverse effects that impair function or quality of life, then there may be ample justification for adding or continuing them. This is included among the benefits of a rational multimodal therapeutic strategy. Attempting to achieve additional pain relief at the cost of inducing untoward adverse effects such as sedation or cognitive impairment is not acceptable practice in patients who desire a more active lifestyle but may be appropriate for those who seek comfort as the only goal of treatment.

Positioning of Treatment

As described in Section IV, opioids are first-line analgesics for severe acute pain and moderate to severe persistent pain related to active cancer or other advanced illnesses (Hanks, Cherny, Fallon, 2004; Lussier, Portenoy, 2004). Opioids remain controversial in the treatment of persistent noncancer pain, and first-line use should be considered only when the severity of the pain or the urgency of treatment is such that aggressive opioid dosing is perceived to be the most likely way to help promptly (Dworkin, Backonja, Rowbotham, et al., 2003).

For patients with persistent noncancer pain, the NSAIDs or adjuvant analgesics are usually viewed as the first-line therapies. For those with acute postoperative pain, an adjuvant analgesic, such as an anticonvulsant, may be considered for preoperative or immediate postoperative administration, as an adjunct to an opioid regimen.

The adjuvant analgesics, as a group, are considered to be adjunctive to opioid therapy in the setting of moderate to severe pain related to active cancer or other serious illnesses, because extensive experience supports the conclusion that analgesic effects from opioids are both more reliable and faster in onset (Lussier, Huskey, Portenoy, 2004; Lussier, Portenoy, 2004). This observation has not been contradicted in the literature, which generally lacks well-designed, controlled trials in cancer populations. Slower onset of analgesic effects for most adjuvant agents and the need to initiate therapy at low doses to avoid adverse effects also may be responsible for achieving inconsistent benefits (Lussier, Portenoy, 2004).

Survey data demonstrate satisfactory pain relief within days for 70% to 90% of cancer patients who receive opioid therapy (Lussier, Huskey, Portenoy, 2004; Lussier, Portenoy, 2004; Ripamonti, Dickerson, 2001); however, more time may be needed to adjust the dose of an adjuvant analgesic and judge its effects (Maizels, McCarberg, 2005; Saarto, Wiffen, 2007). Studies of TCAs show that these drugs may require treatment for weeks to obtain optimal results; with adequate dosing, pain may be relieved by more than 50% in 50% to 75% of patients with neuropathic pain (Lussier, Huskey, Portenoy, 2004; Lussier, Portenoy, 2004).

Although the extant data are insufficient to conclude that all adjuvant analgesics perform less well than an opioid in every type of pain experienced by cancer patients, the safest and most efficient approach in patients with serious medical illness usually involves the addition of an adjuvant analgesic to an opioid regimen that is not producing adequate analgesia despite dose escalation to limiting adverse effects (Lussier, Huskey, Portenoy, 2004; Lussier, Portenoy, 2004). Unless another indication for an earlier trial exists (e.g., a co-morbidity that may also respond to the drug, a history of problems with opioids, or a type of pain that may be particularly responsive to a specific adjuvant), it is reasonable to initiate treatment with the adjuvant analgesic after the opioid dose has been optimized. In practice, some clinicians attempt to improve patient response by initiating therapy with an opioid and an adjuvant analgesic concurrently, but it must be recognized that this approach increases the risk of additive toxicity and may make it difficult to determine which drug is responsible for the resulting analgesia or adverse effects.

Conclusion

The adjuvant analgesic group is the largest group of analgesics, representing drugs that vary widely in their underlying mechanisms of action and indications for use. Selection of the optimal adjuvant analgesic is strongly influenced by the type of pain to be treated as well as a number of patient factors, including age, coexisting disease, and potential for drug-drug interactions. Cost of the drug is another major consideration. Almost all of the adjuvant analgesics require titration of dose to find a balance between pain relief and adverse effects.

Chapter 22 Multipurpose Adjuvant Analgesics

nonopioid analgesics (Portenoy, 2000). The multipurpose adjuvant analgesics that are currently considered to be among the more useful in clinical practice include antidepressants, corticosteroids, and alpha$_2$-adrenergic agonists (e.g., clonidine). Many of the multipurpose adjuvant analgesics are appropriate for both acute pain and persistent pain. Antidepressants have a delayed onset of analgesia, making them inappropriate for acute pain. Other drug classes, such as the sodium channel blockers and cannabinoids, have evidence to suggest broad applicability, but conventional use continues to position them solely for neuropathic pain (Lussier, Portenoy, 2004). Although the use of topical drugs is restricted by the location of pain, there are many types, and, combined, they too may be considered to have multiple purposes (see Chapter 24). See Table V-1, pp. 748-756, at the end of Section V for the characteristics and dosing guidelines for many of the multipurpose adjuvant analgesics.

Antidepressant Drugs

Antidepressant adjuvant analgesics are usually divided into two major groups: the tricyclic antidepressants (TCAs) and the newer biogenic amine reuptake inhibitors (Table 22-1). Of the latter group, the serotonin and norepinephrine reuptake inhibitors (SNRIs) are clearly analgesics, whereas research is lacking or inconsistent regarding the analgesic potential of the selective serotonin reuptake inhibitors (SSRIs) (Arnold, 2007; Collins, Moore, McQuay, et al., 2000; Kroenke, Krebs, Bair, 2009; Saarto, Wiffen, 2007; Veves, Backonja, Malik, 2008).

The multipurpose nature of antidepressants is demonstrated in their efficacy as analgesics in neuropathic pain states, such as painful diabetic neuropathy and postherpetic neuralgia, and other types of persistent pain states, such as headache, fibromyalgia, and some types of back pain. A meta-analysis of 18 randomized controlled trials concluded that there is strong evidence for the use of antidepressants in the treatment of fibromyalgia, with impressive improvements in pain, depression, fatigue, sleep disturbances, and health-related quality of life (Hauser, Bernardy, Uceyler, et al., 2009). These data have

DATA supporting the analgesic efficacy of some adjuvant drug classes are derived from numerous studies of very diverse syndromes. These drugs may be termed *multipurpose* and can be considered for any type of pain, fundamentally similar in this way to the opioids and

Table 22-1	Antidepressant Adjuvant Analgesics: Classes with Examples of Drugs	

Classes	Examples
Tricyclic Antidepressants	
Tertiary amines	Amitriptyline (Elavil)
	Clomipramine (Anafranil)
	Doxepin
	Imipramine (Tofranil)
Secondary amines	Desipramine (Norpramin)
	Nortriptyline (Pamelor)
Triazolopyridine	Trazodone
"Newer" Second-Generation Antidepressants	
Serotonin norepinephrine reuptake inhibitors (SNRIs)	Bupropion (Wellbutrin)
	Duloxetine (Cymbalta)
	Milnacipran (Savella)
	Venlafaxine (Effexor)
Tetracyclic compound	Mirtazapine (Remeron)
Selective serotonin reuptake inhibitors (SSRIs)	Fluoxetine (Prozac)
	Paroxetine (Paxil)
	Sertraline (Zoloft)

From Pasero, C., & McCaffery, M. *Pain assessment and pharmacologic management,* p. 637, St. Louis, Mosby. © 2011, Pasero C, McCaffery M. May be duplicated for use in clinical practice.

influenced treatment guidelines for fibromyalgia, which now include the early use of antidepressants (Hauser, Thieme, Turk, 2009). Guidelines also suggest that antidepressants should be considered an option for persistent low back pain, notwithstanding the lack of research focused on the newer drugs, specifically the SNRIs (Chou, Qaseem, Snow, et al., 2007).

An early systematic review of randomized controlled trials summarized the compelling evidence that antidepressants are efficacious in varied types of neuropathic pain (McQuay, Tramer, Nye, et al., 1996). Antidepressants are now identified as first-line analgesics in neuropathic pain guidelines (Dworkin, Backonja, Rowbotham, et al., 2003; Dworkin, O'Connor, Backonja, et al., 2007; Moulin, Clark, Gilron, et al., 2007). Anticonvulsants are another first-line choice for neuropathic pain and are discussed later in this section (see Chapter 23). Several excellent systematic reviews, some with related evidence-based guidelines for drug selection, provide additional support for the use of antidepressants in the management of neuropathic pain (Finnerup, Otto, McQuay, et al., 2005; Saarto, Wiffen, 2007; Kroenke, Krebs, Bair, et al., 2009). Data from another systematic review showed that there is no difference between antidepressants and anticonvulsants in the likelihood of achieving pain control (Chou, Carson, Chan, 2009).

Tricyclic Antidepressants (TCAs)

Evidence is compelling that the TCAs produce analgesia for a variety of chronic (persistent) pain syndromes including both neuropathic and other types of persistent pain (Argoff, Backonja, Belgrade, et al., 2006; Arnold, 2007; Hauser, Bernardy, Uceyler, et al., 2009; Dworkin, Backonja, Rowbotham, et al., 2003; Dworkin, O'Connor, Backonja, et al., 2007; Moulin, Clark, Gilron, et al., 2007; Perrot, Javier, Marty, et al., 2008; Tomkins, Jackson, O'Malley, et al., 2001; Verdu, Decosterd, Buclin, et al., 2008). The efficacy of the tertiary amine compounds has been demonstrated in a large number of controlled and uncontrolled trials (see each TCA listed below). Amitriptyline (Elavil), a tertiary amine, has an abundance of research showing efficacy and has been used for many years to treat a variety of types of persistent pain. Adverse effects are common, however, and the risk of more serious adverse effects, such as orthostatic hypotension, is relatively high (Curtis, Ostbye, Sendersky, et al., 2004; Dworkin, O'Connor, Backonja, et al., 2007).

Although research is more limited with the secondary amines, such as desipramine (Norpramin) and nortriptyline (Aventyl, Pamelor), they have also been shown to be efficacious in a variety of painful conditions and usually are better tolerated (American Geriatrics Society, 2002; Dworkin, Backonja, Rowbotham, et al., 2003; Dworkin, O'Connor, Backonja, et al., 2007; Gore, Dukes, Rowbotham, et al., 2006; Simon, Lipman, Caudill-Slosberg, et al., 2002). Some neuropathic guidelines recommend the use of a tertiary amine TCA only if a secondary amine TCA is unavailable (Dworkin, Backonja, Rowbotham, et al., 2003; Dworkin, O'Connor, Backonja, et al., 2007). This recommendation is particularly appropriate in high-risk populations, such as older adults who are at greater risk for antidepressant adverse effects, especially when they are administered in high doses and in combination with other CNS-acting medications (Wright, Roumani, Boudreau, et al., 2009). An increasingly popular alternative to the secondary amine TCAs is the SNRI antidepressants, all of which have a better toxicity profile than the TCAs (see adverse effects).

The best evidence for the use of TCAs for the treatment of neuropathic pain is summarized in several clinical reviews (Collins, Moore, McQuay, et al., 2000; Dobecki, Schocket, Wallace, 2006; Jensen, Finnerup, 2007; Dworkin, Backonja, Rowbotham, et al., 2003; Verdu, Decosterd, Buclin, et al., 2008). Agents in this class are useful for managing all types of dysesthesias (abnormal unpleasant sensations), such as burning, electrical-like, shock-like, shooting, and lancinating (stabbing). A Cochrane Collaboration Review of 61 randomized controlled trials documented the efficacy of TCAs and reported the following additional findings (Saarto, Wiffen, 2007):

- The number-needed-to-treat (NNT) when TCAs are studied as analgesics for varied types of neuropathic pain averages 3.6 (95% CI 3 to 4.5), which means that it is necessary to treat 3 to 4 patients to find one who gets at least a 50% reduction in pain; in other words, one-third of patients with neuropathic pain who take TCAs achieve moderate pain relief.

- Amitriptyline has been the best studied TCA, and in a range of doses up to 150 mg/day (10 studies, 588 patients), this drug has an NNT of 3.1 (95% CI 2.5 to 4.2).
- Studies of painful HIV-related neuropathy have not confirmed the efficacy of the TCAs.
- Analgesic doses for TCAs are typically less than antidepressant doses, and the effect on pain can be independent of any effect on depression.
- Although several small studies have suggested that analgesic efficacy correlates with dose, dose-response data have not been established; nonetheless, TCAs must be titrated in individual patients to identify responders and, within the group of responders, achieve the most effective dose (gradual titration also reduces the risk of adverse effects and is especially important in older patients).
- Across studies (N = 453), 13% of participants dropped out of active groups for a variety of reasons including intolerable adverse effects; discontinuation of dosing due to adverse effects is likely to be more prevalent in clinical populations, and prescribers usually attempt to select specific drugs based on relatively more favorable adverse effect profiles.

Amitriptyline

Amitriptyline (Elavil) is a tertiary amine TCA and has been extensively studied as an analgesic. The following are among the pain syndromes for which this drug has established analgesic efficacy:

- Postherpetic neuralgia (Argoff, Backonja, Belgrade, et al., 2006; Bowsher, 2003; Collins, Moore, McQuay, et al., 2000; Dubinsky, Kabbani, El-Chami, et al., 2004; Rowbotham, Reisner, Davies, et al., 2005)
- Painful diabetic neuropathy (Boulton, Vinik, Arezzo, et al., 2005; Collins, Moore, McQuay, et al., 2000; Duby, Campbell, Setter, et al., 2004; Max, Culnane, Schafer, et al., 1987; Max, Lynch, Muir, et al., 1992)
- Fibromyalgia (Arnold, 2007; Nishishinya, Urrutia, Walitt, et al., 2008; Hauser, Bernardy, Uceyler, et al., 2009; Heymann, Helfenstein, Feldman, 2001; Uceyler, Hauser, Sommer, 2008) (see also Hauser, Thieme, Turk, 2009)
- Migraine and other types of headache (Ashina, Bendtsen, Jensen, 2004; Descombes, Brefel-Courbon, Thalamas, et al., 2001; Keskinbora, Aydinli, 2008; Krymchantowski, Silva, Barbosa, et al., 2002)
- Arthritis (Frank, Kashini, Parker, et al., 1988; Katz, Rothenberg, 2005; Simon, Lipman, Caudill-Slosberg, et al., 2002)
- Central spinal cord injury pain (Cardenas, Warms, Turner, et al., 2002)
- Central post-stroke pain (Frese, Husstedt, Ringelstein, et al., 2006; Kumar, Kalita, Kumar, et al., 2009)
- Persistent facial pain (List, Axelsson, Leijon, 2003)

- Cancer-related neuropathic pain (Miaskowski, Cleary, Burney, et al., 2005; Ventafridda, Bonezzi, Caraceni, et al., 1987)
- Chemotherapy-induced neuropathy (Note: 50 mg/day was thought to be too low to produce positive effects) (Kautio, Haanpaa, Saarto, et al., 2008)
- Interstitial cystitis (van Ophoven, Pokupic, Heinecke, et al., 2004)
- As mentioned, antidepressants are not appropriate for treatment of acute pain because of the delay in time before appreciable analgesia. However, although not approved for use in the United States at the time of publication, a phase I trial of IV amitriptyline established the safety of a 25 mg to 50 mg preoperative infusion (Fridrich, Colvin, Zizza, et al., 2007). (See amitriptyline patient medication information, Form V-1 on pp. 759-760, at the end of Section V).

Desipramine

Desipramine (Norpramin) is a secondary amine TCA. It has relatively more effect on norepinephrine reuptake than amitriptyline and usually causes fewer adverse effects. (See desipramine patient medication information, Form V-5 on pp. 767-768, at the end of Section V). Clinical reviews and single studies have shown its efficacy in the following:

- Postherpetic neuralgia (Collins, Moore, McQuay, et al., 2000; Dubinsky, Kabbani, El-Chami, et al., 2004; Max, Lynch, Muir, et al., 1992; O'Connor, Noyes, Holloway, 2007; Zin, Nissen, Smith, et al., 2008)
- Painful diabetic neuropathy (Argoff, Backonja, Belgrade, et al., 2006; Boulton, Vinik, Arezzo, et al., 2005; Collins, Moore, McQuay, et al., 2000; Duby, Campbell, Setter, et al., 2004; Zin, Nissen, Smith, et al., 2008)
- Cancer-related neuropathic pain (Miaskowski, Cleary, Burney, et al., 2005)
- Arthritis (Simon, Lipman, Caudill-Slosberg, et al., 2002)

Nortriptyline

Nortriptyline (Aventyl, Pamelor) also is a secondary amine compound. (See nortriptyline patient medication information, Form V-10 on pp. 777-778, at the end of Section V). It has been researched for the following types of pain:

- Fibromyalgia (Heyman, Helfenstein, Feldman, 2001) (See also Hauser, Thieme, Turk, 2009.)
- Postherpetic neuralgia (Dubinsky, Kabbani, El-Chami, et al., 2004)
- Painful diabetic neuropathy (Boulton, Vinik, Arezzo, et al., 2005)
- Persistent lumbar radiculopathy (Khoromi, Cui, Nackers, et al., 2007)
- Cancer-related neuropathic pain (Miaskowski, Cleary, Burney, et al., 2005)
- Chemotherapy-induced neuropathy (Hammack, Michalak, Loprinzi, et al., 2002)
- Arthritis (Simon, Lipman, Caudill-Slosberg, et al., 2002)

"Newer" Antidepressants

Evidence of analgesic efficacy is compelling for the drugs that are synaptic reuptake blockers of both serotonin and norepinephrine. The SNRIs have a better adverse effect profile than TCAs (Zin, Nissen, Smith, et al., 2008). Duloxetine (Cymbalta) has been most studied, and milnacipran (Savella), an SNRI recently released in the United States, also has been approved for the treatment of fibromyalgia pain. There is limited evidence that venlafaxine (Effexor) is analgesic and, as yet, no evidence in support of the newer desvenlafaxine (Pristiq).

Bupropion (Aplenzin, Budeprion, Wellbutrin) and mirtazapine (Remeron) are relatively older drugs and have structures and actions distinct from the TCAs and SNRIs. Both increase activity in the pathways that use biogenic amines, including serotonin, norepinephrine, and dopamine. Evidence of analgesia from these drugs is very limited, but they are sometimes considered for patients with persistent pain, particularly when a concurrent symptom, such as fatigue or insomnia, would benefit from targeted treatment.

Guidelines for the treatment of neuropathic pain that recommend the analgesic antidepressants as possible first-line or second-line drugs suggest that consideration be given to the use of the SNRIs over the TCAs because of a more favorable adverse effect profile (Dworkin, Backonja, Rowbotham, et al., 2003; Moulin, Clark, Gilron, et al., 2007). There have been no comparative effectiveness trials, and the decision to select one or another is based on risk assessment and best clinical judgment. The newer antidepressants are discussed in alphabetical order in the following paragraphs.

Bupropion

Bupropion (Aplenzin, Budeprion, Wellbutrin) is distinguished from the TCAs and SNRIs because it inhibits neuronal norepinephrine reuptake and, less potently, dopamine reuptake (Katz, Penella-Vaughn, Hetzel, et al., 2005). The drug can be useful in the management of neuropathic pain (Semenchuk, Davis, 2000; Semenchuk, Sherma, Davis, 2001), but was found ineffective for relief of non-neuropathic persistent low back pain (Katz, Pennella-Vaughan, Hetzel, et al., 2005). An extensive review suggested bupropion as an option for painful diabetic neuropathy (Duby, Campbell, Setter, et al., 2004), but guidelines list it as a drug with limited evidence for this condition (Argoff, Backonja, Belgrade, et al., 2006). Reported case series indicate that this agent can help relieve pain associated with persistent headache (Pinsker, 1998).

Bupropion has a low risk of somnolence and sexual dysfunction, adverse effects that may be limiting with other antidepressants. Some patients report increased energy that appears to be unrelated to mood effects. This has led to empirical use of this drug for fatigue.

Duloxetine

Duloxetine (Cymbalta) is an established analgesic based on the results of numerous controlled trials (Dworkin, Backonja, Rowbotham, et al., 2003; Kroenke, Krebs, Bair, 2009). In the United States, it is approved for the treatment of fibromyalgia, and randomized controlled studies have shown its effectiveness for this type of pain (Arnold, Lu, Crofford, et al., 2004; Arnold, Rosen, Pritchett, et al., 2005; Hauser, Bernardy, Ucelyler, et al., 2009). A large (N = 520) randomized controlled 6-month trial of patients with fibromyalgia with or without major depression demonstrated improvements in both pain severity and Patient Global Impressions of Improvement (PGI-I) scores regardless of whether or not the patients were depressed (Russell, Mease, Smith, et al., 2008). Others have observed similar findings (Arnold, Hudson, Wang, et al., 2009). A 1-year trial established the long-term safety and efficacy of duloxetine in 350 women with fibromyalgia (Chappell, Littlejohn, Kajdasz, et al., 2009).

A number of randomized controlled studies also report that duloxetine is efficacious for depression-associated pain (Brecht, Courtecuisse, Debieuvre, et al., 2007; Perahia, Pritchett, Raskin, 2006; Raskin, Wiltse, Siegal, et al., 2007). In older depressed patients, duloxetine can improve mood, cognition, and pain (Raskin, Wiltse, Siegal, et al., 2007). However, a meta-analysis of five randomized controlled trials observed a lack of consistency in research findings and suggested that reports of pain relief in patients with depression may be overestimated (Spielmans, 2008).

Duloxetine also is approved for treatment of painful diabetic neuropathy. Numerous randomized controlled trials have shown its efficacy for this type of pain (Goldstein, Lu, Detke, et al., 2005; Kajdasz, Iyengar, Desaiah, et al., 2007; Pritchett, McCarberg, Watkin, et al., 2007; Raskin, Pritchett, Wang, et al., 2005), and some guidelines recommend it as a first-line analgesic for this condition (Argoff, Backonja, Belgrade, et al., 2006). One study suggested that relatively high pain intensity, but no other variable (e.g., age, type and duration of diabetes, or severity of neuropathy), predicted the efficacy of duloxetine (Ziegler, Pritchett, Wang, et al., 2007). A meta-analysis concluded that duloxetine had efficacy and tolerability comparable to gabapentin and pregabalin in diabetic peripheral neuropathic pain (Quilici, Chancellor, Lothgren, et al., 2009).

A study conducted in the United Kingdom concluded that duloxetine is a cost-effective and efficacious agent for the pain of diabetic peripheral neuropathy (Beard, McCrink, Le, et al., 2008). Similar results were found in a study in the United States, in which patients who participated in a previous randomized controlled study of painful diabetic neuropathy were re-randomized for a 52-week trial of 60 mg of duloxetine compared with routine treatment, which most often included gabapentin, venlafaxine, or amitriptyline (Wu, Birnbaum, Mareva, et al., 2006). Duloxetine was found to be more cost-effective than routine treatment from both employer and societal perspectives, which included patients' out-of-pocket expenses.

Other studies have shown that the benefits produced by duloxetine can be sustained over time (Mease, Russell, Kajdasz, et al., 2009; Russell, Mease, Smith, et al., 2008; Wernicke, Wang, Pritchett, et al., 2007) and that improved functional outcomes accompany analgesia (Armstrong, Chappell, Le, et al., 2007; Arnold, Lu, Crofford, et al., 2004; Arnold, Rosen, Pritchett, et al., 2005; Russell, Mease, Smith, et al., 2008; Sullivan, Benlety, Fan, et al., 2009; Wernicke, Wang, Pritchett, et al., 2007). In summary, these favorable data support recent guidelines for the treatment of neuropathic pain, which designate the SNRIs as either first-line analgesics (Dworkin, O'Connnor, Backonja, et al., 2007) or second-line analgesics (Moulin, Clark, Gilron, et al., 2007).

Duloxetine may be effective for central pain as well. An open-label study revealed beneficial effects of duloxetine for the treatment of pain associated with Parkinson disease (Djaldetti, Yust-Katz, Kolianov, et al., 2007).

Although an early review concluded that research does not provide convincing support for the use of antidepressants for musculoskeletal pain (Curatolo, Bogduk, 2001), later research calls for further evaluation of duloxetine for osteoarthritis (OA) pain (Sullivan, Bentley, Fan, et al., 2009). Patients in the latter study were given two weeks of placebo followed by 10 weeks of duloxetine. Self-reported function improved, and pain intensity was reduced 30% as measured on the Western Ontario and McMaster Universities Osteoarthritis Index (WOMAC) between 2 and 12 weeks of treatment. Similarly, improvements in pain (30%) and physical function were found in patients who received duloxetine in another randomized, placebo-controlled trial (Chappell, 2009). More and larger studies on the use of duloxetine for this type of pain are needed. (See duloxetine patient medication information, Form V-6 on pp. 769-770, at the end of Section V).

Milnacipran

Milnacipran (Savella) is another SNRI that has been used for many years in Europe and Japan and was approved for use in the United States in 2009 for the treatment of fibromyalgia (12.5 mg to 100 mg/day). A 15-week multicenter randomized, placebo-controlled trial (N = 1196) reported significant improvements in pain, physical functioning, and fatigue associated with fibromyalgia (Clauw, Mease, Palmer, et al., 2008). A 27-week randomized, placebo-controlled trial (N = 888) found similar improvements in pain, fatigue, cognition, and other functional domains in patients with fibromyalgia (Mease, Clauw, Gendreau, et al., 2009). The drug is well tolerated even at high doses (Vitton Gendreau, Gendreau, et al., 2004), and response to treatment is reported to have a durability of up to one year (Owen, 2008). An interesting case report described the complete resolution of phantom limb pain with the use of milnacipran (50 mg/day) (Sato, Higuchi, Hishikawa, 2008). Further research on the use of this drug for this and other types of pain is needed.

Mirtazapine

Mirtazapine (Remeron) is distinguished from the other antidepressants by its tetracyclic chemical structure. Its antidepressant efficacy is similar to the SSRIs, such as fluoxetine (Prozac) (Howland, 2008). A meta-analysis of 12 new-generation antidepressants concluded that mirtazapine is similar to venlafaxine and more efficacious than duloxetine, fluoxetine, and paroxetine (Paxil) for the treatment of depression (Cipriani, Furukawa, Salanti, et al., 2009). It may be better tolerated than TCAs with fewer anticholinergic effects.

Well-controlled trials that fully evaluate the analgesic effects of the drug are lacking at this time; however, a randomized, placebo-controlled trial in 10 healthy adults found that a single dose of mirtazapine (30 mg) significantly increased pain tolerance during electrical stimulation (Arnold, Vuadens, Kuntzer, et al., 2008). A 4-week prospective, open-label study of cancer patients reported rapid improvements in pain, nausea, sleep disturbance, depression, and quality of life (Kim, Shin, Kim, et al., 2008). However, a study of cancer patients with major depression, anxiety, or adjustment disorders found that mirtazapine was effective in resolving insomnia, anxiety, and depressive symptoms, but not pain (Cankurtaran, Ozalap, Soygur, et al., 2008). Mirtazapine has been suggested as an option for treatment of tension-type headaches (Bigal, Rapoport, Hargreaves, 2008). It was also reported to resolve postdural puncture headache, but the authors of this paper noted that the drug has unknown fetal effects and cannot be routinely recommended for the headache that follows inadvertent dural puncture in the laboring patient (Sheen, Ho, 2008). Preoperative administration of mirtazapine has been shown to reduce preoperative anxiety and postoperative nausea and vomiting (Chen, Lin, Ko, et al., 2008).

Venlafaxine

In a study of experimental pain, venlafaxine (Effexor) increased pain tolerance (Enggaard, Klitgaard, Gram, et al., 2001), and in a study of patients with neuropathic pain, the drug reduced hyperalgesia and temporal summation (repeated neuronal stimulation and action potentials) but not intensity and pain detection thresholds (Yucel, Ozyalcin, Talu, et al., 2005). Electrocardiogram (ECG) changes have been associated with venlafaxine, so cautious use in patients with high cardiovascular (CV) risk is recommended (Dworkin, Backonja, Rowbotham, et al., 2003). (See venlafaxine patient medication information, Form V-12 on pp. 781-782, at the end of Section V). Among the studies of venlafaxine for the treatment of pain are the following:

- Persistent pain and associated depression (Bradley, Barkin, Jerome, et al., 2003)
- Painful diabetic neuropathy (Davis, Smith, 1999; Duby, Campbell, Setter, et al., 2004; Dworkin, Backonja, Rowbotham, et al., 2003)
- Postherpetic neuralgia (Dworkin, Backonja, Rowbotham, et al., 2003)

- Chemotherapy-induced peripheral neuropathy (Durand, Alexandre, Guillevin, et al., 2005)
- Neuropathic back pain (Pernia, Mico, Calderon, et al., 2000; Sumpton, Moulin, 2001)
- Persistent pelvic pain (Karp, 2004)
- Tension headaches (Zissis, Harmoussi, Vlaikidis, et al., 2007)
- Central pain (Dworkin, Backonja, Rowbotham, et al., 2003)

Selective Serotonin Reuptake Inhibitors (SSRIs)

The evidence of analgesic efficacy for both the TCAs and the SNRIs far exceeds the SSRIs. Favorable anecdotal reports of fluoxetine (Prozac) analgesia (Diamond, Frietag, 1989; Geller, 1989) were refuted in a controlled trial, which showed no benefit in patients with painful diabetic neuropathy (Max, Lynch, Muir, et al., 1992). Other studies of fluoxetine yielded mixed results. A double-blind comparison of fluoxetine, desipramine, and amitriptyline in patients with postherpetic neuralgia revealed that all three were analgesic; although fluoxetine produced the fewest adverse effects, the dropout rate during fluoxetine treatment was highest (Davies, Reisner-Keller, Rowbotham, 1996). Another controlled study of 59 patients with rheumatic pain revealed that both amitriptyline 25 mg and fluoxetine 20 mg produced significant pain relief compared with placebo during 4 weeks of treatment; fluoxetine was considered superior to amitriptyline because of fewer adverse effects (Rani, Naidu, Prasad, et al., 1996).

Paroxetine (Paxil), another SSRI, has some benefit in the control of pain from diabetic neuropathy (Sindrup, Gram, Brosen, et al., 1990), and while one study reported that the drug was effective in improving mood and reducing anxiety in 116 patients with fibromyalgia, its pain relieving properties were far less apparent (Patkar, Masand, Krulewicz, et al., 2007). In contrast, a later meta-analysis found strong evidence for both paroxetine and fluoxetine in reducing pain but just small effects for mood and no effects on fatigue and sleep (Hauser, Bernardy, Uceyler, et al., 2009).

Fewer clinical trials have specifically compared the efficacy of antidepressants as analgesics for cancer pain. Nonetheless, there are general recommendations to advocate for the use of TCAs and SRNIs rather than SSRIs for treatment of neuropathic pain syndromes caused by progressive cancer and cancer treatments (Dworkin, O'Connor, Backonja, et al., 2007).

Summary

Substantial evidence exists that antidepressant drugs (both TCAs and SNRIs) have analgesic effects for diverse types of persistent pain. Given the range of pain syndromes that are potentially responsive, it is appropriate to classify these drugs as nonspecific, multipurpose analgesics. These agents are especially useful for the treatment of neuropathic pain states. The strongest evidence of analgesic efficacy is found in the numerous controlled trials of the tertiary amine drugs, of which amitriptyline is the best studied. There is less abundant data to support efficacy for the secondary amine TCAs nortriptyline and desipramine. Nevertheless, guidelines recommend the use of a tertiary amine TCA only if a secondary amine is unavailable because of a more favorable adverse effect profile (Argoff, Backonja, Belgrade, et al., 2006; Dworkin, O'Connor, Backonja, et al., 2007).

Antidepressants with more norepinephrine selective actions are also analgesic, and very impressive data have been generated for the SNRIs, with evidence mounting for their role in the treatment of numerous pain syndromes. Clinical interest is less for SSRIs despite their relatively good adverse effect profile. Among the SSRIs, limited evidence supports the analgesic efficacy of paroxetine and fluoxetine, but data are equivocal or absent for the others.

Mechanism of Action

The antidepressants presumably produce analgesic effects through increased activity in endogenous monoaminergic pain modulating pathways. Specific pathways originate from neuronal pools in the brainstem and descend to the spinal cord, where they release substances, such as the amines serotonin (5HT), and norepinephrine (NE), that inhibit the transmission of nociceptive impulses (see Section I and Figure I-2, *D* on pp. 4-5). By blocking the reuptake (resorption) of serotonin and norepinephrine at the synapse, the antidepressants presumably increase activity in these pathways (Maizels, McCarberg, 2005; Veves, Backonja, Malik, 2008). Norepinephrine is thought to play a more significant role than other amines in the endogenous analgesia pathways, which helps to explain the greater analgesic effectiveness of the SNRIs compared with the SSRIs (Veves, Backonja, Malik, 2008). Conversely, serotonin may be the more powerful mediator of depression, and low serotonin levels are associated with depression.

Other mechanisms also may be involved in antidepressant-mediated analgesia. Some of these drugs block peripheral sodium channels, but the extent to which this effect contributes to analgesia is uncertain (Gerner, 2004; Strumper, Durieux, 2004). The SSRIs are less potent sodium channel blockers than the TCAs and SNRIs (Dick, Brochu, Purohit, et al., 2007). Some of the antidepressants also block histamine (H_1) receptors, and this, too, could contribute to analgesic effects (Mays, 2006).

Although effective treatment of concurrent depression can contribute to a favorable outcome from antidepressant therapy in patients with persistent pain, the analgesic effect of these drugs is not dependent on their antidepressant activity. Many controlled studies of TCAs, for example, have demonstrated that they are effective in relieving pain often at lower doses than those required to treat depression, and that the onset of analgesia typically occurs much sooner than the antidepressant effect, usually within one week. Moreover, patients who are not depressed can experience analgesia, and depressed patients can report pain relief without a change in mood (Kishore-Kumar, Max, Schafer, et al., 1990; Max, Lynch, Muir, et al., 1992).

Adverse Effects

Although serious adverse effects associated with the TCAs are uncommon at the doses usually administered for pain, less serious adverse effects are frequent and include dry mouth, sedation, dizziness, mental clouding, weight gain, and constipation, especially with the more anticholinergic TCAs such as amitriptyline. Even at low doses, patients with major organ dysfunction or those who might be taking multiple other drugs may experience troublesome adverse effects (Kurella, Bennett, Chertow, 2003). Moreover, some patients who receive low doses of the TCAs actually attain relatively high plasma drug concentrations. Rarely, serious anticholinergic toxicity can occur, including precipitation of acute angle closure glaucoma, tachycardia, severe constipation, or urinary retention. Amitriptyline is not recommended in older patients as they have increased sensitivity to its anticholinergic and sedative effects (see Table 13-4 on p. 336). Nevertheless the drug continues to be used in older adults. An extensive review of a health insurance claims database in the United States revealed that 20% of patients ages 65 years and older with a diagnosis of painful diabetic neuropathy were prescribed TCAs, primarily amitriptyline, and over half of these had co-morbidities or were taking other medications that could render the prescribing of a TCA potentially inappropriate and dangerous (Berger, Dukes, Edelsberg, et al., 2007).

When relatively mild, the anticholinergic adverse effects, such as dry mouth, blurred vision, or constipation, can usually be managed or tolerated. In a double-blind study of 26 older patients receiving nortriptyline, adverse effects of dry mouth and blurred vision were safely reduced with bethanechol (Urecholine) 10 mg three times a day (Rosen, Pollock, Altieri, et al., 1993). The drug was well tolerated except for causing an increase in orthostatic hypotension. The decrease in salivation caused by TCAs is especially troublesome for patients with dentures. Precautions should be taken to ensure that all patients practice good oral hygiene, keep well hydrated, and have regular dental examinations.

Of the TCAs, the secondary amines, desipramine and nortriptyline, are less anticholinergic than the tertiary amines, so are preferred particularly in populations who are at high risk for anticholinergic adverse effects, such as older adults, individuals who are otherwise predisposed to these symptoms, and those who have experienced distressing adverse effects during a trial of a tertiary amine drug.

Orthostatic hypotension is a potentially serious TCA adverse effect. Of the TCAs, nortriptyline and desipramine are the least likely to cause this. Orthostatic hypotension appears to be much more likely in older adults and, combined with the sedative effects of these drugs, probably accounts for an increased risk of hip fracture in this population (Ray, Griffin, Schaffner, et al., 1987). It is prudent to consider an SNRI before a TCA for patients who are predisposed to orthostasis. Care should always focus on preventing adverse events, and patients receiving TCAs should be advised to get up slowly from a supine position and rely on assistance if they are feeling dizzy or lightheaded.

The most serious adverse effect of TCAs is cardiotoxicity, which was recognized decades ago (Glassman, Bigger, 1981). While extremely rare, the potential for cardiotoxicity should always be considered when selecting an antidepressant (Dworkin, O'Connor, Backonja, et al., 2007). Patients at risk are those who have significant heart disease, including conduction disorders, dysrhythmias, or heart failure. Conduction abnormalities and a recent cardiac event are contraindications for TCAs (Maizels, McCarberg, 2005). Doses higher than 100 mg/day have been associated with sudden cardiac death (Ray, Meredith, Thapa, et al., 2004). If patients with known heart problems are treated with TCAs, initial doses should be low, dose escalation should be gradual, and the ECG should be regularly assessed as doses reach relatively high levels. SNRIs and SSRIs do not carry the same risk for cardiotoxic effects, and therefore, are acceptable alternatives for antidepressant analgesia in high-risk patients.

Both SNRIs and SSRIs have a more favorable adverse effect profile than the TCAs. They are less likely to cause mental clouding, confusion, or somnolence, and overall, appear to be better tolerated. The most common adverse effects of the SNRIs and SSRIs are nausea, headache, sedation, insomnia, weight gain, impaired memory, sweating, tremor, and sexual dysfunction. Of the SNRIs, duloxetine and milnacipran appear better tolerated than venlafaxine (Stahl, Grady, Moret, et al., 2005). Venlafaxine can cause dose-related hypertension, and, if appropriate, blood pressure (BP) monitoring should be done during initiation of treatment. A meta-analysis of four randomized controlled trials concluded that SSRIs taken alone and in combination with NSAIDs substantially increases upper gastrointestinal (GI) hemorrhage (Loke, Trivedi, Singh, 2008).

A troubling adverse effect for many patients taking any of the antidepressants is sexual dysfunction. Haberfellner (2007) provides an extensive review of 79 clinical trials describing this adverse effect and can be referred to for guidance related to specific antidepressants. Of interest is a suggestion to add bupropion to SSRI treatment for major depression as a means of reversing sexual adverse effects and bolstering antidepressant effects (Zisook, Rush, Haight, et al., 2006). Other strategies include: (1) switching to another antidepressant, (2) selecting an antidepressant with reduced likelihood for sexual dysfunction, (3) selecting an antidepressant with a short half-life, and (4) watchful waiting to see if this adverse effect may improve over time (Taylor, 2006). The use of a phosphodiesterase (PDE) inhibitor (e.g., sildenafil [Viagra], tadalafil [Cialis]) for men with erectile dysfunction can be considered as well (Rudkin, Taylor, Hawton, 2004; Taylor, 2006). Low-dose psychostimulant therapy, such as dextroamphetamine or methylphenidate 5 mg sublingually, one or more hours before intercourse, has been anecdotally reported to enhance sexual performance (Bartlik, Kaplan, Kaplan, 1995).

Drug-drug interactions are relatively common with antidepressants because they inhibit the various isoenzymes in the cytochrome P450 enzyme system (Virani, Mailis, Shapiro, et al., 1997) (see Chapter 11). Each antidepressant has a unique profile, and it is important for the clinician to become familiar with the potential for drug-drug interactions and toxicity associated with the particular antidepressant being administered. Patients must be told to report adverse effects promptly, and in some cases, serum drug concentrations should be monitored when adding a new drug or changing the dose of a drug in an existing regimen.

Caution is warranted when drugs that increase CNS levels of serotonin, such as antidepressants, monoamine oxidase inhibitors (MAOIs), and tramadol or tapentadol, are combined. This can precipitate serotonin syndrome (serotonin toxicity), which is characterized by nausea, agitation, confusion, tremulousness, hyperreflexia, and hyperthermia. Diagnosis can be challenging, particularly when medications in the inpatient setting are added to preconsumed outpatient prescriptions (Altman, Jahangiri, 2010). Treatment of serotonin syndrome depends on the severity of symptoms but can include reducing or discontinuing the causative medications, symptom management, and administering antiserotonergic drugs such as chlorpromazine (Thorazine) (Skinner, Epstein, Pappagallo, 2009). Rarely, patients are treated for respiratory failure, renal failure, and coagulopathy (Altman, Jahangiri, 2010).

All of the TCAs are metabolized in the liver so must be used with caution in individuals with hepatic impairment (Mays, 2006). An increase in hepatotoxicity has been linked to the use of duloxetine in individuals with pre-existing liver disease, suggesting that the drug may aggravate the disease (United States Food and Drug Administration [U.S. FDA], 2005a). All patients taking antidepressants should be told to report pruritus, dark urine, jaundice, right upper-quadrant tenderness, or unexplained flu-like symptoms, and prescribers should investigate these symptoms promptly. It is also important to recommend smoking cessation in patients taking duloxetine, as the drug's bioavailability is reduced by as much as one-third in smokers (U.S. FDA, 2007a). Antidepressants are generally considered safe in patients with renal disease; however, their metabolites rely on renal clearance, and patients should be watched for signs of metabolite accumulation, such as increased sedation and anticholinergic effects (Leo, 2008; Mays, 2006).

Rapid discontinuation of the SNRIs or SSRIs after an extended period of dosing can cause a discontinuation syndrome characterized by both somatic (dizziness, lightheadedness, nausea, fatigue, lethargy, sleep disturbances) and psychologic (anxiety, agitation, crying, irritability) symptoms (Rosenbaum, Zajecka, 1997). If discontinued, all antidepressants that have been taken for more than 6 weeks should be tapered over 2 weeks to reduce the risk of any withdrawal phenomena.

Indications

As multipurpose analgesics, antidepressant drugs could potentially be considered for the treatment of any persistent pain syndrome. Opioids are first-line therapy for moderate or severe persistent pain in populations with active cancer or other serious advanced illness, and in these populations, analgesic antidepressants usually are considered for opioid-refractory neuropathic pain. In other types of persistent neuropathic pain, antidepressants are widely considered first-line or second-line treatment (e.g., after a trial of gabapentin or pregabalin) (Dworkin, O'Connor, Backonja, et al., 2007; Moulin, Clark, Gilron, et al., 2007). Similar guidelines can be applied to fibromyalgia. The positioning of the analgesic antidepressants in other types of persistent pain is a matter of clinical judgment.

Great variability exists in the range of symptoms presented by patients with neuropathic pains. Conceivably, specific symptoms may indicate the existence of mechanisms that respond differently to drugs with varying modes of action (Jensen, Baron, 2003). Statements in older literature suggest that antidepressants are more useful for neuropathic pains characterized by continuous dysesthesias (e.g., "burning" pain or hypersensitivity to stimuli) than pains described as lancinating ("stabbing" pain). This impression is not supported by individual controlled trials (Kishore-Kuman, Max, Schafer, et al., 1990; Mishra, Bhatnagar, Gupta, et al., 2009) or a systematic review (McQuay, Tramer, Nye, et al., 1996). At this time, symptom-specific drug selection remains a future goal.

In a recent meta-analysis of randomized clinical trials, it was not possible to find appreciable differences in the effectiveness of TCAs compared with the anticonvulsant gabapentin for the treatment of diabetic neuropathy and postherpetic neuralgia (Chou, Carson, Chan, 2009). However, TCAs are often preferred for initial treatment of neuropathic pain if the patient has coexisting insomnia, anxiety, or depression, or if cost is a consideration. In the treatment of postherpetic neuralgia in older adults, desipramine was shown to be more effective and less expensive compared with the gabapentenoids (gabapentin and pregabalin) (O'Connor, Noyes, Holloway, 2007). However, duloxetine has been shown to be more cost-effective than some of the other drugs used for neuropathic pain, including amitriptyline, in cost comparison studies (Beard, McCrink, Le, et al., 2008; Wu, Birnbaum, Mareva et al., 2006). As mentioned, multiple factors must be considered when determining the most cost-effective drug for a given patient.

In terminally ill patients, early use of an adjuvant analgesic is also considered when pain is accompanied by other symptoms that may respond to a nonanalgesic effect of the drug. For example, antidepressants are commonly used when pain is complicated by depression, and TCAs are especially useful when pain is accompanied by the inability to sleep or insomnia.

Drug Selection

A systematic review could not identify significant differences in analgesic efficacy across TCAs (McQuay, Tramer, Nye, et al., 1996). This conclusion is tentative, however, because very few studies have directly compared these drugs (Kroenke, Krebs, Bair, 2009). Although the extensive data from controlled clinical trials suggests that amitriptyline might be considered first when an antidepressant is indicated, despiramine and nortriptyline usually are better tolerated and may be more appropriate first-line options (Dworkin, O'Connor, Backonja, et al., 2007). Doxepin is sometimes used for intractable itching (pruritus), and an oral doxepin rinse has been shown to be effective in reducing the pain associated with oral mucositis due to cancer therapy (Epstein, Epstein, Epstein, et al., 2006).

There is sufficient evidence of analgesic efficacy for some of the SNRIs that a recent guideline on the treatment of neuropathic pain considers these drugs as first-line options (Dworkin, O'Connor, Backonja, et al., 2007). Other guidelines have recommended them as second-line treatment, to be tried if a TCA is ineffective, poorly tolerated, or relatively contraindicated (Moulin, Clark, Gilron, et al., 2007). Of the SNRIs, duloxetine has the most supporting data from randomized trials.

Substantial variability exists in the analgesic response to the different antidepressants. Failure of one drug might reasonably be followed by a trial of an alternative. No guidelines exist for drug selection during these sequential trials, and the process usually proceeds by trial and error.

Dose Selection

The starting dose of the TCAs should be low, 10 mg in older adults and 25 mg in younger adults (Dworkin, O'Connor, Backonja, et al., 2007). Beginning with a low initial dose and titrating relatively slowly thereafter, with intervals between dose changes as long as every 1 to 2 weeks, has been recommended for patients with organ failure (Kurella, Bennett, Chertow, 2003). Based on clinical experience, the interval between dose changes can be shorter—several days to one week—in those without significant medical illness.

The usual early dose increases are the same size as the starting dose; as the baseline dose increases, the increments can be greater, but usually no more than one-third of the baseline dose. For example, an older adult patient may begin with 10 mg of desipramine. Every 3 to 5 days, the dose may be increased by 10 mg until 50 mg is reached. In the absence of any adverse effects, the next increment may be 25 mg, and these 25 mg increments every few days may continue until the dose is 125 mg to 150 mg. Above this, the increments may be 50 mg.

The usual effective analgesic dose range for all of the commonly used TCAs is 50 to 150 mg, and the maximum recommended dose usually is 150 mg daily (Dworkin, O'Connor, Backonja, et al., 2007). Some patients will benefit from doses less than or greater than these parameters, however, and at doses above 100 mg it is prudent to obtain an ECG and to measure the plasma drug concentration, if possible. If the concentration of drug and metabolites is below the reported upper range for antidepressant effects, cautious titration may be continued (Dworkin, O'Connor, Backonja, et al., 2007). This evaluation of plasma concentration is not to imply that antidepressant blood levels are needed for analgesia; in fact, the doses of TCAs used for analgesia are usually lower than those used for depression (Kroenke, Krebs, Bair, 2009). A check of the concentration can be reassuring, however, and allow dose escalation to explore the analgesic potential of the drug.

Duloxetine can be started at 20 mg to 30 mg once daily and increased after 1 week to 40 mg to 60 mg once daily. The effective dose in clinical trials was 60 mg daily (Dworkin, O'Connor, Backonja, et al., 2007). Although doses of 60 mg twice daily do not appear to produce significantly better pain relief and are associated with increased adverse effects, individual patients benefit and dose escalation to this limit is appropriate if outcomes are not favorable and adverse effects are not a problem.

Milnacipran is started at a dose of 12.5 mg daily, rapidly titrated to 12.5 mg twice daily, and then 25 mg twice daily. The dose can then be gradually increased to a dose as high at 100 mg twice daily. Venlafaxine can be initiated using the long-acting formulation at a dose of 37.5 mg daily (Dworkin, O'Connor, Backonja, et al., 2007). The dose can be increased as tolerated each week, up to a maximum dose of 225 mg to 375 mg/day. Most patients who obtain pain relief achieve it at a dose lower than this maximum. Reductions in doses of venlafaxine, duloxetine, and milnacipran by 25% for mild-to-moderate renal or hepatic function impairment and 50% for those with moderate-to-severe renal or hepatic insufficiency are needed to minimize adverse effects (Leo, 2008). The manufacturer of duloxetine does not recommend its use in dialysis-dependent patients.

In the use of all the analgesic antidepressants, a dose lower than the usual antidepressant dose is expected to yield analgesic effects in responding patients, but it is impossible to know whether those who initially fail to respond at a lower dose than the antidepressant dose would in fact attain benefit if the dose were increased. Accordingly, a patient who does not benefit from the usual analgesic dose and has no adverse effects should have the dose titrated upward until the antidepressant dose is reached. This course is clearly justified in patients with a coexistent depression but should be considered even in patients without depression. As noted previously, laboratory measurement of plasma drug concentration is possible for most of the TCAs, and monitoring of these levels may reveal that typical doses are yielding low levels, indicating rapid metabolism of the drug or the possibility that the patient is not taking all doses. If adherence is not an issue, rapid metabolizers can undergo dose titration beyond the usual dose range, with repeated monitoring of the plasma concentration.

Most patients take a single nighttime dose of the TCAs to prevent excessive daytime sedation. The less sedating SNRIs and SSRIs are usually taken in a single daytime dose, or twice daily. If pain relief is adequate throughout the day during treatment with a TCA but the patient experiences "hangover" or double vision in the morning, the total daily dose may be divided into two doses given in the early and late evening. Similarly, if the patient has increased pain in the afternoon, the total daily dose may be divided into two doses, one given in the morning and one in the evening.

As noted, dose tapering is important when planning to discontinue an analgesic, particularly if treatment has continued for more than 6 weeks. In the absence of serious toxicity, slow tapering over 2 weeks reduces the risk of any withdrawal phenomena. Table V-1, pp. 748-756, at the end of Section V contains dosing recommendations for all of the commonly used antidepressants.

Monitoring Therapy

Changes in pain, mood, cognitive status, sleep pattern, and other effects must be carefully monitored during antidepressant analgesic dose escalation. Although favorable analgesic effects are usually observed within 1 week after achieving an effective dosing level, some patients accrue benefit over a longer period, and antidepressant effects may be further delayed in onset. The potential delay to realize the full benefit from these drugs, combined with the period required for dose titration, may result in a relatively lengthy period during which patients experience unsatisfactory effects from the therapy. Unless the patient is well-informed about this potential, the patient is likely to discontinue the drug.

Corticosteroids

Corticosteroids are considered multipurpose analgesics. Their use in this capacity is largely limited to the cancer population. (See Chapter 30 for a discussion of their use in the treatment of malignant bowel obstruction.) In the heterogeneous population with persistent noncancer

pain, corticosteroids often are used as analgesics for a brief trial, based on the goal of "breaking the cycle" of pain, or they are used on a prolonged basis in inflammatory conditions as disease-modifying agents.

In the cancer population, corticosteroids are used to treat many pain syndromes, including bone pain and pain from stretching of the liver capsule due to metastasis, neuropathic pain from infiltration or compression of neural structures, headache caused by increased intracranial pressure, arthralgia, and pain caused by obstruction of hollow viscera (e.g., bowel or ureter) (Knotkova, Pappagallo, 2007; Lussier, Portenoy, 2004; Lussier, Huskey, Portenoy, 2004; Miaskowski, Cleary, Burney, et al., 2005). An evidence-based review of analgesic options for cancer pain evaluated the available data and also found support for the administration of steroids for spinal cord compression (Dy, Asch, Naeim, et al., 2008).

A limited course of corticosteroids has been recommended for pain associated with complex regional pain syndrome (CRPS) (Quisel, Gill, Witherell, 2005). Short-term administration for analgesic and disease-modifying purposes often is used as well in patients with inflammatory arthritis (Simon, Lipman, Caudill-Slosberg, et al., 2002). Intraarticular corticosteroids are used to alleviate pain associated with intense flares of OA and rheumatoid arthritis (RA) (Furtado, Oliveira, Natour, 2005; Lavelle, Lavelle, Lavelle, 2007; Simon, Lipman, Caudill-Slosberg, et al., 2002). Long-term corticosteroid use, which is conventional practice in some populations with chronic autoimmune disease, is not an accepted therapy for the pain of OA.

In the cancer population, dexamethasone (Decadron and others) 8 mg given before radiation therapy can effectively reduce the incidence of pain flare (Chow, Loblaw, Harris et al., 2007), as well as improve functional outcomes (Loblaw, Perry, Chambers, et al., 2005). Pain flare occurs in as many as 25% of patients following palliative radiation therapy and can persist for several days (Loblaw, Wu, Kirkbride, et al., 2007).

Multiple symptoms occur among those with advanced illnesses, and corticosteroid therapy is favored because of the potential benefit of these drugs on anorexia, nausea, malaise, and overall quality of life (Lussier, Portenoy, 2004; Lussier, Huskey, Portenoy, 2004; Mercadante, Fulfaro, Casuccio, 2001; Mercadante, Berchovich, Casuccio, et al., 2007; Shih, Jackson, 2007). These drugs are also particularly useful in alleviating symptoms associated with primary brain tumors and metastases to the brain (Newton, 2007).

Corticosteroids are seldom used in the setting of acute, self-limited pain, but a randomized controlled trial that compared intraarticular dexamethasone and intraarticular morphine found that both reduced pain for 5 days following knee surgery in patients with chronic OA (Stein, Yassouridis, Szopko, et al., 1999). Numerous guidelines and systematic reviews also recommend that corticosteroids be considered for the prevention and treatment of postoperative nausea and vomiting (PONV) (Gan, Meyer, Apfel, et al., 2003, 2007; Habib, Gan, 2004; Habib, El-Moalem, Gan, 2004), and they are often included in multimodal postoperative treatment plans that identify prevention of PONV as a primary goal (Kehlet, Wilmore, 2008) (see Chapter 19). Coating endotracheal tubes with topical betamethasone may help to decrease edema and inflammation with a subsequent reduction in sore throat, hoarseness, and cough after tracheal intubation (Ayoub, Ghobashy, Koch, et al., 1998).

Mechanism of Action

Steroids bind to glucocorticoid receptors in cells to produce antiinflammatory and immunosuppressive effects (Buvanendran, Kroin, 2007). The relationship between these effects and analgesia is poorly understood. Any of several processes may be involved. Compression of pain-sensitive structures may be relieved by reduction of inflammation and edema or, in the case of steroid-responsive neoplasms, by shrinkage of a tumor mass (Lussier, Portenoy, 2004). Activation of nociceptors may be lessened by reduced tissue concentrations of some inflammatory mediators, specifically prostaglandins and leukotrienes. Aberrant electrical activity in damaged nerves may also be tempered by these agents (Lussier, Portenoy, 2004).

Adverse Effects

Well-recognized adverse effects are associated with short-term and long-term administration of corticosteroids and with withdrawal of these drugs after long-term use (Lussier, Portenoy, 2004). The risk of serious toxicity increases with the dose, duration of therapy, and predisposing factors associated with the medical condition of the patient (Buvanendran, Kroin, 2007). Concern about toxicity is the reason that long-term use of these drugs generally is considered only when they are required as disease-modifying agents or when the target population has advanced disease and short life expectancies.

Acute, short-term use of corticosteroids is generally well tolerated. Potential adverse effects include hyperglycemia, fluid retention, and GI disturbances ranging from dyspepsia to ulceration (Lussier, Portenoy, 2004). Similar to short-term use, long-term use in low doses is usually well-tolerated; however, long-term use can cause cushingoid habitus, skin changes, weight gain, hypertension, osteoporosis, myopathy, increased risk of serious infection, and GI toxicity (Lussier, Portenoy, 2004). Dexamethasone (16 mg to 24 mg/day) produces the least mineralcorticoid effect, which may reduce the risk of fluid overload and hypertension (Miaskowski, Cleary, Burney, et al., 2005). Treatment with a bisphosphonate, calcium, and vitamin D should be considered to lower the risk of corticosteroid-induced osteoporosis. Long-term co-administration of an NSAID is not recommended, if it can be avoided, given the increased risk of peptic ulcer

disease (Lussier, Portenoy, 2004). If combined therapy is used, concomitant administration of a proton pump inhibitor is recommended (see Chapter 6).

Neuropsychologic toxicity can occur with short- or long-term corticosteroid administration and ranges from changes in mood and cognitive functioning to delirium. Mood changes may be at either end of the spectrum, that is, depression to euphoria (Jenkins, Bruera, 2000; Lussier, Portenoy, 2004). Those at highest risk are cognitively impaired patients and older patients (Jenkins, Bruera, 2000). Several mechanisms are thought to be responsible for neuropsychologic changes including their interaction at the neurotransmitter level at multiple receptor sites and enhanced catecholamine synthesis (Jenkins, Bruera, 2000). Neuropsychologic toxicity usually occurs early during treatment and when relatively high doses are administered. No specific steroid has been identified as more likely than another to produce the effect. This adverse effect can be difficult to evaluate and diagnose in patients with multisystem disease, such as those with advanced cancer (Jenkins, Bruera, 2000). Patients must be monitored for changes in mood and cognition during corticosteroid therapy, and the occurrence of these adverse effects typically requires a change in therapy. In some settings, the problem is best treated by the addition of an antidepressant, a mood-stabilizing drug, or a neuroleptic (Jenkins, Bruera, 2000). In others, the steroid should be tapered, and ultimately discontinued, or treatment should be switched to another corticosteroid to determine whether toxicities are different.

Systematic assessment of response to steroid therapy should include neurologic examination of muscle strength, in an effort to identify a steroid-induced myopathy at an early point in its course. Changes in mood, appetite, fluid status, and blood glucose levels associated with high-dose steroids also should be evaluated regularly during therapy. Depending on the context, any of these toxicities may necessitate tapering and discontinuation of the drug.

Withdrawal after long-term corticosteroid use can produce myalgia and arthralgia ("pseudorheumatism"), headache, and mood disturbance. Flares of symptoms for which steroid treatment was initiated may be experienced as well (Lussier, Portenoy, 2004). The rate at which to taper corticosteroids to prevent severe withdrawal phenomena is not known (Jenkins, Bruera, 2000). Slow dose reduction from long-term therapy is prudent. Some corticosteroids have a long half-life (e.g., dexamethasone), and elimination of the drug and resolution of adverse effects may take weeks (Jenkins, Bruera, 2000).

Indications

In the cancer population, corticosteroid administration is strongly indicated in the management of spinal cord compression, superior vena cava syndrome, and increased intracranial pressure (Dy, Asch, Naeim, 2008; Jenkins, Bruera, 2000; Lussier, Portenoy, 2004).

The purpose in these conditions is to modify the disease process by reducing peritumoral edema, as well as providing pain relief. In an early survey of 83 patients given high doses of dexamethasone (96 mg/day for 2 weeks) for malignant epidural spinal cord compression, pain relief was observed in 64% of patients within hours of the initial dose (Greenberg, Kim, Posner, 1980). A relatively high-dose regimen of this type usually is considered in the setting of emerging spinal cord or cauda equina signs; a lower dose regimen (e.g., 8 mg dexamethasone twice daily) often is used to reduce symptoms when epidural disease is present or suspected, but emerging cord or cauda equina signs do not exist (Rolles, 2005). Radiation therapy for appropriately selected patients is included in evidence-based guidelines for the treatment of spinal cord compression and associated pain (Abrahm, 2004; McQuay, Collins, Caroll, et al., 1999; Miaskowski, Cleary, Burney, et al., 2005), and as mentioned earlier, prophylactic dexamethasone may help to prevent pain flares following radiotherapy (Chow, Loblaw, Harris, et al., 2007).

On the basis of anecdotal experience, corticosteroids are also administered for many other cancer pain syndromes, including metastatic bone pain, neuropathic pain caused by compression or infiltration of peripheral nerves or nerve plexus, painful lymphedema, pain caused by obstruction of hollow viscera, and pain caused by organ capsule dissention (Lussier, Portenoy, 2004). The usual approach is a relatively low-dose regimen, typically equivalent to 1 mg to 4 mg of dexamethasone 2 to 4 times per day.

In patients with advanced illness, corticosteroids are usually added to an opioid regimen after the opioid dose has been increased to dose-limiting adverse effects. Patients with these pain syndromes commonly have other symptoms that could potentially be improved by steroid therapy such as nausea or malaise, and corticosteroid therapy may be considered earlier if primarily indicated by these other symptoms (Lussier, Portenoy, 2004). The low-dose regimen also is preferred in this setting.

Drug Selection

The relative risks and benefits of the various corticosteroids are unknown. In the United States, dexamethasone usually is a first choice and one that gains theoretical support from the relatively low mineralocorticoid effects (less fluid and electrolyte retention) (Lussier, Portenoy, 2004). Prednisone (Sterapred) and methylprednisolone (Depo-Medrol, Medrol, Solu-Medrol) have also been used. For convenience in prescribing, many clinicians consider these equivalencies: methylprednisolone 8 mg = prednisone 10 mg = dexamethasone 2 mg (see Table 22-2 for equivalent doses of corticosteroids).

Dose Selection

As noted, corticosteroids are usually administered either in a high-dose regimen or a low-dose regimen. These

Table 22-2	Equivalent Doses of Corticosteroids	
Corticosteroid	**Equivalent Dose (mg)**
Cortisone	25
Hydrocortisone	20
Prednisolone	5
Prednisone	5
Methylprednisolone	4
Triamcinolone	4
Dexamethasone	0.75-1
Betamethasone	0.6

From Pasero, C., & McCaffery, M. *Pain assessment and pharmacologic management*, p. 647, St. Louis, Mosby. Data from Clinical Pharmacology Online. Gold Standard, Inc. Available at http://clinicalpharmacology.com. Accessed August 1, 2009. © 2011, Pasero C, McCaffery M. May be duplicated for use in clinical practice.

recommendations derive from very few data and mostly reflect clinical experience. Table V-1, pp. 748-756, at the end of Section V contains dosing recommendations for corticosteroids.

High-Dose Regimen

A high-dose regimen (e.g., dexamethasone, 100 mg, followed initially by 96 mg/day in divided doses, usually 24 mg every 6 hours) has been used for oncologic emergencies, such as emerging spinal cord or cauda equina compression or worsening superior vena cava obstruction, and also has been advocated for patients who experience an acute episode of very severe pain that cannot be promptly reduced with opioids, such as that associated with a rapidly worsening malignant plexopathy (Lussier, Portenoy, 2004). The dose can be tapered over weeks, concurrent with the initiation of other analgesic approaches, such as radiotherapy.

Low-Dose Regimen

A low-dose corticosteroid regimen (e.g., usually dexamethasone, 1 to 2 mg twice daily, with a range of 1 mg twice daily to 4 mg every 6 hours) has been used for patients with advanced medical illness who continue to have pain despite optimal dosing of opioid drugs. In most cases, long-term therapy is planned. Although the risks associated with prolonged steroid use in this setting are more than balanced by the need for enhanced comfort, repeated assessments are required to ensure that benefits are sustained (Lussier, Portenoy, 2004). Ineffective regimens should be tapered and discontinued and, in all cases, the lowest dose that yields the desired results should be sought.

As mentioned, short-term and long-term corticosteroid therapy also is administered for other types of pain. A brief "pulse" of an oral drug, e.g., for 1 to 2 weeks, may be used to treat an acute flare of an inflammatory disorder, such as RA, or acute neuropathic pains of various types (e.g., acute herpes zoster). The dose selected is variable and may range from prednisone 15 mg/day to 80 mg/day, or the equivalent dose of another steroid. Long-term treatment usually is undertaken as a disease-modifying therapy appropriate for chronic inflammatory conditions. The dose usually is equivalent to prednisone 10 mg/day, or less (Simon, Lipman, Caudill-Slosberg, et al., 2002).

Alpha$_2$-Adrenergic Agonists

Animal and human studies have led to the classification of alpha$_2$-adrenergic agonists as nonspecific, multipurpose analgesics for a variety of types of acute and persistent pain (Lussier, Portenoy, 2004). The most commonly used alpha$_2$-adrenergic agonists are clonidine (Catapres, Duraclon), dexmedetomidine (Precedex), and tizanidine (Zanaflex). Each has unique properties and indications, adverse effect profiles, and preferable routes of administration. Following is a discussion of clonidine and tizanidine for persistent pain treatment. See Chapter 24 for more on transdermal clonidine use for persistent pain, Chapter 26 for perioperative clonidine use, and Chapter 27 for the use of dexmedetomidine for intravenous (IV) procedural sedation and goal-directed sedation in the critically ill.

Clonidine

Clonidine (Catapres, Duraclon) is a centrally-acting alpha$_2$-adrenergic agonist that has been used for years to treat hypertension and more recently has been used as an aid in smoking cessation. Clonidine is approved in the United States for epidural administration, and both epidural and intrathecal administration are commonplace when it is used in neuraxial analgesia (Ackerman, Follett, Rosenquist, 2003; Christo, Mazloomdoost, 2008; Eisenach, Hood, Curry, 2000; Nielsen, Sjogren, 2008). Its use as a systemic analgesic (administered as a tablet or transdermal patch) is limited (see the paragraphs that follow).

An early meta-analysis reported that successful outcomes with systemic clonidine can only be expected in pain states associated with increased sympathetic nervous system activity (Motsch, Kamler, 1997). Indeed, clonidine has been specifically suggested as an option for complex regional pain syndrome (CRPS) (Berthelot, 2006). Although some have reported less benefit with intrathecal clonidine for this condition (Ackerman, Follett, Rosenquist, 2003), methodologic problems and the need for improvements in the research of this very complex pain syndrome have been cited as a challenge in interpreting observations of this type (Perez, Kwakkel, Zuurmond, et al., 2001).

Despite the suggestion that systemic clonidine may have particular usefulness in syndromes characterized by sympathetically-maintained pain, it has been explored

for other types of persistent pain, including persistent headaches, various neuropathic pains, and some cancer pain syndromes (Ackerman, Follett, Rosenquist, 2003; Christo, Mazloomdoost, 2008; Eisenach, Du Pen, Dubois, et al., 1995; Lussier, Portenoy, 2004; Tumber, Fitzgibbon, 1998). Some recommend a trial of clonidine for intractable central pain, such as following spinal cord injury (Devulder, Crombez, Mortier, 2002).

Systemic therapy using the commercially-available transdermal clonidine patch was studied in a randomized controlled trial that included 41 patients with painful diabetic neuropathy; there was little effect overall, but a secondary analysis suggested that patients with sharp and shooting pain may benefit (Byas-Smith, Max, Muir, et al., 1995). Others have found benefit with clonidine cream for orofacial neuropathic pain described as lancinating and sharp more than burning and aching (Epstein, Grushka, Le, 1997).

The transdermal clonidine patch also was tested in postoperative pain. The clonidine patch or a placebo patch was applied to patients the evening before undergoing abdominal hysterectomy followed by an IV clonidine or placebo infusion before anesthesia induction (Dimou, Paraskeva, Papilas, et al., 2003). Although those in the clonidine group required less analgesia during the first 24 hours postoperatively, there were no differences in pain relief or analgesic requirements thereafter.

Oral or transdermal clonidine is started at 0.1 mg/day (tablet) or TTS-1 patch (equivalent to 0.1 mg twice daily) and then is titrated upward until benefit occurs or adverse effects supervene (Elliott, 2009). If the patch is used, it is changed weekly. If doses lower than those commercially available are desirable, the transdermal system can be cut into pieces without changing its delivery properties.

Tizanidine

Tizanidine (Zanaflex), another centrally-acting alpha$_2$-adrenergic agonist, is approved in the United States for the treatment of spasticity (Lussier, Portenoy, 2004). A Cochrane Collaboration Review concluded that there is not enough evidence to adequately compare the effectiveness of the various antispasmodics for treatment of multiple sclerosis spasticity (Shakespeare, Boggild, Young, 2003). However, a systematic review of various skeletal muscle relaxants used to treat spasticity related to multiple sclerosis found that tizanidine was more effective than placebo and had efficacy and toxicity comparable to baclofen (Lioresal) (Chou, Peterson, Helfand, 2004) (see Chapter 24 for a discussion of baclofen). Other systematic reviews have reported similar limited evidence for the effectiveness of tizanidine and many of the other commonly-used agents for spasticity associated with multiple sclerosis (Beard, Hunn, Wight, 2003; Paisley, Beard, Hunn, et al., 2002).

Conclusions were similar for a Cochrane Collaboration Review of the use of the various antispasmodics used to treat spasticity associated with spinal cord injury (Taricco,

Adone, Pagliacci, et al., 2000). A cross-over, randomized controlled trial (N = 19) found tizanidine, titrated to a maximum tolerated dose over a 6-week period, also reduced spasticity associated with acquired brain injury, such as from stroke or trauma (Meythaler, Guin-Renfroe, Johnson, 2001).

Tizanidine has been reported to relieve neuropathic pain (Knotkova, Pappagallo, 2007; Semenchuk, Sherman, 2000), persistent neck and lower back pain that has a myofascial component (Malanga, Reiter, Garay, 2008), and myofascial pain syndrome (Malanga, Gwynn, Smith, et al., 2002). A combination of tizanidine and amitriptyline was found to be more effective for prevention of persistent tension headache than amitriptyline alone (Bettuci, Testa, Calzoni, et al., 2006).

Mechanism of Action

Alpha$_2$ receptors are located in presynaptic sympathetic nerve endings and noradrenergic nerve endings in the dorsal horn of the spinal cord (Pandharipande, Ely, Maze, et al., 2006). When alpha$_2$-adrenergic agonists bind to the latter receptor sites, the endogenous inhibitory pathway is activated and pain is diminished (Phillips, Gadiraju, Dickey, et al., 2007) (see Section I).

The ability of the alpha$_2$-adrenergic agonists to block the sympathetic nervous system, which regulates CV functions, explains the efficacy of these drugs for the treatment of hypertension, although the introduction of angiotensin-converting enzyme (ACE) inhibitors and β-adrenergic antagonists has relegated clonidine to a third-line treatment option today (Jones, Maze, 2001). This also explains the adverse effects of bradycardia and hypotension that can occur with administration of alpha$_2$-adrenergic agonists (see the discussion on adverse effects in the following paragraphs). Research is beginning to uncover the potential ability of some of the alpha$_2$-adrenergic agonists to provide renal, cardiac, and neurocognitive protection (Sanders, Maze, 2007; Kamibayashi, Mace, 2000).

The capacity of alpha$_2$-adrenergic agonists to inhibit nociceptive input to the CNS may indicate a role in the prevention of different types of pain syndromes. For example, by reducing sympathetic tone, clonidine may produce analgesia for pain that is sustained, at least in part, by circulating catecholamines or efferent activity in the sympathetic nervous system (so-called *sympathetically-maintained* pain) (Lussier, Portenoy, 2004). Although exact mechanisms are unclear, antihyperalgesia properties have been noted with both clonidine and dexmedetomidine (Kamibayashi, Mace, 2000) (see Section I for more on hyperalgesia).

The alpha$_2$ receptors are thought to influence spatial memory (recording information about the environment). Dexmedetomidine is the most highly selective in this class for the alpha$_2$ receptors, possessing a receptor affinity eight times that of clonidine. This strong affinity

for this receptor subtype underlies its unique characteristic of enhancing, rather than diminishing, cognitive performance during sedation (Kamibayashi, Mace, 2000). This intense binding also has implications for its administration, i.e., the loading dose must be infused very slowly (e.g., over 20 minutes) to minimize bradycardia and hypotension (Phillips, Gadiraju, Dickey, et al., 2007). Dexmedetomidine is also shorter acting than clonidine, making it more appropriate for short-procedure sedation (see Chapter 27 for more on dexmedetomidine).

Adverse Effects

The most common adverse effects of the alpha$_2$-adrenergic agonists are excessive sedation, hypotension, bradycardia, and dry mouth (Lussier, Portenoy, 2004). However, sedation is not accompanied by respiratory depression, and delayed sedation has not been observed. The occurrence of sedation can be more common and pronounced in patients who are debilitated or at the end of life. Cautious use of clonidine is recommended in older adults as orthostatic hypotension and CNS adverse effects can be more pronounced in this population.

Alpha$_2$-adrenergic agonists can produce either hypotension or hypertension (Kamibayashi, Mace, 2000). With high doses or rapid bolus dosing of dexmedetomidine, there is an initial peripheral vasoconstriction and hypertension caused by activation of the alpha$_2$ receptors located in the smooth muscle cells in vessels (Golembiewski, 2005; Kamibayashi, Mace, 2000). Reflex bradycardia can occur as well. These effects are transient and can be reduced or managed by decreasing the rate of administration or stopping infusion if they persist. An initial low heart rate that returns to baseline after administration is discontinued has been noted (Venn, Grounds, 2001). An early controlled trial of epidural clonidine in cancer pain demonstrated that this drug produced sustained hypotensive effects in almost 50% of patients but was considered serious in only 2 patients (Eisenach, Du Pen, Dubois, et al., 1995). Although most patients experience no hypotension, or mild and transient changes in BP, alpha$_2$-adrenergic agonists generally should be avoided in patients who are hemodynamically unstable or predisposed to serious hypotension (e.g., autonomic neuropathy, intravascular volume depletion, or concurrent therapy with potent hypotensive agents).

The most frequent adverse effects of tizanidine are dry mouth and excessive sedation. The drug is often compared to baclofen and possesses similar adverse effects except that tizanidine produces more dry mouth and baclofen produces more muscle weakness (Chou, Peterson, Helfand, 2004). Liver function should be checked during administration of tizanidine as elevated liver function tests have been reported (Semenchuk, Sherman, 2000), and the drug should be stopped if hepatotoxicity occurs. Tizanidine is not recommended in patients with severe hepatic dysfunction, and the dose should be reduced with renal impairment, especially if creatinine clearance is less than 25 mL/min (Elliott, 2009). A number of drugs, including oral contraceptives, some antibiotics, some histamine receptor type-2 (H_2) antagonists, and several antiarrhythmic drugs affect clearance of the drug (Elliott, 2009).

Indications

Clonidine and tizanidine can be considered for the treatment of all types of intractable persistent pain (Lussier, Portenoy, 2004). Both systemic administration (by the oral or transdermal route) and intraspinal administration can yield favorable effects. A trial of a systemic formulation (oral or transdermal clonidine or oral tizanidine) typically is considered only after therapeutic trials of many other adjuvant analgesics have proved ineffective. This is appropriate given the limited supporting data, adverse effect liability, and observations suggesting that a minority of those with intractable pain (less than 25%) are likely to respond. The limited experience with the use of alpha$_2$-adrenergic agonists in advanced illness suggests that these drugs are appropriate only after titrated opioids and other adjuvant analgesics have failed to provide acceptable pain relief (Lussier, Portenoy, 2004).

Although clonidine has more evidence of analgesic efficacy than tizanidine, the latter drug may be preferable if hypotension is a concern (Lussier, Portenoy, 2004). Tizanidine also is preferred for the treatment of pain associated with spasm caused by multiple sclerosis or spinal cord or brain injury (Chou, Peterson, Helfand, 2004; Meythaler, Guin-Renfroe, Johnson, 2001).

Alpha$_2$-adrenergic agonists blunt the signs of drug withdrawal, which include sympathetic hyperactivity (e.g., hypertension and tachycardia), anxiety, agitation, and generalized pain. Withdrawal may accompany cessation or dose reduction of diverse drug classes, including opioids, benzodiazepines, nicotine, and alcohol. Reports of the successful use of clonidine and dexmedetomidine to reduce these symptoms can be found in the literature (Bamgbade, 2006; Multz, 2003; Jones, Maze, 2001; Kamibayashi, Maze, 2000; Moss, Glick, 2005; Pandharipande, Ely, Maze, 2006; Westfall, Westfall 2006). If the clinical scenario suggests that pain could be related to substance withdrawal, an earlier trial of clonidine would be justified.

Routes of Administration

Clonidine can be administered via the oral, transdermal, IV, and intraspinal routes. Tizanidine is available in oral capsules and tablets.

Although evidence is strong that neuraxial clonidine administration is an effective therapy for some patients with refractory pain, this route of administration may not be possible in clinical settings that might lack pain specialists who can insert catheters and implantable devices or nursing support to manage therapy. An alternative may

be the oral or transdermal route (see Chapter 24 for more on transdermal clonidine). As mentioned, the drug is well-absorbed by the oral route and has 100% bioavailability. Tizanidine, on the other hand, undergoes significant first-pass effect and has an oral bioavailability of 40% (Elliott, 2009) (see Chapter 11 for discussion of first-pass effect).

Because clonidine is lipophilic, it is rapidly absorbed into the systemic circulation after epidural administration. However, it is approximately twice as effective given epidurally as intravenously, a reflection of its spinal site of action for analgesia. The relative potency of epidural to intrathecal clonidine has been shown to differ depending on type of pain. Twenty-four healthy volunteers were randomized to receive either intrathecal or epidural clonidine in various doses and were subjected to thermal noxious stimuli (acute pain model [nociception]) or intradermal capsaicin (central hypersensitivity model [neuropathic]) (Eisenach, Hood, Curry, 2000). Intrathecal clonidine was found to be at least 10 times more potent than epidural clonidine to relieve acute thermal pain but two or less times more potent than epidural clonidine for capsaicin-induced mechanical hyperalgesia and allodynia. For acute thermal pain, intrathecal clonidine produced a dose-dependent analgesia with a lumbar > thoracic > cervical gradient; however, only one dose of epidural clonidine reduced thermal pain and only at the thoracic testing site.

Intraspinal clonidine is administered via implanted and external infusion devices and is usually combined with other drugs. Research has established the stability and compatibility of admixtures containing clonidine and other agents, including baclofen (Alvarez, de Mazancourt, Chartier-Kastler et al., 2004), bupivacaine (Classen, Wimbish, Kupiec, 2004; Wulf, Gleim, Mignat, 1994), hydromorphone (Rudich, Peng, Dunn, et al., 2004), meperidine (Vranken, van Kan, van der Vegt, 2006), and morphine (Classen, Wimbish, Kupiec, 2004; Hildebrand, Elsberry, Hassenbusch, 2003) (see Chapter 15).

Dose Selection

To limit the risk of adverse effects, doses of the alpha$_2$-adrenergic agonists should be started low and increased slowly. Monitoring of both pain and adverse effects, particularly BP, is necessary during gradual dose escalation. An analgesic ceiling dose has not been determined for systemic clonidine therapy, but there appears to be a ceiling on intrathecal clonidine at 75 mcg (Eisenach, Hood, Curry, 2000). Table V-1, pp. 748-756, at the end of Section V contains dosing recommendations for the commonly used alpha$_2$-adrenergic agonists.

Cannabinoids

Although the use of cannabinoids for pain is still very limited, emerging preclinical and clinical data suggest that they are best categorized as multipurpose drugs.

Historically, these agents sparked considerable controversy, prejudice, and confusion concerning their appropriateness as medicinal agents, mostly because cannabinoids have some relation to the cannabis plant—also known as marijuana.

A synthesized form of one of marijuana's active ingredients is delta-9-tetrahydrocannabinol (THC), which is marketed as dronabinol (Marinol), available in 2.5, 5, and 10 mg capsules, and approved for medical use in the United States, Canada, and the United Kingdom. Nabilone, another derivative, also is available in the United States for the indication of nausea. In the United Kingdom and Canada, a cannabis extract (Sativex), a spray that contains THC and cannabidiol and is delivered under the tongue, has been approved for the treatment of neuropathic pain from multiple sclerosis and advanced cancer pain. In the United States, some states already have legislation or ballot initiatives for crude herbal cannabis for medical use with specific indications (McCarberg, 2007).

Cannabinoids exert effects on the endogenous cannabinoid system to produce a wide variety of effects, including analgesia, psychologic effects, sedation, and appetite stimulation (Martin, Wiley, 2004). The analgesic effects of cannabinoids are mediated through the cannabinoid-1 (CBI) and cannabinoid-2 (CB2) receptors in the periphery and CNS (McCarberg, 2007; Hosking, Zajicek, 2008; Huskey, 2006). CBI stimulation modulates central neurotransmission in the serotonergic, dopaminergic, and glutamatergic systems as well as other systems (see Section 1). It is also believed that cannabinoids enhance the endogenous opioid system. The CB2 receptor is involved in the inflammatory response.

Smoking marijuana or cannabis rapidly increases plasma levels of THC, but the amount is highly variably, primarily dependent on the composition of the marijuana cigarette and inhalation technique. Thus, this form of use is both illegal and associated with unpredictable and less reliable results in relieving pain and symptoms (Hosking, Zajicek, 2008); it cannot be recommended. It also carries risks associated with any smoked substance.

Commercially available oral preparations offer better absorption and bioavailability, and are much more reliable and predictable. In an early single-dose study of patients with cancer pain, THC, 10 mg orally, was well tolerated and produced analgesic effects similar to 60 mg codeine, but a higher dose yielded severe adverse effects in many patients (Noyes, Brunk, Avery, et al., 1976). Thus, the therapeutic window for this drug appears to be narrow, and maximal efficacy at tolerable doses is limited (Martin, Wiley, 2004). A more recent crossover study randomized 32 patients with fibromyalgia to receive 0.5 mg of nabilone or 10 mg of amitriptyline before sleep; after 1 week, the dose was doubled based on whether or not the physician thought the patient might benefit from an increase in dose (Ware, Fitzcharles, Joseph, et al., 2010). More patients taking amitriptyline (26 of 28) required a dose increase at 1 week than patients

taking nabilone (21 or 29). Both drugs improved the quality of sleep, but nabilone was superior. There were no effects on pain, mood, or quality of life. Nabilone adverse effects were mild to moderate and included dizziness, nausea, and dry mouth.

Recent studies of nabilone also suggest limited utility from this drug. Although an observational study in 112 cancer patients yielded promising results (Maida, Ennis, Irani, et al., 2008), a randomized, cross-over trial (N = 96) indicated that the drug was no more effective than dihydrocodeine and was less well-tolerated (Frank, Serpell, Hughes, et al., 2008).

In contrast, recent large and well-controlled studies of the THC-cannabidiol mixture (Sativex) yielded positive outcomes. A randomized controlled study of 125 patients with neuropathic pain of peripheral origin showed a significant reduction in pain and allodynia, favorable effects that persisted during an open-label extension study for 52 weeks (Nurmikko, Serpell, Hoggart, et al., 2007). Another controlled study of 66 patients with central pain from multiple sclerosis (Rog, Nurmikko, Friede, et al., 2005) revealed that the drug was well-tolerated and was effective in reducing pain and sleep disturbance. Other studies in patients with refractory cancer pain led to the approval of the drug for this indication in two countries, with development proceeding in the United States and elsewhere.

The reason that a mixture of cannabinoid alkaloids is more effective than single compounds is not known. The studies with the extract confirm that cannabinoids are analgesic and can benefit patients with diverse types of pain. The utility of these drugs will increase with the availability of the THC-cannabidiol formulation and other formulations on the market. At this time, trials of THC or nabilone should be considered only in the situation of pain that has not responded to many other, more established drug therapies.

Dizziness, somnolence, and dry mouth are the most common adverse effects associated with the cannabinoids. With pharmaceutical preparations, the incidence of adverse effects with short-term use involving euphoria, disorientation, confusion, dissociation, or depressed mood is relatively low. Studies of the THC-cannabidiol mixture suggest that better outcomes occur with drugs that include a combination of cannabinoid compounds.

There are many other beneficial effects for cannabinoids, such as alleviation of nausea and increased appetite (Martin, Wiley, 2004). In addition to some pain relief, they may also have opioid dose-sparing effects, possibly reduce opioid tolerance, and even ameliorate symptoms of opioid withdrawal (Svendsen, Jensen, Bach, 2004; McCarberg, 2007). Additional studies may provide new agents for clinical use and hopefully clarify the relative benefits and burdens.

Some authors have explored the controversial elements inherent in the use of cannabis substances for medical purposes (Degenhardt, Hall, 2008). First, the approval of cannabis for treatment of medical conditions in certain states and countries has occurred without strong evidence for its safety and efficacy. Second, the review of evidence from clinical trials involving cannabinoids and cannabis extracts for medical indications shows that the short-term benefits of this therapy and adverse effects have been limited for the drugs that have been available, although this is likely to change with new formulations. Last, there is a compelling need for more rigorous and scientific research to evaluate adverse effects, especially with long-term use for conditions such as multiple sclerosis and persistent pain. A systematic review and meta-analysis of cannabis treatment for persistent pain concluded that beneficial effects of the treatment may be partially or completely offset by potentially serious harms and urged more research to clarify the true balance of benefits to harms (Martin-Sanchez, Furukawa, Taylor et al., 2009).

Conclusion

Multipurpose adjuvant analgesic drugs have been shown to be effective for a variety of diverse pain syndromes and can be considered for the treatment of any type of pain. The multipurpose agents that are currently thought to be among the more useful in clinical practice include antidepressants, corticosteroids, and alpha$_2$-adrenergic agonists. Except for antidepressants, the multipurpose adjuvant analgesics are appropriate for both acute and persistent pain. Antidepressants are not appropriate for acute pain because of their delayed onset of action.

Chapter 23 Adjuvant Analgesics for Persistent (Chronic) Neuropathic Pain

SOME of the adjuvant analgesic classes are conventionally used solely for persistent neuropathic pain. The drugs in these classes, combined with the drugs in classes subsumed under the category of multipurpose analgesics, offer a very large group of individual agents that might be useful for pains of this type. Antidepressants and anticonvulsants are the first-line adjuvant analgesics for a wide variety of neuropathic pain syndromes. The multipurpose antidepressants were discussed earlier in Chapter 22, and the anticonvulsants will be discussed in detail here. Refractory neuropathic pain, which has not responded to these first-line approaches, may be considered for trials of the other so-called multipurpose drugs, or other agents classified as drugs used conventionally for neuropathic pain. Other adjuvant agents used for refractory neuropathic pain include sodium channel blockers, several topical agents, gamma aminobutyric acid (GABA) agonists (baclofen [Lioresal]), N-methyl-D-aspartate (NMDA) receptor antagonists (e.g., dextromethorphan and ketamine), and the relatively new intrathecal drug, ziconotide (Prialt). In addition to persistent pain, certain adjuvant agents are used to manage the neuropathic component of some types of acute pain and for the purpose of preventing persistent neuropathic pain, such as persistent neuropathic postsurgical pain. These are discussed later in this section.

Recent systematic reviews, some with evidence-based guidelines for drug selection, provide information about a range of therapies used for neuropathic pain (Finnerup, Otto, McQuay, et al., 2005; Saarto, Wiffen, 2007; Kroenke, Krebs, Bair, 2009). Table 23-1 lists many of these drugs, and Table V-1 at the end of Section V provides dosing guidelines and other characteristics of many of the adjuvant analgesics for the treatment of neuropathic pain. See also Section II for assessment of neuropathic pain.

Anticonvulsant Drugs

Several systematic reviews of randomized controlled trials of anticonvulsants for pain management have demonstrated strong evidence to support the efficacy of anticonvulsants in the management of both acute and

Table 23-1 | Adjuvant Analgesics for Neuropathic Pain

Class	Examples
Usually Tried First	
Tricyclic antidepressants	Despiramine, nortriptyline
Serotonin Norepinephrine Reuptake Inhibitors (SNRIs)	Duloxetine, venlafaxine, bupropion
Anticonvulsants	Gabapentin, pregabalin
Topical agents	Lidocaine patch 5%
For Refractory Cases	
Tricyclic antidepressants	Amitriptyline may be tried if a secondary amine is unavailable
Anticonvulsants	Lamotrigine, lacosamide, oxcarbazepine, tiagabine, topiramate, zonisamide *First generation:* Carbamazepine, clonazepam, divalproex, phenytoin, valproate
Alpha$_2$-adrenergic agonists	Clonidine, tizanidine
Systemic sodium channel blockers	Mexiletine, tocainide,[1] flecainide, IV lidocaine
NMDA receptor antagonists	Ketamine
Baclofen	Lioresal
Ziconotide	Prialt
Cannabinoids	Sativex
Topical agents	Capsaicin, local anesthetics, others
Neuroleptics	Olanzapine, haloperidol

IV, Intravenous; *NMDA*, N-methyl-D-aspartate.
[1]No longer marketed in the United States.
This table provides the classes of adjuvant analgesics for neuropathic pain and examples of those that should be used first and for refractory pain. See text for discussion and references.
From Pasero, C., & McCaffery, M. *Pain assessment and pharmacologic management*, p. 654, St. Louis, Mosby. © 2011, Pasero C, McCaffery M. May be duplicated for use in clinical practice.

persistent neuropathic pain (Backonja, Glanzman, 2003; Backonja, Serra, 2004; Goodyear-Smith, Halliwell, 2009; Serpell, Neuropathic Pain Study Group, 2002; Wiffen, Collins, McQuay, et al., 2005; Wiffen, McQuay, Rees, et al., 2005; Wiffen, McQuay, Moore, 2005). They are listed as first-line agents in several evidence-based neuropathic pain treatment guidelines (Argoff, Backonja, Belgrade, et al., 2006; Dworkin, Backonja, Rowbotham, et al., 2003; Dworkin, O'Connor, Backonja, et al., 2007; Moulin, Clark, Gilron, et al., 2007). There is good

evidence to support the clinical impression that anticonvulsants may be effective for all qualities of neuropathic pain, including neuropathic pain that does not have a dysesthetic component, neuropathic pain described as continuous dysesthesia (e.g., burning), and neuropathic pain that is lancinating, sharp, shooting, stabbing, or knife-like (Backonja, Glanzman, 2003; Krafft, 2008; Serpell, Neuropathic Pain Study Group, 2002; Wiffen, McQuay, Rees, et al., 2005; Wiffen, McQuay, Moore, 2005).

Anticonvulsants are discussed today in terms of the length of time they have been available (Gilron, 2006). The "older" or "first-generation" anticonvulsants include carbamazepine (Tegretol), phenytoin (Dilantin), clonazepam (Klonopin), divalproex sodium (Depakote), and valproic acid or valproate (Depacon, Depakene). Anticonvulsants that are referred to as "newer" or "second-generation" include the alpha-2-delta-1 modulators gabapentin (Neurontin) and pregabalin (Lyrica), lamotrigine (Lamictal), oxcarbazepine (Trileptal), tiagabine (Gabitril), topiramate (Topamax), zonisamide (Zonegran), lacosamide (Vimpat), and felbamate (Felbatol). One group of researchers commented that the quality of research, and hence of the evidence, tends to be higher with the newer anticonvulsants (Goodyear-Smith, Halliwell, 2009). With the exception of felbamate, which has the potential for serious bone marrow toxicity, the newer anticonvulsants generally have better safety profiles and now are prescribed as the first-line drugs for epilepsy and neuropathic pain.

"Newer" Second-Generation Anticonvulsants

Following is a discussion of several of the "newer" second-generation anticonvulsants. See Chapter 26 for their use in acute pain treatment.

Gabapentin

Gabapentin (Neurontin) has been demonstrated to be analgesic in many types of neuropathic pain, some other types of persistent pain, and acute perioperative pain (Knotkova, Pappagallo, 2007; Kong, Irwin, 2007; Seib, Paul, 2006; Tiippana, Hamunen, Kontinen, et al., 2007; Wiffen, McQuay, Rees, et al., 2005). (See Chapter 26 for perioperative use of gabapentin.) For example, a large randomized, placebo-controlled study of 305 patients with diverse neuropathic pain syndromes, including postherpetic neuralgia, complex regional pain syndrome (CRPS), central pain, and persistent postsurgical pain, found that gabapentin in doses up to 2400 mg were well-tolerated and improved pain intensity by 21% compared with 14% with placebo (Serpell, Neuropathic Pain Study Group, 2002). Improvements were noted in patient-reported quality of life and functional indicators as well.

Other studies confirmed the potential utility of gabapentin in specific syndromes. A large, multicenter 7-week study randomized 334 patients with postherpetic neuralgia to receive 1800 or 2400 mg of gabapentin or placebo daily in three divided doses (Rice, Maton, Postherpetic

Neuralgia Study Group, 2001). Within 1 week, pain scores were reduced, with a final improvement difference from baseline pain of approximately 34.5% for the 1800 mg dose and 34.4% for the 2400 mg dose. The drug was well-tolerated, with the worst adverse effects being dizziness and sedation, which were especially bothersome during the titration phase. Additional studies in the population with postherpetic neuralgia observed similar results (Backonja, Glanzman, 2003).

Guidelines recommend gabapentin as a first-line (Dworkin, O'Connor, Backonja, et al., 2007) or second-line (Argoff, Backonja, Belgrade, et al., 2006) analgesic for treatment of painful diabetic neuropathy. A 12-week open-label pilot study of 25 patients with type-II diabetes and neuropathy demonstrated greater pain reduction, decreased paresthesia, and less frequent adverse effects with gabapentin than with amitriptyline (Elavil) (Dallocchio, Buffa, Mazzarello, et al., 2000). Other studies in this condition have confirmed these positive results (Backonja, Glanzman 2003).

A randomized controlled trial evaluated gabapentin for the treatment of fibromyalgia (Arnold, Goldenberg, Stanford, et al., 2007). Patients received either gabapentin (1200 to 2400 mg/day) or placebo for 12 weeks. Those who took gabapentin experienced significant improvements in quality of life and functional outcomes and a 51% reduction in pain compared with 31% in the placebo group.

Central neuropathic pain such as from stroke or spinal cord injury can be particularly difficult to treat. An 18-week trial randomized 20 patients with traumatic spinal cord injury to receive gabapentin or placebo during a 4-week titration period followed by a 4-week stable dosing period. After a 2-week washout period, patients were crossed over to the alternative treatment for 4 weeks of titration followed by a 4-week stable dosing period (Levendoglu, Ogun, Ozerbil, et al., 2004). During the period of treatment with the active drug, an effort was made to titrate the dose to 900 mg/day by the end of the first week, 1800 mg/day by the second week, 2400 mg/day by the third, and 3600 mg/day by the fourth. Patients received the maximum tolerated dose during the 4 weeks of stable dosing. All patients completed the study, and gabapentin was shown to be efficacious for neuropathic pain, including all types of neuropathic phenomena except sensations described as itchy, sensitive, dull, and cold. Quality of life was also improved.

A retrospective study of 38 patients with central pain found similar dramatic results during gabapentin treatment, with improvements in sharp, burning pain and numerous quality of life and functional indicators such as ability to sleep and participate in domestic activities (To, Lim, Hill, et al., 2002). Some patients in this study reported that life would be unbearable without gabapentin. The range of dosing was 900 to 4800 mg/day. Follow-up interviews with 21 patients with traumatic spinal cord injury who were treated with gabapentin found that 67% reported a favorable response at 6-month interview, and 91% of these continued to report effective pain relief at 36-month interview (Putzke, Richards, Kezar, et al., 2002).

Gabapentin is also effective as an adjuvant to opioid analgesia for neuropathic pain treatment. A randomized controlled trial of 57 patients with postherpetic neuralgia or diabetic neuropathy administered placebo, gabapentin alone, morphine alone, or gabapentin plus morphine (Gilron, Bailey, Tu, et al., 2005). Pain relief was best with the combination of morphine plus gabapentin, and the maximum tolerated doses of gabapentin and morphine were lower with the combination than for each drug alone. Similar results have been found when gabapentin is added to opioids for neuropathic cancer pain, particularly if the patient has allodynia and burning, shooting pain (Caraceni, Zecca, Martini, et al., 1999; Keskinbora, Pekel, Aydinli, 2007). Its effectiveness for these symptoms was supported in a systematic review of randomized controlled trials that concluded that the drug was particularly effective in relieving the neuropathic symptoms of allodynia, burning pain, shooting pain, and hyperesthesia (Backonja, Glanzman, 2003).

Not all studies in neuropathic pain have yielded positive results. In an 8-week 3-phase crossover trial (N = 38) that compared gabapentin, amitriptyline, and diphenhydramine (Benadryl) for spinal cord injury–related pain, gabapentin was no more effective than diphenhydramine in patients who had the highest baseline pain scores; amitriptyline was more effective than diphenhydramine (Rintala, Holmes, Courtade, et al., 2007) (see Chapter 31 for more on antihistamines).

Although gabapentin frequently is given to patients with chemotherapy-induced peripheral neuropathy (Mao, Chen, 2000a), few controlled trials have been conducted, and investigations have shown conflicting results. A phase III multicenter, placebo-controlled, randomized trial (N = 115) using gabapentin for this type of pain failed to show any significant benefits (Rao, Michalak, Sloan, et al., 2007). However, another study grouped 75 patients with chemotherapy-induced neuropathy into three categories according to the severity of their pain (mild, moderate, or severe) and administered all of them a fixed dose of 800 mg/day of gabapentin (Tsavaris, Kopterides, Kosmas, et al., 2008). Results in these groups were compared with a control group that received naproxen and codeine plus acetaminophen. Of those who received gabapentin, approximately 25% had complete relief, 44% had partial relief, 25% had minor relief, and 5% had no relief. Of those in the control group, none had complete relief, approximately 5% had partial relief, 46% had minor relief, and 49% had no relief.

Small trials in phantom pain produced generally favorable results. A 14-week, randomized controlled trial that included 19 patients with phantom limb pain noted that gabapentin (titrated to 2400 mg) reduced pain but had no significant effect on mood, sleep interference, or activities of daily living compared with placebo (Bone, Critchley, Buggy, 2002). A report on 7 children and young adults with phantom limb pain revealed that 6 of the 7 had resolution of their phantom limb pain within 2 months of gabapentin treatment (Rusy, Troshynski, Weisman, 2001).

Some types of back pain may be responsive to anticonvulsants such as gabapentin (Backonja, Glanzman, 2003). One guideline suggests that gabapentin may provide short-term benefit for painful radiculopathy, but also concludes that evidence is limited and all but lacking for other anticonvulsants (Chou, Qaseem, Snow, et al., 2007).

The foregoing describes a small proportion of the large number of clinical trials, case reports, and reviews that have addressed the analgesic potential of gabapentin. A broader review of this literature reveals publications on the following conditions:

- Postherpetic neuralgia (Backonja, Glanzman, 2003; Chou, Carson, Chan, 2009; Dubinsky, Kabbani, El-Chami, et al., 2004; Mao, Chen, 2000a; Rosenberg, Harrell, Ristic, et al., 1997; Rice, Maton, Postherpetic Neuralgia Study Group, 2001; Rosner, Rubin, Kestenbaum, 1996; Rowbotham, Harden, Stacey, et al., 1998; Serpell, Neuropathic Pain Study Group, 2002)
- Painful diabetic neuropathy (Argoff, Backonja, Belgrade, et al., 2006; Backonja, Beydoun, Edwards, et al., 1998; Backonja, Glanzman, 2003; Boulton, Vinik, Arezzo, et al., 2005; Chou, Carson, Chan, 2009; Dallocchio, Buffa, Mazzarello, et al., 2000; Duby, Campbell, Setter, et al., 2004; Gilron, Bailey, Tu, et al., 2005; Hemstreet, Lapointe, 2001; Jensen, Larson, 2001; Mao, Chen, 2000a; Serpell, Neuropathic Pain Study Group, 2002; Veves, Backonja, Malik, 2008)
- Fibromyalgia (Arnold, Goldenberg, Stanford, et al., 2007) (see also Hauser, Thieme, Turk, 2009)
- Neuropathic cancer pain (Caraceni, Zecca, Martini, et al., 1999; Keskinbora, Pekel, Aydinli, 2007)
- Chemotherapy-induced pain (Mao, Chen, 2000a; Tsavaris, Kopterides, Kosmas, et al., 2008)
- Central pain from spinal cord injury (To, Lim, Hill, et al., 2002; (Levendoglu, Ogun, Ozerbil, et al., 2004)
- Central poststroke pain (Frese, Husstedt, Ringelstein, et al., 2006; Kumar, Kalita, Kumar, et al., 2009; Serpell, Neuropathic Pain Study Group, 2002)
- Multiple sclerosis (Mao, Chen, 2000a)
- Phantom limb pain (Bone, Critchley, Buggy, 2002; Serpell, Neuropathic Pain Study Group, 2002)
- CRPS (Backonja, Glanzman, 2003; Mao, Chen, 2000a; Mellick, Mellick, 1995; Serpell, Neuropathic Pain Study Group, 2002)
- Radiculopathy (Serpell, Neuropathic Pain Study Group, 2002)
- HIV-related neuropathy (Rosner, Rubin, Kestenbaum, 1996; Hahn, Arendt, Braun, et al., 2004)
- Spinal stenosis (Yaksi, Ozgonenel, Ozgonenel, 2007)
- Atypical facial pain and trigeminal neuralgia (Mao, Chen, 2000a; Serpell, Neuropathic Pain Study Group, 2002)
- Cluster and migraine headache (Kaniecki, 2008; Mathew, 2001; Tay, Ngan Kee, Chung, 2001)
- Neuroma of peripheral nerve (Serpell, Neuropathic Pain Study Group, 2002)

- Persistent neuropathic postsurgical pain syndromes (e.g., postmastectomy, postthoractomy, post inguinal hernia, cholecystectomy) (Backonja, Glanzman, 2003; Mao, Chen, 2000a; Pandey, Patra, Pant, et al., 2006; Serpell, Neuropathic Pain Study Group, 2002; Tiippana, Hamunen, Kontinen, et al., 2007)
- Persistent back pain (Backonja, Glanzman, 2003; Chou, Qaeem, Snow, et al., 2007; Serpell, Neuropathic Pain Study Group, 2002)
- Persistent masticatory muscle pain (Kimos, Biggs, Mah, et al., 2007)
- Guillain-Barré syndrome (Mao, Chen, 2000a; Pandey, Bose, Garg, et al., 2002)
- Vulvodynia (Ben-David, Friedman, 1999)

Pregabalin

Pregabalin (Lyrica) is a newer gabapentinoid and a precursor to gabapentin. It has a similar mechanism of action and many of the same pharmacologic properties, but has different pharmacokinetics and can exert a different profile of effects than gabapentin in the individual patient.

The oral bioavailability of gabapentin is 27% to 60%, depending on dose (Lacy, Armstrong, Goldman, et al., 2008), and 90% for pregabalin (Gajraj, 2007). Similar to gabapentin, pregabalin is not metabolized and is essentially unchanged with renal elimination. Neither drug has known drug-drug interactions.

The onset of pregabalin analgesia is approximately 25 minutes (Hill, Balkenohl, Thomas, et al., 2001), compared with 1 to 3 hours for gabapentin (Twycross, Wilcock, Charlesworth, et al., 2003). This faster onset of analgesic action may be clinically relevant in some cases (Blommel, Blommel, 2007). Equally important, pregabalin can be more rapidly titrated to the typical effective dose range than gabapentin. The time to effective dose for pregabalin may be as brief as 1 to 2 days (Gajraj, 2007; Portenoy, Murphy, Young, et al., 2006), compared to approximately 9 days for gabapentin (Gajraj, 2007). (See Chapter 26 for the perioperative use of pregabalin.)

Gabapentin is not a controlled substance, but pregabalin is designated a Schedule V drug. The Drug Enforcement Administration (DEA) reportedly designated pregabalin as a Schedule V drug because it produces some pharmacologic effects similar to diazepam (Valium) and alprazolam (Xanax); however, the data to support this conclusion are limited, and the effects are not sustained over time (Blommel, Blommel, 2007).

Pregabalin is approved in the United States for treatment of postherpetic neuralgia, painful diabetic neuropathy, and fibromyalgia. In the latter condition, studies have shown that the drug improves several core symptoms including pain, fatigue, and overall health and function (Arnold, Russell, Diri, et al., 2008; Crofford, Rowbotham, Mease, et al., 2005; Lyseng-Williamson, Siddiqui, 2008).

Although pregabalin may have effects on co-morbid anxiety, as suggested in a positive trial in patients with central pain from spinal cord injury (Murphy, Siddall, Griesing, 2007), a controlled trial in fibromyalgia patients demonstrated that anxiolysis was not necessary for pain reduction (Arnold, Crofford, Martin, et al., 2007). Studies show that pregabalin also can reduce pain-related sleep interference (Freynhagen, Grond, Schupfer, et al., 2007; Lesser, Sharma, LaMoreaux, et al., 2004; Sabatowski, Galvez, Cherry, et al., 2004; van Seventer, Feister, Young, 2006). Compared with alprazolam (Xanax) and placebo in healthy volunteers without pain, pregabalin produced improvements in features of disturbed sleep that have been reported in patients with fibromyalgia and anxiety disorders (Hindmarch, Dawson, Stanley, 2005).

Recent evidence-based guidelines indicate that pregabalin (or gabapentin) should be considered the first-line drug for the treatment of postherpetic neuralgia, painful diabetic neuropathy, and other neuropathic pains, unless a co-morbid depression suggests that an analgesic antidepressant should be tried first (Argoff, Backonja, Belgrade, et al., 2006; Dworkin, O'Connor, Backonja, et al., 2007) (see Chapter 22). This conclusion gains support from the consistent results observed in randomized controlled trials.

A 4-week randomized, placebo-controlled trial (N = 269) showed that pregabalin produced significant reductions in the spontaneous pain and allodynia caused by postherpetic neuralgia (Stacey, Barrett, Whalen, et al., 2008). An interesting finding was that improvements in pain and allodynia were correlated, which led the researchers to suggest allodynia could serve as an outcome measure in future research of this type. This trial compared fixed (300 mg/day) and flexible (150 to 600 mg/day) dosing regimens, and the latter was recommended as a way to reduce discontinuations, facilitate higher final doses, and improve ultimate pain relief. Flexible dosing of pregabalin has been recommended by others as well (Baron, Brunnmuller, Brasser, et al., 2007; Freynhagen, Grond, Schupfer, et al., 2007; Freynhagen, Strojek, Griesing, et al., 2005; Rowbotham, Stacey, Phillips, et al., 2007; Vranken, Dijkgraaf, Kruis, et al., 2008) (see later discussion of dosing recommendations).

In a recent meta-analysis of placebo-controlled trials in populations with painful diabetic neuropathy, pregabalin treatment yielded pain reduction; higher quality of life scores; and increased risk of dizziness, sedation, and edema (Hurley, Lesley, Adams, et al., 2008). Others have found similar results (Richter, Portenoy, Sharma, et al., 2005; Rosenstock, Tuchman, LaMoreaux, et al., 2004). A systematic review of research conducted between 1966 and 2005 concluded that pregabalin had a lower number-needed-to-treat (NNT = 3.24) for achieving greater than 50% analgesia in patients with painful diabetic neuropathy than any other anticonvulsants studied (Gutierrez-Alvarez, Beltran-Rodriguez, Moreno, 2007).

Positive findings also have been demonstrated in the treatment of central pain caused by spinal cord injury or stroke. A 4-week randomized, placebo-controlled trial of a flexible dosing regimen of pregabalin in 40 patients with central pain from brain or spinal cord injury demonstrated significant decreases in mean pain score and improvements in health status, but no difference in Pain Disability Index scores on follow-up evaluation compared with placebo (Vranken, Dijkgraaf, Kruis, et al., 2008).

The safety and effectiveness of pregabalin was evaluated in several open-label trials. A study of 55 patients with diverse types of refractory pain in which each patient's physician prescribed pregabalin with or without other analgesics according to their own preferences observed a reduction in the mean pain score from 6.5 at baseline to 5.5 on day 14 and to 4.9 on day 28; associated improvements in quality of life, sleep, and functional outcomes; and no serious adverse effects (Freynhagen, Grond, Schupfer, et al., 2007). A review of the open-label extension phases following 7 placebo-controlled trials reported that pain levels remained constant without clinically meaningful dose variations over a 2-year follow-up period (Portenoy, Murphy, Young, et al., 2006). A 15-month open-label trial that incorporated flexible dosing of pregabalin demonstrated persistent positive drug effects in a subset of patients (N = 81) with postherpetic neuralgia or painful diabetic neuropathy refractory to other adjuvant analgesics (e.g., gabapentin and antidepressants) (Stacey, Dworkin, Murphy, et al., 2008). Almost half of the patients had a greater than 30% reduction in pain, and the prevalence of severe pain declined from 63% on admission to the trial to only 23% after 15 months of pregabalin treatment; when pregabalin was stopped during the study drug holidays, pain rapidly returned. Because patients were allowed to continue to take their other analgesics during this study, pregabalin was seen as an add-on therapy, and the researchers cautioned that the results should be interpreted with this in mind.

The prior studies are representative of a larger literature documenting the clinical trials, case reports, and reviews that have evaluated the analgesic potential of pregabalin. Recent studies also suggest that the drug may have utility in several nonpainful conditions (Ehrchen, Stander, 2008; Porzio, Aielli, Verna, et al., 2006) and restless leg syndrome pain (Sommer, Bachmann, Liebetanz, et al., 2007). A broad review of the literature on pregabalin reveals publications on the following conditions:

- Painful diabetic neuropathy (Argoff, Backonja, Belgrade, et al., 2006; Baron, Brunnmuller, Brasser, et al., 2007; Boulton, Vinik, Arezzo, et al., 2005; Frampton, Scott, 2004; Frank, Cousins, 2008; Freeman, Durso-Decruz, Emir, 2008; Freynhagen, Strojek, Griesing, et al., 2005; Freynhagen, Grond, Schupfer, et al., 2007; Richter, Portenoy, Sharma, et al., 2005; Rosenstock, Tuchman, LaMoreaux, et al., 2004; Tolle, Freynhagen, Versavel et al., 2008; Veves, Backonja, Malik, 2008)

- Fibromyalgia (Arnold, Crofford, Martin, et al., 2007; Arnold, Russell, Diri, et al., 2008; Crofford, Rowbotham, Mease, et al., 2005) (see also Hauser, Thieme, Turk, 2009.)
- Postherpetic neuralgia (Baron, Brunnmuller, Brasser, et al., 2007; Dubinsky, Kabbani, El-Chami, et al., 2004; Dworkin, Corbin, Young, et al., 2003; Frampton, Foster, 2005; Freynhagen, Strojek, Griesing, et al., 2005; Rowbotham, Stacey, Phillips, et al., 2007; Stacey, Barrett, Whalen, et al., 2008; van Seventer, Feister, Young, et al., 2006)
- Central pain from brain or spinal cord injury (Siddall, Cousins, Otte, et al., 2006; Vranken, Dijkgraaf, Kruis, et al., 2008)
- Trigeminal neuralgia (Obermann, Yoon, Sensen, et al., 2008)
- Glossopharyngeal neuralgia (Guido, Specchio, 2006)
- Restless leg syndrome with or without neuropathic pain (Sommer, Bachmann, Liebetanz, et al., 2007).

Lamotrigine

A recent meta-analysis of clinical trials evaluating lamotrigine (Lamictal) for acute and persistent pain showed limited efficacy for neuropathic pain states and no studies on its use for acute pain (Wiffen, Rees, 2007). In practice, the drug may be tried in those with persistent neuropathic pain that has not responded to the gabapentinoids and one or more of the analgesic antidepressants. The limited data supporting the potential for analgesic efficacy includes randomized trials for trigeminal neuralgia (Zakrzewska, Chaudhry, Nurmikko, et al., 1997), HIV painful neuropathy (Simpson, Olney, McArthur, et al., 2000), and central poststroke pain (Frese, Husstedt, Ringelstein, et al., 2006; Kumar, Kalita, Kumar, et al., 2009; Vestergaard, Andersen, Gottrup, et al., 2001). Open-label trials suggest analgesic effects in trigeminal neuralgia (Canavero, Bonicalzi, 1997; Rosen, 2001), sciatic pain (Eisenberg, Damunni, Hoffer, et al., 2003), and pain associated with multiple sclerosis (Cianchetti, Zuddas, Randazzo, et al., 1999). In contrast, studies in populations with painful diabetic neuropathy have yielded conflicting results (Duby, Campbell, Setter, et al., 2004; Eisenberg, Alon, Ishay, et al., 1998; Jose, Bhansali, Hota, et al., 2007; Vinik, Tuchman, Safirstein, et al., 2007), and a controlled study that evaluated the addition of lamotrigine (up to 400 mg/day) to either a nonopioid analgesic, gabapentin, or a tricyclic antidepressant (TCA) for a variety of different types of neuropathic pains did not reveal an analgesic response (Silver, Blum, Grainger, et al., 2007).

Lamotrigine carries a relatively high risk of rash—up to 7% of patients in some studies—and serious cutaneous hypersensitivity (e.g., Stevens-Johnson syndrome or toxic epidermal necrolysis). This adverse effect occurs far more frequently with lamotrigine than during treatment with other adjuvant analgesics. The latter risk is increased in younger patients, and the drug should not be used in patients younger than 15 years old. Although the risk of serious rash in adults is low overall (less than 1%), the availability of other agents (e.g., antidepressants and other anticonvulsants) with less of this risk suggests that lamotrigine may best be relegated to a trial only after several other drugs have failed to provide benefit. If a lamotrigine trial is undertaken, dosing should follow the manufacturer's recommendation for gradual titration from a low dose, which has been determined to reduce the risk of cutaneous toxicity.

Oxcarbazepine

Another relatively new anticonvulsant is oxcarbazepine (Trileptal), which structurally is a metabolite of carbamazepine (Tegretol). It is approved in the United States for the treatment of trigeminal neuralgia and has been described as the drug of choice for this condition (Carrazana, Mikoshiba, 2003; Jensen, 2002). Simple dose titration and dose adjustments and convenient twice-daily dosing are cited among the advantages of this drug. A meta-analysis supports effectiveness comparable to carbamazepine but with fewer adverse effects; 62% reported good to excellent tolerability with oxcarbazepine compared with 48% who took carbamazepine (Beydoun, Schmidt, D'Souza, et al., 2002). Open-label studies support these findings as well (Carrazana, Mikoshiba, 2003).

In contrast to the studies in trigeminal neuralgia, studies in diabetic painful neuropathy have yielded equivocal results. A 16-week randomized, placebo-controlled study (N = 146) titrated patients with painful diabetic neuropathy to a maximum dose of 1800 mg/day and reported a larger decrease in average visual analog scale (VAS) score (–24.3) compared with placebo (–14.7) (Dogra, Beydoun, Mazzola, et al., 2005). More patients had a greater than 50% reduction in pain with oxcarbazepine (35.2%) than with placebo (18.4%), and there were fewer arousals from sleep because of pain in those who took the active drug. Another large placebo-controlled trial (N = 347) evaluating the drug for painful diabetic neuropathy found a trend toward meaningful changes in pain scores from baseline to the last week of the study with oxcarbazepine 1200 mg/day and 1800 mg/day compared with placebo, but the changes did not reach statistical significance (Beydoun, Shaibani, Hopwood, et al., 2006). A 9-week open-label trial in 30 patients with painful diabetic neuropathy found that oxcarbazepine (highest dose of 1200 mg/day) produced significant improvements in pain relief, with a decrease in mean VAS score from 66.3 at baseline to 34.3 at the end of the trial (Beydoun, Kobetz, Carrazana, 2004). The most common adverse effects were sedation and dizziness, similar to other anticonvulsants.

The efficacy of oxcarbazepine has been studied in other conditions as well. A randomized controlled trial of 32 patients with colon cancer undergoing chemotherapy found a dramatically lower incidence of chemotherapy-induced neuropathy when oxcarbazepine was administered prior to chemotherapy (31.2%) compared with chemotherapy without oxcarbazepine (75%) (Argyriou,

Chroni, Polychronopoulos, 2006). In contrast, a controlled study of patients with frequent migraine was negative, demonstrating no reduction in the number of attacks over 28 days of prophylactic treatment (Silberstein, Saper, Berenson, et al., 2008). Efficacy in postherpetic neuralgia and CRPS has been suggested in published case reports (Criscuolo, Auletta, Lippi, et al., 2004; Lalwani, Shoham, Koh, et al., 2005). Further research and clinical experience with this drug are needed to better evaluate its safety and what types of pain will benefit most (Guay, 2003).

Topiramate

Topiramate (Topamax) is approved in the United States for migraine prevention. A multicenter, double-blind study randomized 487 people with persistent migraine to receive placebo, or 50, 100, or 200 mg of topiramate daily for 26 weeks to determine efficacy and optimal dose (Silberstein, Neto, Schmitt et al., 2004). The percent of individuals who experienced 50% or greater reduction in monthly migraine were: 23% (placebo), 36% (50 mg), 54% (100 mg), and 52% (200 mg) (see dosing guidelines later in this chapter). Topiramate treatment also resulted in a reduction in the use of acute headache treatment medications in this study. The most frequent adverse effects were paresthesia, fatigue, nausea, anorexia, and abnormal taste. Weight loss, a common effect of topiramate, was experienced in those taking 100 and 200 mg. Other randomized controlled trials similarly support 100 mg/day as the most efficacious and best-tolerated dose of topiramate for migraine prevention (Brandes, Saper, Diamond, et al., 2004; Silberstein, 2005; Silberstein, Diener, Lipton, et al., 2008; Silberstein, Lipton, Dodick, et al., 2007).

Topiramate also has been shown to be effective for persistent cluster headache (Lainez, Pascual, Pascual, et al., 2003), idiopathic trigeminal neuralgia (Solaro, Uccelli, Brichetto, et al., 2001), and trigeminal autonomic cephalalgias, which is a grouping of headache syndromes that include paroxysmal hemicrania and short-lasting unilateral neuralgiform headache with conjunctival injection and tearing (SUNCT) syndrome in addition to cluster headache (Cohen, Matharu, Goadsby, 2007; May, Leone, Afra, et al., 2006).

Topiramate has been studied for other types of persistent pain, with equivocal outcomes. A 10-week randomized placebo-controlled trial (N = 96) demonstrated that topiramate titrated to a maximum dose of 300 mg/day was safe and significantly improved pain, quality of life, and functional outcomes in a group of patients with persistent low back pain (Muehlbacher, Nickel, Kettler, et al., 2006). Again, weight loss was notable in this study, which may be a significant benefit in some patients with persistent pain who are also overweight. A small pilot study of 4 patients with phantom limb pain showed that 3 of the 4 experienced significant decreases in pain with topiramate (Harden, Houle, Remble, et al., 2005); the peak effect was noted at 800 mg/day, but such high doses are not recommended (United States Food and Drug Administration [U.S. FDA],

2004). Topiramate has not been shown to be effective for painful diabetic neuropathy (Jensen, 2002), and guidelines list it as a drug with limited evidence for treatment of this condition (Argoff, Backonja, Belgrade, et al., 2006).

Metabolic acidosis caused by renal wasting of bicarbonate has been linked to the use of topiramate. Mild to moderate decreases in serum bicarbonate are most likely at doses of 400 mg/day and usually occur early in treatment; however, these effects have also been noted in doses as low as 50 mg/day (U.S. FDA, 2004). These effects are of particular concern when the drug is used on a long-term basis (Welch, Graybeal, Moe, et al., 2006). Nephrolithiasis also has been noted.

Other Second-Generation Anticonvulsants

Very few studies have evaluated the analgesic potential of zonisamide (Zonegran). A study that randomized 25 patients with painful diabetic neuropathy to receive placebo or zonisamide found that a mean dose of 540 mg/day over 6 weeks was associated with a nonsignificant improvement in pain (Atli, Dogra, 2005). A larger sample size would have likely demonstrated analgesic efficacy in this trial, but the dropout rate was high due to a variety of adverse effects (e.g., irritability, insomnia, metallic taste, and rash) in those taking zonisamide. Given the limited data, this drug is rarely tried for patients with neuropathic pain or migraine (Kaniecki, 2008), and further research is needed to evaluate its efficacy and safety for these conditions (Duby, Campbell, Setter, et al., 2004; Guay, 2003).

Lacosamide (Vimpat) was recently approved in the United States for the indication of seizures. There are data suggesting analgesic efficacy in painful diabetic neuropathy. A randomized controlled trial (N = 119) found lacosamide titrated to 100 to 400 mg/day or maximum tolerated dose produced significantly better pain relief and improvements in quality of life compared with placebo in patients with moderate to severe intensity painful diabetic neuropathy (Rauck, Shaibani, Bilton, et al., 2007). An open-label trial (N = 69) demonstrated both short-term and long-term (2.5 years) safety and efficacy at maximum titrated doses of 400 mg/day in patients with painful diabetic neuropathy (Shaibani, Biton, Rauck, et al., 2009). Other studies have produced similar findings (Hidvegi, Bretschneider, Thierfelder, et al., 2008; Kenney, Simpson, Koch, et al., 2006; Shaibani, Fares, Selam, et al., 2009). Long-term safety and efficacy was established for 400 mg/day of lacosamide for 18 weeks in a double-blind, randomized, placebo-controlled trial of 370 patients with painful diabetic neuropathy (Wymer, Simpson, Sen, et al., 2009). The lower dose of 200 mg/day reduced pain but failed to significantly dissociate from placebo for primary and secondary outcome measures.

No substantial metabolism, low or no inhibition of cytochrome P450 isoenzymes, and low protein binding contribute to a low incidence of drug-drug interactions with lacosamide (Kropeit, Scharfenecker, Schiltmeyer, et al., 2006). There is no interaction between lacosamide and the oral antidiabetic drug metformin, which is an advantage in patients who take that drug for diabetes and also have painful diabetic neuropathy (Schiltmeyer, Kropeit, Cawello, et al., 2006).

Tiagabine (Gabitril) is used for treatment of a wide variety of conditions including epilepsy and other seizure disorders, depression, anxiety, posttraumatic stress syndrome, and substance withdrawal symptoms. There has been little investigation of its analgesic potential. A 3-month, open-label study comparing tiagabine and gabapentin in 91 patients with persistent pain, such as back pain, musculoskeletal headache, and fibromyalgia, found that both drugs significantly reduced pain, but tiagabine showed greater improvements in sleep quality (Todorov, Kolchev, Todorov, 2005). The drug has been linked to new-onset seizures, which have occurred at doses as low as 4 mg/day and usually occur after dose increases; this adverse effect led the United States Food and Drug Administration (2005b) to recommend discontinuation of the drug in nonepileptic patients who develop seizures.

Felbamate (Felbatol) has been used anecdotally to treat hemifacial spasm (Mellick, 1995), a painless syndrome characterized by paroxysmal contraction of facial muscles. Although this observation and treatment of a small number of patients initially raised expectations, no follow-up studies have been done in populations with pain. The potential for lethal aplastic anemia from this drug has tempered enthusiasm for these trials (see adverse effects).

First-Generation Anticonvulsants

The older anticonvulsants have been used as analgesics for several decades. Although the newer drugs are now preferred, patients with refractory pain may be offered trials of these drugs.

Carbamazepine

Carbamazepine (Tegretol) has been reported to be effective for many pain syndromes, including diabetic neuropathy, postherpetic neuralgia, poststroke pain, and CRPS (Dobecki, Schocket, Wallace, 2006; Harke, Gretenkort, Ladleif, et al., 2001; Vurdelja, Budincevic, Prvan, 2008; Zin, Nissen, Smith, et al., 2008). It is approved for treatment of trigeminal neuralgia, and based on years of positive experience in this syndrome, often is selected as a first-line drug (Jensen, 2002; Jensen, Finnerup, 2007; Krafft, 2008; Sindrup, Jensen, 2002) (see also oxcarbazepine). Carbamazepine also has been used to treat cancer-related pruritus (Korfitis, Trafalis, 2008). A systematic review of controlled trials concluded that carbamazepine has analgesic properties for varied acute and persistent pains and can treat lancinating neuropathic pain, regardless of the specific pathologic condition contributing to the presence of this pain characteristic (Wiffen, McQuay, Moore, 2005). Although the numbers of patients in these

clinical trials were small, clinicians wanting to use this agent as a second-line anticonvulsant can access important information as to how effective it is with certain types of pain from this review.

Clonazepam

Clonazepam (Klonopin) is a benzodiazepine and has been used primarily as an anticonvulsant. It has been suggested to be analgesic in the lancinating pain associated with phantom limb pain, neuropathic cancer-related pain, and myofascial pain (Bartusch, Sanders, D'Alessio, et al., 1996; Hugel, Ellershaw, Dickman, 2003; Fishbain, Cutler, Rosomoff, et al., 2000). The supporting evidence is very limited, however, and its use may be more related to its potential to help co-morbid anxiety than to its established analgesic efficacy. Given its long half-life, the potential for accumulation with repeated dosing must be recognized, and it must be used very cautiously in patients predisposed to adverse effects, including the cognitively impaired (particularly older adults) and patients with sleep apnea syndrome or advanced cardiopulmonary disease. (See clonazepam patient medication information, Form V-3 on pp. 763-764, at the end of Section V.)

Divalproex Sodium and Valproic Acid

Divalproex sodium (Depakote) is approved and widely used for migraine prevention (Freitag, Diamond, Diamond, et al., 2001; Silberstein, Collins, 1999). The drug is closely related to valproic acid and shares the same pharmacology, but differs in that it is available in gastro-resistant sprinkles and modified-release formulation. In a 12-month, open-label study of 241 adolescents with migraines who were given a titrated dose of modified-release divalproex to a maximum dose of 1000 mg/day, the median number of migraine attacks decreased 75% between the first and fourth month of the study and remained at or below this level for the remainder of the study (Apostol, Lewis, Laforet et al., 2009). The most common adverse effects were nausea, vomiting, and weight gain; 17% discontinued therapy because of an adverse event.

Divalproex sodium has not been studied in neuropathic pain, and the evidence for valproic acid is mixed. Whereas one study showed improvements in painful diabetic neuropathy (Kochar, Rawat, Agrawal, et al., 2004), another found no benefit in pain from polyneuropathy (Otto, Bach, Jensen, et al., 2004). Based on the limited data (Chong, Hester, 2007), divalproex sodium is rarely tried for neuropathic pain, and the IV formulation of valproic acid (Depacon) is only occasionally used in an effort to quickly reverse severe pain, typically in an inpatient setting.

Phenytoin

Similar to carbamazepine, phenytoin (Dilantin) has been used as an analgesic for decades, but has been largely supplanted by newer anticonvulsants (Jensen, 2002; Vanotti, Osio, Mailland, et al., 2007). In early controlled trials, phenytoin was shown to be an effective analgesic for neuropathic pain, particularly pains characterized by a prominent lancinating component (McCleane, 1999). Isolated case reports illustrate its use, and one in particular that shows it has benefits for treating crescendo pelvic cancer–related pain with lancinating quality (Chang, 1997). IV phenytoin, like IV valproate, is sometimes suggested as an option for treatment of acute attacks of neuropathic pain (Jensen, 2002; McCleane, 1999). An extensive review (Duby, Campbell, Setter, et al., 2004) and guidelines (Argoff, Backonja, Belgrade, et al., 2006) list phenytoin as a drug with limited evidence for treatment of painful diabetic neuropathy.

Summary

At present, gabapentin and pregabalin share with selected antidepressants first-line status for the treatment of neuropathic pain. Numerous other anticonvulsants have some evidence of efficacy, but in all cases, this evidence is limited or conflicting. Nonetheless, patients with neuropathic pain that has not responded to trials of the gabapentinoids and appropriate antidepressants should be considered candidates for trials of those anticonvulsants with some supporting data. Sequential trials are appropriate for patients with severe and intractable pain. Each anticonvulsant has a unique pharmacodynamic and pharmacokinetic profile (LaRoche, 2007), and their use as analgesics largely mirrors the prescribing guidelines employed for their primary indication.

Mechanism of Action

The specific mechanisms of the analgesia produced by anticonvulsant drugs are not known, but presumably relate to those actions underlying anticonvulsant effects (Lussier, Portenoy, 2004). Most of the anticonvulsants have multiple mechanisms of action (Gilron, 2006), and these may differ among the various anticonvulsants (Lussier, Portenoy, 2004).

One of the mechanisms is blockade of presynaptic voltage-gated ion channels, which prevents the generation of spontaneous ectopic discharges (Beydoun, Backonja, 2003; Taylor, 2009) (see Section I and Figure I-2, *B* on pp. 4-5). Some anticonvulsants (e.g., carbamazepine, felbamate, lamotrigine, oxcarbazepine, phenytoin, topiramate, and zonisamide) relieve pain, in part, by prolonging the recovery phase of sodium channels after their activation (Gilron, 2006; Soderpalm, 2002). Some (e.g., carbamazepine, felbamate, gabapentin, lamotrigine, pregabalin, valproic acid, and zonisamide) bind to presynaptic voltage-gated calcium channels and inhibit calcium influx and the release of excitatory neurotransmitters from primary afferent nerve fibers (Dickenson, Matthews, Suzuki, 2002; Gajraj, 2007; Gilron, 2006; Taylor, 2009; Tiippana, Hamunen, Kontinen, et al., 2007). Pregabalin has an even higher calcium-channel affinity than gabapentin and has no effect on sodium channels (Gilron, Watson, Cahill,

et al., 2006; Mao, Chen, 2000a; Nicholson, 2000). Recent research confirmed that gabapentin had no effect on transient sodium currents but inhibited persistent sodium currents in a dose-dependent way (Yang, Wang, Chen, et al., 2009). The clinical significance of these findings is unknown.

Other mechanisms also may be important. Inhibition of glutamate, an excitatory neurotransmitter that promotes the transmission of pain through increased activity at the NMDA receptor and other receptors, may be relevant for some drugs (Jensen, 2002; Soderpalm, 2002) (see Section I and Figure I-2, *B* on pp. 4-5). Others may indirectly or directly augment inhibitory GABAergic neurotransmission (Gilron, 2006; Soderpalm, 2002). For example, gabapentin is a GABA analogue, and although it does not bind to GABA receptors or modulate GABA reuptake, it does enhance overall GABA-mediated inhibitory tone (Dickenson, Matthews, Suzuki, 2002; Jensen, 2002; Mao, Chen, 2000). Gabapentin and pregabalin share a specific high affinity drug binding site (calcium channel α_2-δ ligands) localized at synapses and sufficient in amount to account for their analgesic action (Taylor, 2009).

Interestingly, there is evidence that some of the anticonvulsants have peripheral effects that may be involved in pain. For example, carbamazepine and phenytoin produce antiinflammatory effects, and local injection of gabapentin and lamotrigine in animals exerts an analgesic effect (Gilron, 2006).

The central effects of anticonvulsants have been evaluated in experimental studies. Animal and human research has shown that gabapentin selectively reduces nociception in a sensitized (damaged) nervous system but not in a normal nervous system (Gilron, 2002). Healthy volunteers in two separate randomized, placebo-controlled studies were subjected to experimental thermal injury (acute pain model [nociception]) (Werner, Perkins, Holte, et al., 2001) and heat-capsaicin sensitization (central hypersensitivity model [neuropathic]) (Dirks, Petersen, Rowbotham, et al., 2002). Gabapentin was found to have no effect on pain transmission on normal skin but significantly reduced hyperalgesia. Gilron (2002) pointed out that the clinical value of these findings is that gabapentin may reduce pathologic (neuropathic) pain while leaving other protective nociceptive mechanisms intact.

Adverse Effects

Anticonvulsants usually are well-tolerated (Collins, Moore, McQuay, et al., 2000). The most common adverse effects are dizziness and sedation. These are usually transient and most notable during the titration phase of treatment (Serpell, Neuropathic Pain Study Group, 2002). GI upset (e.g., nausea) can occur but usually decreases with time. Occasionally, patients report changes in mood, such as dysphoria or cognitive impairment, which may be subtle.

There is a long history of concern about the association between anticonvulsant use and loss of bone mineral density (Sheth, 2005), particularly during treatment with enzyme-inducing anticonvulsants, such as carbamazepine and phenytoin (Petty, Paton, O'Brien, et al., 2005). Risk factors for this adverse effect are ages 40 years and older and anticonvulsant use for more than 2 years. Gabapentin, pregabalin, lamotrigine, and topiramate are examples of non–enzyme-inducing anticonvulsants (Novy, Stupp, Rossetti, 2009). Valproate is a non–enzyme-inducing anticonvulsant but it is associated with reduced bone mineralization (Novy, Stupp, Rossetti, 2009).

Although there have been case reports of hepatotoxicity with gabapentin (Richardson, Williams, Kingham, 2002), they are rare. Neither gabapentin nor pregabalin undergo hepatic metabolism, a positive effect of which is a minimal risk of drug-drug interactions (Frank, Cousins, 2008). The new anticonvulsant, lacosamide, produces low or no inhibition of cytochrome P450 isoenzymes and also may have a reduced risk of interactions (Kropeit, Scharfenecker, Schiltmeyer, et al., 2006). Other anticonvulsants inhibit various isoenzymes of the cytochrome P450 enzyme system, which can result in drug-drug interactions (Virani, Mailis, Shapiro, et al., 1997) (see Chapter 11, for more on the cytochrome P450 enzyme system). Each anticonvulsant has a unique profile (LaRoche, 2007), and it is important for the clinician to become familiar with the potential for drug-drug interactions associated with the particular anticonvulsant being administered. Patients must be told to report adverse effects promptly, and in some cases serum drug concentrations should be closely monitored to prevent toxicity, such as in patients who take multiple other medications and those who take anticonvulsants during chemotherapy (Yap, Chui, Chan, 2008). Following is a more detailed discussion of adverse effects associated with selected anticonvulsants.

Gabapentin

Gabapentin has a relatively low adverse effect profile, and in clinical practice dizziness and sedation seem to be the most dose-limiting adverse effects. A meta-analysis of 36 randomized, placebo-controlled studies of several of the second-generation anticonvulsants used for seizure control confirmed that gabapentin was significantly associated with sedation and dizziness; however, comparisons between drugs were not possible (Zaccara, Gangemi, Cincotta, 2008). Gabapentin is reported to produce more sedation but less dry mouth than amitriptyline (Mao, Chen, 2000).

Confusion and weight gain are other less common effects of gabapentin (Mao, Chen, 2000). Ataxia and other movement disorders have been reported and appear to cease when the drug is discontinued (Buetefisch, Guiterrez, Gutmann, et al., 1996; Reeves, So, Sharbrough, et al., 1996). The most commonly reported adverse gabapentin effects in surgical patients are nausea, sedation, dizziness, and urinary retention (Tiippana, Hamunen, Kontinen, et al., 2007).

As mentioned, a major benefit of gabapentin is that it is not hepatically metabolized. This results in minimal drug-drug interactions and hepatic adverse effects. The drug is excreted entirely by the renal system. Gabapentin toxicity was reported in a case describing its use during an episode of acute renal failure (Miller, Price, 2009). The importance of recognizing the need to adjust the dose downward during acute illness, particularly when there is a decline in renal clearance, must be recognized. (See gabapentin patient medication information, Form V-7 on pp. 771-772, at the end of Section V.)

Pregabalin

Pregabalin also has a low adverse effect profile and is well tolerated (Gajraj, 2007). As with gabapentin, dizziness and somnolence are common, and these are typically dose related, transient, and mild to moderate in severity (Gajraj, 2007; Arnold, Russell, Diri, et al., 2008; Lyseng-Williamson, Siddiqui, 2008). Pregabalin has a documented low risk for blurred vision. Patients should be told to report this to their health care provider should it occur. Weight gain also has been noted.

Also, like gabapentin, pregabalin does not undergo hepatic metabolism and has no reported drug interactions of concern (Frank, Cousins, 2008). Additive pharmacodynamic effects of the type that may occur whenever two or more centrally-acting drugs are taken also occurs during pregabalin dosing; patients may report effects on cognitive and gross-motor function when the drug is co-administered with other drugs or alcohol (Blommel, Blommel, 2007). Being a relatively new drug, evaluation of the impact of its adverse effects in older patients requires further research and clinical experience (Guay, 2005). (See pregabalin patient medication information, Form V-11 on pp. 779-780, at the end of Section V.)

Oxcarbazepine

Oxcarbazepine has a better adverse effect profile and is better tolerated than the older anticonvulsants, such as carbamazepine (Jensen, 2002). Rare cases of anaphylactic reactions and angioedema resulted in postmarketing labeling changes for oxcarbazepine (U.S. FDA, 2007b). The drug should be discontinued permanently should these occur. Potentially serious skin reactions, including Stevens Johnson syndrome and toxic epidermal necrolysis, have been reported with the use of oxcarbazepine and also require prompt discontinuation of the drug (Lacy, Armstrong, Goldman, et al., 2008). Hyponatremia should be recognized as a rare adverse effect of this drug, and other effects, such as edema, diplopia, abnormal gait, cognitive slowing, and speech difficulties, have been noted (Guay, 2005; Lacy, Armstrong, Goldman, et al., 2008).

Topiramate

Topiramate is generally well tolerated. Dose-related paresthesia is the most common adverse effect (Adleman, Freitag, Lainez, et al., 2008). Fatigue, nausea, and difficulty concentrating are usually mild to moderate in severity, if they occur. Serious adverse effects are rare

(2%) and include abdominal pain, vomiting, dehydration, anorexia, venous thrombosis, and renal calculi. Language disturbances (i.e., difficulty finding the right word) also have been associated with the drug (Coppola, Rossi, Mancini, et al., 2008). Weight loss has been observed during treatment with this drug; it is generally modest and yields clinically noticeable effects in a minority of patients (Adleman, Freitag, Lainez, et al., 2008).

Other Second-Generation Anticonvulsants

Other second-generation anticonvulsant drugs also are usually well tolerated but present a range of potential toxicities (Walia, Khan, Ko, et al., 2004). As noted, all of these drugs can produce the spectrum of adverse effects common to centrally-acting agents, including dizziness, cognitive slowing, mood change, and related experiences. Other adverse effects are more specific to one or another of the drugs. Felbamate, for example, has been associated with rare fatal aplastic anemia and liver failure, which has limited its use to patients with refractory epilepsy. It is generally not considered for neuropathic pain. Lamotrigine has been associated with a relatively high incidence of serious cutaneous hypersensitivity, both Stevens Johnson syndrome and toxic epidermal necrolysis (Lacy, Armstrong, Goldman, et al., 2008). The dropout rate in a clinical trial of zonisamide was high due to a variety of causes including irritability, insomnia, metallic taste, and rash (Atli, Dogra, 2005).

Carbamazepine

Carbamazepine commonly causes sedation, dizziness, nausea, and unsteadiness. These effects can be minimized by low initial doses and gradual dose titration. The intensity diminishes in most patients maintained on the drug for several weeks. Of much greater concern, carbamazepine may cause aplastic anemia, agranulocytosis, or thrombocytopenia in a very small percentage of patients (Hart, Easton, 1982). Therefore, it is critical to obtain a complete hematologic profile prior to therapy, after several weeks, and every 3 to 4 months thereafter. A leukocyte count less than 4000 is usually considered to be a contraindication to treatment, and a decline to less than 3000 (or an absolute neutrophil count of less than 1500) during therapy should lead to discontinuation of the drug. Patients need to be told to report any signs or symptoms of infection, easy bruising, or fatigue.

Other extremely rare adverse effects of carbamazepine include hepatic damage and hyponatremia caused by inappropriate secretion of antidiuretic hormone (Van Amelsvoort, Bakshi, Devaux, et al., 1994). Liver and renal function tests should be routinely evaluated at the start and during the course of therapy. Treatment with carbamazepine may be complicated in older patients who are at risk for cardiac disease, water retention, decreased osmolality, and hyponatremia (Jensen, 2002). Balancing adverse effects with optimal effects in this population can be challenging. Careful monitoring during therapy is recommended.

Clonazepam

Drowsiness is the most common and troubling adverse effect of clonazepam. Tolerance to the effect often develops within weeks after dosing is begun. Occasional patients develop ataxia, particularly at higher doses. Idiosyncratic reactions, including dermatitis, hepatotoxicity, and hematologic effects, appear to be very rare. Like other benzodiazepine drugs, a withdrawal syndrome may occur with abrupt discontinuation of relatively high doses, so tapering gradually for 2 weeks or more is recommended.

Phenytoin

Most of the common adverse effects of phenytoin are dose dependent and usually occur at plasma concentrations greater than the therapeutic range for seizure control. These include sedation or mental clouding, dizziness, unsteadiness, and diplopia. Occasional patients experience toxicity with lower concentrations of the drug in the blood. Of the idiosyncratic effects, the most serious are hepatotoxicity and exfoliative dermatitis. The occurrence of a maculopapular rash, which can be the harbinger of the more severe cutaneous reactions, should lead to discontinuation of the drug.

Valproic Acid

At therapeutic doses, the adverse effects of valproate are usually mild, and include sedation, nausea, tremor, and sometimes increased appetite. An enteric-coated tablet minimizes GI disturbances, and dose-dependent adverse effects are reduced by the use of low initial doses and gradual upward dose titration. Hepatotoxicity, encephalopathy, dermatitis, alopecia, and a rare hyperammonemia syndrome are among the reported idiosyncratic reactions. Because the idiosyncratic hyperammonemia syndrome can occur without abnormalities in other liver function tests, the occurrence of confusion during therapy should be evaluated with both liver function tests and serum ammonia level.

Indications

All types of neuropathic pain are generally considered the primary indication for trying an anticonvulsant drug. Neuropathic pain guidelines recommend gabapentin and pregabalin as first-line choices (Dubinsky, Kabbani, El-Chami, et al., 2004; Dworkin, O'Connor, Backonja, et al., 2007; Moulin, Clark, Gilron, et al., 2007).

Drug Selection

For patients with neuropathic pain, the widely accepted first-line drugs are either the anticonvulsants gabapentin or pregabalin, or antidepressants in the tricyclic antidepressant (TCA) or serotonin norepinephrine reuptake inhibitor (SNRI) classes (Dworkin, Backonja, Rowbotham, et al., 2003; Dworkin, O'Connor, Backonja, et al., 2007; Moulin, Clark, Gilron, et al., 2007). There are few comparative trials, and a recent meta-analysis could not find appreciable differences in the effectiveness of TCAs compared with the anticonvulsant gabapentin for the treatment of diabetic neuropathy and postherpetic neuralgia (Chou, Carson, Chan, 2009). A reasonable guideline would be to consider one of the gabapentinoids first, unless there is a concurrent indication for antidepressant therapy, such as depressed mood, anxiety, or insomnia. The variability in responses to anticonvulsant adjuvant analgesics is great, and sequential trials in patients with refractory pain are amply justified by clinical experience.

Various influences may bear on the selection of an anticonvulsant, particularly in the setting of neuropathic pain that has been poorly responsive to gabapentin and pregabalin and one or more of the analgesic antidepressants. These factors include the pain diagnosis, patient characteristics, prior response to a particular drug, issues with convenience and adherence to therapy, cost and availability of agents, and access to care and follow-up treatment.

Occasionally, a drug is selected based on the type of pain. This is most typical in the case of trigeminal neuralgia, for which treatment with carbamazepine or oxcarbazepine often is preferred, even before trials of the usual first-line drugs for neuropathic pain. Similarly, a trial of topiramate, valproate, or lamotrigine may be considered early if neuropathic pain is accompanied by frequent headache with migranous features.

Unique patient characteristics must be considered as well. For example, a trial of topiramate, which can lead to weight loss (Adleman, Freitag, Lainez, et al., 2008), may be preferred in the obese patient and discouraged in the very thin patient.

Dose Selection

Dosing guidelines used in the treatment of seizures are typically extrapolated for the management of pain. As with all of the adjuvant analgesics, doses of anticonvulsants must be tailored to meet the patient's individual needs. Titration is almost always required. Dose escalation should continue until favorable effects occur, intolerable and unmanageable adverse effects supervene, or plasma drug concentration has reached some arbitrary level (customarily at the upper end of the therapeutic range for seizure control). Table V-1, pp. 748-756, at the end of Section V contains dosing recommendations for all of the commonly used anticonvulsants. Following is a discussion of dosing considerations for selected anticonvulsants.

Gabapentin

Although a comprehensive review of available data recommends treatment of persistent pain with a maintenance gabapentin dose of 900 mg/day (Backonja, Glanzman, 2003), clinical experience indicates that analgesic effectiveness often requires a higher dose, and some patients have good outcomes at lower amounts. A low starting dose gradually titrated upward is recommended, for example, starting with 300 mg/day for most patients and 100 mg/day for

those with significant renal insufficiency advanced age, or serious medical co-morbidities. In most cases, the dose can be increased every 3 to 4 days, initially by an amount equal to the starting dose. The doses should be divided into twice-daily administration; some patients experience better outcomes with three divided doses and this should be explored if patients report adverse effects at the peak effect of a twice-daily dose. Dose titration usually continues with a target of 1800 mg/day to 3600 mg/day in two or three divided doses. The dose required to maintain analgesia varies widely, and one study reported good results with a dose range between 900 mg/day and 4800 mg/day (median dose 2400 mg/day) in patients with spinal cord injury (To, Lim, Hill, et al., 2002). Doses as high as 6000 mg/day have been taken for cancer pain (Farrar, Portenoy, 2001). Patients with renal insufficiency should be titrated to a lower level and observed more carefully. Table 23-2 provides recommendations for dosing adjustments in patients with renal impairment.

GUIDELINES

Table 23-2 | Gabapentin and Pregabalin Dosing Adjustments in Renal Impairment

Drug	Creatinine Clearance (mL/min)	Daily Dose Range (mg/day)	Dosing Frequency
Gabapentin[1,2]	≥60	300-1200	Three times daily
	>30-59	200-700	Twice daily
	>15-29	200-700	Single daily dose
	15	100-300	Single daily dose
Pregabalin[3]	≥60	150-600	2-3 divided doses
	30-59	75-300	2-3 divided doses
	15-29	25-150	1-2 divided doses
	<15	25-75	Single daily dose

[1]**Gabapentin posthemodialysis:** Single supplemental dose of 125 to 300 mg administered after each 4 hours of hemodialysis.
[2]Reduce daily dose in proportion to creatinine clearance for creatinine clearance less than 15 mL/min.
[3]**Pregabalin posthemodialysis:**
25 mg/day schedule: Single supplemental dose of 25 to 50 mg
25 to 50 mg/day schedule: Single supplemental dose of 50 to 75 mg
50 to 75 mg/day schedule: Single supplemental dose of 75 to 100 mg
75 mg/day schedule: Single supplemental dose of 100 to 150 mg
From Pasero, C., & McCaffery, M. *Pain assessment and pharmacologic management,* p. 664, St. Louis, Mosby. Data from Lacy, C. F., Armstrong, L. L., Goldman, M. P., et al (Eds.). (2008). *Drug information handbook,* ed. 17, Hudson, OH, Lexi-Comp Inc. © 2011, Pasero C, McCaffery M. May be duplicated for use in clinical practice.

The oral bioavailability of gabapentin is affected by a saturable absorption mechanism, such that doses above a certain level are characterized by a declining bioavailability. In one study, the drug was 60% bioavailable at 900 mg/day, 47% at 1200 mg/day, 34% at 2400 mg/day, 33% at 3600 mg/day, and 27% at 4800 mg/day (Lacy, Armstrong, Goldman, et al., 2008; Twycross, Wilcock, Charlesworth, et al., 2003). Dose escalation can be accompanied by a ceiling effect, which in the case of this drug, may be either pharmacokinetic or pharmacodynamic, or possibly both. If an increment in dose does not yield improved outcomes, titration should stop (the dose usually lowered) and a decision should be made about the value of the therapy overall. Dose escalation also can be limited by adverse effects, and should an increment produce intolerable effects, the same decision is required.

Gabapentin should be administered at least 2 hours after intake of antacids that contain aluminum, as concurrent administration decreases the bioavailability of gabapentin by 10% to 25% (Twycross, Wilcock, Charlesworth, et al., 2003). Capsules of gabapentin may be opened and contents mixed with juice or water for patients who have difficulty swallowing capsules or tablets.

The future may hold simpler dosing regimens for patients who take gabapentin. A modified-release formulation of gabapentin had been studied but not released at the time of this publication. The formulation was described as having a unique gastric-retentive characteristic made possible by polymer-based technology (Irving, Jensen, Cramer, et al., 2009). Administered with food, the modified-release tablet swells and is retained in the stomach for up to 8 hours, allowing gradual release of the drug over 10 hours. Patients (N = 158) with postherpetic neuralgia of at least 3 months duration were randomized to receive a placebo or the modified-release gabapentin once daily (1800 mg) or twice daily (600 mg in the morning and 1200 mg in the evening) (Irving, Jensen, Cramer, et al., 2009). A 50% or greater reduction in pain was reported in 25.5% (gabapentin once daily), 28.8% (gabapentin twice daily), and 11.8% (placebo) of the patients. The drug was well-tolerated, with dizziness and sedation being the most common adverse effects and experienced most often by those who received gabapentin once daily.

Pregabalin

Pregabalin is typically started at a dose of 75 mg/day or 150 mg/day. Older patients or those who are medically frail or have renal insufficiency typically are started at an even lower dose (e.g., 25 mg/day or 50 mg/day). The dose usually is titrated every 3 to 4 days by an amount equal to the starting dose (or higher as the dose goes up), and the total dose is divided. The usual effective dose is between 150 mg twice daily and 300 mg twice daily, but some patients have good outcomes at doses that are higher or lower than this range. A 15-month open-label trial of patients with refractory neuropathic pain showed that doses between 150 mg/day and 600 mg/day

significantly improved pain (Stacey, Dworkin, Murphy, et al., 2008). The discontinuation rate for adverse effects was low (12.3%). Others have found similar results with doses of 150 to 600 mg/day (Frampton, Foster, 2005; Frampton, Scott, 2004; Freynhagen, Strojek, Griesing, et al., 2005). Pregabalin doses must be adjusted downward for patients with renal impairment, as the drug is eliminated almost entirely by renal excretion (Gajraj, 2007) (see Table 23-2 for dosing adjustments in patients with renal impairment).

Other Anticonvulsants

There is a general lack of research to guide dosing of other anticonvulsants. Following is information to consider related to specific agents.

- An initial dose of 100 mg/day of lacosamide followed by weekly increases of 100 mg/day to a maximum of 400 mg/day proved to be safe and effective in a study of patients with painful diabetic neuropathy (Shaibani, Biton, Rauck, et al., 2009). Clinical experience is limited with this drug, and it is prudent to initiate dosing at 50 mg/day in older or medically frail patients.

- To reduce the risk of cutaneous hypersensitivity, lamotrigine should be started at a relatively low dose for 1 month, after which the dose can be more rapidly increased (Jensen, 2002; Maizels, McCarberg, 2005). For example, one strategy administers the drug at 25 mg/day for the first week, 25 mg twice daily for the second, 25 mg in the morning and 50 mg at night for the third, and 50 mg twice daily for the fourth. Starting with the fifth week, the dose can be increased by 50% to 100% weekly, until the usual effective dose of 300 mg/day to 500 mg/day is reached. Another strategy for initiating treatment uses 25 mg twice daily for the first 2 weeks followed by 50 mg twice daily for the next 2 weeks, after which the dose is increased quickly.

- The recommended starting dose of oxcarbazepine for treatment of trigeminal neuralgia is 600 mg/day (300 mg twice daily) with increases of 150 to 300 mg every few days (Carrazana, Mikoshiba, 2003). Again, older or medically frail patients should be started at a dose as low as 150 mg/day. The drug has been shown to be efficacious at doses between 900 mg/day and 2100 mg/day, producing pain relief equivalent to carbamazepine at doses of 400 to 1200 mg/day. The effective dose range for most patients was 600 to 1200 mg/day (Carrazana, Mioshiba, 2003).

- Topiramate is often started at 25 mg twice daily followed by weekly increases of 25 mg as tolerated (Lacy, Armstrong, Goldman, et al., 2008). A 26-week trial of patients with migraine administered topiramate in daily doses of 50 mg, 100 mg, and 200 mg and found little difference between 50 mg and placebo; 100 mg and 200 mg doses resulted in significant reductions in migraine attacks (Silberstein, Neto, Schmitt, et al., 2004).

Other research supports 100 mg/day as the most efficacious and best-tolerated dose of topiramate for migraine prevention (Brandes, Saper, Diamond, et al., 2004; Silberstein, 2005). Doses as high as 400 mg/day may be beneficial in some patients.

- Low initial doses are appropriate for carbamazepine, valproate, and clonazepam, but the administration of phenytoin often begins with the presumed therapeutic dose (e.g., 300 mg/day) or a prudent oral loading regimen (e.g., 400 mg followed by another 400 mg 2 to 3 hours later).

Sodium Channel Blockers

By far, the largest clinical use of traditional sodium channel blockers is as local anesthetics, drugs that are deposited adjacent to peripheral nerves and inhibit transduction or transmission of afferent input to the CNS, including information about noxious stimuli (see Section I and Figure I-2 on pp. 4-5). Local anesthetics at high concentration can block sensory and motor nerves and produce regional anesthesia; at lower concentrations, they may provide pain relief without blocking other nerve functions.

In pain management, local anesthetics may be delivered via direct injection or placement of a catheter into the tissues adjacent to major nerves or a nerve plexus (neural blockade), or by neuraxial (epidural or intrathecal) administration. In this way, they produce regional anesthesia or analgesia. Local anesthetics are effective by surgical site infiltration for postoperative pain associated with minor surgery, and an excellent systematic review provides data on this technique for control of pain following a variety of major surgical procedures as well (Dahl, Moiniche, 2009). Scalp infiltration of ropivacaine has been used to reduce both postoperative pain and the incidence of persistent postsurgical pain in patients following intracranial tumor resection (Batoz, Verdonck, Pellerin, et al., 2009). Local anesthetics have been administered by intraperitoneal instillation for postoperative pain treatment after minor surgery (Callesen, Hjort, Mogensen, et al., 1999; Hazinedaroglu, Kayaoglu, Ates, et al., 2006; Visalyaputra, Lertakyamanee, Pethpaisit, et al., 1999). These drugs also may be given by topical application, allowing absorption into the skin and underlying tissues (e.g., patches, gels, creams). Topical anesthetics produce analgesia or anesthesia depending on the amount absorbed.

Drugs that block sodium channels also have a long history as systemic analgesics, which may be administered orally or parenterally. The following text reviews this systemic use of traditional sodium channel blockers for the treatment of persistent neuropathic pain. The use of IV lidocaine for acute and postoperative pain and continuous neural blockade are discussed in Chapter 26. See also Chapter 24 for topical local anesthetics including the lidocaine patch 5%, and local anesthetics for procedural pain. Neuraxial (epidural and intrathecal) local anesthetics are discussed in Chapter 15. Table V-1, pp. 748-756, at the end of Section V presents the characteristics of the commonly used systemic local anesthetics.

Systemic (Oral and Parenteral) Sodium Channel Blockers

The systemic local anesthetics used most often for persistent neuropathic pain treatment are IV lidocaine and oral mexiletine (Mexitil). Mexiletine is described as an oral sodium channel antagonist that is structurally similar to lidocaine (Wallace, Magnuson, Ridgeway, 2000) and is classified as a cardiac antiarrhythmic. Other drugs in this class, such as flecainide (Tambocor) and tocainide (Tonocard), are similarly classified but rarely used for pain treatment (Wallace, Galer, Gammaitoni, 2006). Both IV lidocaine and mexiletine have efficacy for neuropathic pain, but the evidence of analgesic effects varies, and their respective roles in practice differ (Galer, Harle, Rowbotham, 1996). Both are considered third-line (Dworkin, O'Connor, Backonja, et al., 2007) or fourth-line (Moulin, Clark, Gilron, et al., 2007) options for neuropathic pain. A new drug in the United States, lacosamide (Vimpat), is a first-in-class sodium channel modulator that is now classified as an anticonvulsant (and is discussed earlier in the chapter).

There is relatively strong evidence of analgesic efficacy for IV lidocaine and little evidence of this effect for the oral compounds. Tremont-Lukats and colleagues (2005) conducted a systematic review of 9 mexiletine and 10 parenteral lidocaine trials and found that their therapeutic benefit was more consistent for neuropathic pain from trauma, diabetes, and cardiovascular (CV) disease and less for neuropathic pain from HIV, cancer, and infectious etiology. These researchers also conducted a more extensive Cochrane Collaboration Review of 32 controlled clinical trials (two of these were duplicate studies) (Challapalli, Tremont-Lukats, McNicol, et al., 2005), which included studies of IV lidocaine (16 trials), mexiletine (12 trials), IV lidocaine plus mexiletine sequentially (1 trial), and tocainide (1 trial). Lidocaine and mexiletine showed superior efficacy compared with placebo, and while data were limited for comparison, no differences in efficacy between these systemic sodium channel blockers and other more commonly used drugs for neuropathic pain (e.g., carbamazepine, gabapentin, morphine) were noted. The systemic sodium channel antagonists were found to be safe, and no deaths or life-threatening toxicities were associated with their use.

Some patients experience immediate analgesia from an IV lidocaine infusion, and this potential suggests that the utility of this approach is the management of "pain crises" or crescendo neuropathic pain. Some patients experience favorable effects that continue for a long enough time period after the infusion is completed that repeated IV infusions can be adopted as part of the long-term plan of care. Most patients, however, appear to experience relatively short-lasting relief after the infusion is discontinued, and this is a limitation of the therapy (Sharma, Rajagopal, Palat, et al., 2009). Other limitations are the incidence of adverse effects at optimal dose ranges and wide variations in response among patients and different pain conditions.

Information is lacking about the long-term safety and effectiveness of these drugs (see adverse effects). Given this limited experience, a trial of a systemic sodium channel blocker generally is reserved for pain that has not responded to the more typical first-line adjuvant analgesics. The exception, as noted, is the specific use of IV lidocaine in an effort to address unrelenting severe or progressive dysesthesias (a crescendo pain pattern).

Oral Sodium Channel Blockers

Of the oral sodium channel blockers, mexiletine has been used most often for pain treatment and should be tried before flecainide and tocainide (the latter is no longer marketed in the United States). Although there is some evidence of analgesic efficacy from mexiletine, data from controlled trials are very limited (Caroll, Kaplan, Mackey, 2008; Wallace, Magnuson, Ridgeway, 2000). For example, a small (N = 20) randomized controlled trial titrated oral mexiletine to a maximum dose of 900 mg/day or dose-limiting adverse effects in patients with allodynic neuropathic pain (Wallace, Magnuson, Ridgeway, 2000). The treatment had a significant effect on pain induced (evoked) by stroking but no effect on the area of allodynia or quality of life measurements. Peak lidocaine plasma levels (0.54 mcg/mL), reached on day 10, were below those associated with cardiac antiarrhythmic activity (1.5 mcg/mL) and toxicity (5 mcg/mL) (Lema, 1996).

Wallace and colleagues (2006) reported that although two double-blind, placebo-controlled trials of mexiletine for neuropathic pain showed positive results, four others showed no significant effect on painful diabetic neuropathy, spinal cord dysesthetic pain, and allodynic neuropathic pain. In contrast, a comprehensive critical review of research on analgesics for painful diabetic neuropathy listed mexiletine among those showing some benefit in alleviating this pain (Adriaensen, Plaghki, Mathieu et al., 2005). Mexiletine has been reported anecdotally to provide sustained pain relief for some patients with poststroke pain (Edmondson, Simpson, Stubler et al., 1993) and has been used to effectively treat alcoholic neuropathy, peripheral nerve injury pain, and thalamic pain (Wallace, Galer, Gammaitoni, 2006). Mexiletine was studied in 9 patients with refractory persistent headaches deriving some benefit (Marmura, Passero, Young, 2008). Of these, 7 had adverse effects; nevertheless, the investigators concluded that this agent may be useful for the management of daily headaches.

These studies of mexiletine have had small sample sizes and, in some cases, conflicting results. One review of four controlled trials suggested that there is no clear evidence of mexiletine superiority over placebo (Duby, Campbell,

Setter, et al., 2004). Overall, it is more reasonable to conclude that there is evidence of analgesic effect, but compared to other groups of adjuvant analgesics, such as the antidepressants and the gabapentinoids, and compared to IV lidocaine, this evidence is sparse.

Some studies indicate that mexiletine has a relatively high adverse effect liability. The incidence of nausea and dizziness may prevent dose titration to levels that optimize positive clinical outcomes related to pain (Wallace, Magnuson, Ridgeway, 2000; Wallace, Galer, Gammaitoni, 2006).

Flecainide, another antiarrhythmic agent, has properties similar to mexiletine. Animal research demonstrated that the drug could suppress ectopic discharge from injured nerves (Ichimata, Kitano, Ikebe et al., 2001), and a phase II exploratory clinical trial of 14 patients with neuropathic pain demonstrated a 30% response rate after weeklong courses of flecainide (50 mg twice daily followed by 100 mg twice daily) (von Gunten, Eappen, Cleary, et al., 2007). In another study, significant improvement in pain was demonstrated in 15 patients with postherpetic neuralgia who, following a positive response to IV flecainide, were treated with the oral formulation (Ichimata, Ikebe, Yoshitake, et al., 2001). In contrast, flecainide has been shown to be ineffective in treating neuropathic cancer pain (Wallace, Galer, Gammaitoni, 2006), and paranoid psychosis from flecainide toxicity was reported in a patient with cancer-related neuropathic pain (Bennett, 1997).

Although tocainide, another antiarrhythmic agent, has analgesic activity, there is a lack of research supporting its use in humans (Wallace, Galer, Gammaitoni, 2006). In an early study, it showed efficacy similar to carbamazepine for trigeminal neuralgia (Lindstrom, Lindblom, 1987). The drug has also been found to reduce pain from postherpetic neuralgia (Ichimata, Ikebe, Yoshitake, et al., 2001). Withdrawal arrhythmias have been reported with sudden cessation of the drug (McCleane, 2009a)

On the basis of clinical experience and the limited data from studies, a trial of a systemic sodium channel blocker, specifically mexiletine, can be considered for refractory neuropathic pain. If administration yields meaningful partial analgesia, it should be continued. If a risk of drug interaction or additive toxicities exists, dosing must be very cautious and monitoring intensified.

Given the chemical similarities between IV lidocaine and the oral sodium channel blockers, there has been interest in determining whether the results of an IV infusion of lidocaine could be used to assess the potential benefit from long-term oral therapy (Carroll, 2007; Carroll, Kaplan, Mackey, 2008; Cohen, Kapoor, Rathmell, 2009; Galer, Harle, Rowbotham, 1996; McCleane, 2008). In an early study of 9 patients with persistent neuropathic pain of peripheral origin, a moderate or better response to IV lidocaine infusion correlated with a subsequent equal or better response to a 4-week trial of oral mexiletine (Galer, Harle, Rowbotham, 1996). In a case series of 37 patients with neuropathic pain, patients were given mexiletine after showing a benefit from IV lidocaine and were evaluated to determine predictors of a response (Carroll, Kaplan, Mackey, 2008). The median time to discontinuing mexiletine was 43 days, and fewer than 20% of the patients continued therapy for a year. The reasons for discontinuation were unknown; however, those who had a positive response to the IV lidocaine infusion prior to mexiletine therapy were more likely to accept and continue mexiletine after it was started. Younger age and male gender also predicted acceptance of mexiletine therapy. These data are too limited to conclude that the response to IV lidocaine adequately predicts the outcome of mexiletine therapy.

IV Lidocaine

Over the past several years, IV lidocaine has been widely studied and shown to be effective for a variety of painful conditions (McCleane, 2009a; Tremont-Lukats, Challapalli, McNicol, et al., 2005; Challapalli, Tremont-Lukats, McNicol, et al., 2005; Wallace, Galer, Gammaitoni, 2006). (See Chapter 26 for use of IV lidocaine for acute and postoperative pain.) McCleane (2009a) suggests that anecdotal reports of its use in over 7000 cases without untoward CV adverse effects should increase confidence in the use of IV lidocaine for pain treatment. The reader is referred again to the systematic reviews discussed above (Tremont-Lukats, Challapalli, McNicol, et al., 2005; Challapalli, Tremont-Lukats, McNicol, et al., 2005).

IV lidocaine appears to be more effective in relieving neuropathic pain arising from a lesion or damage of the peripheral nervous system than pain from CNS damage (Kawamata, Sugino, Narimatsu, et al., 2006; Kingery, 1997; McCleane, 2009a; Tremont-Lukats, Challapalli, McNicol, et al., 2005; Wallace, Galer, Gammaitoni, 2006; Wu, Tella, Staats, et al., 2002). A randomized, double-blind, active placebo-controlled, cross-over trial (N = 31) provided clues to a better understanding of the underlying mechanisms of stump and phantom limb pain and the effect of IV lidocaine on different types of neuropathic pain (Wu, Tella, Staats, et al., 2002). Individuals with both stump pain and phantom limb pain (N = 11) and those with either stump pain (N = 11) or phantom limb pain (N = 9) were titrated off all medications except acetaminophen and NSAIDs, and then admitted and randomly assigned to receive a series of three IV infusions: An initial bolus of lidocaine, morphine, or the active placebo diphenhydramine (Benadryl) was followed by an infusion of the same drug. The maximum infusion dose of lidocaine was 400 mg, and the maximum dose of morphine was 25 mg. There were 24-hour intervals between infusions, and doses were decreased for adverse effects. Compared with placebo, morphine significantly reduced both stump and phantom limb pain, and lidocaine reduced stump but not phantom limb pain. This suggests that the underlying mechanisms of stump and phantom pain differ and reinforces the suggestion that IV lidocaine is more effective in treating peripherally-mediated pain syndromes than centrally-mediated pain syndromes.

The relatively smaller effect of IV lidocaine in studies of central pain syndromes may reflect a need for a higher dose to address the underlying pathophysiology. A randomized study demonstrated that 5 mg/kg infused over 30 minutes resulted in reduction of spontaneous pain at and below the level of spinal cord injury, independent of the presence of evoked (induced) pain (Finnerup, Biering-Sorensen, Johannesen, et al., 2005), and an earlier study reported a similar reduction in spontaneous central poststroke pain at this dose (Attal, Gaude, Brasseur, et al., 2000). A small randomized controlled study (N = 10) found that lidocaine (2.5 mg/kg) had no significant effect on spinal cord injury pain (Kvarnstrom, Karlsten, Quiding, et al., 2004). These data suggest that the different responses between peripheral and central neuropathic pain observed in some studies may not reflect the inefficacy of sodium channel blockade in the latter syndromes, but instead, a need for higher serum concentration relative to peripherally-generated neuropathic pain. Evaluation of serum level to determine this may be helpful, and it has been suggested that serum levels of at least 4 mcg/mL may be required for reduction in central pain (Kingery, 1997).

Although it is possible that IV lidocaine is relatively less useful in the management of cancer-related neuropathic pain than other types of neuropathic pain, the data are conflicting. A previously discussed systematic review of mexiletine and parenteral lidocaine trials concluded this (Tremont-Lukats, Challapalli, McNicol, et al., 2005), but a phase II pilot study (N = 88) found that an IV lidocaine bolus (2 mg/kg) followed by infusion (2 mg/kg) produced significant improvements in pain relief for patients with opioid-refractory cancer pain (Sharma, Rajagopal, Palat, et al., 2009). Mean onset of analgesia was 40 minutes after initiation of infusion, and mean duration of analgesia was 9 days after infusion was completed.

As noted, there is extensive literature describing the response of varied populations with pain to IV lidocaine treatment. Following is a list of research, case reports, and reviews on the use of IV lidocaine for a variety of types of persistent pain and pain-related conditions.

- Painful diabetic neuropathy and other peripheral neuropathies (Kingery, 1997; McClean, 2009; Tremont-Lukats, Challapalli, McNicol, et al., 2005; Tremont-Lukats, Hutson, Backonja, 2006; Wallace, Galer, Gammaitoni, 2006)
- Postherpetic neuralgia (Baranowski, De Courcey, Bonello, 1999; Kingery, 1997; Tremont-Lukats, Challapalli, McNicol, et al., 2005; Wallace, Galer, Gammaitoni, 2006)
- Central pain (stroke, spinal cord injury) (Attal, Gaude, Brasseur, et al., 2000; Frese, Hustedt, Ringelstein, et al., 2006; Finnerup, Biering-Sorensen, Johannesen, et al., 2005; Kumar, Kalita, Kumar, et al., 2009; Kvarnstrom, Karlsten, Quiding, et al., 2004; Tremont-Lukats, Challapalli, McNicol, et al., 2005; Wallace, Galer, Gammaitoni, 2006)

- Phantom limb pain; stump pain (Wu, Tella, Staats, et al., 2002)
- CRPS (Kingery, 1997; Schwartzman, Patel, Grothusen, et al., 2009; Tremont-Lukats, Hutson, Backonja, 2006)
- Fibromyalgia (McClean, 2009; Wallace, Galer, Gammaitoni, 2006)
- Brachial plexopathy (Tremont-Lukats, Hutson, Backonja, 2006)
- Radicular pain (Tremont-Lukats, Hutson, Backonja, 2006)
- Sciatica (Medrik-Goldberg, Lifschitz, Pud, et al., 1999)
- Migraine and other headaches (Hand, Stark, 2000; Wallace, Galer, Gammaitoni, 2006)
- Cancer-related neuropathic pain (Brose, Cousins, 1991; Bruera, Ripamonti, Brenneis, et al., 1992; Ferrini, 2000; Galer, Harle, Rowbotham, 1996; Sharma, Rajagopal, Palat, et al., 2009; Tremont-Lukats, Challapalli, McNicol, et al., 2005)

Mechanism of Action

Peripheral nerve injury causes changes in the number and location of ion channels, particularly sodium channels. These channels, which abnormally accumulate in injured peripheral nociceptors, may lead to ectopic discharges and other phenomena that initiate and maintain neuropathic pain (Beydoun, Backonja, 2003; Bridges, Thomson, Rice, 2001). IV lidocaine, mexiletine, and the other drugs in this class relieve pain by blocking sodium channels, stabilizing nerve membranes, slowing depolarization, and reducing ectopic discharges (McCleane, 2009a) (see Section I and Figure I-2 on pp. 4-5).

Lidocaine also has significant antiinflammatory effects, which may account for its effectiveness in postoperative pain treatment (Martin, Cherif, Gentili, et al., 2008). Research in animals (Kawamata, Sugino, Narimatsu, et al., 2006) and humans (Kingery, 1997; McClean, 2009; Tremont-Lukats, Challapalli, McNicol, et al., 2005; Wallace, Galer, Gammaitoni, 2006; Wu, Tella, Staats, et al., 2002) as well as clinical experience support a peripheral analgesic action site for systemic local anesthetics.

Although peripherally-mediated effects appear to be very important in the analgesic effect of the sodium channel blockers, supraspinal and spinal mechanisms of action have been suggested for many years. IV lidocaine may activate the endogenous opioid system (Bach, Jensen, Kastrup, et al., 1990; Kastrup, Bach, Petersen, et al., 1989), and more recent research has demonstrated expression of sodium channels on dorsal horn neurons near spinal cord lesions, which were linked to central pain behaviors (Finnerup, Biering-Sorensen, Johannesen, et al., 2005; Hains, Klein, Saab, et al., 2003). This may help to explain the effectiveness of IV lidocaine for some types of central pain. Further research is needed, but the ability of IV lidocaine to reduce several features of pain caused by CNS injuries suggests a central action in the mechanisms underlying these types

of pain (Attal, Gaude, Brasseur, et al., 2000; Finnerup, Biering-Sorensen, Johannesen, et al., 2005). Many questions remain, however, in light of other research that shows IV lidocaine was effective in relieving stump pain (peripherally mediated) but not phantom limb pain (centrally mediated) (Wu, Tella, Staats, et al., 2002).

Adverse Effects

The most common adverse effects of the systemic sodium channel blockers are nausea, vomiting, abdominal pain, diarrhea, dizziness, and perioral numbness (numbness and tingling inside and surrounding the mouth) (Tremont-Lukats, Challapalli, McNicol, et al., 2005). Although reviews are reassuring about the adverse effects associated with these drugs (Challapalli, Tremont-Lukats, McNicol, et al., 2005; Tremont-Lukats, Challapalli, McNicol, et al., 2005), they potentially can produce serious and even life-threatening effects involving the CNS and the CV system. These are directly related to serum concentration (Gordon, 2008). Lidocaine levels above 1.5 mcg/mL and 5 mcg/mL are associated with cardiac antiarrhythmic activity and toxicity, respectively (Lema, 1996). Observable CNS effects generally occur at a lower serum concentration than cardiac changes and are more common with IV lidocaine than with mexiletine (Tremont-Lukats, Challapalli, McNicol, et al., 2005). Dizziness, perioral numbness, other paresthesias (abnormal sensations), and tremor usually occur first (Catterall, Mackie, 2006). At higher plasma concentrations, progressive encephalopathy develops and seizures may occur. At concentrations above this, cardiac conduction disturbances and myocardial depression can occur.

All the sodium channel antagonists must be used cautiously in patients with pre-existing heart disease, and patients who have significant heart disease should undergo cardiologic evaluation before therapy is administered. It is prudent to avoid this therapy in patients with cardiac rhythm disturbances, those who are receiving alpha agonists or beta blockers, and those who have cardiac insufficiency (Gordon, 2008). Lidocaine infusion can aggravate and increase first- and second-degree heart conduction blocks. Periodic ECG evaluation is recommended during mexiletine therapy (Argoff, Backonja, Belgrade, et al., 2006). Withdrawal arrhythmias have been reported with sudden cessation of tocainide (McClean, 2009).

A bolus over 20 minutes and infusion over no less than 1 hour has been suggested to lower the risk of serious adverse effects with IV lidocaine (Sharma, Rajagopal, Palat, et al., 2009). Large-dose infusions have been safely administered via longer infusion times. A 5 mg/kg lidocaine infusion administered over 6 hours for persistent neuropathic pain was tolerated without serious adverse effects (Tremont-Lukats, Hutson, Backonja, 2006) (see the following paragraphs). Bolus doses and infusions should be administered via an infusion device that does not allow free flow to help ensure accurate dose delivery.

Should adverse effects occur during IV lidocaine therapy, the clinician should stop the infusion; monitor blood pressure closely; assess for the presence of associated symptoms including pain; obtain a stat blood sample for serum lidocaine level; and notify the primary prescriber, anesthesia provider, or pain service (Gordon, 2008). In the case of a life-threatening overdose, treatment may include (as indicated by patient condition) airway support, oxygenation and hyperventilation to raise seizure threshold, diazepam (Valium) for seizure, IV fluids and Trendelenburg position to increase fluid volume, and CV depression treatment including IV fat emulsion as an antidote (Gordon, 2008). Lipid emulsion has been used to successfully resuscitate several patients from cardiac arrest from local anesthetic-induced cardiotoxicity (Clark, 2008); however, this appears to be related to the type of local anesthetic administered. The effects appear to be positive for bupivacaine-induced but not ropivacaine- or mepivacaine-induced cardiac arrest (Espinet, Emmerton, 2009; Zausig, Zink, Keil, et al., 2009). Large doses of epinephrine are also reported to be required for reversal of bupivacaine-induced cardiotoxicity (Mulroy, 2002). These findings have implications for local anesthetics administered via neuraxial and regional techniques (see Chapters 19 and 26 for more information).

IV lidocaine therapy should not be administered to individuals who are allergic to amide local anesthetics such as bupivacaine or ropivacaine (Gordon, 2008). (Procaine [Novocaine] is not a contraindication, as procaine is an ester local anesthetic.) Patients with liver dysfunction, pulmonary disease with a prominent feature of carbon dioxide retention, or congestive heart failure are at higher risk for lidocaine-induced adverse effects (Gordon, 2008).

A less serious but common adverse effect of IV lidocaine is painful inflammation of the vein upon injection (McCleane, 2008). This is unrelated to the pH or presence of preservatives and is thought to be caused primarily by the concentration of the lidocaine infusion. The use of dilute solutions and a glyceryl trinitrate (GTN, nitroglycerine) patch above the infusion site are suggested to reduce the pain (McCleane, 2008). The nitrate patch is reported to have sufficient local antiinflammatory properties to negate this complication.

Adverse effects on postoperative wound healing during continuous IV lidocaine infusion have not been reported. One study described healing disturbances in one patient who received IV lidocaine and had minor skin wound irritation and one patient who received placebo and had a much more serious subphrenic abscess (Herroeder, Pecher, Schonherr, et al., 2007).

A few publications have reported the safety of long-term IV lidocaine therapy. Although there are no controlled studies, there are case reports of hospice patients tolerating in-home IV lidocaine infusions for as long as 240 days prior to death (Ferrini, 2000). Anecdotally, long-term subcutaneous administration of lidocaine was also reported to yield sustained relief of refractory neuropathic pain in cancer patients (Brose, Cousins, 1991).

Indications

Data from controlled trials and clinical experience suggest that any one of a variety of persistent pains can be considered a potential indication for systemic therapy with a sodium channel blocker. Although peripherally-generated neuropathic pain may be more likely to respond than central pain (Backonja, Arndt, Gombar, 1994; Galer, Miller, Rowbotham, 1993; Wallace, Galer, Gammaitoni, 2006; Kvarnstrom, Karlsten, Quiding, et al., 2004; Kingery, 1997; McClean, 2009; Tremont-Lukats, Challapalli, McNicol, et al., 2005; Wu, Tella, Staats, et al., 2002), the data are not clear-cut and patients with central pain may respond favorably (Galer, Miller, Rowbotham, 1993). It has also been suggested that IV lidocaine may reduce sympathetic activity, resulting in a subsequent reduction in sympathetically-mediated pain (Wallace, Galer, Gammaitoni, 2006). Further research is needed to confirm this.

On the basis of clinical experience, a trial of a brief lidocaine infusion is sometimes implemented in patients with severe neuropathic pain that has not responded promptly to other interventions and requires immediate relief. This technique, therefore, may be a useful approach to the uncommon circumstance of crescendo neuropathic pain.

As mentioned, some studies suggest that a brief IV infusion may predict response to oral therapy (Galer, Harle, Rowbotham, 1996), particularly in younger and male patients (Carroll, Kaplan, Mackey, 2008). However, if the IV infusion fails to provide pain relief, a trial of oral therapy is still appropriate. Older age and higher pain severity may be important predictors of a positive response to IV lidocaine for the treatment of neuropathic pain (Carroll, Gaeta, Mackey, 2007).

On the basis of the limited data available concerning long-term safety and efficacy, it is appropriate to position the oral sodium channel blockers as third-line (Dworkin, O'Connor, Backonja, et al., 2007) or fourth-line (Moulin, Clark, Gilron, et al., 2007) drugs for neuropathic pain. A trial is warranted in patients with neuropathic pain who do not respond adequately or who cannot tolerate first-line adjuvant analgesics (e.g., antidepressants and anticonvulsants). In the palliative care setting, therapy usually is considered only for the long-term management of opioid-refractory neuropathic pain. In all settings, a trial of IV lidocaine may be considered at any point in time if the indication of crescendo pain is present.

Drug Selection

On theoretical grounds (less potency at the sodium channel), mexiletine may be the oral local anesthetic least likely to produce serious toxicity. Although intraindividual variability in the response to different drugs in this class has not been systematically assessed, such variability has been observed commonly with other drug classes and is likely to exist with the oral sodium channel blockers as well.

Thus if mexiletine does not provide relief to a patient with severe neuropathic pain that has already proved refractory to other drugs, a trial with an alternative oral sodium channel blocker may be justified. Lidocaine is currently the primary parenteral local anesthetic.

Dose Selection

IV lidocaine and mexiletine in varying doses for some types of persistent pain have been proven to be generally safe and efficacious in placebo-controlled trials (Tremont-Lukats, Challapalli, McNicol, et al., 2005; Challapalli, Tremont-Lukats, McNicol, et al., 2005). Low initial doses followed by slow titration reduce the likelihood of adverse effects.

Mexiletine

In the absence of contrary information, overall dosing should conform to that used in the treatment of cardiac arrhythmias. For example, mexiletine usually should be started at 150 to 200 mg once or twice per day (Guay, 2001). Doses are better tolerated when taken with food. If intolerable adverse effects do not occur, the dose can be increased by a like amount every few days until the usual dose of 300 mg three times per day is reached. A maximum daily dose of 1200 mg is recommended (Guay, 2001). (See the following paragraphs for a discussion of optimal serum levels.) (See mexiletine patient medication information, Form V-9 on pp. 775-776, at the end of Section V.)

IV Lidocaine

It is not possible to specify an exact dose of parenteral lidocaine that will be both safe and effective for treatment of neuropathic pain (Tremont-Lukats, Hutson, Backonja, 2006). Brief lidocaine infusions for persistent pain have been administered at varying doses, typically within a range of 1 to 5 mg/kg infused over 30 to 45 minutes (Guay, 2001; Tremont-Lukats, Hutson, Backonja, 2006). Slow bolus administration (over 20 minutes) and infusion rates (1 hour) have been suggested as a way to reduce the risk of serious adverse effects (Sharma, Rajagopal, Palat et al., 2009). One randomized controlled trial administered doses of 1, 3, and 5 mg/kg via IV infusion over a 6-hour period to patients with peripheral neuropathic pain and found the 5 mg/kg dose to be the most effective in relieving pain (Tremont-Lukats, Hutson, Backonja, 2006). This large dose given over an extended time produced no serious adverse effects, and pain relief lasted for 4 hours after administration. Although the speed of administration appears to affect the adverse effect profile of IV lidocaine, studies are needed to determine if the speed of administration also influences analgesic effectiveness (Baranowski, De Courcey, Bonello, 1999).

Dose must be individualized according to the patient's condition and type of pain. In the medically frail patient, it may be prudent to start much lower than the usual starting dose, for example, 0.5 mg/kg of IV lidocaine infused over 45 to 60 minutes. Central neuropathic pain may require larger doses of IV lidocaine than the more responsive peripheral neuropathic pain (Galer, Miller, Rowbotham, 1993; Kingery, 1997; McClean, 2009; Tremont-Lukats, Challapalli, McNicol, et al., 2005). Whereas a small randomized controlled study conducted in patients with spinal cord injury pain found no significant relief with lidocaine at a dose of 2.5 mg/kg infused over 40 minutes (Kvarnstrom, Karlsten, Quiding, et al., 2004), randomized controlled studies demonstrated that a larger dose of 5 mg/kg of IV lidocaine resulted in significant reductions in spinal cord injury pain (Finnerup, Biering-Sorensen, Johannesen, et al., 2005) and poststroke pain (Attal, Gaude, Brasseur, et al., 2000) (see Table V-1 on pp. 748-756).

Dosing and Serum Lidocaine Levels

Evaluation of serum concentration to determine adequate levels may provide guidance in dosing for some types of pain or when pain relief is not apparent despite what is thought to be adequate dosing. For example, it has been suggested that relatively higher serum lidocaine levels (greater than 4 mcg/mL) may be required to relieve central pain, ischemic pain, or thermally-evoked pain, and that levels of 1.5 to 2 mcg/mL are sufficient to relieve allodynia and peripheral neuropathic pain (Kingery, 1997). Gradual dose escalation through repeated brief infusions should be considered if treatment initially fails (Ferrante, Paggioli, Cherukuri, et al., 1996). However, upward titration is always a balancing act, as increased doses bring increased adverse effects; cardiac antiarrhythmic activity and toxicity are associated with lidocaine serum levels of 1.5 mcg/mL and 5 mcg/mL, respectively (Lema, 1996; Groudine, Fisher, Kaufman, et al., 1998).

Serum lidocaine levels during IV lidocaine infusion vary widely among studies in large part because of different dosing protocols (dose administered, infusion with or without bolus, speed of bolus or infusion). One older study of patients with postherpetic neuralgia administered 1 and 5 mg/kg IV lidocaine infusions over a 2-hour period and observed that patients reported relief of pain and allodynia with the 1 mg/kg infusion and had a mean serum level of 1.7 mcg/mL (Baranowski, De Courcey, Bonello, 1999). The mean serum levels for those who received 5 mg/kg were significantly higher, with no appreciable benefits noted. Several patients reached toxic levels, but there were no CV complications, and only two patients in the higher-dose group reported symptoms (circumoral paresthesia). A later study reported a mean plasma concentration of 4.2 mcg/mL in patients with spinal cord injury who had significantly improved pain following a 5 mg/kg lidocaine 30-minute infusion; the majority of these patients rated adverse effects, such as sedation and dizziness, as mild (Finnerup, Biering-Sorensen, Johannessen, et al., 2005).

A summary of long-term, in-home lidocaine infusions in hospice patients reported effective pain control with a serum lidocaine level as high as 9.3 mcg/mL in a patient receiving a lidocaine infusion of 10 to 15 mg/h plus bolus doses (Ferrini, 2000). The patient experienced lightheadedness that resolved when the infusion rate was reduced. A letter to the editor described two cases of lidocaine toxicity during low-dose lidocaine infusion in medically ill patients (Tei, Morita, Shishido, et al., 2005). Both were older adults with advanced cancer and normal liver and renal function. One received a daily dose of 300 mg of IV lidocaine, and the other received 200 mg. Both developed somnolence within 1 week, which resolved within 24 to 48 hours after infusion was discontinued. Serum concentration in both cases was 8.4 mcg/mL, and the patients experienced acceptable pain control.

Higher doses and higher blood levels of mexiletine had no association with greater degrees of pain relief in an early study of patients with peripheral neuropathic pain and allodynia (Galer, Harle, Rowbotham, 1996). Dose-limiting adverse effects rather than a true lack of a dose-response relationship were proposed as an explanation for this finding. The highest tolerated mexiletine dose (878 mg/day) during the study produced a mean serum level of 0.76 mcg/mL. Following completion of the study, one patient eventually achieved complete pain relief with a very high mexiletine dose (1750 mg/day with a serum level of 1.3 mcg/mL). Another study reported a low peak plasma level of 0.54 mcg/mL but no effect on pain with a maximum mexiletine dose of 900 mg/day (Wallace, Magnuson, Ridgeway, 2000). The researchers concluded that adverse effects might preclude higher doses. Experts suggest that serum levels indicate a mexiletine dose of 1200 to 1500 mg daily are needed for optimal pain relief but are unlikely to be achieved without significant adverse effects (Wallace, Galer, Gammaitoni, 2006). This helps to explain mexiletine's lack of efficacy for many neuropathic pain syndromes.

See Chapter 26 for a discussion of serum lidocaine levels during perioperative IV lidocaine infusions. Also see Table V-1, pp. 748-756, at the end of Section V for dosing recommendations for the commonly used systemic local anesthetics.

Gamma Aminobutyric Acid (GABA) Agonists

Among the GABA agonists used as adjuvant analgesics are the anticonvulsant tiagabine, the benzodiazepines (specifically clonazepam), and baclofen. Other GABA agonists, such as propofol (Diprivan) and fospropofol (Lusedra), are IV sedative hypnotics (anesthetics) used for anesthesia induction, sedation and analgesia in the critically ill, and procedural sedation. The latter two drugs are discussed in Chapter 27.

Baclofen

Baclofen (Lioresal) is an agonist at the GABA type B receptor and may be administered by the oral or intrathecal route. It is considered another alternative for the treatment of neuropathic pain that might be refractory to other adjuvant agents. GABA is the most abundant inhibitory neurotransmitter in the CNS (Dickenson, Matthews, Suzuki, 2002) and comprises a major inhibitory neurotransmitter system (Bridges, Thompson, Rice, 2001); when GABA inhibition is suppressed, abnormal pain processing occurs (Bridges, Thompson, Rice, 2001) (see Section I). As an agonist at GABA B receptors in the spinal cord, baclofen relieves pain by inhibiting excitatory neurotransmitters and enhancing the GABA inhibitory pathway.

Oral baclofen is an accepted second-line drug for trigeminal neuralgia (Lussier, Portenoy, 2004), and headache treatment guidelines list baclofen (15 to 30 mg orally) as a preventive drug for cluster headache (May, Leone, Afra, et al., 2006). Although studies are lacking in other persistent pain states (Siddall, 2005), oral baclofen also has been used empirically to treat other types of refractory neuropathic pain (Lussier, Portenoy, 2004). One early study showed that baclofen enhanced morphine analgesia for postoperative pain (Gordon, Gear, Heller et al., 1995), but its use is limited in this setting because of a lack of sufficient evidence of effectiveness and the potential for adverse effects, particularly sedation and confusion (Fitzgerald, Buggy, 2006).

Generally speaking, baclofen is reserved for intractable persistent neuropathic pain or muscle spasm–induced pain that is refractory to other adjuvant agents (Slonimski, Abram, Zuniga, 2004). Similarly, intrathecal baclofen usually is reserved for patients who have implanted infusion devices and are experiencing inadequate analgesia or intolerable and unmanageable adverse effects from opioids, local anesthetics, or clonidine (Slonimski, Abram, Zuniga, 2004; Zuniga, Schlicht, Abram, 2000). Intrathecal baclofen doses vary widely from 50 mcg/day to 460 mcg/day (Hassenbusch, Portenoy, Cousins, et al., 2004). Therapy must be individualized according to patient response.

Intrathecal baclofen may be administered alone (Harmer, Larson, 2002; Zuniga, Schlicht, Abram, 2000) or in combination with other drugs, including morphine (Zuniga, Schlicht, Abram, 2000), clonidine (Slonimski, Abram, Zuniga, 2004; Zuniga, Perera, Abram, 2002), and ziconotide (Saulino, Burton, Danyo, et al., 2009) (see later in this chapter for more on ziconotide). Compatibility and stability of baclofen with clonidine (Alvarez, Mazancourt, Chartier-Kastler, et al., 2004) and morphine are established (Slonomski, Abram, Zuniga, 2004) (see Chapter 15).

Baclofen has been reported to relieve sympathetically-mediated pain by inhibiting sympathetic nervous system activity (Slonimski, Abram, Zuniga, 2004). A double-blind, randomized, cross-over study found numerous dramatic improvements in pain, paresthesias, and dystonia following administration of intrathecal baclofen to 7 women with CRPS, in whom the distinguishing clinical feature was multifocal or generalized fixed dystonia (van Hilten, van de Beek, Hoff, et al., 2000). The effects were more prominent in the arms than in the legs. A study of 36 patients with CRPS demonstrated that intrathecal baclofen via implanted pump improved dystonia (abnormal involuntary muscle contractions that cause twisting or repetitive movements or sustained postures), pain, disability, and quality of life indices over a period of 1 year, but complications related to the drug or infusion pump or catheter were common (van Rijn, Munts, Marinus, et al., 2009). Case reports described the use of intrathecal baclofen alone and in combination with clonidine to improve pain, allodynia, and autonomic function in two patients with well-established and refractory lower-extremity CRPS (Zuniga, Perera, Abram, 2002).

An excellent case series described pain relief following intrathecal baclofen for a variety of neuropathic pain conditions including stump pain, low back pain, cerebral palsy–related back pain and radiculopathy, and persistent lower extremity pain (Zuniga, Schlicht, Abram, 2000). All involved patients had been previously unable to achieve pain relief with an exhaustive list of analgesics and interventions.

Intrathecal baclofen also has been used for many years for refractory cancer pain, alone or in combination with other analgesics, most often by implanted infusion technology (Newsome, Frawley, Argoff, 2008).

Two excellent references are recommended for clinicians and pharmacists who are involved in the care of patients receiving intrathecal baclofen: (1) A comprehensive review by Ghafoor and colleagues (2007) that includes pharmacology of the various medications, adverse effects and complications, and information about the implanted devices including information on compounding drugs for administration, and (2) nursing care guidelines by Bhimani (2008), which include patient monitoring and management of implantable devices used to administer baclofen intrathecally. Nurses are also referred to the American Society for Pain Management Nursing's position paper, which describes the nurse's responsibilities in administering analgesics by catheter techniques (Pasero, Eksterowicz, Primeau, et al., 2007).

Baclofen for Spasticity

A primary indication for baclofen is the treatment of spasticity of spinal origin, such as that associated with spinal cord injury or multiple sclerosis. As mentioned, it has also been given intrathecally for treatment of dystonia associated with CRPS (van Rijn, Munts, Marinus, et al., 2009). At least 50% of patients with these disorders experience muscle spasm, and oral baclofen is reported to improve spasticity in 70% to 87% of patients (Dario, Tomei, 2004; Slonomski, Abram, Zuniga, 2004). Intrathecal baclofen, which is approved in the United States for treatment of spasticity, is thought to be even more effective (Dario, Tomei, 2004). Oral baclofen reduced lower extremity but not upper extremity spasms in patients with acquired brain injury (Meythaler, Clayton, Davis, et al., 2004), and intrathecal baclofen significantly reduced spasms resulting from stroke (Meythaler, Guin-Renfroe, Brunner,

et al., 2001) and cerebral palsy (Meythaler, Guin-Renfroe, Law, et al., 2001). A small (N = 11) prospective, placebo-controlled trial found intrathecal baclofen significantly improved function and comfort in patients with cerebral palsy (Van Schaeybroeck, Nuttin, Lagae, et al., 2000).

Oral Baclofen Dosing

The administration of oral baclofen for pain is undertaken in a manner similar to the use of the drug for its primary indication—spasticity (Lussier, Portenoy, 2004). A starting dose of 5 mg two to three times per day is gradually escalated to the range of 30 to 90 mg/day and sometimes higher if adverse effects do not occur. Occasionally patients require more than 200 mg/day to benefit maximally; however, doses greater than 60 mg are associated with a higher incidence of adverse effects (Dario, Tomei, 2004). It is appropriate to continue dose escalation until pain is relieved or limiting adverse effects occur. (See baclofen patient medication information, Form V-2 on pp. 761-762, at the the end of Section V.)

Adverse Effects

The common adverse effects of baclofen are dizziness, sedation, excessive weakness, GI distress, and cognitive disturbances (Dario, Tomei, 2004) that may range from mild confusion to rare transient global amnesia (Grande, Loeser, Samii, 2008). Others include headache, loss of deep-tendon reflexes, hypotension, slurred speech, urinary frequency, and sexual dysfunction (Slonomski, Abram, Zuniga, 2004). The incidence of adverse effects associated with oral baclofen ranges from 10% to 75%, and as many as 35% of patients experience adverse effects from intrathecal baclofen; an evaluation of risk and benefit prior to therapy and throughout the course of administration is recommended (Dario, Tomei, 2004). Although there are reports of the need for dose escalation during therapy, this appears to be rare (Slonomski, Abram, Zuniga, 2004).

Baclofen's adverse effects are dose-related. Administration of the lowest effective dose is essential, and this dose is identified by using a low starting dose and gradual dose escalation (Dario, Tomei, 2004; Lussier, Portenoy, 2004).

The potential for a serious withdrawal syndrome, including delirium and seizures, exists with abrupt discontinuation of baclofen after prolonged use; therefore, doses should always be tapered before the drug is discontinued (Dario, Tomei, 2004; Hansen, Gooch, Such-Neibar, 2007; Lussier, Portenoy, 2004). Baclofen withdrawal syndrome following abrupt discontinuation of intrathecal baclofen is sometimes confused with malignant hyperthermia and neuroleptic malignant syndrome. If untreated, baclofen withdrawal syndrome can progress to rhabdomyolysis, hepatic and renal failure, and disseminated intravascular coagulation (DIC). Treatment is high-dose IV benzodiazepines and restoration of intrathecal baclofen delivery (Slonomski, Abram, Zuniga, 2004). (See Chapter 15 for intraspinal complications that can occur with intrathecal drug administration.)

N-Methyl-D-Aspartate (NMDA) Receptor Antagonists

The evidence of analgesic efficacy for the several oral NMDA receptor antagonists on the market is limited and conflicting, and these drugs—dextromethorphan, memantine and amantadine, and magnesium—play a limited role in pain management. The data supporting the analgesic efficacy of ketamine are more robust, and this parenteral drug is gaining increasing acceptance in the management of carefully selected patients. The NMDA receptor antagonists, particularly ketamine, may have a role in preventing neuropathic pain states, such as persistent postsurgical pain, by suppressing secondary hyperalgesia and central sensitization (De Kock, Lavand'homme, 2007; Manning, Jianren, Frenk, et al., 1996; Xuerong, Yuguang, Xia, et al., 2008) (see Section I).

Following is a discussion of the research and clinical use of the NMDA receptor antagonists for persistent noncancer pain, cancer pain, and a variety of neuropathic types of pain. Perioperative use of dextromethorphan and ketamine is presented in Chapter 26.

Ketamine

Ketamine is a so-called dissociative anesthetic with dose-dependent analgesic, sedative, and amnestic properties. Preclinical data support its analgesic efficacy (Kosson, Klinowiecka, Kosson, et al., 2008; Pelissier, Laurido, Kramer, et al., 2003). At the low doses typically used for analgesia, the psychomimetic effects of ketamine are minimized; analgesia occurs at lower doses than psychomimetic effects (Panzer, Moitra, Sladen, 2009). Case reports, open-label and randomized controlled trials, and systematic reviews have reported that ketamine has analgesic efficacy in a variety of acute and persistent pains. The data are mixed, however, and more work is needed to clarify the analgesic potential in varied clinical settings. The drug is typically given intravenously, but it is possible to treat using the oral, rectal, intranasal, or subcutaneous routes (see Chapter 24 for a discussion of topical and see following discussion or research on intranasal ketamine). A discussion of ketamine's role in preventing persistent neuropathic pain syndromes by suppressing secondary hyperalgesia and central sensitization is found in Chapter 26. See Box 23-1 for guidelines on the administration of low-dose ketamine.

A systematic review of ketamine studies between 1966 and 2002 described the drug's efficacy in the treatment of persistent pain as moderate to weak (Hocking, Cousins, 2003). The most frequent use was as a third-line analgesic for the management of acute episodes of pain superimposed on persistent neuropathic pain, particularly when opioid-induced hyperalgesia was believed to be present. A more recent review concluded that a short course of ketamine might benefit some patients with refractory

neuropathic pain, but there is insufficient research to support longer use (Bell, 2009). The drug is not mentioned as an option in general neuropathic pain treatment guidelines (Dworkin, O'Connor, Backonja, et al., 2007; Moulin, Clark, Gilron, et al., 2007). Treatment guidelines for postherpetic neuralgia consider ketamine an unproven option (Dubinsky, Kabbani, El-Chami, et al., 2004).

Although a 2003 Cochrane Collaboration Review of randomized controlled trials concluded that further research is needed to establish ketamine's efficacy in improving opioid analgesia for cancer pain (Bell, Eccleston, Kalso, 2003a, 2003b), some studies and case reports attest to benefits when ketamine is added to the treatment plan for some patients with intractable cancer-related neuropathic pain (Chung, Pharo, 2007; Jackson, Ashby, Martin, et al., 2001; Kannan, Saxena, Bhatnagar, et al., 2002; Kotlinska-Lemieszek, Luczak, 2004; Mercadante, Villari, Ferrara, et al., 2009; Sen, Aydin, Aydin, 2006; Tarumi, Watanabe, Bruera, et al., 2000). The administration of ketamine to improve cancer pain that is refractory to opioid treatment is called *burst* ketamine therapy and has been shown to be effective when other options have failed (Hocking, Viser, Schug, et al., 2007; Jackson, Ashby, Martin, et al., 2001). For example, a case report described the successful use of ketamine burst infusion (100 mg/day) for 2 consecutive days to relieve excruciating movement-related pain caused by bony metastases that was unresponsive to aggressive opioid administration in 2 patients (Mercadante, Villari, Ferrera et al., 2009). Both patients experienced excessive sedation and nausea during IV morphine titration and were switched to an IV methadone infusion with concomitant IV ketamine burst infusion. Within approximately 2 days of infusion, the patients were able to resume daily activities. The ketamine was discontinued, and both patients were switched to oral methadone and discharged with well-controlled baseline and movement-related pain.

Analgesic efficacy of ketamine in acute pain has been established in several contexts. It is useful as part of a multimodal plan for treatment of pain associated with major surgery, burns, trauma, and during painful procedures in the ICU (Panzer, Moitra, Sladen, 2009). A placebo-controlled trial of transdermal ketamine in gynecologic surgery revealed that patients who received ketamine experienced a longer time to first request for analgesia and consumed less supplemental analgesia compared with those who received a placebo (Azevedo, Lauretti, Pereira, et al., 2000). A controlled trial of intranasal ketamine for breakthrough pain demonstrated both safety and analgesic efficacy (Carr, Goudas, Denman, et al., 2004a). The latter study led to two excellent letters to the editor about misunderstandings related to the potential for abuse of ketamine (and other agents) by patients with pain (Carr, Goudas, Denman, et al., 2004b; Lynch, Clark, 2004), which were written in response to a critical editorial (Bell, Kalso, 2004).

Box 23-1 | Low-Dose Ketamine Administration

INDICATIONS

- Refractory neuropathic pain (third-line agent; see text)
- Postoperative pain
  - Synergy with other analgesics
  - Opioid dose-sparing effects
- Prevention of persistent neuropathic postsurgical pain
- Treatment of opioid-induced hyperalgesia (OIH) (see Chapters 11 and 26)
- Procedural sedation and analgesia

IMPORTANT CONSIDERATIONS

- Ketamine therapy should be prescribed and coordinated only by those with a thorough understanding of the drug's adverse effects and the management of related complications, such as those skilled in pain management, anesthesia, or palliative care.
- Some hospitals restrict the administration of ketamine to specific clinical areas, such as the intensive care unit, emergency department, and palliative care.[1]
- An infusion device that does not allow free flow must be used to administer IV ketamine infusions (no exceptions), and doses must be verified by an independent double-check process to help insure accurate dose delivery (see Chapter 17).
- Co-administration of a benzodiazepine, such as midazolam or lorazepam, or low-dose haloperidol is recommended to prevent or minimize psychomimetic effects.[2]
- Try to maintain a quiet patient care environment to reduce excessive stimulation.

CONTRAINDICATIONS (CONSIDER CASE BY CASE)

- Head trauma
- Post intracranial surgery
- Increased intracranial pressure
- Intracranial bleeding
- Intracranial mass
- Seizure disorder, e.g., epilepsy

PRECAUTIONS (CONSIDER CASE BY CASE)

- Hypertension or hypotension
- Pulmonary disease associated with hypercarbia
- Posttraumatic stress disorder
- Psychosis or schizophrenia
- Recent psychiatric hospitalization
- History of stroke or myocardial infarction

OPIOID TAPERING

- Ketamine administration produces a significant opioid dose-sparing effect. Patients should be systematically

assessed for the need to decrease the dose of concurrent opioid analgesics. Excessive sedation may indicate the need for a decrease in opioid dose.
- Some clinicians decrease the opioid dose by 25% to 50% at initiation of ketamine therapy and then by 25% every 12 to 24 hours as tolerated, but this must be done on an individual basis based on patient response.
- Signs of abstinence syndrome indicate too rapid reduction in opioid dose. These include diaphoresis, abdominal cramps, diarrhea, or rhinorrhea. This can be treated by slowing opioid taper and low-dose ketamine bolus administration.

DOSING RECOMMENDATIONS

Note: Dosing recommendations in the literature and clinical practice vary widely and must be individualized. The starting dose should be low and titrated based on patient response.

Refractory persistent (chronic) pain

- IV[3,4]
  - Initial loading bolus (optional and physician-administered only): 0.25 to 0.5 mg/kg over 10 minutes
  - Continuous infusion: Start at 0.1 mg/kg/h and increase gradually as needed and tolerated. A maximum dose of 600 mg/day has been suggested (see text).
  - Intermittent bolus-only therapy: 0.1 to 0.2 mg/kg every 30 minutes PRN for breakthrough pain
  - IV burst therapy: 100 to 500 mg/24 h (given by infusion; dose titrated per patient response) for 2 to 5 days (duration of treatment adjusted per patient response)
- Oral[5,6]
  - 0.25 to 0.5 mg/kg or 10 to 25 mg at bedtime. May be increased as tolerated to 50 mg three times daily
  - Intermittent: 5 to 10 mg every 60 minutes PRN for breakthrough pain

Refractory acute pain (e.g., severe trauma pain in prehospital or emergency department setting; see contraindications)

- IV ketamine doses of 0.2 to 0.5 mg/kg are reported to produce analgesia for refractory acute pain.
- One study protocol for opioid dose-sparing effect: IV bolus dose of 0.2 mg/kg of ketamine over a 10-minute period with IV morphine titration to comfort with an initial IV morphine dose of 0.1 mg/kg followed by 3 mg of IV morphine (or equivalent) every 5 minutes (see Chapter 26 text for discussion of research).

Critically ill

- 0.06 to 0.12 mg/kg/h IV combined with opioid

Continued

Box 23-1 | Low-Dose Ketamine Administration—cont'd

Perioperative

- IV[3,4]
  - Intraoperative: 0.5 mg/kg bolus followed by a 5 mcg/kg/min infusion until skin closure
  - Postoperative: 2 mcg/kg/min infusion for 48 hours
  - Intermittent bolus-only therapy: 0.1 to 0.2 mg/kg every 30 minutes PRN for breakthrough pain
- Oral[5,6]
  - 25 to 50 mg twice daily
  - Breakthrough pain: 5 to 10 mg every 60 minutes PRN

Procedural

- IV: 0.2 to 0.8 mg/kg bolus (slow administration over 2 to 3 minutes)[3,4]
- Oral: 4 to 6 mg/kg[6]

A benzodiazepine, such as midazolam or lorazepam, is often combined with ketamine to reduce ketamine's dose-dependent adverse effects during procedural sedation and analgesia.[2] Following are two examples of dosing protocols that combine agents.

- 0.07 mg/kg of IV midazolam followed by IV ketamine 2 mg/kg over a 2-minute period
- Procedural IV PCA: 10 mg ketamine plus 0.5 mg of midazolam per 1 mL PCA bolus dose[4]

ADVERSE EFFECTS

- Hypotension or hypertension
- Psychotomimetic effects such as hallucinations or dreamlike feelings (these may be reduced or prevented by co-administration of a benzodiazepine; see monitoring below[6])
- Increased intracranial pressure
- Excessive sedation
- Excessive salivation
- Nausea, vomiting
- Tonic-clonic movements, tremors
- Apnea (with rapid IV administration)
- Diplopia

MONITORING[7,8]

- Vital signs including respiratory status, pain, sedation, and adverse effects 15 minutes after initial IV dose and 30 minutes after oral dose and with any bolus or dose increase. Monitor these parameters every 15 minutes for a total of 1 hour after initiation of therapy, then every 2 hours for 2 hours, then every 4 hours if stable. Adjust monitoring as needed based on patient response.
- Immediate effects of ketamine (e.g., pupil dilation, lacrimation, nystagmus, and increased muscle tone) are seen within 1 minute and are not necessarily adverse.
- Stop administration and notify prescriber if systolic blood pressure is less than 85 mmHg, heart rate is less than 60 beats per minute (check baseline), respiratory rate is less than 10 breaths per minute, or intolerable psychomimetic effects occur.

Note: Psychomimetic effects are often present and tolerable when the clinician stays with the patient and provides reassurance that these effects will resolve quickly or with a decrease in dose. For example, usually mild psychomimetic effects occur after a bolus dose but resolve quickly.

DISCONTINUATION OF THERAPY

- No formal weaning process is needed when the decision to discontinue ketamine is made.
- Systematic pain assessment should continue to ensure adequate control.

PATIENT TEACHING

- Discuss psychotomimetic effects prior to therapy and that measures are taken to avoid or minimize them; tell patients to expect dreamlike feelings.

Continued

The many studies and reviews and related literature about ketamine do not answer important questions about the analgesic potential of ketamine, but in aggregate, indicate that the drug should play a role as an adjuvant analgesic, particularly for refractory neuropathic pain of diverse types. The following is a list of case reports, reviews, and placebo-controlled research on the use of ketamine for cancer pain and other persistent pain states:

- Cancer-related pain (Bell, Eccleston, Kalso, 2003a, 2003b; Ben-Ari, Lewis, Davidson, 2007; Edmonds, Davis, 1996; Grande, O'Donnell, Fitzgibbon, et al., 2008; Jackson, Ashby, Martin, et al., 2001; Kannan, Saxena, Bhatnagar, et al., 2002; Lussier, Portenoy, 2004; Mercadante, Arcuri, Tirelli, et al., 2000; Mercadante, Villari, Ferrera, et al., 2009; Sen, Aydin, Aydin, 2006; Tarumi, Watanabe, Bruera, et al., 2000; Wood, 2006)
- Fibromyalgia (Graven-Nielsen, Aspegren, Henriksson, et al., 2000; Hocking, Cousins, 2003)
- Postherpetic neuralgia (Ben-Ari, Lewis, Davidson, 2007; Cvrcek, 2008; Eide, Stubhaug, Oye, et al., 1995; Hempenstall, Nurmikko, Johnson, et al., 2005; Hocking, Cousins, 2003)
- Painful diabetic neuropathy (Cvrcek, 2008)
- CRPS (Ben-Ari, Lewis, Davidson, 2007; Correll, Maleki, Gracely, et al., 2004; Hocking, Cousins,

- Tell patient to inform staff if psychotomimetic effects or any other adverse effects occur and if they are bothersome or frightening.
- Warn patients about the bitter taste of oral ketamine, and tell them this can be lessened by taking it with sweet juice or gelatin.

---

[1]Nurses are referred to their scope of practice as defined by their individual state board of nursing with regard to ketamine administration.

[2]Check with pharmacy department for compatibility of selected benzodiazepine with IV ketamine.

[3]Ketamine is administered subcutaneously in the palliative care setting in particular (e.g., 0.1 to 0.15 mg/kg by brief infusion or 0.1 to 0.15 mg/kg/h by continuous infusion) but can be irritating and may require frequent infusion site changes; the intramuscular route is discouraged for ketamine administration.

[4]If administered by IV PCA, combining ketamine with the PCA opioid in the same drug reservoir could result in an unnecessarily high ketamine dose; separate infusion solutions are recommended (see text).

[5]Conversion to oral ketamine can be achieved without loss of pain control at doses 30% to 40% lower than those required by the parenteral route.

[6]Oral ketamine can produce a bitter taste and irritation of the throat. When the injectable formulation is used orally, the bitter taste may be masked with orange juice or cola drinks.

[7]This protocol is also used in terminally ill patients, and monitoring and actions should be adjusted accordingly.

[8]Continuous pulse oximetry or capnography is recommended in nonpalliative care areas when ketamine and high-dose opioids are co-administered (see Chapter 19 for more on monitoring modalities).

From Pasero, C., & McCaffery, M. *Pain assessment and pharmacologic management*, pp. 675-677, St. Louis, Mosby. Data from e-mail communication and review on April 22, 2009, by Laura Trexor, MSN, RNC, APRN, BC, Clinical Nurse Specialist, Pain Service, St. Luke's Hospital, Kansas City, MO; e-mail communication and review on May 27, 2009, by Kathleen Colfer MSN, RN-BC, Acute Pain Management Clinical Nurse Specialist, Department of Anesthesiology, Thomas Jefferson University Hospital, Philadelphia. © 2004, Pasero C. May be duplicated for use in clinical practice.

Additional references: Chudnofsky, C. R., Weber, J. E., Stoyanoff, P. J., et al. (2000). A combination of midazolam and ketamine for procedural sedation and analgesia in adult emergency department patients. *Acad Emerg Med, 7*(3), 228-235; De Kock, M., & Lavand'homme, P. (2007). The clinical role of NMDA receptor antagonists for the treatment of postoperative pain. *Best Prac Res Clin Anaesthes, 21*(1), 85-98; Fine, P. (1999). Low-dose ketamine in the management of opioid nonresponsive terminal cancer pain. *J Pain Symptom Manage, 17*(4), 296-300; Friedman, R., Jallo, J., & Young, W. F. (2001). Oral ketamine for opioid-resistant acute pain. *J Pain, 2*(1), 75-76; Galinski, M., Dolveck, F., Combes, X., et al. (2007). Management of severe acute pain in emergency settings: Ketamine reduces morphine consumption. *Am J Emerg Med, 25*(4), 385-390; Guillou, N., Tanguy, M., Seguin, P., et al. (2003). The effects of small-dose ketamine on morphine consumption in surgical intensive care unit patients after major surgery. *Anesth Analg, 97*(3), 843-847; Hocking, G., & Cousins, M. J. (2003). Ketamine in chronic pain management: An evidence-based review. *Anesth Analg, 97*(6), 1730-1739; Jackson, K., Ashby, M., Martin, P., et al. (2001). "Burst" ketamine for refractory cancer pain: An open-label audit of 39 patients. *J Pain Symptom Manage, 22*(4), 834-842; Lussier, D., & Portenoy, R. K. (2004). Adjuvant analgesics in pain management. In D. Doyle, G. Hanks, N. I. Cherny, et al. (Eds.), *Oxford textbook of palliative medicine*, ed. 3, New York, Oxford Press; MacPherson, R. D., Woods, D., & Penfold, J. (2008). Ketamine and midazolam delivered by patient-controlled analgesia in relieving pain associated with burns dressings. *Clin J Pain, 24*(7), 568-571; Mercadante, S., Villari, P., Ferrera, P., et al. (2009). Opioid switching and burst ketamine to improve the opioid response in patients with movement-related pain due to bone metastases. *Clin J Pain, 25*(7), 648-649; Panzer, O., Moitra, V., & Sladen, R. N. (2009). Pharmacology of sedative-analgesic agents: Dexmedetomidine, remifentanil, ketamine, volatile anesthetics and the role of peripheral mu antagonists. *Crit Care Clin, 25*(3), 451-469; Pasero, C., & McCaffery, M. (2005). Ketamine: Low doses may provide relief for some painful conditions. *Am J Nurs, 105*(4), 60-64; Portenoy, R., & Rowe, G. (2003). Adjuvant analgesic drugs. In E. Bruera, & R. Portenoy. (Eds.), *Cancer pain*, New York, Cambridge University Press; Reves, J., Glass, P. S. A., Lubarsky, D. A., et al. (2005). Intravenous nonopioid anesthetics. In R. Miller (Ed.), *Miller's anesthesia*, ed 6, Philadelphia, Churchill Livingstone; Svenson, J. E., & Abernathy, M. K. (2007). Ketamine for prehospital use: New look at an old drug. *Am J Emerg Med, 25*(8), 977-980.

2003; Kiefer, Rohr, Ploppa, et al., 2008; Schwartzman, Alexander, Grothusen, et al., 2009; Sigtermans, van Hilten, Bauer, et al., 2009)
- Ischemic pain (Capel, Jenkins, Jefferson, et al., 2008; Hocking, Cousins, 2003; Mitchell, Fallon, 2002)
- Phantom limb pain (prevention and treatment) (Ben-Ari, Lewis, Davidson, 2007; Eichenberger, Neff, Sveticic, et al., 2008; Hayes, Armstrong-Brown, Burstal, et al., 2004; Hocking, Cousins, 2003; Mitchell, 2001)
- Spinal cord injury pain (Hocking, Cousins, 2003; Kvarnstrom, Karlsten, Quiding, et al., 2004)
- Central poststroke pain (Kumar, Kalita, Kumar, et al., 2009)
- Multiple sclerosis (Sakai, Tomiyasu, Ono, et al., 2004)
- Burn pain (Gregoretti, Decaroli, Piacevoli, et al., 2008)
- Acute exacerbation of chronic pain; high-dose, opioid-related hyperalgesia (Hocking, Cousins, 2003)
- Restless leg syndrome (Kapur, Friedman, 2002)
- Various types of refractory pain of neuropathic origin (Bell, 2009; Ben-Ari, Lewis, Davidson, 2007; Chung, Pharo, 2007; Edmonds, Davis, 1996; Jackson, Ashby, Martin, et al., 2001; Kannan, Saxena, Bhatnagar, et al., 2002; Persson, Axelsson, Hallin, et al., 1995; Tarumi, Watanabe, Bruera, et al., 2000; Visser, Schug, 2006)

Other NMDA Receptor Antagonists

Although basic research conducted largely in the 1990s increased optimism that NMDA receptor antagonism could be a means by which many types of pain could be addressed, clinical trials of other commercially-available drugs with this mechanism yielded mixed results. Preclinical evidence suggested that dextromethorphan, the antitussive, is analgesic (Chow, Huang, Ho, et al., 2004). Clinical trials of oral dextromethorphan have not yielded impressive results, however. In one study, the drug was shown to produce dose-related analgesia for patients with painful diabetic neuropathy (N = 23) or postherpetic neuralgia (N = 21); median dose for both types of pain was 400 mg (Sang, Booher, Gilron, et al., 2002). Doses of 100 mg had no effect on the relief produced by IV morphine in another study (Heiskanen, Hartel, Dahl, et al., 2002), and others indicated no meaningful effect in trigeminal neuralgia or anesthesia dolorosa (Gilron, Booher, Rowan, et al., 2000). Although early research of a novel oral formulation that combined morphine with dextromethorphan (MorphiDex) suggested that the addition of dextromethorphan might inhibit the development of tolerance to morphine (Chevlen, 2000), three subsequent controlled studies evaluating 3-month use of the formulation or morphine alone failed to show enhanced analgesia or reduction in opioid tolerance in patients with persistent noncancer, non-neuropathic pain (Galer, Lee, Ma, et al., 2005).

Memantine (Ebixa, Namenda), a long-acting oral NMDA receptor antagonist, is approved for the treatment of Alzheimer's disease. Randomized controlled trials have produced disappointing results as an analgesic (Buvanendran, Kroin, 2008). It was ineffective for phantom limb pain in one placebo-controlled, randomized trial (Wiech, Kiefer, Topfner, et al., 2004), and a later placebo-controlled trial that administered memantine immediately after traumatic upper limb amputation and for 4 weeks postoperatively demonstrated a four-fold decrease in the incidence of phantom limb pain at 4 weeks and 6 months but not at 12 months (Schley, Topfncr, Wicch, et al., 2007). Case reports described very positive responses in patients with treatment-refractory phantom limb pain (Hackworth, Tokarz, Fowler, et al., 2008) and cancer pain (Grande, O'Donnell, Fitzgibbon, ct al., 2008).

Amantadine (Symmetrel) is another NMDA receptor antagonist that has been used for treatment of Parkinson's disease and spasticity but is rarely used for pain. A randomized controlled trial administered amantadine or placebo to women the day before mastectomy and axillary lymph node dissection and continued treatment for 14 days (Eisenberg, Pud, Koltun, et al., 2007). There were no differences between the groups in any of the neuropathic pain outcome measures. A preoperative dose of 200 mg of IV amantadine failed to enhance postoperative analgesia in women undergoing abdominal hysterectomy (Gottschalk, Schroeder, Ufer, et al., 2001).

Magnesium, another agent that blocks NMDA receptor activity, has been used for the treatment of pain but with disappointing or mixed results. A randomized controlled trial (N = 200) showed no analgesic or dose-sparing effects from a single 4 g IV bolus of magnesium after anesthesia induction in ambulatory surgery patients (Tramer, Glynn, 2007). A systematic review of research on the perioperative use of NMDA receptor antagonists showed promise with dextromethorphan and ketamine but no effect with magnesium (McCartney, Sinha, Katz, 2004). Another systematic review of 14 trials evaluated its effect on postoperative pain and concluded a lack of convincing evidence that the drug provides effective analgesia for this type of pain (Lysakowski, Dumont, Czarnetzki, et al., 2007). A placebo-controlled, cross-over study found improved pain scores in 7 patients with postherpetic neuralgia 20 to 30 minutes following IV infusion of magnesium (30 mg/kg) (Brill, Sedgwick, Hamann, et al., 2002), and a single IV dose of 500 mg or 1000 mg of magnesium was found to be effective in most of 12 patients with cancer pain that was refractory to opioid analgesics (Crosby, Wilcock, Corcoran, 2000). A pilot study reported improved pain, impairment level, and quality of life with 4-hour IV magnesium infusions (70 mg/kg; 25 mL/h/day) for 5 days in 8 patients with CRPS type 1 (Collins, Zurrmond, de Lange, et al., 2009). The treatment was well-tolerated with infusion site pain, flushing, burning eyes, and fatigue being the most common adverse effects.

Mechanism of Action

Research regarding the underlying mechanisms of action of the NMDA receptor antagonists is ongoing and believed to be complex (Hocking, Visser, Schug, et al., 2007). Afferent input caused by tissue injury causes a series of events, including changes in calcium channels, which facilitates the transmission of pain (De Kock, Lavand'homme, 2007) (see Section I and Figure I-2, *B* on pp. 4-5). This facilitation of transmission, or "wind up," is thought to be associated with the development of neuropathic pain. NMDA antagonizes this facilitated response. The binding of antagonists to the NMDA receptor can produce analgesia in this way, and also can reduce the desensitization of the mu opioid receptor that follows binding to opioid compounds. In animal models, the latter effect is associated with the reversal of opioid tolerance. Other mechanisms also may be important. Ketamine, for example, inhibits serotonin and dopamine uptake and influences other ion channel activity (Hocking, Visser, Shug, et al., 2007), effects that could further explain its role in suppressing hyperalgesia and central sensitization (De Kock, Lavand'homme, 2007).

Adverse Effects

The most common adverse effects of the NMDA receptor antagonists are dose-related and include sedation, confusion that can progress to delirium, severe nightmares, hallucinations, and dysphoria (Pasero, McCaffery, 2005).

Psychotomimetic effects and other adverse effects are rare with dextromethorphan and are minimized with ketamine by administration of low (subanesthetic) doses.

Even at low doses, sedation is common with ketamine, which is one reason it is sometimes used for procedural sedation. The drug increases muscle tone, and purposeless movements may occur. Other adverse effects are hypotension, tachycardia, and nausea and vomiting. Ketamine should not be used in patients with increased intracranial or intraocular pressure as it may worsen these pathologies. Slow IV administration of ketamine does not produce respiratory depression, which is a major advantage. Although hypotension can occur, CV function, hepatic blood flow, laryngeal protective reflexes, and bowel function are generally not depressed with low doses.

When administered intravenously (the usual approach), the risks associated with ketamine have led some experts to recommend that its use be limited to those skilled in pain management and anesthesiology (Bell, 2009; Cvrcek, 2008). Palliative care specialists are also among those knowledgeable in the safe administration of the drug. Co-administration of a benzodiazepine or a neuroleptic has been recommended to reduce the risk of psychotomimetic effects (Fitzgibbon, Hall, Schroder, et al., 2002; Mercadante, 1996). Some hospitals restrict the administration of ketamine to specific clinical areas, such as the intensive care unit (ICU), emergency department (ED), and palliative care. Nurses should be aware of their scope of practice, state board of nursing's opinions, and institutional policies and procedures regarding the administration and monitoring of agents such as ketamine as these vary widely.

Ketamine's adverse effect profile also makes it a less favorable therapy for long-term use (Cvrcek, 2008). A case series reported severe ulcerative cystitis associated with long-term recreational use of ketamine that has implications also for individuals using ketamine for persistent pain (Shahani, Streutker, Dickson, et al., 2007).

Other NMDA antagonists also can cause CNS toxicity, including dizziness, confusion, and dysphoria. The adverse effects are more pronounced in frail medically ill patients. Dextromethorphan inhibits the cytochrome P450 2D6 isoenzyme, an effect that has been associated with serious drug-drug interactions (Forget, le Polain de Waroux, Wallemacq, et al., 2008) (see Chapter 11 for more on the cytochrome P450 enzyme system). These drug-drug interactions, such as the potential for higher-than-expected TCA levels when co-administered with dextromethorphan, must be anticipated and monitored if the latter drug is added to an existing regimen.

Indications

Although two trials suggest that a brief IV infusion of ketamine may be a predictor of response to an oral agent, specifically dextromethorphan (Cohen, Verdolin, Chang, 2006; Cohen, Wang, Chen, et al., 2009), it remains uncertain that this novel use has sufficient predictive validity, or

is widely enough available, to be useful. As an avenue of research leading to a more rational "mechanism-based" selection of analgesic therapy, it is interesting, and in the future, may be helpful in identifying patients with pain that is mediated by NMDA receptor activation.

At the present time, brief IV ketamine infusion is gaining increased acceptance as an approach to treat severe neuropathic pain that has been refractory to conventional oral therapies. Experience probably is greatest in the treatment of CRPS. Brief ketamine infusion also is a strategy considered for "crescendo" pain, and it may be selected to provide pain relief and sedation for intolerable distress at the end of life (in a treatment approach known as *palliative sedation*). Some patients are offered repeated brief infusions as a long-term strategy for persistent pain, and some pain specialists provide ongoing treatment by compounding an oral formulation (or having the patient take the injectable formulation by mouth). Finally, small numbers of patients with refractory CRPS have been treated with high-dose ketamine, with intriguing early observations (see list of case studies and research provided earlier in the chapter).

Trials of the oral NMDA receptor antagonists are occasionally considered for patients with refractory neuropathic pain. Memantine is most often tried.

Dose Selection

To date, there are no universally agreed-upon guidelines or protocols for ketamine, but there is available literature based on clinical experience that can be used to guide practice. See Box 23-1 for suggested dosing.

Ketamine

Several different dosing regimens have been used for ketamine treatment of refractory persistent pain, including IV boluses (0.25 to 0.5 mg/kg), continuous low- or high-dose IV infusion (up to 600 mg/24 h), IV burst infusion therapy (100 to 500 mg/24 h for 2 to 5 days [see the paragraphs that follow]), and oral doses (0.5 mg/kg three times daily) (Jackson, Ashby, Martin, et al., 2001; Lussier, Portenoy, 2004) (see Chapter 26 and Box 23-1 for dosing recommendations for acute pain). A titrated continuous infusion of ketamine is used to induce sedation in imminently dying patients. Ketamine infusions should be administered via an infusion device that does not allow free flow to insure accurate dose delivery.

A case report of patients with refractory pain recommended an initial low parenteral ketamine dose of 40 to 60 mg over 24 hours (Fitzgibbon, Hall, Schroder, et al., 2002). Conversion to oral ketamine was achieved without loss of pain control at doses 30% to 40% lower than those required by the parenteral route.

For oral therapy, an initial dose of 50 mg at bedtime increased as tolerated to 50 mg 3 times daily has been suggested for central types of refractory neuropathic pain (Hocking, Cousins, 2003). Another source suggests 0.5

mg/kg taken at bedtime (Reves, Glass, Lubarsky, et al., 2005). As with other adjuvant analgesics, low initial doses followed by titration upward to optimal pain relief with minimal adverse effects is recommended. The case reports of 21 patients with intractable persistent pain described a starting dose of oral ketamine of 100 mg/day (40 mg/day in sensitive individuals) and titration with 40 mg/day doses every 2 days until efficacy or adverse effects were encountered; the final median dose was 220 mg/day (range 40 to 500 mg/day) (Enarson, Hays, Woodruffe, 1999).

Outpatient treatment of persistent pain with ketamine followed by close monitoring during and after treatment with home health visits is possible (Webster, Walker, 2006). Experience with multi-day dosing for outpatients with CRPS has been described (Goldberg, Domsky, Scaringe, et al., 2005).

Oral and intranasal ketamine can produce a bitter taste and burning of the throat. When the injectable formulation is used orally, the bitter taste may be masked with orange juice or cola drinks.

Other NMDA Antagonists

In one study, the median dose of dextromethorphan for treatment of painful diabetic neuropathy or postherpetic neuralgia was 400 mg, much higher than the usual antitussive dose (Sang, Booher, Gilron, et al., 2002). Dextromethorphan has an extremely good safety profile and has been administered at doses higher than 1 g/day; however, sedation and confusion can occur with higher doses. The drug is available in cough suppressant products only in the United States, and at present, the most concentrated source is in a suspension of 30 mg/5 mL (e.g., Delsym 12-Hour). A trial of dextromethorphan may be initiated using a proprietary cough suppressant (ensuring that the product contains no alcohol or other active drugs). A prudent starting dose is 45 to 60 mg daily, which can be gradually escalated until favorable effects occur, adverse effects supervene, or a conventional maximum daily dose of 1 g is achieved (Lussier, Portenoy, 2004).

If memantine or amantadine is offered as a trial for neuropathic pain, dosing typically starts in a range similar to the primary indication for these drugs, such as memantine 10 mg/day. The dose is then gradually titrated upward until favorable effects occur or adverse effects develop. Dosing of IV magnesium usually takes the form of a bolus or brief infusion, usually at a 1 g dose. There is no experience with the use of oral magnesium for the longer-term management of neuropathic pain, but several products are available over the counter and provide guidelines for administration.

Ziconotide

Ziconotide (Prialt) is a nonopioid intrathecal analgesic currently approved for the treatment of intractable pain. The preparation is a synthetic peptide that is obtained from the marine snail Conus magus (Vitale, Battelli, Gasperoni, et al., 2008). Intrathecal ziconotide exerts its effects through blockade of the N-type calcium channel in the dorsal horn of the spinal cord (see Section I). It is administered via an implanted intrathecal infusion device, usually following a trial to assess its potential to relieve pain without toxicity. Ziconotide can be administered alone or with other analgesics, such as morphine (Wallace, Kosek, Staats, et al., 2008), hydromorphone (Deer, Krames, Hassenbusch, et al., 2007), and baclofen (Saulino, Burton, Danyo, et al., 2009).

Early studies of ziconotide revealed a high incidence of significant cognitive adverse effects, including hallucinations and psychosis. These studies evaluated a dose range higher than is now recommended (see the paragraphs that follow).

A phase II open-label study of 26 patients with primarily severe persistent low back pain demonstrated a 14.5% mean percentage improvement of baseline VAS scores (Wallace, Kosek, Staats, et al., 2008). The initial dose was 0.60 mcg/day, which was titrated to a median dose of 4.80 mcg/day (maximum 7.2 mcg/day) by week 5. Adverse effects were described as mild to moderate in most patients and included confusion, dizziness, abnormal gait, hallucinations, and anxiety. One patient experienced hallucinations for 57 days, and another had memory impairment for 163 days; these resolved in both patients after therapy was discontinued.

In a multicenter, open-label trial of 78 patients with persistent noncancer pain, the median ziconotide dose was 6.48 mcg/day at the start of the study and ranged from 5.52 to 7.20 mcg/day across all study visits (Webster, Fisher, Charapata, et al., 2009). With this dosing range and stable pain scores for the treatment duration of 3 years, the type and frequency of adverse events included memory impairment (11.3%); dizziness, nystagmus, and speech disorder (8.5% each); nervousness and somnolence (7.0% each); and abnormal gait (5.6%). Pain relief seemed to be relatively disappointing, with VAS improvements of just greater than 10% above baseline at most evaluation periods (see Section II for discussion of meaningful pain relief).

A 12-month study showed that ziconotide was effective for long-term treatment of a wide variety of persistent cancer and noncancer types of pain (Ellis, Dissanayake, McGuire, et al., 2008). Other research has also demonstrated efficacy for refractory cancer and AIDS-related pain (Staats, Yearwood, Charapata, et al., 2004) and refractory neuropathic pain and spasticity (Saulino, Burton, Danyo, et al., 2009).

Based on this research and clinical experience with ziconotide, the expert panel of the 2007 Polyanalgesic Consensus Conference suggested that ziconotide may be considered a first-line intrathecal agent, with indications beyond intractable pain in patients who had exhausted all other therapeutic options (Deer, Krames, Hassenbusch, et al., 2007). Given the cost and short history of this drug, its appropriate positioning within the armamentarium of

Box 23-2 | Administration of Intrathecal Ziconotide[1]

Indications: Intractable persistent (chronic) pain

IMPORTANT CONSIDERATIONS

- Ziconotide therapy should be prescribed and coordinated only by those with a thorough understanding of the drug's adverse effects and the management of related complications, such as those who specialize in pain management.
- Ziconotide has a lag time (9 to 14 days) before optimal pain relief, which is achieved through slow dose titration to effect. Therapy should be initiated at low doses and titrated very slowly.
- There is wide variability in analgesic response to ziconotide. A ziconotide trial is recommended, and although a trial does not determine optimal post-trial dose, it does help to determine if the agent will be analgesic in a specific patient.

ZICONOTIDE TRIAL

Supplies

- 100 mcg/mL in 1 mL vial—to be used for trialing purposes only
- Bag #1: 20 mcg of ziconotide per 100 mL of normal saline = 0.2 mcg/mL
- Bag #2: 100 mcg of ziconotide per 100 mL of normal saline = 1.0 mcg/mL
- An infusion device will be used to administer a ziconotide trial (no exceptions), and doses will be verified by independent double-check process (see Chapter 17)
- The ziconotide trial infusion should be delivered by an infusion pump that has the following capabilities:
  - Capacity to deliver 0.1 mL/h
  - Will not allow free flow of fluid
  - Can be locked to prevent tampering

Procedure

- An intrathecal catheter is placed and externalized
- Patients who live more than 100 miles from the prescribing pain management specialist are encouraged to remain in the hospital for an inpatient trial but may be discharged to home if monitoring by a physician familiar with the characteristics of ziconotide is possible. During outpatient trial, the patient should be accompanied by a family member, significant other, or friend to monitor adverse effects (see the following dosing recommendations).

Trial dosing recommendations

- Start with 0.5 mcg/day
- First increase is 0.5 mcg/day

- Then increase by 0.5 to 1.0 mcg every 12 to 24 hours
- Trial may be extended 1 to 2 weeks

Trial monotherapy

- Use 25 mcg/mL in a 20 mL vial (undiluted) when dose is 1.2 mcg/day or greater
  - Stability data supports a pump refill every 90 days
- Use 100 mcg/mL in a 5 mL vial (undiluted) when dose is 10 mcg/day or greater
  - Stability data supports pump refill every 150 days

Trial combination therapy

- Use 25 mcg/mL in a 20 mL vial (undiluted) to combine with hydromorphone, bupivacaine, clonidine, or baclofen (stability data supports pump refill every 60 days—see text)

ZICONOTIDE THERAPY POST TRIAL PROCEDURE

Implanted intrathecal pumps are used to administer long-term ziconotide therapy (see Chapter 15 for more on intrathecal analgesia).

Flushing of intrathecal pump

- Due to the binding of ziconotide to the internal titanium of the intrathecal pumps, all pumps must be rinsed (flushed) with ziconotide before therapy is initiated.
- The flushing is done just once.
- Only ziconotide-naïve pumps need to be flushed as the binding is permanent
- A kit ("Prialt Rinse Kit," usually ordered by the pharmacy department) is used to flush the intrathecal pump. The kit includes three 2 mL syringes filled with undiluted ziconotide (25 mcg/mL = total of 6 mL of ziconotide).
- Upon initiation of therapy (before infusion), the intrathecal pump is accessed and one syringe-full of ziconotide (2 mL) is instilled, then withdrawn, then discarded. This process is repeated until all three syringes are used.

Dosing recommendations

- Start at 25% of the dose used in trial.
- The concentration and dose per day of ziconotide are calculated so that no less than 0.2 mL volume is delivered per day.
- Doses are slowly titrated over several weeks according to patient response.
- Intrathecal pump refills are every 2 to 4 weeks, and doses are increased at the time of refill.
- Dose increases should be made no more frequently than every 14 days and preferably 21 days due to the characteristic slow uptake of ziconotide.

Continued

Box 23-2   Administration of Intrathecal Ziconotide—cont'd

Calculation of dose

- Dosing patients after trial (new implanted intrathecal pump)
  - Patients who had a ziconotide trial are dosed at 25% of the total trial dose that provided adequate pain relief.

Example of procedure in patient who was receiving 8 mcg/day at the end of the trial:

1. The intrathecal pump is rinsed at the time of the intrathecal pump implant (see flushing procedure).
2. The initial solution is calculated to deliver a dose of 2 mcg/day (25% of 8 mcg/day).
3. The dose will remain the same until the first pump refill.
4. The dose per day is increased 0.5 to 1.0 mcg every 21 to 40 days thereafter until satisfactory pain control is achieved or adverse effects occur.

- Dosing patients with implanted pump who were not trialed
  - Patients with an existing intrathecal pump can be trialed with ziconotide by adding ziconotide to the patient's current intrathecal solution when the patient comes for a refill visit.
  - Ziconotide may be added to the existing intrathecal solution as combination therapy.

Example:

1. The intrathecal pump is rinsed (see flushing procedure).
2. The existing intrathecal solution will remain the same but with the addition of ziconotide.
3. The dose per day of ziconotide is calculated to start at 0.5 mcg/day for the first two pump refills.
4. At every intrathecal pump refill thereafter, the solution is adjusted to allow dose increases by increments of 0.5 to 1 mcg until satisfactory pain control is achieved or adverse effects occur.
5. As pain control is achieved, the opioid solution is adjusted with each refill to reduce the opioid dose per day by 10% to 20% until it is removed from the solution.

MANAGEMENT OF ADVERSE EFFECTS

Mild adverse effects: Auditory hallucinations, nausea, diarrhea, and dizziness.

Action: Reduce the daily dose of ziconotide by 0.5 to 1.0 mcg. These adverse effects will usually resolve within 2 to 8 hours. Titration can be resumed thereafter with increases in dose by increments of 0.1 to 0.2 mcg until pain control is achieved.

Moderate adverse effects: Nervous system impairment, such as gait disturbance, ataxia, increased dizziness, and somnolence.

Action: Reduce daily dose by 50% until adverse effects resolve. Titration can be resumed thereafter by increments of 0.2 to 0.5 mcg. Close monitoring of adverse effects is required.

Severe adverse effects: Cognitive changes, mental slowing, confusion, aphasia, memory loss, and/or psychosis.

Action: Stop ziconotide administration until adverse effects are gone. Ziconotide may be restarted at 0.5 mcg/day and titrated slowly at increments of 0.2 mcg. Close monitoring of adverse effects is required.

---

[1]Nurses are referred to their scope of practice as defined by their individual state board of nursing for their role in the administration of intrathecal analgesia. They should also see the American Society for Pain Management Nursing's Position Paper on the Role of the Registered Nurse in the Management and Monitoring of Analgesia by Catheter Techniques (Pasero, Eksterowicz, Primeau, et al., 2007; www.aspmn.org).

As appears in Pasero, C., & McCaffery, M. (2011). *Pain assessment and pharmacologic management*, pp. 681-682, St. Louis, Mosby. Contributed by Michael D. Stanton-Hicks, MD and Anne J. Sapienza-Crawford, CNP; Cleveland Clinic Foundation, Department of Pain Management, Cleveland, OH. © 2009, Cleveland Clinic Foundation. May be duplicated for use in clinical practice.

---

agents that may be explored for intrathecal use remains uncertain, however. It is likely that a larger proportion of trials of neuraxial analgesia will include a specific ziconotide trial in the future.

Ziconotide has a lag time before optimal pain relief (e.g., 9 to 14 days), which is achieved through slow dose titration to effect. One study reported a mean time to onset of analgesia as 15 weeks at a mean dose of 3.7 mcg/day (Saulino, Burton, Danyo et al., 2009). The therapeutic and safety dosing range is narrow. Further research is needed to determine ideal catheter tip location for optimal analgesic response (Deer, Krames, Hassenbusch, et al., 2007). The maximum recommended ziconotide dose is 19.2 mcg/day, although higher doses have been safely administered (Webster, Fisher, Charapata, et al., 2009). More research is needed with regard to the molecular stability of ziconotide. It appears to have stability at concentrations higher than 1 mcg/mL (Deer, Krames, Hassenbusch, et al, 2007). The rate of ziconotide degradation is accelerated when the agent is compounded with morphine and hydromorphone, so combinations of ziconotide with lower concentrations of the compounded opioid are expected to be more stable. Gradual dose escalation can reduce the occurrence and severity of CNS adverse effects, such as dizziness, nausea, and confusion (Klotz, 2006). Intolerable and unmanageable adverse effects are reported to resolve with dose reduction or termination of treatment (Webster, Fisher, Charapata, et al., 2009). Ziconotide does not cause respiratory depression or physical dependence, and tolerance has not been reported (Klotz, 2006).

Ziconotide must be administered by pain management specialists who are familiar with the drug, indications, dose ranges, adverse events, dose titration, and follow-up care. Patients receiving this agent must be closely followed for a treatment response and the occurrence of adverse effects. It is critical that patients have easy access to their care providers. They must be informed about the potential CNS adverse events and instructed to promptly report these if any are experienced. See Box 23-2 for guidelines on the administration of ziconotide.

Conclusion

There are several adjuvant analgesics that are used solely for persistent neuropathic pain. Along with the multipurpose adjuvant analgesics these drugs offer many options for the treatment of this type of pain. Among those discussed in this chapter are the anticonvulsants, which are first-line for neuropathic pain, and the sodium channel blockers, GABA agonists, NMDA receptor antagonists, and relatively new intrathecal drug ziconotide, which are options for neuropathic pain that is refractory to the recommended first-line options.

Chapter 24 Topical Analgesics for Persistent (Chronic) Pain

IT is important to distinguish between the terms *topical* and *transdermal* (Stanos, 2007). Although both routes require a drug to cross the stratum corneum to produce analgesia (Figure 24-1), transdermal drug delivery (e.g., long-acting transdermal fentanyl patch) requires absorption to achieve systemic effects, whereas topical agents (e.g., lidocaine patch 5% and other local anesthetics, capsaicin) are intended to produce effects in the tissues immediately under the site of application (Stanos, 2007). Transdermal analgesic drugs provide systemic analgesia, and topical analgesics provide what is referred to as "targeted peripheral analgesia," or pain relief achieved by "dampening" pain mechanisms within the peripheral nervous system (Argoff, 2003). Transdermal delivery systems typically have a slow onset and extended duration of analgesia. Topical analgesics are faster acting and dissipate relatively soon after removal of the drug.

There are significant benefits to using topical analgesics, including patient acceptance, ease of administration, reductions in systemic adverse effects, and fewer drug interactions (Argoff, 2003; McCleane, 2008; Stanos, 2007). Some preparations (e.g., capsaicin, L.M.X.4) can be obtained without a prescription; others (e.g., lidocaine patch 5%, clonidine, EMLA, diclofenac patch) require a prescription. Some topical analgesics (e.g., antidepressants, anticonvulsants, ketamine) are not commercially available but may be prepared by a compounding pharmacy. The topical therapies discussed here are those used primarily for persistent pain and include the lidocaine patch 5% and other local anesthetics, capsaicin, antidepressants, anticonvulsants, clonidine, and ketamine. A bupivacaine patch (Eladur) was under development at the time of publication. Local anesthetics used for procedural pain are discussed in Chapter 28. Topical formulations containing aspirin or NSAIDs are discussed in Chapter 7. A list of topical agents can be found in Table 24-1.

Lidocaine Patch 5%

The topical lidocaine patch 5% (Lidoderm) is 10 cm by 14 cm and contains 700 mg of lidocaine in an aqueous base. After removing a polyethylene terephthalate film release liner, the patch is placed directly over or adjacent to the painful area (Pasero, 2003b) (see Box 24-1 for guidelines on the use of the lidocaine patch 5%). The patch is not sterile so should not be placed in wounds, but they are often placed around painful wounds. They may be cut to fit smaller areas as well. For example, a patch can be cut into strips and wrapped around painful fingers or toes. A trial period of three weeks is recommended to determine effectiveness of lidocaine patch 5% (Dworkin, O'Connor, Backonja, et al., 2007).

Lidocaine and other local anesthetics relieve pain primarily by suppressing the activity of peripheral sodium channels thereby reducing ectopic, paroxysmal discharges and pathologic pain transmission (see Section I and Figure I-2 on pp. 4-5). A major advantage of analgesics such as the lidocaine patch 5% is that they work peripherally rather than systemically, and thus are associated with a low incidence of systemic adverse effects (Stanos, 2007). Although lidocaine is a local anesthetic, penetration of the drug following topical application is sufficient to produce an analgesic effect but not a sensory block. Patients

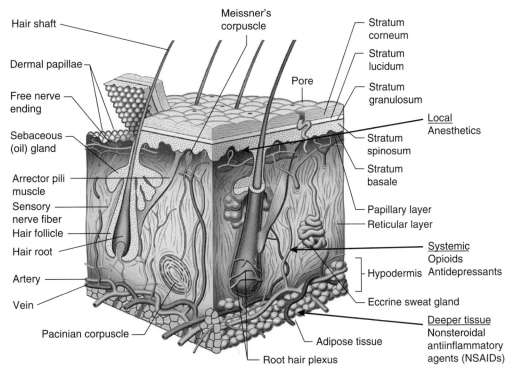

Figure 24-1 | Anatomy and physiology of the skin: potential analgesic action sites.

Adapted from Brown, M. B., Martin, G. P., Jones, S. A., et al. (2006). Dermal and transdermal drug delivery systems: Current and future prospects. *Drug Deliv, 13*(3), 175-187. In S. P. Stanos. (2007). Topical agents for the management of musculoskeletal pain. *J Pain Symptom Manage, 33*(3), 345.

GUIDELINES

Table 24-1 | Topical Analgesics

Type	Example	Indications/Comments
Local anesthetics	Lidocaine patch 5% (Lidoderm)	Approved for postherpetic neuralgia; used for a wide variety of types of persistent (chronic) and acute pain
	Eutectic mixture of local anesthetics (EMLA) (2.5 mg lidocaine + 2.5 mg prilocaine)	Cream used primarily for dermal procedural local anesthesia; some data on long-term use
	Lidocaine 4% cream (L.M.X.4)	Cream for dermal procedural local anesthesia
	Lidocaine 70 mg + tetracaine 70 mg (Synera)	Patch for dermal procedural local anesthesia
	J-tip	Needless delivery under pressure of local anesthetic for dermal procedures
	Benzocaine 20% Spray (Hurricaine)	Associated with methemoglobinemia
Capsaicin	Qutenza 8% patch, Arthritis Formula Capiscum, Capzasin, Trixaicin, Zostrix, and others	Patient must be warned of burning sensation on application and that this will subside with regular, uninterrupted applications; patch requires a prescription, and supervised application is recommended
Antidepressants	Tricyclic antidepressants (amitriptyline, doxepin)	No commercially available preparations
Anticonvulsants	Clonazepam (Klonopin)	No commercially available preparations
Clonidine	Catapres TTS	Transdermal formulation
Ketamine	Ketalar	No commercially available preparations

This table provides guidelines for the use of the several of the topical analgesics.
From Pasero, C., & McCaffery, M. *Pain assessment and pharmacologic management*, p. 685, St. Louis, Mosby. © 2011, Pasero C, McCaffery M. May be duplicated for use in clinical practice.

Box 24-1 Use of Topical Lidocaine Patch 5%[1]

DESCRIPTION
10 cm by 14 cm patch containing 700 mg of lidocaine in an aqueous base

INDICATIONS
Targeted peripheral neuropathic and other pains (see text for research on specific types of pain and Figure 24-1 for action site)

CONTRAINDICATIONS
- Allergy to amide local anesthetics
- Lack of skin integrity at site of application

Safety warning: May produce additive effects in patients taking antiarrhythmic medications (e.g., mexiletine, IV lidocaine)

DOSING RECOMMENDATIONS
Up to 3 patches worn for 12 hours, then removed and followed by a period of wearing no patch for 12 hours (12 hours on, 12 hours off). This application process may be repeated as needed for continued analgesia.

Note: Although the manufacturer recommends no more than 3 patches in a 24-hour period, up to 4 patches worn continuously for 24 hours has been shown to be safe. Further, long-term use of 3 to 4 patches for 12 to 24 hours has been shown to be safe (see text).

TRIAL PERIOD TO DETERMINE EFFECTIVENESS
3 weeks

PATCH STORAGE
- Keep patch at room temperature of 15° to 30°C (59° to 86°F).
- Keep patch in sealed package until ready to use.
- Apply promptly after removal from sealed package.

APPLICATION INSTRUCTIONS
1. Ensure that area of application is clean and dry.

Note: Application of the patch after daily hygiene activities (e.g., bathing or showering) is recommended. Do not apply cream or powder to the targeted area prior to application. Protect patch from becoming wet during wear (e.g., cover with waterproof material such as ordinary plastic [polyethylene] wrap if bathing is necessary while patch is in place).

Patients should be told to avoid putting heat (e.g., heating pads, hot packs) directly on the patch as this increases absorption of the lidocaine and can lead to toxicity.

2. Slowly remove the film release liner from the back of the patch.

Note: The patch may be cut before removal of the release liner to fit the targeted area. Cutting the patch does not affect absorption of the drug.

3. Warn the patient that the patch may feel cool when first applied.
4. Place the patch (or patches) directly on or beside (e.g., around wound) the painful area.

Note: The patch is not sterile and should be placed on intact skin only. Although the patch may be used in patients with acute herpes zoster (near affected area), it should not be placed on open vesicles.

5. Smooth out the patch over the targeted area making sure all edges adhere.
6. The patch may be covered with clothing to prevent accidental displacement, e.g., patches placed on a foot or calf may be covered with a sock or stocking.
7. After 12 to 24 hours, remove the patch.
8. Repeat application process for continued pain relief.

DISPOSAL INSTRUCTIONS
1. Fold the used patch on top of itself.

Note: Only 2% of the drug in the patch is absorbed; at least 95% is left in the patch when removed after 12 hours. Proper disposal is essential to prevent exposure to others, such as children and pets.

2. Discard in the same manner as other pharmaceutical waste in health care institutions.

Note: Most health care institutions do not consider the lidocaine patch 5% to be hazardous waste.

[1]The lidocaine patch 5% should not be confused with other patch systems such as the fentanyl transdermal patch (see text for distinction between topical and transdermal delivery systems).

should be told to expect pain relief, not anesthesia. At this time, the lidocaine patch 5% is available only by prescription. (See lidocaine patch 5% patient medication information, Form V-8 on pp. 773-774, at the end of Section V.)

Guidelines on the treatment of neuropathic pain recommend the lidocaine patch 5% as a first-line (Dubinsky,

Kabbani, El-Chami, et al., 2004; Dworkin, O'Connor, Backonja, et al., 2007) or second-line (Moulin, Clark, Gilron, et al., 2007) drug for postherpetic neuralgia. However, a Cochrane Collaborative Review called for further research comparing it with other medications for the treatment of this condition (Khaliq, Alam, Puri,

2007). Nevertheless, it is approved for postherpetic neuralgia, and the safety, effectiveness, and convenience of this drug for treatment of this condition led to its use for a wide variety of other types of pain and pain syndromes. Below is a list of case reports, reviews, and research.

- Postherpetic neuralgia (Argoff, 2000; Argoff, Galer, Jensen et al., 2004; Dubinsky, Kabbani, El-Chami, et al., 2004; Dworkin, Schmader, 2003; Gammaitoni, Alvarez, Galer, 2003; Galer, Rowbotham, Perander, 1999; Katz, Gammaitoni, Davis, et al., 2002; Khaliq, Alam, Puri, 2007; Pasero, 2003b; Rowbotham, Davies, Verkempinck et al., 1996)
- Acute herpes zoster (within 4 weeks of infection onset) (Lin, Fan, Huang, et al., 2008)
- Variety of other focal peripheral neuropathic pain syndromes (see list in Meier, Wasner, Faust, et al., 2003)
- Painful diabetic neuropathy (Argoff, Backonja, Belgrade, et al., 2006; Argoff, Galer, Jensen, et al., 2004; Barbano, Herrmann, Hart-Gouleau, et al., 2004; Devers, Galer, 2000; Veves, Backonja, Malik, 2008)
- Idiopathic distal sensory polyneuropathy (Hermann, Barbano, Hart-Gouleau et al., 2005)
- Myofascial pain (Argoff, 2002; Dalpiaz, Dodds, 2002; Gammaitoni, Alvarez, Galer, 2003)
- Neuroma (Devers, Galer, 2000)
- Meralgia paresthetica (Devers, Galer, 2000)
- Intercostal neuralgia (Devers, Galer, 2000)
- Traumatic rib fracture (Ingalls, Horton, Bettendorf, et al., 2009)
- Erythromelalgia (Davis, Sandroni, 2002)
- Complex regional pain syndrome (CRPS types 1 and 2) (Devers, Galer, 2000)
- Cervical pain (Gammaitoni, Alvarez, Galer, 2003)
- Back pain (Gammaitoni, Alvarez, Galer, 2003; Gimbel, Linn, Hale, et al., 2005; Hines, Keaney, Moskowitz, et al., 2002)
- Radiculopathy (Devers, Galer, 2000)
- Variety of persistent pains (head, neck, extremity, back, knee) (Fishbain, Lewis, Cole, et al., 2006)
- Cancer-related neuropathic pain (Wilhelm, Griessinger, Koppert, et al., 2005)
- Osteoarthritis (OA) (Gammaitoni, Galer, Onawola, et al., 2004)
- Carpal tunnel syndrome (Nalamachu, Crockett, Gammaitoni, et al., 2006)
- Laparoscopic ventral hernia repair (postoperative pain) (Saber, Elgamal, Rao, et al., 2008)
- Radical retropubic prostatectomy (Habib, Polascik, Weizer, et al., 2009)
- Inguinal hernia repair (Lockhart, 2006)
- Persistent neuropathic postsurgical pain (thoracotomy, mastectomy) (Devers, Galer, 2000)

Many patients with neuropathic pain experience allodynia, or pain with a nonnoxious stimulus (see Section I). Allodynia can be so severe in some patients that even air currents and wearing clothing are excruciatingly painful. Understandably, individuals who suffer allodynia can become housebound in an effort to avoid wearing clothing or being exposed to other elements that increase pain (Rowbotham, Davies, Verkempinck, et al., 1996). In addition to relief of pain, after the initial patch application, the protective nature of the lidocaine patch 5% over allodynic skin is often cited as a reason for patient satisfaction with this method of analgesia.

Common misconceptions are that topical analgesics are capable of relieving only surface neuropathic pain, such as allodynia, and systemic analgesics are required to relieve other types of neuropathic pain (e.g., sharp, hot, or deep-quality pain). Research has refuted this thinking. A randomized controlled trial of patients with postherpetic neuralgia with and without allodynia (Galer, Jensen, Ma, et al., 2002) and another randomized controlled trial of patients with painful diabetic neuropathy with or without allodynia (Dworkin, Hart-Gouleau, Galer, et al., 2003) demonstrated that the lidocaine patch 5% relieved both types of neuropathic pain.

Older individuals are at highest risk for developing some of the conditions most responsive to treatment with the lidocaine patch 5%, such as postherpetic neuralgia, painful diabetic neuropathy, and OA. They are also among the highest risk for adverse effects related to systemic analgesics that are often used to treat these conditions (e.g., antidepressants, anticonvulsants, NSAIDs). A follow-up survey of older adults with postherpetic neuralgia who used the lidocaine patch 5% on a long-term basis after participating in its research revealed a mean duration of usage of 7.6 years and a high rate of satisfaction overall and in all subcategories, including convenience and ability to do normal activities (Galer, 2003). Erythema was the most common adverse effect, but most (75%) reported no adverse effects whatsoever. Pooled analysis of data from three open-label trials showed that the lidocaine patch 5% reduced pain intensity and pain interference and improved sleep and other quality of life indicators with a low risk of systemic adverse effects in geriatric patients (Gammaitoni, Onawola, Galer, 2005). Again, the most common adverse effect was dermal reactions.

The lidocaine patch 5% has been used safely in patients as early as 4 weeks after the onset of acute herpes zoster. Patients with moderate to severe acute pain were randomized to receive a vehicle patch (placebo) or lidocaine patch 5% applied on the torso or limbs with intact skin (without vesicles) by a 12-hours-on, 12-hours-off regimen (Lin, Fan, Huang, et al., 2008). Improvements in pain during rest and movement and patients' global impression were greater in those who received the lidocaine patch 5%. Adverse effects were similarly low in both groups.

The lidocaine patch 5% can be used with a systemic drug regimen, potentially providing additive relief. For example, it can provide further relief when response to gabapentin and other systemic analgesics is only partial (Meier, Wasner, Faust, et al., 2003).

Although the risks associated with the lidocaine patch 5% are very small, it should be used with caution in patients taking antiarrhythmic medications (e.g., mexiletine, IV lidocaine) to prevent the potential for additive toxicity (Pasero, 2003b). Patients who are sensitive to amide local anesthetics (e.g., bupivacaine, ropivacaine) should not use the lidocaine patch 5%. The product has not been tested in pregnant or nursing women. Patients must be told to avoid putting heat (e.g., heating pads, hot packs) directly on the lidocaine patch because this will increase absorption of lidocaine and can lead to toxicity (Shemirani, Tang, Friedland, 2010) (see Chapter 23 for local anesthetic adverse effects).

Pharmacokinetics

Patients typically report feeling the onset of analgesia within 30 minutes of application of the lidocaine patch 5% and significant improvements in pain within days of regular use (Pasero, 2003b). The majority of patients in one study responded within the first week of continuous treatment, reporting better pain relief on day 7 than on day 0 (Katz, Gammaitoni, Davis, et al., 2002). Steady-state lidocaine plasma concentrations are reached by the second day of patch application. Pharmacokinetic studies show that maximal lidocaine plasma concentrations ranged from 0.13 mcg/mL (three patches 12-hours-on, 12-hours-off regimen) to 0.225 mcg/mL (four patches 12-hours-on, 12-hours-off regimen) (Gammaitoni, Alvarez, Galer, 2003). These levels are well below those associated with cardiac antiarrhythmic activity (1.5 mcg/mL) and toxicity (5 mcg/mL) (Lema, 1996), and lidocaine concentration does not increase with daily use. Every-12-hour administration of four patches was associated with slightly higher minimum and maximum plasma concentrations at steady state compared with every-24-hour administration of four patches. The plasma half-life of the lidocaine patch 5% is approximately 6 to 8 hours.

Dosing Regimen

The manufacturer of the lidocaine patch 5% (Endo) recommends a dosing regimen of up to 3 patches worn for 12 hours, then removed and not replaced until another 12 hours has elapsed (12 hours on, 12 hours off). The pharmacokinetic studies have established the safety of continuous daily use of three to four patches worn 12 hours/day (Devers, Galer, 2000; Gammaitoni, Alvarez, Galer, 2002), 18 hours/day (Gammaitoni, Davis, 2002), and 24 hours/day (Gammaitoni, Alvarez, Galer, 2002). In an open-label trial of 332 patients with postherpetic neuralgia, 28 days of treatment (12 hours on, 12 hours off) was shown to be safe (Katz, Gammaitoni, Davis, et al., 2002). The most common adverse effect was localized rash, which was a reason for discontinuation of treatment in three patients (1%). No systemic adverse effects were reported. A case report described the safe and effective use of up to four lidocaine

patches 5% for 19 months followed by 10 patches for 4 months, worn continuously (24 hours/day), in a patient with cancer-related neuropathic pain (Wilhelm, Griessinger, Koppert, et al., 2005). Serum lidocaine plasma levels were low throughout treatment (less than 0.5 mcg/mL) (see discussion of serum lidocaine levels in Chapter 23).

EMLA

Eutectic mixture of local anesthetics (EMLA) is used most often for procedural pain management (see Chapter 28). It has limited use in persistent pain because of its relatively short duration of action, and there are very few studies on its use for this type of pain. Some studies reported that EMLA could provide pain relief for 5 to 6 hours for postherpetic neuralgia (Wallace, Galer, Gammaitoni, 2006). A case report described reduction in painful neuropathy of a forearm and improvement in hand function when EMLA was applied to the patient's forearm (Rosen, Bjorkman, Lundborg, 2008). This led the authors to randomize 40 volunteers to receive a 2-hour application of EMLA or placebo cream to a lower leg (Rosen, Bjorkman, Weibull, et al., 2009). EMLA produced significant improvement in touch thresholds and sensation, which suggests therapeutic potential for neuropathies that cause disturbances in sensitivity.

Further research is needed to determine a potential role for EMLA in the prevention of persistent neuropathic postsurgical pain. A randomized controlled trial of women undergoing breast surgery demonstrated no differences between EMLA and placebo treatment on pain at rest and movement; however, analgesic consumption was reduced on the second to fifth day, and the incidence of persistent pain was less in those who received EMLA (Fassoulaki, Sarantopoulos, Melemeni, et al., 2000).

As explained in a more detailed discussion in Chapter 28, a relatively thick application of EMLA is needed for at least 1 hour to create an area of dense sensory loss. The effect is enhanced by application of an occlusive dressing over the cream. A 5 gm tube of EMLA can be used to spread 2.5 gm over a 20 to 25 cm^2 [2 inch by 2 inch] area. Clinical experience suggests that an application time of 90 to 120 minutes produces better results, particularly for treatment of persistent pain states. These guidelines are difficult if the area of pain is larger or is adjacent to the face or a mobile region of the body.

No evidence exists that cutaneous anesthesia is necessary to gain benefit from a topical local anesthetic and, anecdotally, some patients seem to respond favorably to a thin application applied without a dressing. In the absence of any systematic evaluation of dosing techniques, the patient should be encouraged to try various modes of administration in an effort to identify a salutary approach. If possible, one of these trials should include EMLA for a duration of at least 1 hour under an occlusive dressing of some type (ordinary plastic wrap can be used for large areas).

Other Local Anesthetics

Novel approaches have been used to administer local anesthetics for persistent pain. A case report described the use of a 5% lidocaine plaster applied via a 12-hours-on, 12-hours-off regimen for 2 weeks in combination with an oral antidepressant and anticonvulsant to reduce persistent postorchiectomy pain by 70% (DeMello, Desai, 2009). A randomized, cross-over trial administered a metered dose of 8% lidocaine spray (not available in the United States) or saline placebo spray to completely cover the painful skin in 24 patients with postherpetic neuralgia (Kanai, Kumaki, Niki, et al., 2009). After 7 days, the patients crossed over to the alternative treatment. The lidocaine spray produced significantly greater decreases in pain compared with placebo, and the median analgesic duration was 4.5 hours after application. A second part of this study included an open-label trial of 100 patients who were given metered doses of 8% lidocaine spray as previously described for 2 weeks. These patients also experienced significant pain relief and no systemic adverse effects. Convenience and rapid analgesia were cited as benefits of the topical lidocaine spray. A topical bupivacaine patch (Eladur), intended to provide 3 days of pain relief from a single application, was in development at the time of publication.

A wide variety of other topical local anesthetics are available over the counter (OTC). Local anesthetics in various concentrations (e.g., lidocaine, benzocaine, tetracaine) are formulated alone and with other ingredients, such as aloe and hydrocortisone, in creams, ointments, gels, lozenges, and sprays. Lidocaine patches are commercially available without a prescription. For example, MediPad-L Plus is a 3 inch by 5 inch pad containing 4% lidocaine with 0.2% menthol. Anecdotal experience with commercially available, relatively low concentrations of local anesthetic topical ointments (e.g., Foille Plus Medicated First Aid with benzocaine 5%) and sprays (e.g., Medi-Quick First Aid with lidocaine 2%) has not been favorable, however, unless the painful area involves mucosal surfaces. The effectiveness and safety of these products vary widely (Zilbert, 2002), and research is needed to establish a role in relieving persistent pain. An excellent resource for available nonprescription products is the American Pharmacists Association's *Handbook of Nonprescription Drugs* (Berardi, Kroon, McDermott, et al., 2006). See Chapter 28 for topical local anesthetics that are used for procedural pain treatment.

Capsaicin

Capsaicin (e.g., Qutenza 8%, Arthritis Formula Capiscum, Capzasin, Trixaicin, Zostrix, and others) is a naturally-occurring constituent of the chili pepper that produces its pungent taste. The mechanism of action of capsaicin is not entirely understood, but when applied topically, it affects function in primary afferent nociceptive neurons by inhibiting the release of substance P and other inflammatory neurochemicals (Argoff, Backonja, Belgrade, et al., 2006; Alvarez, Galer, Gammaitoni, 2006; Knotkova, Pappagallo, Szallasi, 2008; Lussier, Portenoy, 2004) (see Section I and Figure I-2, *A* and *B* on pp. 4-5). Regular application of capsaicin to the skin stimulates the release of substance P until it is eventually depleted from the C-fiber terminals. When depleted, desensitization occurs and pain transmission is diminished. Depending on concentration, capsaicin can selectively activate, desensitize, or produce a neurotoxic effect on the small diameter afferent C fibers while leaving larger diameter afferent fibers unaffected (Sawynok, 2003). Animal research suggests that capsaicin has a central mechanism, affecting prostaglandins at the spinal cord level as well (Minami, Bakoshi, Nakano, et al., 2001).

Cream preparations of capsaicin are available in varying concentrations to be applied to intact skin, usually three to five times daily. Pain relief is dependent on regular application, and the rubbing required for application may contribute to an analgesic effect (Simon, Lipman, Caudill-Slosberg, et al., 2002). A capsaicin skin patch (Qutenza patch 8%) containing 8% capsaicin (179 mg/patch) was approved in the United States in 2009 for the treatment of postherpetic neuralgia. The drug requires a prescription, and the manufacturer recommends application only by health care professionals under the supervision of a physician (NeurogesX, Inc, 2009). Local anesthetic cream (e.g., EMLA, L.M.X.4) should be applied to the painful intact skin prior to patch application. Nitrile (not latex) gloves are worn to apply up to 4 patches for 60 minutes every 3 months. (Application should be no more frequent than every 3 months; see the package insert). After the patch is removed, a cleansing gel (included with each patch) is applied for 1 minute then removed, and the skin is wiped dry (NeurogesX, Inc, 2009) (see research later in chapter).

Capsaicin has been used in a variety of persistent pain conditions including arthritis pain, postmastectomy pain, myofascial pain, simple back pain, postherpetic neuralgia, painful diabetic neuropathy, and HIV-related peripheral neuropathy (Argoff, 2002; Argoff, Backonja, Belgrade, et al., 2006; Paice, Ferrans, Lashley, et al., 2000; Robbins, 2000; Sawynok, 2003; Simon, Lipman, Caudill-Slosberg, et al., 2002; Simpson, Estanislao, Brown, et al., 2008; Stanos, 2007). A systematic review of the use of capsaicin concluded that although the drug is better than placebo, it has moderate to poor efficacy for treatment of persistent musculoskeletal and neuropathic pain but might be appropriate in some patients with pain refractory to other treatments (Mason, Moore, Deery, et al., 2004).

The United Kingdom's National Collaborating Centre for Chronic Conditions discussed the research to date, including economic analysis, and suggested capsaicin as a second-line pharmacologic option for OA pain (National Collaborating Centre for Chronic Conditions, 2008). Others have similarly supported its use for OA (Hunter, Lo, 2008). One study showed efficacy for knee pain from both rheumatoid arthritis (RA) and

OA (Deal, Schnitzer, Lipstein, et al., 1991), and another supported its use for hand pain of OA but not RA (McCarthy, McCarty, 1992). It is noted to be more effective than analgesic balms, such as menthol preparations, for arthritis pain (Simon, Lipman, Caudill-Slosberg, et al., 2002).

An early randomized controlled trial of patients with HIV distal symmetrical peripheral neuropathy assessed a variety of pain outcomes and found no significant differences between those who received capsaicin 0.025% and those who received placebo; those who received capsaicin had higher current pain scores and a higher withdrawal rate (Paice, Ferrans, Lashley, et al., 2000).

An open-label study was conducted to examine a single, 1-hour application of the high-concentration capsaicin patch (Qutenza) (640 mcg/cm²) in 12 HIV patients with peripheral neuropathy (Simpson, Estanislao, Brown, et al., 2008). There was a significant reduction (mean 40%) in pain throughout the 12-week study period, and one-third of the patients experienced 50% or greater reduction. Pretreatment with a local anesthetic cream was applied 1 hour prior to capsaicin patch application to address treatment-associated pain in this study, and all patients were able to complete at least 90% of the application time. One patient was hospitalized for severe pain after patch application that was thought to be related to the capsaicin, and 67% of the patients reported at least one pain score 30% higher than baseline, but application-related increased pain resolved within 1 week, and treatment was generally well-tolerated by the majority of patients. It is unlikely that this treatment with high concentration capsaicin and the usual topical treatment with 0.025% or 0.075% cream can be meaningfully compared.

Capsaicin is listed as a topical analgesic option in a consensus guideline on the treatment of painful diabetic neuropathy (Argoff, Backonja, Belgrade, et al., 2006) but is not listed in other neuropathic pain treatment guidelines (Dworkin, O'Connor, Backonja, et al., 2007; Moulin, Clark, Gilron, et al., 2007). Nonetheless, a large randomized controlled trial of patients (N = 200) with a variety of types of persistent neuropathic pain (McCleane, 2000) noted that topical capsaicin 0.025% yielded similar results as topical doxepin 3.3%, and the combination of the two drugs, when applied daily. Pain ratings were unchanged for placebo but decreased by 0.9, 1.12, and 1.07 in the doxepin, capsaicin, and combination groups, respectively. Burning pain decreased for all three treatment groups after 4 weeks of treatment, and sensitivity ratings and shooting pain decreased in those who received capsaicin or the combination cream.

Topical capsaicin also has been discussed as an option for postoperative pain and prevention of persistent neuropathic postsurgical pain. One randomized, placebo-controlled trial instilled ultrapurified capsaicin intraoperatively into the wound after hernia repair in 41 men and found significantly lower pain scores for the first 3 postoperative days but no difference at 1 and 4 weeks postoperatively (Aasvang, Hansen, Malmstrom, et al., 2008). There were no significant adverse effects except a mild, transient elevation in liver enzymes in those who received capsaicin. Further research is needed to define a role in this setting.

Adverse Effects

Topical capsaicin is associated with a minimal risk of systemic toxicity (Argoff, Backonja, Belgrade et al., 2006; Simon, Lipman, Caudill-Slosberg et al., 2002) but a larger risk of localized burning, pricking, or itching sensation. This may be caused by vasodilation at the site of application (Mason, Moore, Deery, et al., 2004), as well as the direct neurostimulatory effects of substance P release in the periphery. Although the effect can wane over time with repeated administration, it can be severe enough to force discontinuation of the therapy, and even if mild, can be quite bothersome to some patients (Alvarez, Galer, Gammaitoni, 2006; Argoff, 2002). As a result, there may be poor adherence with treatment. One in three patients experience local adverse effects, which contribute to a high withdrawal rate from capsaicin studies (Mason, Moore, Deery, et al., 2004).

Unfortunately, decreased doses in the capsaicin cream do not reduce the burning associated with capsaicin application (Argoff, Backonja, Belgrade, et al., 2006). Co-administration of topical local anesthetics has been reported to have no effect on the burning (Sawynok, 2003); however, as mentioned, the application of L.M.X.4 (local anesthetic) cream 1 hour prior to application is recommended to reduce burning associated with the high concentration formulation (Simpson, Estanislao, Brown, et al., 2008), and, anecdotally, some patients report benefit from this strategy. As mentioned, application of local anesthetic cream is advised prior to application of the capsaicin 8% patch.

Transient increases in blood pressure (BP) may occur during and shortly after application of the capsaicin 8% patch. The manufacturer recommends monitoring BP during and following the treatment procedure. Further research and clinical use are needed to more fully evaluate both the safety and effectiveness of this formulation. The full prescribing information should be read prior to the use of this product (NeurogesX, Inc, 2009).

Patient teaching is essential to successful treatment with capsaicin. Prior to application, patients must be told about the burning sensation and not to be alarmed by it. They can be reassured that it probably will subside and be replaced with analgesia as the substance P is depleted; however, it is important for them to understand that depletion of neurotransmitters is dependent on regular, uninterrupted application of the cream and that repeated application after a holiday from therapy may result in renewed burning.

Another key teaching point is that pain relief is not achieved rapidly; it is gradual and can take several days to weeks to be realized. A trial application three to four times daily for at least 4 weeks may be necessary to fully evaluate effect.

Capsaicin should never be applied to eyes, mouth, nostrils, genitals, or open or broken skin areas or close to areas where skin breakdown is present. This is especially important when it is used for herpes zoster pain; it should be used only after the skin lesions are fully healed. Patients should be told to wash their hands well after application. Cotton tip applicators or gloves may be used to apply the cream formulation but are not necessary if hands are washed well. If the hands are the site being treated, the cream should be applied and hands washed at least 30 seconds later.

Antidepressants

Although not listed in neuropathic guidelines as a pharmacologic option, the tricyclic antidepressants doxepin (Prudoxin, Zonalon) and amitriptyline (Elavil) have been claimed to be somewhat effective when applied topically for treatment of persistent pain (de Leon-Casasola, 2007; Lockart, 2004; Mays, 2006; McCleane, 2000). As with other topical analgesics, there is minimal systemic absorption and adverse effects (McCleane, 2008). The underlying mechanism of antidepressants was discussed earlier in Chapter 22 (also see Section I). Doxepin cream 5% is commercially available, but topical preparations of amitriptyline 1% to 5% are not and must be compounded for use.

The first use of amitriptyline applied to skin was reported in a patient with depression and pain from inflammatory bowel disease who could no longer take oral medications (Scott, Letrent, Hager, et al., 1999). The patient's mood, but not pain, improved with the use of amitriptyline gel, suggesting systemic absorption. This was followed by several animal studies and research in healthy volunteers that demonstrated topical effects with little systemic absorption (Gerner, Kao, Srinivasa, et al., 2003).

A trial comparing topical amitriptyline 1%, topical ketamine 0.5%, or a combination of the two in patients with postherpetic neuralgia, painful diabetic neuropathy, or posttrauma neuropathic pain found no differences in pain relief following the 2-day application phase, but significant reductions after the 7-day open trial, which suggested a longer duration of treatment was indicated for effective analgesia (Lynch, Clark, Sawynok, 2003). A larger randomized, placebo-controlled trial using higher doses of these drugs applied three times daily for 3 weeks in patients (N = 92) with these same types of neuropathic pain observed no difference in pain relief between groups (Lynch, Clark, Sawynok, et al., 2005). The researchers speculated that even higher concentrations of the drugs are needed for effect, which may be consistent with observations suggesting that amitriptyline 4% and ketamine 2% are efficacious in patients with postherpetic neuralgia (Lockart, 2004).

Other studies also yielded mixed results. In a crossover study of 35 patients with postherpetic neuralgia, painful diabetic neuropathy, or postsurgical neuropathic pain who received 7-day treatments of twice-daily topical amitriptyline 5%, lidocaine 5%, or placebo in randomized sequence with 7-day washout periods between treatments, topical amitriptyline was not effective in relieving pain (Ho, Huh, White, et al., 2008).

Doxepin 5% cream applied three times daily has been suggested to relieve chemotherapy-induced polyneuropathy (Mays, 2006). It has also been reported to reduce pain associated with complex regional pain syndrome (CRPS) (McCleane, 2002). Topical doxepin 3.3%, capsaicin 0.025%, a combination of the two, or placebo applied three times daily produced similar improvements in pain ratings in all treatment groups in a large (N = 200) randomized controlled trial of patients with a variety of types of persistent neuropathic pain (McCleane, 2000). Pain ratings were unchanged for placebo but decreased by 0.9, 1.12, and 1.07 in the doxepin, capsaicin, and combination groups, respectively. Burning pain decreased for all three treatment groups after 4 weeks of treatment, and sensitivity ratings and shooting pain decreased in those who received capsaicin or the combination cream.

Animal research and the presence of oral numbness following doxepin oral rinse suggests that the drug has a local anesthetic effect (de Leon-Casasola, 2007). A study of 51 patients with painful oral mucositis from cancer and cancer therapy found that 90% of the patients experienced pain reduction (oral numbness) following oral doxepin rinse (5 mg/mL doxepin in a solution containing 0.1% alcohol and sorbitol) (Epstein, Epstein, Epstein, et al., 2006). The maximum effect was 70% reduction in pain, and relief lasted over 4 hours in 37% of the patients.

Anticonvulsants

There are no commercially available preparations of topical anticonvulsants and little research regarding their use. A randomized controlled study instructed 41 patients with spontaneous burning oral mucosal pain associated with stomatodynia to suck a tablet of clonazepam (Klonopin) 1 mg or placebo and hold the saliva near the site of pain inside the mouth without swallowing for 3 minutes, then spit out the contents (Gremeau-Richard, Woda, Navez, et al., 2004). This was repeated 3 times daily for 14 days. Pain scores at 2 weeks were significantly reduced in those receiving clonazepam (2.4 points on 0 to 10 scale) compared with placebo (0.6 points).

Clonidine

The potential systemic mechanisms of clonidine analgesia were discussed in Chapter 22. Clonidine is available as a transdermal (Catapres-TTS) formulation, which is approved for treatment of hypertension and smoking cessation, and can be used to provide systemic clonidine as a treatment for pain.

The clonidine patch has been suggested to have topical analgesic effects when applied to areas of pain (Davis, Treede, Raja, et al., 1991; McCleane, 2008). Early research in patients with persistent noncancer pain and hyperalgesia utilized clonidine patches (30 mcg/cm²/day) for 7 days and found significant reductions or complete resolution of hyperalgesia (Davis, Treede, Raja, et al., 1991). The clonidine patch was studied in a randomized controlled trial that included 41 patients with painful diabetic neuropathy; there was little effect overall, but a secondary analysis suggested that patients with sharp and shooting pain may benefit (Byas-Smith, Max, Muir, et al., 1995). Others have found benefit with clonidine cream for orofacial neuropathic pain described as lancinating and sharp more than burning and aching (Epstein, Grushka, Le, 1997). Given the size of the patch and the occurrence of systemic absorption, the utility of topical clonidine is very limited.

Ketamine

Although research is generally lacking, case reports describe compounding the NMDA receptor antagonist ketamine into a gel for treatment of various types of pain. It is thought that topical ketamine acts on a variety of receptors and calcium, sodium, and potassium channels to produce analgesia (de Leon-Casasola, 2007; Sawynok, 2003). A randomized controlled trial of 20 patients with CRPS demonstrated inhibition of allodynia but no pain reduction after application of topical ketamine to the symptomatic limb (Finch, Knudsen, Drummond, 2009). Topical ketamine also has been administered as an oral rinse preoperatively to reduce posttonsillectomy pain in children (Canbay, Celebi, Uzun, et al., 2008). Research in healthy volunteers found that ketamine gel had no effect on immediate burning after injection of capsaicin but produced a significant reduction in mechanical hyperalgesia; this suggests a central mechanism of action, rather than a clear topical effect (Poyhia, Vainio, 2006).

Various compounded formulations of ketamine have been developed and used in cancer-related pain (Wood, 2000). Clinical observations have suggested that other types of persistent pain also may respond favorably. Five patients with CRPS, lumbar radiculopathy, or postherpetic neuralgia applied varying amounts of ketamine gel (0.093 mg/kg to 9.33 mg/kg) depending on involved surface area and reported dose-related changes (Gammaitoni, Gallagher, Welz-Bosna, 2000). At lower doses, patients reported alterations in temperature sensation, and as the dose was increased, feelings of relaxation and decreased tension in the painful area were reported. At higher doses, patients felt significant reductions in pain. Others have reported similar results for CRPS (Sawynok, 2003; Ushida, Tani, Kanbara, et al., 2002) and postherpetic neuralgia (Quan, Wellish, Gilden, 2003).

As mentioned earlier, topical ketamine has also been co-administered with topical amitriptyline for postherpetic neuralgia and CRPS (de Leon-Casasola, 2007; Lockart, 2004; Lynch, Clark, Sawynok, 2003; Lynch, Clark, Sawynok, et al., 2005). These studies yielded uncertain results.

A remarkable case report described immediate relief of refractory chemotherapy-induced neuropathic pain with three-times-daily applications of a gel combining ketamine 5%, clonidine 0.5%, and gabapentin 6% (Prommer, 2009). An increased dose of ketamine to 10% resulted in further improvement. Ultimately, all other analgesics could be discontinued.

Summary of Indications for Topical Analgesics for Persistent Pain

On the basis of these data, a trial of lidocaine patch 5% should be considered for well-localized pain, particularly peripherally-mediated neuropathic pain, such as postherpetic neuralgia and painful diabetic neuropathy. A number of other types of pain may be responsive to this drug as well. The other topical drugs discussed in this section may be considered for pains that are refractory to other treatments. With the exception of topical capsaicin in the treatment of pain caused by disease of small joints, the usefulness of the topical analgesics for nociceptive pains caused by injury of the skin, subcutaneous tissues, muscles, or joints is limited.

Summary of Adverse Effects of Topical Analgesics for Persistent Pain

The adverse effects associated with topical analgesic therapy are rare because they are associated with minimal systemic absorption. The most common are cutaneous reactions. As explained, capsaicin can cause local burning, which is sometimes intense. Although this symptom is not related to tissue damage and poses no risk to the patient, it can create significant discomfort and lead to discontinuation of the treatment.

Conclusion

Topical drug delivery produces effects in the tissues immediately under the site of application, whereas transdermal drug delivery requires absorption to achieve systemic effects. Topical analgesics are also faster acting and dissipate relatively soon after removal of the drug compared with transdermal analgesics. Benefits of topical analgesics include high patient acceptance and satisfaction, ease of administration, reductions in systemic adverse effects, and fewer drug interactions.

Chapter 25 Adjuvant Analgesics for Musculoskeletal Pain

IN the management of acute traumatic sprains or strains in the nonmedically ill, nonopioid and opioid analgesics are commonly supplemented by treatment with so-called muscle relaxant drugs or benzodiazepines (Table 25-1). Although pains that originate from injury to muscle or connective tissue are also prevalent in medically ill patients, the role of these drugs remains ill-defined.

Skeletal Muscle Relaxants

The group of drugs known as skeletal muscle relaxants are a heterogeneous group of drugs that are not chemically related (Chou, Peterson, Helfand, 2004) but are grouped together under this classification because they have been approved by the United States Food and Drug Administration (FDA) for treatment of musculoskeletal conditions or spasticity (Chou, Huffman, American Pain Society [APS], et al., 2007). Two groups must be distinguished. The first are drugs used to treat spasticity from upper motor neuron syndromes, such as multiple sclerosis, spinal cord injury, and poststroke syndrome. These drugs include tizanidine [Zanaflex], baclofen [Lioresal], and dantrolene [Dantrium]. The second group consists of drugs used to treat muscular pain or spasms from peripheral musculoskeletal conditions, such as myofascial pain syndrome and mechanical low back or neck pain. This group includes drugs that are antihistamines, such as orphenadrine (Norflex); tricyclic compounds structurally similar to the tricyclic antidepressants, such as cyclobenzaprine (Flexeril); and other types of drugs, such as carisoprodol (Soma), chlorzoxazone (Parafon Forte DSC), methocarbamol (Robaxin), and metaxalone (Skelaxin). Midazolam (Versed) is used primarily for procedural sedation (see Chapter 27).

The musculoskeletal relaxants are administered primarily by the oral route. Because they are chemically unrelated, there are differences in efficacy among the various drugs, but comparative research is lacking (Chou, Peterson, Helfand, 2004). See Table 25-1 for examples of skeletal muscle relaxants, Chapter 23 for a more detailed discussion of baclofen, Chapter 22 for tizanidine, and Chapter 31 for antihistamines. The reader is also referred to extensive reviews of the many skeletal muscle relaxants used for spasticity and musculoskeletal pain (Chou, Huffman, APS, et al., 2007; Chou, Peterson, Helfand, 2004).

When clinicians use the term *muscle relaxant*, they most often are referring to the heterogeneous drugs that are frequently used to treat acute musculoskeletal conditions. Ironically, there is little high-quality evidence that these drugs actually relax skeletal muscle. Although they do inhibit myogenic reflexes in animal models, the relationship between this action and analgesia is not known. The common muscle relaxant drugs can relieve musculoskeletal pain, but these effects may not be specific and do not depend on relaxation of skeletal muscle.

Evidence that the muscle relaxants used to treat common musculoskeletal pain are analgesic derives from studies of variable quality. Poor methodologic designs, insensitive assessment methods, and small numbers of patients are responsible for the inability to demonstrate high efficacy with muscle relaxants (Chou, Peterson, Helfand, 2004; See, Ginzburg, 2008). A Cochrane Collaboration Review concluded that muscle relaxants provide effective symptomatic relief of acute and persistent low back pain on the short term, but with a high incidence of drowsiness, dizziness, and other adverse effects (van Tulder, Touray, Furlan, et al., 2003). A later review of guidelines for the treatment of low back pain concluded that muscle relaxants offer fair relief of acute back pain, but did not recommend them for long-term use (Chou, Huffman, APS, et al., 2007). The review also noted that tizanidine (which, as discussed in Chapter 22, is an alpha$_2$-adrenergic agonist and a multipurpose analgesic) has evidence of efficacy in low back pain. In contrast, little evidence was found to support the effectiveness of baclofen and dantrolene, the other two drugs approved for spasticity. This review provides diagnostic steps and a decision-making algorithm that help to guide appropriate treatment of acute and persistent low back pain.

In a systematic review of 101 clinical trials focused on the common muscle relaxants used for musculoskeletal pain, none of the studies was rated of good quality, and there was little evidence of rigorous assessments of adverse effects (Chou, Peterson, Helfand, 2004). This review also confirmed that there is fair evidence that tizanidine, baclofen, and dantrolene are efficacious for spasticity and that tizanidine and baclofen are equi-effective. While the overall rate of adverse effects between tizanidine and baclofen is similar, tizanidine seems to be associated with more dry mouth and baclofen with more muscle weakness. The researchers also noted that there is insufficient evidence for the relative efficacy or safety of several muscle relaxants for musculoskeletal conditions.

Orphenadrine is combined with aspirin and caffeine and marketed as an analgesic and muscle relaxant. This drug is derived from diphenhydramine (Benadryl) and acts on multiple targets, including histamine and NMDA receptors, the norepinephrine reuptake system, and voltage-gated sodium channels (see Section I) (Desaphy, Dipalma, De Bellis, et al., 2009). Although these actions have implications for analgesia, further research is needed to more clearly define orphenadrine's role in pain management. Significant adverse effects, such as anticholinergic effects and the potential for seizures and arrhythmias, limit its use.

Cyclobenzaprine has been shown to be more favorable than placebo for fibromyalgia and musculoskeletal disorders (Kroenke, Krebs, Bair, 2009). A meta-analysis of five randomized, placebo-controlled trials of cyclobenzaprine in patients with fibromyalgia revealed that reports of overall improvement and moderate reductions in symptoms, especially sleep disturbances, were three times greater with cyclobenzaprine treatment compared with placebo (Tofferi, Jackson, O'Malley, 2004). A meta-analysis concluded that cyclobenzaprine is efficacious for the treatment of acute back pain, but its effects may be short-lived, with the greatest response occurring within 4 days and slowly diminishing with continued therapy (Browning, Jackson, O'Malley, 2001).

Although the results from clinical studies seem to support the short-term use of skeletal muscle relaxants in clinical practice for various indications, there are no efficacy data from comparator trials to favor one agent over another (Chou, Huffman, APS, et al., 2007). Studies have demonstrated that the analgesic effects of muscle relaxants are superior to those produced by aspirin or acetaminophen, but there have been no controlled trials or investigations that have directly compared the efficacy and adverse effect profiles of these drugs with NSAIDs or opioids. These drugs have no antiinflammatory properties, and it is possible that the combination of a muscle relaxant and an NSAID may provide better analgesia than either drug alone (McCleane, 2009b). Given the limited data available, it may be most appropriate to view the common muscle relaxants as add-on therapy for acute musculoskeletal pain, complementing acetaminophen, NSAIDs, or opioids (Chou, Huffman, APS, et al., 2007).

The muscle relaxant drugs are generally well-tolerated but have sedative effects that may be additive to other centrally-acting drugs, including opioids. Muscle relaxants are not recommended in older adults as this age group has increased sensitivity to the anticholinergic and sedating effects of the drugs, and the muscle relaxant effect may contribute to falls (see Section IV, Table 13-4 on p. 336).

Anecdotally, some patients report differences among drugs in analgesic efficacy or sedative adverse effects, and it is reasonable to switch to an alternative drug if treatment is initially ineffective. Although the dose-response relationships of the muscle relaxant drugs have not been systematically explored, dose-dependent effects probably exist, and the use of a low initial dose followed by gradual dose escalation can be recommended as a means to identify the most salutary balance between analgesia and adverse effects. Experience with these drugs is too limited to pursue dose escalation beyond the usual recommended range. A report of severe withdrawal syndrome in a patient who abruptly stopped taking carisoprodol after long-term use has led to the recommendation to gradually taper doses before discontinuing treatment (Reeves, Beddingfield, Mack, 2004). This is probably good advice for all of the skeletal muscle relaxants. (See cyclobenzaprine patient medication information, Form V-5 on pp. 765-766, at the end of Section V.)

Benzodiazepines

Benzodiazepines bind to benzodiazepine receptors in the terminals of primary afferent fibers, causing an influx of chloride and increasing GABA receptor inhibition (McCleane, 2009b) (see Section I). This class of drugs produces sedation, hypnosis, decreased anxiety, anterograde amnesia, centrally-mediated muscle relaxation, and anticonvulsant activity (Olkkola, Ahonen, 2008). There is clearly a role for benzodiazepines in the management of symptoms, such as anxiety, and to provide sedation (Devlin, Roberts, 2009), but their role in the treatment of muscle pain is less defined. The APS (2003) concludes that, with the exception of pain related to muscle spasm, benzodiazepines are not effective analgesics.

Diazepam (Valium) is a widely used benzodiazepine for acute musculoskeletal pain, particularly those characterized by spasm. This is so despite the uncertainty about the efficacy of the orally-administered drug for these conditions (Charney, Mihic, Adron, et al., 2006). Clonazepam (Klonopin) in nonsedating doses produces muscle relaxation, but it has a long half-life and can accumulate (McCleane, 2009b). Lorazepam (Ativan) has a shorter half-life and is preferred, particularly in the older adult patient (McCleane, 2009b).

Despite the uncertainty, it is common clinical practice to use either a skeletal muscle relaxant or a benzodiazepine to supplement analgesic therapy in the management of acute traumatic sprains or strains in the nonmedically ill. Although pains that originate from injury to muscle or connective tissue are prevalent in the medically ill, there has been no systematic evaluation of analgesic therapies for this problem. The role of these drugs for opioid-refractory musculoskeletal pain in populations with advanced medical illness remains ill-defined. Of interest, benzodiazepines given preoperatively exerted ongoing antianalgesic effects with opioids (Gear, Miaskowski, Heller, et al., 1997).

The usual oral dose of diazepam is 5 to 10 mg three to four times a day. The usual oral dose of clonazepam is 0.5 mg three times a day. Because of their marked sedative effects, the use of benzodiazepines for muscle spasm should usually be limited to short courses (McCleane, 2009b). Other less-sedating analgesics are more appropriate for patients in whom functional restoration is the goal. They must also be used with caution in older adults as this age group has increased sensitivity to the CNS effects of benzodiazepines (see Section IV, Table 13-4 on p. 336). Withdrawal can occur if benzodiazepines are abruptly discontinued, and dose tapering is recommended. See Chapter 27 for benzodiazepine use for procedural sedation.

Conclusion

The so-called muscle relaxants and benzodiazepine are common as supplements to analgesics in the management of acute traumatic sprains or strains in the nonmedically ill; their role in the medically ill is not well defined. There is little high-quality evidence that these drugs actually relax skeletal muscle. With the exception of pain related to muscle spasm, benzodiazepines are not considered to be effective analgesics. Their primary adverse effect is excessive sedation, and they are not recommended in older patients for that reason.

Chapter 26 Adjuvant Analgesics for Postoperative and Other Acute Pain

MANY of the adjuvant analgesics used to treat persistent pain are also used for acute pain. Most are combined with other analgesics as part of a multimodal plan to attack various underlying mechanisms of action (see Chapters 12 and 21 for more on multimodal analgesia). This chapter will present selected adjuvant agents for acute pain, including local anesthetic continuous peripheral nerve block and wound infusion; IV lidocaine; the anticonvulsants gabapentin and pregablin; clonidine; corticosteroids; and ketamine. Antidepressants, which compose another major adjuvant analgesic group, are not discussed here because they have not been shown to be effective for acute pain, including acute experimental pain (Wallace, Barger, Schulteis, 2002), and their delayed onset of analgesia makes them inappropriate for acute pain (Lussier, Portenoy, 2004) (see Chapter 22 for discussion of antidepressantes). See Table V-1, pp. 748-756, at the end of Section V for dosing guidelines and other characteristics of selected adjuvant analgesics.

Continuous Peripheral Nerve Block

For many years, regional anesthesia has been administered via single injection peripheral nerve blocks using a long-acting local anesthetic, such as bupivacaine (Marcaine) or ropivacaine (Naropin), to target a specific nerve or nerve plexus. This technique is highly effective in producing pain relief, but the effect is temporary (Rawal, 2007). The short duration of pain relief of the single-injection technique (4 to 12 hours duration for bupivacaine and ropivacaine) limits its use to a brief period, e.g., during and immediately after surgery (Richman, Liu, Courpas, et al., 2006). However, a relatively new pain management approach, continuous peripheral nerve block (also called *perineural regional analgesia*), offers an alternative. A continuous peripheral nerve block involves establishment of an initial block followed by the placement of a catheter through which an infusion of local anesthetic is administered continuously, with or without PCA capability. When PCA capability is added, this is referred to as PCRA (patient-controlled regional analgesia) (see dosing regimens that follow). In the acute pain setting, the therapy typically is continued during the first 24 to 72 hours postoperatively, depending on the type of surgery.

The first continuous peripheral nerve blocks were used for surgical pain several decades ago (Ilfeld, Morey, Enneking, 2002a). Over the years, the technique has been perfected, and reports of excellent pain relief, opioid dose-sparing effects, improved rehabilitation, and earlier discharge in the late 1990s sparked an increase in its use (Rawal, Axelsson, Hylander, et al., 1998; Singelyn, Deyaert, Joris, et al., 1998). More recent advances in operator skill and catheters and infusion devices made specifically for continuous peripheral nerve block have resulted in the widespread use of this technique for a variety of types of pain, particularly surgical pain, in both the inpatient and outpatient setting.

Catheter Placement

To place a peripheral nerve catheter, the anesthesiologist inserts a needle into the targeted nerve site, injects incremental doses of local anesthetic to block the desired nerve or nerves, and then threads the catheter through the needle (see Figure 26-1 for the site of lumbar plexus catheter placement). The needle is then removed, the catheter is secured, and the site is dressed. In the inpatient setting, continuous peripheral nerve blocks can be administered by the same infusion devices that are used to administer IV PCA or epidural analgesia. In the outpatient setting, portable disposable pumps (elastomeric or vacuum-driven syringe types) are usually used (Skryabina, Dunn, 2006). These latter pumps offer the benefits of being very small and easily discarded after use, avoiding the need for the patient to return the pump and the hospital to develop

a pump tracking system. Some pumps allow patient-controlled capability for breakthrough pain so that PCRA may be administered. Some can be programmed to deliver automated bolus delivery in addition to PCRA capability (Taboada, Rodriguez, Bermudez, et al., 2009). The pumps also have simple mechanisms for stopping the infusion if adverse effects occur or at the end of therapy. Catheters are easily removed by clinicians, patients, or family members (Ilfeld, Enneking, 2002; Rawal, Axelsson, Hylander, et al., 1998; Swenson, Bay, Loose, et al., 2006).

There are a number of excellent resources for detailed information on catheters and the placement procedure for continuous peripheral nerve block. For this, the reader is referred to the texts by Cousins, M. J., & Bridenbaugh, P. O. (Eds.). (1998). *Neural blockade in clinical anesthesia and management of pain*, Philadelphia, Lippincott-Raven; Miller, R. D. (Ed.). (2005). *Miller's anesthesia*, ed 6, Philadelphia, Churchill Livingstone; Sinatra, R. S., de Leon-Casasola, O. A., Ginsberg, B., et al. (Eds.). (2007). *Acute pain management*, Cambridge, NY, Cambridge University Press; Meier, G., & Buttner, J. (2007). *Peripheral regional anesthesia: An atlas of anatomy and techniques*, ed 2, English translation available, New York, Thieme; and Waldman, S. (2009). *Pain review*, Philadelphia, Saunders; as well as any one of the research articles cited in this section. Capdevila and colleagues (2009) offer excellent suggestions for proper sterile technique for placement and site dressing. The various pumps used to administer continuous peripheral nerve blocks have been compared and discussed elsewhere (Capdevila, Macaire, Aknin, et al., 2003; Wedel, Horlocker, 2005).

Nurses are referred to their scope of practice as defined by their individual state board of nursing for their role in the administration of continuous peripheral nerve block, and

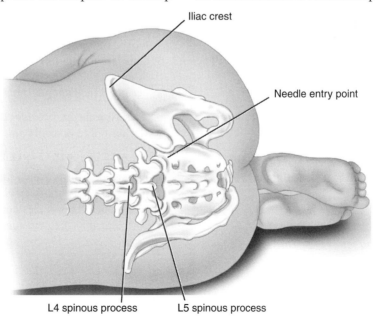

Iliac crest

Needle entry point

L4 spinous process   L5 spinous process

Figure 26-1 | Needle entry point for lumbar plexus catheter insertion.

Box 26-1 | Continuous Peripheral Nerve Block[1]

INDICATIONS

Postoperative pain control (see text for research on specific types of pain and Figure 26-1 for an example of catheter placement)

GENERAL CONTRAINDICATIONS

- Patient refusal
- Allergy to local anesthetic
- Blood dyscrasias
- Infection in the region of puncture

KEY POINTS TO ADDRESS IN THERAPY ADMINISTRATION ORDERS

- The anesthesia provider will write all analgesic and anesthetic orders as long as the patient has a nerve block infusion.
- Pain management is provided by the primary service when nerve block infusion is discontinued.
- An infusion device that does not allow free flow will be used to administer continuous peripheral nerve blocks (no exceptions), and doses will be verified by independent double-check process (see Chapter 17).[1]
- Tubing without injection ports will be used, and infusion tubing will be labeled with the site of the nerve block infusion.
- Ambulation will be done with assistance if indicated by block site.

Note: Supplemental analgesia should be administered prior to painful activities, such as ambulation and physical therapy (e.g., oral opioid 30 to 60 minutes prior); patients receiving PCRA therapy and those receiving IV PCA for breakthrough pain during continuous nerve block (basal-only) therapy should be taught to self-administer a dose prior to these activities (see examples of supplemental analgesia).

- Continuous peripheral nerve block infusion rate in premixed solution (type and concentration of local anesthetic varies depending on anesthesia provider preference and type of nerve block; see text)
  - Bupivacaine 0.625% at _____ mL/h
  - Bupivacaine 0.125% at _____ mL/h
  - Ropivacaine 0.1% at _____ mL/h
  - Ropivacaine 0.2% at _____ mL/h
  - Lidocaine 0.5% at _____ mL/h

- PCRA: _____ Use basal rate (continuous infusion) above; _____ No basal rate; PCRA bolus _____ mL; lockout (delay) _____ minutes

Note: The decision to administer a peripheral nerve block via continuous infusion (basal rate) only, PCRA with basal rate, or PCRA bolus-only mode varies depending on anesthesia provider preference (see text).

- Examples of supplemental analgesia that are used with continuous peripheral nerve blocks are as follows (see text):
  - IV PCA (often used when continuous peripheral nerve block is administered without PCRA boluses)
  - Acetaminophen every 6 hours PRN for mild pain[2,3]
  - NSAID (e.g., ketorolac, celecoxib) in scheduled doses
  - Nonopioid-opioid combination analgesics (e.g., various strengths of acetaminophen + hydrocodone or oxycodone) every 4 hours PRN for moderate pain[2,3]
  - Oxycodone (various strengths) every 4 hours PRN for moderate to severe pain[3]
  - Anticonvulsant (e.g., gabapentin, pregabalin) in scheduled doses (see text)

Note: Protocols sometimes vary the type of supplemental analgesic depending on day of surgery and number of postoperative days.

- Management of breakthrough pain:
  - Bolus via nerve block catheter with _____ mL of local anesthetic from pump every 1 hour PRN for a maximum of 2 doses for each breakthrough pain episode.
  - If above bolus is ineffective, administer opioid (e.g., morphine 2 to 3 mg or equivalent) by IV push or clinician-administered bolus via IV PCA pump every 30 minutes PRN, not to exceed a total of 3 bolus doses per breakthrough pain episode.

Note: Anesthesia provider should be notified if these approaches fail to control pain.

LOCAL ANESTHETIC (SYSTEMIC) ADVERSE EFFECTS

- Mild adverse effects are an early sign of toxicity and can progress to fatal cardiovascular collapse and death if unattended. All local anesthetic adverse effects should be reported promptly to the anesthesia provider.

Continued

they should see the American Society for Pain Management Nursing's Position Paper on the Nurse's Role in the Management and Monitoring of Analgesia by Catheter Techniques for additional guidance (Pasero, Eksterowicz, Primeau, et al., 2007). See also Box 26-1 for guidelines on the care of patients receiving continuous peripheral nerve block.

Research on the Use of Continuous Peripheral Nerve Block

There is now an impressive body of research supporting continuous peripheral nerve block as a primary analgesic technique for postoperative pain, particularly following orthopedic surgery. The following is a list of case reports,

- Tell patient to notify a nurse if any of the adverse effects described below are detected.

Mild: Numbness and tingling in the fingers and toes, numbness and unusual sensations around and inside the mouth (perioral), metallic taste, ringing in the ears, light-headedness, dizziness, visual disturbances, and confusion

Moderate: Nausea and vomiting, severe dizziness, decreased hearing, tremors, changes in blood pressure and pulse, and confusion

Severe: drowsiness, confusion, muscle twitching, convulsions, loss of consciousness, cardiac arrhythmias, cardiac arrest

MONITORING ON CLINICAL UNIT

- Assess pain and vital signs at least every 4 hours for duration of nerve block infusion (see Chapter 19 for guidelines on monitoring during opioid therapy if opioids are administered concomitantly).
- Perform neurovascular assessment of affected (nerve block) area every 4 hours for duration of therapy: Sensory and motor function, and skin temperature, color, and capillary refill

Note: Numbness and weakness are expected; it is particularly important to assess for changes.

- Assess for adverse effects and complications at least every 4 hours (see adverse effects above).
- Inspect catheter insertion site for dressing integrity, signs of infection or hematoma, excessive drainage of infusate, and catheter stability at least every 8 hours and following any activity.

Note: Drainage of infusate is expected with shallow insertion of some peripheral nerve catheters; notify if excessive.

NOTIFY ANESTHESIA PROVIDER

- Presence of frank blood or clear fluid upon aspiration of catheter prior to initiation of infusion

Note: Initial local anesthetic doses are administered by the anesthesia provider; infusion is usually started by the nurse.[1]

- If patient is to be started on any anticoagulants other than subcutaneous heparin
- If patient is to be started on any pain medications ordered by another physician

- If another physician requests that nerve block infusion be discontinued
- Inadequate pain relief; not responding to prescribed treatment for breakthrough pain
- Change in level of sensory or motor function of the nerve block area (e.g., extremity)
- Signs of site infection
- Signs of local anesthetic toxicity
- Change in neurologic status: Confusion, slurred speech
- Opioid administration: Opioid-induced adverse effects unrelieved by prescribed treatment (see Chapter 19)

EXAMPLE ORDERS TO DISCONTINUE CONTINUOUS NERVE BLOCK INFUSION THERAPY

- Stop nerve block infusion at 0600.
- Remove nerve block catheter 2 hours after infusion is stopped if pain is 4/10 or less.
- Obtain orders from primary service for ongoing analgesia after nerve block catheter is discontinued
- Administer analgesia as soon as patient reports sensation returning in affected area.

Note: Orders to discontinue therapy are influenced by many factors, including type of surgery, type of nerve block, and patient's general status.

PATIENT TEACHING (SEE PP. 757-758)

PCRA, Patient-controlled regional analgesia; *PRN,* as needed

[1]Nurses are referred to their scope of practice as defined by their individual state board of nursing with regard to the administration of continuous peripheral nerve block. They should also see the American Society for Pain Management Nursing's Position Paper on the Role of the Registered Nurse in the Management and Monitoring of Analgesia by Catheter Techniques (Pasero, Eksterowicz, Primeau, et al., 2007; www.aspmn.org).

[2]Do not exceed 4000 mg of acetaminophen in a 24-hour period (see Section III).

[3]Sometimes given in scheduled doses to prevent breakthrough pain.

From Pasero, C., & McCaffery, M. (2011). *Pain assessment and pharmacologic management,* pp. 698-699, St. Louis, Mosby. Developed with input from Jacques Chelly, MD, PhD, MBA and Lois Pizzi, RN from University of Pittsburgh Medical Center, UPMC Presbyterian—Shadyside Hospital, Pittsburgh, and Lex Hubbard MD, Willis-Knighton Medical Center, Pierremont, Shreveport, LA. © 2009, Pasero C. May be duplicated for use in clinical practice.

reviews, and placebo-controlled research on the use of this method for a variety of types of pain. Note that continuous peripheral nerve blocks have been used for some types of persistent noncancer and cancer-related pain as well.

- Breast surgery (Buckenmaier, Klein, Nielsen, et al., 2003)
- Radical prostatectomy (Ben-David, Swanson, Nelson, et al., 2007)

- Hand surgery (Rawal, Allvin, Axelsson, et al., 2002)
- Wrist, elbow surgery (Grant, Nielsen, Greengrass, et al., 2001; Ilfeld, Morey, Enneking, 2002b)
- Shoulder surgery (Borgeat, Kalberer, Jacob, et al., 2001; Borgeat, Perschak, Bird, et al., 2000; Fredrickson, Ball, Dalgleish, 2008; Gottschalk, Burmeister, Radtke, et al., 2003; Grant, Nielsen,

Greengrass, et al., 2001; Hofmann-Kiefer, Eiser, Chappell, et al., 2008; Ilfeld, Enneking, 2002; Ilfeld, Morey, Wright, et al., 2003; Ilfeld, Wright, Enneking, et al., 2005; Mariano, Afra, Loland, et al., 2009; Singelyn, Seguy, Gouverneur, 1999; Stevens, Werdehausen, Golla, et al., 2007)

- Hip surgery (Chelly, 2007; Hebl, Kopp, Ali, et al., 2005; Ilfeld, Ball, Gearen, et al., 2009; Siddiqui, Cepeda, Denman, et al., 2007; Singelyn, Ferrant, Malisse, et al., 2005; Singelyn, Vanderelst, Gouverneur, 2001)
- Knee surgery (Barrington, Olive, Low, et al., 2005; Brodner, Buerkle, Van Aken, et al., 2007; Chelly, Greger, Gebhard, et al., 2001; Dauri, Fabbi, Mariani, et al., 2009; Door, Raya, Long, et al., 2008; Duarte, Fallis, Slonowsky, et al., 2006; Eledjam, Cuvillon, Capdevila, et al., 2002; Fowler, Symons, Sabato, et al., 2008; Grant, Nielsen, Greengrass, et al., 2001; Hayek, Ritchey, Sessler, et al., 2006; Hebl, Kopp, Ali, et al., 2005; Ilfeld, Gearen, Enneking, et al., 2006; Morin, Kratz, Eberhart, et al., 2005; Pulido, Colwell, Hoenecke, et al., 2002; Salinas, Liu, Mulroy, 2006; Syngelyn, Gouverneur, 2000; Zaric, Boysen, Christiansen, et al., 2006)
- Lower extremity distal to knee (Ilfeld, Morey, Wang, et al., 2002)
- Ankle surgery (Grant, Nielsen, Greengrass, et al., 2001; Ilfeld, Loland, Gerancher, et al., 2008; Ilfeld, Thannikary, Morey, et al., 2004)
- Foot surgery (di Benedetto, Casati, Bertini, 2002; Ilfeld, Thannikary, Morey, et al., 2004)
- Amputation (Grant, Nielsen, Greengrass, et al., 2001)
- Multiple combat casualties, amputation (Stojadinovic, Auton, Peoples, et al., 2006)
- Inguinal hernia repair (Schurr, Gordon, Pellino, et al., 2004)
- Cancer-related neuropathic pain (Vranken, van der Vegt, Zuurmond, et al., 2001)
- Burn pain during skin grafting (Cuignet, Pirson, Boughrouph, et al., 2004)
- Complex regional pain syndrome (CRPS Type I) (Wang, Chen, Chang, et al., 2001)
- Trigeminal neuralgia (Umino, Kohase, Ideguchi, et al., 2002)

Inpatient Use

A prospective analysis of nearly 1500 patients who had received continuous peripheral nerve block following inpatient orthopedic procedures found that this approach, supplemented with nonopioid or opioid analgesia as needed, provided effective pain relief in 96.3% of patients, with a very low incidence of complications (Capdevila, Pirat, Bringuier, et al., 2005). The technique is often incorporated into multimodal protocols, with the goal of improving functional outcomes following major orthopedic surgery. A total joint (hip and knee) clinical pathway that utilized a minimally invasive surgical technique and progressive daily recovery goals aggressively

addressed pain with continuous peripheral nerve block in addition to preoperative and PRN postoperative opioids and nonopioids (Hebl, Kopp, Ali, et al., 2005). Patients in this study were matched with control patients who underwent the same surgery (non–minimally invasive) in the past 5 years and were managed with conventional opioid-based pain treatment methods. Those who were managed via the pathway had lower pain scores, required 50% less supplemental opioid, and experienced fewer opioid-induced adverse effects, increased ability to ambulate, and a shorter length of hospital stay (2.8 days compared with 5.0 days). There were no local anesthetic or catheter-related complications. Of note, 15% and 0% of those in the control group and the pathway group, respectively, experienced postoperative cognitive dysfunction.

Others have found positive results with this approach. A prospective study randomized patients undergoing total knee arthroplasty via a clinical pathway to receive a single-injection peripheral nerve block or a continuous peripheral nerve block infusion postoperatively and found lower pain scores during physical therapy and reduced supplemental analgesic requirements in those who received continuous peripheral nerve block but no differences in hospital length of stay and long-term functional outcomes (Salinas, Liu, Mulroy, 2006). The authors concluded that analgesia with continuous peripheral nerve block was superior to single-injection nerve block, but suggested that the somewhat disappointing functional results could have been related to the use of clinical pathways that dictate specific daily goals, which may overshadow the ability of improvements in the quality and duration of postoperative analgesia to affect recovery following total knee replacement.

Outpatient Use

The phenomenal growth in ambulatory surgery is described as one of the most significant changes in surgical practice in the past two decades (Rawal, 2007). However, patients in this setting are discharged rapidly following painful surgery, usually with a prescription for an oral nonopioid-opioid analgesic, and their postoperative pain may be poorly controlled. A systematic review revealed that 45% of patients undergoing ambulatory surgery experience moderate to severe pain and a high incidence of other distressing symptoms, such as nausea (17%) and sedation (42%), during the first 48 hours postoperatively (Wu, Berenholtz, Pronovost, et al., 2002).

Numerous studies have demonstrated the value of continuous peripheral nerve block for a variety of ambulatory surgical procedures (Richman, Liu, Courpas et al., 2006). Randomized controlled trials report excellent pain control with minimal adverse effects and complications, and patients and their families are able to manage the infusions at home without difficulty (Evans, Nielsen, Tucker, et al., 2009; Ilfeld, Morey, Enneking, 2002a, 2002b, 2002c; Ilfeld, Morey, Wright, et al., 2003; Rawal, Allvin, Axelsson, et al., 2002; Swenson, Bay, Loose, et al., 2006).

An observational study described the outcomes of 620 patients who received continuous peripheral nerve blocks in the home setting following ambulatory surgery (Swenson, Bay, Loose, et al., 2006). The patients underwent a variety of different ambulatory surgical procedures, and all received continuous peripheral nerve blocks with a fixed infusion of 5 mL of bupivacaine 0.25% (without PCRA capability) and a prescription of a nonopioid-opioid analgesic for breakthrough pain. A very small number (1.1%) experienced inadequate pain control, usually related to catheter problems. Two patients had complications, both following popliteal fossa catheterization—one developed CRPS and one experienced weakness and sensory loss; both resolved within weeks. A small number of patients (26 patients, 4.2%) required additional interventions, such as for inadequate pain control, additional patient teaching, and pump malfunction. Anesthesiologists were able to manage many of the problems by providing telephone instructions.

A randomized controlled trial of patients undergoing anterior cruciate ligament repair demonstrated that continuous femoral nerve block (4-day) infusion, as part of a multimodal plan that included standardized spinal anesthesia and NSAID and ketamine administration, significantly reduced pain scores for 7 days postoperatively, compared with placebo infusion (Williams, Kentor, Vogt, et al., 2006). However, analysis of patient-reported health status and functional outcomes between 7 days and 12 weeks found no differences among the groups (Williams, Dang, Bost, et al., 2009).

Efficacy Compared with Other Analgesic Approaches

A meta-analysis of research (19 randomized controlled trials, 603 patients) comparing postoperative opioid analgesia (variety of agents and routes) and continuous peripheral nerve block (variety of catheter locations and regimens) concluded that the latter provided superior analgesia (approximately a 50% VAS score reduction) at all evaluation time periods through postoperative day 3, fewer adverse effects (e.g., sedation, nausea), and higher patient satisfaction compared with opioid-based analgesic approaches (Richman, Liu, Courpas, et al., 2006). A later randomized controlled study comparing IV PCA alone with continuous peripheral nerve block plus IV PCA following hip arthroplasty observed similar findings (Siddiqui, Cepeda, Denman, et al., 2007). Those who received a continuous lumbar plexus block combined with IV PCA had improved analgesia, reduced opioid requirements and adverse effects, and enhanced patient satisfaction. One patient in the IV PCA-only group experienced clinically significant respiratory depression and required ventilator support for 6 hours. One patient in the continuous nerve block group developed quadricep weakness, which was discovered 4 weeks following surgery. Although the cause of the deficit was not determined, its occurrence led the researchers to speculate that it could have been related to the use of regional anesthesia in the presence of anticoagulation (see following discussion of adverse effects). A later study comparing IV PCA and continuous peripheral nerve block after open shoulder surgery reported better analgesia with the block but no differences in functional outcomes (Hofmann-Kiefer, Eiser, Chappell, et al., 2008).

Epidural analgesia has long been a first-line approach for the management of pain after total knee replacement. A meta-analysis of research comparing peripheral nerve block with epidural analgesia did not distinguish between single-injection and continuous peripheral nerve blocks and emphasized the urgent need for more research comparing the two techniques; the researchers concluded that peripheral nerve blocks appear to represent the best balance between analgesia and adverse effects for major knee surgery (Fowler, Symons, Sabato, et al., 2008). Patients undergoing knee replacement in one study were randomized to receive continuous epidural (ropivacaine + fentanyl) or continuous peripheral nerve block (femoral nerve = ropivacaine + fentanyl; sciatic nerve = ropivacaine) (Zaric, Boysen, Christansen, et al., 2006). Adverse effects, such as sedation and nausea, were more common in the epidural group, but pain was equally well-controlled in both groups, and there were no differences in mobilization and other rehabilitation outcomes or length of hospital stay between the two groups. Another study concluded that IV PCA morphine, continuous femoral nerve block, and continuous epidural analgesia provided similar pain relief, rehabilitation, and hospital stay but recommended continuous femoral nerve block as the best choice following hip arthroplasty given its more favorable adverse effect profile (Singelyn, Ferrant, Malisse, et al., 2005) (see Chapter 17 for IV PCA and Chapter 15 for epidural analgesia). An interesting study used an aggressive multimodal plan that included preoperative and postoperative nonopioid and opioid analgesics; preoperative pericapsular ropivacaine, steroid, and morphine; and epidural anesthesia for patients undergoing total knee arthroplasty (Dorr, Raya, Long, et al., 2008). Patients were given continuous femoral nerve block (N = 35) or continuous epidural analgesia (N = 35) postoperatively. Those receiving continuous peripheral nerve block consumed less oral opioid; walking distance on day 0 and day 1 was better for patients with epidural analgesia; length of stay was comparable between the groups; and adverse effects and complications were minimal in both groups. No patients had ileus or respiratory depression, which the researchers attributed to the avoidance of parenteral opioids in almost all patients in the study.

Other methods of local anesthetic administration have been compared as well. A prospective, randomized study of patients undergoing anterior cruciate ligament repair found that continuous femoral nerve block produced better pain relief during rest and activity and greater nonopioid and opioid dose-sparing effects compared with intraarticular and wound infusions of local anesthetic (see later in the chapter for these methods) (Dauri, Fabbi, Mariani, et al., 2009).

Dosing and Administration Regimens

Continuous peripheral nerve blocks are administered via three basic regimens: continuous infusion only (basal rate only), PCRA with basal rate, and PCRA with bolus doses only (Boezaart, 2006). Similar to PCA by other routes of administration, PCRA allows patients to take an active role in the management of their pain and individualize therapy to meet their unique analgesic needs. Some clinicians prefer to use PCRA with a basal rate rather than use a basal rate-only mode for continuous peripheral nerve block because it allows the lowest effective continuous infusion dose (Ilfeld, Morey, Enneking, 2002b, 2004; Ilfeld, Thannikary, Morey, et al., 2004). Practice varies widely, however (see later in the chapter).

As mentioned, automated bolus doses have been administered in addition to PCRA capability. A study randomized 50 patients to receive a continuous popliteal nerve block by automated bolus doses or a continuous infusion; both had PCRA capability (Taboada, Rodriguez, Bermudez, et al., 2009). The quality of analgesia and need for rescue analgesia were similar among the two groups, but those who received automated bolus doses required fewer PCRA doses and consumed less local anesthetic.

A variety of multimodal strategies are used with continuous peripheral nerve block therapy. Nonopioids, such as acetaminophen and an NSAID, and/or anticonvulsants, such as gabapentin or pregabalin (see later in this chapter), may be provided in scheduled doses. IV (opioid) PCA (usually without basal rate) is sometimes used to provide supplemental analgesia for patients receiving continuous peripheral nerve block by basal rate only (i.e., without PCRA capability). Alternately, oral opioid or nonopioid-opioid combination analgesics are provided as needed for breakthrough pain. These are sometimes administered in scheduled doses to prevent breakthrough pain. Supplemental analgesia is also provided prior to ambulation and physical therapy to maximize comfort during these painful activities; when PCRA is used, patients are taught to self-administer a dose prior to these activities to improve their ability to participate.

The most commonly used local anesthetics and concentrations for continuous peripheral nerve block are ropivacaine 0.1% to 0.2% and bupivacaine 0.0625% to 0.125%. (The initial block is established with incremental doses of a higher concentration, usually of the same local anesthetic.) Some clinicians report efficacy with higher concentrations, e.g., a fixed infusion of 0.25% bupivacaine at 5 mL/h (Swenson, Bay, Loose, et al., 2006). One study found that 0.1% ropivacaine provided ineffective analgesia and 0.2% and 0.3% ropivacaine provided similarly effective analgesia (Brodner, Buerkle, Van Aken, et al., 2007). There were no adverse effects among the various concentrations, and the researchers suggested

0.2% concentration at an initial infusion rate of 15 mL/h. Clonidine is sometimes added to peripheral nerve block infusions to enhance the duration and effectiveness of the local anesthetic (Ilfeld, Morey, Enneking, 2003) (see Chapter 22 for more on clonidine).

Randomized studies have evaluated various dosing strategies in an attempt to determine an optimal regimen. It appears to vary depending on type of surgery and location of catheter. One compared 0.2% ropivacaine administered by: (1) a basal rate of 12 mL/h plus a low PCRA bolus dose of 0.05 mL (designated the basal group), (2) a basal rate of 8 mL/h plus a PCRA bolus dose of 4 mL (designated the basal-bolus group), or (3) a low basal rate of 0.3 mL/h plus a large PCRA bolus dose of 9.9 mL (designated the bolus group) in patients following foot or ankle surgery (Ilfeld, Thannikary, Morey, et al., 2004). PCRA bolus doses were available once every hour. The patients in the bolus group (PCRA only) had a higher incidence of inadequate pain control, increased supplemental opioid requirements, and more sleep disturbances compared with the basal groups. The basal-bolus group experienced the best overall outcome. The same mode was recommended following upper extremity surgery at or distal to the elbow (Ileld, Morey, Enneking, 2004). However, another group of researchers found no benefit with the addition of a ropivacaine basal rate, and they recommended PCRA bolus-only mode after major knee surgery (Eledjam, Cuvillon, Capdevila, et al., 2002). Others have conducted similar studies with bupivacaine 0.125%, and recommended PCRA bolus-only following total knee replacement (Singelyn, Gouverneur, 2000) and hip replacement (Singelyn, Vanderelst, Gouverneur, 2001) and a basal rate plus PCRA boluses for shoulder surgery (Singelyn, Seguy, Gouverneur, 1999).

The relationship between concentration and volume has also been studied and varies depending on catheter location. One study recommended a more concentrated solution (0.4% versus 0.2% of ropivacaine) in a smaller volume (4 mL/h versus 8 mL/h) for popliteal sciatic nerve block (Ilfeld, Loland, Gerancher, et al., 2008). Another recommended further research but suggested that a lower concentration in a larger volume provided superior analgesia for interscalene nerve blocks (Le, Loland, Mariano, et al., 2008) and for infraclavicular nerve blocks (Ilfeld, Le, Ramjohn, et al., 2009).

The duration of continuous peripheral nerve block therapy depends on many factors, including type of surgical procedure, location of catheter, and patient status (e.g., NPO, chest tubes still in place). A review of the data of nearly 1500 patients who received continuous peripheral nerve block for inpatient orthopedic surgeries revealed a median duration of 56 hours (Capdevila, Pirat, Bringuier, et al., 2005). Generally, the duration ranges from 24 to 72 hours. A secondary analysis of a double-blind, randomized controlled study found that extending the duration of therapy to 96 hours (4 days) had no effect on patients' functional status and well-being between 7 days and 1 year following knee arthroplasty (Ilfeld, Meyer, Le, et al., 2009).

Adverse Effects and Complications

The adverse effects of local anesthetics delivered by continuous peripheral nerve block are similar to those by other routes of administration (see Box 26-1 and Chapter 15). Intravascular catheter migration is rare but has been reported (Capdevila, Pirat, Bringuier, et al., 2005) and would produce signs of local anesthetic toxicity, such as metallic taste, perioral numbness, and tinnitus. Patients receiving this technique should be evaluated systematically for these signs, and those who receive continuous peripheral nerve block in the home setting must be given verbal and written instructions that include the signs and symptoms of adverse effects and what to do if detected (see pp. 757-758 at the end of Section V). Intravascular injection and undetected early signs of local anesthetic toxicity can progress to cardiovascular collapse. Lipid emulsion has been used to successfully resuscitate several patients from cardiac arrest from local anesthetic-induced cardiotoxicity (Clark, 2008); however, the effectiveness of this treatment depends on the type of local anesthetic administered. That is, intralipid treatment appears to be effective for bupivacaine-induced but not ropivacaine- or mepivacaine-induced cardiac arrest (Espinet, Emmerton, 2009; Zausig, Zink, Keil, et al., 2009). Large doses of epinephrine are also reported to be required for reversal of bupivacaine-induced cardiotoxicity (Mulroy, 2002).

All local anesthetics produce both motor and sensory blockade (Wilson, 2009). The ability to participate in physical therapy early and effectively during the postoperative course for orthopedic patients is critical. Despite the administration of low concentrations of local anesthetic, motor block can present a problem, but adjustments in dose and technique, multimodal approaches, and the use of assistive devices have contributed to improved outcomes in these patients (Dorr, Raya, Long et al., 2008; Ilfeld, Gearden, Enneking, et al., 2006; Wilson, 2009) (see later discussion of Local Infiltration Analgesia).

As mentioned, opioids and nonopioids are often used for breakthrough pain during continuous peripheral nerve block therapy; however, the significant dose-sparing effects of the therapy reduce the incidence of adverse effects associated with these other analgesics, such as GI disturbances from nonopioids, and nausea, sedation, and respiratory depression from opioids. Research suggests that there is less cognitive dysfunction with this technique as well, which has implications particularly in older adult patients (Hebl, Kopp, Ali, et al., 2005). Still, patients must be assessed for these adverse effects whenever these other analgesics are co-administered with the therapy (see Chapters 6 and 19).

Complications are rare with continuous peripheral nerve blocks (Capdevila, Pirat, Bringuier, et al., 2005; Cuvillon, Ripart, Lalourcey, et al., 2001; Swenson, Bay, Loose, et al., 2006) and are thought to be less common than with single-injection blocks (Boezaart, 2006). Transient or permanent nerve injury can be caused by the nerve block as well as by inadvertent intraoperative or postoperative pressure applied to a nerve or postoperatively from traction injury (Boezaart, 2006) or hematoma compression (Siddiqui, Cepeda, Denman, et al., 2007). Transient nerve damage has been reported most often with interscalene blocks (Capdevila, Pirat, Bringuier, et al., 2005) and axillary blocks (Boezaart, 2006). Low incidences of persistent sensory blockade (3%), persistent motor blockade (2.2%), and paresthesias or dysesthesias (1.5%) during the postoperative period were described in one prospective analysis (Capdevila, Pirat, Bringuier, et al., 2005). All resolved without sequelae.

The use of anticoagulation therapy has significantly improved morbidity and mortality following some major surgeries, such as total knee or hip replacement, but this practice has presented a challenge to those who must find strategies that provide both effective and safe management of the associated pain. Peripheral nerve blocks provide exceptional pain relief but are not without a low risk (0.019% to 1.7%) of nerve damage and deficits from complications (Meier, Buttner, 2007), such as hematoma formation and compression (Siddiqui, Cepeda, Denman, et al., 2007). It is essential that patients be regularly assessed for signs of compression syndrome, such as changes in skin color in the affected area indicating poor circulation or increased numbness, tingling, or weakness in an affected extremity, and to be aware that these may be masked by the effects of local anesthetics (see Box 26-1). The reader is referred to the American Society of Anesthesiologists (ASA) guideline for the use of regional anesthetic techniques in anticoagulated patients, which describes the safe use of peripheral nerve blocks in these patients (Horlocker, Wedel, Benzon, et al., 2003) (see Chapter 15 and Table 15-8 on p. 439).

As with any indwelling catheter technique, there is a risk of infection and localized inflammation with continuous peripheral nerve blocks. Risk factors include a stay in the ICU with a possible association with catheter placement in patients who have sustained traumatic injury, duration of the indwelling catheter for greater than 48 hours, site of catheter (e.g., higher risk with femoral than with popliteal), male sex, and absence of antibiotic prophylaxis (Capdevila, Bringuier, Borgeat, 2009). Capdevila and colleagues (2009) recommend the same maximal sterile precautions used for epidural catheter placement to anesthesia providers placing peripheral nerve catheters (see Chapter 15). A prospective study of the experiences of nearly 1500 patients who had received continuous peripheral nerve blocks provided bacterial analysis of the catheters placed in 68% of the patients (Capdevila, Pirat, Bringuier et al., 2005). Positive bacterial colonization occurred in 28.7% of the cases, most often from the staphylococcus species (*staphylococcus epidermidis* [61%], gram-negative bacillus [21.6%], and *staphylococcus aureus* [17.6%]). The reader is referred to this study for a breakdown of the incidence and type of bacteria depending on type of peripheral nerve block. One patient in this study experienced symptomology from a staphylococcus aureus infection that resolved with antibiotic treatment. Another study found a 57% rate of bacterial colonization (primarily staphylococcus epidermidis) of femoral catheters; three transitory bacteremias occurred but resolved with catheter removal and no antibiotics (Cuvillon, Ripart, Llaourcey, et al., 2001). The authors recommended close monitoring of patients for signs of infection but did not recommend systematic bacterial analysis of catheters (see Box 26-1). Subcutaneous tunneling of the catheter is suggested as a means of further reducing risk, but well-controlled research is needed to confirm the effectiveness of this approach for this purpose (Compere, Legrand, Guitard, et al., 2009).

Technical difficulties in placement and maintaining the placement of catheters are reported in nearly every study but are relatively rare (Capdevila, Pirat, Bringuier, et al., 2005; Swenson, Bay, Loose, et al., 2006). As with any therapy that utilizes infusion devices, equipment malfunction is described as well.

Continuous Local Anesthetic Wound Infusion

Continuous local anesthetic wound infusions involve the surgeon's placement of a catheter subcutaneously into the surgical wound at the end of the surgical procedure to be used for continuous infusion of local anesthetics, such as bupivacaine or ropivacaine, to control postoperative pain (Rawal, 2007). For some orthopedic surgeries, the wound catheter may be placed intraarticularly (Axelsson, Gupta, Johanzon, et al., 2008; Vintar, Rawal, Veselko, 2005). Intraarticular local anesthetics have also been administered by single injections (Convery, Milligan, Quinn, et al., 2001; Moiniche, Mikkelsen, Wetterslev, et al., 1999; Muittari, Kirvela, 1998; Ng, Nordstrom, Axelsson, et al., 2006). Single-dose intra-wound local anesthetic instillation has been used as well (Goldstein, Grimault, Henique, et al., 2000; Labaille, Mazoit, Paqueron, et al., 2002; Ng, Swami, Smith, et al., 2002). Just as with continuous peripheral nerve blocks, supplemental opioid or nonopioid-opioid combination analgesics must be provided in addition to these therapies.

The same analgesic infusion devices used for continuous peripheral nerve blocks can be used for continuous wound infusions. Advantages of this modality include that it is a simple and efficient technique and is less labor-intensive and expensive than some of the other methods used to manage postoperative pain, such as epidural analgesia and peripheral nerve blocks. A quantitative and qualitative systematic review of randomized controlled trials conducted between 1983 and 2006 showed that continuous local anesthetic wound infusions produced effective analgesia with a consistent and significant opioid dose-sparing effect, which was linked to a 30% to 80% reduction in postoperative nausea and vomiting (Liu, Richman, Thirlby, et al., 2006). Other findings were high patient satisfaction, reduced length of hospital stay, a low incidence of technical failure

(1%), and no cases of local anesthetic toxicity. There were similar wound infection rates among those who received wound infusion and those who did not. In contrast, a more recent systematic review of the literature on local anesthetic infiltration for major abdominal and orthopedic surgeries concluded that a variety of techniques are used to administer continuous wound infusions, effectiveness is inconsistent, and none of the techniques described thus far in the literature could be recommended for routine use (Dahl, Moiniche, 2009).The reader is referred to this review and the review by Liu and colleagues (2006) for the many studies that have been conducted using this technique. Some of the research and surgical procedures for which the technique has been used are listed below.

- Shoulder repair (Axelsson, Gupta, Johanzon, et al., 2008; Axelsson, Nordenson, Johanzon, et al., 2003; Barber, Herbert, 2002; Gottschalk, Burmeister, Radtke, et al., 2003; Park, Lee, Kim, et al., 2002)
- Hip surgery (Bianconi, Ferraro, Traina, et al., 2003)
- Knee surgery (Alford, Fadale, 2003; Bianconi, Ferraro, Traina, et al., 2003; Vintar, Rawal, Veselko, 2005)
- Iliac crest bone graft (Blumenthal, Dullenkopf, Rentsch, et al., 2005; Singh, Samartzis, Strom, et al., 2005)
- Thoracotomy (Karakaya, Baris, Ozkan, et al., 2004; Tetik, Islamoglu, Ayan, et al., 2004)
- Mastectomy (Sidiropoulou, Buonomo, Fabbi, et al., 2008)
- Coronary bypass, cardiac surgery (Dowling, Thielmeier, Ghaly, et al., 2003; Magnano, Montalbano, Lamarra, et al., 2005; White, Rawal, Latham, et al., 2003)
- Inguinal hernia (Lau, Patil, Lee, 2003; LeBlanc, Bellanger, Rhynes, et al., 2005; Sanchez, Waxman, Tatevossian, et al., 2004)
- Colectomy (Baig, Zmora, Derdemezi, 2006)
- Cesarean section (Fredman, Shapiro, Zohar, et al., 2000; Givens, Lipscomb, Meyer, 2002)
- Abdominal hysterectomy (Gupta, Perniola, Axelsson, et al., 2004; Leong, Lo, Chiu, 2002)
- Major abdominal surgeries, e.g., colectomy, gastrectomy, cholecystectomy (Fredman, Zohar, Tarabykin, et al., 2001)
- Abdominoplasty (Bray, Nguyen, Craig, et al., 2007)

Local Infiltration Analgesia

The concept of local infiltration analgesia is based on the long history of infiltration of wounds with single injections of local anesthetics, but it differs in that local infiltration analgesia administers boluses of local anesthetic in a systematic fashion via a catheter placed in the wound prior to wound closure (Wilson, 2009). The administration of local infiltration analgesia was first introduced as part of a fast track program for lower limb surgery with a goal of aggressive ambulation in the immediate postoperative period and early discharge (Kerr, Kohan, 2008). Patients in this study (N = 325) underwent hip resurfacing or total hip or total knee arthroplasty and were given systematic infiltrations of ropivacaine, ketorolac, and epinephrine via single injections followed by a catheter placed in a manner that would ensure delivery of the mixture to the joint, tissue planes, and under the wound. (The reader is referred to the publication of this study [Kerr, Kohan, 2008] for direction for catheter placement depending on surgical procedure.) The researchers used other measures to localize the local anesthetic mixture to the surgical site and prevent motor blockade, such as extremity splinting, cooling, and compression. Before removal of the catheter at 15 to 20 hours postoperatively, it was reinjected with 15 mL of the local anesthetic mixture. Oral nonopioid and IV opioid supplemental analgesia was provided as needed. More than 80% of the patients in each group reported pain ratings of 3/10 or less at 4 hours (time of highest pain score) during both rest and mobilization; mean time to mobilization ranged from 9 (hip resurfacing) to 13 (knee arthroplasty) hours; 89%, 51%, and 41% of the patients receiving hip resurfacing, knee arthroplasty, and hip arthroplasty, respectively, were discharged directly home after a 1-night stay; and there were no serious adverse effects or complications. A systematic review of the literature on local anesthetic infiltration techniques for major abdominal and orthopedic surgeries emphasized the need for more research into local infiltration analgesia and discussed the difficulties in concluding effectiveness (i.e., many other variables must be factored in when a multimodal approach such as was described in the above study is used) (Dahl, Moiniche, 2009).

IV Lidocaine

As discussed earlier in Chapter 23, IV lidocaine is an option for refractory persistent neuropathic pain. It is also occasionally used for acute pain treatment. One of its primary benefits is its ability to reduce postoperative GI complications (Wright, Durieux, Groves, 2008). Early research demonstrated that IV lidocaine was effective in reducing postoperative ileus (Rimback, Cassuto, Tollesson, 1990), a major cause of morbidity after surgery (Kehlet, 2005) (see Chapter 19 for more on ileus). This effect is a primary reason for the occasional use of IV lidocaine in the perioperative setting as part of a multimodal pain treatment plan. It is usually combined with a nonopioid, such as ketorolac or celecoxib, and an opioid. A meta-analysis of eight studies involving patients who underwent abdominal surgery revealed that IV lidocaine compared with placebo was associated with better pain control as well as decreases in the duration of ileus, nausea and vomiting, and length of hospital stay (Marret, Rolin, Beaussier, et al., 2008). Although more research is needed, it has also been shown to attenuate surgery-induced suppression of immune function (Yardeni, Beilin, Mayburd, et al., 2009). Perioperative IV lidocaine reduced opioid requirement but did not reduce time to discharge

in ambulatory surgery patients (McKay, Gottschalk, Ploppa, et al., 2009). More research and clinical experience are needed to define the role of IV lidocaine in this setting (Wu, Liu, 2009) (see Chapter 23 for mechanisms of action and adverse effects of IV lidocaine and Box 26-2 for administration guidelines).

A randomized controlled study administered a preoperative loading bolus dose of IV lidocaine (1.5 mg/kg) followed by a 4-hour lidocaine infusion (2 mg/minute) after skin closure or a placebo bolus and 4-hour placebo infusion for colorectal surgery (Herroeder, Pecher, Schonherr, et al., 2007). Return of bowel function and other GI parameters were significantly better and length of hospital stay was shorter for those who received IV lidocaine, but pain relief and opioid consumption did not differ between the two groups. Serum lidocaine levels were acceptable for all patients except one who presented with a peak value of 5.8 mcg/mL after lidocaine bolus (see later in the chapter for a discussion of serum lidocaine levels). All patients who were started on the lidocaine infusion finished it without adverse cardiac effects. Other studies have shown similar positive results with IV lidocaine (Groudine, Fisher, Kaufman, et al., 1998; Koppert, Weigand, Neumann, et al., 2004). Co-administration of the $alpha_2$-adrenergic agonist dextromethorphan (see Chapter 23) and IV lidocaine demonstrated a synergistic effect and resulted in better pain relief and improved bowel function compared with placebo after laparoscopic cholecystectomy (Wu, Borel, Lee, et al., 2005).

In contrast, a randomized, placebo-controlled study showed a preoperative bolus of lidocaine (1.5 mg/kg) followed by an intraoperative lidocaine infusion (1.5 mg/kg/h) had no effect on postoperative pain control, opioid consumption, or hip flexion following hip arthroplasty (Martin, Cherif, Gentili, et al., 2008). However, another randomized controlled study used a more aggressive treatment protocol that consisted of a preoperative IV lidocaine bolus (1.5 mg/kg) followed by intraoperative (2 mg/kg/h) and 24-hour postoperative (1.33 mg/kg/h) lidocaine infusions or placebo administration in the same manner to patients undergoing colectomy (Kaba, Laurent, Detroz, et al., 2007). Compared with placebo, the patients who received lidocaine had significantly better results in consumption of opioid, pain and fatigue scores, return of bowel function, and hospital stay. Serum lidocaine levels remained well below toxic levels during infusion and for 24 hours after. Although lidocaine did not inhibit the stress response in this study, obvious major benefits to patient outcomes were attained. The researchers pointed out that a more profound blockade (e.g., epidural analgesia) may be required to alter stress response. Thoracic epidural lidocaine has been shown to produce better pain relief, less opioid consumption, and an earlier return of bowel function compared with IV lidocaine following colon surgery (Kuo, Jao, Chen, et al., 2006), but studies comparing the two therapies for effects on stress response could not be found.

Box 26-2 | IV Lidocaine for Postoperative Pain[1]

INDICATIONS

Adjuvant analgesia for multimodal postoperative pain treatment (see text)

CONTRAINDICATIONS

- First- and second-degree heart conduction blocks could be aggravated and progress to a higher degree of heart block with lidocaine administration.
- Cardiovascular instability and concomitant use of alpha agonists or beta blockers are relative contraindications.
- Allergies to other amide local anesthetics (e.g., bupivacaine, ropivacaine); allergy to procaine (Novocaine) is not a contraindication as procaine is an ester local anesthetic.

SUPPLIES

- Solution of 4 mg/mL (0.4% solution) of preservative-free lidocaine prepared as 2 g in 500 mL will be supplied by the pharmacy department for IV infusion.
- Infusion pump

Note: An infusion device that does not allow free flow will be used to administer IV lidocaine (no exceptions), and doses will be verified by an independent double-check process (see Chapter 17).[1]

ADMINISTRATION

1. Anesthesiologist will administer a bolus dose (e.g., 1.5 mg/kg) followed by initiation of a continuous infusion (e.g., 2 mg/kg/h) in the operating room.

2. A continuous infusion (e.g., 1.33 mg/kg/h) will be administered in the PACU and for approximately 24 hours postoperatively.[1]
3. The infusion will be delivered for 24 hours or until the 500 mL bag is empty, whichever comes first.[1]

Safety warning: Bupivacaine and ropivacaine are *never* given intravenously.

ADVERSE EFFECTS

- Adverse effects are rare at serum lidocaine levels of 2 to 6 mcg/mL.
- Mild adverse effects are an early sign of toxicity and can progress to fatal cardiovascular collapse and death if unattended. All lidocaine adverse effects should be reported promptly to the anesthesia provider.
- Tell patient to notify a nurse if any of the adverse effects described below are detected.
- Patients with liver dysfunction, pulmonary disease with a prominent feature of carbon dioxide retention, or congestive heart failure are at higher risk for lidocaine-induced adverse effects.

Mild (serum levels 3 to 8 mcg/mL): Numbness and tingling in the fingers and toes, numbness and unusual sensations around and inside the mouth (perioral numbness), metallic taste, ringing in the ears, lightheadedness, dizziness, visual disturbances, confusion

Moderate (serum levels 8 to 12 mcg/mL): Nausea and vomiting, severe dizziness, decreased hearing, tremors, changes in blood pressure and pulse, confusion

Continued

Anecdotal experience suggests that IV lidocaine may be efficacious for burn pain, but a Cochrane Collaboration Review showed no significant benefits of systemic lidocaine compared with placebo and other pain therapies for this type of pain (Wasiak, Cleland, 2007). A lack of effectiveness for burn pain may be related to inadequate dosing. It has been noted that serum lidocaine levels higher than 4 mcg/mL are required to relieve thermally-evoked pain (Kingery, 1997). Monitoring serum lidocaine levels during therapy to determine optimal dose may be helpful for some types of pain (see Chapter 23).

Dosing and Serum Lidocaine Levels

Published IV lidocaine dosing regimens have varied (see Box 26-2). Most studies have produced good results with a preoperative bolus of 1.5 to 3 mg/kg followed by a continuous infusion of 1.33 to 3 mg/kg/h (Kaba, Laurent, Detroz, et al., 2007; Koppert, Weigand, Neumann,

et al., 2004; Kuo, Jao, Chen, et al., 2006) or 2 to 3 mg/min (Groudine, Fisher, Kaufman, et al., 1998; Herroeder, Pecher, Schonherr, et al., 2007). If administered, intraoperative infusions of 2 mg/kg/h (Kaba, Laurent, Detroz, et al., 2007) and 2 to 3 mg/min have been used (Gordon, 2008; Herroeder, Pecher, Schonherr, et al., 2007; Wu, Borel, Lee, et al., 2005). Bolus doses are usually administered over a few minutes (e.g., 10 minutes). The length of infusion time varies widely among studies, with some administered only through surgery and others lasting between 1 hour and 24 hours postoperatively (Marret, Rolin, Beaussier, et al., 2008). Bolus doses and infusions should be administered via an infusion device to help ensure accurate dose delivery.

Cardiac antiarrhythmic activity and toxicity are associated with lidocaine serum levels of 1.5 mcg/mL and 5 mcg/mL, respectively (Lema, 1996; Groudine, Fisher, Kaufman, et al., 1998). Concentrations below toxicity levels (range 1.3 to 4.6 mcg/mL) have been reported in

Severe (serum levels greater than 12 mcg/mL): drowsiness, confusion, muscle twitching, convulsions, loss of consciousness, cardiac arrhythmias, cardiac arrest

MONITORING DURING THERAPY

Note: Telemetry is not necessary.

- Assess pain and adverse effects every 1 hour × 2 hours, every 2 hours × 2 hours, then every 4 hours if stable.
- If any adverse effects occur during infusion:
  - Stop infusion
  - Obtain blood pressure reading
  - Assess associated symptoms including pain
  - Obtain stat blood sample for serum lidocaine level (draw 6 mL in royal blue- or red-top tube)
  - Notify anesthesia provider or pain service
- Life-threatening overdose (in addition to the above actions, one or all of the following actions should be taken as indicated by patient condition):
  - Airway support
  - Oxygenation and hyperventilation to raise seizure threshold
  - Diazepam for seizure
  - IV fluids and Trendelenburg position to increase fluid volume
  - Cardiovascular depression treatment including IV fat emulsion as an antidote

Note: Half-life of lidocaine is 30 to 60 minutes, which means adverse effects typically dissipate within this time frame after stopping an infusion. The analgesic effect of lidocaine may last longer than the pharmacologic half-life.

[1]Nurses are referred to their scope of practice as defined by their individual state board of nursing for their role in the administration of local anesthetics.

As appears in Pasero, C., & McCaffery, M. (2011). *Pain assessment and pharmacologic management,* pp. 706-707, St. Louis, Mosby. Used with permission: Fast Facts—5 Minute Inservice, University of Wisconsin Hospital, Clinics, Madison, WI. Data from Gordon, D. B. (2008). Intravenous lidocaine for postoperative analgesia: Renewed interest in an old strategy. *APS Bulletin, 18*(3), 3-5; Groudine, S. B., Fisher, H. A., Kaufman, R. P. Jr, et al. (1998). Intravenous lidocaine speeds the return of bowel function, decreases postoperative pain, and shortens hospital stay in patients undergoing retropubic prostatectomy. *Anesth Analg, 86*(2), 235-239; Herroeder, S., Pecher, S., Schonherr, M. E., et al. (2007). Systemic lidocaine shortens length of stay after colorectal surgery: A double-blinded, randomized, placebo-controlled trial. *Ann Surg, 246*(2), 192-200; Kaba, A., Laurent, S. R., Detroz, B. J., et al. (2007). Intravenous lidocaine infusion facilitates acute rehabilitation after laparoscopic colectomy. *Anesthesiology, 106*(1), 11-18; Koppert, W., Weigand, M., Neumann, F., et al. (2004). Perioperative intravenous lidocaine has preventive effects on postoperative pain and morphine consumption after major abdominal surgery. *Anesth Analg, 98*(4), 1050-1055; Kuo, C. P., Jao, S. W., Chen, K. M., et al. (2006). Comparison of the effects of thoracic epidural analgesia and IV infusion with lidocaine on cytokine response, postoperative pain and bowel function in patients undergoing colonic surgery. *Br J Anaesth, 97*(5), 640-646; Marret, E., Rolin, M., Beaussier, M., et al. (2008). Meta-analysis of intravenous lidocaine and postoperative recovery after abdominal surgery. *Br J Surg, 95*(11), 1331-1338; Martin, F., Cherif, K., Gentili, M. E., et al. (2008). Lack of impact of intravenous lidocaine on analgesia, functional recovery, and nociceptive pain threshold after total hip arthroplasty. *Anesthesiology, 109*(1), 118-123; Wu, C. L., Tella, P., Staats, P. S., et al. (2002). Analgesic effects of intravenous lidocaine and morphine on postamputation pain. *Anesthesiology, 96*(2), 841-848; Wu, C. T., Borel, C. O., Lee, M. S., et al. (2005). The interaction effect of perioperative cotreatment with dextromethorphan and intravenous lidocaine on pain relief and recovery of bowel function after laparoscopic cholecystectomy. *Anesth Analg, 100*(2), 448-453. May be duplicated for use in clinical practice.

postoperative studies with the dosing previously described (Groudine, Fisher, Kaufman, et al., 1998; Kaba, Laurent, Detroz et al., 2007; Koppert, Weigand, Neumann, et al., 2004). One postoperative study reported that serum levels were within a range of 1.1 to 4.2 mcg/mL during IV lidocaine infusion in all of the patients except one who had a peak level of 5.8 mcg/mL following a lidocaine bolus (Herroeder, Pecher, Schonherr, et al., 2007). See Table V-1 on pp. 748-756 for dose selection for persistent neuropathic pain.

Anticonvulsants

The anticonvulsants gabapentin and pregabalin are first-line analgesics for neuropathic pain (see Chapter 23) and are increasingly being added to postoperative pain treatment plans. They have been shown to improve analgesia, allow lower doses of other analgesics, and help to

prevent persistent neuropathic postsurgical pain syndromes (Dauri, Faria, Gatti, et al., 2009). Following is a discussion of the use of these two drugs for acute pain. See Chapter 23 for detailed discussion of their mechanisms of action and adverse effects.

Gabapentin

Several years before gabapentin was used in the clinical setting for acute pain treatment, it was studied in volunteers for its effects in an acute inflammatory pain model (Werner, Perkins, Holte, et al., 2001). The subjects in this study were randomized to receive placebo or 1200 mg of gabapentin 3 hours before delivery of a first-degree experimental thermal injury. Gabapentin diminished both the decrease in mechanical pain threshold in the burn area and the secondary hyperalgesia. Another study in healthy volunteers using heat-capsaicin sensitization showed similar results (Dirks, Petersen,

Rowbotham, et al., 2002). The researchers in both groups concluded that gabapentin might have clinical potential in the treatment of acute pain disorders involving neuronal sensitization.

Animal research has shown that gabapentinoids work synergistically with the nonopioid naproxen to reverse peripheral inflammation and hyperalgesia (Hurley, Chatterjea, Feng, et al., 2002). Although more human research is needed to define the association between the gabapentinoids and other analgesics, these studies support a role for gabapentin (and pregabalin) in acute pain management. The practice of adding gabapentin to multimodal pain treatment plans to improve postoperative analgesia and prevent persistent neuropathic postsurgical pain is increasing (Ho, Gan, Habib, 2006; Tiippana, Hamunen, Kontinen, et al., 2007) and should be considered for other types of acute inflammatory pain as well (Gray, Williams, Cramond, 2008).

A meta-analysis of 18 studies concluded that gabapentin improved postoperative analgesia at rest and movement, and reduced opioid dose requirements and opioid-induced adverse effects (Peng, Wijeysundera, Li, 2007). Several other reviews have yielded similar conclusions (Gilron, 2006; Ho, Gan, Habib, 2006; Hurley, Cohen, Williams, et al., 2006; Seib, Paul, 2006; Tiippana, Hamunen, Kontinen, et al., 2007). All have called for more research with larger numbers of patients to establish optimal dose and titration for acute pain. Nonanalgesic effects, such as anxiolysis, and the impact of dizziness and sedation require further study as well (Peng, Wijeysundera, Li, 2007).

Numerous randomized controlled trials were identified for the first procedure-specific review of the literature on perioperative gabapentin (Mathiesen, Moiniche, Dahl, 2007). Surgical procedures included in this review were abdominal hysterectomy, breast surgery, spinal surgery, laparoscopic surgeries, orthopedic surgeries, ear-nose-throat surgeries, and others. Of these, only abdominal hysterectomy and spinal surgery offered enough studies to perform a quantitative procedure-specific analysis, which underscores the need for more research. The researchers concluded that perioperative use of gabapentin improved pain control and produced a significant opioid dose-paring effect for both abdominal hysterectomy and spinal surgery.

A meta-analysis of 18 clinical trials that combined gabapentin with other analgesics or placebo was undertaken to evaluate analgesic consumption as an efficacy outcome measure of analgesics (McQuay, Poon, Derry, et al., 2008). The authors concluded that it was difficult to precisely measure treatment gains by adding gabapentin to opioid or combination analgesic therapy and called for further analysis of analgesic consumption as a measure of analgesic efficacy in clinical trials. Nonetheless, the use of gabapentin preoperatively (400 mg to 1200 mg) and postoperatively (400 to 600 mg every 6 to 8 hours for at least 24 hours) is gaining favor as a therapeutic option for postoperative pain control (see dose selection). Following

is a list of the research, case reports, and reviews on the use of gabapentin for acute pain.

- Craniotomy (Ture, Sayin, Karlikaya, et al., 2009)
- Abdominal hysterectomy (Dierking, Duedahl, Rasmussen, et al., 2004; Fassoulaki, Stamatakis, Petropoulos, et al., 2006; Gilron, Orr, Tu, et al., 2005; Mathiesen, Moiniche, Dahl, 2007; Sen, Sizlan, Yanarates, et al., 2009; Tiippana, Hamunen, Kontinen, et al., 2007; Turan, White, Karamanlioglu, et al., 2006)
- Vaginal hysterectomy (Rorarius, Mennander, Suominen, et al., 2004)
- Mastectomy and lumpectomy (Dirks, Fredensborg, Christensen, et al., 2002; Mathiesen, Moiniche, Dahl, 2007; Tiippana, Hamunen, Kontinen, et al., 2007)
- Spinal surgeries; laminectomy (Mathiesen, Moiniche, Dahl, 2007; Pandey, Navkar, Giri, et al., 2005; Pandey, Sahay, Gupta, et al., 2004; Radhakrishnan, Bithal, Chaturvedi, 2005; Turan, Karamanlioglu, Memis, et al., 2004; Van Elstraete, Tirault, Lebrun, et al., 2008)
- Laparoscopic cholecystectomy (Gilron, Orr, Tu, et al., 2009; Pandey, Priye, Ambesh, et al., 2004; Pandey, Priye, Singh, et al., 2004)
- Nephrectomy (Pandey, Singhal, Kumar, et al., 2005)
- Breast surgery (Dirks, Fredensborg, Christensen, et al., 2002; Fassoulaki, Patris, Sarantopoulos, et al., 2002; Fassoulaki, Triga, Melemeni, et al., 2005)
- Hand surgery (enhanced IV regional anesthesia) (Turan, White, Karamanlioglu, et al., 2007)
- Hip surgery (Rasmussen, Mathiesen, Dierking, et al., 2009)
- Knee surgery (Clarke, Pereira, Kennedy, et al., 2009; Dietrich, Kinney, Pulido, et al., 2009; Menigaux, Adam, Guignard, et al., 2005)
- Lower limb scar revision, skin graft (Turan, Kaya, Karamanlioglu, et al., 2006)
- Shoulder surgery (Adam, Menigaux, Sessler, et al., 2006)
- Ear-nose-throat surgery (Turan, Memis, Karamanlioglu, et al., 2004)
- Thyroidectomy (Al-Mujadi, A-Refai, Katzarov, et al., 2006; Brogly, Wattier, Andrieu, et al., 2008)
- Varicocele (Koc, Memis, Sut, 2007)
- Acute neuropathic burn pain (Gray, Williams, Cramond, 2008)

Prevention of Persistent Neuropathic Postsurgical Pain

The use of gabapentin preoperatively may be justified on the empirical basis that this drug can potentially reduce the likelihood of acute pain leading to persistent pain (Gilron, 2006; Tiippana, Hamunen, Kontinen et al., 2007) (see Section I for more on the incidence and underlying mechanisms of persistent postsurgical pain). With this goal in mind, it has been administered to patients undergoing surgical procedures that pose considerable risk for the development of persistent neuropathic postsurgical pain syndromes (e.g., thoracotomy, mastectomy, hernia repair, limb amputation, abdominal hysterectomy, and cholecystectomy).

A randomized controlled trial of patients undergoing thyroidectomy found that preoperative gabapentin (1200 mg) did not impact the quality of immediate postoperative pain or analgesic intake; however, it was associated with a significant reduction in the incidence of persistent neuropathic pain at a 6-month evaluation (Brogly, Wattier, Andrieu, et al., 2008). Another study found similar results, with a reduction in the incidence of persistent post–abdominal surgery pain (Fassoulaki, Stamatakis, Petropoulos, et al., 2006). In this study, treatment involved 400 mg of gabapentin or placebo given every 6 hours, beginning 18 hours preoperatively and continuing for 5 days.

An interesting blinded study randomized 50 patients undergoing cancer breast surgery to receive placebo or a multimodal treatment plan (Fassoulaki, Triga, Melemeni, et al., 2005). The treatment group received gabapentin 400 mg preoperatively and every 6 hours for 8 postoperative days, EMLA (eutectic mixture of local anesthetics) cream applied to the surgical wound area on the day of surgery and for 3 postoperative days, and intraoperative irrigations of ropivacaine 0.75% to the brachial plexus and adjacent intercostal spaces. The control group received placebo oral capsules, placebo cream, and saline irrigations administered as described for the treatment group. Those who received the multimodal treatment had better postoperative pain control and consumed less supplemental analgesia. A major finding was a significant reduction in persistent pain in the multimodal treatment group. Whereas 82% and 57% of those in the control group reported pain at 3 and 6 months, respectively, 45% and 30% of those in the treatment group reported persistent pain at 3 and 6 months, respectively. A later study found similar results with ropivacaine 0.75% wound irrigation and 400 mg gabapentin every 6 hours for 7 days postoperatively in women undergoing abdominal hysterectomy (Fassoulaki, Melemeni, Stamatakis, et al., 2007). An interesting placebo-controlled study compared preoperative gabapentin and ketamine and found that both drugs improved pain control and reduced opioid consumption; however, gabapentin, but not ketamine, prevented persistent pain in the first 6 months after abdominal hysterectomy (Sen, Sizlan, Yanarates, et al., 2009).

Not all studies have produced positive results with regard to prevention of persistent neuropathic postsurgical pain with gabapentin. One trial randomized 75 patients to receive gabapentin (1200 mg/day for 10 days) or the oral local anesthetic mexiletine (600 mg/day for 10 days) or placebo after cancer breast surgery (Fassoulaki, Patris, Sarantopoulos, et al., 2002). Those who were given gabapentin or mexiletine experienced less pain, reduced acetaminophen intake, and a 50% reduction in opioid requirement during the postoperative period compared with those who received placebo. Although burning pain was less frequent at 3 months in those who were given gabapentin or mexiletine, the incidence of persistent pain,

its intensity, and the need for analgesia was similar among the three groups. A randomized controlled trial in which gradually increased doses (to 2400 mg/day) of gabapentin were administered for 30 days following elective lower amputation failed to demonstrate an effect on the incidence of phantom limb pain (Nikolajsen, Finnerup, Kramp, et al., 2006). More research with well-designed patient groups (surgical procedure and adjuvant therapy), more detailed follow-up evaluations, and sufficient numbers of patients has been encouraged (Kehlet, 2006).

Dose Selection

There is no consensus on an optimal perioperative gabapentin dosing regimen, and they vary widely in studies. An extensive review of the research on the use of gabapentin for postoperative pain treatment described both single- and multiple-dose regimens (Ho, Gan, Habib, 2006). Generally, preoperative doses range between 400 mg and 1200 mg. Postoperative doses are typically 400 mg to 600 mg administered every 6 to 8 hours. The duration of postoperative administration also varies widely and ranges from 24 hours to several days. The reader is referred to the systematic reviews that describe the various studies and dosing regimens (Gilron, 2006; Ho, Gan, Habib, 2006; Hurley, Cohen, Williams, et al., 2006; Peng, Wijeysundera, Li, 2007; Seib, Paul, 2006; Tiippana, Hamunen, Kontinen, et al., 2007).

Pregabalin

As a newer anticonvulsant, more research is needed to fully evaluate the effects of pregabalin on postoperative and other types of acute pain. Although a 2007 systematic review concluded that gabapentin and pregabalin effectively reduce postoperative pain, the researchers identified only one randomized controlled trial on the use of pregabalin for acute pain (Tiippana, Hamunen, Kontinen, et al., 2007). Patients in this study were randomized to receive placebo, ibuprofen (400 mg), pregabalin (50 mg), or pregabalin (300 mg) following third-molar extraction (Hill, Balkenohl, Thomas, et al., 2001). Onset of analgesia was rapid for pregabalin (23.5 minutes) but slightly slower than ibuprofen (16 minutes). Those who received the larger 300 mg dose of pregabalin or ibuprofen experienced superior pain relief compared with placebo. Pregabalin at the 50 mg dose did not differ from placebo in outcome parameters. Pregabalin 300 mg exhibited a significantly longer duration of analgesia compared with ibuprofen, pregabalin 50 mg, and placebo. The group who received pregabalin 300 mg had the highest patient global impression scores but also experienced adverse effects (e.g., dizziness, sedation, vomiting) most frequently (48%).

A randomized, placebo-controlled trial in which a single dose of 100 mg of pregabalin was administered preoperatively to women undergoing minor gynecologic surgery failed to show any reduction in postoperative pain or improvement in quality of recovery (Paech, Goy, Chua, et al., 2007). Given the findings of the previous study, in which 50 mg was essentially equivalent to placebo (Hill, Balkenohl, Thomas, et al., 2001), the lack of positive results in this study may have been due to the administration of too low a dose.

Patients undergoing upper or lower limb amputation were randomized to receive placebo or 300 mg or 600 mg of pregabalin 2 hours before surgery, followed by placebo or 300 mg or 600 mg of pregabalin 8, 16, and 24 hours after the preoperative dose (Azer, Abdelhalim, Elsayed, 2006). Both pregabalin doses significantly reduced pain and supplemental morphine consumption compared with placebo. The most common adverse effect was sedation, but this was not statistically significant. A single preoperative dose of pregabalin has been shown to produce similar opioid-dose sparing effects (Murcia Sanchez, Orts Castro, Perez Doblado, et al., 2006).

Another study of 91 women undergoing laparoscopic hysterectomy used the maximum recommended pregabalin dose (600 mg) and found that the drug produced a dose-dependent opioid dose-sparing effect, but the incidence of headache, dizziness, and blurred vision was highest with this dose compared with diazepam 10 mg and pregabalin 300 mg (Jokela, Ahonen, Tallgren, et al., 2008). A dose-ranging study randomized 108 patients undergoing a variety of outpatient surgical procedures to receive placebo or pregabalin 75, 150, or 300 mg 60 to 90 minutes prior to surgery (White, Tufanogullari, Taylor, et al., 2009). There were no differences in anxiety scores, pain scores, patient satisfaction, tolerance of normal diet, or return of bowel activity among the four groups. Sedation scores were higher and reports of dizziness more common in those who received 300 mg of pregabalin; some patients were reported to be difficult to arouse in this group. Length of hospital stay was also longer in this group, but this did not reach statistical significance. Others found similar results in patients following laparoscopic cholecystectomy (Chang, Lee, Kim, et al., 2009).

Pregabalin was studied as a component of a multimodal analgesia treatment plan but with disappointing results. Patients (N = 116) undergoing abdominal hysterectomy were randomized to receive preoperative acetaminophen (1000 mg) plus placebo alone, or with pregablin (300 mg), or with pregabalin (300 mg) plus dexamethasone (8 mg) (Mathieson, Rasmussen, Dierking, et al., 2009). Morphine consumption and pain scores at rest and activity did not differ among the groups. The incidence of nausea was significantly lower in the group that received dexamethasone, and vomiting was less in both of the groups that received pregabalin. Other adverse effects did not differ among the groups. An earlier placebo-controlled study by these researchers used the same protocol but without acetaminophen in patients undergoing hip arthroplasty (N = 120) and reported a reduction in morphine consumption but no differences in pain scores, no reduction in nausea and vomiting, and increased sedation in those who received pregabalin (Mathiesen, Jacobsen, Holm, et al., 2008).

Like gabapentin, pregabalin may have a role in the prevention of persistent postsurgical pain. A prospective, randomized controlled trial (N = 240) administered placebo or 300 mg of pregabalin preoperatively and 150 mg twice daily postoperatively through day 10; 75 mg twice daily on days 11 and 12; and 50 mg twice daily on days 13 and 14 to patients undergoing total knee arthroplasty; all patients received epidural analgesia postoperatively (Buvanendran, Kroin, Della Valle, et al., 2010). Those who received pregablin experienced significantly less persistent neuropathic postsurgical pain at 6 months than placebo (0% and 5.2%, respectively). Other positive results in those who received pregabalin in this study were greater knee flexion, less epidural analgesia consumption, better sleep, and faster time to meeting discharge criteria; however, the patients who received pregabalin also experienced more sedation and confusion on the day of surgery and the first postoperative day compared with those who received placebo.

These studies provide information similar to that obtained about gabapentin. Some, but not all, indicated benefit for treatment in the acute pain setting, and dose effects are likely to be important. Overall, more research is needed to determine the role of the gabapentinoids as adjuvant agents in multimodal postoperative pain treatment plans.

Clonidine

In the perioperative setting, the alpha$_2$-adrenergic agonist clonidine has been used via multiple routes of administration to enhance pain relief, produce an opioid dose-sparing effect, and prolong anesthesia (Buvandendran, Kroin, 2007). Studies have suggested that it can reduce dose requirements for both general and IV anesthesia (Moss, Glick, 2005). When used for pain or anesthesia, it must be appreciated that hemodynamic effects of both spinal and systemic clonidine begin within 30 minutes of administration, reach a peak at 1 to 3 hours, and last approximately 6 to 8 hours after injection. Bioavailability by the oral route is almost 100%, and half-life ranges from 6 to 24 hours (Westfall, Westfall, 2006). A meta-analysis of randomized controlled trials comparing the various alpha$_2$-adrenergic agonists (e.g., clonidine, dexmedetomidine) with controls concluded that the alpha$_2$-adrenergic agonists reduce mortality and myocardial infarction after vascular surgery, and that during cardiac surgery, they may reduce ischemia and have effects on mortality and myocardial infarction (Wijeysundera, Naik, Beattie, 2003).

Dexmedetomidine (Precedex), another alpha$_2$-adrenergic agonist, is used primarily for perioperative management and sedation in the critically ill. Similar to clonidine, dexmedetomidine has been shown to act synergistically with opioids, exert an opioid dose-sparing effect, and enhance anesthesia (Pandharipande, Ely, Maze, 2006). This drug is discussed in more detail in Chapter 27. (See Chapter 22

Table 26-1 | Perioperative Use of Alpha₂-Adrenergic Agonists: Efficacy and Major Adverse Effects

Drug	Route of Administration	Time of Administration	Primary Analgesic	Efficacy	Major Adverse Effects
Clonidine	Oral	Preoperative, perioperative	Opioid	o - +	Sedation
	Epidural	Perioperative	Opioid or LA	++	Sedation, hypotension
	Intrathecal	Perioperative	LA	+	Hypotension
	Nerve block	Perioperative	LA	++	None
	Intraarticular	Perioperative	LA	++	None
Dexmedetomidine	Intravenous	Perioperative	Opioid	+	None
	Intravenous	Perioperative	Epidural LA	+	Hypotension

LA, Local anesthetic

This table shows the efficacy and major adverse effects of some of the alpha₂-adrenergic agonists used in the perioperative setting.

From Pasero, C., & McCaffery, M. *Pain assessment and pharmacologic management*, p. 711, St. Louis, Mosby. ©2011, Pasero C, McCaffery M. May be duplicated for use in clinical practice.

for underlying mechanisms and adverse effects of the alpha₂-adrenergic agonists and Table 26-1 for a summary of the efficacy and adverse effects specifically with perioperative use of clonidine and dexmedetomidine.)

Intraspinal clonidine has been shown to work synergistically with opioids to produce improved postoperative pain outcomes. A randomized controlled trial of 85 patients undergoing coronary artery bypass surgery administered intrathecal morphine with or without clonidine (Nader, Li, Dosluoglu, et al., 2009). Those who received clonidine experienced a significant morphine dose-sparing effect, lower pain intensity, and shorter ventilation time. A trend toward increased vasopressin use was noted in the clonidine group, but this was not statistically significant. Intrathecal remifentanil and clonidine produced similar results in this same high-risk population (Lena, Balarac, Lena, et al., 2008). Another randomized controlled trial administered an epidural infusion of clonidine or placebo to patients following decompressive spinal surgery; all patients received IV PCA morphine postoperatively (Farmery, Wilson-MacDonald, 2009). Those who received clonidine used less morphine and experienced less nausea than those who received placebo. Other studies have shown similar positive results (Paech, Pavy, Orlikowski, et al., 2004; Schug, Saunders, Kurowski, et al., 2006). Compared with intrathecal morphine alone, the addition of clonidine to intrathecal morphine resulted in less intraoperative sufentanil, a longer time to first request for analgesia, and improved analgesia with rest and coughing in patients following radical prostatectomy (Andrieu, Roth, Ousmane, et al., 2009).

Timing of administration may be an important factor in determining efficacy of intraspinal clonidine. Epidural clonidine administered before abdominal surgery resulted in a greater opioid dose-sparing effect, better pain scores at 6 and 24 hours, and less sedation than epidural

clonidine administered at the end of surgery (Persec, Persec, Bukovic, et al., 2007).

Other research has combined clonidine with an opioid and local anesthetic intraspinally (Forster, Rosenberg, 2004; Huang, Lin, Huh, et al., 2007; Schug, Saunders, Kurowski, et al., 2006). A systematic review of 22 randomized controlled trials concluded that clonidine prolonged the analgesic action and sensory and motor blockade of a variety of intrathecal local anesthetics in a dose-dependent manner, but was unable to establish the optimal dose of clonidine for these effects (Elia, Culebras, Mazza, et al., 2008) (see Chapter 15 for more on intraspinal clonidine).

An abundance of research has shown the benefits of adding clonidine to local anesthetic peripheral nerve blockade. An early systematic review of 24 studies concluded that clonidine as an adjunct to brachial plexus block produced improved analgesia and minimal adverse effects in single doses up to 150 mcg (Murphy, McCartney, Chan, 2000). A later review of 27 studies found that clonidine improved the duration of anesthesia and analgesia of continuous local anesthetic peripheral block, again with a low incidence of adverse effects in single doses up to 150 mcg (McCartney, Duggan, Apatu, 2007).

Randomized controlled trials have shown that intraarticular administration of clonidine alone (Gentili, Enel, Szymskiewicz, et al., 2001) or a combination of clonidine, opioids, and local anesthetics (Armellin, Nardacchione, Ori, 2008; Joshi, Reuben, Kilaru, et al., 2000) improved pain relief and reduced supplemental analgesic intake following knee surgery.

Systemic Clonidine

Systemic (oral and IV) clonidine has also been administered in the perioperative setting. Preoperative oral clonidine produced an anxiolytic effect and reduced postoperative morphine consumption by 30% in one study (Caumo, Levandovski, Hidalgo, 2009). An interesting study administered oral clonidine (2 mcg/kg) or placebo to patients with obstructive sleep apnea the night before ear-nose-throat surgery (Pawlik, Hansen, Waldhauser, et al., 2005). Those who received clonidine had significantly lower pain scores and consumed significantly less opioid postoperatively than those who received placebo. Another important finding was that minimal postoperative oxygen saturation was lower in the placebo group than in the clonidine group. Similar effects have been noted with the use of IV clonidine in this high-risk population. One study randomly assigned morbidly obese patients undergoing bariatric surgery to receive a preoperative IV infusion of clonidine and ketamine or standard anesthesia protocol and demonstrated reduced analgesic requirements and earlier extubation in those who received clonidine and ketamine (Sollazzi, Modesti, Vitale, et al., 2009). Given the need to find methods that allow reduced opioid doses in morbidly obese patients, who may be at higher risk for postoperative respiratory depression (ASA, 2006), the results of these studies of systemic clonidine are noteworthy (see Chapter 19 for more on postoperative respiratory depression).

Clonidine has also been added to opioids for IV PCA administration (Lehman, 2005). Patients (N = 60) undergoing lower abdominal surgery were randomized to receive a 20-minute IV infusion of clonidine (4 mcg/kg) at the end of surgery followed by postoperative PCA bolus doses of morphine (1 mg) plus clonidine (20 mcg) or a placebo infusion followed by postoperative PCA bolus doses of morphine (1 mg) alone (Jeffs, Hall, Morris, 2002). Although morphine consumption was similar between the groups, those who received clonidine had better pain relief during the first 12 hours postoperatively, less nausea during the first 24 hours, and were more satisfied with their pain relief.

Finally, IV clonidine has been used to effectively prevent and treat postanesthesia shivering (Kranke, Eberhart, Roewer, et al., 2004). A randomized controlled trial found that 100% of patients who received a single dose of 150 mcg of IV clonidine administered in the postanesthesia care unit (PACU) stopped shivering; a single dose of 25 mg of meperidine, which is the most common treatment for shivering in the PACU, stopped shivering in 18 of 20 patients with 2 patients requiring a second dose to cease shivering (Schwarzkopf, Hoff, Hartmann, et al., 2001).

Prevention of Persistent Neuropathic Postsurgical Pain

Clonidine may have a role in preventing persistent neuropathic postsurgical pain as well. A randomized controlled study found that an intraoperative intrathecal injection of clonidine (300 mcg) was more effective than an intraoperative intrathecal injection of bupivacaine or placebo in influencing several postoperative outcomes in patients undergoing colonic surgery (De Kock, Lavand'homme, Waterloos, 2005). Patients in the clonidine group had a longer time to first request for analgesia, lower pain scores and supplemental analgesic consumption, and a lower incidence of persistent pain at 6 and 12 months following colonic surgery compared with those in the other groups. No adverse events occurred in any of the groups. Intraoperative hemodynamic adverse effects, e.g., hypotension and bradycardia, occurred most often in the clonidine group but were corrected without incident. No one experienced excessive sedation.

Corticosteroids

Corticosteroids, particularly dexamethasone (Decadron), have been suggested as adjuvant agents in multimodal treatment plans for some types of postoperative pain (Buvanendran, Kroin, 2007; Gilron, 2004; Salerno, Hermann, 2006) (see Chapter 22 for underlying mechanisms and adverse effects). In experimental research in healthy volunteers, IV dexamethasone was not found to reduce inflammatory changes and pain when administered 2 hours prior to burn injury (Werner, Lassen, Kehlet, 2002). This finding supports the clinical impression that the drug does not provide sufficient analgesia acutely to be designated a primary analgesic. Nonetheless, it may contribute to positive outcomes when combined with other analgesics for acute pain. For example, a single dose of 40 mg IV dexamethasone administered as part of a multimodal treatment plan reduced pain with movement post–hip arthroplasty (Kardash, Beng, Tessler, et al., 2008), and 0.1 mg/kg dexamethasone IV given preoperatively enhanced intrathecal opioid analgesia following abdominal surgery (Movafegh, Soroush, Navi, et al., 2007).

Corticosteroids have a well-established role in the prevention and treatment of postoperative nausea and vomiting (PONV). Doses of 4 to 8 mg of dexamethasone are widely recommended for prevention of PONV (Fujii, Nakayama, 2007, 2008; Gan, Meyer, Apfel, et al., 2007; Golembiewski, Tokumaru, 2006) (see Chapter 19 for more on PONV).

A randomized controlled trial compared intraarticular dexamethasone and intraarticular morphine and found that both reduced pain for 5 days following knee surgery in patients with persistent osteoarthritis (Stein, Yassouridis, Szopko, et al., 1999). Further research is required to establish the efficacy of intraarticular corticosteroids for postoperative pain control (Lavelle, Lavelle, Lavelle, 2007).

N-Methyl-D-Aspartate (NMDA) Receptor Antagonists

The NMDA receptor antagonists, dextromethorphan and ketamine, were discussed in Chapter 23 for the treatment of persistent neuropathic pain. The discussion here will focus on their use for acute and postoperative pain. (See Chapter 23 for mechanisms of action and adverse effects.)

Dextromethorphan

Dextromethorphan has been administered by the oral or parenteral (IM, IV) routes with opioids and NSAIDs to enhance analgesia after surgery. The drug is available in cough suppressant products only in the United States. Some formulations are combined with alcohol and other additives, and, at present, the most concentrated source is in a 30 mg/5 mL suspension (e.g., Delsym 12-Hour). The lack of an IV formulation is problematic in postoperative patients who are often unable to take oral medications. This, in addition to unpredictable efficacy and no clear benefit over other analgesics, has resulted in limited use of dextromethorphan in the postoperative setting in the United States; however, it is used in countries where other formulations are available.

A systematic review of 28 randomized, placebo-controlled trials concluded that although there is potential for dextromethorphan to be a safe adjuvant to opioid analgesia for postoperative pain, the extant research has demonstrated inconsistent opioid dose-sparing and analgesic effects (Duedahl, Romsing, Moiniche, et al., 2006). Parenteral dextromethorphan produced more consistent reductions in opioid requirements than oral formulations, and adverse effects were minimal with the drug. Benefits appear to be greater when dextromethorphan is initiated before rather than after surgical incision (Helmy, Bali, 2001).

One study randomized patients (N = 100) undergoing abdominal hysterectomy to receive 30 mg of oral dextromethorphan or oral placebo preoperatively and three times during the first 24 hours after surgery (Chau-In, Sukmuan, Ngamsangsirisapt, et al., 2007). IV PCA morphine was administered postoperatively. Those who received dextromethorphan consumed less opioid intraoperatively and in the PACU and had significantly lower pain scores and a longer time to first analgesic use in the PACU, but there were no differences in pain scores, analgesic requirements, or adverse effects at later postoperative evaluations (6 and 24 hours). Others found similar disappointing results when the drug was added to a multimodal plan that included intrathecal morphine (Choi, Kliffer, Douglas, 2003).

Large doses of dextromethorphan were evaluated in a two-part randomized controlled trial of patients following knee surgery (Wadhwa, Clarke, Goodchild, et al., 2001). The first part of the study was undertaken to determine a maximum tolerated oral dextromethorphan dose, which was accomplished by administering titrated doses in the PACU. Some patients experienced unacceptable adverse effects of slurred speech and sedation followed by deep sedation, and one patient experienced frightening hallucinations with doses of 800 mg. This led the researchers to identify 750 mg as the maximum tolerated oral dextromethorphan dose. The second phase of the study randomized another group of patients undergoing knee surgery to receive 400 mg of dextromethorphan preoperatively followed by 200 mg at 8 and 16 hours postoperatively, or placebo at the same intervals. Those who received dextromethorphan consumed 30% less morphine but experienced no other benefits. Another important finding was that both the preoperative and postoperative doses of dextromethorphan were associated with a significantly high incidence of postoperative nausea. A placebo-controlled trial that administered preoperative dextromethorphan (150 mg) also found no benefits except a 30% reduction in opioid requirements but only for the first 3 hours postoperatively in patients following total abdominal hysterectomy (Ilkjaer, Bach, Nielsen, et al., 2000). This lower dose most likely contributed to a similar adverse effect profile compared with placebo. There were no differences between the placebo and dextromethorphan groups in hyperalgesia at 24 hours and 3 months postoperatively.

A different dosing regimen led to better results in a double-blind, placebo-controlled study in patients (N = 120) undergoing lower body bone and soft-tissue cancer surgery (Weinbroum, Bender, Nirkin, et al., 2004). The patients in this study had preoperative pain that was well controlled with NSAIDs. They were randomized to receive 90 mg of oral dextromethorphan or placebo 90 minutes before surgery and 90 mg daily for two days postoperatively. These patients were further randomized to one of two methods of postoperative pain control: IV PCA or patient-controlled epidural analgesia (PCEA). All patients were given the same general anesthetic approach for surgery. Overall, the patients who received IV PCA had the worst pain, sedation, and well-being scores. Analgesic consumption and pain and sedation scores were lowest and well-being scores the highest in the patients receiving PCEA and dextromethorphan. Other important benefits were that those given dextromethorphan ambulated earlier and experienced a two- to three-fold lower incidence of adverse effects compared with those who were given placebo. Lower pain scores, shorter time to first analgesic request, lower analgesic requirements, and earlier bowel function were also found with preincisional IM dextromethorphan (40 mg) in patients undergoing colon surgery (Yeh, Jao, Huh, et al., 2005).

In summary, until further research is conducted and more IV and oral formulations are available in the United States, the use of dextromethorphan cannot be recommended for acute pain management.

Ketamine

Ketamine has been administered in low (subanesthetic) doses for the treatment of postoperative pain and other types of acute pain. A low dose of ketamine is defined as an IV or epidural bolus less than 1 mg/kg and an infusion of 1.2 mg/kg/h (DeKock, Lavand'homme, 2007). Subanesthetic doses help to diminish the concerning psychotomimetic effects that can occur with higher ketamine doses. Ketamine may also have a role in treating acute opioid-related hyperalgesia and tolerance (Edrich, Friedrich, Eltzschig, et al., 2004; Gurfinkel, Czeiger, Douvdevani, et al., 2006; Svenson, Abernathy, 2007), and it has been studied for prevention of persistent neuropathic postsurgical pain syndromes (Remerand, Le Tendre, Baud, et al., 2009).

Although ketamine has been given alone for acute pain, the existing data suggest that its best use may be in combination with other analgesics, particularly opioids, to produce a dose-sparing effect. The versatility of routes by which it can be administered is an advantage, along with the fact that it does not produce respiratory depression. The primary routes of administration for perioperative ketamine are IV and epidural. The nurse has an important role in the administration and monitoring of ketamine (see Chapter 23 for mechanism of action and adverse effects and Box 23-1 on pp. 675-677 for administration guidelines).

Research on the use of ketamine for acute postoperative pain is more abundant and favorable than it is for persistent pain. An extensive review of the literature evaluated the use of ketamine as an adjuvant to opioid analgesia (Subramaniam, Subramaniam, Steinbrook, 2004). Only studies that compared an opioid alone with an opioid plus ketamine were included in the review. Nearly as many trials found improvement (20) as no improvement (17) in analgesia with the addition of ketamine. However, a later Cochrane Collaboration Review concluded that perioperative ketamine in subanesthetic doses reduces opioid requirements and PONV during the first 24 hours after surgery, and adverse effects at the doses used in this setting were found to be mild or absent (Bell, Dahl, Moore, et al., 2006). Another review found similar benefits (Elia, Tramer, 2005).

IV Ketamine

Practice varies considerably with IV ketamine use in the perioperative setting. It has been administered preoperatively, intraoperatively, and postoperatively via single bolus technique, continuous infusion, and added to IV PCA regimens. As part of a multimodal analgesic treatment plan, IV ketamine administered pre-incision, and then again postoperatively, produced a morphine dose-sparing effect, facilitated rehabilitation at 1 month, and was associated with reduced postoperative persistent pain at 6 months following total hip arthroplasty (Remerand, Le Tendre, Baud, et al., 2009). A low-dose ketamine infusion initiated immediately after anesthesia induction and completed before the end of surgery decreased opioid requirements both during and after

open colorectal surgery (Guignard, Coste, Costes, et al., 2002). A combination approach whereby ketamine was administered intraoperatively followed by a postoperative infusion for 2 days resulted in significantly better pain control and less morphine consumption and postoperative nausea compared with just intraoperative ketamine or placebo (Zakine, Samarcq, Lorne, et al., 2008). A randomized, placebo-controlled study administered a single dose of 0.15 mg/kg ketamine or placebo IV 10 minutes after anesthesia induction for anterior cruciate ligament repair (Menigaux, Fletcher, Dupont, et al., 2000). Those who received ketamine consumed lower opioid doses and had improved mobilization postoperatively compared with those who received placebo. A systematic review concluded that there are no differences in postoperative effects based on the timing of ketamine administration (Subramaniam, Subramaniam, Steinbrook, 2004).

The addition of ketamine to IV PCA after surgery has produced excellent results and significant opioid dose-sparing effects in some studies (Guillou, Tanguy, Seguin, et al., 2003; Michelet, Guervilly Helaine, et al., 2007; Nesher, Ekstein, Paz, et al., 2009; Yamauchi, Asano, Watanabe, et al., 2008); however, a systematic review concluded that, although its addition to IV PCA therapy does not increase adverse effects, it does not improve analgesia either (Subramaniam, Subramaniam, Steinbrook, 2004). A fixed PCA combination, as occurs when the drugs are combined in the same drug reservoir, should be avoided in opioid-tolerant patients who may require large and rapidly increased opioid doses to control pain. This could result in unnecessarily high ketamine doses and a subsequent increase in adverse psychotomimetic effects (De Kock, Lavand'homme, 2007).

Continuous IV infusion of ketamine as an adjunct to opioid therapy produced somewhat better results in the previously mentioned review (Subramaniam, Subramaniam, Steinbrook, 2004). It was suggested that the small infrequent doses that are administered via PCA may be less effective than a continuous infusion, which produces a steady state. Three trials showed no difference, but four showed improvement when continuous ketamine was added to a postoperative opioid treatment plan; the research was strongest for the use of this method of delivery following major abdominal surgery.

Ketamine and Other Therapies

Ketamine has also been administered as part of a multimodal postoperative plan that included midazolam (Versed) (Wang, Xie, Wang, 2006) and tramadol (Webb, Skinner, Leong, et al., 2007) and also has been found to work synergistically with propofol to produce significant reductions in postoperative opioid requirement (Badrinath, Avramov, Shadrick, et al., 2000; Kakinohana, Higa, Sasara, et al., 2004). One study found that intraoperative co-administration of ketamine with propofol attenuated hypoventilation and produced positive mood effects without perceptual changes after ambulatory surgery (Mortero, Clark, Tolan, et al., 2001). The researchers suggested that ketamine might facilitate earlier recovery of postoperative cognition. In another study, patients with preexisting major depression who were undergoing orthopedic surgery were induced with propofol and fentanyl plus ketamine or placebo (Kudoh, Takahira, Katagai, et al., 2002). Those who received ketamine had significantly lower scores in pain, depressed mood, suicidal tendencies, somatic anxiety, and hypochondriasis. It has also been shown to attenuate delirium in patients following cardiac surgery with cardiopulmonary bypass (Hudetz, Patterson, Iqbal, et al., 2009).

IV ketamine has been administered with opioid-local anesthetic epidural analgesia and produced excellent results. A randomized controlled trial administered an intraoperative IV ketamine or placebo bolus and infusion and postoperative epidural morphine-bupivacaine analgesia to patients who underwent renal surgery (Kararmaz, Kaya, Karaman, et al., 2003). Both resting and coughing pain scores were lower, analgesic consumption was less, time to first analgesia was longer, and incidence of adverse effects was lower in those who received ketamine. Others have found this same synergistic effect between IV ketamine and epidural opioid–local anesthetic infusions (Suzuki, Haraguti, Sugimoto, et al., 2006).

Epidural Ketamine

Ketamine is not approved in the United States for epidural administration because of a lack of availability of a preservative-free ketamine and concerns about neurotoxicity from the preservative chlorbutanol and from the drug itself (Wilson, Nimmo, Fleetwood-Walker, et al., 2008). Nevertheless, its administration by the epidural route has been studied extensively, and a systematic review reported impressive results when administered by a single bolus technique or added to a continuous infusion with PCEA (Subramaniam, Subramaniam, Steinbrook, 2004). Systemic (not epidural) ketamine reduces hyperalgesia (see the paragraphs that follow) and appears to be more effective than epidural ketamine; therefore, the parenteral (IV) route of administration is the preferred route for postoperative pain treatment (De Kock, Lavand'homme, 2007).

Ketamine for Other Types of Acute Pain

Ketamine has shown good results for treatment of other types of acute pain as well. A retrospective study of 40 patients transported by a regional aeromedical program found IV ketamine to be an ideal drug in the prehospital setting (Svenson, Abernathy, 2007). Ketamine provided effective sedation and improved analgesia for burn pain and trauma pain that was refractory to opioid and sedative treatment in combative patients. Other benefits were maintenance of ventilatory response in patients with a difficult airway, and hemodynamic stability in patients who were hypotensive or had experienced hypotension with propofol sedation. A multicenter clinical trial randomized

trauma patients with severe acute pain admitted to the emergency department to receive an IV ketamine or placebo infusion over 10 minutes followed by titration to comfort with IV morphine (Galinski, Dolveck, Combes, et al., 2007). Pain scores were similar, but morphine consumption was significantly less in those who received ketamine.

Animal research has shown that ketamine can interfere with the inflammatory cascade associated with burn injury and can improve survival in the presence of sepsis (Gurfinkel, Czeiger, Douvdevani, et al., 2006). As discussed, it can also produce effective analgesia for burn pain that is refractory to high doses of opioid analgesics (Svenson, Abernathy, 2007). A case report described long-term use of ketamine for sedation and analgesia in a patient with second- to third-degree facial and neck burns (Edrich, Friedrich, Eltzschig, et al., 2004). Prior to the addition of ketamine, the patient was receiving large doses of diazepam, midazolam, propofol, hydromorphone, and fentanyl without adequate sedation and comfort. He also developed bowel obstruction. The addition of a ketamine infusion (2.7 mg/kg/h) allowed tapering of opioid and sedative doses within 12 hours and eventual resolution of the severe ileus. The patient maintained good pain control and denied any psychotomimetic effects, was tapered from ketamine over a 2-day period, and was discharged after 37 days in the ICU.

Secondary Hyperalgesia and Central Sensitization

The role of the NMDA receptor in central sensitization suggests that NMDA receptor antagonists may be able to reduce the CNS changes following acute trauma that result in spreading or persistent pain (see Section I). Following surgical incision or similar tissue injury, there is primary hyperalgesia (immediate hypersensitivity and pain at the site of injury) and secondary hyperalgesia (pain felt in uninjured adjacent tissues). Secondary hyperalgesia may be related to the changes associated with NMDA-mediated central sensitization. Ketamine's effect on experimental central sensitization suggests that it may be a drug that could be used to reduce the clinical phenomena associated with this pathophysiology. Studies show conflicting results, and more research is needed to identify underlying mechanisms and best prevention regimens (Duale, Sibaud, Guastella, et al., 2008; Wilson, Nimmo, Fleetwood-Walker, et al., 2008). It is possible that systemic (not epidural) therapy is needed to obtain these putative benefits (De Kock, Lavand'homme, Waterloos, 2001). If so, systemic (i.e., IV) ketamine would be the preferred route of administration as part of a balanced multimodal perioperative pain treatment plan (De Kock, Lavand'homme, 2007).

Opioid-Induced Hyperalgesia

Opioid-induced hyperalgesia (OIH) is a paradoxical situation in which increasing doses of opioid result in increasing sensitivity to pain (Compton, 2008) (see Chapter 11 for more on OIH). It is easily demonstrated in animal models and is thought to be an uncommon but potentially serious consequence of opioid administration (Angst, Clark, 2006; Chu, Angst, Clark, 2008). It is closely related to tolerance, in which increasing doses of opioid are needed to provide the same level of pain relief (Angst, Clark, 2006). Tolerance involves decreased sensitivity to opioids as a result of opioid exposure, whereas OIH represents increased sensitivity to pain in response to opioid exposure (DuPen, Shen, Ersek, 2007). OIH can be demonstrated in animals after minimal opioid exposure, but it is very rarely considered a phenomenon of interest during short-term opioid use in the acute pain setting.

OIH is suspected when increasing doses (usually high, rapidly escalating doses) of opioid fail to "catch up" with escalating pain; pain and skin sensitivity may occur at sites remote from the original pain (Chu, Angst, Clark, 2008; Mitra, 2008). There may be diffuse pain, and diffuse allodynia (Compton, 2008; Chu, Angst, Clark, 2008; Mitra, 2008), and this syndrome may be associated with agitation and tremulousness.

To assess the possible presence of OIH, other reasons for failure of the opioid to relieve pain must be ruled out. These include increase in pain pathology, opioid tolerance, opioid withdrawal, pseudoaddiction, and opioid addiction (Compton, 2008) (see Table 11-3, p. 296, for a brief description of these conditions compared with OIH). If the conditions outlined in Table 11-3 have been ruled out, OIH should be considered.

Several strategies have been suggested for the treatment of OIH. Though more research and clinical experience are needed, there may be a role for the NMDA receptor antagonists, particularly ketamine, when OIH occurs during pain treatment (De Kock, Lavand'homme, 2007). When added to the treatment plan, dramatic reductions in opioid dose have been reported (Edrich, Friedrich, Eltzschig, et al., 2004; Gurfinkel, Czeiger, Douvdevani, et al., 2006; Svenson, Abernathy, 2007).

Indications

The NMDA receptor antagonists are not first-line analgesics for any type of pain but may be considered in patients with severe pain refractory to first-line analgesics. Low-dose perioperative ketamine should be considered in patients at high risk for persistent neuropathic postsurgical pain, such as those undergoing hernia repair, thoracotomy, mastectomy, or elective limb amputation. A trial of a subanesthetic dose of ketamine may be appropriate in patients who are strongly suspected of having OIH. The decision to use NMDA receptor antagonists should be made by experienced pain management clinicians or anesthesiologists who are aware of their indications, patient populations who may benefit most, dosing regimens, administration techniques, adverse effects, and monitoring parameters to ensure patient safety.

Dose Selection

There are no consistent dosing recommendations for dextromethorphan. A preoperative dose of 90 mg administered 90 minutes before surgery then 90 mg daily for 2 days postoperatively produced good results in one study (Weinbroum, Bender, Nirkin, et al., 2004). On the other hand, another study found reduced opioid consumption but no other benefits with 400 mg of dextromethorphan preoperatively followed by 200 mg at 8 and 16 hours postoperatively (Wadhwa, Clarke, Goodchild, et al., 2001). An initial arm of this study established a maximum tolerated oral dose of 750 mg in the PACU.

Dosing guidelines have not been established for IV ketamine either. Typically treatment of acute pain is initiated with very low (subanesthetic) doses and titrated according to response (pain relief and adverse effects). IV ketamine doses of 0.2 to 0.5 mg/kg are reported to produce analgesia (Svenson, Abernathy, 2007). Severe trauma-related acute pain was treated in one study with an IV ketamine bolus dose of 0.2 mg/kg over a 10-minute period and IV morphine titration to comfort with an initial IV morphine dose of 0.1 mg/kg followed by 3 mg of IV morphine every 5 minutes (Galinski, Dolveck, Combes, et al., 2007). Although this ketamine protocol produced a significant morphine dose-sparing effect, pain scores were not significantly different than those who received a placebo bolus infusion and the same morphine titration protocol in this study.

The reader is referred to systematic reviews that provide the range of doses for perioperative ketamine that were effective and safe in research (e.g., Bell, Dahl, Moore, et al., 2006; Subramaniam, Subramaniam, Steinbrook, 2004). In general, intraoperative IV ketamine dosing recommendations are to give a 0.5 mg/kg bolus followed by a 5 mcg/kg/min infusion until skin closure then a 2 mcg/kg/min infusion for 48 hours (De Kock, Lavand'homme, 2007). Others have found good results with similar dosing (Guillou, Tanguy, Seguin, et al., 2003). Still others recommend a wider intraoperative dose range, i.e., 0.5 to 2 mg/kg at induction of general anesthesia followed by PRN or low-dose infusion depending on general anesthetic agent (Reves, Glass, Lubarsky, et al., 2005). Ketamine infusions should be administered via an infusion device that does not allow free flow to ensure accurate dose delivery.

It is believed that higher ketamine doses are no better than lower doses in providing pain relief. One early study found no significant differences in pain relief between IV doses of 5, 10, and 20 mg/h in older adults following surgery, and effects such as dreaming increased with increased doses (Edwards, Fletcher, Cole, et al., 1993).

The drug has been administered with the opioid in the same drug reservoir for IV PCA or has been infused concurrently but via a separate infusion. A novel study analyzed 12 combinations of morphine and ketamine for IV PCA and found a 1:1 ratio of morphine to ketamine and a lockout (delay) interval of 8 minutes to be optimal (Sveticic, Gentilini, Eichenberger, et al., 2003). However, a fixed combination is not recommended and is particularly important to avoid in opioid-tolerant patients who may require large and rapidly increased opioid doses to control pain. A fixed combination in this case could result in unnecessarily high ketamine doses and a subsequent increase in adverse psychotomimetic effects (De Kock, Lavand'homme, 2007).

There are no guidelines for epidural ketamine dosing. A randomized controlled trial administered 3.3 mg/kg/L ketamine in combination with 0.125% bupivacaine epidurally at 15 mL/h to patients prior to limb amputation; infusion rates were adjusted (range 10 to 20 mL/h) and bolus doses (10 to 15 mL) were administered postoperatively to provide optimal pain control (Wilson, Nimmo, Fleetwood-Walker, et al., 2008). The researchers described their previous experience with frequent and safe administration of 2 to 4 mg/h of epidural ketamine and noted that 500 mcg/kg or higher epidural ketamine bolus doses were associated with excessive sedation. Another study administered a single epidural ketamine bolus dose of 1 mg/kg combined with 50 mcg/kg of morphine and found no significant difference in pain or adverse effects compared with epidural placebo combined with 50 mcg/kg of morphine (Subramaniam, Subramaniam, Pawar, et al., 2001). A randomized controlled trial found that low epidural ketamine doses of 0.5 mg/kg provided better analgesia compared with low IV ketamine doses of 0.5 mg/kg or placebo (Xie, Wang, Liu, et al., 2003).

Oral ketamine is rarely used in the postoperative setting, but following a well-tolerated subcutaneous test dose of 0.1 mg/kg of ketamine, 50 mg of oral ketamine given twice daily in juice was added to other analgesics to treat an opioid-tolerant patient with severe refractory acute postoperative pain following spinal fusion (Friedman, Jallo, Young, 2001). Pain was stabilized at a pain rating of 3/10, and significant reductions in opioid were possible. Pain ratings remained stable after the ketamine was discontinued on the day of discharge 12 days after surgery.

As mentioned, the undesirable effects of ketamine have led some experts to recommend its prescription and management only by those skilled in pain management and anesthesiology (Bell, 2009; Cvrcek, 2008). Palliative care specialists are also among those knowledgeable in the safe administration of the drug. Some hospitals restrict the administration of ketamine to specific clinical areas, such as ICU, palliative care, and the emergency department. Nurses should be aware of their scope of practice, state board of nursing's opinions, and institutional policies and procedures regarding the administration and monitoring of agents such as ketamine. See Box 23-1 on pp. 675-677 for guidelines on ketamine administration.

Conclusion

Many of the adjuvant analgesics can be combined with other analgesics as part of a multimodal plan for the treatment of acute pain. Among the most common are local anesthetics given by the IV or perineural routes of administration, gabapentinoids, clonidine, and ketamine. Each of these agents has a different underlying mechanism of action, and many work synergistically with other analgesics to produce significant dose-sparing effects.

Chapter 27 Adjuvant Agents for Goal-Directed Sedation in the Critically Ill and for Procedural Sedation

CHAPTER OUTLINE

THE intravenous (IV) sedative/hypnotics have become first-line agents for the administration of purposeful, goal-directed sedation such as in ventilated critically ill patients. These agents are also increasingly used for procedural pain management. Benzodiazepines have been first-line drugs for procedural sedation for many years, and ketamine has been used extensively for pediatric sedation and is increasingly used in adults for procedural sedation. Following is a discussion of selected drugs used for these purposes. See Table V-1, pp. 748-756, for dosing and other general information about some of these agents.

Propofol

Propofol (Diprivan) is a gamma aminobutyric acid (GABA) type A agonist with sedative and hypnotic effects. It is the most frequently used IV anesthesia induction agent (Reves, Glass, Lubarsky, et al., 2005) and a primary sedative for goal-directed sedation in the critically ill (Barr, Egan, Sandoval, et al., 2001; Devlin, Roberts, 2009); it has been associated with shorter ventilator time than when benzodiazepines are used for this purpose (Carson, Kress, Rodgers, et al., 2006) (see also discussion on dexmedetomidine later in this chapter). It is also increasingly administered for procedural sedation (Odom-Forren, 2008; Zed, Abu-Laban, Chan, et al., 2007) primarily because it has a significantly faster onset and shorter duration than the commonly used benzodiazepines and has amnestic properties at low doses (Devlin, Roberts, 2009). Advantages of propofol over traditional sedation with benzodiazpines include less nausea and faster recovery and discharge (Odom-Forren, 2008). Other uses are as an adjunct in the treatment of refractory metastatic cancer-related abdominal and hip pain (Graves, Moran, Porter, et al., 1996) and to relieve nausea (Kim, Han, Kil, et al., 2000; Odom-Forren, Watson, 2005) and intrathecal morphine-induced pruritus (Charuluxananan, Kyokong, Somboonviboon, et al., 2001). The drug can reduce intracranial pressure after traumatic brain injury and decreases cerebral blood flow and metabolism (Devlin, Roberts, 2009). A single IV propofol infusion (2.4 mg/kg) did not reduce pain or analgesic use and produced statistically significant, but not clinically meaningful, reduction in disability associated with chronic daily headache, which led the researchers in one study to recommend against its use for this type of pain (Simmonds, Rashiq, Sobolev, et al., 2009). The reader is referred to a comprehensive practical guide on the administration of moderate sedation/analgesia, which includes pharmacology, management of adverse effects and complications, and administration protocols

(Odom-Forren, Watson, 2005). Following is an overview of the drug.

Propofol has an extremely rapid onset of sedation (30 to 45 seconds) and peak sedative effect (90 to 100 seconds) (Odom-Forren, Watson, 2005; Reves, Glass, Lubarsky, et al., 2005). The drug undergoes rapid hepatic metabolism, has no known active metabolites, and is excreted renally (Reves, Glass, Lubarsky, et al., 2005). Clearance of the drug is very high, exceeding hepatic blood flow, suggesting extrahepatic metabolism of the drug, probably via the lungs. Studies using a 3-compartment distribution model show initial and slower distribution half-lives of 1 to 8 minutes and 30 to 70 minutes, respectively (Reves, Glass, Lubarksy, et al., 2005). Its terminal half-life varies from 3 to 9 hours (Odom-Forren, Watson, 2005; Reves, Glass, Lubarksy, et al., 2005).

The drug is given intravenously only and can be administered by intermittent dosing or infusion. Because intermittent doses must be administered frequently, infusion is preferred when used for an extended period (Reves, Glass, Lubarksy, et al., 2005). Bolus doses also can cause severe hypotension, and if administered, caution is recommended (see the following material on adverse effects). Propofol infusion should be administered via an infusion device that does not allow free-flow delivery; to help ensure accurate dose delivery, programming should be verified by the independent double-check process (see Chapter 17). Propofol has been administered by patient-controlled sedation technique; however, one group of researchers concluded that although this approach was effective, the risk of oversedation is too high for such unsupervised use (Thorpe, Balakrishnan, Cook, 1999).

Some anesthesiologists administer a small dose to test for allergic reactions; however, a loading dose of propofol usually is not administered prior to goal-directed sedation in the intensive care unit (ICU). Dosing of propofol varies, but 5 mcg/kg/min for at least 5 minutes (0.3 mg/kg/h) via IV infusion with subsequent increases of 5 to 10 mcg/kg/min (0.3 to 0.6 mg/kg/h) every 5 to 10 min is used to achieve desired level of sedation in the intubated and ventilated critically ill (Clinical Pharmacology, 2010). The usual maintenance dose with this regimen is 5 to 50 mcg/kg/min (mean 27 mcg/kg/min) depending on the clinical situation and coadministration of other sedating agents. An infusion of 50 to 150 mg titrated by 50 mg increments as needed to a maximum of 300 mg/h in a 70 kg adult is a common propofol regimen for light to moderate sedation in the ICU (Odom-Forren, Watson, 2005).

There is no consensus on propofol dosing regimens for procedural sedation either. One group of researchers administered an initial dose of 0.25 to 0.5 mg/kg administered over 60 seconds followed by 10 to 20 mg/min in subsequent doses (mean dose required was 1.6 mg/kg) to achieve procedural sedation in the emergency department (ED); this dosing resulted in adequate sedation in 90% of the patients and was well tolerated (Zed, Abu-Laben, Chan, et al., 2007) (see following material on adverse effects).

The propofol dose should be lowered for older adults because they are more sensitive to the hypnotic and cardiovascular (CV) effects of propofol than younger adults (Odom-Forren, Watson, 2005; Olmos, Ballester, Vidarte, et al., 2000; Reves, Glass, Lubarksy, et al., 2005; Schnider, Minto, Shafer, et al., 1999). The dose should also be lowered when propofol is combined with other agents, such as opioids and benzodiazepines, because these drugs (particularly benzodiazepines) produce additive sedative and hemodynamic (e.g., hypotensive) effects (Odom-Forren, Watson, 2005; Olmos, Ballester, Vidarte, et al., 2000). Reves, et al. (2005) noted that marked reductions in propofol dose are possible when patients are premedicated with an opioid or benzodiazepine prior to surgery (see the following material on propofol analgesia). Abrupt discontinuation of propofol can result in rapid awakening with anxiety and agitation, so the dose should be tapered prior to the end of therapy.

Adverse Effects

Common adverse effects associated with propofol administration are nausea, vomiting, abdominal cramping, headache, dizziness, twitching and myoclonic movement, hypertension and hypotension, bradycardia, respiratory depression, and apnea. Patients and families should be warned that the drug causes some patients to experience vivid sexual dreams (Odom-Forren, Watson, 2005). Reports of tolerance to the drug have not been supported by research; the need for individualized titration is stressed (Reves, Glass, Lubarksy, et al., 2005).

Propofol is formulated in a 10% lipid solution, which has been associated with elevated triglyceride and glucose levels in some patients (Odom-Forren, Watson, 2005). This formulation also heightens the risk of bacteremia, one of the most serious complications of propofol. Strict aseptic technique when handling the medication, infusion tubing changes every 12 hours, and regular assessment for signs of local and systemic infection are essential for safe administration of the drug (Odom-Forren, Watson, 2005).

Propofol injection may cause pain at the injection site, which occurs in as many as 70% of those who receive the drug (Schaub, Kern, Landau, 2004). Very slow injection is recommended to reduce this. Various other approaches to reduce injection pain have been successful and include pretreatment with injected lidocaine (Schaub, Kern, Landau, 2004; Zed, Abu-Laben, Chan, et al., 2007) or ondansetron (Ambesh, Dubey, Sinha, 1999). The 10% emulsion lipid formulation of propofol is reported to be less painful on injection than other formulations; however, this solution was associated with a higher incidence of propofol injection pain than pretreatment with 40 mg of IV lidocaine prior to administration of propofol 1% for Bier's block (Schaub, Kern, Landau, 2004). The addition of lidocaine to propofol infusion solutions was reported to produce antibacterial activity (Gajraj, Hodson, Gillespie, et al., 1998); however, this practice has been associated with a higher incidence of CV reactions and is discouraged (Wild, Shinde, Newton, 1999).

Deaths have occurred with the use of propofol for purposeful sedation in critically ill patients. A systematic review of reported deaths in the United States with "long-term" nonprocedural propofol use concluded that higher doses and concentrations and longer durations of therapy increase the risk of what is referred to as "propofol syndrome" (mean duration of use was 7.3 days; peak propofol dose was 7.2 mg/kg/h) (Wysowski, Pollock, 2006). Propofol syndrome is described as a CV and metabolic derangement characterized by progressive cardiac dysfunction, bradycardia, hypotension, cardiac failure, rhabdomyolysis, and metabolic acidosis. Risk factors associated with propofol syndrome include a dose higher than 83 mcg/kg/min, duration of therapy longer than 48 hours, concomitant use of catecholamine vasopressors or glucocorticoids, and patient age older than 18 years (Devlin, Roberts, 2009). It is important to note that there is no antidote for propofol.

Analgesia During Propofol Sedation

Subanesthetic doses of propofol produce only negligible analgesia (Frolich, Price, Robinson, et al., 2005; Odom-Forren, Watson, 2005; Zacny, Coalson, Young, et al., 1996). It is, therefore, essential to address the analgesic needs of patients receiving propofol sedation. Research supports the co-administration of analgesics (e.g., opioids, nonopioids) with drugs such as propofol because the conditions under which the propofol is administered are painful. For example, mechanical ventilation is required in patients receiving propofol for goal-directed sedation, and mechanical ventilation and endotracheal suctioning in addition to multiple other procedures ICU patients undergo while receiving propofol sedation have been shown to be painful (Konstantatos, Silvers, Myers, 2008; Puntillo, White, Morris, et al., 2001; Stanik-Hutt, Soeken, Belcher, et al., 2001). As mentioned, propofol is also used in lower doses for procedural sedation in non-ventilated patients. These procedures are clearly painful (see following discussion), justifying the need for analgesia. Further, as mentioned, the addition of an opioid may allow lower propofol doses and thus fewer adverse effects. (See Section II for pain assessment in the nonverbal critically ill.)

Propofol Outside of the ICU

Propofol is being used with increasing frequency for procedures performed outside of the ICU setting. A prospective, observational study (N = 113) evaluated the use of a propofol protocol for painful procedures in the ED

and found the drug to be safe and effective in this setting (Zed, Abu-Laban, Chan, et al., 2007). The study protocol required an attending physician to be responsible for the procedure; a registered nurse (RN) to initiate the IV, administer the drug, and monitor patient response; and a respiratory therapist to monitor ventilation and oxygenation throughout the procedure. Administration involved the administration of a low initial propofol dose of 0.25 to 0.5 mg/kg followed by 10 to 20 mg/min until adequate sedation was achieved. Lidocaine to prevent injection pain and fentanyl for procedural pain control were administered at the discretion of the treating physician. Sedation was reached and procedures were completed in 90% of the patients. Reasons were not given for failure to complete 10% of the procedures. Nine patients experienced hypotension, but there were no major complications. Interestingly, while lidocaine was administered to 78% of patients to prevent injection pain, fentanyl was administered to only 17% despite treatment of known painful procedures, such as orthopedic manipulation, cardioversion, and abscess incision and drainage. Reluctance to use opioids may have been for fear of additive respiratory depressant effects as the authors mentioned this opioid characteristic. Further, they noted that only 6.2% of the patients had procedural recall, confirming amnesia in the majority and implying that most patients experienced no pain. However, patients were not asked specifically about pain; when they returned to baseline mental status postprocedure, they were asked if they remembered the procedure and to rate overall satisfaction but were not asked about whether or not they experienced pain during the procedure, and no follow-up information (e.g., next day pain recall) was provided. Most patients (92%) and physicians (85%) reported that they were very satisfied with the use of propofol; however, the process for obtaining patient satisfaction was not clear.

Another prospective, observational 6-month study (N = 82) administered propofol by a less well-defined protocol and also found it to be safe and effective for sedation during painful procedures in the ED (Weaver, Hauter, Brizendine, et al., 2007). The most common procedures were incision and drainage, joint reduction, and fracture care. Adverse sedation events occurred in 21% of the patients. Clinical hypoventilation and transient, brief hypoxemia were the most common. Simple corrective measures, such as increased physical stimulation and head repositioning, were implemented to treat hypoventilation; no patients required assisted ventilation or intubation. More fentanyl analgesia was administered in this study (61%) than in the previous study, but those who received fentanyl were more likely to experience an adverse event. However, it is unknown if the adverse events in those who received fentanyl might have been less common if the dose of propofol had been reduced. The addition of opioid analgesia is known to allow lower and potentially safer doses of sedative agents (Olmos, Ballester, Vidarte, et al., 2000; Reves, Glass, Lubarsky, et al., 2005), but no adjustments in propofol dose were made for those who received fentanyl (i.e., there were no significant differences in the mean initial and cumulative amounts of propofol administered to those who had an adverse event and those who did not). ASA classification is another important consideration when evaluating the incidence of adverse events in this study. Of those who experienced an adverse event, 24% were classified ASA III, and only 5% of those who did not experience an adverse event were classified ASA III. The ASA classification of those who received fentanyl is unknown, so that relationship cannot be fully evaluated either. The researchers appropriately concluded that an association between opioid use and hypoxia should not be interpreted as proving a cause-effect relationship.

Of concern is the apparent general lack of attention to analgesia during propofol sedation for very painful procedures. Some of the studies suggest that providing analgesia increases adverse events, but not enough information is provided to adequately evaluate this or to determine whether the noted adverse events have a detrimental effect on patient outcomes. That is, further research is needed to determine if transient hypoventilation and brief hypoxemia that are as easily corrected as they appear to have been in the previously discussed studies are harmful.

In summary, it is important for those who provide procedural sedation to remember that low doses of propofol do not provide sufficient analgesia (Frolich, Price, Robinson, et al., 2005; Odom-Forren, Watson, 2005; Zacny, Coalson, Young, et al., 1996). Protocols for propofol administration for procedures thought to be painful should include the administration of analgesia regardless of the amnestic qualities of the sedative agent used. At all times, the goals of procedural sedation are to provide both pain control and sedation (Peck, Down, 2009).

The Propofol Controversy

The studies described above demonstrate that propofol is increasingly being administered for procedural sedation outside of the operating room and monitored settings; however, its administration by professionals who are not trained anesthesia providers is controversial (Institute for Safe Medication Practices, 2006; Odom-Forren, 2006; Sullivan, 2006). Concerns over the safety of this practice are based on the unique pharmacokinetics and pharmacodynamics of the drug as well as reports of near-fatal and fatal respiratory events (Institute for Safe Medication Practices, 2006). Anesthesia provider groups, such as the American Association of Nurse Anesthetists (AANA) and the American Society of Anesthesiologists (ASA) oppose propofol administration by non-anesthetists because of the rapid and profound changes in depth of sedation that can occur with the drug and a lack of antagonistic agents to reverse its effects (AANA, ASA, 2004). A survey conducted of monitoring practices

during sedation by non-anesthetists revealed alarming findings including a failure to follow guidelines and protocols in 30%, inadequate monitoring (e.g., 47% failure to use ECG monitoring, 0% use of capnography), Advanced Cardiac Life Support (ACLS) certification in only 29% of providers, and a 22% incidence of adverse effects during procedures (Fanning, 2008). Nevertheless, the American College of Gastroenterology (ACG) and others have petitioned the United States Food and Drug Administration to change propofol labeling to allow non-anesthetists to administer the drug (United States Food and Drug Administration, (U.S. FDA), 2005c). In an effort to better control the quality of non-anesthetist administration of propofol during endoscopy, the American Association for the Study of Liver Diseases, ACG, American Gastroenterological Association, and American Society for Gastrointestinal Endoscopy issued a joint position statement that discusses the safety of this practice and provides recommendations for non-anesthetists' training prior to administration (Vargo, Cohen, Rex, et al., 2009).

Research has shown no major complications with nurse-administered propofol sedation (NAPS) in 11,000 patients in the GI setting (Odom-Forren, 2008). However, the studies that have been conducted so far on non-anesthetist propofol administration for procedural sedation make it difficult to adequately evaluate its safety. The authors of the joint position statement described in the preceding paragraph concluded that sedation administered by non-anesthetists appears to be as safe as that of standard sedation, but that the worldwide experience with this practice is insufficient to draw definitive conclusions about its safety (Vargo, Cohen, Rex, et al., 2009). Randomized, placebo-controlled trials are lacking, and there are no well-defined and agreed-upon criteria of what signifies an adverse sedation event. Further, the clinical significance of transient hypoxemia that can occur during propofol administration is unknown (Weaver, Hauter, Brizendine, et al., 2007). Safe dosing guidelines are also lacking. As discussed, the administration of sedation without analgesia for painful procedures is a serious error, yet this practice appears to be widely accepted in part because the impact of analgesic administration on propofol dosing and adverse effects has not been fully evaluated. The ability of non-anesthetists to adequately address analgesia during propofol sedation is a concern and requires further examination.

Boards of nursing have confirmed that the administration of moderate sedation by competent RNs is within the scope of RN practice; however, Odom-Forren (2006) emphasizes that propofol sedation is often deep (not moderate) sedation and borders on anesthesia. Regardless of the outcome of this controversy and the FDA decision regarding labeling, RN scope of practice is determined ultimately by the nurse's individual state board of nursing. Nurses should be aware of their scope of practice, state board of nursing's opinions, and institutional policies and procedures regarding the administration and monitoring of agents such as propofol.

Fospropofol

Fospropofol (Lucedra) is a relatively new GABA agonist approved for use in adults undergoing diagnostic or therapeutic procedures in a monitored care setting. It is a prodrug of propofol with very similar pharmacokinetic and pharmacodynamic characteristics. The same concerns about safety apply to fospropofol as apply to propofol, and like propofol, it is approved for administration only by trained anesthesia providers, such as nurse anesthetists and anesthesiologists. Research and clinical experience with this drug were lacking at the time of publication.

Dexmedetomidine

Dexmedetomidine (Precedex) is an alpha$_2$-adrenergic agonist that was initially approved in the United States for IV sedation in intubated patients and later approved for IV sedation before and during surgery and other procedures in nonintubated patients. It is used perioperatively as an adjunct to general and IV regional anesthesia (Kamibayashi, Maze, 2000; Reves, Glass, Lubarsky, et al., 2005) and has been shown to produce a significant opioid dose-sparing effect (Akin, Aribogan, Arslan, 2008; Arain, Ruehlow, Uhrich, et al., 2004; Buvandendran, Kroin, 2007; Golembiewski, 2005; Takrouri, Seraj, Channa, et al., 2002; Panzer, Moitra, Sladen, 2009). It has been added to morphine for administration via IV patient-controlled analgesia (PCA) (no basal rate) to produce superior analgesia, less nausea, and no sedation and adverse hemodynamic effects compared with morphine-only IV PCA (no basal rate) in 100 women following hysterectomy (Lin, Yeh, Lin, et al., 2009). Reports of remarkable reductions in high opioid doses without loss of pain control have implications for the treatment of opioid-induced hyperalgesia (OIH) (Kamibayashi, Maze, 2000) (see Chapter 11 for more on OIH).

The drug has demonstrated a median onset of IV analgesia of 7.8 minutes (Gomez-Vasquez, Hernandez-Salazar, Hernandez-Jimenez, et al., 2007). By the intranasal route, dexmedetomidine had a 45-minute onset of sedation with a peak at 90 to 150 minutes and no effect on pain pressure threshold in 18 healthy volunteers (Yuen, Irwin, Hui, et al., 2007). It is metabolized in the liver by the cytochrome P450 enzyme system and excreted in the urine and feces. It has a very rapid distribution phase (half-life of 6 minutes) and a terminal half-life of 2 hours. Its pharmacokinetic properties are unchanged by age, weight, or renal or hepatic failure (Reves, Glass, Lubarsky, et al., 2005), which indicates that dose adjustment may not be necessary for these factors.

Goal-Directed Sedation in the Critically Ill

Benzodiazepines, such as lorazepam (Ativan) and midazolam (Versed) (see pp. 724-725), and the IV sedative/hypnotic propofol (Diprivan) (see pp. 718-722) have been the most commonly used sedation agents in critically ill patients in the ICU for many years; however, dexmedetomidine may be a better choice for this purpose (Riker, Shehabi, Bokesch, et al., 2009). The drug does not produce respiratory depression, and it has both analgesic and anxiolytic properties (Golembiewski, 2005; Takrouri, Seraj, Channa, et al., 2002; Wunsch, Kress, 2009). It has also been found to provide hemodynamic stability, cause minimal postsedation cognitive impairment, and allow easy arousal of the patient such that coherent communication between caregiver and patient is possible (Venn, Grounds, 2001). It is reported to be the only drug to both reduce the development of delirium and improve the resolution of delirium in the ICU (Riker, Shehabi, Bokesch, et al., 2009).

Recommended dexmedetomidine dosing for goal-directed sedation in the critically ill is an initial IV bolus dose of 1 mcg/kg over 10 minutes followed by a maintenance infusion of 0.2 to 0.7 mcg/kg/h for 24 hours (Pandharipande, Ely, Maze, 2006; Clinical Pharmacology, 2010). The drug is administered by an infusion device that does not allow free-flow delivery, and to help ensure accurate dose delivery, programming should be verified by the independent double-check process (see Chapter 17).

A barrier to more common use of dexmedetomidine in the United States is the U.S. FDA–imposed maximum dose of 0.7 mcg/kg/h and use of the drug for up to 24 hours only. Research suggests that these restrictions should be reconsidered (Brush, Kress, 2009; Panzer, Moitra, Sladen, 2009). A study conducted in two tertiary ICUs obtained approval to administer dexmedetomidine for longer than 24 hours and randomized 106 mechanically ventilated adults to receive either dexmedetomidine or lorazepam sedation for up to 120 days (Pandharipande, Pun, Herr, et al., 2007). Patients who received dexmedetomidine experienced more days alive without delirium or coma, a lower prevalence of coma, more time at their sedation goal, and a better 28-day mortality rate. The 12-month time to death was 363 days in the dexmedetomidine group compared with 188 days in the lorazepam group. A large multicenter, 2-year, randomized controlled trial compared midazolam and dexmedetomidine in ventilated ICU patients (Riker, Shehabi, Bokesch, et al., 2009). The researchers received approval to administer dexmedetomidine in up to twice the approved dose for up to 30 days (Wunsch, Kress, 2009). While time at targeted sedation level did not differ, those who received dexmedetomidine experienced less time on the ventilator and less delirium, tachycardia, and hypertension than those who received midazolam. There was a greater incidence of bradycardia in the dexmedetomidine group, and 4.9% of the bradycardic patients required treatment that included titration or interruption of the study drug and use of atropine.

Dexmedetomidine is also used for monitored anesthesia care. A prospective, double-blind, multicenter trial randomized 326 patients prior to elective surgery or procedure to receive dexmedetomidine 0.5 mcg/kg, or dexmedetomidine 1 mcg/kg, or placebo for an initial loading dose administered over 10 minutes followed by a maintenance (titrated) infusion of 0.2 to 1 mcg/kg/h of dexmedetomidine in all of the patients (Candiotti, Bergese, Bokesch, et al., 2010). All patients were given a local anesthetic block for their surgery or procedure. Those who received dexmedetomidine (in either dose) required lower midazolam and fentanyl doses compared with placebo. The anesthesiologists reported greater ease of achieving and maintaining targeted sedation and higher satisfaction with dexmedetomidine. Patient satisfaction was also higher with dexmedetomidine. The most common dexmedetomidine-induced adverse effects were bradycardia and hypotension, which were described as mild to moderate, and there were fewer episodes of bradypnea and oxygen desaturation in those treated with dexmedetomidine.

Dexmedetomidine has also been compared with propofol. One study randomized critically ill postoperative patients to receive either propofol or dexmedetomidine and found no differences between the groups in time of ideal sedation and time to extubation, and there were no clinically significant adverse effects in either group (Venn, Grounds, 2001). However, those who received propofol required three times more opioid than those who received dexmedetomidine. Patients who received dexmedetomidine also had lower heart rates during infusion, which the researchers proposed may help to protect against myocardial infarction (MI). An early meta-analysis called for more randomized trials but concluded that alpha$_2$-adrenergic agonists reduce mortality and MI following vascular surgery (Wijeysundera, Naik, Beattie, 2003); however, a later meta-analysis of dexmedetomidine's effect on CV outcomes after noncardiac surgery showed a trend but no statistically significant improvement in cardiac outcomes (Biccard, Goga, de Beurs, 2008). Further research is needed to draw conclusions (Panzer, Moitra, Sladen, 2009).

The lack of a respiratory depressant effect with dexmedetomidine has implications for its use during weaning from mechanical ventilation and extubation as administration can be continued throughout these processes (Panzer, Moitra, Sladen, 2009). A study of patients who had failed previous attempts at ventilator weaning secondary to agitation unresponsive to traditional sedatives described successful extubation of 14 of the 20 patients who were given dexmedetomidine (Arpino, Klafatas, Thompson, 2008). Dexmedetomidine has also been reported to facilitate terminal weaning and withdrawal of ventilatory support at end of life in palliative care (Kent, Kaufman, Lowy, 2005).

In addition to the previously discussed studies, numerous others have reported that dexmedetomidine allows a reduction in concomitant sedative and analgesic use and produces minimal adverse effects (Arpino, Klaftas, Thompson, 2008; Bulow, Barbosa, Rocha, 2007; Gurbet, Basagan-Mogol, Turker, et al., 2006; Siobal, Kallet, Kivett, et al., 2006; Unlugenc, Gunduz, Guler et al., 2005). These findings have implications in particular for patients at high risk for respiratory depression, such as older surgical patients (Akin, Aribogan, Arslan, 2008) and obese patients undergoing bariatric surgery (Ramsay, 2006).

Analgesia

Dexmedetomidine has analgesic properties but is not appropriate as a sole analgesic for painful conditions or procedures, and it should not be used alone in patients receiving a neuromuscular blocking agent (Venn, Grounds, 2001). A study comparing dexmedetomidine (0.3 mcg/kg for 50 minutes) to propacetamol (IV acetaminophen, 2 g for 10 minutes) following knee surgery found dexmedetomidine produced comparable analgesia but higher total morphine requirements at 8 hours postoperatively (Gomez-Vasquez, Hernandez-Salazar, Hernandez-Jimenez, et al., 2007). A cross-over study randomized six healthy volunteers to receive infusions of the opioid remifentanil or dexmedetomidine during painful heat stimuli (Cortinez, Hsu, Sum-Ping, et al., 2004). Withdrawal from painful stimuli was recorded for any subject who was unarousable and unable to report pain using the VAS. The magnitude of the analgesic effect of dexmedetomidine was smaller than that of remifentanil, confirming that alpha$_2$-agonists are not as effective analgesics as opioids. This research supports the observation that dexmedetomidine has an analgesic ceiling (Kent, Kaufman, Lowy, 2005).

An exception to this was described in an interesting letter to the editor that reported profound analgesia with a dexmedetomidine loading dose (1 mcg/kg) and infusion (0.5 mcg/kg/h) in two adults with severe pain associated with sickle cell vaso-occlusive crisis (VOC) that was refractory to opioid analgesia (Phillips, Gadiraju, Dickey, et al., 2007). Complete pain relief was achieved with dexmedetomidine without opioid analgesia. The infusion was gradually reduced by 0.1 mcg/kg/h and discontinued after 4 hours. There were no adverse effects, and both patients were discharged reporting no pain. An observational study reported that patients' memories of their ICU experiences were better in patients who received dexmedetomidine than in those who received propofol, and patients in both groups recalled "discomfort" but no pain during mechanical ventilation (Venn, Grounds, 2001). Nevertheless, until research and more clinical experience with the drug demonstrate otherwise, opioid analgesia should always be provided when dexmedetomidine is administered to patients with painful pathology and those undergoing painful procedures.

Procedural Sedation

Research on dexmedetomidine for sedation during painful procedures has contributed to a better understanding of the limitations of the drug's analgesic effectiveness and its adverse effect profile in this setting. One study randomized 64 patients to receive an initial IV dose (1 mcg/kg) followed by IV infusion (0.2 mcg/kg) of dexmedetomidine, or an initial IV dose of meperidine (1 mg/kg) plus midazolam (0.05 mg/kg), or an initial IV dose of fentanyl (0.1 to 0.2 mg) for outpatient colonoscopy (Jalowiecki, Rudner, Gonciarz, et al., 2005). Supplemental fentanyl was required in 47%, 42.8%, and 79.2% of those who received dexmedetomidine, meperidine plus midazolam, and fentanyl, respectively. Adverse effects, such as nausea and vertigo, were greatest, and time to discharge readiness was longest in those who received dexmedetomidine. Dose-dependent adverse effects have been noted by others, reinforcing the importance of administering the lowest effective dexmedetomidine dose (Riker, Shehabi, Bokesch, et al., 2009; Venn, Grounds, 2001). This research suggests that lower loading doses and continuous infusion rates should be administered for patients undergoing procedures than for ventilated patients undergoing goal-directed sedation in the ICU.

A cross-over, placebo-controlled study found that intranasal dexmedetomidine provided effective, well-tolerated, and convenient sedation in 18 healthy volunteers (Yuen, Irwin, Hui, et al., 2007). More research and clinical experience with the use of dexmedetomidine by this noninvasive route of administration for procedural pain is needed.

Adverse Effects

Dexmedetomidine is generally well-tolerated. The most common adverse effects are bradycardia and hypotension (Gomez-Vasquez, Hernandez-Salazar, Hernandez-Jimenez, et al., 2007). It has been shown to blunt perioperative hypertensive responses without causing hypotension or bradycardia in patients undergoing craniotomy, a procedure frequently complicated by hypertensive episodes (Bekker, Sturaitis, Bloom, et al., 2008). As discussed, some researchers have proposed that lower heart rates during dexmedetomidine infusion may help to protect against MI (Venn, Grounds, 2001); however, further research is needed (Panzer, Moitra, Sladen, 2009).

The beneficial respiratory effect profile of dexmedetomidine was demonstrated in a study comparing it with the ultra-short–acting opioid analgesic remifentanil in 6 healthy volunteers (Hsu, Cortinez, Robertson, et al., 2004). Remifentanil decreased respiratory rate and minute ventilation and produced respiratory acidosis and apneic episodes resulting in desaturation. In contrast, dexmedetomidine did not produce any respiratory depression and, in fact, decreased the apnea/hypopnea index and exhibited similarities to natural sleep.

A case report described pyrexia of 39° C (102.2° F) in a 59-year-old man who was receiving dexmedetomidine and that resolved when the drug was discontinued (Okabe, Takeda, Akada, et al., 2009). All other potential causes of fever, such as infection, had been eliminated.

As mentioned, dexmedetomidine causes minimal post-sedation cognitive impairment (Venn, Grounds, 2001) and reduces ICU delirium (Riker, Shehabi, Bokesch, et al., 2009). Research has shown excellent tolerability in older patients and a very high satisfaction rate with dexmedetomidine (Akin, Aribogan, Arslan, 2008).

Indications

Dexmedetomidine is indicated for purposeful, goal-directed sedation to control agitation and anxiety in the critically ill ventilated patient in the ICU setting (Brush, Kress 2009). It is also approved for sedation during procedures in nonintubated patients outside of the ICU. Dexmedetomidine is not adequate as a sole analgesic; therefore, an appropriate analgesic, such as an opioid, must be administered when the drug is used in patients who have painful underlying pathology and prior to and during any procedure thought to be painful.

Many hospitals restrict the administration of dexmedetomidine to specific clinical areas, such as the ICU and ED. Nurses should be aware of their scope of practice, state board of nursing's opinions, and institutional policies and procedures regarding the administration and monitoring of agents such as dexmedetomidine.

Benzodiazepines

Benzodiazepines, such as midazolam (Versed), lorazepam (Ativan), and diazepam (Valium), have been used for procedural sedation for many years. An extensive systematic review of the various agents used for moderate sedation during endoscopic procedures found marked variability in studies and problems in pooling data but established benzodiazepines as first-choice agents for these procedures (McQuaid, Laine, 2008). At the time of the review, 85% of endoscopists in the United States used midazolam, and 10% used diazepam. Physicians cited their preference for midazolam based on its faster onset, shorter duration, and a belief that the drug has sufficient amnestic properties. There was high physician satisfaction with the level of sedation achieved and a high patient satisfaction rate with the use of midazolam. However, the researchers concluded that midazolam-based regimens have longer sedation and recovery times than propofol-based regimens (see earlier in the chapter for propofol).

Of interest, 3 patients experienced transient apnea in a study that administered a combination of ketamine and midazolam for procedural sedation (Chudnofsky, Weber, Stoyanoff, et al., 2000) (see discussion in following paragraphs on ketamine). All 3 of these patients weighed in excess of 97 kg and received large doses of midazolam, which led the researchers to recommend midazolam dosing based on ideal rather than actual weight.

As mentioned throughout this chapter, pain control should be a primary goal during painful procedures. Benzodiazepines can diminish pain associated with musculoskeletal spasm, reduce anxiety, and at high doses produce amnesia; however, they lack analgesic properties for acute tissue injury (American Pain Society, 2003; Pasero, McCaffery, 1999). The benzodiazepine dose required to produce amnesia varies widely among patients. Many individuals recall pain and other unpleasant procedural experiences when benzodiazepines are used as a sole agent during painful procedures. It is encouraging to note that most endoscopists believe a combination of a benzodiazepine and opioid is superior to either drug alone; however, it is concerning that 25% of procedures were performed with just a benzodiazepine (McQuaid, Laine, 2008). This is likely due to a fear of opioid-induced respiratory depression. Research is lacking regarding the effectiveness of combining the two types of drugs for procedural sedation; however, several studies have established efficacy and opioid dose-sparing effects with the use of multimodal strategies (e.g., adding ketorolac or celecoxib to opioids) for acute pain, and the same principles of providing the lowest effective opioid dose can be applied during procedures (see Chapter 12). The importance of providing adequate analgesia cannot be overemphasized. This is especially important for patients who must endure repetitive procedures (Pasero, McCaffery, 1999).

Ketamine

Ketamine has been discussed elsewhere in this section for its use in treating various types of intractable persistent pain (see Chapter 23) and postoperative and other types of acute pain (see Chapter 26). See Chapter 23 for mechanisms and adverse effects and Box 23-1 on pp. 675-677 for administration guidelines. Following is a brief discussion of its use for sedation and analgesia during painful procedures.

Low doses of ketamine have been administered for many years to provide procedural sedation, particularly in children (Mistry, Nahata, 2005). For procedural sedation, ketamine is usually combined with other agents, such as opioids or benzodiazepines. A drawback of opioids and benzodiazepines is that they can produce dose-dependent respiratory depression. In contrast, ketamine produces dose-sparing effects and is rarely associated with respiratory depression. Its addition allows lower doses of these other agents and reduces the likelihood of respiratory depression.

Midazolam is one of the most common benzodiazepines combined with ketamine for sedation. The drug can both enhance sedation and minimize psychotomimetic

and other adverse effects (Deng, Xiao, Luo, et al., 2001). Patients (N = 77) undergoing painful procedures in the ED setting were given 0.07 mg/kg of IV midazolam followed by IV ketamine 2 mg/kg over a 2-minute period (Chudnofsky, Weber, Stoyanoff, et al., 2000). Procedures were begun immediately after ketamine administration. The mean dose of midazolam administered was 5.6 mg, and the mean dose of ketamine was 159.1 mg. Adverse effects were considered minimal; 5 patients reported unpleasant dreaming, 3 experienced transient apnea, and 2 experienced emergence anxiety. As mentioned earlier, all 3 of the patients who experienced apnea weighed in excess of 97 kg and received large doses of midazolam. The mean time to discharge alertness was 63.4 minutes. All patients in this study, including those who experienced an adverse effect, stated that they would choose the same drugs to sedate them for future painful procedures.

A midazolam-ketamine combination has also been administered via IV PCA. A PCA dose of 10 mg of ketamine and 0.5 mg of midazolam per mL was self administered by 44 adult patients during painful burn dressing changes (MacPherson, Woods, Penfold, 2008). The incidence of adverse effects was low; hallucinations were the most common adverse effect, occurring in 11 of the 44 patients. Both patients and staff rated the method as highly effective.

The undesirable effects of ketamine have led some experts to recommend its prescription and management only by those skilled in pain management and anesthesiology (Bell, 2009; Cvrcek, 2008). Palliative care specialists are also among those knowledgeable in the safe administration of the drug. Some hospitals restrict the administration of ketamine to specific clinical areas, such as the ICU, palliative care, and the ED. Nurses should be aware of their scope of practice, state board of nursing's opinions, and institutional policies and procedures regarding the administration and monitoring of agents such as ketamine.

Conclusion

Benzodiazepines have a long history as first-line drugs for procedural sedation, and ketamine has been used extensively for pediatric sedation and is increasingly used in adults for procedural sedation. Propofol and dexmedetomidine have become first-line agents for the administration of purposeful, goal-directed sedation such as in ventilated critically ill patients. They are also used with increasing frequency for procedural pain management. A major objective of goal-directed sedation and procedural sedation is to provide both analgesia and sedation. This underscores the importance of carefully considering the analgesic properties of the agents to be administered and providing appropriate analgesia such as opioids whenever indicated by the presence of a painful pathology, condition, or procedure.

Chapter 28 Local Anesthetics for Procedural Pain

RESEARCH shows that many procedures are painful and distressing to patients, and that greater attention to relieving procedural pain is needed. Clinicians are encouraged to form task forces to establish policies and procedures that address the provision of adequate analgesia and anesthesia prior to painful procedures, including minor procedures, such as venipuncture. Local anesthetics are first-line analgesics and anesthetics for procedural pain. They are versatile and well-tolerated by most patients. The local anesthetics discussed in this chapter include lidocaine infiltration, topical formulations of lidocaine alone or in combination with other local anesthetics, and other less used local anesthetics. All of the topical local anesthetics vary in the length of application time and duration of local anesthetic action, making these characteristics important considerations when determining the best formulation for the specific procedure. The mechanisms of action underlying local anesthetics have been discussed in Chapter 23.

Infiltrated Lidocaine

Lidocaine 1% to 2% is the local anesthetic of choice when administered by infiltration at the site prior to painful procedures, ranging from IV starts to skin suturing, because it has a fast onset and can be administered in a wide range of doses with minimal risk of toxicity (Pasero, Wong, 1997). The onset of analgesia is rapid (i.e., within 2 minutes), and anesthesia lasts 1.5 to 2 hours (Achar, Kundu, 2002; Strichartz, Berde, 2005). The maximum recommended adult dose is 4 mg/kg, not to exceed 280 mg (Achar, Kundu, 2002).

Research shows that many patients fear dermal procedures, particularly venipuncture and IV catheter placement (Windle, Kwan, Warwick, et al., 2006). Lidocaine 1% given intradermally to anesthetize the site prior to venous or arterial puncture is an inexpensive, easy, and effective way of addressing this fear by minimizing the associated pain (see Figure 24-1 on p. 685 for intradermal site of action). All state boards of nursing in the United States approve this nursing function, and the Infusion Nurses Society Standards of Practice call for the nurse to consider providing local anesthesia prior to venipuncture (Infusion Nurses Society, 2006). Despite this, nurses, who perform a large number of venipunctures, rarely use local anesthetic even though they would prefer a local anesthetic if they were to undergo this type of procedure (Valero Marco, Martinez Castillo, Macia Solera, 2008). A lack of knowledge is the most common reason for failure to provide dermal local anesthetic, which underscores the need for nurse managers and educators to develop policies and procedures that support the nurse's use of local anesthetics and to teach nurses who perform painful dermal procedures how to competently use them (Brown, 2002).

To administer intradermal local anesthesia, a wheal of approximately 1-cm diameter (approximately 0.05 to 0.1 mL) of lidocaine 1% is injected intradermally with a 29- or 30-gauge needle over or just distal to the vein or artery (Pasero, McCaffery, 1999). Patients often report burning and stinging with intradermal injection of lidocaine. This is caused by the acidic nature of the lidocaine solution and can be reduced by adding sodium bicarbonate to normalize the pH (buffering) (Strichartz, Berde, 2005; Wong, Pasero, 1997) (Box 28-1). Administration of buffered lidocaine 1% is recommended 2 minutes prior to venipuncture and has been shown to produce superior anesthesia compared with unbuffered lidocaine 1%, diphenhydramine 1%, and 0.9% saline placebo (Xia, Chen, Tibbits, et al., 2002). Warming the lidocaine by rolling the syringe between the hands several times and

Box 28-1 | Preparation and Use of Buffered Lidocaine

SUPPLIES

- 8.4% sodium bicarbonate (1 mEq/mL)
- 1% lidocaine
- TB syringe with removable needle (use larger syringe for larger doses), 30-gauge needle

INSTRUCTIONS

- Use 1 part sodium bicarbonate to 10 parts lidocaine (e.g., draw up 1 mL of lidocaine and 0.1 mL of sodium bicarbonate).
- Change needle used to withdraw BL to 30-gauge needle for intradermal injection.
- For venipuncture or port access, inject 0.1 mL or less (child) or 0.5 mL or less (adult) BL intradermally directly over intended puncture site; anesthesia occurs almost immediately.
- Suggested maximum dose of lidocaine for local anesthesia is 4.5 mg/kg.
- If buffering lidocaine vial (e.g., 20 mL lidocaine with 2 mL sodium bicarbonate), use solution for 7 days or less and preferably when freshly prepared.

BL, Buffered lidocaine; *TB*, tuberculin.

Modified from Wong, D. L. (1997). *Whaley and Wong's essentials of pediatric nursing*, ed. 5, St Louis, Mosby.

slowing the speed of injection can also reduce the pain associated with intradermal lidocaine. Lidocaine has been warmed to 40° to 42° C in a controlled warm-water bath but should never be warmed in a microwave (Achar, Kundu, 2002; Pasero, McCaffery, 1999).

Intradermal lidocaine was shown to produce superior anesthesia compared with another antihistamine (chlorpheniramine) and midazolam in healthy volunteers (Orhan, Yuksel, Bilgin, et al., 2007). However, bacteriostatic saline may be an even better choice than lidocaine to anesthetize the site prior to a venous or arterial puncture. A randomized controlled trial administered lidocaine 1%, bacteriostatic normal saline, or no intradermal anesthesia to 221 adults prior to outpatient or same-day surgery (Windle, Kwan, Warwick, et al., 2006). Venipuncture was significantly less painful with both lidocaine and bacteriostatic saline compared with placebo, and bacteriostatic saline produced better anesthesia than lidocaine. It is important to note that the saline must be bacteriostatic, because it is the 0.9% benzyl alcohol preservative that produces the local anesthetic effect (Pasero, McCaffery, 1999).

Infiltrated lidocaine, particularly when buffered, provides an excellent option for controlling pain during more extensive procedures as well. A randomized controlled trial administered buffered lidocaine or unbuffered lidocaine to patients prior to posterior iliac crest bone marrow biopsy (Ruegg, Curran, Lamb, 2009). Those who received buffered lidocaine reported significantly lower pain scores leading the researchers to conclude that the use of unbuffered lidocaine for such a procedure should be questioned. Others have found similar results with buffered lidocaine (Vossinakis, Stavroulaki, Paleochorlidis, et al., 2004; Younis, Bhutiani, 2004) and warmed lidocaine (Yiannakopoulos, 2004) for other procedures.

Femoral artery sheath removal is a painful procedure, but there is no consensus on how best to manage the pain. Infiltrated lidocaine may not be the best choice for this particular procedure. Patients in one study were randomized to receive IV fentanyl and midazolam, or lidocaine 1% infiltrated around the femoral sheath, or both treatments, or neither treatment (Kiat Ang, Leung, Lo, et al., 2006). The highest pain scores and the highest incidence of vasovagal reactions were in the group who received local anesthesia only. These findings led the researchers to caution against the use of lidocaine infiltration prior to femoral sheath removal and suggest IV fentanyl and midazolam instead.

Adverse effects are rare with infiltrated local anesthetics such as lidocaine because there is minimal systemic absorption when they are given in small amounts for minor procedures. However, at low doses, local anesthetics have been known to produce vasoconstriction and hypertension in some patients (Achar, Kundu, 2002). The addition of epinephrine can slow absorption but can also further increase vasoconstriction and should not be used on tissues with end arteriole blood supply, such as fingers, toes, the penis, nose, or ears (Pasero, McCaffery, 1999). Signs of systemic toxicity include metallic taste, tinnitus, perioral numbness, lightheadedness, and confusion. If not detected, this can proceed to tremors, shivering, and ultimately seizures and respiratory and cardiovascular collapse (Achar, Kundu, 2002). Allergy to amide local anesthetics is rare but is a contraindication to use.

EMLA

Eutectic mixture of local anesthetics (EMLA), available only by prescription in the United States (nonprescription in some other countries, e.g., Canada), combines lidocaine 2.5% and prilocaine 2.5% in a cream for topical application. Most anesthetic agents exist as solids preventing efficient skin penetration (Kundu, Achar, 2002). However, a eutectic mixture, which has a melting point lower than that of the two anesthetics alone, permits the drug to penetrate the skin (see Figure 24-1 on p. 685 for action site).

To create an area of dense sensory loss using EMLA, a relatively thick application must remain in contact with the skin for at least 1 hour (2.5 g [½ of a 5 g tube] per 20 to 25 cm² [2 inch by 2 inch] area to a maximum of 10 g). This is usually covered with an occlusive dressing, but occlusion is optional and intended to help keep the drug in place. The application site can be expanded as needed for major dermal procedures. Clinical experience suggests that a 90- to 120-minute application time produces the best results. This time should be reduced significantly and the drug removed promptly when EMLA is applied to male genital skin and female genital mucous membranes (see EMLA drug package insert). The depth of anesthesia is approximately 3 mm after a 60-minute application and 5 mm after 120 minutes (Kundu, Achar, 2002). The 60- to 120-minute application time is a noted drawback of the drug because it requires preplanning (Eidelman, Weiss, Lau, et al., 2005); however, most procedures are not emergencies and allow for this. A benefit of EMLA is a comparatively long duration of anesthesia, reaching maximal anesthesia at 2 to 3 hours and lasting up to 2 hours after the cream is removed (Wong, 2003). This is an advantage for longer procedures or when pain is expected after the procedure is completed. Another commonly used topical local anesthetic, L.M.X.4, has a shorter duration of up to 60 minutes (see later in the chapter).

The manufacturer (AstraZeneca) recommends that EMLA be applied to intact skin and genital mucous membranes only; however, it has also been applied to or around extremity lacerations and other types of open wounds (Briggs, Nelson, 2003; Kundu, Achar, 2002). Variable penetration is reported when EMLA is applied to hands and soles of the feet (Kundu, Achar, 2002), and it should not be applied to eyes as this can result in severe irritation and corneal abrasion.

An extensive systematic review of research on local anesthetics for painful dermal procedures reported inconsistent findings with regard to comparisons between EMLA and infiltrated local anesthetic; half of the research favored EMLA, and half favored infiltrated local anesthetic (Eidelman, Weiss, Lau, et al., 2005). EMLA and L.M.X.4 were equally efficacious in this review, but the latter was described as preferable because it is commercially available, has a more rapid onset of action (L.M.X.4 = 30-minute application time), and is less expensive (Eidelman, Weiss, Lau, et al., 2005).

EMLA has been shown to reduce pain of needle puncture when applied prior to local anesthetic blockade (Raber, Scattoni, Roscigno, et al., 2008; Samson, Minville, Chassery, et al., 2007), IV catheter placement, and lab blood tests (Eidelman, Weiss, Lau, et al., 2005). A Cochrane Collaboration Review concluded that EMLA produced effective pain relief for venous leg ulcer debridement, but suggested further research to determine its impact on ulcer healing (Briggs, Nelson, 2003). A case report described the development of hemorrhagic margins around leg ulcers that led to ischemia and necrosis following application of EMLA for debridement (Stahl, Meyer, Haas, et al., 2008). EMLA was ineffective for treatment of pain during vasectomy (Thomas, Nguyen, Dhar, et al., 2008) and amniocentesis (Pongrojpaw, Somprasit, Chanthasenanont, 2008).

The use of topical analgesics is strongly encouraged in pediatric patients undergoing painful procedures. As a result, the vast majority of research showing EMLA to be safe and effective for painful procedures has been conducted in that population and findings extrapolated to adults. The reader is referred to the pediatric literature for more research. Some of the studies showing efficacy in adults are listed as follows.

- Fine-needle aspiration biopsy (Gursoy, Ertugrul, Sahin, et al., 2007)
- Transrectal prostate biopsy (Giannarini, Autorino, Valent, et al., 2009; Tiong, Liew, Samuel, et al., 2007)
- Hysterosalpingography (Liberty, Gal, Halevy-Shalem, et al., 2007)
- Shockwave lithotripsy (Kumar, Gupta, Hemal, et al., 2007)
- Perineal repair (Franchi, Cromi, Scarperi, et al., 2009)
- Hemorrhoidectomy (Shiau, Hung, Chen, et al., 2007; Shiau, Su, Chen, et al., 2008)
- Chest tube removal (Valenzuela, Rosen, 1999)
- Fiberoptic endotracheal intubation (Larijani, Cypel, Gratz, et al., 2000)
- Variety of cosmetic dermatologic procedures (Kaweski, 2008; Railan, Alster, 2007).

The most common adverse effects associated with EMLA are mild, transient local skin reactions, including erythema, blanching, edema, and rare blistering. Several studies have shown that when EMLA is applied as recommended, serum lidocaine and prilocaine concentrations are approximately 0.12 mcg/mL and 0.07 mcg/mL, respectively, which are well below toxicity levels. (The signs of local anesthetic toxicity are described in Chapter 23.) Caution is recommended when EMLA is used concomitantly with other local anesthetics or antiarrhythmics, such as mexiletine and tocainide, which can result in an additive effect. Methemoglobinemia, which impairs the ability of hemoglobin to transport oxygen, has been linked to the use of EMLA, caused by systemic absorption of prilocaine. Some patients, such as premature infants, are predisposed to methemoglobinemia, and co-administration of certain medications, such as phenytoin and nitroglycerin, can increase the incidence of this condition. The incidence is minimized when precautions are taken such as not exceeding the maximum recommended dose and removing EMLA promptly after use (Shachor-Meyouhas, Galbraith, Shavit, 2008). A rare adverse effect is petechial and purpuric eruption following EMLA application (Roldan-Marin, de-la Barreda Becerril, 2009). Allergy to amide local anesthetics is a contraindication to the use of EMLA.

L.M.X.4

L.M.X.4 (lidocaine cream 4%, formerly ELAMax) is another commonly used topical local anesthetic for procedural pain management. Advantages of this drug over EMLA are that it is commercially available in the United States and has a shorter 30-minute application time. This shorter application time is a major benefit given the current focus on reduced length of stay in all health care settings.

L.M.X.4 is applied by rubbing a small amount into the site for about 30 seconds followed by application of a 2-cm-thick coating. Although optional, this is usually covered with an occlusive dressing to keep the drug in place for the 30-minute application time. As with EMLA, depth of anesthesia increases as application time increases, and the drug should be removed promptly after use. A drawback of L.M.X.4 is a relatively short duration of anesthesia of 30 to 60 minutes after removal (Wong, 2003). Maximum serum concentration following recommended topical application is low at 0.3 mcg/mL. Adverse effects and signs of local anesthetic toxicity associated with L.M.X.4 are similar to other topical local anesthetics except that it does not contain prilocaine so is not associated with methemoglobinemia (see discussion of EMLA regarding this condition).

L.M.X.4 is an appropriate alternative to EMLA. A review of research conducted primarily in children comparing L.M.X.4 and EMLA showed similar efficacy (Wong, 2003). A more recent systematic review of topical anesthetics for dermal pain concluded that although the two are essentially equally efficacious, L.M.X.4 has the previously mentioned advantages of being commercially available, faster acting, and less expensive (Eidelman, Weiss, Lau, et al., 2005).

EMLA's 60- to 120-minute application time has long been cited as a reason for not using it in the emergency department (ED) setting where time is often of the essence. A prospective, double-blind study randomized patients admitted to the ED to receive L.M.X.4 or placebo 30 minutes prior to IV catheter placement (Valdovinos, Reddin, Bernard, et al., 2009). Those who received L.M.X.4 reported significantly lower pain scores even after adjustments were made for difficulty of cannulation.

Synera

Synera (also called S-Caine in some studies) is a 6.25 cm by 7.5 cm (approximately 2.5 inch by 3 inch) oval patch containing lidocaine 70 mg and tetracaine 70 mg that is approved for dermal procedural pain. The patch is unique in that it has an integrated oxygen-activated heating component that enhances the absorption of the local anesthetics. As soon as the patch is removed from its pouch, the component is exposed to air and begins to warm the drug. The backing is peeled off, and the patch is simply placed on the target site (similar to placing an adhesive bandage) and left in place for 20 to 30 minutes. This short appli-

cation time and the ease of application compared with local anesthetic cream formulations are major advantages of this drug. Similar to other topical local anesthetics, serum local anesthetic levels are low when the drug is used as directed (Sethna, Verghese, Hannallah, et al., 2005). Adverse effects and signs of local anesthetic toxicity are similar to other topical local anesthetics (see previous discussion).

Research is lacking on the use of Synera because it is a relatively new topical local anesthetic formulation. A randomized, double-blind, paired study compared Synera with a placebo patch in 40 adult volunteers (Curry, Finkel, 2007). Subjects received simultaneous Synera and placebo patch applications for 20 minutes followed by a vascular access procedure. All subjects favored Synera over placebo; 49% had lower pain scores with Synera compared with 17% with placebo; 63% reported having no pain with Synera compared with 33% with placebo. Adverse effects were mild dermal reactions in 2 patients, which resolved within 3 hours of patch removal. A randomized, double-blind trial applied Synera or a placebo patch 20 minutes prior to venipuncture in children at two different medical centers (Sethna, Verghese, Hannallah, et al., 2005). More than half (59%) of the children who received Synera reported no pain during the procedure compared with 20% of those who received a placebo patch. The most common adverse effects were mild, transient erythema and edema at the application site, which occurred with similar frequency in both groups.

In a double-blind, paired study, 82 volunteers were randomized to receive Synera or EMLA cream prior to vascular access (Sawyer, Febbraro, Masud, et al., 2009). Application time was shorter (as short as 10 minutes in some patients), and analgesia was best with Synera. EMLA was associated with more blanching, and Synera was associated with more erythema.

Synera has major advantages over other topical anesthetic products for superficial procedures such as vascular access in that the product is easy to use (peel and stick), nonmessy, allows uniform distribution of the drug, and has a short application time. Research comparing it with other topical local anesthetics for penetration, duration of anesthesia, patient satisfaction, and cost is needed.

Jet Injection

Jet injection (J-Tip) is a needless device that delivers 0.25 to 0.5 mL lidocaine under pressure into the subcutaneous tissue. It provides rapid (0.2 seconds) anesthesia at a depth of 3 to 8 mm so is appropriate only for very brief dermal procedures such as IV catheter placement or venipuncture for lab work. This product is increasingly used for brief vascular access-type procedures; well-controlled studies comparing it with other local anesthetics for penetration, duration of analgesia, patient satisfaction, and cost are needed. One early study of 72 adults who were consecutively admitted for surgery compared 0.3 mL of 1% plain lidocaine given subcutaneously by J-tip or by conventional syringe and 25-gauge needle prior to large-bore IV cannulation and found significant reductions in pain with J-tip and no difference in number of failed cannulations between the two groups (Cooper, Bromley, Baranowski, et al., 2000). However, these researchers suggested that J-tip appears to be less effective when subcutaneous access is small and recommended its use when the subcutaneous space is deeper. A study of 116 children found J-Tip application before IV cannulation was not painful and produced better anesthesia than EMLA (average EMLA application time was 69 minutes) (Jimenez, Bradford, Seidel, et al., 2006). A later study of 70 children found J-tip produced better anesthesia than a 30-minute application of L.M.X.4 prior to IV cannulation (Spanos, Booth, Koenig, et al., 2008).

A randomized, double-blind study of children undergoing needle insertion in the ED found no difference in local anesthesia between jet-injection lidocaine and jet-injection normal saline, and the researchers concluded that both treatments may provide superior analgesia compared with no pretreatment (Auerbach, Tunik, Mojica, 2009). The majority of patients in the study said they would request the jet device for future needle insertions, and clinicians reported similar visualization with or without the use of a jet device. (See discussion previously in the chapter regarding the anesthetic effect of bacteriostatic normal saline.) A randomized controlled trial of 400 children undergoing peripheral IV cannulation in the ED involved administration of jet injection of saline or jet injection of lidocaine and reported lower pain scores compared with no intervention but no differences in effectiveness between lidocaine and saline jet injection (Lysakowski, Dumont, Tramer, et al., 2003). The researchers also noted that the use of jet injection was not painless (patients reported at least moderate pain because of the treatment itself) and the number of technical failures was large. The researchers suggested carefully considering costs and identifying patients who would benefit most when deciding to routinely use local anesthetic prior to this procedure.

LET, TLC, and TAC

Various mixtures of local anesthetics, including tetracaine, lidocaine, and cocaine (TLC); tetracaine, adrenaline (epinephrine) and cocaine (TAC); and lidocaine, epinephrine, and tetracaine (LET), have been compounded and applied topically for dermal anesthesia. The maximum safe total doses for healthy 70 kg adults are 50 mg of tetracaine, 500 mg of lidocaine, and 200 mg of cocaine (Pasero, McCaffery, 1999).

These combinations are used most often before wound cleaning and repairing uncomplicated facial and scalp

lacerations. The gel form is preferred because it is easier to control the application (see Box 28-2 for preparation and use of LET topical gel). It is recommended that the gel or solution be painted into and around the wound with cotton-tipped applicators and left for a minimum of 10 minutes and a maximum of 30 minutes; then the wound is irrigated to remove the LET. Peak anesthetic effect after topical mixtures that contain cocaine or lidocaine is 2 to 5 minutes and 3 to 8 minutes for tetracaine combinations. Anesthesia is superficial and does not extend to submucosal structures (Pasero, McCaffery, 1999). These mixtures are used less today with the introduction and more widespread availability of the other previously discussed topical local anesthetics; however, an advantage is that they can be applied to a wound.

Other Local Anesthetic Approaches for Procedural Pain

Although other products are used for procedural pain, there is a general lack of research to adequately evaluate their safety and effectiveness. Some examples follow.

- Refrigerant sprays (e.g., Pain Ease) provide anesthesia by rapid cooling of the skin. The target site is sprayed 4 to 10 seconds from a distance of 3 to 7 inches just until the skin begins to blanch. Care must be taken not to freeze (frost) the skin. The anesthetic effect lasts just 60 seconds, so refrigerant sprays are appropriate only for very brief and superficial dermal procedures such as injections and immunizations. They are ideal for settings such as the ED where a topical anesthetic with a rapid onset of analgesia is particularly important. One randomized, placebo-controlled study showed that vapocoolant spray used immediately prior to venipuncture produced effective and safe anesthesia for IV catheter placement in adults in the ED (Hijazi, Taylor, Richardson, 2009). Successful IV start rates were similar between groups, and 62% of the patients said they would choose the vapocoolant spray again. Vapocoolant spray was shown to be ineffective in reducing intramuscular immunization pain in children (Cohen, MacLaren, DeMore, et al., 2009).

- Topical benzocaine 20% spray (Hurricane) is used for some procedures. A meta-analysis concluded that topical anesthetic sprays (e.g., lidocaine, tetracaine, and benzocaine) used prior to endoscopic procedures improves ease of endoscopy and patient tolerance but cited concerns about related adverse effects, such as methemoglobinemia (see previous discussion), anaphylactic reactions, and aspiration (Evans, Saberi, Kim, et al., 2006). It was shown to be safe but had

Box 28-2 | Preparation and Use of LET Topical Gel

PREPARATION A

Concentrations

- 4% lidocaine
- 0.05% epinephrine
- 0.5% tetracaine

Ingredients

- 0.90 g of lidocaine powder
- 0.15 g of tetracaine powder
- 15.0 mL of epinephrine 1:1000 multidose injections
- qs ad 30.0 mL of 2% Xylocaine jelly (in hydroxyproplymethylcellulose)

Procedure

- Weigh 0.9 g lidocaine powder and 0.15 tetracaine powder.
- Combined weighed powders in a graduate or calibrated amber bottle.
- With a syringe, draw up 15 mL epinephrine 1:1000 injection from multidose vial.
- Add to graduate or calibrated bottle and stir until dissolved.
- Draw this solution through a 5 mcm filter and place in a calibrated amber bottle.
- Slowly add 2% Xylocaine jelly to a volume of 30 mL and mix thoroughly.
- Dispense in an airtight amber bottle and refrigerate.
- Store up to 30 days.

PREPARATION B

Concentrations

- 4% lidocaine
- 0.1% epinephrine
- 0.5% tetracaine

Ingredients

- 40 mL of 20% lidocaine
- 15 mL of 2.25% racemic epinephrine
- 1.72 g of tetracaine added to 0.26 g of sodium bisulfate

Procedure

- To make a gelatinous form, use 300 mL of 2% lidocaine jelly.
- This preparation yields 114 doses of LET (3 mL/dose).
- Refrigerate and protect from light.

Directions for applying LET

1. Review LET order for correct dose, time, and route.
2. Inspect LET for discoloration or broken seal.
3. Gather supplies needed for application: nonsterile gloves, sterile cotton-tipped applicator, LET gel/solution in 3 mL syringe, and bacteriostatic normal saline for irrigation.
4. Inform patient/family members of the application procedure for LET and why it is needed.
5. Wash hands and put on nonsterile gloves.
6. Apply LET with sterile cotton-tipped applicator into the wound bed and around its edges (1.5 to 3 mL, depending on the size of the laceration), or squirt LET into and around laceration with syringe tip.
7. Avoid contact with or application near mucous membranes because these membranes may more readily absorb LET than a wound bed.
8. Allow LET to remain on wound for at least 10 minutes but no more than 30 minutes. (It may be covered with gauze secured in place.)
9. Practitioner may choose to check laceration after 10 minutes to assess degree of anesthesia. Skin may blanch because of vasoconstriction as LET takes effect.
10. If a wound is still sensitive after 20 minutes, more LET may be applied and left on for an additional 10 minutes.
11. Once anesthesia is achieved, irrigate wound to remove LET and any remaining dirt or foreign bodies. Laceration is then sutured.
12. Wash hands and discard supplies.

---

ad, Increase; *qs,* quantity sufficient.
From Pasero, C., & McCaffery, M. *Pain assessment and pharmacologic management,* p. 731, St. Louis, Mosby. Data from United Healthcare System, Department of Pharmacy, Newark, NJ, 1996 (Preparation A); Jacqueline Oschsenreither, RN, Rita Jew, Pharm D, Children's Hospital of Philadelphia, Philadelphia, personal communication, October 1996 (Preparation B); Ochsenreither, J. M. (1996). Better topical anesthetic. *Am J Nurse,* 96(5), 21-22. © 2011, Pasero C, McCaffery M. May be duplicated for use in clinical practice.

---

limited effectiveness as an anesthetic prior to minor gynecologic surgery (Einarsson, Henao, Young, 2005). Numerous cases of methemoglobinemia have been linked to the use of topical benzocaine and attributed to a lack of precise dosing such as might be possible with a metered dose; stricter labeling and very cautious use are recommended (Moore, Walsh, Cohen, 2004).

- Viscous lidocaine (e.g., 2%) is sometimes used for inflamed oral mucosa or on gums prior to dental procedures and prior to ureteral catheterization (Pasero, McCaffery, 1999). Attention to dosing is recommended as amounts greater than 240 mg/day have been associated with lidocaine toxicity (Yamashita, Sato, Kakiuchi, et al., 2002).

Conclusion

The distress and pain associated with procedures are often underestimated and ignored by those who perform them. Clinicians are encouraged to establish policies and procedures that address the provision of adequate analgesia and anesthesia with first-line agents, such as local anesthetics, prior to painful procedures, including minor procedures such as venipuncture. Local anesthetics are versatile and well-tolerated by most patients. There are several formulations to choose from, and more are in development.

Chapter 29 Adjuvant Analgesics for Persistent (Chronic) Bone Pain

BONE pain is a common problem in the palliative care setting, especially for patients with progressive cancer. Radiation therapy is usually considered for cancer patients when bone pain is focal and poorly controlled by an opioid or is associated with a lesion that appears to be prone to fracture on radiographic examination. Anecdotally, multifocal bone pain has been observed to benefit from treatment with a nonsteroidal antiinflammatory drug (NSAID) or a corticosteroid (Lussier, Huskey, Portenoy, 2004; Lussier Portenoy, 2004; Mercadante, Casuccio, Agnello, et al., 1999). Other adjuvant analgesics that are potentially useful in this setting include calcitonin, bisphosphonate compounds, gallium nitrate, and selected radiopharmaceuticals (Table 29-1). Because there arc limited data comparing the advantages and disadvantages of these adjuvant analgesics for bone pain, selection of one agent over another is usually made on the basis of convenience, cost, patient preference, and clinical setting. See Table V-1 for characteristics and dosing of some of the adjuvant analgesics used for persistent bone pain.

Calcitonin

Calcitonin has been shown to ameliorate bone pain in some but not all patients with and without cancer. Clinical experience with this drug suggests that it is relatively safe and can produce substantial pain relief for some patients (Lussier, Portenoy, 2004). Optimal doses and dosing frequency for calcitonin remain unknown, and the durability of favorable effects, if they occur, has not been evaluated systematically. For bone pain associated with cancer metastases, a systematic review of two studies showed variable results and emphasized that calcitonin did not slow disease progression in the bone (Martinez-Zapata, Roque, Alonso-Coello, et al., 2006).

More favorable outcomes have been noted in the treatment of osteoporosis. In patients with this disorder, calcitonin may help in maintaining bone density, but its efficacy in fracture prevention is not known (Cranney, Welch, Adachi, et al., 2000; Karsdal, Henriksen, Arnold, et al., 2008). It can provide significant analgesia for acute osteoporotic vertebral compression fractures (Lussier, Portenoy, 2004), and the use of calcitonin in older women with osteoporosis is an acceptable practice with perceived benefits in reducing pain and improving bone health (Mehta, Malootian, Gilligan, 2003; Miller, 2006).

When used for relief of malignant bone pain, calcitonin is administered most often by the intranasal or subcutaneous routes (Lussier, Portenoy, 2004). It is available as a nasal spray (Miacalcin Nasal Spray) with a recommended dose of one puff in one nostril daily, providing 200 IU. If this does not produce adequate results, an increase in dose (400 IU, two sprays/day) can be tried. Subcutaneous therapy is usually initiated with a low dose, such as 25 IU daily. This may reduce the incidence of nausea, the major adverse effect. Skin testing with 1 IU before the start of therapy is sometimes recommended because of the small risk for serious hypersensitivity reactions. After therapy begins, gradual dose escalation may identify a minimal effective dose. The usual maximum dose, which is recommended solely on the basis of clinical experience, is in the range of 100 to 200 IU/day subcutaneously. The dosing frequency is usually daily at the start of therapy, then reduced, if possible, to the fewest weekly doses required to sustain effects. Calcitonin therapy is associated with a relatively high incidence of the most common adverse effects, facial flushing and nausea (Cranney, Welch, Adachi, et al., 2000).

Table 29-1 | Adjuvant Analgesics Used for Malignant Bone Pain

Class	Comment
Calcitonin	Reduces bone pain; decreases rate of bone turnover; useful in osteoporosis; used most often by subcutaneous injection or nasal spray
Bisphosphonates (e.g., pamidronate, clodronate, zolendronate)	Reduces malignant bone pain and risk for skeletal morbidity
Radionuclides (e.g., strontium-89, samarium-153, rhenium-186, hydroxyethylene diphosphonic acid, gallium nitrate)	Slow onset; used only if no further chemotherapy is planned
Corticosteroids	Anecdotal reports of effectiveness in bone pain
NSAIDs	Anecdotal reports of effectiveness in bone pain

NSAIDs, Nonsteroidal antiinflammatory drugs.
Note: This table lists the classes of adjuvant analgesics for malignant bone pain with comments on their use. See text for discussion and references.
From Pasero, C., & McCaffery, M. *Pain assessment and pharmacologic management,* p. 734, St. Louis, Mosby. © 2011, Pasero C, McCaffery M. May be duplicated for use in clinical practice.

Bisphosphonates

Bisphosphonates (previously known as diphosphonates) are analogs of inorganic pyrophosphate that inhibit osteoclast activity and, consequently, reduce bone resorption in a variety of illnesses causing pathologic effects on bone (Lussier, Portenoy, 2004). Bone metastases cause an imbalance between bone formation and resorption, and this process may be involved in the development of pain (Catala, Martinez, 2006). It is reported that more than half of all cancer pain is caused by metastases to bone (Halvorson, Sevcik, Ghilardi, et al., 2008). Hypercalcemia, caused in part by the release of mediators such as cytokines and prostaglandins, is another common complication of bone metastases and can affect 10% to 20% of patients with these lesions (Mehrotra, 2009).

Bisphosphonates are widely used to prevent and treat the complications of bone metastases (Gainford, Dranitsaris, Clemons, 2005). Although recent concerns about an uncommon toxicity, osteonecrosis of the jaw (see adverse effects) has tempered enthusiasm for long-term or prophylactic use, bisphosphonates continue to be used for symptoms and may provide analgesia and improve function and quality of life (Knotkova, Pappagallo, 2007). The underlying mechanisms of analgesia are not clear but

are thought to be related to inhibition of osteoclasts and macrophages (Knotkova, Pappagallo, 2007). Commonly used bisphosphonate agents for cancer-related bone pain include pamidronate (Aredia), clodronate (Bonefos in Canada), zolendronate (Zometa), and the more recent, ibandronate (Boniva). Readers are referred to a 2009 journal supplement devoted to bisphosphonate treatment (*J Oral Maxillofac Surg,* 67[5, Suppl 1], 1-120).

A systematic review of 95 articles found that bisphosphonates significantly reduced skeletal morbidity except in the outcomes of spinal cord compression and time to first skeletal-related event (Ross, Saunders, Edmonds, et al., 2003). Pain relief was not included in this review but this analysis points to the importance of the role of bisphosphonates in reducing factors that influence the pain experience. A Cochrane Collaboration Review evaluated 30 randomized trials (including open trials) and concluded that bisphosphonates provide some pain relief for bone metastases, but there was insufficient evidence to recommend them as first-line analgesic therapy (Wong, Wiffen, 2002). The researchers generally recommended their use when other analgesics or radiotherapy are inadequate for the management of cancer-related bone pain (Wong, Wiffen, 2002). Concomitant administration of other analgesics with bisphosphonates treatment is recommended (Catala, Martinez, 2006).

A synthesis of findings from 10 randomized controlled trials found that reductions in pain were associated with bisphosphonate therapy in men with bone metastases resulting from advanced prostate cancer, but there was no effect on disease progression or survival rates (Yuen, Shelley, Sze, et al., 2006). There was an increase in nausea with bisphosphonates compared with placebo. Other systematic reviews have demonstrated similar results (Catala, Martinez, 2006; Santangelo, Testai, Barbagallo, et al., 2006).

A 44-week randomized controlled trial administered mitoxantrone chemotherapy and prednisone plus the bisphosphonate clodronate (1500 mg IV every 3 weeks) or mitoxantrone and prednisone plus placebo to men with hormone-resistant prostate cancer and bone metastases (Ernst, Tannock, Winquist, et al., 2003). There were no significant differences in palliative response and overall quality of life; however, subgroup analysis revealed that the best response rate in terms of pain relief was in those who had entered the study with moderate pain. The researchers concluded that clodronate may be beneficial in patients with this level of pain.

Animal research demonstrated rapid attenuation of bone pain both with a single dose and with three consecutive daily doses of ibandronate (Halvorson, Sevcik, Ghilardi, et al., 2008). This research also established that the bisphosphonate prevented bone destruction and produced tumor necrosis. Further, ibandronate treatment attenuated neurochemical reorganization of the peripheral and central nervous systems, a discovery that helps to clarify previously unknown underlying mechanisms of action.

Bisphosphonates may be helpful for other types of pain as well. An open-label pilot study administered 6-mg infusions of ibandronate on 3 consecutive days to patients with complex regional pain syndrome (CRPS) type I (Breuer, Pappagallo, Ongseng, et al., 2008). The treatment was well tolerated and resulted in significant improvements in several of the neuropathic pain qualities (e.g., sensitive, deep, intense, and surface). Results were more impressive in hand than in foot CRPS. Others have found similar results in this painful condition (Knotkova, Pappagallo, 2007).

Dose Selection

Several generations of bisphosphonates have evolved over the years, and each new generation seems to provide increased effectiveness (Catala, Martinez, 2006). Etidronate (Didronel), a first-generation bisphosphonate, has no efficacy for bone-related pain treatment. The second-generation agent pamidronate is recommended in doses of 60 to 90 mg IV for 2 hours once a month (Catala, Martinez, 2006). A 2-year study showed that a single 60-mg dose of pamidronate improved pain scores, patients' global assessments of disease severity, and function scores in patients with CRPS (Robinson, Sandom, Chaptman, 2004). The third-generation bisphosphonates are used more often and include ibandronate and zolendronate. Ibandronate is given in 4 to 6 mg IV doses over a 2-hour period once per month. Zolendronate, which is 100 times more potent than pamidronate, was recommended by the American Society of Clinical Oncology as the bisphosphonate of choice for patients with bone cancer (Berenson, Hillner, Kyle, et al., 2002). Its benefits, when compared to other bisphosphonates, include faster onset, shorter infusion time, and greater efficacy (Maxwell, Swift, Goode, et al., 2003). Dosing is 4 mg IV over 15 minutes once a month (Catala, Martinez, 2006). The IV route is preferred for administration of bisphosphonates because it produces faster onset and better effectiveness. There is evidence of effectiveness with oral clodronate, so its use is justified in countries where it is available (Catala, Martinez, 2006).

Adverse Effects

The incidence of adverse effects varies among bisphosphonate agents, routes of administration, and lengths of therapy. The most common acute-phase adverse effects are flulike symptoms of nausea and vomiting, fever, and diarrhea (Maxwell, Swift, Goode, et al., 2003). Anemia, myalgia and arthralgia, constipation, headache, and anorexia can also occur during therapy. Gastrointestinal effects occur primarily with oral agents and may be avoided by adhering to dosing instructions. Renal toxicity is a potentially serious event and is more likely with IV administration and when drug delivery is faster than recommended (Catala, Martinez, 2006). Renal function should be checked prior to administration of these drugs and monitored during the course of therapy.

More recently, anecdotal reports and observations in studies of cancer patients have linked long-term bisphosphonate therapy to what is called bisphosphonate-related osteonecrosis of the jaw (BRONJ), a concerning and severe adverse event that can significantly affect quality of life (Adamo, Caristi, Sacca, et al., 2008; Knotkova, Pappagallo, 2007). This has also been a growing problem among noncancer populations treated with bisphosphonates and is more prevalent when IV bisphosphonate is administered (Gutta, Louis, 2007). Although BRONJ is rare, it is important that all patients receiving bisphosphonates be warned of this adverse effect and the need to practice good oral hygiene and preventive dental care. If patients develop BRONJ, they should be referred promptly for dental medicine evaluation.

The United States Food and Drug Administration (U.S. FDA) (2008) issued an informational bulletin to health care professionals regarding the possibility of severe and sometimes incapacitating bone, joint, or muscle pain in patients taking bisphosphonates. Risk factors are unknown, and some patients report complete relief after discontinuing bisphosphonates. The bulletin encourages health care professionals to consider whether bisphosphonate use might be responsible for any reports of severe musculoskeletal pain.

Radiopharmaceuticals

Radionuclides that are absorbed at areas of high bone turnover have been evaluated as potential therapies for metastatic bone disease (Lussier, Portenoy, 2004). The first radionuclide introduced into clinical practice was phosphorus-32 orthophosphate. Early data suggest that treatment with a radiopharmaceutical can yield meaningful pain relief in approximately 80% of patients, and 10% can expect complete relief of pain (Robinson, Preston, Baxter, et al., 1993; Robinson, Preston, Schiefelbein, et al., 1995). A Cochrane Collaboration Review of seven trials concluded that radioisotopes alone provided effective pain relief comparable to external-beam radiotherapy (McQuay, Collins, Carroll, et al., 1999). A later review of four trials reported a small effect on short-term (1 to 6 months) pain control, but treatment was associated with an increased risk of leukocytopenia and thrombocytopenia (Roque, Martinez-Zapata, Alonso-Coello, et al., 2003). Data were insufficient to evaluate long-term effects. A more recent systematic review of trials with single-agent radiopharmaceuticals (strontium-89 and samarium-153) shows that there are benefits to using these agents, and treatment should be considered for the palliation of multiple sites of bone pain resulting from metastatic cancer when pain control cannot be achieved by means of conventional analgesic regimens (Bauman, Charette, Reid, et al., 2005).

The clinical response to a radiopharmaceutical occurs in 7 to 21 days, and peak response may be delayed for a month or more. Approximately 5% to 10% of patients experience a transitory pain flare immediately after treatment. The usual duration of benefit is 3 to 6 months, after which retreatment may regain favorable effects. Leukopenia or thrombocytopenia peaks a few weeks after treatment and occurs to a clinically significant degree in approximately 10% and 33% of patients, respectively (Porter, McEwan, Powe, et al., 1993). Bone marrow effects usually wane by 12 weeks after treatment. Bone marrow suppression is the major toxicity, and the desire for a compound with a better therapeutic index has spurred the development of several new radionuclides.

Treatment Considerations

The newer radionuclides, strontium chloride-89, samarium-153 ethylenediamine tetramethylene phosphonic acid, rhenium-186, and hydroxyethylene diphosphonic acid, have been most promising thus far (Lussier, Portenoy, 2004). Observational studies of patients with bone metastases resulting from a variety of tumor types have provided strong evidence that these compounds can reduce bone pain without undue risk to bone marrow or other vital structures. A prospective evaluation of 64 patients with breast or prostate cancer who were receiving rhenium-188 hydroxyethylidene diphosphonate (188Re-HEDP); rhenium-186 hydroxyethylidene diphosphonate (186Re-HEDP); or strontium-89 (89Sr) showed that all of the drugs were effective in palliating pain symptoms and improving quality of life, but functional status was significantly better with 188Re-HEDP (Liepe, Runge, Kotzerke, 2005).

Strontium-89 and samarium-153, which are commercially available in the United States, have been most extensively evaluated as treatments for bone pain (Akerley, Butera, Wehbe, et al., 2002; Lussier, Portenoy, 2004; Nilsson, Strang, Ginman, et al., 2005; Porter, McEwan, Powe, et al., 1993; Tripp, Kuettel, 2006). Like other radiopharmaceuticals, they are potentially effective in the treatment of pain due to osteoblastic bone lesions or lesions with osteoblastic components. Prior to treatment, an osteoblastic component should be confirmed by positive bone scintigraphy.

Given the delayed onset and peak effects, treatment with these agents should not be considered unless patients have life expectancies greater than 3 months. The delay also implies that this treatment should not be considered as the sole approach for patients with severe pain. Because of the potential for bone marrow toxicity, treatment should not be considered unless adequate bone marrow reserve has been documented (Lussier, Portenoy, 2004). In the case of strontium-89, this is usually considered to be a platelet count above 60,000 and a white blood cell count above 2400 (Robinson, Preston, Schiefelbein, et al., 1995). Impending pathologic fracture is another contraindication to use of radiopharmaceuticals (Tripp, Kuettel, 2006). Patients who continue to be candidates for myelosuppressive chemotherapy should not be treated because the effects on bone marrow may worsen the toxicity of later cytotoxic therapy or limit the ability to rebound after therapy (Lussier, Portenoy, 2004).

Limited data are available for comparative studies of strontium-89 and samarium-153. Unlike strontium-89, samarium-153 can be imaged and provides a scintigraphic picture of bone metastases at the same time treatment is given. In a small case series of 57 patients with metastatic prostate cancer (38 treated with strontium-89 and 19 with samarium-153), no differences were observed in effects on pain or time to disease progression (Dickie, Macfarlane, 1999). For now, the indications and safety issues should be assumed to be similar for both of these radiopharmaceuticals.

Radiopharmaceuticals are not widely used in the United States because of relatively disappointing results; however, these results may be related to the low maximum allowed dose of 4 mCi in the United States (Tripp, Kuettel, 2006). Trials in other countries that used higher doses (e.g., 10.8 mCi in Canada) have yielded more positive results (Porter, McEwan, Powe, et al., 1993).

Conclusion

Radiation therapy is usually considered for patients with progressive cancer who have bone pain that is focal and poorly controlled by an opioid or is associated with a lesion that appears to be prone to fracture on radiographic examination. Adjuvant analgesics that may be useful in this setting include calcitonin, bisphosphonate compounds, gallium nitrate, and selected radiopharmaceuticals. Because there are limited data comparing the advantages and disadvantages of these adjuvant analgesics for bone pain, selection of one agent over another is usually made on the basis of convenience, cost, patient preference, and clinical setting.

Chapter 30 Adjuvant Analgesics for Malignant Bowel Obstruction

BOWEL obstruction can occur in any patient with cancer but is most common in those with ovarian or GI cancers (Davis, Hinshaw, 2006). This complication occurs most frequently in the advanced stages of the illness (Mercadante, Casuccio, Mangione, 2007). Malignant bowel obstruction (MBO) is caused usually by external compression of the bowel lumen by an adjacent tumor or masses of the mesentery or omentum, or by abdominal or pelvic adhesions. Surgical correction of MBO is usually not an option for patients with advanced cancer (Mercadante, Casuccio, Mangione, 2007). If surgical decompression or endoscopic interventions such as stent placement for upper and lower bowel obstructions are not feasible, then the need to control pain and other obstructive symptoms, including distension, nausea, and vomiting, becomes paramount (Davis, Hinshaw, 2006; Davis, Nouneh, 2001; Lussier, Portenoy, 2004). Various analgesics, anticholinergics, antisecretory agents, and antiemetics play important roles (Figure 30-1).

The management of symptoms associated with MBO can be extremely challenging, and there is surprisingly very little well-designed research to guide treatment decisions (Mercadante, Casuccio, Mangione, 2007). International experts have begun to address this issue by reaching a consensus on two research protocols based on location of bowel obstruction, with the hope that well-designed studies will provide better direction for clinical treatment in the future (Anthony, Baron, Mercadante, 2007).

Opioid administration is appropriate to treat abdominal pain, even in the context of suspected bowel obstruction. Opioids will not hinder diagnosis and may facilitate physical examination (Davis, Hinshaw, 2006). If initial examination suggests that mechanical obstruction is not likely, treatment may include efforts to reduce drugs that can adversely influence bowel motility, including opioids. Adding nonopioids, such as ketorolac, during the acute phase may help to reduce the opioid dose; the lowest effective opioid dose should be given.

If constipation is contributing to the MBO, this must be addressed as part of the approach to symptom management. The first step is to exclude or treat fecal impaction. Unless obstruction is complete, treatment with laxatives should be initiated, and consideration should be given to treatment with an opioid antagonist with limited or no penetration into the CNS (Davis, Hinshaw, 2006). In the United States, methylnaltrexone (Relistor) is now approved for refractory opioid-induced constipation. Oral naloxone or another nonabsorbable opioid antagonist, such as alvimopan (Entereg), also can be considered for this purpose. (See Chapter 19 for more on these drugs for constipation and ileus.)

Other drugs are used to treat both the lower and upper GI symptoms associated with MBO. Metoclopramide (Reglan), for example, may be given to increase GI activity if there is no colic and the bowel is partially obstructed; however, metoclopramide should not be given if obstruction is complete as it can increase colic under those circumstances (Davis, Hinshaw, 2006; Mercadante, Ferrera, Villari, et al., 2004).

Clinical reviews and case series suggest that anticholinergic drugs, the somatostatin analogue octreotide (Sandostatin), and corticosteroids may be useful as adjuvant analgesics for palliative management of MBO (Mercadante, Casuccio, Mangione, 2007; Mercadante, Ferrera, Villari, et al., 2004; Ripamonti, Easson, Gerdes, et al., 2008; Weber, Zulian, 2009). The use of these drugs may also ameliorate nonpainful symptoms and minimize the need for chronic drainage using nasogastric or percutaneous catheters (Mercadante, Casuccio, Mangione,

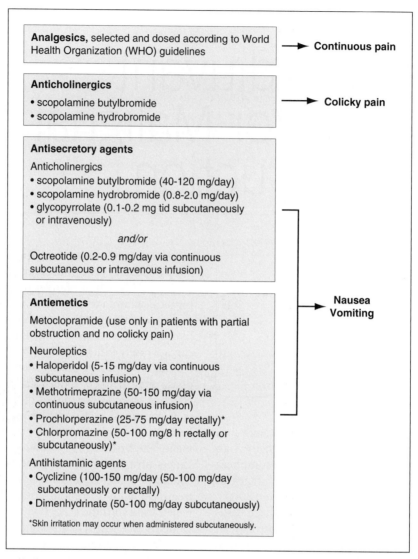

Figure 30-1 | Pharmacologic management of malignant bowel obstruction.

From Ripamonti, C., & Mercadante, S. (2004). How to use octreotide for malignant bowel obstruction. *J Support Oncol, 2*(4), 357-364.

2007). Following is a discussion of the adjuvant analgesics used to treat MBO.

Anticholinergic Drugs

Anticholinergics are used as antisecretory drugs (reduce water and salt secretion from the bowel lumen) in combination with analgesics and antiemetics to treat MBO (Mercadante, Casuccio, Mangione, 2007). In a small case series evaluating aggressive multimodal pharmacotherapy for MBO, 15 patients were consecutively treated with a combination of metoclopramide, octreotide, dexamethasone (Decadron and others), and an initial oral bolus of amidotrizoic acid, a hyperosmolar solution that promotes shifting of fluid into the bowel lumen, a goal

of treatment (Mercadante, Ferrera, Villari, et al., 2004). Intestinal transit was improved between day 1 and day 5 of therapy, and this fast bowel recovery was attributed to the combination of propulsive and antisecretory agents that can act synergistically.

Scopolamine is a commonly used anticholinergic drug (Ripamonti, Mercadante, Groff, 2000) and is available as a transdermal patch, which is a convenient route of delivery in this setting (see Chapter 19 for more on the scopolamine patch). Problematic adverse effects include somnolence or drowsiness, confusion, loss of balance, headache, and dry mouth. These effects typically subside as patients adjust to the medication, but caution is recommended when the drug is used in older individuals who may be more sensitive to some of the effects. Adverse effects usually subside with patch removal.

If CNS toxicity is problematic, a trial of an anticholinergic that is relatively less likely to pass through the blood-brain barrier, such as glycopyrrolate (Robinul), is reasonable. Along with antisecretory medications, parenteral hydration over 500 mL/day can help to reduce nausea and drowsiness (Ripamonti, Mercadante, Groff, 2000).

Octreotide

The somatostatin analog octreotide (Sandostatin) is desirable for rapid, aggressive management of MBO. It is a potent antisecretagogue that controls endogenous fluid losses and reduces gastric and intestinal secretion and bile flow (Mercadante, Casuccio, Mangione, 2007; Mercadante, Ferrera, Villari, et al., 2004). Octreotide

has also been used to manage severe diarrhea caused by enterocolic fistula, high output jejunostomies or ileostomies, or secretory tumors of the GI tract. In a prospective randomized clinical trial, 17 patients with inoperable MBO and decompression nasogastric tube were randomized to receive octreotide 0.3 mg/day or scopolamine butylbromide 60 mg/day for 3 days through a continuous subcutaneous infusion (Ripamonti, Mercadante, Groff, et al., 2000). Pain relief was achieved in all patients, and there was no difference in the common adverse effect of dry mouth between groups.

Octreotide has a good safety profile but can be expensive. In some settings, however, the cost may be balanced by an excellent clinical response or avoidance of the costs associated with a GI drainage procedure. See Box 30-1 for an algorithm to guide the use of octreotide for bowel obstruction.

GUIDELINES

Box 30-1 | Treatment Algorithm for the Management of Bowel Obstruction with Octreotide

PATIENTS UNDERGOING SURGERY FOR BOWEL OBSTRUCTION—PREOPERATIVE USE

- Octreotide 0.3 mg/day (0.1 mg three times a day) intravenously until surgery
- Intravenous hydration with plasma expanders and electrolyte correction
- Decompressive nasogastric tube
- Antibiotics, including a cephalosporin and metronidazole

Maintain octreotide for the first 24 to 48 hours postoperatively.

PATIENTS WITH RECENT GASTROINTESTINAL SYMPTOMS—POTENTIALLY REVERSIBLE BOWEL OBSTRUCTION

- Octreotide 0.3 mg/day (0.1 mg three times a day) intravenously or subcutaneously
- Dexamethasone 4 mg three times a day intravenously or subcutaneously
- Metoclopramide 60 to 120 mg intravenously or subcutaneously
- Amidotrizoate 30 to 50 mL orally

Maintain metoclopramide-octreotide regimen according to the clinical evolution.

PATIENTS WITH PERSISTENT GASTROINTESTINAL SYMPTOMS, INOPERABLE—EARLY TREATMENT UNSUCCESSFUL—DEFINITIVE OBSTRUCTION

- Stop metoclopramide
- Octreotide 0.3 mg/day (0.1 mg three times a day) intravenously or subcutaneously; increase dose up to 0.9 mg/day, if partially successful
- Haloperidol 2 to 5 mg/day intravenously or subcutaneously
- Parenteral or transdermal opioid analgesics
- Also consider venting gastrostomy, if surgically feasible.

From Ripamonti, C., & Mercadante, S. (2004). How to use octreotide for malignant bowel obstruction. *J Support Oncol*, 2(4), 357-364.

Corticosteroids

Corticosteroids have long been used to reduce inflammatory intestinal edema and promote intestinal transit, which can have immediate effects of reducing obstruction and promoting relief (Mercadante, Casuccio, Mangione, 2007). They act as antisecretory agents and are inexpensive and well-tolerated. The mode of action is unclear, and the most effective drug, dose, and dosing regimen have not been established. A broad range of doses have been described anecdotally. A systematic review demonstrated a trend toward IV dexamethasone doses of 6 to 16 mg/day for MBO (Feuer, Broadley, 1999). The previously discussed multimodal approach to aggressive treatment of MBO administered 12 mg/day of dexamethasone as an IV infusion (Mercadante, Ferrera, Villari, et al., 2004). Methylprednisolone (Depo-Medrol and others) has been administered in a dose range of 30 to 50 mg/day (Farr, 1990). In a small case series of 4 patients, subcutaneous dexamethasone doses of 4 to 40 mg/day or oral prednisone 50 mg/day along with analgesics and antiemetics were effective in managing symptoms associated with MBO (Weber, Zulian, 2009). The potential for complications during long-term therapy, including an increased risk of bowel perforation, may limit this approach to patients with life expectancies that are likely to be short (see Chapter 22 for more on corticosteroids and their adverse effects).

Conclusion

Bowel obstruction can occur in any patient with cancer, particularly in the advanced stages of the illness, and is considered a major complication. If surgical decompression or endoscopic interventions are not feasible, then the need to control pain and other obstructive symptoms is critical. Various analgesics, anticholinergics, antisecretory agents, and antiemetics play important roles in the treatment of this serious condition.

Chapter 31 Adjuvants Less Often Used

THIS chapter presents a few agents that are sometimes added to the treatment plan in some patients with pain. Their use as analgesics is limited, but they may provide other benefits.

Psychostimulants and Anticholinesterases

Psychostimulant drugs and drugs that block the effects of acetylcholinesterase (an enzyme that degrades acetylcholine) are sometimes used to counteract opioid-induced sedation associated with both short-term and long-term therapy. The psychostimulant medications used most often include dextroamphetamine (Dexedrine), methylphenidate (Concerta, Metadate, Methylin, Ritalin, others), modafinil (Provigil), and caffeine. Others include amphetamine (Addaral), armodafinil (Nuvigil), atomoxetine (Strattera), and dexmethylphenidate (Focalin).

The acetylcholinesterase inhibitor used most often is donepezil (Aricept); others include rivastigmine (Exelon) and galantamine (Razadyne).

There is substantial evidence that psychostimulants may be analgesic (Lussier, Portenoy, 2004). However, with the exception of caffeine, which is a constituent of many proprietary analgesic products, these drugs are generally used only when pain is accompanied by another symptom such as sedation or fatigue. Nevertheless, their effect on pain relief should be monitored to identify if and when a dose of analgesics can be lowered. Although there are no specific clinical guidelines available to direct therapy, clinicians often prescribe psychostimulants when it is difficult to titrate analgesics to pain relief or when patients report unresolved sleepiness from the sedating effects of analgesics. Opioid-induced sedation usually improves within 7 days of regular dosing; however, this varies, and some individuals will benefit from either short-term or long-term treatment with a psychostimulant (Harris, Kotob, 2006). From clinical experience, these drugs can improve concentration and physical activity. In addition, psychostimulants can be helpful with depression (Macleod, 1998; Menza, Kaufman, Castellanos, 2000) and fatigue (Fishbain, Cutler, Lewis, et al., 2004a). Table V-1, pp. 748-756, at end of Section V contains dosing recommendations for selected psychostimulants.

Methylphenidate (Sarhill, Walsh, Nelson, 2001) and the newer agent modafinil (Prommer, 2006) are most commonly used to counteract sedation and fatigue in cancer populations. Clinical reviews discuss their usefulness in reducing opioid-induced sedation and improving fatigue and overall well-being, but more studies are needed to measure their efficacy in the treatment plans of individuals with pain (Bruera, Neumann, 1998; Fishbain, Cutler, Lewis, et al., 2004a; Reissig, Rybarczyk, 2005; Shaiova, 2005). This was confirmed in a Cochrane Collaboration Review that concluded that methylphenidate has been shown to improve concentration and is effective for fatigue in cancer patients based on studies with small sample sizes, and further research was encouraged (Minton, Stone, Richardson, et al., 2008). A review of the literature between 1996 and 2002 concluded that methylphenidate effectively attenuated opioid-induced somnolence, augmented opioid analgesia, treated depression, and improved cognitive function in cancer patients and recommended its use in palliative care (Rozans, Dreisbach, Lertora, et al., 2002).

Methylphenidate has also been used in the acute care setting. An interesting publication reported that methylphenidate facilitated the weaning from mechanical ventilation in 5 of 7 patients who exhibited psychomotor retardation associated with markedly depressed mood (Rothenhausler, Ehrentraut, von Degenfeld, et al., 2000). The drug has also been researched for treatment of postanesthesia shivering, though it is rarely used for this purpose as more effective drugs are available (Kranke, Eberhart, Roewer, et al., 2004).

The use of modafinil is gaining more popularity in practice, most likely because the drug has been shown to be very effective in treating fatigue and increasing alertness (Prommer, 2006). One randomized controlled trial found that modafinil decreased fatigue and increased "alertness" and "energy" in 71% of those given the drug, compared with 18% of those given a placebo, in the immediate postoperative period following general anesthesia (Larijani, Goldberg, Hojat, et al., 2004). The drug was well-tolerated, and those in the modafinil group experienced less pain and nausea. The drug is especially effective for cognitive impairment that can accompany both analgesic therapy and chemotherapy in cancer patients (Biegler, Chaoul, Cohen, 2009). A comprehensive evidence-based review of modafinil provides several indications and guidelines for its use (Kumar, 2008). Further research is needed to establish its analgesic potential.

Dextroamphetamine is used less today than in the past as the newer and better-tolerated psychostimulants have become available. A placebo-controlled study comparing dextroamphetamine, caffeine, and modafinil in healthy volunteers who were subjected to 44 hours of continuous wakefulness found that duration of vigilance and wakefulness were shortest with caffeine and longest with dextroamphetamine (Killgore, Rupp, Grugle, et al., 2008). Adverse effects with modafinil were similar to placebo, caffeine was associated with the most adverse effects, and restorative sleep was adversely affected by dextroamphetamine. A randomized controlled trial administered dextroamphetamine 10 mg or placebo to fatigued older adults with advanced cancer receiving palliative care (Auret, Schug, Bremner, et al., 2009). Although improvements in fatigue were noted on the second day, there were no significant differences in fatigue or quality of life at the end of the 8-day study period.

Caffeine has been used for many years to treat opioid-induced sedation or somnolence related to other adjuvant analgesics. It also can reduce general fatigue associated with drug therapies or disease states. More importantly, research has shown that caffeine has analgesic properties, for example, in the treatment of headaches. Clinical trials indicate that caffeine in doses of more than 65 mg may enhance the analgesia of other agents (Zhang, 2001). Caffeine is widely available in both medications and food items, particularly coffee and tea. See Chapter 9 for a more detailed discussion of the use of caffeine as an adjuvant analgesic, and refer to Table 9-1 (p. 241) for dietary sources of caffeine and Table 9-2 (pp. 242-245) for nonopioid analgesics that contain caffeine.

Patients who require psychostimulants to counteract sedation caused by their opioid and adjuvant therapy should be monitored for benefits. These include assessing for a decrease in daytime sleepiness, reduction in the number of daytime naps, feelings of having more energy, improved physical stamina during the day, better mental concentration, and ability to engage in social activities. It is equally important to watch for adverse effects such as insomnia, nervousness, feelings of uneasiness, tachycardia, decreased appetite, and weight loss. If any of these occur, depending on how severe, dose adjustments can always be made to the therapy.

Donepezil, an oral acetylcholinesterase inhibitor approved for the treatment of Alzheimer's disease, is the drug in this class that is most frequently tried as a strategy to reduce opioid-induced sedation. In one case series, 6 patients with cancer pain who were experiencing marked sedation from their pain therapy (opioid doses higher than 200 mg of morphine equivalents per day) had notable improvements after taking donepezil (Slatkin, Rhiner, Bolton, 2001). Patients indicated fewer episodes of spontaneous sleeping during the day, fewer myoclonic twitches, and better function and social interaction. Sleep at night also improved. Clearly, more research is needed to measure the benefits of this agent for opioid- and adjuvant-induced sedation.

Calcitonin

The use of calcitonin for bone pain has been previously addressed in Chapter 29. Additionally, this agent has also been used for the treatment of other types of pain syndromes. Unfortunately, there are insufficient data to support widespread use beyond bone pain. It has little to no effectiveness for phantom limb pain (Albazaz, Wong, Homer-Vanniasinkam, 2008; Halbert, Crotty, Cameron, 2003; Smith, Dubin, Parikh, 2009). However, intranasal calcitonin was shown to relieve pain with movement and rest and improve ability to work in patients with complex regional pain syndrome (Gobelet, Waldburger, Meier, et al., 1992; Perez, Kwakkel, Zuurmond, 2001). It has also been used to effectively treat intractable painful diabetic neuropathy (Quatraro, Minei, De Rosa, et al., 1992; Zieleniewski, 1990). The literature suggests that it may be useful for acute neuropathic pain (Gray, 2008) and pain from trigeminal neuralgia (Qin, Cai, Yang, 2008). The exact mechanisms for possible analgesic effects for neuropathic pain remain unknown. The optimal dose and dosing frequency for calcitonin are not established (Perez, Kwakkel, Zuurmond, 2001). Dosing recommendations discussed previously in relation to bone pain may be used for neuropathic pain (see Chapter 39).

Neuroleptics

In an evidence-based review, it was concluded that some neuroleptics, including at least one of the newer, so-called atypical neuroleptics, may have analgesic activity, but there are far too few randomized controlled and other clinical trials to draw definitive conclusions (Fishbain, Cutler, Lewis, et al., 2004b). There is no clear evidence that the phenothiazines (e.g., chlorpromazine [Thorazine], fluphenazine [Prolixin]) specifically either relieve pain or potentiate opioid analgesia (American Pain Society [APS], 2003).

Olanzapine (Zyprexa) is a newer, so-called *atypical* neuroleptic and has a somewhat better safety profile than the traditional neuroleptics. This drug may have some benefit when added to opioid therapy in those with severe cancer pain associated with cognitive impairment or anxiety (Khojainova, Santiago-Palma, Kornick, et al., 2002). In a case series, olanzapine also was reported to be effective in rapidly aborting episodic and persistent cluster headache (Rozen, 2001) and relieving refractory fibromyalgia symptoms, including pain (Kiser, Cohen, Freedenfeld, et al., 2001).

Evidence that traditional neuroleptics other than methotrimeprazine are analgesic is equally sparse. Pimozide (Orap) was effective in patients with trigeminal neuralgia, and this has suggested a role for neuroleptics in patients with refractory neuropathic pain (Lussier, Portenoy, 2004). Given its adverse effect liability, pimozide specifically is not considered. Other neuroleptics, such as haloperidol (Haldol) and fluphenazine, would be preferred in this rare circumstance.

Mechanism of Action

The mechanism of neuroleptic analgesia is unknown, but may involve the effect of dopaminergic blockade on endogenous pain-modulating systems (Lussier, Portenoy, 2004) (see Section I). Dopamine receptors, specifically the D2 subtype, are represented among the numerous pathways that subserve pain modulation (Yaksh, 2006). Studies in animals have suggested that selective dopamine antagonists can potentiate morphine analgesia, and controlled clinical trials have demonstrated that metoclopramide, a relatively selective blocker of the D2 receptor, is mildly analgesic in humans (Kandler, Lisander, 1993; Rosenblatt, Cioffi, Sinatra, et al., 1991). This evidence, however, does not confirm that a dopaminergic mechanism underlies the analgesic effects of neuroleptic drugs, because all these drugs interact with other receptors that could potentially mediate analgesic effects. Metoclopramide has a dopaminergic mechanism, and there is no strong evidence that this drug is analgesic (Gupta, 2006).

Indications

Given the lack of supporting data, neuroleptics are very rarely considered for a primary pain indication. For patients with advanced illness who have pain associated with agitation, anxiety, or nausea, the use of one of these drugs is separately indicated and its effects on pain can be tracked. Among those without these other indications, the use of a neuroleptic for pain would only be considered after many trials of other drug strategies proved ineffective.

Dose Selection

The neuroleptics are started at low doses and increased to whatever dose the literature suggests is usually analgesic, and then discontinued if no analgesia ensues (Lussier, Portenoy, 2004). For example, low initial doses of fluphenazine can be escalated to 1 to 2 mg 3 times daily, and the dose of haloperidol can be slowly increased to 2 to 5 mg 2 to 3 times a day.

Adverse Effects

Common adverse effects of neuroleptic drugs include sedation, orthostatic dizziness, and anticholinergic effects (Lussier, Portenoy, 2004). Some patients experience mental clouding or confusion. Phenothiazines, such as chlorpromazine and fluphenazine, are more likely to produce these effects than other subclasses, such as the butyrophenones (e.g., haloperidol). The sedation produced by the neuroleptics can be additive to other CNS depressants.

The possibility of extrapyramidal adverse effects is perhaps the greatest concern in the clinical use of neuroleptic drugs (Lussier, Portenoy, 2004). The incidence of these disorders varies with the drug, duration of therapy, and dose. Fluphenazine and haloperidol are more likely to produce these effects than olanzapine (Tardy, Baldessarini, Tazari, 2002). The most serious extrapyramidal reaction is the neuroleptic malignant syndrome that is characterized by rigidity, autonomic instability, and encephalopathy. Successful management requires prompt diagnosis, discontinuation of the neuroleptic, and intensive supportive measures. The use of dantrolene (Dantrium) and bromocriptine (Parlodel) has been suggested in severe cases.

Other extrapyramidal effects can be distressing or seriously impair function. These include acute dystonic reactions (muscle contraction and jerking movements), akathisia (restlessness), parkinsonism, and tardive dyskinesia. The management of these complications usually involves discontinuation of the neuroleptic, with or without the administration of an anticholinergic drug, such as benztropine (Lussier, Portenoy, 2004).

Benzodiazepines

The benzodiazepines, clonazepam (Klonopin) (Fishbain, Cutler, Rosomoff, et al., 2000; Wiffen, Collins, McQuay, et al., 2005) and alprazolam (Xanax) (Fernandez, Adams, Holmes, 1987) have been used in the management of both musculoskeletal pains and neuropathic pains. Although clonazepam often is considered specifically for neuropathic pain, a critical review finds little support (Dellemijn, Fields, 1994; Reddy, Patt, 1994) (see Chapter 23 for more research and discussion of clonazepam). Negative findings also have been reported in an early controlled trial of lorazepam (Ativan) for postherpetic neuralgia (Max, Schafer, Culnane, et al., 1988) and in a small controlled repeated-dose study of oral chlordiazepoxide (Librium) for persistent pain (Yosselson-Superstine, Lipman, Sanders, 1985). Thus, the evidence for benzodiazepine analgesia is limited and conflicting, leading the APS (2003) to conclude that benzodiazepines are not effective analgesics except for muscle spasm (see Chapter 25).

Nonetheless, it must be acknowledged that clonazepam, and sometimes alprazolam, are tried in cases of refractory neuropathic pain on the basis of anecdotal experience, the relative safety of these drugs, and the common coexistence of pain and anxiety. If this is considered, clinicians should recognize the limited supporting evidence. The wider use of benzodiazepines as adjuvant analgesics is not warranted.

As discussed previously, the evidence for use of benzodiazepines as muscle relaxants also is minimal (see Chapter 25). Diazepam (Valium) and other benzodiazepines are widely used for this purpose, but benefits are limited, especially when given orally.

Adenosine

Adenosine (Adenocard, Adenoscan) is an antiarrhythmic agent commercially available for IV administration. The basis for its analgesic potential lies within the fact that adenosine is an important modulator of neurotransmission associated with many physiologic functions, including the regulation of arousal and sleep, anxiety, cognition, and memory, and may contribute to the etiology of pathologic pain (Ribeiro, Sebastiao, de Mendonca, 2002; Sawynok, Liu, 2003). Early research of adenosine suggested that the drug had analgesic effects for postoperative pain (Segerdahl, Ekblom, Sandelin, et al., 1995) and neuropathic pain (Sollevi, Belfrage, Lundeberg, et al., 1995). A later comprehensive review of adenosine also supported a role in relieving both postoperative and persistent neuropathic pain states (Hayashida, Fukuda, Fukunaga, 2005). Although adenosine has been identified as having potential as an intrathecal analgesic, further research is needed to more clearly define its place in pain management by this route of administration (Schug, Saunders, Kurowski, et al., 2006).

Antihistamines

Many antihistamines are available, including diphenhydramine (Benadryl), hydroxyzine (Vistaril parenterally), phenyltoloxamine (Phenylgesic, a nonprescription cold remedy), pyrilamine (an ingredient in several cold remedies [e.g., Codimal PH syrup, ND-Gesic tablets]), and orphenadrine (Norflex). Orphenadrine is an analogue of diphenhydramine and is combined with aspirin and caffeine for analgesia but is classified as a skeletal muscle relaxant (see Chapter 25). There is little evidence that this drug, or other antihistamines, relax muscles or effectively relieve pain.

A randomized study of women undergoing hysterectomy found a lower incidence of severe nausea with perioperative diphenhydramine but no differences in pain or opioid consumption compared with placebo (Lin, Yeh, Yeh, et al., 2005). At best, diphenhydramine has been observed anecdotally to augment the treatment of pain that has failed to respond to opioids and other adjuvant analgesics (Santiago-Palma, Fischberg Kornick, et al., 2001). Suggested therapy can start at 25 mg of oral or parenteral diphenhydramine every 6 to 8 hours, and be titrated to effect. However, the coadministration of diphenhydramine with opioids is problematic in the postoperative setting because this can increase the risk of excessive sedation and respiratory depression (Anwari, Iqbal, 2003); increased monitoring of sedation levels is required with this practice (see Chapter 19 for more information).

The purported analgesic properties of hydroxyzine, which has been traditionally combined with an opioid for an opioid dose-sparing effect, have never been confirmed (Gordon, 1995). Studies reporting analgesic activity for this agent suffer from major methodologic flaws, including the lack of placebo-controlled trials and scientific rigor in analyzing results. These have compromised the ability to draw definitive conclusions about its benefits (Glazier, 1990). With doses that may contribute to pain relief, hydroxyzine would have the potential for inducing significant sedation, which adds to the adverse effects of opioids, but would not be reversed with naloxone (Gordon, 1995). Further, when given parenterally, it can cause significant local pain and tissue damage. Antihistamines must also be used with caution in older patients as they have increased sensitivity to the anticholinergic and sedative effects of these drugs (see Table 13-4 on p. 336). Clinical experience suggests that treatment with antihistamines should be reserved for treating anxiety and opioid-induced nausea and pruritus in some patients (see Chapter 19).

Botulinum Toxin Type A

Botulinum toxin type A (Botox) is a fermented product derived from *Clostriduium botulinum,* an anaerobic spore-forming bacterium (Setler, 2002). It is approved for administration by injection for several conditions, including cervical dystonia, hemifacial spasm, and blepharospasm (Lew, 2002). Injection of botulinum produces partial chemical denervation and localized reduction in muscle activity. The toxin is used to treat spasticity (O'Brien, 2002), and clinical reports, open-label trials, and a few randomized controlled studies have shown that it may be effective for some types of persistent pain when more conservative approaches fail to provide relief (Arezzo, 2002; Gajraj, 2005; Smith, Audette, Royal, 2002). When effective, the toxin provides long-term (weeks) relief with a relatively low incidence of adverse effects (Smith, Audette, Royal, 2002). Adverse effects are usually transient but can last for months and include localized muscle weakness and pain at the injection site, skin rash, pruritus, and flu-like symptoms. Prompted by reports that the botulinum toxin may spread from the area of injection to other parts of the body, the United States Food and Drug Administration (U.S. FDA) announced label changes in 2009 for all botulinum toxin products, which included a boxed warning. Reported symptoms were similar to those of botulism, including unexpected loss of strength or muscle weakness, hoarseness or trouble talking, trouble saying words clearly, loss of bladder control, trouble breathing, trouble swallowing, double vision, blurred vision, and drooping eyelids.

Myofascial pain syndrome and fibromyalgia have been shown to be responsive to botulinum toxin injection into trigger points or tender points (Smith, Audette, Royal, 2002). A case report described successful use of botulinum injection for persistent perineal pain (Gajraj, 2005). It has been suggested as a possible treatment for chronic whiplash-associated disorder (Freund, Schwartz, 2002). A small randomized trial of postwhiplash neck pain found the best efficacy if the toxin is administered within 1 year of the injury (Braker, Yariv, Adler, et al., 2008). Whereas botulinum treatment has been used to relieve back pain in select patients (Difazio, Jabbari, 2002), a placebo-controlled, randomized study found that single-dose treatment without physical therapy is ineffective for persistent neck pain (Wheeler, Goolkasian, Gretz, 2001). Those who were injected experienced a high incidence of adverse effects in this study; further research on multidose therapy was encouraged.

Botulinum treatment also has been considered a viable option for persistent headaches, with the advantage of a lack of systemic effects associated with conventional treatments (Loder, Biondi, 2002). However, a randomized, double-blind, placebo-controlled trial found it ineffective for the treatment of tension-type headaches (Schulte-Mattler, Krack, BoNTTH Study Group, 2004), and another well-controlled study showed that it had no efficacy for episodic migraine headaches (Saper, Mathew, Loder, et al., 2007).

The underlying mechanism of the analgesic action of botulinum toxin type A is not entirely clear but is thought to be related to its ability to inhibit the release of the neurotransmitter acetylcholine from cholinergic

nerve terminals (Setler, 2002). A study of human volunteers found that botulinum toxin type A preferentially targets C-fibers, blocks neurotransmitter release, and subsequently reduces pain and neurogenic inflammation (Gazerani, Pendersen, Staahl, et al., 2009). A decrease in active tender trigger points is suggested as an underlying mechanism for pain relief with soft-tissue pain syndromes (Smith, Audette, Royal, 2002). The reader is referred to a journal supplement devoted to botulinum toxin treatment for specific types of pain that might best respond, dosing guidelines, administration technique, expected responses, and adverse effects (*Clinical Journal of Pain*, *18*[Suppl 6], 2002).

Vitamin D

Interest in vitamin D supplementation as an analgesic approach began when a number of studies suggested a link between inadequate levels of vitamin D and a higher incidence of persistent pain. A prospective study found a prevalence of vitamin D inadequacy in 26% of patients (N = 267) seeking help for diverse types of persistent pain (Turner, Hooten, Schmidt, et al., 2008). Other findings were that among patients taking opioids in this study, those with vitamin D deficiency were taking approximately twice the opioid dose and had been taking opioids 60% longer than those without a vitamin D deficiency. The underlying mechanisms of these relationships are unknown. The idea that an intervention as simple as vitamin supplementation could be used to treat persistent pain is very attractive; however, a systematic review (22 relevant studies) concluded that the well-controlled studies thus far are too small and that supporting studies are insufficient to support the hypothesis that vitamin D might be helpful for treatment of persistent pain (Straube, Moore, Derry, et al., 2009). Clearly, more research is needed to better understand how deficiencies in vitamin D might initiate and maintain pain and whether or not supplementation is helpful.

Nicotine

Antinociceptive effects of nicotine via nicotinic acetylcholine receptors distributed throughout the nervous system have been observed for many years in animal and human experimental research (Habib, White, El Gasim, et al., 2008; Perkins, Grobe, Stiller, et al., 1994; Shapiro, Jarvik, 1998); however, the use of nicotine for pain management has been limited because of associated gastrointestinal and cardiovascular (CV) adverse effects (Rowbotham, Duan, Thomas, et al., 2009). Nevertheless, a small placebo-controlled trial randomized 20 healthy women who underwent gynecologic surgery to receive an intranasal spray of saline or nicotine (3 mg) after surgery and before emergence from anesthesia and found that those who received the intranasal nicotine had no CV adverse effects, lower pain scores, and consumed less supplemental opioid during the first 24 postoperative hours than those who received placebo (Flood, Daniel, 2004).

Later studies have reported less impressive results. Patients (N = 90 nonsmokers) undergoing radical retropubic prostatectomy were randomized to receive a 7 mg transdermal nicotine patch or placebo patch behind the ear 30 to 60 minutes prior to anesthesia induction (Habib, White, El Gasim, et al., 2008). All patients received morphine IV patient-controlled analgesia (PCA) and IV ketorolac 15 mg every 6 hours postoperatively. Although those who received the nicotine patch consumed significantly less morphine, there were no differences in pain scores and incidences of nausea and vomiting compared with placebo. Another randomized control trial of nonsmokers undergoing various general surgery procedures reported transdermal nicotine patches (5 to 15 mg) applied preoperatively reduced postoperative pain scores but did not decrease the need for opioid analgesics and did not reduce the incidence of opioid-induced adverse effects (Hong, Conell-Price, Cheng, et al., 2008). An interesting study of patients undergoing surgery showed that preoperatively applied transdermal nicotine (5 to 15 mg) did not relieve postoperative pain or reduce opioid use in smokers (Olson, Hong, Conell-Price, et al., 2009). A high-dose (21 mg) transdermal nicotine patch did not improve analgesia or decrease analgesic requirements postoperatively in patients after hysterectomy, and adverse effects did not differ significantly from those associated with placebo (Turan, White, Koyuncu, et al., 2008). In contrast, the nicotine patch was associated with a reduced incidence of postoperative nausea and vomiting in another study (Ionescu, Badescu & Acalovschi, 2007).

Alcohol (Ethanol)

For centuries, alcohol has served as an analgesic in the absence of other more effective alternatives. It has been referred to as the "poor man's pain reliever." This practice continues today as a socially, although not medically, accepted remedy for dealing with pain. For example, according to Kotarba's (1983) observations of social drinking in neighborhood cocktail lounges, many pain-afflicted working-class bar drinkers use alcohol as an analgesic. Some drinkers consciously take advantage of the relationship between drinking alcohol and "feeling no pain." Years ago IV alcohol in 5% to 10% solution was used to relieve mild to moderate pain (Cutter, O'Farrell, Whitehouse, et al., 1986). The effects of IV administration appear to be the same as those that occur with oral administration.

Early research based on experimentally-induced pain suggests that the analgesia of alcohol is related to increased pain tolerance rather than decreased pain perception (Woodrow, Eltherington, 1988). The alcohol equivalent of two cocktails induced analgesia (in the form of pain tolerance) that was comparable to that of 11.6 mg of subcutaneous morphine. This occurred at a blood concentration of approximately 70 mg/100 mL. More recently, investigators proposed that G protein-activated inwardly rectifying potassium (GIRK) channels are likely involved in ethanol-induced analgesia (Ikeda, Kobayashi, Kumanishi, et al., 2002).

The therapeutic value of alcohol is extremely limited because of the intoxicating effects that accompany acute consumption and the medical problems associated with long-term use. Furthermore, alcohol used in conjunction with opioids increases sedation and may decrease respirations. Long-term use of alcohol in conjunction with acetaminophen increases the risk of hepatic damage. Use with NSAIDs increases the risk of gastric injury. Thus alcohol is not recommended as an adjuvant analgesic. However, clinicians should be aware of why patients with pain may consume alcohol and should attempt to replace the perceived benefits of alcohol with other pain relief methods.

Conclusion

The agents discussed in this chapter are rarely added to the pain treatment plan because research is lacking to support their use as analgesics. Although their use as analgesics is limited, some may provide other benefits, such as relief of anxiety and treatment of opioid-induced adverse effects, in selected patients.

Section V | Conclusion

A review of the literature revealed numerous reasons why patients do not adhere to a variety of medications prescribed for pain (Monsivais, McNeil, 2007). In addition to an introductory review of the literature, these authors examined 42 abstracts and 17 full-text articles. Some of the concerns revealed are pertinent to adjuvant analgesics and may be diminished by providing the patient with written information about their medications. (See pp. 757-758 and Patient Medication Information Forms V-1 to V-12 on pp. 759-782.) A common reason for nonadherence was high levels of concern about the medication, such as adverse effects, "dependency," and questions about the real need for the medication. Patients also had misconceptions about how long it should take for the drug to be effective, and they would stop taking it if no benefits occurred by the expected time. Patients also feared tolerance, that is, that the medication might cease to work if taken on a regular basis.

The information in the "Patient Medication Information" forms is based on content from this section and the following four references:

- Clinical Pharmacology Online. Gold Standard, Inc. Available at http://clinicalpharmacology.com.
- Drug inserts, available online for each medication.
- Lacy, C. F., Armstrong, L. L., Goldman, M. P., et al. (Eds). (2009-2010). *Drug information handbook*, ed 18, American Pharmacists Association, Lexi-Comp.

- Fox Chase Cancer Center/Pain Management. *Patient Education Forms*, Philadelphia, PA (baclofen, 2007; clonazepam, 2007; desipramine, 2007; gabapentin, 2007; licodaine patch 5%, 2007; mexiletine, 2007; nortriptyline, 2007).

There is an abundance of evidence to support the use of some of the adjuvant analgesics for acute and persistent pain states; however, the use of others remains largely guided by anecdotal experience. Future investigations of nociceptive processes and pain pathophysiology will undoubtedly lead to the development of novel drugs.

For many patients with pain, particularly those in the palliative care settings, opioid drugs continue to be the mainstay of analgesia. However, adjuvant analgesics offer opportunities for improved outcomes in those patients who cannot attain an acceptable balance between pain relief and opioid or NSAID-induced adverse effects. For many patients with persistent noncancer pain, adjuvants are the primary analgesics and may offer an alternative to opioids or more invasive therapies. The future of adjuvant analgesics for acute pain requires more research, but already it is clear that they have a role in multimodal pain management. Table V-1 provides guidelines for the use of the more common adjuvant analgesics discussed in this section.

Table V-1 | Selected Adjuvant Analgesics[1-4]

Drug Class	Indications	Drugs/Routes	Usual Starting Dose	Usual Effective Dose Range	Dosing Schedule	Comments
Alpha$_2$-adrenergic agonist	Multipurpose for persistent (chronic) and acute pain; treatment of substance withdrawal symptoms	Clonidine (Catapres) PO	0.1 mg qd	0.2-0.6 mg/day	qd	Dose may be increased by 0.1-0.2 mg/day increments weekly as tolerated. Taper dose 0.1 mg-0.2 mg/day before discontinuing after use for withdrawal symptoms.
	Persistent neuropathic pain; treatment of substance withdrawal symptoms	Clonidine (Catapres-TTS) Transdermal	0.1 mg/24 h strength patch	0.2-0.6 mg/day	q week patch change	Dose may be increased by 0.1 mg/day q 3-5 days. Apply to hairless skin on upper extremity or torso; alternate application site if possible. 2-3 day lag time until onset of action. Taper dose 0.1 mg-0.2 mg/day before discontinuing after use for withdrawal symptoms.
	Persistent (chronic) and acute pain treatment; treatment of postanesthesia shivering	Clonidine (Duraclon) IV	4-8 mcg/kg (analgesia); 150 mcg (shivering)	2 mcg/kg/h	Infusion or bolus	Administered with IV opioids to enhance analgesia and produce opioid dose-sparing effect. See text for clonidine added to IV opioid PCA.
	Persistent (chronic) and acute pain treatment	Clonidine Epidural	30 mcg/h; 150 mcg or less single dose	1-2 mcg/kg/h	Infusion or single injection	Enhances and prolongs local anesthetic effect; produces opioid dose-sparing effect. Single doses greater than 150 mcg associated with high incidence of adverse effects, e.g., hypotension. Maximum single dose 700 mcg.
	Persistent (chronic) and acute pain treatment	Clonidine Intrathecal	30-225 mcg/day	To 400 mcg/day	Infusion or single injection	Dose range varies widely. Long-term use of doses as high as 950 mcg/day have been reported.
	Agent in multimodal postoperative pain treatment plan	Clonidine in Continuous Peripheral Nerve Block	1 mcg/mL in solution with local anesthetic infused per block rate	1 mcg/mL in solution with local anesthetic infused per block rate	Infusion	Enhances and prolongs local anesthetic effect.
	Goal-directed sedation in the critically ill; procedural sedation	Dexmedetomidine (Precedex) IV	1 mcg/kg over 10-20 min	0.2-0.7 mcg/kg/h for 24 h	Infusion	At the time of publication, dexmedetomidine was restricted to a maximum dose of 0.7 mcg/kg/h for up to 24 h (see text). Slow titration minimizes hypotension and bradycardia.

		Starting dose	Usual dose range	Interval	Comments
	Multipurpose for persistent (chronic) pain and spasticity	Tizanidine (Zanaflex) PO	2-4 mg q8h	6-12 mg/day	q 8 h	Dose may be increased 2-8 mg/day weekly as tolerated to 36 mg/day. Limited information on the long-term use of single doses greater than 8-12 mg or total daily doses greater than 24-36 mg. Monitor liver function during administration. Several drugs affect clearance of tizanidine (see text).
Anticonvulsants	First line for neuropathic pain	Gabapentin (Neurontin) PO	100-300 mg/day	1800-3600 mg/day	q 8 h	In most cases, the dose can be increased every 3-4 days, initially by an amount equal to the starting dose. Doses should be divided into twice-daily administration; some patients experience better outcomes with three divided doses. Dose titration usually continues with a target of 1800 mg/day to 3600 mg/day in two or three divided doses. Trial of 3-8 weeks for titration plus 2 weeks at maximum dose is suggested. Oral bioavailability of gabapentin is inversely proportional to dose, e.g., 900 mg/day (60%); 2400 mg/day (34%); 4800 mg/day (27%). Adjust dose for renal impairment (see Table 23-2).
		Pregabalin (Lyrica) PO	50-75 mg q12h or 150 mg at hs	150-600 mg/day	q 12 h	In most cases, the dose is titrated every 3-4 days by an amount equal to the starting dose; the usual effective dose is between 150 mg twice daily and 300 mg twice daily, but some patients have good outcomes at doses that are higher or lower than this range. 600 mg/day can be tried, but there may be no clinical advantage over 300 mg/day; allow 4-week trial. Flexible (dose and time of dose) rather than fixed regimen is preferred by many (see text). Adjust dose for renal impairment (see Table 23-2).
	Second or third line for neuropathic pain	Carbamazepine (Tegretol) PO	200 mg/day	600-1200 mg/day	q 6-8 h	Effective particularly for trigeminal neuralgia. Leukocyte count less than 4000 is possible contraindication to use; discontinue if decline to less than 3000 (or absolute neutrophil count of less than 1500).

Continued

Table V-1 | Selected Adjuvant Analgesics[1-4]—cont'd

Drug Class	Indications	Drugs/Routes	Usual Starting Dose	Usual Effective Dose Range	Dosing Schedule	Comments
		Clonazepam (Klonopin) PO	0.5 mg/day	0.5-3 mg/day	q 8 h	Classified as both anticonvulsant and benzodiazepine; may be helpful for both pain and anxiety related to disease process.
		Divalproex sodium (Depakote Sprinkle, Depakote DR, ER) PO	500 mg/day	1000 mg/day	q 8-12 h	Closely related to valproic acid. Also used for persistent hiccups.
		Lamotrigine (Lamictal) PO	50 mg/day	50-200 mg/day	q 12 h	Used for migraine prevention. Start low and increase slowly every 2 weeks up to 200 mg/day (400 mg/day has been given; see text). Associated with life-threatening rashes; do not administer higher than recommended doses, and do not co-administer with valproic acid.
		Oxcarbazepine (Trileptal) PO	300 mg q12h	600-1200 mg/day	q 12 h	Dose may be increased 150-300 mg every few days (increase by no more than 600 mg/day/week) to 2400 mg/day.
		Phenytoin (Dilantin) PO	300 mg/day	300 mg/day	hs	Loading doses may be used (e.g., 400 mg × 2; see text).
		Phenytoin (Dilantin) IV	500-1000 mg/day	ND	Infusion	IV dose used for rapidly escalating neuropathic pain. Adjust rate according to response.
		Topiramate (Topamax) PO	25-50 mg/day	100-400 mg/day	q 12 h	Dose may be increased by 25 mg weekly; reported dose range of 25-800 mg/day (see text).
		Valproic acid (Depakene Stavzor DR) PO	500 mg/day	1000 mg/day	q 8-12 h	Closely related to divalproex sodium. Also used for persistent hiccups. Do not co-administer with lamotrigine. Available in oral solution.
		Valproic acid (Depacon, Valproate Sodium) IV	Maximum 20 mg/kg over 5 min	ND	ND	IV (Depacon) dose used for rapidly escalating neuropathic pain followed by PO doses; oral solution available.
	Agent in multimodal postoperative pain treatment plan	Gabapentin (Neurontin) PO	400-1200 mg 1 h preoperatively	1200-2400 mg/day postoperatively	q 8 h	No consensus on optimal dose or dosing regimen in this setting.
		Pregabalin (Lyrica) PO	Less than 300 mg 1 h preoperatively	150-300 mg/day postoperatively	q 12 h	No consensus on optimal dose or dosing regimen in this setting; 300 mg preoperatively and 600 mg postoperatively have been associated with increased adverse effects.

Category		Drug	Starting dose	Maximum dose	Interval	Comments
Antidepressants: (secondary amines)	First line for neuropathic pain	Desipramine (Norpramin) PO	10-25 mg/day	50-150 mg/day	hs	Preferred over amitriptyline. Increase weekly by 10-25 mg/day; allow 6-8 week trial with 2 weeks at maximum tolerated dose.
		Nortriptyline (Aventyl, Pamelor) PO	10-25 mg/day	50-150 mg/day	hs	Preferred over amitriptyline. Increase weekly by 10-25 mg/day; allow 4- to 6-week trial with 2 weeks at maximum tolerated dose.
Antidepressants: (serotonin norepinephrine reuptake inhibitors [SNRIs])	First line for neuropathic pain	Bupropion (Aplenzin, Budeprion, Wellbutrin, Zyban)	100 mg q12h or 150 mg once daily of modified-release	400 mg/day	q 12 h	Increase by 100 mg/week to 450 mg maximum dose. Modified-release formulations available.
		Duloxetine (Cymbalta)	30 mg/day	60 mg/day	q 12 h or qd	Increase to 60 mg/day after 1 week; allow 4-week trial; 120 mg/day can be tried, but there may be no clinical advantage. Reduce dose 50% in hepatic or renal insufficiency; do not use in dialysis-dependent patients.
		Milnacipran (Savella)	12.5-25 mg/day	50-100 mg/day	q 12 h	Initiate with once-daily dosing, then increase to twice-daily dosing. Doses greater than 200 mg/day have not been studied. Reduce dose 50% in hepatic or renal insufficiency.
		Venlafaxine (Effexor)	37.5 mg/day	150 mg/day	q 12 h	Available in 75 mg modified-release formulation. May increase dose by 37.5 mg/week to 300 mg as tolerated. Reduce dose 50% in hepatic or renal insufficiency.
Antidepressants (tertiary amines)	Second line for neuropathic pain (use tertiary amine only if secondary amine is unavailable)	Amitriptyline (Elavil) PO	10-25 mg/day	50-150 mg/day	hs	Amitriptyline is no longer listed as first line for neuropathic pain; because of a better adverse effect profile and evidence of comparable analgesia, desipramine is preferred for many patients, especially older adults. Less hypotension with nortriptyline. Evaluate and titrate upward every 3-5 days. Some patients may prefer divided doses (e.g., q8h).
		Clomipramine (Anafranil) PO	10-25 mg/day	50-150 mg/day	hs	Maximum dose 250 mg/day.

Continued

Table V-1 | Selected Adjuvant Analgesics[1-4]—cont'd

Drug Class	Indications	Drugs/Routes	Usual Starting Dose	Usual Effective Dose Range	Dosing Schedule	Comments
		Doxepin PO	10-25 mg/day	50-150 mg/day	hs	Oral doxepin rinse is effective for oral mucositis due to cancer therapy. Frequently used for intractable itching (pruritus).
		Imipramine (Tofranil) PO	10-25 mg/day	50-150 mg/day	hs	Maximum dose 250 mg/day.
Antidepressants (tetracyclic amine)	Third line for neuropathic pain	Mirtazapine (Remeron) PO	15 mg/day	15-45 mg/day	hs	Available in 15, 30, and 45 mg oral disintegrating tablet. Effective for depression, fatigue, and intractable itch (pruritus), but research on analgesia is lacking.
Antidepressants (selective serotonin reuptake inhibitors [SSRIs])	Third line for neuropathic pain	Fluoxetine (Prozac) PO	10-20 mg/day	20-40 mg/day	qd	Increase dose weekly as tolerated and needed to 80 mg/day. Fewer adverse effects than TCAs but less evidence of analgesic effectiveness.
		Paroxetine (Paxil) PO	20 mg/day	20-50 mg/day	qd	Increase dose weekly as tolerated and needed to 80 mg/day. Fewer adverse effects than TCAs but less evidence of analgesic effectiveness. Modified-release formulation available.
		Sertraline (Zoloft) PO	25-50 mg/day	150-200 mg/day	qd	Increase dose weekly as tolerated and needed to maximum 200 mg/day. Used for intractable itch (pruritus).
Bisphosphonates	Persistent (chronic) bone pain	Ibandronate (Boniva) IV	4-6 mg IV over 2-h period	4-6 mg q month	q month	Available in oral tablet formulations, but IV route is preferred for faster onset and better efficacy.
		Pamidronate (Aredia)	60-90 mg IV over 2-h period	60-90 mg q month	q month	
		Zolendronate (Zometa) IV	4 mg IV over 15-min period	4 mg q month	q month	Faster onset, shorter infusion time than other bisphosphonates.

Class	Indication	Drug	Dose		Route/Interval	Comments
Corticosteroids	Multipurpose analgesics	Dexamethasone (Baycadron, Decadron, Dexamethasone Intensol) PO	Low-dose regimen: 2-16 mg/day	Same	q 6-12 h	See text for discussion of dosing and Table 22-2 for equivalent corticosteroid doses. May also improve appetite, nausea, and malaise. In patients with advanced medical illness, long-term treatment with low doses is generally well-tolerated; used when pain persists after optimal opioid dosing. See text and Figure 30-1 and Box 30-2 for treatment of malignant bowel syndrome.
			High-dose regimen: 100 mg/day, then 96 mg/day in 4 divided doses	Same	q 6 h	See text for discussion of dosing and Table 22-2 for equivalent corticosteroid doses. High doses used for acute episode of severe pain unresponsive to opioids. Risk of serious toxicity increases with dose, duration of therapy, and co-administration of an NSAID.
		Prednisone PO	15-80 mg/day for brief "pulse" treatment for 1-2 wk	Long term: 10 mg/day for chronic antiinflammatory conditions		A brief "pulse" of oral corticosteroid (see Table 22-2 for equivalent corticosteroid doses) for 1-2 wk for acute flare of an inflammatory disorder, such as rheumatoid arthritis, or acute neuropathic pains of various types (e.g., acute herpes zoster). See text.
Gamma aminobutyric acid agonists (GABAergic)	Refractory neuropathic pain, particularly "shooting" neuropathic pain	Baclofen (Lioresal) PO	5-15 mg/day	30-200 mg/day	q 8 h	May be useful for prevention of cluster headaches (15-30 mg/day). Doses greater than 60 mg/day associated with more adverse effects. See text for intrathecal administration.
	Goal-directed sedation in critically ill ventilated patients	Propofol (Diprivan) IV	No loading dose necessary	5 mcg/kg/min for at least 5 min (0.3 mg/kg/h) with subsequent increases of 5-10 mcg/kg/min (0.3-0.6 mg/kg/h) every 5-10 min to achieve desired level of sedation	Infusion	Dosing regimens vary (see text for more). Must be administered via infusion device. Low doses do not produce sufficient analgesia; therefore, co-administration of appropriate analgesics (e.g., an opioid) is essential. Taper dose before discontinuation. Adverse effects are more likely with high doses, bolus doses, and use in hypovolemic patients and older adults.

Continued

Table V-1 | Selected Adjuvant Analgesics[1-4]—cont'd

Drug Class	Indications	Drugs/Routes	Usual Starting Dose	Usual Effective Dose Range	Dosing Schedule	Comments
	Procedural sedation	Propofol (Diprivan) IV	Initial dose of 0.25-0.5 mg/kg administered over 3-5 min	Subsequent dosing with this initial protocol: 10-20 mg/min until adequate sedation is achieved	Infusion or incremental doses	Dosing regimens vary (see text for more). Low doses do not produce sufficient analgesia; therefore, co-administration of appropriate analgesics, e.g., an opioid, is essential. Infusion recommended especially for longer procedures. Adverse effects are more likely with high doses, bolus doses, and in hypovolemic patients and older adults. Nurses must be aware of scope of practice issues (see text).
Local anesthetics	Third line for persistent neuropathic pain of any type	Mexiletine (Mexitil) PO	150-200 mg/day	900-1200 mg/day	q 8 h	Plasma concentrations should be followed to reduce risk of toxicity. Periodic ECG evaluation recommended.
		Flecainide (Tambocor) PO	50 mg/day	50-100 mg/day	q 12 h	Mexiletine should be tried first. Dosing recommendations are based on doses used to treat cardiac arrhythmias. Titration by 50 mg increments every 4 days is recommended. Periodic ECG evaluation recommended.
	Persistent neuropathic pain (See Box 26-2 for IV lidocaine for postoperative pain).	Lidocaine IV	Brief infusion (see comments): 1-5 mg/kg over 30-45 min	—	Infusion	Analgesia occurs within 15-30 min. Extended infusion of 5 mg/kg/h over 6-h period was safe and effective (see text); 5 mg/kg was more effective than 1 and 3 mg/kg. May be appropriate for rapidly escalating neuropathic pain. Dose should be decreased significantly for medically ill, e.g., 0.5 mg/kg/h infusion.
		SC, IV	Continuous infusion 2.5-5 mg/kg/h over 1 h	—	Infusion	Doses may depend on type of pain (see text). Dose should be decreased significantly for medically ill, e.g., 0.5 mg/kg/h infusion.
Psychostimulants[5]	Multipurpose for acute or persistent pain; neuropathic or physiologic (nociceptive) pain; conventionally used to reverse somnolence caused by opioids	Caffeine PO	50-150 mg per dose of opioid or NSAID	ND	ND	Used in combination products for headache. (See Chapter 9 for detailed discussion of caffeine.)

	Drug	Starting Dose	Usual Dose Range	Frequency	Comments
	Dextroamphetamine (Dexedrine)[6] PO	2.5-5 mg with first meal of day	10-30 mg/day	Once or twice daily	Available in oral solution and modified-release formulation (Dexedrine Spansule); see comments below (PO methylphenidate) regarding dosing and modified-release formulations.[6]
	Methylphenidate (Ritalin, Methylin) (see comments for modified-release formulations)[6] PO	2.5-5 mg 30-45 minutes before first meal of day	10-30 mg/day	Once or twice daily	Short-acting methylphenidate is available in tablets, chewable tablets, oral solution, and powder for compounding. Time of dose administration of short-acting drug should be based on patient's activity/sleep pattern; the first dose should be taken upon awakening, and doses right before sleep are discouraged. Monitor quality of sleep, and adjust as needed, e.g., a formulation that allows twice- or once-daily dosing may be preferable if sleep is adversely affected with three-times-daily dosing. There are a variety of modified-release formulations (Concerta; Metadate CD, ER; Methylin ER; Ritalin LA, SR) in different dose strengths that allow every 8, 12, and 24-h dosing. The reader is advised to review all options and the manufacturer's dosing recommendations.[6] Do not crush modified-release formulations.
	Methylphenidate (Daytrana) Transdermal	10 mg/day (one 9-h patch)	20 mg/day	qd	Apply patch to hip in morning or 2 h before effect is desired, and remove patch after 9 h. May increase dose 5 mg/day weekly to 20 mg/day; 30 mg/day can be tried, but there may be no clinical advantage.
	Modafinil (Provigil)	100 mg/day	100-400 mg/day	qd with first meal of day	There may be no clinical advantage of doses >200 mg/day. Doses of 800 mg resulted in discontinuation of the drug due to elevated blood pressure and heart rate (see text).
	Donepezil (Aricept)	2.5 mg/day	2.5-5 mg/day	qd with first meal of day	Available in disintegrating tablet.
Miscellaneous					
Various neuropathic pains; persistent (chronic) bone pain; osteoarthritis; osteoporosis	Calcitonin IV, SC	25 IU/day	100-200 IU/day	qd	Assess need daily. Can be given by slow infusion over 20 minutes (see text).

Continued

Table V-1 | Selected Adjuvant Analgesics[1-4]—cont'd

Drug Class	Indications	Drugs/Routes	Usual Starting Dose	Usual Effective Dose Range	Dosing Schedule	Comments
Neuroleptics	Trigeminal neuralgia; persistent cluster headache, refractory, paroxysmal (sudden) onset, or "shooting" neuropathic pain	Calcitonin Nasal Spray (Miacalcin)	200 IU/day	200-400 IU/day	qd	One puff in one nostril; alternate nostril daily. 400 IU is taken in two (200 IU) sprays/day.
		Olanzapine (Zyprexa; Zydis) PO	5 mg/day	5-10 mg/day	qd	Atypical neuroleptic available in tablet, disintegrating tablet, and injectable formulation; may be beneficial in addition to opioid for severe cancer pain with co-existing anxiety or cognitive impairment in some patients; has been used for refractory fibromyalgia; less likely than other neuroleptics to produce extrapyramidal effects (see text).
		Haloperidol (Haldol, Decanoate) PO	2 mg	4-15 mg/day	q 8-12 h	Available in tablet, oral solution, and injectable formulations.
		Pimozide (Orap) PO	2 mg/day	4-10 mg/day	q 8 h	Extrapyramidal effects are concerning; other adjuvant analgesics are preferred (see text).

IU, International unit; ND, no data; PO, oral; q, every; qd, every day; SC, subcutaneous

[1]Older adults are more sensitive than younger adults to adverse effects of many of the adjuvant agents; initiate therapy with lower starting doses, and titrate slowly.

[2]Dose escalation should be gradual and individualized based on assessment of both pain and adverse effects.

[3]Doses should be gradually tapered before discontinuation of most adjuvant analgesics.

[4]Take single doses or largest dose of sedating medication before longest sleep period.

[5]Take single or first dose of psychostimulant upon awakening or after longest sleep period.

[6]It is generally recommended that titration with a short-acting formulation be done before switching to a modified-release formulation of a drug. Switching may be done when the available dosage of the modified-release formulation corresponds with the titrated dose of the short-acting formulation (e.g., 8-hour dose of the modified-release formulation corresponds with the 8-hour titrated dose of the short-acting formulation).

From Pasero, C., & McCaffery, M. *Pain assessment and pharmacologic management*, pp. 748-756, St. Louis, Mosby. Data from Ackerman, L. L., Follett, K. A., & Rosenquist, R. W. (2003). Long-term outcomes during treatment of chronic pain with intrathecal clonidine or clonidine/opioid combinations. *J Pain Symptom Manage*, 26(1), 668-677; Argoff, C. E., Backonja, M. M., Belgrade, M. J., et al. (2006). Consensus guidelines: Treatment planning and options. Diabetic peripheral neuropathic pain. *Mayo Clin Proc*, 81(Suppl 4), S12-S25; Backonja, M., & Glanzman, R. L. (2003). Gabapentin dosing for neuropathic pain: evidence from randomized, placebo-controlled clinical trials. *Clin Ther*, 25(1), 81-104; Brush, D. R., & Kress, J. P. (2009). Sedation and analgesia for the mechanically ventilated patient. *Clin Chest Med*, 30(1), 131-141; Carrazana, E., & Mikoshiba, I. (2003). Rationale and evidence for the use of oxcarbazepine in neuropathic pain. *J Pain Symptom Manage*, 25(Suppl 5), S31-S35; Clinical Pharmacology Online. Gold Standard, Inc. Available at http://clinicalpharmacology.com. Accessed March 1, 2009; Dworkin, R. H., O'Connor, A. B., Backonja, M., et al.: Pharmacologic management of neuropathic pain: evidence-based recommendations, *Pain*, 132, 237-251, 2007; Eisenach, J. C., Hood, D. D., & Curry, R. (2000). Relative potency of epidural to intrathecal clonidine differs between acute thermal pain and capsaicin-induced allodynia. *Pain*, 84(1), 57-64; Elliott, J. A. (2009). α2-agonists. In H. S. Smith (Ed.), *Current therapy in pain*, Philadelphia, Saunders; Epstein, J. B., Epstein, J. D., Epstein, M. S., et al. (2006). Oral doxepin rinse: The analgesic effect and duration of pain reduction in patients with oral mucositis due to cancer therapy. *Anesth Analg*, 103(2), 465-470; Gilron, I. (2006). Review article: The role of anticonvulsant drugs in postoperative pain management: A bench-to-bedside perspective. *Can J Anesth*, 53(6), 562-571; Guay, D. R. (2001). Adjunctive agents in the management of chronic pain. *Pharmacotherapy*, 21(9), 1070-1080; Harris, J. D., & Kotob, F. (2006). Management of opioid-related side effects. In O. A. de Leon-Casasola (Ed.), *Cancer pain. Pharmacological, interventional and palliative care approaches*, Philadelphia, Saunders; Ho, K. Y., Gan, T. J., & Habib, A. S. (2006). Gabapentin and postoperative pain—A systematic review of randomized controlled trials. *Pain*, 126(1-3), 91-101; Ilfeld, B. M., Morey, T. E., & Enneking, F. K. (2003). Continuous infraclavicular perineural infusion with clonidine and ropivacaine compared with ropivacaine alone: A randomized, double-blinded, controlled study. *Anesth Analg*, 97(3), 706-712; Kim, S. W., Shin, I. S., Kim, J. M., et al. (2008). Effectiveness of mirtazapine for nausea and insomnia in cancer patients with depression. *Psychiatry Clin Neurosci*, 62(1), 75-83; Lacy, C. F., Armstrong, L. L., Goldman, M. P., et al. (Eds.). (2008). *Drug information handbook*, ed 17, Hudson, OH, Lexi-Comp Inc; Maizels, M., & McCarberg, B. (2005). Antidepressants and antiepileptic drugs for chronic non-cancer pain. *Am Fam Physician*, 71(3), 483-490; May, A., Leone, M., Afra, J., et al. (2006). EFNS guidelines on the treatment of cluster headache and other trigeminal-autonomic cephalalgias. *Eur J Neurol*, 13(10), 1066-1077; Moss, J., & Glick, D. (2005). The autonomic nervous system. In R. D. Miller (Ed.), *Miller's anesthesia*, ed 6, Philadelphia, Elsevier; Moulin, D. E., Clark, A. J., Gilron, I., et al. (2007). Pharmacological management of chronic neuropathic pain—Consensus statement and guidelines from the Canadian Pain Society. *Pain Res Manag*, 12(1), 13-21; Odom-Forren, J., & Watson, D. (2005). Practical guide to moderate sedation/analgesia. St. Louis, Mosby; Reves, J., Glass, P. S. A., Lubarsky, D. A., et al. (2005). Intravenous nonopioid anesthetics. In R. D. Miller (Ed.), *Miller's anesthesia*, ed 6, Philadelphia, Churchill Livingstone; Semenchuk, M. R., & Sherman, S. (2000). Effectiveness of tizanidine in neuropathic pain: An open-label study. *J Pain*, 1(4), 285-292; Sharma, S., Rajagopal, M. R., Palat, G., et al. (2009). A phase II pilot study to evaluate use of intravenous lidocaine for opioid-refractory pain in cancer patients. *J Pain Symptom Manage*, 37(1), 85-93; Silberstein, S. D., Neto, W., Schmitt, J., et al. (2004). Topiramate in migraine prevention: Results of a large, controlled trial. *Arch Neurol*, 61(4), 490-495; Stacey, B. R., Dworkin, R. H., Murphy, K., et al. (2008). Pregabalin in the treatment of refractory neuropathic pain: Results of a 15-month open-label trial. *Pain Med*, 9(8), 1202-1208; Tremont-Lukats, I. W., Challapalli, V., McNicol, E. D., et al. (2005). Systemic administration of local anesthetics to relieve neuropathic pain: A systematic review and meta-analysis. *Anesth Analg*, 101(6), 1738-1749; Tremont-Lukats I.W., Hutson, P. R., & Backonja, M. (2006). A randomized, double-masked, placebo-controlled pilot trial of extended IV lidocaine infusion for relief of ongoing neuropathic pain. *Clin J Pain*, 22(3), 266-271; White, P. F., Tufanogullari, B., Taylor, J., et al. (2009). The effect of pregabalin on postoperative anxiety and sedation levels: A dose-ranging study. *Anesth Analg*, 108(4), 1140-1145; Zed, P. J., Abu-Laban, R. B., Chan, W. W. Y., et al. (2007). Efficacy, safety and patient satisfaction of propofol for procedural sedation and analgesia in the emergency department: A prospective study. *Can J Emerg Med*, 9(6), 421-427. © 2011, Pasero C, McCaffery M. May be duplicated for use in clinical practice.

Patient Information Brochure: Continuous Peripheral Nerve Block Infusion

HOW DOES PAIN AFFECT MY BODY?

When you are injured, pain warns you to protect yourself and avoid further injury. However, unrelieved pain can be harmful, especially when you are sick or after surgery. Pain can make it difficult to take a deep breath and interferes with your ability to move and walk. This can result in complications and a long stay in the hospital.

HOW WILL OTHERS KNOW HOW MUCH PAIN I HAVE?

- Your nurses will check you often while you are receiving the continuous nerve block infusion. They will ask you to rate your pain on a 0 to 10 scale. A rating of 0 means you feel no pain at all, 5 means you feel a moderate (medium) amount of pain, and 10 means you feel the worst pain you can imagine.

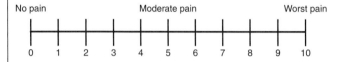

- Your comfort-function goal is _____ _____. If you are unable to maintain this level of comfort, especially during activities such as physical therapy, let your nurse know. The dose of pain medicine usually can be increased to keep you as comfortable as possible.

WHAT ARE SOME OF THE GOALS OF PAIN MANAGEMENT WITH CONTINUOUS PERIPHERAL NERVE BLOCK INFUSION?

- To keep pain from becoming severe and out of control.
- To keep comfortable so that you can sleep, visit with others, and participate in physical therapy.
- To decrease the length of time spent in the hospital.

HOW DOES A CONTINUOUS PERIPHERAL NERVE BLOCK INFUSION WORK?

- Pain medicine, called local anesthetic, will be given by a small pump through a tiny tube that the anesthesiologist will insert near a nerve or nerves in the area of your surgery. This will be done before surgery.
- The pump is set to deliver a specific dose of local anesthetic continuously. This medicine will numb the area of your body for as long as the infusion is running.
- You may have some pain even though you are receiving the local anesthetic infusion. If you do, let your nurse know. The dose of local anesthetic may need to be increased, or you may be given oral pain medicine.

IS CONTINUOUS PERIPHERAL NERVE BLOCK INFUSION SAFE?

- The pump will be programmed to give you an amount of pain medicine that is typically safe for someone your sex, size, age, and diagnosis or type of surgery. If this is too much, the dose of the pain medicine can be reduced.
- Let the nurse know before you take any other medicines, including the ones you usually take at home.

WILL I BE ABLE TO WALK AND DO PHYSICAL THERAPY EXERCISES WHILE I HAVE THE CONTINUOUS PERIPHERAL NERVE BLOCK INFUSION?

- You will have a heavy, numb feeling in the area of the body where the local anesthetic is infusing. It will feel similar to the numbness you feel when the dentist numbs your gums before dental work. Because of this numbness, the muscles in that area will feel weak. *It is very important that you always ask for assistance when getting in and out of bed to prevent you from falling*, especially if the numbed area is in the legs.
- The dose is sometimes decreased if the numbness bothers you.
- The numbness will also go away after the infusion is stopped.
- The pump that infuses the local anesthetic is small and can be carried easily when you get out of bed and during physical therapy.

Continued

Patient Information Brochure: Continuous Peripheral Nerve Block Infusion—cont'd

WHEN SHOULD I CALL THE NURSE?

- If you are experiencing pain
- If the numb feeling is bothering you
- If you want to turn or get out of bed
- If you experience any of the following:
  - A metallic taste in your mouth
  - Numbness of your tongue, lips, or gums
  - Dizziness
  - Ringing in your ears
  - Blurred vision
  - Shaking or jitteriness

HOW LONG WILL THE CONTINUOUS PERIPHERAL NERVE BLOCK INFUSION BE USED?

- As your condition improves, your pain will decrease.
- The infusion will be used for 2 to 3 days depending on the type of surgery you have.
- If you are in the hospital, the nurse will stop the pump and remove the tube when it is time. If you are home, you or a family member will be told when and how to do these things. This is a simple and painless procedure.
- You will be able to take oral pain medicine to keep your pain under control after the infusion is stopped. Take a dose of oral pain medicine as soon as you start to feel sensation returning in the area that was previously numb. Remember to stay on top of your pain by taking pain medicine before pain is severe or out of control.

In addition to talking with patients about therapies and their adverse effects, providing written information reinforces explanations about the method of delivery and other important points the patient will need to remember. Box 26-1 provides an example of a patient information brochure on continuous peripheral nerve block infusion.

From Pasero, C., & McCaffery, M. *Pain assessment and pharmacologic management,* pp. 757-758, St. Louis, Mosby. Data from Peripheral Nerve Block Infusion Information for Patients. University of Pittsburgh Medical Center, UPMC Presbyterian—Shadyside Hospital, Pittsburgh, PA. © 2011, Pasero C, McCaffery M. May be duplicated for use in clinical practice.

PATIENT MEDICATION INFORMATION

Amitriptyline (generic name)

BRAND NAME: Elavil

TYPE OF PAIN MEDICINE: Antidepressant

DESCRIPTION: Tablets come in 6 strengths: 10 mg, 25 mg, 50 mg, 75 mg, 100 mg, 150 mg

USES:
- Relieves pain caused by nerve damage.
- Relieves depression.
- Improves sleep.

DOSAGE AND ADMINISTRATION:
- <u>Take only as directed</u>.
- The starting dose is usually 10 mg or 25 mg per day. The dose may need to be increased every 3 to 7 days until relief is satisfactory.
- Pain relief usually takes 2 to 4 weeks or longer if the dose needs to be increased.
- Take with a glass of water. May be taken with or without food.
- Avoid grapefruit juice because it may increase the effects of amitriptyline.
- If you miss a dose, take the missed dose as soon as possible. Skip the missed dose if it is almost time for the next dose.
- If the only dose you take in one day is at bedtime and you miss this dose, you may take the missed dose when you awaken. But do not take this dose if it is ordered for sleep or if it makes you so drowsy that it interferes with your normal activities.
- Do not take two doses at the same time.
- Before taking amitriptyline tell your pharmacist, nurse, or doctor if you are taking:
  - MAOIs like selegiline (Eldepryl®) or phenelzine (Nardil®)
  - other antidepressants
  - St. John's wort or other herbs
  - heart medicines
  - clonidine
  - bupropion
  - anti-seizure medicines, such as barbiturates
- Tell your pharmacist, nurse, or doctor if you have any of these conditions:
  - difficulty passing urine, prostate trouble
  - liver disease
  - thoughts of suicide
  - heart disease
  - heavy consumer of alcohol
  - pregnancy, trying to get pregnant, or breast-feeding
  - glaucoma
  - seizures
  - diabetes

Continued

Form V-1 | Patient medication information: amitriptyline.

PATIENT MEDICATION INFORMATION—cont'd

Amitriptyline (generic name)

POSSIBLE SIDE EFFECTS:
- Drowsiness—May occur initially or as your dose is increased. If this happens your dose may need to be lowered.
- Dizziness—May occur when moving from lying to sitting or sitting to standing. Change position slowly. If this does not help, call your nurse or doctor.
- Dry mouth—May be relieved by chewing sugarless gum, sucking sugarless or sour hard candy, or drinking fluids frequently.
- Constipation—Can be controlled with daily laxatives.
- Dry eyes or blurred vision—If your wear contact lenses, lubricating drops may help.
- Nausea or vomiting
- Change in sex drive or performance
- Weight gain or loss
- Tell your nurse or doctor at once if you have:
  - difficulty starting your urine
  - increased depression or thoughts of suicide
  - increased anxiety or panic
  - fast or irregular heart beat
  - allergic reactions like skin rash, swelling of the face
  - abnormal breast enlargement in either male or female; abnormal production of milk in females

PRECAUTIONS:
- Avoid alcohol. It may increase dizziness or drowsiness.
- If you are dizzy or drowsy, do not do anything that may be dangerous such as operating machinery or driving a car, until this goes away.
- If you are a diabetic, check your blood sugar level more often than usual during the first few weeks, since amitriptyline can affect your blood sugar levels.
- Amitriptyline makes you sensitive to sunlight. If you cannot avoid sunlight, wear protective clothing or sunscreen.
- Should be discontinued several days before elective surgery because of the risk of high blood pressure.

STOPPING MEDICATIONS: Do not suddenly stop taking your amitriptyline. Suddenly stopping amitriptyline can cause severe side effects such as nausea, vomiting, or diarrhea. Call your pharmacist, nurse, or doctor for directions on how to decrease the dose gradually.

REMEMBER!
- Keep count of your medicine.
- Do not run out of medicine.
- Do not mix medicines in the same container.
- Get a **new** prescription filled a few days before you will run out of medicine.
- **Call** your nurse or doctor if side effects occur or if pain changes or does not go away. Your medicine may need to be changed.
- Take unused, unneeded, or expired medicines out of their original containers and flush them down the toilet. Do not put them in the trash.

COMMENTS:

WARNING: Keep this and all medicines out of reach of children!

Form V-1 | Cont'd.

PATIENT MEDICATION INFORMATION

Baclofen (generic name)

BRAND NAME: Lioresal

TYPE OF PAIN MEDICINE: Muscle relaxant

DESCRIPTION: Baclofen comes in 2 strengths: 10 mg and 20 mg.

USES:
- Relaxes muscle spasms.
- Decreases hiccups.
- Relieves pain caused by nerve damage.
- Treats trigeminal neuralgia.

DOSAGE AND ADMINISTRATION:
- <u>Take only as directed</u>.
- May be taken with or without food.
- If baclofen upsets your stomach try taking it with food.
- If you miss a dose take the missed dose as soon as possible. Skip the missed dose if it is almost time for the next dose.
- Do not take two doses at the same time.
- The initial doses usually do not produce pain relief for 3 to 5 days or longer. The initial dose may need to be increased until relief is satisfactory.
- Before taking baclofen tell your pharmacist, nurse, or doctor if you are taking:
  - cold or allergy medicines
  - alcohol
  - medicines for depression, anxiety, and other mental conditions
  - medicines for sleep
  - phenobarbital
  - medicines for pain such as codeine, oxycodone, or tramadol
  - St John's wort
- Tell your pharmacist, nurse, or doctor if you have any of these conditions:
  - kidney disease
  - stroke
  - seizures
  - pregnant, trying to get pregnant, or breast-feeding
  - diabetes
  - an unusual or allergic reaction to baclofen, foods, dyes, or preservatives

POSSIBLE SIDE EFFECTS:
The following should be reported to your nurse or doctor if they persist:
- Dizziness or drowsiness—Do not do anything that may be dangerous such as operating machinery or driving a car, until this goes away. Stand up or sit up slowly.
- Nausea and vomiting

Continued

Form V-2 | Patient medication information: baclofen.

PATIENT MEDICATION INFORMATION—cont'd

Baclofen (generic name)

- Weakness
- Fatigue
- Headache
- Difficulty sleeping
- Confusion
- Numbness in arms and legs
- In diabetes, blood sugar may rise
- <u>Report the following side effects to your nurse or doctor as soon as possible</u>:
  - allergic reactions such as a rash
  - chest pain
  - hallucinations
  - seizure.
  - numbness in arms or legs

PRECAUTIONS:
- Avoid alcohol while taking baclofen.
- If you are a diabetic, monitor your blood sugar carefully.

STOPPING MEDICATIONS: Do not suddenly stop taking your baclofen. Suddenly stopping baclofen can cause confusion, hallucinations, and other severe symptoms. Call your pharmacist, nurse, or doctor before you stop taking your medicine. <u>Doses should always be decreased gradually over 1 to 2 weeks or longer.</u>

REMEMBER!
- Keep count of your medicine.
- Do not run out of medicine.
- Do not mix medicines in the same container.
- Get a **new** prescription filled a few days before you will run out of medicine.
- **Call** your nurse or doctor if side effects occur or if pain changes or does not go away. Your medicine may need to be changed.
- Take unused, unneeded, or expired medicines out of their original containers and flush them down the toilet. Do not put them in the trash.

COMMENTS:

WARNING: Keep this and all medicines out of reach of children!

Form V-2 │ Cont'd.

PATIENT MEDICATION INFORMATION

Clonazepam (generic name)

BRAND NAME: Klonopin (a type of benzodiazepine)

TYPE OF PAIN MEDICINE: Anti-seizure; anti-anxiety, muscle relaxant

DESCRIPTION: Oral tablets come in 3 strengths: 0.5 mg, 1 mg, 2 mg. Oral disintegrating tablets (wafers) come in 5 strengths: 0.125 mg, 0.25 mg, 0.5 mg, 1 mg, 2 mg.

USES:
- Controls seizures.
- Relieves anxiety or panic.
- Relaxes muscle jerks.
- Relieves pain caused by nerve damage.
- Improves sleep.
- Helps with restless leg syndrome.

DOSAGE AND ADMINISTRATION:
- <u>Take only as directed</u>.
- <u>Do not take with alcohol</u>.
- Conventional oral tablets may be taken with a glass of water, with or without food.
- Begins to take effect in 20-60 minutes. If it does not relieve your pain, the dose may need to be adjusted.
- Orally disintegrating tablets (wafer) may be taken with or without water. Open the pouch by peeling back the foil on the blister pack. Do not push the tablet through the foil. Using dry hands, immediately remove the tablet and place in mouth. Tablet disintegration occurs rapidly. Use immediately. You don't need to take it with a glass of water but you may take it with water if you wish.
- You may be told to take one dose during the day and a different dose at bedtime.
- If you miss a dose, take the missed dose as soon as possible. Skip the missed dose if it is almost time for the next dose. Do not take 2 doses at the same time.
- Before taking clonazepam tell your pharmacist, nurse, or doctor if you are taking:
  - medicines for depression, anxiety, or any other mental condition
  - medicines for fungal infections such as fluconazole (Diflucan®)
  - medicines for HIV infection or AIDS
  - medicines for sleep
  - medicines for seizures
  - prescription pain medicines
  - propantheline (Pro-Banthine®)
  - rifampin (Rifadin®)
  - sevelamer (Renagel®)
  - herbal or dietary supplements such as kava kava or St. John's wort
- Tell your pharmacist, nurse, or doctor if you have any of these conditions:
  - liver disease
  - pregnant, trying to get pregnant, or breast-feeding
  - glaucoma
  - kidney disease
  - mental health condition such a depression, suicidal thoughts
  - seizures, past or present

Continued

Form V-3 | Patient medication information: clonazepam.

PATIENT MEDICATION INFORMATION—cont'd

Clonazepam (generic name)

- lung or breathing disease, such as chronic obstructive pulmonary disease (COPD) or sleep apnea
- myasthenia gravis
- Parkinson's disease
- heavy use of alcohol

POSSIBLE SIDE EFFECTS:

- Dizziness or drowsiness—May occur when moving from lying to sitting or sitting to standing. Change position slowly. If this does not help, call your nurse or doctor. Your dose may need to be lowered.
- Difficulty sleeping or nightmares
- Constipation or diarrhea
- Headache
- Increased saliva from your mouth
- Nausea or vomiting
- Lightheadedness
- Tell your nurse or doctor at once if you have:
  - allergic reactions like skin rash, swelling of the face
  - changes in vision
  - confusion
  - mood changes such as depression, thoughts of suicide, excitability, or anger
  - hallucinations
  - movement difficulty such as falling, staggering, or jerky movements
  - muscle cramps, weakness
  - tremors
  - unusual eye movements

PRECAUTIONS:

- If you are dizzy, unsteady, or drowsy, do not do anything that may be dangerous such as operating machinery or driving a car, until this goes away.
- Avoid alcohol since it can increase symptoms such as dizziness and drowsiness.

STOPPING MEDICATIONS: Do not suddenly stop taking your clonazepam because you may experience irritability, nervousness, or difficulty thinking. Call your pharmacist, nurse, or doctor for directions on how to decrease the dose gradually.

REMEMBER!

- Keep count of your medicine.
- Do not run out of medicine.
- Do not mix medicines in the same container.
- Get a **new** prescription filled a few days before you will run out of medicine.
- **Call** your nurse or doctor if side effects occur or if pain changes or does not go away. Your medicine may need to be changed.
- Take unused, unneeded, or expired medicines out of their original containers and flush them down the toilet. Do not put them in the trash.

COMMENTS:

WARNING: Keep this and all medicines out of reach of children!

Form V-3 | Cont'd.

PATIENT MEDICATION INFORMATION

Cyclobenzaprine (generic name)

BRAND NAMES: Flexeril (short acting; sometimes referred to as immediate release or IR), Amrix (extended release)

TYPE OF PAIN MEDICINE: Skeletal muscle relaxant

DESCRIPTION: Capsules (extended release) are available in 2 strengths: 15 mg, 30 mg. Tablets (short acting) are available in 2 strengths: 5 mg, 10 mg.

USES:
- Relieves skeletal muscle spasm.
- Relieves fibromyalgia.

DOSAGE AND ADMINISTRATION:
- <u>Take only as directed</u>.
- Take with a glass of water. If cyclobenzaprine upsets your stomach, take it with food or milk.
- If you miss a dose, take the missed dose as soon as possible. Skip the missed dose if it is almost time for the next dose. Do not take two doses at the same time.
- An initial dose of 15 mg extended release capsule is usually ordered once a day. An initial dose of short-acting 5 mg tablet is usually ordered 3 times a day. Doses may be increased.
- Take extended release capsules at the same time each day, usually bedtime. Do not crush or chew capsule,
- Usually used for 2 to 3 weeks for skeletal muscle injury, such as low back pain, since effectiveness decreases. Used longer for fibromyalgia.
- Before taking cyclobenzaprine tell your pharmacist, nurse, or doctor if you are taking:
  - MAOIs like selegiline (Eldepryl®) or phenelzine (Nardil®) within 14 days
  - tricyclic antidepressants such as desipramine (Norpramin®) and amitriptyline (Elavil®)
  - bupropion (Wellbutrin®)
  - phenothiazines such as prochlorperazine (Compazine®)
  - clonidine
  - tramadol (Ultram®)
  - cisapride (Propulcid®)
  - pimozide (Orap®)
  - flecainide (Tambocar®)
- Tell your pharmacist, nurse, or doctor if you have any of these conditions:
  - hyperthyroidism
  - heart disease
  - liver disease
  - pregnant, trying to get pregnant, or breast-feeding
  - heavy use of alcohol
  - glaucoma
  - difficulty passing urine or prostate trouble

POSSIBLE SIDE EFFECTS:
- Dizziness, especially during the first week or after a dose increase. May occur when moving from lying to sitting or sitting to standing. Change position slowly. If this does not help, call your nurse or doctor.
- Drowsiness, especially initially
- Dry mouth—May be relieved by chewing sugarless gum, sucking sugarless or sour hard candy, or drinking fluids frequently.

Continued

Form V-4 | Patient medication information: cyclobenzaprine.

PATIENT MEDICATION INFORMATION—cont'd

Cyclobenzaprine (generic name)

- Dry eyes or blurred vision—If your wear contact lenses, lubricating drops may help.
- Headache
- <u>Tell your nurse or doctor at once if you have</u>:
  - allergic reactions such a skin rash or swelling of the face
  - chest pain
  - fast heartbeat
  - hallucinations
  - seizures
  - vomiting

PRECAUTIONS:
- Avoid alcohol because it may increase some side effects such as drowsiness.
- If you are dizzy or drowsy, do not do anything that may be dangerous such as operating machinery or driving a car, until this goes away.
- Cyclobenzaprine may cause increased sensitivity to sunburn. When exposed to sunlight, use sunscreens or protective clothing.

STOPPING MEDICATIONS: Do not suddenly stop taking your cyclobenzaprine if you have been taking it for a long time. Although the possibility of withdrawal symptoms is not known, suddenly stopping your medicine may cause nausea, headache, and fatigue. Call your pharmacist, nurse, or doctor for directions on how to decrease the dose gradually.

REMEMBER!
- Keep count of your medicine.
- Do not run out of medicine.
- Do not mix medicines in the same container.
- Get a **new** prescription filled a few days before you will run out of medicine.
- **Call** your nurse or doctor if side effects occur or if pain changes or does not go away. Your medicine may need to be changed.
- Take unused, unneeded, or expired medicines out of their original containers and flush them down the toilet. Do not put them in the trash.

COMMENTS:

WARNING: Keep this and all medicines out of reach of children!

Form V-4 | Cont'd.

PATIENT MEDICATION INFORMATION

Desipramine (generic name)

BRAND NAME: Norpramin®

TYPE OF PAIN MEDICINE: Antidepressant

DESCRIPTION: Desipramine tablets come in 6 strengths: 10 mg, 25 mg, 50 mg, 75 mg, 100 mg, 150 mg

USES:
• Relieves pain caused by nerve damage.
• Relieves depression.
• Improves sleep.

DOSAGE AND ADMINISTRATION:
• <u>Take only as directed.</u>
• The starting dose is usually 10 mg or 25 mg per day. The dose may need to be increased every 3 to 4 days until relief is satisfactory.
• Pain relief usually takes 2 to 4 weeks or longer if the dose needs to be increased.
• Take with a glass of water. May be taken with or without food.
• Avoid grapefruit juice because it may increase the effects of desipramine.
• Tablet may be crushed if difficult to swallow.
• Usually taken at bedtime. May be ordered 3 times a day.
• If you miss a dose, take the missed dose as soon as possible. Skip the missed dose if it is almost time for the next dose.
• If the only dose you take in one day is at bedtime and you miss this dose, you may take the missed dose when you awaken. But do not take this dose if it is ordered for sleep or if it makes you so drowsy that it interferes with your normal activities.
• Do not take two doses at the same time.
• Before taking desipramine tell your pharmacist, nurse, or doctor if you are taking:
  - MAOIs like selegiline (Eldepryl®) or phenelzine (Nardil®)
  - other antidepressants
  - St. John's wort or other herbs
  - heart medicines
  - cold or allergy medicines
  - clonidine
• Tell your pharmacist, nurse, or doctor if you have any of these conditions:
  - kidney disease
  - liver disease
  - diabetes
  - heavy consumer of alcohol
  - pregnancy, trying to get pregnant, or breast-feeding
  - glaucoma
  - seizures

POSSIBLE SIDE EFFECTS:
• Drowsiness initially or as the dose is increased. Your dose may need to be lowered.
• Dry mouth—May be relieved by chewing sugarless gum, sucking sugarless or sour hard candy, or drinking fluids frequently.

Continued

Form V-5 | Patient medication information: desipramine.

PATIENT MEDICATION INFORMATION—cont'd

Desipramine (generic name)

- Constipation (can be controlled with daily laxatives) or diarrhea
- Nausea or vomiting
- Dry eyes or blurred vision—If you wear contact lenses, lubricating drops may help.
- Weight gain or loss
- Change in sex drive or performance
- Dizziness may occur when moving from lying to sitting or sitting to standing. Change position slowly. If this does not help, call your doctor or nurse.
- <u>Tell your nurse or doctor at once if you have:</u>
  - difficulty starting your urine
  - increased depression or thoughts of suicide
  - increased anxiety or panic
  - fast or irregular heart beat
  - allergic reactions like skin rash, swelling of the face
  - abnormal breast enlargement in either male or female; abnormal production of milk in female

PRECAUTIONS:
- Avoid alcohol. It may increase dizziness or drowsiness.
- If you are dizzy or drowsy, do not do anything that may be dangerous such as operating machinery or driving a car, until this goes away.
- If you are a diabetic, check your blood sugar level more often than usual during the first few weeks, since desipramine can affect your blood sugar levels.
- Desipramine makes you sensitive to sunlight. If you cannot avoid sunlight, wear protective clothing or sunscreen.
- Should be discontinued several days before elective surgery because of the risk of high blood pressure.

STOPPING MEDICATIONS: Do not suddenly stop taking your desipramine. Suddenly stopping desipramine can cause severe side effects such as nausea, vomiting, or diarrhea. Call your pharmacist, nurse, or doctor for directions on how to decrease the dose gradually.

REMEMBER!
- Keep count of your medicine.
- Do not run out of medicine.
- Do not mix medicines in the same container.
- Get a <u>**new**</u> prescription filled a few days before you will run out of medicine.
- <u>**Call**</u> your nurse or doctor if side effects occur or if pain changes or does not go away. Your medicine may need to be changed.
- Take unused, unneeded, or expired medicines out of their original containers and flush them down the toilet. Do not put them in the trash.

COMMENTS:

WARNING: Keep this and all medicines out of reach of children!

Form V-5 | Cont'd.

PATIENT MEDICATION INFORMATION

Duloxetine (generic name)

BRAND NAME: Cymbalta

TYPE OF PAIN MEDICINE: Antidepressant

DESCRIPTION: Capsules (delayed release) come in 3 strengths: 20 mg, 30 mg, 60 mg

USES:
- Relieves pain, particularly diabetic neuropathy and fibromyalgia.
- Relieves depression.
- Relieves anxiety.

DOSAGE AND ADMINISTRATION:
- <u>Take only as directed</u>.
- The starting dose is usually 30 mg to 60 mg once a day. The 30 mg dose may be increased to 60 mg after one week. Sometimes the dose is given twice a day.
- Pain relief generally occurs over 1 week and may continue to increase for weeks.
- Take with a glass of water. May be taken with or without food.
- Do not cut, break open, crush, or chew the capsule.
- If you miss a dose, take the missed dose as soon as possible. Skip the missed dose if it is almost time for the next dose.
- Stopping smoking is recommended since smoking reduces duloxetine's effectiveness.
- Before taking duloxetine tell your pharmacist, nurse, or doctor if you are taking:
  - MAOIs like selegiline (Eldepryl®) or phenelzine (Nardil®) within 14 days
  - antidepressants called SSRIs, such as sertraline (Zoloft®), paroxetine (Paxil®), or citalopram (Celexa®)
  - venlafaxine (Effexor®)
  - thioridazine (Mellaril®)
  - St. John's wort or other herbs
  - certain diet drugs
  - tryptophan
  - medicines for colds or allergies
- Tell your pharmacist, nurse, or doctor if you have any of these conditions:
  - thoughts of suicide
  - seizures
  - liver disease
  - moderate to severe kidney impairment
  - diabetic
  - heavy consumer of alcohol
  - glaucoma
  - pregnant, trying to get pregnant, or breast-feeding
  - difficulty passing urine

POSSIBLE SIDE EFFECTS:
- Dizziness, especially during the first week or after a dose increase. May occur when moving from lying to sitting or sitting to standing. Change position slowly. If this does not help, call your nurse or doctor.
- Fatigue

Continued

Form V-6 | Patient medication information: duloxetine.

PATIENT MEDICATION INFORMATION—cont'd

Duloxetine (generic name)

- Drowsiness
- Headache
- Nausea
- Difficulty sleeping
- Diarrhea or constipation
- Dry mouth—May be relieved by chewing sugarless gum, sucking sugarless or sour hard candy, or drinking fluids frequently
- Blurred vision
- Change in appetite
- Increased sweating
- Sore throat
- <u>Tell your nurse or doctor at once if you have</u>:
  - unusual bleeding or bruising
  - thoughts of suicide
  - allergic reactions such as rash or swelling of the face
  - confusion
  - fast talking, excited feelings or actions that are out of control
  - loss of contact with reality
  - fast, irregular heartbeat
  - fever or stomach flu-like symptoms

PRECAUTIONS:

- Avoid alcohol since it may interfere with duloxetine.
- If you are dizzy or drowsy, do not do anything that may be dangerous such as operating machinery or driving a car, until this goes away.
- If you are a diabetic, check your blood sugar level more often than usual during the first few weeks, since duloxetine can affect your blood sugar levels.

STOPPING MEDICATIONS: Do not suddenly stop taking your duloxetine. Suddenly stopping duloxetine can cause your symptoms to get worse or can cause severe side effects such as abnormal dreams, headache, inability to sleep and others. Call your pharmacist, nurse, or doctor for directions on how to decrease the dose gradually.

REMEMBER!

- Keep count of your medicine.
- Do not run out of medicine.
- Do not mix medicines in the same container.
- Get a **new** prescription filled a few days before you will run out of medicine.
- **Call** your nurse or doctor if side effects occur or if pain changes or does not go away. Your medicine may need to be changed.
- Take unused, unneeded, or expired medicines out of their original containers and flush them down the toilet. Do not put them in the trash.

COMMENTS:

WARNING: Keep this and all medicines out of reach of children!

Form V-6 | Cont'd.

PATIENT MEDICATION INFORMATION

Gabapentin (generic name)

BRAND NAME: Neurontin

TYPE OF PAIN MEDICINE: Anticonvulsant

DESCRIPTION: Capsules and tablets come in 3 strengths: 100 mg, 300 mg, 400 mg. Tablets come in 2 additional strengths: 600 mg, 800 mg.
Oral liquid comes in 250 mg/teaspoon (5 ml).

USES:
• Helps relieve seizures.
• Relieves various types of nerve pain.

DOSAGE AND ADMINISTRATION:
• <u>Take only as directed</u>.
• Take with a glass of water, with or without food. If it upsets your stomach, take it with food.
• The first dose is usually taken at bedtime. As the dose increases, the second dose is taken in the morning and the third dose mid-day. Dose increases are usually done every week until the desired effect occurs.
• Usually taken in 3 doses a day. Time between doses should not be longer than 12 hours.
• If tablets are scored (line down the middle) they may be cut in half for ease of swallowing or for purposes of increasing or decreasing the dose. The 600 mg and 800 mg tablets are scored. If a tablet is split in half, the extra half should be used for the next dose or discarded within 3 days.
• Oral solution of gabapentin should be refrigerated.
• If you miss a dose, take the missed dose as soon as possible. Skip the missed dose if it is almost time for the next dose. Do not take 2 doses at the same time.
• If you take antacids, take gabapentin at least 2 hours following the antacid.
• Before taking gabapentin tell your pharmacist, nurse, or doctor if you are taking:
  - antacids
  - hydrocodone (may increase the effectiveness of gabapentin; gabapentin decreases the effectiveness of hydrocodone)
  - morphine (may increase the effect of gabapentin)
  - naproxen (may increase the effect of gabapentin)
  - other anticonvulsants
• Tell your pharmacist, nurse, or doctor if you have any of these conditions:
  - kidney disease
  - depression or thoughts of suicide
  - pregnant, trying to get pregnant, or breast-feeding
  - epilepsy

POSSIBLE SIDE EFFECTS:
• Visual disturbances such as blurred vision, double vision, and unusual movement of the eyeball
• Dizziness—May occur when moving from lying to sitting or sitting to standing. Change position slowly.
• Drowsiness
• Fatigue

Continued

Form V-7 | Patient medication information: gabapentin.

From Pasero, C., & McCaffery, M. *Pain assessment and pharmacologic management*, pp. 771-772, St. Louis, Mosby. © 2011, McCaffery M, Pasero C. May be duplicated for use in clinical practice.

PATIENT MEDICATION INFORMATION—cont'd

Gabapentin (generic name)

- Decreased coordination, such as stumbling or staggering
- Slurred speech
- Swelling of hands or feet
- Nausea
- Dry mouth—May be relieved by chewing sugarless gum, sucking sugarless or sour hard candy, or drinking fluids frequently
- Tell your nurse or doctor at once if you have:
  - thoughts of suicide. This is especially a concern if you are taking other anticonvulsants
  - allergic reactions such as a skin rash

PRECAUTIONS:
- If you are dizzy or drowsy, do not do anything that may be dangerous such as operating machinery or driving a car, until this goes away.
- Avoid alcohol because gabapentin may increase the effects of alcohol.

STOPPING MEDICATIONS: Do not suddenly stop taking your gabapentin. It should be discontinued slowly, over at least a week. Call your pharmacist, nurse, or doctor for directions on how to decrease the dose gradually.

REMEMBER!
- Keep count of your medicine.
- Do not run out of medicine.
- Do not mix medicines in the same container.
- Get a **new** prescription filled a few days before you will run out of medicine.
- **Call** your nurse or doctor if side effects occur or if pain changes or does not go away. Your medicine may need to be changed.
- Take unused, unneeded, or expired medicines out of their original containers and flush them down the toilet. Do not put them in the trash.

COMMENTS:

WARNING: Keep this and all medicines out of reach of children!

Form V-7 | Cont'd.

PATIENT MEDICATION INFORMATION

Lidocaine Patch 5% (generic name)

BRAND NAME: Lidoderm®

TYPE OF PAIN MEDICINE: Local anesthetic patch to make the skin less sensitive. The patch is about the size of an adult's hand.

DESCRIPTION: Soft pliable patch containing a local anesthetic

USES:
- Relieves nerve pain and may relieve other types of pain such as arthritis.
- Relieves itch.

DOSAGE AND ADMINISTRATION:
- <u>Take only as directed.</u>
- The patch does not numb the skin, but it makes the skin under it less sensitive to touch, pain, and other sensations.
- Do not reuse a patch.
- Usually 1 to 3 patches are applied for 12 hours and taken off for 12 hours (12 hours on, 12 hours off). However, evidence suggests that up to 4 patches may be applied continuously for up to 24 hours a day.
- Most people begin to feel pain relief within 30 minutes of application of the patch. Pain relief tends to improve with daily use. It may be 1 to 3 weeks until the full benefit is felt.
- Keep the patches at room temperature in the sealed package until ready to use. Apply promptly after removal from the sealed package.
- <u>Instructions for application of the lidocaine patch 5%:</u>
    1. Plan to apply the patch(es) over the most painful area(s) of skin. Be sure the skin is clean (such as after a shower), dry, and does not have any open sores or rashes. Do not apply cream or powder under where the patch(es) will be applied. If the painful area has open sores or a rash, patches may be placed around the open skin instead of over it.
    2. Cut the outer seal from the package along the dotted line, and pull apart the zipper seal.
    3. Remove the desired number of patches. Reseal the package using pressure on the zipper seal. The patches will dry out if the package is left open. Be prepared to use the patch immediately.
    4. A patch may be cut to fit an area before removing the adhesive liner. For example, the patch may be cut in strips to fit around fingers.
    5. Slowly remove the adhesive liner from the back of the patch.
    6. Apply over or beside the most painful areas. Smooth out the patch making sure all edges stick to the skin.
    7. The patch may feel cool when first applied. If mild skin reactions such as stinging, swelling, or burning occur, they may go away within a few minutes. If not, remove the patch and call your nurse or doctor.
    8. Clothing may be worn over the patch.
    9. Protect the patch from getting wet. If bathing is necessary, place plastic wrap over the patch.
    10. When the patch is removed, fold the sticky sides together and discard it out of reach of children or animals.
    11. After applying the patch and removing it, wash your hands so you do not get lidocaine in your eyes or mouth. This can be irritating. If it gets in your eye, flush the eye with water and protect the eye until sensation returns.

Continued

Form V-8 | Patient medication information: lidocaine patch 5%.

PATIENT MEDICATION INFORMATION—cont'd

Lidocaine Patch 5% (generic name)

- Before using lidocaine patch 5% tell your pharmacist, nurse, or doctor if you are taking:
  - dofetilide (Tikosyn®)
  - MAOIs like selegiline (Eldepryl®) or phenelzine (Nardil®)
- Tell your pharmacist, nurse, or doctor if you have any of these conditions:
  - skin rash or irritation in the area where the patches are to be placed
  - allergy to local anesthetics

POSSIBLE SIDE EFFECTS:
- Most people have no side effects.
- The most common side effects are mild skin reactions that go away in a few minutes. If they do not go away or are more severe such as blisters, remove the patch(es) and call your nurse or doctor. Sometimes a medicine can be applied to relieve or prevent the irritation.

PRECAUTIONS:
- If you are going to have an MRI, let your MRI technician know if you are wearing the lidocaine patch. The patch must be removed before the MRI. Bring another patch with you to put on after the MRI.

REMEMBER!
- Keep count of your patches.
- Do not run out of your patches.
- Get a **new** prescription filled a few days before you will run out of patches.
- **Call** your nurse or doctor if side effects occur or if pain changes or does not go away.
- Discard unused, unneeded, or expired patches in a place where children and animals cannot get to them. Do not put them in the trash.

COMMENTS:

WARNING: Keep this and all medicines out of reach of children!

Form V-8 | Cont'd.

PATIENT MEDICATION INFORMATION

Mexiletine (generic name)

BRAND NAME: Mexitil

TYPE OF PAIN MEDICINE: Oral local anesthetic; anti-arrhythmic

DESCRIPTION: Mexiletine capsules come in 3 strengths: 150 mg, 200 mg, 250 mg.

USES:
- Relieves pain caused by nerve damage.
- Controls irregular heartbeats.

DOSAGE AND ADMINISTRATION:
- <u>Take only as directed</u>.
- <u>Do not smoke when using this medicine</u>.
- Take this with a glass of water and with food or antacid.
- Take every 8 hours (not simply 3 times a day) to maintain steady level of medicine in your body.
- If you miss a dose, take the missed dose as soon as possible. Skip the missed dose if it is almost time for the next dose. Do not take 2 doses at the same time.
- Mexiletine is usually not effective immediately. It is started at a low dose and then increased slowly.
- If you have surgery, tell your doctor or dentist you are taking this medicine.
- Before taking mexiletine tell your pharmacist, nurse, or doctor if you are taking:
  - caffeine, such as coffee
  - heart medicines, especially those that control heart rhythm such as dofetilide (Tikosyn®)
  - cimetidine (Tagamet®)
  - medicines for depression, anxiety, or psychotic disturbances
  - phenobarbital
  - phenytoin (Dilantin®)
  - rifampin (Rifadin®)
  - theophylline (TheoCap®, Uniphyl®)
  - lidocaine such as in a patch or gel
  - EMLA cream
  - metoclopramide (Reglan®)
- Tell your pharmacist, nurse, or doctor if you have any of these conditions:
  - liver disease
  - heart problems, past or present
  - pregnant, trying to get pregnant, or breast-feeding
  - slow heart rate
  - kidney disease
  - smoking tobacco—If you smoke and decide to cut down or quit, inform your nurse or doctor
  - low blood pressure

POSSIBLE SIDE EFFECTS:
- Stomach irritation or heartburn—Be sure you are taking mexiletine with food or an antacid.
- Nausea or vomiting—Can be controlled with medication; call your nurse or doctor.
- Diarrhea or constipation—Can be controlled with medication; call your nurse or doctor.

Continued

Form V-9 | Patient medication information: mexiletine.

PATIENT MEDICATION INFORMATION—cont'd

Mexiletine (generic name)

- Dizziness or lightheadedness—May occur when moving from lying to sitting or sitting to standing. Change position slowly.
- Fatigue or weakness
- Numbness or tingling of fingers or toes
- Lack of coordination of legs and arms, such as stumbling
- Blurred vision
- Nervousness
- <u>Tell your nurse or doctor at once if you have</u>:
  - chest pain, pounding in chest, or shortness of breath
  - allergic reactions such as rash, swelling of face or tongue
  - redness, blistering, or peeling of the skin or mouth
  - unsteady hands, trembling, or shaking
  - unusual bleeding or bruising
  - seizures

PRECAUTIONS:
- If you are dizzy, unsteady, or drowsy, do not do anything that may be dangerous such as operating machinery or driving a car, until this goes away.
- Avoid alcohol since it can increase symptoms such as dizziness, flushing, and rapid heartbeats.

STOPPING MEDICATIONS: Do not suddenly stop taking your mexiletine or change the dose or frequency. Call your pharmacist, nurse, or doctor for directions on how to decrease the dose gradually.

REMEMBER!
- Keep count of your medicine.
- Do not run out of medicine.
- Do not mix medicines in the same container.
- Get a **new** prescription filled a few days before you will run out of medicine.
- **Call** your nurse or doctor if side effects occur or if pain changes or does not go away. Your medicine may need to be changed.
- Take unused, unneeded, or expired medicines out of their original containers and flush them down the toilet. Do not put them in the trash.

COMMENTS:

WARNING: Keep this and all medicines out of reach of children!

Form V-9 | Cont'd.

PATIENT MEDICATION INFORMATION

Nortriptyline (generic name)

BRAND NAMES: Aventyl, Pamelor

TYPE OF PAIN MEDICINE: Antidepressant

DESCRIPTION: Nortriptyline capsules come in 4 strengths: 10 mg, 25 mg, 50 mg, 75 mg. Nortriptyline comes in liquid: 10 mg/teaspoon (5 ml).

USES:
- Relieves pain caused by nerve damage.
- Relieves depression.
- Improves sleep.

DOSAGE AND ADMINISTRATION:
- Take only as directed.
- The starting dose is usually 10 mg or 25 mg per day. The dose may need to be increased every 3 to 4 days until relief is satisfactory.
- Pain relief usually takes 2 to 4 weeks or longer if the dose needs to be increased.
- Take with a glass of water. May be taken with or without food.
- Usually taken at bedtime. Sometimes it is ordered 3 or 4 times a day.
- If you miss a dose, take the missed dose as soon as possible. Skip the missed dose if it is almost time for the next dose.
- If the only dose you take in 1 day is at bedtime and you miss this dose, you may take the missed dose when you awaken. Do not take this dose if it is ordered for sleep or if it makes you so drowsy that it interferes with your normal activities.
- Do not take 2 doses at the same time.
- Before taking nortriptyline tell your pharmacist, nurse, or doctor if you are taking:
  - MAOIs like selegiline (Eldepryl®) or phenelzine (Nardil®)
  - other antidepressants
  - St. John's wort or other herbs
  - heart medicines
  - barbiturate medicines for sleep or seizures
  - clonidine
  - cold or allergy medicines
- Tell your pharmacist, nurse, or doctor if you have any of these conditions:
  - difficulty passing urine, prostate trouble
  - liver disease
  - thoughts of suicide
  - heart disease
  - heavy consumer of alcohol
  - pregnancy, trying to get pregnant, or breast-feeding
  - glaucoma
  - seizures
  - diabetes

Continued

Form V-10 | Patient medication information: nortriptyline.

PATIENT MEDICATION INFORMATION—cont'd

Nortriptyline (generic name)

POSSIBLE SIDE EFFECTS:

- Drowsiness—May occur initially or as your dose is increased. If this happens, your dose may need to be lowered.
- Dizziness—May occur when moving from lying to sitting or sitting to standing. Change position slowly. If this does not help, call your nurse or doctor.
- Dry mouth—May be relieved by chewing sugarless gum, sucking sugarless or sour hard candy, or drinking fluids frequently.
- Constipation—Can be controlled with daily laxatives.
- Dry eyes or blurred vision—If you wear contact lenses, lubricating drops may help.
- Nausea or vomiting
- Change in sex drive or performance
- Weight gain or loss
- Tell your nurse or doctor at once if you have:
  - difficulty starting your urine
  - increased depression or thoughts of suicide
  - increased anxiety or panic
  - fast or irregular heart beat
  - allergic reactions like skin rash, swelling of the face
  - abnormal breast enlargement in either male or female; abnormal production of milk in females

PRECAUTIONS:

- Avoid alcohol. It may increase dizziness or drowsiness.
- If you are dizzy or drowsy, do not do anything that may be dangerous such as operating machinery or driving a car, until this goes away.
- If you are a diabetic, check your blood sugar level more often than usual during the first few weeks, since nortriptyline can affect your blood sugar levels.
- Nortriptyline makes you sensitive to sunlight. If you cannot avoid sunlight, wear protective clothing or sunscreen.
- Should be discontinued several days before elective surgery because of the risk of high blood pressure.

STOPPING MEDICATIONS:
Do not suddenly stop taking your nortriptyline. Suddenly stopping nortriptyline can cause severe side effects such as nausea, vomiting, or diarrhea. Call your pharmacist, nurse, or doctor for directions on how to decrease the dose gradually.

REMEMBER!

- Keep count of your medicine.
- Do not run out of medicine.
- Do not mix medicines in the same container.
- Get a **new** prescription filled a few days before you will run out of medicine.
- **Call** your nurse or doctor if side effects occur or if pain changes or does not go away. Your medicine may need to be changed.
- Take unused, unneeded, or expired medicines out of their original containers and flush them down the toilet. Do not put them in the trash.

COMMENTS:

WARNING: Keep this and all medicines out of reach of children!

Form V-10 | Cont'd.

PATIENT MEDICATION INFORMATION

Pregabalin (generic name)

BRAND NAME: Lyrica

TYPE OF PAIN MEDICINE: Analgesic; anticonvulsant

DESCRIPTION: Capsules are available in 8 strengths: 25 mg, 50 mg, 75 mg, 100 mg, 150 mg, 200 mg, 225 mg, 300 mg.

USES:
• Helps control seizures.
• Relieves various types of nerve pain.

DOSAGE AND ADMINISTRATION:
• <u>Take only as directed.</u>
• Take with a glass of water, with or without food.
• Taken in 2 to 3 doses a day. Doses are not effective immediately and may need to be increased after 1 week.
• If you miss a dose, take the missed dose as soon as possible. Skip the missed dose if it is almost time for the next dose. Do not take 2 doses at the same time.
• Before taking pregabalin tell your pharmacist, nurse, or doctor if you are taking:
  - medicines for diabetes, such as pioglitazone (Duetact®) or rosiglitazone (Avandia®)
  - medicines to help you sleep or to relieve anxiety
  - prescription pain medicines
  - medicines for seizures
  - ACE inhibitors such as ramipril (Altace®) and fosinopril (Monopril®)
• Tell your pharmacist, nurse, or doctor if you have any of these conditions:
  - kidney disease
  - bleeding problems
  - heart disease
  - diabetes
  - history of drug abuse or heavy use of alcohol
  - thoughts of suicide
  - glaucoma
  - history of rapid swelling of areas beneath the skin
  - pregnant, trying to get pregnant, or breast-feeding

POSSIBLE SIDE EFFECTS:
• Difficulty sleeping
• Drowsiness
• Fatigue
• Nausea
• Headache
• Constipation or diarrhea
• Dry mouth—May be relieved by chewing sugarless gum, sucking sugarless or sour hard candy, or drinking fluids frequently.

Continued

Form V-11 | Patient medication information: pregabalin.

PATIENT MEDICATION INFORMATION—cont'd

Pregabalin (generic name)

- Dizziness—May occur when moving from lying to sitting or sitting to standing. Change position slowly.
- Blurred vision
- Swelling of hands or feet
- Weight gain
- Confusion
- Decreased coordination, such as stumbling or staggering
- <u>Tell your nurse or doctor at once if you have</u>:
  - thoughts of suicide
  - anxiety, confusion
  - allergic reactions such as a skin rash
  - breathing problems
  - swelling of the face, mouth, or throat
  - changes in vision such as blurred vision
  - chest pain
  - a heart condition and notice that you have swelling in your hands or feet
  - tremors, jerking, or unusual movements of any part of your body
  - loss of memory
  - unexplained muscle pain, tenderness, or weakness
  - unusual bruising or bleeding

PRECAUTIONS:
- If you are dizzy or drowsy, do not do anything that may be dangerous such as operating machinery or driving a car, until this goes away.
- Avoid alcohol since it may interfere with the effect of pregabalin and increase drowsiness.
- If possible, avoid medications that may cause drowsiness because drowsiness may increase.

STOPPING MEDICATIONS: Do not suddenly stop taking your pregabalin. The dose should be tapered over at least a week to avoid symptoms such as insomnia, nausea, headache, or diarrhea. Call your pharmacist, nurse, or doctor for directions on how to decrease the dose gradually.

REMEMBER!
- Keep count of your medicine.
- Do not run out of medicine.
- Do not mix medicines in the same container.
- Get a **new** prescription filled a few days before you will run out of medicine.
- **Call** your nurse or doctor if side effects occur or if pain changes or does not go away. Your medicine may need to be changed.
- Take unused, unneeded, or expired medicines out of their original containers and flush them down the toilet. Do not put them in the trash.

COMMENTS:

WARNING: Keep this and all medicines out of reach of children!

Form V-11 | Cont'd.

PATIENT MEDICATION INFORMATION

Venlafaxine (generic name)

BRAND NAMES: Effexor (short acting, sometimes referred to as immediate release or IR), Effexor XR (extended release)

TYPE OF PAIN MEDICINE: Antidepressant

DESCRIPTION: Extended release capsules and tablets come in 3 strengths: 37.5 mg, 75 mg, 150 mg. Extended release tablets also come in 225 mg.
Short acting tablets come in 5 strengths: 25 mg, 37.5 mg, 50 mg, 75 mg, 100 mg.

USES:
• Relieves depression.
• Relieves anxiety.
• Relieves pain caused by nerve damage.

DOSAGE AND ADMINISTRATION:
• <u>Take only as directed</u>.
• Short acting tablets are usually taken 2 to 3 times a day. Extended release is taken once a day. Doses may be increased every 4 to 7 days.
• Take venlafaxine with food and a glass of water.
• Do not crush, cut, place in water, or chew the extended tablets or capsules.
• If you miss a dose, take the missed dose as soon as possible. Skip the missed dose if it is almost time for the next dose. Do not take 2 doses at the same time.
• If necessary, carefully open the extended release capsule and sprinkle the entire contents on a spoonful of applesauce and swallow immediately without chewing. Follow with a glass of water.
• Before taking venlafaxine tell your pharmacist, nurse, or doctor if you are taking:
  - MAOIs like selegiline (Eldepryl®) or phenelzine (Nardil®) within 14 days
  - St John's wort or other herbs
  - tryptophan
  - duloxetine (Cymbalta®)
  - weight control medicines
  - nefazodone (Serzone®)
  - cold or allergy medicines
  - antidepressants called SSRIs such as sertraline (Zoloft®), paroxetine (Paxil®), or citalopram (Celexa®)
  - pentazocine (Talwin®)
• Tell your pharmacist, nurse, or doctor if you have any of these conditions:
  - weight loss
  - glaucoma
  - heart disease
  - high blood pressure
  - high cholesterol levels or receiving treatment for this
  - kidney disease
  - liver disease
  - manic symptoms, mental disorders, or thoughts of suicide
  - seizures
  - thyroid problems
  - pregnant, trying to get pregnant, or breast-feeding

Continued

Form V-12 | Patient medication information: venlafaxine.

PATIENT MEDICATION INFORMATION—cont'd

Venlafaxine (generic name)

POSSIBLE SIDE EFFECTS:
- Headache
- Difficulty sleeping
- Drowsiness
- Nervousness/anxiety
- Dizziness—Some people adapt to this after 6 weeks; may occur when moving from lying to sitting or sitting to standing. Change position slowly.
- Nausea/vomiting
- Decreased appetite
- Constipation—Some people adapt to this over a few weeks
- Dry mouth—May be relieved by chewing sugarless gum, sucking sugarless or sour hard candy, or drinking fluids frequently
- Decrease in sexual desire or arousal, unusual ejaculation or orgasm (absent or delayed)
- Weakness
- Blurred vision
- Increased sweating
- Tremor
- <u>Tell your nurse or doctor at once if you have</u>:
  - unusual bleeding or bruising
  - fast heart beat
  - loss of contact with reality
  - thoughts of suicide
  - trouble passing urine
  - allergic reactions such as a skin rash, swelling of the face
  - seizures
  - changes in vision

PRECAUTIONS:
- If you are dizzy or drowsy, do not do anything that may be dangerous such as operating machinery or driving a car, until this goes away.
- Avoid alcohol because it may increase dizziness or drowsiness.

STOPPING MEDICATIONS: Do not suddenly stop taking your venlafaxine because you may experience side effects such as difficulty sleeping, agitation/anxiety, headache, and dizziness. Call your pharmacist, nurse, or doctor for directions on how to decrease the dose gradually.

REMEMBER!
- Keep count of your medicine.
- Do not run out of medicine.
- Do not mix medicines in the same container.
- Get a **new** prescription filled a few days before you will run out of medicine.
- **Call** your nurse or doctor if side effects occur or if pain changes or does not go away. Your medicine may need to be changed.
- Take unused, unneeded, or expired medicines out of their original containers and flush them down the toilet. Do not put them in the trash.

COMMENTS:

WARNING: Keep this and all medicines out of reach of children!

Form V-12 | Cont'd.

References

Aasvang, E. K., Hansen, J. B., Malmstrom, J., et al. (2008). The effect of wound instillation of a novel purified formulation on postherniotomy pain: A double-blind, randomized, placebo-controlled study. *Anesthesia and Analgesia, 107*(1), 282–291.

Abrahm, J. L. (2004). Assessment and treatment of patients with malignant spinal cord compression. *The Journal of Supportive Oncology, 2*(5), 377–388, 391.

Achar, S., & Kundu, S. (2002). Principles of office anesthesia: Part II. Infiltrative anesthesia. *American Family Physician, 66*(1), 91–94.

Ackerman, L. L., Follett, K. A., & Rosenquist, R. W. (2003). Long-term outcomes during treatment of chronic pain with intrathecal clonidine or clonidine/opioid combinations. *Journal of Pain and Symptom Management, 26*(1), 668–677.

Adam, F., Menigaux, C., Sessler, D. I., et al. (2006). A single preoperative dose of gabapentin (800 milligrams) does not augment postoperative analgesia in patients given interscalene brachial plexus blocks for arthroscopic shoulder surgery. *Anesthesia and Analgesia, 103*(5), 1278–1282.

Adamo, V., Caristi, N., Sacca, M. M., et al. (2008). Current knowledge and future directions on bisphosphonate-related osteonecrosis of the jaw in cancer patients. *Expert Opinion on Pharmacotherapy, 9*(8), 1351–1361.

Adelman, J., Freitag, F. G., Lainez, M., et al. (2008). Analysis of safety and tolerability data obtained from over 1,500 patients receiving topiramate for migraine prevention in controlled trials. *Pain Medicine (Malden, Mass.), 9*(2), 175–185.

Adriaensen, H., Plaghki, L., Mathieu, C., et al. (2005). Critical review of oral drug treatments for diabetic neuropathic pain-clinical outcomes based on efficacy and safety data from placebo-controlled and direct comparative studies. *Diabetes Metabolism Research and Reviews, 21*(3), 231–240.

Akerley, W., Butera, J., Wehbe, T., et al. (2002). A multiinstitutional, concurrent chemoradiation trial of strontium-89, estramustine, and vinblastine for hormone refractory prostate carcinoma involving bone. *Cancer, 94*(9), 1654–1660.

Akin, S., Aribogan, A., & Arslan, G. (2008). Dexmedetomidine as an adjunct to epidural analgesia after abdominal surgery in elderly intensive care patients: A prospective, double-blind, clinical trial. *Current Therapeutic Research, Clinical and Experimental, 69*(1), 16–28.

Albazaz, R., Wong, Y. T., & Homer-Vanniasinkam, S. (2008). Complex regional pain syndrome: A review. *Annals of Vascular Surgery, 22*(2), 297–306.

Alford, J. W., & Fadale, P. D. (2003). Evaluation of postoperative bupivacaine infusion for pain management after anterior cruciate ligament reconstruction. *Arthroscopy, 19*(8), 855–1561.

Al-Mujadi, H., A-Refai, A. R., Katzarov, M. G., et al. (2006). Preemptive gabapentin reduces postoperative pain and opioid demand following thyroid surgery. *Canadian Journal of Anaesthesia, 53*(3), 268–273.

Altman, C. S., & Jahangiri, M. F. (2010). Serotonin syndrome in the perioperative period. *Anesthesia and Analgesia,* (11092), 526–528.

Alvarez, J. C., de Mazancourt, P., Chartier-Kastler, E., et al. (2004). Drug stability testing to support clinical feasibility investigations for intrathecal baclofen-clonidine admixture. *Journal of Pain and Symptom Management, 28*(3), 268–272.

Alvarez, N. A., Galer, B. S., & Gammaitoni, A. R. (2006). In O. A. de Leon-Casasola (Ed.), *Cancer pain. Pharmacological, interventional and palliative care approaches* (pp. 123–137). Philadelphia: Saunders.

Ambesh, S. P., Dubey, P. K., & Sinha, P. K. (1999). Ondansetron pretreatment to alleviate pain on propofol injection: A randomized, controlled, double-blinded study. *Anesthesia and Analgesia, 89*(1), 197–199.

American Association of Nurse Anesthetists—American Society of Anesthesiologists. (2004). *Joint statement regarding propofol administration.* http://www.asahq.org/news/propofolstatement.htm. Accessed March 22, 2009.

American Geriatrics Society (AGS) Panel on Persistent Pain in the Older Person. (2002). The management of persistent pain in older persons. *Journal of the American Geriatrics Society, 50*(Suppl. 6), S205–S224.

American Pain Society (APS). (2003). *Principles of analgesic use in the treatment of acute and cancer pain* (5th ed.). Glenview IL: APS.

American Society of Anesthesiologists (ASA) (2006). Practice guidelines for the perioperative management of patients with obstructive sleep apnea. *Anesthesiology, 104*(5), 1081–1093.

Andrieu, G., Roth, B., Ousmane, L., et al. (2009). The efficacy of intrathecal morphine with or without clonidine for postoperative analgesia after radical prostatectomy. *Anesthesia and Analgesia, 108*(6), 1954–1957.

Angst, M. S., & Clark, D. (2006). Opioid-induced hyperalgesia. *Anesthesiology, 104*(3), 570–587.

Anthony, T., Baron, T., Mercadante, S., et al. (2007). Report of the clinical protocol committee: Development of randomized trials for malignant bowel obstruction. *Journal of Pain and Symptom Management, 34*(Suppl. 1), S49–S59.

Apostol, G., Lewis, D. W., Laforet, G. A., et al. (2009). Divalproex sodium extended-release for the prophylaxis of migraine headache in adolescents: Results of a stand-alone, long-term open-label safety study. *Headache, 49*(1), 45–53.

Arain, S. R., Ruehlow, R. M., Uhrich, T. D., et al. (2004). The efficacy of dexmedetomidine versus morphine for postoperative analgesia after major inpatient surgery. *Anesthesia and Analgesia, 98*(1), 153–158.

Arezzo, J. C. (2002). Possible mechanisms for the effects of botulinum toxin on pain. *The Clinical Journal of Pain, 18*(Suppl. 6), S125–S132.

Argoff, C. E. (2000). New analgesics for neuropathic pain: The lidocaine patch. *The Clinical Journal of Pain, 16*(Suppl. 2), S62–S66.

Argoff, C. E. (2002). A review of the use of topical analgesics for myofascial pain. *Current Pain and Headache Reports, 6*(5), 375–378.

Argoff, C. E. (2003). Targeted topical peripheral analgesics in the management of pain. *Current Pain and Headache Reports, 7*(1), 34–38.

Argoff, C. E. (2006). Topical agents for the treatment of chronic pain. *Current Pain and Headache Reports, 10*(1), 11–19.

Argoff, C. E., Albrecht, P., Irving, G., et al. (2009). Multimodal analgesia for chronic pain: Rationale and future directions. *Pain Medicine (Malden, Mass.)*, 10(Suppl. 2), S53–S66.

Argoff, C. E., Backonja, M. M., Belgrade, M. J., et al. (2006). Consensus guidelines: Treatment planning and options. Diabetic peripheral neuropathic pain. *Mayo Clinic Proceedings*, 81(Suppl. 4), S12–S25.

Argoff, C. E., Galer, B. S., Jensen, M. P., et al. (2004). Effectiveness of the lidocaine patch 5% on pain qualities in three chronic pain states: Assessment with the Neuropathic Pain Scale. *Current Medical Research Opinion*, 20(Suppl. 2), S21–S28.

Argyriou, A., Chroni, E., Polychronopoulos, P., et al. (2006). Efficacy of oxcarbazepine for prophylaxis against cumulative oxaliplatin-induced neuropathy. *Neurology*, 67(12), 2253–2255.

Armellin, G., Nardacchione, R., & Ori, C. (2008). Intra-articular sufentanil in multimodal analgesic management after outpatient arthroscopic anterior cruciate ligament reconstruction: A prospective, randomized, double-blinded study. *Arthroscopy*, 24(8), 909–913.

Armstrong, D. G., Chappell, A. S., Le, T. K., et al. (2007). Duloxetine for the management of diabetic peripheral neuropathic pain: Evaluation of functional outcomes. *Pain Medicine (Malden, Mass.)*, 8(3), 410–418.

Arnold, L. M. (2007). Duloxetine and other antidepressants in the treatment of patients with fibromyalgia. *Pain Medicine (Malden, Mass.)*, 8(Suppl. 2), S63–S74.

Arnold, L. M., Crofford, L. J., Martin, S. A., et al. (2007). The effect of anxiety and depression on improvements in pain in a randomized, controlled trial of pregabalin for treatment of fibromyalgia. *Pain Medicine (Malden, Mass.)*, 8(8), 633–638.

Arnold, L. M., Goldenberg, D. L., Stanford, S. B., et al. (2007). Gabapentin in the treatment of fibromyalgia. *Arthritis and Rheumatism*, 56(4), 1336–1344.

Arnold, L. M., Hudson, J. I., Wang, F., et al. (2009). Comparisons of the efficacy and safety of duloxetine for the treatment of fibromyalgia in patients with versus without major depressive disorder. *The Clinical Journal of Pain*, 25(6), 461–468.

Arnold, L. M., Lu, Y., Crofford, L. J., et al. (2004). A double-blind, multicenter trial comparing duloxetine with placebo in the treatment of fibromyalgia with or without major depressive disorder. *Arthritis and Rheumatism*, 50(9), 2974–2984.

Arnold, L. M., Rosen, A., Pritchett, Y. L., et al. (2005). A randomized, double-blind, placebo-controlled trial of duloxetine in the treatment of women with fibromyalgia with or without major depressive disorder. *Pain*, 119(1–3), 5–15.

Arnold, L. M., Russell, I. J., Diri, E. W., et al. (2008). A 14-week, randomized, double-blinded, placebo-controlled monotherapy trial of pregabalin in patients with fibromyalgia. *The Journal of Pain*, 9(9), 792–805.

Arnold, P., Vuadens, P., Kuntzer, T., et al. (2008). Mirtazapine decreases the pain feeling in healthy participants. *The Clinical Journal of Pain*, 24(2), 116–119.

Arpino, P. A., Klafatas, K., & Thompson, B. T. (2008). Feasibility of dexmedetomidine in facilitating extubation in the intensive care unit. *Journal of Clinical Pharmacy and Therapeutics*, 33(1), 25–30.

Ashburn, M. A., Caplan, R. A., Carr, D. B., et al. (2004). Practice guidelines for acute pain management in the perioperative setting: An updated report by the American Society of Anesthesiologists task force on acute pain management. *Anesthesiology*, 100(6), 1573–1581.

Ashina, S., Bendtsen, L., & Jensen, R. (2004). Analgesic effect of amitriptyline in chronic tension-type headache is not directly related to serotonin reuptake inhibition. *Pain*, 108(1–2), 108–114.

Atli, A., & Dogra, S. (2005). Zonisamide in the treatment of painful diabetic neuropathy: A randomized, double-blind, placebo-controlled pilot study. *Pain Medicine (Malden, Mass.)*, 6(3), 225–234.

Attal, N., Gaude, L., Brasseur, L., et al. (2000). Intravenous lidocaine in central pain. *Neurology*, 54(3), 564–574.

Auerbach, M., Tunik, M., & Mojica, M. (2009). A randomized, double-blind controlled study of jet lidocaine compared to jet placebo for pain relief in children undergoing needle insertion in the emergency department. *Emergency Medicine*, 16(3), 388–393.

Auret, K. A., Schug, S. A., Bremner, A. P., et al. (2009). A randomized, double-blind, placebo-controlled trial assessing the impact of dexamphetamine on fatigue in patients with advanced cancer. *Journal of Pain and Symptom Management*, 37(4), 613–621.

Axelsson, K., Gupta, A., Johanzon, E., et al. (2008). Intraarticular administration of ketorolac, morphine, and ropivacaine combined with intraarticular patient-controlled regional analgesia for pain relief after shoulder surgery: A randomized, double-blind study. *Anesthesia and Analgesia*, 106(1), 328–333.

Axelsson, K., Nordenson, U., Johanzon, E., et al. (2003). Patient-controlled regional analgesia with ropivacaine after arthroscopic subacromial decompression. *Acta Anaesthesiologica Scandinavica*, 47(8), 993–1000.

Ayoub, C. M., Ghobashy, A., Koch, M. E., et al. (1998). Widespread application of topical steroids to decrease sore throat, hoarseness, and cough after tracheal intubation. *Anesthesia and Analgesia*, 87(3), 714–716.

Azer, M. S., Abdelhalim, S. M., & Elsayed, G. G. (2006). Preemptive use of pregabalin in postamputation limb pain in cancer hospital: A randomized, double-blind, placebo-controlled, double dose study. (Presentation.) *European Journal of Pain (London, England)*, 10(Suppl. 1), S98.

Azevedo, V. M. S., Lauretti, G. R., Pereira, N. L., et al. (2000). Transdermal ketamine as an adjuvant for postoperative analgesia after abdominal gynecological surgery using lidocaine epidural blockade. *Anesthesia and Analgesia*, 91(6), 1479–1482.

Bach, F. W., Jensen, T. S., Kastrup, J., et al. (1990). The effect of intravenous lidocaine on nociceptive processing in diabetic neuropathy. *Pain*, 40(1), 29–34.

Backonja, M. M. (1994). Local anesthetics as adjuvant analgesics. *Journal of Pain and Symptom Management*, 9(8), 491–499.

Backonja, M. M., Arndt, G., Gombar, K. A., et al. (1994). Response of chronic neuropathic pain syndromes to ketamine: A preliminary study. *Pain*, 56(1), 51–57.

Backonja, M. M., Beydoun, A., Edwards, K. R., et al. (1998). Gabapentin for the treatment of painful neuropathy in patients with diabetes mellitus. *JAMA*, 280(21), 1831–1835.

Backonja, M. M., & Glanzman, R. L. (2003). Gabapentin dosing for neuropathic pain: Evidence from randomized, placebo-controlled clinical trials. *Clinical Therapeutics*, 25(1), 81–104.

Backonja, M. M., & Serra, J. (2004). Pharmacologic management part 1: Better-studied neuropathic pain diseases. *Pain Medicine (Malden, Mass.)*, 5(Suppl. 1), S28–S47.

Badrinath, S., Avramov, M. N., Shadrick, M., et al. (2000). The use of a ketamine-propofol combination during monitored anesthesia care. *Anesthesia and Analgesia*, 90(4), 858–862.

Baig, M. K., Zmora, O., Derdemezi, J., et al. (2006). Use of the On-Q pain management system is associated with decreased postoperative analgesic requirement: A double blind randomized placebo pilot study. *Journal of the American College of Surgeons*, 202(2), 297–305.

Baker, K. (2005). Chronic pain syndromes in the emergency department: Identifying guidelines for management. *Emergency Medicine Australasia*, 17(1), 57–64.

Bamgdade, O. A. (2006). Dexmedetomidine for peri-operative sedation and analgesia in alcohol addiction. *Anaesthesia*, 61(3), 299–300.

Baranowski, A. P., De Courcey, J., & Bonello, E. (1999). A trial of intravenous lidocaine on the pain and allodynia of postherpetic neuralgia. *Journal of Pain and Symptom Management*, 17(6), 429–433.

Barbano, R. L., Herrmann, D. N., Hart-Gouleau, S., et al. (2004). Effectiveness, tolerability, and impact on quality of life of the 5% lidocaine patch in diabetic polyneuropathy. *Archives of Neurology*, 61(6), 914–918.

Barber, F. A., & Herbert, M. A. (2002). The effectiveness of an anesthetic continuous-infusion device on postoperative pain control. *Arthroscopy*, 18(1), 76–81.

Baron, R., Brunnmuller, U., Brasser, M., et al. (2007). Efficacy and safety of pregabalin in patients with diabetic peripheral neuropathy or postherpetic neuralgia: Open-label, noncomparative, flexible-dose study. *European Journal of Pain (London, England)*, 12(1), 850–858.

Barrington, M. J., Olive, D., Low, K., et al. (2005). Continuous femoral nerve blockade or epidural analgesia after total knee replacement: A prospective randomized controlled trial. *Anesthesia and Analgesia*, 101(6), 1824–1829.

Barr, J., Egan, T. D., & Sandoval, N. F. (2001). Propofol dosing regimens for ICU sedation based upon an integrated pharmacokinetic—Pharmacodynamic model. *Anesthesiology*, 95(2), 324–333.

Bartlik, B. D., Kaplan, P., & Kaplan, H. S. (1995). Psychostimulants apparently reverse sexual dysfunction secondary to selective serotonin re-uptake inhibitors. *Journal of Sex & Marital Therapy*, 21(4), 264–271.

Bartusch, S. L., Sanders, B. F., D'Alessio, J. G., et al. (1996). Clonazepam for the treatment of lancinating phantom limb pain. *The Clinical Journal of Pain*, 12(1), 59–62.

Batoz, H., Verdonck, O., Pellerin, C., et al. (2009). The analgesic properties of scalp infiltration with ropivacaine after intracranial tumoral resection. *Anesthesia and Analgesia*, 109(1), 240–244.

Bauman, G., Charette, M., Reid, R., et al. (2005). Radiopharmaceuticals for the palliation of painful bone metastasis—A systemic review. *Radiotherapy and Oncology*, 75(3), 258–270.

Beard, S., Hunn, A., & Wight, J. (2003). Treatments for spasticity and pain in multiple sclerosis: A systematic review. *Health Technology Assessment*, 7(40), iii, ix–x, 1–111.

Beard, S. M., McCrink, L., Le, T. K., et al. (2008). Cost effectiveness of duloxetine in the treatment of diabetic peripheral

neuropathic pain in the UK. *Current Medical Research and Opinion*, 24(2), 385–399.

Bekker, A., Sturaitis, M., Bloom, M., et al. (2008). The effect of dexmedetomidine on perioperative hemodynamics in patients undergoing craniotomy. *Anesthesia and Analgesia*, 107(4), 1340–1347.

Bell, R. F. (2009). Ketamine for chronic non-cancer pain. *Pain*, 141(3), 210–214.

Bell, R. F., Dahl, J. B., Moore, R. A., et al. (2006). Perioperative ketamine for acute postoperative pain. *Cochrane Database Systematic Reviews*, (1), CD004603.

Bell, R. F., Eccleston, C., & Kalso, E. A. (2003a). Ketamine as adjuvant to opioids for cancer pain: A qualitative systematic review. *Cochrane Database Systematic Reviews*, (3), 867–875, Issue 1. Art. No.: CD003351. DOI:10.1002/14651858. CD003351.

Bell, R. F., Eccleston, C., & Kalso, E. A. (2003b). Ketamine as an adjuvant to opioids for cancer pain. *Journal of Pain and Symptom Management*, 26(3), 867–875.

Bell, R. F., & Kalso, K. (2004). Is intranasal ketamine an appropriate treatment for chronic non-cancer breakthrough pain? (Editorial). *Pain*, 108(1), 1–2.

Ben-Ari, A., Lewis, M. C., & Davidson, E. (2007). Chronic administration of ketamine for analgesia. *Journal of Pain & Palliative Care Pharmacotherapy*, 21(1), 7–14.

Ben-David, B., & Friedman, M. (1999). Gabapentin therapy for vulvodynia. *Anesthesia and Analgesia*, 89(6), 1459–1460.

Ben-David, B., Swanson, J., Nelson, J. B., et al. (2007). Multimodal analgesia for radical prostatectomy provides better analgesia and shortens hospital stay. *Journal of Clinical Anesthesia*, 19(4), 264–268.

Bennett, M. I. (1997). Paranoid psychosis due to flecainide toxicity in malignant neuropathic pain. *Pain*, 70(1), 93–94.

Berardi, R. R., Kroon, A. L., McDermott, J. H., et al. (2006). *Handbook of prescription drugs. An interactive approach to self-care.* (15th ed.). Washington, DC: American Pharmacists Association.

Berenson, J. R., Hillner, B. E., Kyle, R. A., et al. (2002). American Society of Clinical Oncology clinical guidelines: The role of biphosphonates in multiple myeloma. *Journal of Clinical Oncology*, 20(17), 3719–3736.

Berger, A., Dukes, E., Edelsberg, J., et al. (2007). Use of tricyclic antidepressants in older patients with diabetic peripheral neuropathy. *The Clinical Journal of Pain*, 23(3), 251–258.

Berthelot, J. M. (2006). Current management of reflex sympathetic dystrophy syndrome (complex regional pain syndrome type I). *Joint Bone Spine*, 73(5), 495–499.

Bettuci, D., Testa, L., Calzoni, S., et al. (2006). Combination of tizanidine and amitriptyline in the prophylaxis of chronic tension-type headache: Evaluation of efficacy and impact on quality of life. *The Journal of Headache and Pain*, 7(1), 34–36.

Beydoun, A., & Backonja, M. M. (2003). Mechanistic stratification of antineuralgic agents. *Journal of Pain and Symptom Management*, 25(Suppl. 5), S18–S30.

Beydoun, A., Kobetz, S. A., & Carrazana, E. J. (2004). Efficacy of oxcarbazepine in the treatment of painful diabetic neuropathy. *The Clinical Journal of Pain*, 20(3), 174–178.

Beydoun, A., Schmidt, D., D'Souza, J., & Oxcarbazepine Study Group. (2002). *Meta-analysis of comparative trials of oxcarbazepine versus carbamazepine in trigeminal neuralgia.* Poster presentation at the 21st American Pain Society Annual Meeting, Baltimore, MD, March 14–17.

Beydoun, A., Shaibani, A., Hopwood, M., et al. (2006). Oxcarbazepine in painful diabetic neuropathy: Results of a dose-ranging study. *Acta Neurologica Scandinavica, 113*(6), 395–404.

Bhimani, R. (2008). Intrathecal baclofen therapy in adults and guideline for clinical nursing care. *Rehabilitation Nursing, 33*(3), 110–116.

Bianconi, M., Ferraro, L., Traina, G. C., et al. (2003). Pharmacokinetics and efficacy of ropivacaine continuous wound instillation after joint replacement surgery. *British Journal of Anaesthesia, 91*(6), 830–835.

Biccard, B. M., Goga, S., & de Beurs, J. (2008). Dexmedetomidine and cardiac protection for non-cardiac surgery: A meta-analysis of randomised controlled trials. *Anaesthesia, 63*(1), 4–14.

Biegler, K. A., Chaoul, M. A., & Cohen, L. (2009). Cancer, cognitive impairment, and meditation. *Acta Oncologica (Stockholm, Sweden), 48*(1), 18–26.

Bigal, M. E., Rapoport, A. M., & Hargreaves, R. (2008). Advances in the pharmacologic treatment of tension-type headache. *Current Pain and Headache Reports, 12*(6), 442–446.

Blommel, M. L., & Blommel, A. L. (2007). Pregabalin: An antileptic agent useful for neuropathic pain. *American Journal of Health-System Pharmacy: AJHP, 64*(14), 1475–1482.

Blumenthal, S., Dullenkopf, A., Rentsch, K., et al. (2005). Continuous infusion of ropivacaine for pain relief after iliac crest bone grafting for shoulder surgery. *Anesthesiology, 102*(2), 392–397.

Boezaart, A. P. (2006). Perineural infusions of local anesthetics. *Anesthesiology, 104*(4), 872–880.

Bone, M., Critchley, P., & Buggy, D. J. (2002). Gabapentin in postamputation phantom limb pain: A randomized, double-blind, placebo-controlled, cross-over study. *Regional Anesthesia and Pain Medicine, 27*(5), 481–486.

Borgeat, A., Kalberer, F., Jacob, H., et al. (2001). Patient-controlled interscalene analgesia with ropivacaine 0.2% versus bupivacaine 0.15% after major open shoulder surgery: The effects on hand motor function. *Anesthesia and Analgesia, 92*(1), 218–223.

Borgeat, A., Perschak, H., Bird, P., et al. (2000). Patient-controlled interscalene analgesia with ropivacaine 0.2% versus patient-controlled intravenous analgesia after major shoulder surgery. *Anesthesiology, 92*(1), 102–108.

Boulton, A. J. M., Vinik, A. I., Arezzo, J. C., et al. (2005). Diabetic neuropathies. A Statement by the American Diabetes Association. *Diabetes Care, 28*(4), 956–962.

Bowsher, D. (2003). Factors influencing the features of postherpetic neuralgia and outcome when treated with tricyclics. *European Journal of Pain (London, England), 7*(1), 1–7.

Bradley, R. H., Barkin, R. L., Jerome, J., et al. (2003). Efficacy of venlafaxine for the long term treatment of chronic pain with associated major depressive disorder. *American Journal of Therapeutics, 10*(5), 318–323.

Braker, C., Yariv, S., Adler, R., et al. (2008). The analgesic effect of botulinum-toxin A on postwhiplash neck pain. *The Clinical Journal of Pain, 24*(1), 5–10.

Brandes, J. L., Saper, J. R., Diamond, M., et al. (2004). Topiramate for migraine prevention: A randomized controlled trial. *JAMA, 291*(8), 965–973.

Bray, D., Nguyen, J., Craig, J., et al. (2007). Efficacy of a local anesthetic pain pump in abdominoplasty. *Plastic and Reconstructive Surgery, 119*(3), 1054–1059.

Brecht, S., Courtecuisse, C., Debieuvre, C., et al. (2007). Efficacy and safety of duloxetine 60 mg once daily in the treatment of pain in patients with major depressive disorder and at least moderate pain of unknown etiology: A randomized controlled trial. *The Journal of Clinical Psychiatry, 68*(11), 1707–1716.

Breuer, B., Pappagallo, M., Ongseng, F., et al. (2008). An open-label pilot trial of ibandronate for complex regional pain syndrome. *The Clinical Journal of Pain, 24*(8), 685–689.

Bridges, D., Thompson, S. W. N., & Rice, A. S. C. (2001). Mechanisms of neuropathic pain. *British Journal of Anaesthesia, 87*(1), 12–26.

Briggs, M., & Nelson, E. A. (2003). Topical agents or dressings for pain in venous leg ulcers. *Cochrane Database Systematic Reviews.*

Brill, S., Sedgwick, M., Hamann, W., et al. (2002). Efficacy of intravenous magnesium in neuropathic pain. *British Journal of Anaesthesia, 89*(5), 711–714.

Brodner, G., Buerkle, H., Van Aken, H., et al. (2007). Postoperative analgesia after knee surgery: A comparison of three different concentrations of ropivacaine for continuous femoral nerve blockade. *Anesthesia and Analgesia, 105*(1), 256–262.

Brodner, G., Van Aken, H., Hertle, L., et al. (2001). Multimodal perioperative management–combining thoracic epidural analgesia, forced mobilization, and oral nutrition–reduces hormonal and metabolic stress and improves convalescence after major urologic surgery. *Anesthesia and Analgesia, 92*(6), 1594–1600.

Brogly, N., Wattier, J. M., Andrieu, G., et al. (2008). Gabapentin attenuates late but not early postoperative pain after thyroidectomy with superficial cervical plexus block. *Anesthesia and Analgesia, 107*(5), 1720–1725.

Brose, W. G., & Cousins, M. J. (1991). Subcutaneous lidocaine for treatment of neuropathic cancer pain. *Pain, 45*(2), 145–148.

Brown, J. (2002). Registered nurses' choices regarding the use of intradermal lidocaine for intravenous insertions: The challenge of changing practice. *Pain Manage Nurs, 3*(2), 71–76.

Brown, M. B., Martin, G. P., Jones, S. A., et al. (2006). Dermal and transdermal drug delivery systems: Current and future prospects. *Drug Delivery, 13*(3), 175–187.

Browning, R., Jackson, J. L., & O'Malley, P. G. (2001). Cyclobenzaprine and back pain: A meta-analysis. *Archives of Internal Medicine, 161*(13), 1613–1620.

Bruera, E., & Neumann, C. M. (1998). The uses of psychotropics in symptom management in advanced cancer. *Psycho-Oncology, 7*(4), 346–358.

Bruera, E., Ripamonti, C., Brenneis, C., et al. (1992). A randomized double-blind crossover trial of intravenous lidocaine in the treatment of neuropathic cancer pain. *Journal of Pain and Symptom Management, 7*(3), 138–140.

Brush, D. R., & Kress, J. P. (2009). Sedation and analgesia for the mechanically ventilated patient. *Clinics in Chest Medicine, 30*(1), 131–141.

Buckenmaier, C. C., Klein, S. M., Nielsen, K. C., et al. (2003). Continuous paravertebral catheter and outpatient infusion for breast surgery. *Anesthesia and Analgesia, 97*(3), 715–717.

Buetefisch, C. M., Guiterrez, M. A., Gutmann, L., et al. (1996). Choreoathetotic movements: A possible side effect of gabapentin. *Neurology, 46*(3), 851–852.

Bulow, N. M., Barbosa, N. V., & Rocha, J. B. (2007). Opioid consumption in total intravenous anesthesia is reduced with dexmedetomidine: A comparative study with remifentanil in gynecologic videolaparoscopic surgery. *Journal of Clinical Anesthesia, 19*(4), 280–285.

Busch, C. A., Shore, B. J., Bhandari, R., et al. (2006). Efficacy of periarticular multimodal drug injection in total knee arthroplasty. *The Journal of Bone and Joint Surgery, 88a*(5), 959–963.

Butterfield, N. N., Schwarz, S. K., Ries, C. R., et al. (2001). Combined pre- and post-surgical bupivacaine wound infiltrations decrease opioid requirements after knee ligament reconstruction. *Canadian Journal of Anaesthesia, 48*(3), 245–250.

Buvanendran, A., & Kroin, J. S. (2007). Useful adjuvants for postoperative pain management. *Best Practice & Research Clinical Anaesthesiology, 21*(1), 31–49.

Buvanendran, A., & Kroin, J. S. (2008). Early use of memantine for neuropathic pain. (Editorial.) *Anesthesia and Analgesia, 107*(4), 1093–1094.

Buvanendran, A., & Kroin, J. S. (2009). Multimodal analgesia for controlling acute postoperative pain. *Current Opinion in Anaesthesiology, 22*(5), 588–593.

Buvanendran, A., Kroin, J. S., Della Valle, C. J., et al. (2010). Perioperative oral pregabalin reduces chronic pain after total knee arthroplasty: A prospective, randomized, controlled trial. *Anesthesia and Analgesia, 110*(1), 199–207.

Byas-Smith, M. G., Max, M. B., Muir, H., et al. (1995). Transdermal clonidine compared to placebo in painful diabetic neuropathy using two-staged "enriched enrollment" design. *Pain, 60*(3), 267–274.

Byers, M. R., & Bonica, J. J. (2001). Peripheral pain mechanisms and nociceptors plasticity. In J. D. Loeser, S. H. Butler, R. C. Chapman, & D. C. Turk (Eds.), *Bonica's management of pain.* (3rd ed., pp. 26–72). Philadelphia: Lippincott, Williams & Wilkins.

Callesen, T., Hjort, D., Mogensen, T., et al. (1999). Combined field block and i.p. instillation of ropivacaine for pain management after laparoscopic sterilization. *British Journal of Anaesthesia, 82*(4), 586–590.

Campbell-Fleming, J. M., & Williams, A. (2008). The use of ketamine as adjuvant therapy to control severe pain. *Clinical Journal of Oncology Nursing, 12*(1), 102–107.

Canavero, S., & Bonicalzi, V. (1997). Lamotrigine control of trigeminal neuralgia: An expanded study. *J Neurology, 244*(8), 527–532.

Canbay, O., Celebi, N., Uzun, S., et al. (2008). Topical ketamine and morphine for post-tonsillectomy pain. *European Journal of Anaesthesiology, 25*(4), 287–292.

Candiotti, K. A., Bergese, S. D., Bokesch, P. M., et al. (2010). Monitored anesthesia care with dexmedetomidine: A prospective, randomized, double-blind, multicenter trial. *Anesthesia and Analgesia, 110*(1), 47–56.

Cankurtaran, E. S., Ozalp, E., Soygur, H., et al. (2008). Mirtazapine improves sleep and lowers anxiety and depression in cancer patients: Superiority over imipramine. *Supportive Care in Cancer, 16*(11), 1291–1298.

Capdevila, X., Bringuier, S., & Borgeat, A. (2009). Infectious risk of continuous peripheral nerve blocks. *Anesthesiology, 110*(1), 182–188.

Capdevila, X., Macaire, P., Aknin, P., et al. (2003). Patient-controlled perineural analgesia after ambulatory orthopedic surgery: A comparison of electronic versus elastomeric pumps. *Anesthesia and Analgesia, 96*(2), 414–417.

Capdevila, X., Pirat, P., Bringuier, S., et al. (2005). Continuous peripheral nerve blocks in hospital wards after orthopedic surgery. *Anesthesiology, 103*(5), 1035–2045.

Capel, M. M., Jenkins, R., Jefferson, M., et al. (2008). Use of ketamine for ischemic pain in end-stage renal failure. *Journal of Pain and Symptom Management, 35*(3), 232–234.

Caraceni, A., Zecca, E., Martini, C., et al. (1999). Gabapentin as an adjuvant to opioid analgesia for neuropathic cancer pain. *Journal of Pain and Symptom Management, 17*(6), 441–445.

Cardenas, D. D., Warms, C. A., Turner, J. A., et al. (2002). Efficacy of amitriptyline for relief of pain in spinal cord injury: Results of a randomized controlled trial. *Pain, 96*(3), 365–373.

Carr, D. B., Goudas, L. C., Denman, W. T., et al. (2004a). Safety and efficacy of intranasal ketamine for the treatment of breakthrough pain in patients with chronic pain: A randomized, double-blind, placebo-controlled, crossover study. *Pain, 108*(1–2), 17–27.

Carr, D. B., Goudas, L. C., Denman, W. T., et al. (2004b). Safety and efficacy of intranasal ketamine in a mixed population with chronic pain. *Pain, 110*(3), 762–769.

Carr, D. B., Reines, H. D., Schaffer, J., et al. (2005). The impact of technology on the analgesic gap and quality of acute pain management. *Regional Anesthesia and Pain Medicine, 30*(3), 286–291.

Carrazana, E., & Mikoshiba, I. (2003). Rationale and evidence for the use of oxcarbazepine in neuropathic pain. *Journal of Pain and Symptom Management, 25*(Suppl. 5), S31–S35.

Carroll, I. R. (2007). Intravenous lidocaine for neuropathic pain: Diagnostic utility and therapeutic efficacy. *Current Pain and Headache Reports, 11*(1), 20–24.

Carroll, I. R., Gaeta, R., & Mackey, S. (2007). Multivariate analysis of chronic pain patients undergoing lidocaine infusions: Increasing pain severity and advancing age predict likelihood of clinically meaningful analgesia. *The Clinical Journal of Pain, 23*(8), 702–706.

Carroll, I. R., Kaplan, K. M., & Mackey, S. C. (2008). Mexiletine therapy for chronic pain: Survival analysis identifies factors predicting clinical success. *Journal of Pain and Symptom Management, 35*(3), 321–326.

Carson, S. S., Kress, J. P., Rodgers, J. E., et al. (2006). A randomized trial of intermittent lorazepam versus propofol with daily interruption in mechanically ventilated patients. *Critical Care Medicine, 34*(5), 1326–1332.

Cassinelli, E. H., Dean, C. L., Garcia, R. M., et al. (2008). Ketorolac use for postoperative pain management following lumbar decompression surgery: A prospective, randomized, double-blinded, placebo-controlled trial. *Spine, 33*(12), 1313–1317.

Catala, E., & Martinez, M. J. (2006). Biphosphonates. In O. A. de Leon-Casasola (Ed.), *Cancer pain. Pharmacological, interventional and palliative care approaches* (pp. 337–347). Philadelphia: Saunders.

Catterall, W. A., & Mackie, K. (2006). In L. L. Brunton, J. S. Lazo, & K. L. Parker (Eds.), *Goodman & Gilman's the pharmacological basis of therapeutics* (11th ed., pp. 369–386). New York: McGraw-Hill.

Caumo, W., Levandovski, R., & Hidalgo, M. P. (2009). Preoperative anxiolytic effect of melatonin and clonidine on postoperative pain and morphine consumption in patients undergoing abdominal hysterectomy: A double-blind, randomized, placebo-controlled study. *The Journal of Pain,* 10(1), 100–108.

Challapalli, V., Tremont-Lukats, I. W., McNicol, E. D., et al. (2005). Systemic administration of local anesthetic agents to relieve neuropathic pain. *Cochrane Database Systematic Reviews,* (4), CD003345.

Chang, S. H., Lee, H. W., Kim, H. K., et al. (2009). An evaluation of perioperative pregabalin for prevention and attenuation of postoperative shoulder pain after laparoscopic cholecystectomy. *Anesthesia and Analgesia,* 109(4), 1284–1286.

Chang, V. T. (1997). Intravenous phenytoin in the management of crescendo pelvic cancer-related pain. *Journal of Pain and Symptom Management,* 13(4), 238–240.

Chappell, A. (2009). *Duloxetine 60-120 mg once daily versus placebo in treatment of patients with osteoarthritis knee pain.* Poster presentation at American Academy of Pain Medicine Annual Meeting, January 29, 2009, Hawaii.

Chappell, A. S., Littlejohn, G., Kajdasz, D. K., et al. (2009). A 1-year safety and efficacy study of duloxetine in patients with fibromyalgia. *The Clinical Journal of Pain,* 25(5), 365–375.

Charney, D. S., Mihic, S. J., Adron, R., et al. (2006). Hypnotics and sedatives. In L. L. Brunton, J. S. Lazo, & K. L. Parker (Eds.), *Goodman & Gilman's the pharmacological basis of therapeutics* (11th ed., pp. 401–427). New York: McGraw-Hill.

Charuluxananan, S., Kyokong, O., Somboonviboon, K., et al. (2001). Nalbuphine versus propofol for treatment of intrathecal morphine-induced pruritus after Cesarean delivery. *Anesthesia and Analgesia,* 93(1), 162–165.

Chau-In, W., Sukmuan, B., Ngamsangsirisapt, K., et al. (2007). Efficacy of pre- and postoperative oral dextromethorphan for reduction of intra- and 24-hour postoperative morphine consumption for transabdominal hysterectomy. *Pain Medicine (Malden, Mass.),* 8(5), 462–467.

Chelly, J. E. (2007). Perineural infusion of local anesthetics: "More to the review" (Letter). *Anesthesiology,* 106(1), 191.

Chelly, J. E., Greger, J., Gebhard, R., et al. (2001). Continuous femoral blocks improve recovery and outcome of patients undergoing total knee arthroplasty. *The Journal of Arthroplasty,* 16(4), 436–445.

Chen, C. C., Lin, C. S., Ko, Y. P., et al. (2008). Premedication with mirtazapine reduces preoperative anxiety and postoperative nausea and vomiting. *Anesthesia and Analgesia,* 106(1), 109–113.

Chevlen, E. (2000). Morphine with dextromethorphan: Conversion from other opioid analgesics. *Journal of Pain and Symptom Management,* 19(Suppl. 1), S42–S49.

Choi, D. M. A., Kliffer, A. P., & Douglas, M. J. (2003). Dextromethorphan and intrathecal morphine for analgesia after Caesarean section under spinal anaesthesia. *British Journal of Anaesthesia,* 90(5), 653–658.

Chong, M. S., & Hester, J. (2007). Diabetic painful neuropathy: Current and future treatment options. *Drugs,* 67(4), 569–585.

Chou, R., Carson, S., & Chan, B. K. (2009). Gabapentin versus tricyclic antidepressants for diabetic neuropathy and post-herpetic neuralgia: Discrepancies between direct and indirect meta-analyses of randomized controlled trials. *Journal of General Internal Medicine,* 24(2), 178–188.

Chou, R., Huffman, L. H., American Pain Society, et al. (2007). Medications for acute and chronic low back pain: A review of the evidence for an American Pain Society/American College of Physicians clinical practice guideline. *Annals of Internal Medicine,* 147(7), 505–514.

Chou, R., Peterson, K., & Helfand, M. (2004). Comparative efficacy and safety of skeletal muscle relaxants for spasticity and musculoskeletal conditions: A systematic review. *Journal of Pain and Symptom Management,* 28(2), 140–175.

Chou, R., Qaseem, A., Snow, V., et al. (2007). Diagnosis and treatment of low back pain: A joint clinical practice guideline from the American College of Physicians and the American Pain Society. *Annals of Internal Medicine,* 147(7), 478–491.

Chow, E., Loblaw, A., Harris, K., et al. (2007). Dexamethasone for the prophylaxis of radiation-induced pain flare after palliative radiotherapy for bone metastases: A pilot study. *Support Cancer Care,* 15(6), 643–647.

Chow, L. H., Huang, E. Y., Ho, S. T., et al. (2004). Dextromethorphan potentiates morphine antinociception at the spinal level in rats. *Canadian Journal of Anaesthesia,* 51(9), 905–910.

Christo, P. J., & Mazloomdoost, D. (2008). Interventional pain treatments for cancer pain. *Annals of the New York Academy of Sciences,* 1138, 299–328.

Chu, L. F., Angst, M. S., & Clark, D. (2008). Opioid-induced hyperalgesia in humans: Molecular mechanisms and clinical considerations. *The Clinical Journal of Pain,* 24(6), 479–496.

Chudnofsky, C. R., Weber, J. E., Stoyanoff, P. J., et al. (2000). A combination of midazolam and ketamine for procedural sedation and analgesia in adult emergency department patients. *Academic Emergency Medicine,* 7(3), 228–235.

Chung, W. J., & Pharo, G. H. (2007). Successful use of ketamine infusion in the treatment of intractable cancer pain in an outpatient. *Journal of Pain and Symptom Management,* 33(1), 2–5.

Cianchetti, C., Zuddas, A., Randazzo, A. P., et al. (1999). Lamotrigine adjunctive therapy in painful phenomena in MS: Preliminary observations. *Neurology,* 53(2), 433.

Cipriani, A., Furukawa, T. A., Salanti, G., et al. (2009). Comparative efficacy and acceptability of 12 new-generation antidepressants: A multiple-treatments meta-analysis. *Lancet,* 373(9665), 746–758.

Clark, M. K. (2008). Lipid emulsion as rescue for local anesthetic-related cardiotoxicity. *Journal of Perianesthesia Nursing,* 23(2), 111–121.

Clarke, H., Pereira, S., Kennedy, D., et al. (2009). Gabapentin decreases morphine consumption and improves functional recovery following total knee arthroplasty. *Pain Research Management,* 14(3), 217–222.

Classen, A. M., Wimbish, G. H., & Kupiec, T. C. (2004). Stability of admixture containing morphine sulfate, bupivacaine hydrochloride, and clonidine hydrochloride in an implantable infusion system. *Journal of Pain and Symptom Management,* 28(6), 603–611.

Clauw, D. F., Mease, P. J., Palmer, R. H., et al. (2008). Milnacipran for the treatment of fibromyalgia in adults: A 15-week, multicenter, randomized, double-blind, placebo-controlled, multi-dose clinical trial. *Clinical Therapeutics,* 30(11), 1988–2004.

Clinical Pharmacology Online. *Gold Standard, Inc.* Available at http://clinicalpharmacology.com. Accessed February 22, 2010.

Cohen, A. S., Matharu, M. S., & Goadsby, P. J. (2007). Trigeminal autonomic cephalagias: Current and future treatments. *J Head Face Pain,* 47(6), 969–980.

Cohen, L. L., MacLaren, J. E., DeMore, M., et al. (2009). A randomized controlled trial of vapocoolant for pediatric immunization distress relief. *The Clinical Journal of Pain*, 25(6), 490–494.

Cohen, S. P., Kapoor, S. G., & Rathmell, J. P. (2009). Intravenous infusion tests have limited utility for selecting long-term drug therapy in patients with chronic pain: A systematic review. *Anesthesiology*, 111(2), 416–431.

Cohen, S. P., Verdolin, M. H., Chang, A. S., et al. (2006). The intravenous ketamine test predicts subsequent response to an oral dextromethorphan treatment regimen in fibromyalgia patients. *The Journal of Pain*, 7(6), 391–398.

Cohen, S. P., Wang, S., Chen, L., et al. (2009). An intravenous ketamine test as a predictive response tool in opioid-exposed patients with persistent pain. *Journal of Pain and Symptom Management*, 37(4), 698–708.

Collins, S. L., Moore, A., McQuay, H. J., et al. (2000). Antidepressants and anticonvulsants for diabetic neuropathy and postherpetic neuralgia: A quantitative systematic review. *Journal of Pain and Symptom Management*, 20(6), 449–458.

Collins, S., Zuurmond, W. W. A., de Lange, J. J., et al. (2009). Intravenous magnesium for complex regional pain syndrome type 1 (CRPS 1) patients: A pilot study. *Pain Medicine (Malden, Mass.)*, 10(5), 930–940.

Compere, V., Legrand, J. F., Guitard, P. G., et al. (2009). Bacterial colonization after tunneling in 402 perineural catheters: A prospective study. *Anesthesia and Analgesia*, 108(4), 1326–1330.

Compton, P. (2008). The OIH paradox: Can opioids make pain worse? *Pain Treatment Topics*. Available at: http://pain-topics.org/pdf/Compton-OIH-Paradox.pdf Accessed Feb. 16, 2009.

Convery, P. N., Milligan, K. R., Quinn, P., et al. (2001). Efficacy and uptake of ropivacaine and bupivacaine after single intra-articular injection in the knee joint. *British Journal of Anaesthesia*, 87(4), 570–576.

Cooper, J. A., Bromley, L. M., Baranowski, A. P., et al. (2000). Evaluation of a needle-free injection system for local anaesthesia prior to venous cannulation. *Anaesthesia*, 55(3), 247–250.

Coppola, F., Rossi, C., Mancini, M. L., et al. (2008). Language disturbances as a side effect of prophylactic treatment of migraine. *J Head Face Pain*, 48(1), 86–94.

Correll, G. E., Maleki, J., Gracely, E. J., et al. (2004). Subanesthetic ketamine therapy: A retrospective analysis of a novel therapeutic approach to complex regional pain syndrome. *Pain Medicine (Malden, Mass.)*, 5(3), 263–275.

Cortinez, L. I., Hsu, Y. W., Sum-Ping, S. T., et al. (2004). Dexmedetomidine pharmacodynamics: Part II. *Anesthesiology*, 101(5), 1077–1083.

Cranney, A., Welch, V., Adachi, J., et al. (2000). Calcitonin for the treatment and prevention of corticosteroid-induced osteoporosis. *Cochrane Database Systematic Reviews*, (2), CD001983.

Criscuolo, S., Auletta, C., Lippi, S., et al. (2004). Oxcarbazepine (Trileptal) monotherapy dramatically improves quality of life in two patients with postherpetic neuralgia refractory to carbamazepine and gabapentin. *Journal of Pain and Symptom Management*, 28(6), 535–536.

Crofford, L. J., Rowbotham, M. C., Mease, P. J., et al. (2005). Pregabalin 1008-105 Study Group: Pregabalin for the treatment of fibromyalgia syndrome: Results of a randomized, double-blind, placebo-controlled trial. *Arthritis and Rheumatism*, 52(4), 1264–1273.

Crosby, V., Wilcock, A., & Corcoran, R. (2000). The safety and efficacy of a single dose (500 mg or 1 g) of intravenous magnesium sulfate in neuropathic pain poorly responsive to strong opioid analgesics in patients with cancer. *Journal of Pain and Symptom Management*, 19(1), 35–39.

Cuignet, O., Pirson, J., Boughrouph, J., et al. (2004). The efficacy of continuous fascia iliaca compartment block for pain management in burn patients undergoing skin grafting procedures. *Anesthesia and Analgesia*, 98(4), 1077–1081.

Curatolo, M., & Bogduk, N. (2001). Pharmacologic pain treatment of musculoskeletal disorders: Current perspectives and future prospects. *The Clinical Journal of Pain*, 17(1), 25–32.

Curry, S. E., & Finkel, J. C. (2007). Use of Synera patch for local anesthesia before vascular access procedures: A randomized, double-blind, placebo-controlled study. *Pain Medicine (Malden, Mass.)*, 8(6), 497–502.

Curtis, L. H., Ostbye, T., Sendersky, V., et al. (2004). Inappropriate prescribing for elderly Americans in a large outpatient population. *Archives of Internal Medicine*, 164(15), 1621–1625.

Cutter, H. S., O'Farrell, T. J., Whitehouse, J., et al. (1986). Pain changes among men from before to after drinking: Effects of expectancy set and dose manipulations with alcohol and tonic as mediated by prior experience with alcohol. *The International Journal of the Addictions*, 21(8), 937–945.

Cuvillon, P., Ripart, J., Lalourcey, L., et al. (2003). The continuous femoral nerve block catheter for postoperative analgesia: Bacterial colonization, infectious rate and adverse effects. *Anesthesia and Analgesia*, 93(4), 1045–1049.

Cvrcek, P. (2008). Side effects of ketamine in the long-term treatment of neuropathic pain. *Pain Medicine (Malden, Mass.)*, 9(2), 253–257.

Dahl, J. B., & Moiniche, S. (2009). Relief of postoperative pain by local anaesthetic infiltration: Efficacy for major abdominal and orthopedic surgery. *Pain*, 143(1–2), 7–11.

Dallocchio, C., Buffa, C., Mazzarello, P., et al. (2000). Gabapentin vs. amitriptyline in painful diabetic neuropathy: An open-label pilot study. *Journal of Pain and Symptom Management*, 20(4), 280–285.

Dalpiaz, A. S., & Dodds, T. A. (2002). Myofascial pain response to topical lidocaine patch therapy: Case report. *Journal of Pain & Palliative Care Pharmacotherapy*, 16(1), 99–104.

Dario, A., & Tomei, G. (2004). A benefit-risk assessment of baclofen in severe spinal spasticity. *Drug safety*, 27(11), 799–818.

Dauri, M., Fabbi, E., Mariani, P., et al. (2009). Continuous femoral nerve block provides superior analgesia compared with continuous intra-articular and wound infusion after anterior cruciate ligament reconstruction. *Regional Anesthesia and Pain Medicine*, 34(2), 95–99.

Dauri, M., Faria, S., Gatti, A., et al. (2009). Gabapentin and pregabalin for the acute post-operative pain management. A systematic-narrative review of the recent clinical evidences. *Current Drug Targets*, 10(8), 716–733.

Davies, P. S., Reisner-Keller, L., & Rowbotham, M. C. (1996). Randomized, double-blind comparison of fluoxetine, despiramine and amitriptyline in postherpetic neuralgia.

(abstract) In *Abstracts: 8th world congress on pain.* (p. 276). Seattle: IASP Press.

Davis, J. L., & Smith, R. L. (1999). Painful peripheral diabetic neuropathy treated with venlafaxine HCl extended release capsules. *Diabetes Care, 22*(11), 1909–1910.

Davis, K. D., Treede, R. D., Raja, S. N., et al. (1991). Topical application of clonidine relieves hyperalgesia in patients with sympathetically maintained pain. *Pain, 47*(3), 309–317.

Davis, M. D. P., & Sandroni, P. (2002). Lidocaine patch for pain of erythromelalgia. *Archives of Dermatology, 138*(1), 17–19.

Davis, M. P., & Hinshaw, D. (2006). Management of visceral pain due to cancer-related intestinal obstruction. In O. A. de Leon-Casasola (Ed.), *Cancer pain. Pharmacological, interventional and palliative care approaches* (pp. 481–495). Philadelphia: Saunders.

Davis, M. P., & Nouneh, C. (2001). Modern management of cancer-related intestinal obstruction. *Current Pain and Headache Reports, 5*(3), 257–264.

Deal, C. L., Schnitzer, T. J., Lipstein, E., et al. (1991). Treatment of arthritis with topical capsaicin: A double-blind trial. *Clinical Therapeutics, 13*(3), 383–395.

Deer, T., Krames, E. S., Hassenbusch, S. J., et al. (2007). Polyanalgesic consensus conference 2007: Recommendations for the management of pain by intrathecal (intraspinal) drug delivery: Report of an interdisciplinary expert panel. *Neuromodulation, 10*(4), 300–329.

Degenhardt, L., & Hall, W. D. (2008). The adverse effects of cannabinoids: Implications for use of medical marijuana. *CMAJ: Canadian Medical Association Journal, 178*(13), 1685–1686.

De Kock, M., & Lavand'homme, P. (2007). The clinical role of NMDA receptor antagonists for the treatment of postoperative pain. *Best Practice & Research. Clinical Anaesthesiology, 21*(1), 85–98.

De Kock, M., Lavand'homme, P., & Waterloos, H. (2001). 'Balanced analgesia' in the perioperative period: Is there a place for ketamine? *Pain, 92*(3), 373–380.

De Kock, M., Lavand'homme, P., & Waterloos, H. (2005). The short-lasting analgesia and long-term antihyperalgesic effect of intrathecal clonidine in patients undergoing colonic surgery. *Anesthesia and Analgesia, 101*(2), 566–572.

de Leon-Casasola, O. A. (2007). Multimodal approaches to the management of neuropathic pain: The role of topical analgesia. *Journal of Pain and Symptom Management, 33*(3), 356–364.

Dellemijn, P. L., & Fields, H. L. (1994). Do benzodiazepines have a role in chronic pain management? *Pain, 57*(2), 137–152.

DeMello, W., & Desai, P. R. (2009). Use of lidocaine plaster for testicular pain. *The Clinical Journal of Pain, 25*(5), 445.

Deng, X. M., Xiao, W. J., Luo, M. P., et al. (2001). The use of midazolam and small-dose ketamine for sedation and analgesia during local anesthesia. *Anesthesia and Analgesia, 93*(5), 1174–1177.

Desaphy, J. F., Dipalma, A., De Bellis, M., et al. (2009). Involvement of voltage-gated sodium channels blockade in the analgesic effects of orphenadrine. *Pain, 142*(3), 225–235.

Descombes, S., Brefel-Courbon, C., Thalamas, C., et al. (2001). Amitriptyline treatment in chronic drug-induced headache: A double-blind comparative pilot study. *Headache, 41*(2), 178–182.

Devers, A., & Galer, B. S. (2000). Topical lidocaine patch relieves a variety of neuropathic pain conditions: An open-label study. *The Clinical Journal of Pain, 16*(3), 205–208.

Devlin, J. W., & Roberts, R. J. (2009). Pharmacology of commonly used analgesics and sedatives in the ICU: Benzodiazepines, propofol, and opioids. *Critical Care Clinics, 25*(3), 431–449.

Devulder, J., Crombez, E., & Mortier, E. (2002). Central pain: An overview. *Acta Neurologica Belgica, 102*(3), 97–103.

Diamond, S., & Frietag, F. G. (1989). The use of fluoxetine in the treatment of headache. *The Clinical Journal of Pain, 5*(2), 200–201.

di Benedetto, P., Casati, A., & Bertini, L. (2002). Continuous subgluteus sciatic nerve block after orthopedic foot and ankle surgery: Comparison of two infusion techniques. *Regional Anesthesia and Pain Medicine, 27*(2), 168–172.

Dick, I. E., Brochu, R. M., Purohit, Y., et al. (2007). Sodium channel blockade may contribute to the analgesic efficacy of antidepressants. *The Journal of Pain, 8*(4), 315–324.

Dickenson, A. H., Matthews, E. A., & Suzuki, R. (2002). Neurobiology of neuropathic pain: Mode of action of anticonvulsants. *European Journal of Pain (London, England), 6*(Suppl. A), 51–60.

Dickie, G. J., & Macfarlane, D. (1999). Strontium and samarium therapy for bone metastases from prostate carcinoma. *Australasian Radiology, 43*(4), 476–479.

Dierking, G., Duedahl, T. H., Rasmussen, M. L., et al. (2004). Effects of gabapentin on postoperative morphine consumption and pain after abdominal hysterectomy: A randomized, double-blind trial. *Acta Anaesthesiologica Scandinavica, 48*(3), 322–327.

Dietrich, C. C., Kinney, M. A., Pulido, J. N., et al. (2009). Preoperative gabapentin in patients undergoing primary total knee arthroplasty. *Acute Pain, 11*(1), 57–63.

Difazio, M., & Jabbari, B. (2002). A focused review of the use of botulinum toxins for low back pain. *The Clinical Journal of Pain, 18*(Suppl. 6), S155–S162.

Dimou, P., Paraskeva, A., Papilas, K., et al. (2003). Transdermal clonidine: Does it affect pain after abdominal hysterectomy. *Acta Anaesthesiologica Belgica, 54*(3), 227–232.

Dirks, J., Fredensborg, B. B., Christensen, D., et al. (2002). A randomized study of the effects of single-dose gabapentin versus placebo on postoperative pain and morphine consumption after mastectomy. *Anesthesiology, 97*(3), 560–564.

Dirks, J., Peterson, K. L., Rowbotham, M. C., et al. (2002). Gabapentin suppresses cutaneous hyperalgesia following heat-capsaicin sensitization. *Anesthesiology, 97*(1), 102–107.

Djaldetti, R., Yust-Katz, S., Kolianov, V., et al. (2007). The effect of duloxetine on primary pain symptoms in Parkinson disease. *Clinical Neuropharmacology, 30*(4), 201–205.

Dobecki, D. A., Schocket, S. M., & Wallace, M. S. (2006). Update on pharmacotherapy guidelines for the treatment of neuropathic pain. *Current Pain and Headache Reports, 10*(3), 185–190.

Dogra, S., Beydoun, S., Mazzola, J., et al. (2005). Oxcarbazepine in painful diabetic neuropathy: A randomized, placebo-controlled study. *European Journal of Pain (London, England), 9*(5), 543–554.

Dorr, L. D., Raya, J., Long, W. T., et al. (2008). Multimodal analgesia without parenteral narcotics for total knee arthroplasty. *Journal of Arthroplasty, 23*(4), 502–508.

Dowling, R., Thielmeier, K., Ghaly, A., et al. (2003). Improved pain control after cardiac surgery: Results of a randomized, double-blind, clinical trial. *The Journal of Thoracic and Cardiovascular Surgery, 126*(5), 1271–1278.

Duale, C., Sibaud, F., Guastella, V., et al. (2008). Perioperative ketamine does not prevent chronic pain after thoracotomy. *European Journal of Pain (London, England), 13*(5), 497–505.

Duarte, V. M., Fallis, W. M., Slonowsky, D., et al. (2006). Effectiveness of femoral nerve blockade for pain control after total knee arthroscopy. *Journal of Perianesthesia Nursing, 21*(5), 311–316.

Dubinsky, R. M., Kabbani, H., El-Chami, Z., et al. (2004). Practice parameter: Treatment of postherpetic neuralgia. An evidence-based report of the quality standards subcommittee of the American Academy of Neurology. *Neurology, 63*(6), 959–965.

Duby, J. J., Campbell, R. K., Setter, S. M., et al. (2004). Diabetic neuropathy: An intensive review. *American Journal of Health-System Pharmacy, 61*(2), 160–173.

Duedahl, T. H., Romsing, J., Moiniche, S., et al. (2006). A qualitative systematic review of peri-operative dextromethorphan in post-operative pain. *Acta Anaesthesiologica Scandinavica, 50*(1), 1–13.

DuPen, A., Shen, D., & Ersek, M. (2007). Mechanisms of opioid-induced tolerance and hyperalgesia. *Pain Management Nursing, 8*(3), 113–121.

Durand, J. P., Alexandre, J., Guillevin, L., et al. (2005). Clinical activity of venlafaxine and topiramate against oxaliplatin-induced disabling permanent neuropathy. *Anti-Cancer Drugs, 16*(5), 587–591.

Dworkin, R. H., Backonja, M., Rowbotham, M. C., et al. (2003). Advances in neuropathic pain: Diagnosis, mechanisms, and treatment recommendations. *Archives of Neurology, 60*(11), 1524–1534.

Dworkin, R. H., Corbin, A. E., Young, J. P., Jr., et al. (2003). Pregabalin for the treatment of postherpetic neuralgia: A randomized, placebo-controlled trial. *Neurology, 60*(8), 1274–1283.

Dworkin, R. H., Hart-Gouleau, S., Galer, B. S., et al. (2003). Effectiveness and impact on quality of life of the lidocaine patch 5% in painful diabetic neuropathy on patients with or without allodynia. *The Journal of Pain, 4*(Suppl. 2), 65.

Dworkin, R. H., O'Connor, A. B., Backonja, M., et al. (2007). Pharmacologic management of neuropathic pain: Evidence-based recommendations. *Pain, 132*(3), 237–251.

Dworkin, R. H., & Schmader, K. E. (2003). Treatment and prevention of postherpetic neuralgia. *Clinical Infectious Diseases, 36*(7), 877–881.

Dy, S. M., Asch, S. M., Naeim, A., et al. (2008). Evidence-based standards for cancer pain management. *Journal of Clinical Oncology, 26*(23), 3879–3885.

Edmonds, P., & Davis, C. (1996). Experience of the use of subcutaneous ketamine in patients with cancer-related neuropathic pain. (Abstract). *Palliative Medicine, 10*, 76–77.

Edmondson, E. A., Simpson, R. K., Stubler, D. K., et al. (1993). Systemic lidocaine therapy for poststroke pain. *Southern Medical Journal, 86*(10), 1093–1096.

Edrich, T., Friedrich, A. D., Eltzschig, H. K., et al. (2004). Ketamine for long-term sedation and analgesia of a burn patient. *Anesthesia and Analgesia, 99*(3), 893–895.

Edwards, N. D., Fletcher, A., Cole, J. R., et al. (1993). Combined infusion of morphine and ketamine for postoperative pain in elderly patients. *Anaesthesia, 48*(2), 124–127.

Ehrchen, J., & Stander, S. (2008). Pregabalin in the treatment of chronic pruritus. *Journal of the American Academy of Dermatology, 58*(Suppl. 2), S36–S37.

Eichenberger, U., Neff, F., Sveticic, G., et al. (2008). Chronic phantom limb pain: The effects of calcitonin, ketamine, and their combination on pain and sensory thresholds. *Anesthesia and Analgesia, 106*(4), 1265–1273.

Eide, K., Stubhaug, A., Oye, I., et al. (1995). Continuous subcutaneous administration of the N-methyl-D-aspartic acid (NMDA) receptor antagonist ketamine in the treatment of post-herpetic neuralgia. *Pain, 61*(2), 221–228.

Eidelman, A., Weiss, J. M., Lau, J., et al. (2005). Topical anesthetics for dermal instrumentation: A systematic review of randomized, controlled trials. *Annals of Emergency Medicine, 46*(4), 343–351.

Einarsson, J. I., Henao, G., & Young, A. E. (2005). Topical analgesia for endometrial biopsy: A randomized controlled trial. *Obstetrics and Gynecology, 106*(1), 128–130.

Eisenach, J. C., Du Pen, S., Dubois, M., et al. (1995). Epidural clonidine analgesia for intractable cancer pain. The Epidural Clonidine Study Group. *Pain, 61*(3), 391–399.

Eisenach, J. C., Hood, D. D., & Curry, R. (2000). Relative potency of epidural to intrathecal clonidine differs between acute thermal pain and capsaicin-induced allodynia. *Pain, 84*(1), 57–64.

Eisenberg, E., Alon, N., Ishay, A., et al. (1998). Lamotrigine in the treatment of painful diabetic neuropathy. *European Journal of Neurology, 5*(2), 167–173.

Eisenberg, E., Damunni, G., Hoffer, E., et al. (2003). Lamotrigine for intractable sciatica: Correlation between dose, plasma concentration and analgesia. *European Journal of Pain (London, England), 7*(6), 485–491.

Eisenberg, E., Pud, D., Koltun, L., et al. (2007). Effect of early administration of the N-methyl-D-aspartate receptor antagonist amantadine on the development of postmastectomy pain syndrome: A prospective pilot study. *The Journal of Pain, 8*(3), 223–229.

Elder, J. B., Hoh, D. J., & Wang, M. Y. (2008). Postoperative continuous paravertebral anesthetic infusion for pain control in lumbar spinal fusion surgery. *Spine, 33*(2), 210–218.

Eledjam, J. J., Cuvillon, P., Capdevila, X., et al. (2002). Postoperative analgesia by femoral nerve block with ropivacaine 0.2% after major knee surgery: Continuous versus patient-controlled techniques. *Regional Anesthesia and Pain Medicine, 27*(6), 604–611.

Elia, N., Culebras, X., Mazza, C., et al. (2008). Clonidine as an adjuvant to intrathecal local anesthetics for surgery: Systematic review of randomized trials. *Regional Anesthesia and Pain Medicine, 33*(2), 159–167.

Elia, N., & Tramer, M. R. (2005). Ketamine and postoperative pain—a quantitative systematic review of randomised trials. *Pain, 113*(1–2), 61–70.

Elliott, J. A. (2009). α2-agonists. In H. S. Smith (Ed.), *Current therapy in pain* (pp. 476–480). Philadelphia: Saunders.

Ellis, D. J., Dissanayake, S., McGuire, D., et al. (2008). Continuous intrathecal infusion if ziconotide for treatment of chronic malignant and non-malignant pain over 12 months: A prospective, open-label study. *Neuromodulation, 11*(1), 40–49.

Enarson, M. C., Hays, H., & Woodruffe, M. A. (1999). Clinical experience with oral ketamine. *Journal of Pain and Symptom Management, 17*(5), 384–386.

Enggaard, T. P., Klitgaard, N. A., Gram, L. F., et al. (2001). Specific effect of venlafaxine on single and repetitive experimental painful stimuli in humans. *Clinical Pharmacology and Therapeutics*, 69(4), 245–251.

Epstein, J. B., Epstein, J. D., Epstein, M. S., et al. (2006). Oral doxepin rinse: The analgesic effect and duration of pain reduction in patients with oral mucositis due to cancer therapy. *Anesthesia and Analgesia*, 103(2), 465–470.

Epstein, J. B., Grushka, M., & Le, N. (1997). Topical clonidine for orofacial pain: A pilot study. *Journal of Orofacial Pain*, 11(4), 346–352.

Ernst, D. S., Tannock, I. F., Winquist, E. W., et al. (2003). Randomized, double-blind, controlled trial of mitoxantrone/prednisone and clodronate versus mitoxantrone/prednisone and placebo in patients with hormone-refractory prostate cancer and pain. *Journal of Clinical Oncology*, 21(17), 3335–3342.

Espinet, A. J., & Emmerton, M. T. (2009). The successful use of intralipid for treatment of local anesthetic-induced central nervous system toxicity. *The Clinical Journal of Pain*, 25(9), 808–809.

Evans, H., Nielsen, K. C., Tucker, M. S., et al. (2009). Regional anesthesia for acute pain management in the outpatient setting. In R. S. Sinatra, O. A. de Leon-Casasola, B. Ginsberg, & E. R. Viscusi (Eds.), *Acute pain management* (pp. 287–301). Cambridge, New York: Cambridge University Press.

Evans, L. T., Saberi, S., Kim, H. M., et al. (2006). Pharyngeal anesthesia during sedated EGDs: Is "the spray" beneficial? A meta-analysis and systematic review. *Gastrointestinal Endoscopy*, 63(6), 761–766.

Fanning, R. M. (2008). Monitoring during sedation given by non-anaesthetic doctors. *Anaesthesia*, 63(4), 370–374.

Farmery, A. D., & Wilson-MacDonald, J. (2009). The analgesic effect of epidural clonidine after spinal surgery: A randomized placebo-controlled trial. *Anesthesia and Analgesia*, 108(2), 631–634.

Farr, W. C. (1990). The use of corticosteroids for symptom management in terminally ill patients. *The American Journal of Hospice Care*, 7(1), 41–46.

Farrar, J. T., & Portenoy, R. K. (2001). Neuropathic cancer pain: The role of adjuvant analgesics. *Oncology*, 15(11), 1435–1445.

Fassoulaki, A., Melemeni, A., Stamatakis, E., et al. (2007). A combination of gabapentin and local anesthetics attenuates acute and late pain after abdominal hysterectomy. *European Journal of Anaesthesia*, 24(6), 521–528.

Fassoulaki, A., Patris, K., Sarantopoulos, C., et al. (2002). The analgesic effect of gabapentin and mexiletine after breast surgery for cancer. *Anesthesia and Analgesia*, 95(4), 985–991.

Fassoulaki, A., Sarantopoulos, C., Melemeni, A., et al. (2000). EMLA reduces acute and chronic pain after breast surgery. *Regional Anesthesia and Pain Medicine*, 25(4), 350–355.

Fassoulaki, A., Stamatakis, E., Petropoulos, G., et al. (2006). Gabapentin attenuates late but not acute pain after abdominal hysterectomy. *European Journal of Anaesthesiology*, 23(2), 136–141.

Fassoulaki, A., Triga, A., Melemeni, A., et al. (2005). Multimodal analgesia with gabapentin and local anesthetics prevents acute and chronic pain after breast surgery for cancer. *Anesthesia and Analgesia*, 101(5), 1427–1432.

Fernandez, F., Adams, F., & Holmes, V. F. (1987). Analgesic effect of alprazolam in patients with chronic, organic pain of malignant origin. *Journal of Clinical Psychopharmacology*, 7(3), 167–169.

Ferrante, F. M., Paggioli, J., Cherukuri, S., et al. (1996). The analgesic response to intravenous lidocaine in the treatment of neuropathic pain. *Anesthesia and Analgesia*, 82(1), 91–97.

Ferrell, B. R., Levy, M. H., & Paice, J. (2008). Managing pain from advanced cancer in the palliative care setting. *Clinical Journal of Oncology Nursing*, 12(4), 575–581.

Ferrini, R. (2000). Parenteral lidocaine for severe intractable pain in six hospice patients continued at home. *Journal of Palliative Medicine*, 3(2), 183–200.

Feuer, D. D. J., & Broadley, K. E. (1999). Corticosteroids for the resolution of malignant bowel obstruction in advanced gynaecological and gastrointestinal cancer. *Cochrane Database Systematic Reviews*, (2), CD001219.

Finch, P. M., Knudsen, L., & Drummond, P. D. (2009). Reduction of allodynia in paitents with complex regional pain syndrome: A double-blind placebo-controlled trial of topical ketamine. *Pain*, 146(1–2), 18–25.

Finnerup, N. B., Biering-Sorensen, F., Johannesen, I. L., et al. (2005). Intravenous lidocaine relieves spinal cord injury pain. *Anesthesiology*, 102(5), 1023–1030.

Finnerup, N. B., Otto, M., McQuay, H. J., et al. (2005). Algorithm for neuropathic pain treatment: An evidence-based proposal. *Pain*, 118(3), 289–305.

Fishbain, D. A., Cutler, R. B., Lewis, J. E., et al. (2004a). Do the second-generation "atypical neuroleptics" have analgesic properties? A structured evidence-based review. *Pain Medicine (Malden, Mass.)*, 5(4), 359–365.

Fishbain, D. A., Cutler, R. B., Lewis, J. E., et al. (2004b). Modafinil for the treatment of pain-associated fatigue: Review and case report. *Journal of Pain & Palliative Care Pharmacotherapy*, 18(2), 39–47.

Fishbain, D. A., Cutler, R. B., Rosomoff, H. L., et al. (2000). Clonazepam open clinical treatment trial for myofascial syndrome associated chronic pain. *Pain Medicine (Malden, Mass.)*, 1(4), 332–339.

Fishbain, D. A., Lewis, J. E., Cole, B., et al. (2006). Lidocaine 5% patch: An open-label naturalistic chronic pain treatment trial and prediction of response. *Pain Medicine (Malden, Mass.)*, 7(2), 135–142.

Fitzgerald, K., & Buggy, D. (2006). Nonconventional and adjunctive analgesia. In G. Shorten, D. B. Carr, D. Harmon, M. M. Puig, & J. Browne (Eds.), *Postoperative pain management: An evidence-based guide to practice* (pp. 197–209). Philadelphia: Saunders.

Fitzgibbon, E. J., Hall, P., Schroder, C., et al. (2002). Low dose ketamine as an analgesic adjuvant in difficult pain syndromes: A strategy for conversion from parenteral to oral ketamine. *Journal of Pain and Symptom Management*, 23(2), 165–170.

Flood, P., & Daniel, D. (2004). Intranasal nicotine for postoperative pain treatment. *Anesthesiology*, 101(6), 1417–1421.

Forget, P., le Polain de Waroux, B., Wallemacq, P., et al. (2008). Life-threatening dextromethorphan intoxication associated with interaction with amitriptyline in poor CYP2D6 metabolizer: A single case re-exposure study. *Journal of Pain and Symptom Management*, 36(1), 92–96.

Forster, J. G., & Rosenberg, P. H. (2004). Small dose of clonidine mixed with low-dose ropivacaine and fentanyl for epidural analgesia after total knee arthroplasty. *British Journal of Anaesthesia*, 93(5), 670–677.

Fowler, S. J., Symons, J., Sabato, S., et al. (2008). Epidural analgesia compared with peripheral nerve blockade after major knee surgery: A systematic review and meta-analysis of randomized trials. *British Journal of Anaesthesia, 100*(2), 154–164.

Frampton, J. E., & Foster, R. H. (2005). Pregabalin: In the treatment of postherpetic neuralgia. *Drugs, 65*(1), 111–118.

Frampton, J. E., & Scott, L. J. (2004). Pregabalin: In the treatment of painful diabetic peripheral neuropathy. *Drugs, 64*(24), 2813–2820.

Franchi, M., Cromi, A., Scarperi, S., et al. (2009). Comparison between lidocaine-prilocaine cream (EMLA) and mepivacaine infiltration for pain relief during perineal repair after childbirth: A randomized trial. *American Journal of Obstetrics and Gynecology, 201*(2), 186, e1–5.

Frank, B., & Cousins, M. J. (2008). Pregabalin in the treatment of neuropathic pain associated with diabetic peripheral neuropathy. *Future Neurol, 3*(6), 631–639.

Frank, B., Serpell, M. G., Hughes, J., et al. (2008). Comparison of analgesic effects and patient tolerability of nabilone and dihydrocodeine for chronic neuropathic pain: Randomised, crossover, double blind study. *BMJ (Clinical Research Ed.), 336*(7637), 199–201.

Frank, R. G., Kashini, J. H., Parker, J. C., et al. (1988). Antidepressant analgesia in rheumatoid arthritis. *The Journal of Rheumatology, 15*(11), 1632–1638.

Fredman, B., Shapiro, A., Zohar, E., et al. (2000). The analgesic efficacy of patient-controlled ropivacaine instillation after cesarean delivery. *Anesthesia and Analgesia, 91*(6), 1436–1440.

Fredman, B., Zohar, E., Tarabykin, A., et al. (2001). Bupivacaine wound instillation via an electronic patient-controlled analgesia device and a double-catheter system does not decrease postoperative pain or opioid requirements after major abdominal surgery. *Anesthesia and Analgesia, 92*(1), 189–193.

Fredrickson, M. J., Ball, C. M., & Dalgleish, A. J. (2008). Successful continuous interscalene analgesia for ambulatory shoulder surgery in a private practice setting. *Regional Anesthesia and Pain Medicine, 33*(2), 122–128.

Freeman, R., Durso-Decruz, E., & Emir, B. (2008). Efficacy, safety and tolerability of pregabalin treatment of painful diabetic peripheral neuropathy: Findings from 7 randomized, controlled trials across a range of doses. *Diabetes Care, 31*(7), 1448–1454.

Freitag, F. G., Diamond, S., Diamond, M. L., et al. (2001). Divalproex in the long-term treatment of chronic daily headache. *Headache, 41*(3), 271–278.

Frese, A., Husstedt, I. W., Ringelstein, E. B., et al. (2006). Pharmacologic treatment of central post-stroke pain. *The Clinical Journal of Pain, 22*(3), 252–260.

Freund, B. J., & Schwartz, M. (2002). Use of botulinum toxin in chronic whiplash-associated disorder. *The Clinical Journal of Pain, 18*(Suppl. 6), S163–S168.

Freynhagen, R., Grond, S., Schupfer, G., et al. (2007). Efficacy and safety of pregabalin in treatment refractory patients with various neuropathic pain entities in clinical routine. *International Journal of Clinical Practice, 61*(12), 1989–1996.

Freynhagen, R., Strojek, K., Griesing, T., et al. (2005). Efficacy of pregabalin in neuropathic pain evaluated in a 12-week, randomized, double-blind, multicentre, placebo-controlled trial of flexible- and fixed-dose regimens. *Pain, 115*(3), 254–263.

Fridrich, P., Colvin, H. P., Zizza, A., et al. (2007). Phase 1A safety assessment of intravenous amitriptyline. *The Journal of Pain, 8*(7), 549–555.

Friedman, R., Jallo, J., & Young, W. F. (2001). Oral ketamine for opioid-resistant acute pain. *The Journal of Pain, 2*(1), 75–76.

Frolich, M. A., Price, D. D., Robinson, M. E., et al. (2005). The effect of propofol on thermal pain perception. *Anesthesia and Analgesia, 100*(2), 481–486.

Fujii, Y., & Nakayama, M. (2007). Reduction of postoperative nausea and vomiting and analgesic requirement with dexamethasone in women undergoing general anesthesia for mastectomy. *The Breast Journal, 13*(6), 564–567.

Fujii, Y., & Nakayama, M. (2008). Dexamethasone for reduction of nausea, vomiting and analgesic use after gynaecological laparascopic surgery. *International Journal of Gynaecology and Obstetrics, 100*(1), 27–30.

Furtado, R. N., Oliveira, L. M., & Natour, J. (2005). Polyarticular corticosteroid injection versus systemic administration in treatment of rheumatoid arthritis patients: A randomized controlled study. *The Journal of Rheumatology, 32*(9), 1691–1698.

Gainford, M. C., Dranitsaris, G., & Clemons, M. (2005). Recent developments in biphosphonates for patients with metastatic breast cancer. *BMJ (Clinical Research Ed.), 330*(7494), 769–773.

Gajraj, N. M. (2005). Botulinum toxin A injection of the obturator internus muscle for chronic perineal pain. *The Journal of Pain, 6*(5), 333–337.

Gajraj, N. M. (2007). Pregabalin: Its pharmacology and use in pain management. *Anesthesia and Analgesia, 105*(6), 1805–1815.

Gajraj, R. J., Hodson, M. J., Gillespie, J. A., et al. (1998). Antibacterial activity of lidocaine in mixtures with Diprivan. *British Journal of Anaesthesia, 81*(3), 444–448.

Galer, B. S. (2003). More than 7 years of consistent neuropathic pain relief in geriatric patients. *Archives of Internal Medicine, 163*(5), 628.

Galer, B. S., Harle, J., & Rowbotham, M. C. (1996). Response to intravenous lidocaine infusion predicts subsequent response to oral mexiletine: A prospective study. *Journal of Pain and Symptom Management, 12*(3), 161–167.

Galer, B. S., Jensen, M. P., Ma, T., et al. (2002). The lidocaine patch 5% effectively treats all neuropathic pain qualities: Results of a randomized, double-blind, vehicle-controlled, 3-week efficacy study with the use of the Neuropathic Pain Scale. *The Clinical Journal of Pain, 18*(5), 297–301.

Galer, B. S., Lee, D., Ma, T., et al. (2005). MorphiDex® (morphine sulfate/dextromethorphan hydrobromide combination) in the treatment of chronic pain: Three multicenter, randomized, double-blind, controlled clinical trials fail to demonstrate enhanced opioid analgesia or reduction in tolerance. *Pain, 115*(3), 284–295.

Galer, B. S., Miller, K. V., & Rowbotham, M. C. (1993). Response to intravenous lidocaine infusion differs based on clinical diagnosis and site of nervous system injury. *Neurology, 43*(6), 1233–1235.

Galer, B. S., Rowbotham, M. C., & Perander, J. (1999). Topical lidocaine patch relieves postherpetic neuralgia more effectively than a vehicle topical patch: Results of an enriched enrollment study. *Pain, 80*(3), 533–538.

Galinski, M., Dolveck, F., Combes, X., et al. (2007). Management of severe acute pain in emergency settings: Ketamine reduces morphine consumption. *The American Journal of Emergency Medicine, 25*(4), 385–390.

Gammaitoni, A. R., Alvarez, N. A., & Galer, B. S. (2002). Pharmacokinetics and safety of continuously applied lidocaine patches 5%. *American Journal of Health-System Pharmacy, 59*(22), 2215–2220.

Gammaitoni, A. R., Alvarez, N. A., & Galer, B. S. (2003). Safety and tolerability of the lidocaine patch 5%, a targeted peripheral analgesic: A review of the literature. *Journal of Clinical Pharmacology, 43*(2), 111–117.

Gammaitoni, A. R., & Davis, M. W. (2002). Pharmacokinetics and tolerability of lidocaine patch 5% with extended dosing. *The Annals of Pharmacotherapy, 36*(2), 236–249.

Gammaitoni, A. R., Galer, B. S., Onawola, R., et al. (2004). Lidocaine patch 5% and its positive impact on pain qualities in osteoarthritis: Results of a pilot 2-week, open-label study using the Neuropathic Pain Scale. *Current Medical Research and Opinion, 20*(Suppl. 2), S13–S19.

Gammaitoni, A. R., Gallagher, R. M., & Welz-Bosna, M. (2000). Topical ketamine gel: Possible role in treating neuropathic pain. *Pain Medicine (Malden, Mass.), 1*(1), 97–100.

Gammaitoni, A. R., Onawola, R., & Galer, B. S. (2005). Lidocaine patch 5% improves sleep, quality of life, and pain intensity in geriatric patients with neuropathic pain: A pooled analysis. *Pain Medicine (Malden, Mass.), 6*(2), 197.

Gan, T. J., Meyer, T. A., Apfel, C. C., et al. (2003). Consensus guidelines for managing postoperative nausea and vomiting. *Anesthesia and Analgesia, 97*(1), 62–71.

Gan, T. J., Meyer, T. A., Apfel, C. C., et al. (2007). Society for ambulatory anesthesia guidelines for the management of postoperative nausea and vomiting. *Anesthesia and Analgesia, 105*(6), 1615–1628.

Gartner, R., Kroman, N., Callesen, T., et al. (2008). Multimodal treatment of pain and nausea in breast cancer surgery. *Ugeskrift for Laeger, 170*(23), 2035–2038.

Gatchel, R. J., & Okifuji, A. (2006). Evidence-based scientific data documenting the treatment and cost-effectiveness of comprehensive pain programs for chronic nonmalignant pain. *The Journal of Pain, 7*(11), 779–793.

Gazerani, P., Pedersen, N. S., Staahl, C., et al. (2009). Subcutaneous botulinum toxin type A reduces capsaicin-induced trigeminal pain and vasomotor reactions in human skin. *Pain, 141*(1–2), 60–69.

Gear, R. W., Miaskowski, C., Heller, P. H., et al. (1997). Benzodiazepine mediated antagonism of opioid analgesia. *Pain, 71*(1), 25–29.

Geller, S. A. (1989). Treatment of fibrositis with fluoxetine hydrochloride (Prozac). *The American Journal of Medicine, 87*(5), 594–595.

Gentili, M., Enel, D., Szymskiewicz, O., et al. (2001). Postoperative analgesia by intraarticular clonidine and neostigmine in patients undergoing knee arthroscopy. *Regional Anesthesia and Pain Medicine, 26*(4), 342–347.

Gerner, P. (2004). Tricyclic antidepressants and their local anesthetic properties: From bench to bedside and back again. *Regional Anesthesia and Pain Medicine, 29*(3), 286–289.

Gerner, P., Kao, G., Srinivasa, V., et al. (2003). Topical amitriptyline in healthy volunteers. *Regional Anesthesia and Pain Medicine, 28*(4), 289–293.

Ghafoor, V. L., Epshteyn, M., Carlson, G. H., et al. (2007). Intrathecal drug therapy for long-term pain management. *American Journal of Health-System Pharmacy, 64*(23), 2447–2461.

Giannarini, G., Autorino, R., Valent, F., et al. (2009). Combination of perianal-intrarectal lidocaine-prilocaine cream and periprostatic nerve block for pain control during transrectal ultrasound guided prostate biopsy: A randomised, controlled trial. *The Journal of Urology, 181*(2), 585–591.

Gilron, I. (2002). Is gabapentin a "broad spectrum" analgesic? *Anesthesiology, 97*(3), 537–539.

Gilron, I. (2004). Corticosteroids in postoperative pain management: Future research directions for a multifaceted therapy. *Acta Anaesthesiologica Scandinavica, 48*(10), 1221–1222.

Gilron, I. (2006). Review article: The role of anticonvulsant drugs in postoperative pain management: A bench-to-bed-side perspective. *Canadian Journal of Anesthesia, 53*(6), 562–571.

Gilron, I., Bailey, J. M., Tu, D., et al. (2005). Morphine, gabapentin, or their combination for neuropathic pain. *The New England Journal of Medicine, 352*(13), 1324–1334.

Gilron, I., Booher, S. L., Rowan, M. S., et al. (2000). A randomized, controlled trial of high-dose dextromethorphan in facial neuralgias. *Neurology, 55*(7), 964–971.

Gilron, I., Orr, E., Tu, D., et al. (2005). A placebo-controlled randomized clinical trial of perioperative administration of gabapentin, rofecoxib and their combination for spontaneous and movement-evoked pain after abdominal hysterectomy. *Pain, 113*(1–2), 191–200.

Gilron, I., Orr, E., Tu, D., et al. (2009). A randomized, double-blind, controlled trial of perioperative administration of gabapentin, meloxicam and their combination for spontaneous and movement-evoked pain after ambulatory laparoscopic cholecystectomy. *Anesthesia and Analgesia, 108*(2), 623–630.

Gilron, I., Watson, P. N., Cahill, C. M., et al. (2006). Neuropathic pain: A practical guide for the clinician. *CMAJ: Canadian Medical Association Journal, 175*(3), 265–275.

Gimbel, J., Linn, R., Hale, M., et al. (2005). Lidocaine patch treatment in patients with low back pain: Results of an open label, nonrandomized study. *American Journal of Therapeutics, 12*(4), 311–319.

Givens, V. A., Lipscomb, G. H., & Meyer, N. L. (2002). A randomized trial of postoperative wound irrigation with local anesthetic for pain after cesarean delivery. *American Journal of Obstetrics and Gynecology, 186*(6), 1188–1191.

Glassman, A. H., & Bigger, J. T. (1981). Cardiovascular effects of therapeutic doses of tricyclic antidepressants. A review. *Arch General Psychiatry, 38*(7), 815–820.

Glazier, H. S. (1990). Potentiation of pain relief with hydroxyzine: A therapeutic myth? *DICP, 24*(5), 484–488.

Gobelet, C., Waldburger, M., & Meier, J. L. (1992). The effect of adding calcitonin to physical treatment on reflex sympathetic dystrophy. *Pain, 48*(2), 171–175.

Goldberg, M. E., Domsky, R., Scaringe, D., et al. (2005). Multi-day low dose ketamine infusion for the treatment of complex regional pain syndrome. *Pain Physician, 8*(2), 175–179.

Goldstein, A., Grimault, P., Henique, A., et al. (2000). Preventing postoperative pain by local anesthetic instillation after laparoscopic gynecologic surgery: A placebo-controlled comparison of bupivacaine and ropivacaine. *Anesthesia and Analgesia, 91*(2), 403–407.

Goldstein, D. J., Lu, Y., Detke, M. J., et al. (2005). Duloxetine vs. placebo in patients with painful diabetic neuropathy. *Pain, 116*(1–2), 109–118.

Golembiewski, J. (2005). Dexmedetomidine—does it have a role in the perioperative setting? *Journal of Perianesthesia Nursing, 20*(4), 289–291.

Golembiewski, J., & Tokumaru, S. (2006). Pharmacological prophylaxis and management of adult postoperative/postdischarge nausea and vomiting. *Journal of Perianesthesia Nursing, 21*(6), 385–397.

Gomez-Vasquez, M. E., Hernandez-Salazar, E., Hernandez-Jimenez, A., et al. (2007). Clinical efficacy and side effects of dexmedetomidine in the early postoperative period after arthroscopic knee surgery. *Journal of Clinical Anesthesia, 19*(8), 576–582.

Goodyear-Smith, F., & Halliwell, J. (2009). Anticonvulsants for neuropathic pain. *The Clinical Journal of Pain, 25*(6), 528–536.

Gordon, D. B. (1995). Hydroxyzine doesn't 'help' opioids. *The American Journal of Nursing, 95*(8), 20.

Gordon, D. B. (2003). Nonopioid and adjuvant analgesics in chronic pain management: Strategies for effective use. *The Nursing Clinics of North America, 3*(3), 447–464.

Gordon, D. B. (2008). Intravenous lidocaine for postoperative analgesia: Renewed interest in an old strategy. *APS Bulletin, 18*(3), 3–5.

Gordon, N. C., Gear, R. W., Heller, P. H., et al. (1995). Enhancement of morphine analgesia by the GABA-B agonist baclofen. *Neuroscience, 69*(2), 345–349.

Gore, M., Dukes, E., Rowbotham, D., et al. (2006). Prevalence of contraindicated medical conditions and use of precluded medications in patients with painful neuropathic disorders prescribed amitriptyline. *Pain Practice, 6*(4), 265.

Gore, M., Sadosky, A., Tai, K. S., et al. (2007). A retrospective evaluation of the use of gabapentin and pregabalin in patients with postherpetic neuralgia in usual-care settings. *Clinical Therapeutics, 29*(8), 1655–1670.

Gottschalk, A., Burmeister, M. A., Radtke, P., et al. (2003). Continuous wound infiltration with ropivacaine reduces pain and analgesic requirement after shoulder surgery. *Anesthesia and Analgesia, 97*(4), 1086–1091.

Gottschalk, A., Schroeder, F., Ufer, M., et al. (2001). Amantadine, a N-methyl-D-aspartate receptor antagonist, does not enhance postoperative analgesia in women undergoing abdominal hysterectomy. *Anesthesia and Analgesia, 93*(1), 192–196.

Gottschalk, A., & Smith, D. S. (2001). New concepts in acute pain therapy: Preemptive analgesia. *American Family Physician, 63*(10), 1979–1984.

Grande, L. A., Loeser, J. D., & Samii, A. (2008). Recurrent transient global amnesia with intrathecal baclofen. *Anesthesia and Analgesia, 106*(4), 1284–1287.

Grande, L. A., O'Donnell, B. R., Fitzgibbon, D. R., et al. (2008). Ultra-low dose ketamine and memantine treatment for pain in an opioid-tolerant oncology patient. *Anesthesia and Analgesia, 107*(4), 1380–1383.

Grant, S. A., Nielsen, K. C., Greengrass, R. A., et al. (2001). Continuous peripheral nerve block for ambulatory surgery. *Regional Anesthesia and Pain Medicine, 26*(3), 209–214.

Graven-Nielsen, T., Aspegren, K. S., Henriksson, K. G., et al. (2000). Ketamine reduces muscle pain, temporal summation, and referred pain in fibromyalgia patients. *Pain, 85*(3), 483–491.

Graves, J. R., Moran, T. J., Porter, B. R., et al. (1996). Propofol as an adjunct in the treatment of cancer-related pain. *Pain Digest, 6*, 371–373.

Gray, P. (2008). Acute neuropathic pain: Diagnosis and treatment. *Current Opinion in Anaesthesiology, 21*(5), 590–595.

Gray, P., Williams, B., & Cramond, T. (2008). Successful use of gabapentin in acute pain management following burn injury: A case series. *Pain Medicine (Malden, Mass.), 9*(3), 371–376.

Greenberg, H. S., Kim, J., & Posner, J. B. (1980). Epidural spinal cord compression from metastatic tumor: Results with a new treatment protocol. *Annals of Neurology, 8*(4), 361–366.

Gregoretti, C., Decaroli, D., Piacevoli, Q., et al. (2008). Analgosedation of patients with burns outside the operating room. *Drugs, 68*(17), 2427–2443.

Gremeau-Richard, C., Woda, A., Navez, M. L., et al. (2004). Topical clonazepam in stomatodynia: A randomized placebo-controlled study. *Pain, 108*(1–2), 51–57.

Groudine, S. B., Fisher, H. A., Kaufman, R. P., Jr., et al. (1998). Intravenous lidocaine speeds the return of bowel function, decreases postoperative pain, and shortens hospital stay in patients undergoing retropubic prostatectomy. *Anesthesia and Analgesia, 86*(2), 235–239.

Guay, D. R. (2001). Adjunctive agents in the management of chronic pain. *Pharmacotherapy, 21*(9), 1070–1080.

Guay, D. R. (2003). Oxcarbazepine, topiramate, zonisamide, and levetiracetam: Potential use in neuropathic pain. *The American Journal of Geriatric Pharmacotherapy, 1*(1), 18–37.

Guay, D. R. (2005). Pregabalin in neuropathic pain: A more "pharmaceutically elegant" gabapentin? *The American Journal of Geriatric Pharmacotherapy, 3*(4), 274–287.

Guido, M., & Specchio, L. M. (2006). Glossopharyngeal neuralgia responding to pregabalin. *Headache, 46*(8), 1307–1308.

Guignard, B., Coste, C., Costes, H., et al. (2002). Supplementing desflurane-remifentanil anesthesia with small-dose ketamine reduces perioperative opioid analgesic requirements. *Anesthesia and Analgesia, 95*(1), 103–108.

Guillou, N., Tanguy, M., Seguin, P., et al. (2003). The effects of small-dose ketamine on morphine consumption in surgical intensive care unit patients after major surgery. *Anesthesia and Analgesia, 97*(3), 843–847.

Gupta, A., Perniola, A., Axelsson, K., et al. (2004). Postoperative pain after abdominal hysterectomy: A double-blind comparison between placebo and local anesthetic infused intraperitoneally. *Anesthesia and Analgesia, 99*(4), 1173–1179.

Gupta, V. K. (2006). Metoclopramide is not an analgesic: Reflection on a premature scientific conclusion. *International Journal of Clinical Practice, 60*(6), 744.

Gurbet, A., Basagan-Mogol, E., Turker, G., et al. (2006). Intraoperative infusion of dexmedetomidine reduces perioperative analgesic requirements. *Canadian Journal of Anaesthesia, 53*(7), 646–652.

Gurfinkel, R., Czeiger, D., Douvdevani, A., et al. (2006). Ketamine improves survival in burn injury followed by sepsis in rats. *Anesthesia and Analgesia, 103*(2), 396–402.

Gursoy, A., Ertugrul, D. T., Sahin, M., et al. (2007). The analgesic efficacy of lidocaine/prilocaine (EMLA) cream during fine-needle aspiration biopsy of thyroid nodules. *Clinical Endocrinology, 66*(5), 691–694.

Gutierrez-Alvarez, A. M., Beltran-Rodriguez, J., & Moreno, C. B. (2007). Antiepileptic drugs in treatment of pain caused by diabetic neuropathy. *Journal of Pain and Symptom Management, 34*(2), 201–208.

Gutta, R., & Louis, P. J. (2007). Bisphosphonates and osteonecrosis of the jaws: science and rationale. *Oral Surgery Oral Medicine Oral Pathology Oral Radiology and Endodontics, 104*(2), 186–193.

Haberfellner, E. M. (2007). A review of the assessment of antidepressant-induced sexual dysfunction used in randomized, controlled clinical trials. *Pharmacopsychiatry, 40*(5), 173–182.

Habib, A. S., & Gan, T. J. (2004a). Evidence-based management of postoperative nausea and vomiting: Review. *Canadian Journal of Anesthesia, 51*(4), 326–341.

Habib, A. S., El-Moalem, H. E., & Gan, T. J. (2004b). The efficacy of the 5-HT receptor antagonists combined with droperidol for PONV prophylaxis is similar to their combination with dexamethasone. A meta-analysis of randomized controlled trials. *Canadian Journal of Anesthesia, 51*(4), 311–319.

Habib, A. S., Polascik, T. J., Weizer, A. Z., et al. (2009). Lidocaine patch for postoperative analgesia after radical retropubic prostatectomy. *Anesthesia and Analgesia, 108*(6), 1950–1953.

Habib, A. S., White, W. D., El Gasim, M. A., et al. (2008). Transdermal nicotine for analgesia after radical retropubic prostatectomy. *Anesthesia and Analgesia, 107*(3), 999–1004.

Hackworth, R. J., Tokarz, K. A., Fowler, I. A., et al. (2008). Profound pain reduction after induction of memantine treatment in two patients with severe phantom limb pain. *Pain Medicine (Malden, Mass.), 107*(4), 1377–1379.

Hahn, K., Arendt, G., Braun, J. S., et al. (2004). German Neuro-AIDS Working Group: A placebo-controlled trial of gabapentin for painful HIV-associated sensory neuropathies. *Journal of Neurology, 251*, 1260–1266.

Hains, B. C., Klein, J. P., Saab, C. Y., et al. (2003). Upregulation of sodium channel Nav1.3 and functional involvement in neuronal hyperexcitability associated with central neuropathic pain after spinal cord injury. *The Journal of Neuroscience, 23*(26), 8881–8892.

Halbert, J., Crotty, M., & Cameron, I. D. (2002). Evidence for the optimal management of acute and chronic phantom pain: A systematic review. *The Clinical Journal of Pain, 18*(2), 84–92.

Halvorson, K. G., Sevcik, M. A., Ghilardi, J. R., et al. (2008). Intravenous ibandromate rapidly reduces pain, neurochemical indices of central sensitization, tumor burden, and skeletal destruction in a mouse model of bone cancer. *Journal of Pain and Symptom Management, 36*(3), 289–303.

Hammack, J. E., Michalak, J. C., Loprinzi, C. L., et al. (2002). Phase III evaluation of nortriptyline for alleviation of symptoms of cis-platinum-induced peripheral neuropathy. *Pain, 98*(1–2), 195–203.

Hand, P. J., & Stark, R. J. (2000). Intravenous lignocaine infusions for severe chronic daily headache. *The Medical Journal of Australia, 172*(4), 157–159.

Hanks, G., Cherny, N. I., & Fallon, M. (2004). Opioid analgesic therapy. In D. Doyle, G. Hanks, N. I. Cherny, & K. Calman (Eds.), *Oxford textbook of palliative medicine.* (3rd ed., pp. 316–341). New York: Oxford Press.

Hanna, M., O'Brien, C., & Wilson, M. C. (2008). Prolonged-release oxycodone enhances the effects of existing gabapentin therapy in painful diabetic neuropathy patients. *European Journal of Pain (London, England), 12*(6), 804–813.

Hansen, C. R., Gooch, J. L., & Such-Neibar, T. (2007). Prolonged, severe intrathecal baclofen withdrawal syndrome: A case report. *Archives of Physical Medicine and Rehabilitation, 88*(11), 1468–1471.

Harden, R. N., Houle, T. T., Remble, T. A., et al. (2005). Topiramate for phantom limb pain: A time-series analysis. *Pain Medicine (Malden, Mass.), 6*(5), 375–378.

Harke, H., Gretenkort, P., Ladleif, H. U., et al. (2001). The response of neuropathic pain and pain in complex regional pain syndrome I to carbamazepine and sustained-release morphine in patients pretreated with spinal cord stimulation: A double-blind randomized study. *Anesthesia and Analgesia, 92*(2), 488–495.

Harmer, J. P., & Larson, B. S. (2002). Pain relief from baclofen analgesia in a neuropathic pain patient who failed opioid and pharmacotherapy: Case report. *Journal of Pain & Palliative Care Pharmacotherapy, 16*(3), 61–64.

Harris, J. D., & Kotob, F. (2006). Management of opioid-related side effects. In O. A. de Leon-Casasola (Ed.), *Cancer pain. Pharmacological, interventional and palliative care approaches* (pp. 207–230). Philadelphia: Saunders.

Hart, R. G., & Easton, J. D. (1982). Carbamazepine and hematological monitoring. *Annals of Neurology, 11*(3), 309–312.

Hassenbusch, S. J., Portenoy, R. K., Cousins, M., et al. (2004). Polyanalgesic consensus conference 2003: An update on the management of pain by intraspinal drug delivery—Report of an expert panel. *J Pain Symptom Manage, 27*(6), 540–563.

Hauser, W., Bernardy, K., Uceyler, N., et al. (2009). Treatment of fibromyalgia syndrome with antidepressants: A meta-analysis. *JAMA, 301*(2), 198–209.

Hauser, W., Thieme, K., & Turk, D. C. (2009). Guidelines on the management of fibromyalgia syndrome—A systematic review. *European Journal of Pain,* Mar 3 [Epub ahead of print].

Hayashida, M., Fukuda, K., & Fukunaga, A. (2005). Clinical application of adenosine and ATP for pain control. *Journal of Anesthesia, 19*(3), 225–235.

Hayek, S. M., Ritchey, R. M., Sessler, D., et al. (2006). Continuous femoral nerve analgesia after unilateral total knee arthroplasty: Stimulating versus nonstimulating catheters. *Anesthesia and Analgesia, 103*(6), 1565–1570.

Hayes, C., Armstrong-Brown, A., Burstal, R., et al. (2004). Perioperative intravenous ketamine infusion for the prevention of persistent post-amputation pain: A randomized, controlled trial. *Anaesthesia and Intensive Care, 32*(3), 330–338.

Hazinedaroglu, S. M., Kayaoglu, H. A., Ates, Y., et al. (2006). Intraperitoneal bupivacaine for postoperative pain after laparascopic cholecystectomy. *Pain Medicine (Malden, Mass.), 7*(6), 539–541.

Hebl, J. R., Kopp, S. L., Ali, M. H., et al. (2005). A comprehensive anesthesia protocol that emphasizes peripheral nerve blockade for total knee and total hip arthroplasty. *The Journal of Bone and Joint Surgery, 87-A*(Suppl, 2), 63–70.

Heiskanen, T., Hartel, B., Dahl, M. L., et al. (2002). Analgesic effects of dextromethorphan and morphine in patients with chronic pain. *Pain, 96*(3), 261–267.

Helmy, S. A. K., & Bali, A. (2001). The effect of the preemptive use of the NMDA receptor antagonist dextromethorphan on postoperative analgesic requirements. *Anesthesia and Analgesia, 92*(3), 739–744.

Hempenstall, K., Nurmikko, T. J., Johnson, R. W., et al. (2005). Analgesic therapy in postherpetic neuralgia: A quantitative systematic review. *PLoS Medicine, 2*(7), e164.

Hemstreet, B., & Lapointe, M. (2001). Evidence for the use of gabapentin in the treatment of diabetic peripheral neuropathy. *Clinical Therapeutics, 23*(4), 520–531.

Hermann, D. N., Barbano, R. L., Hart-Gouleau, S., et al. (2005). An open-label study of the lidocaine patch 5% in painful idiopathic sensory polyneuropathy. *Pain Medicine (Malden, Mass.), 6*(5), 379–384.

Herroeder, S., Pecher, S., Schonherr, M. E., et al. (2007). Systemic lidocaine shortens length of stay after colorectal surgery: A double-blinded, randomized, placebo-controlled trial. *Annals of Surgery, 246*(2), 192–200.

Hess, P., & Aleshi, P. (2008). Pain in pregnancy, childbirth, and the puerperium. In P. E. Macintyre, S. M. Walker, & D. J. Rowbotham (Eds.), *Acute pain.* (2nd ed., pp. 460–476). London, UK: Hodder Arnold.

Heymann, R. E., Helfenstein, M., & Feldman, D. (2001). A double-blind, randomized, controlled study of amitriptyline, nortriptyline and placebo in patients with fibromyalgia: An analysis of outcome measures. *Clinical and Experimental Rheumatology, 19*(6), 697–702.

Hidvegi, T., Bretschneider, M., Thierfelder, S., et al. (2008). Long-term efficacy of lacosamide in subjects with painful distal diabetic neuropathy. *The Journal of Pain, 9*(4), 27.

Hijazi, R., Taylor, D., & Richardson, J. (2009). Effect of topical alkane vapocoolant spray on pain with intravenous cannulation in patients in emergency departments: Randomised double blind placebo controlled trial. *BMJ (Clinical Research Ed.), 338*, b215.

Hildebrand, K. R., Elsberry, D. D., & Hassenbusch, S. J. (2003). Stability and compatibility of morphine—clonidine admixtures in an implantable infusion system. *Journal of Pain and Symptom Management, 25*(5), 464–471.

Hill, C. M., Balkenohl, M., Thomas, D. W., et al. (2001). Pregabalin in patients with postoperative dental pain. *European Journal of Pain (London, England), 5*(2), 119–124.

Hindmarch, I., Dawson, J., & Stanley, N. (2005). A double-blind study in healthy volunteers to assess the effects on sleep of pregabalin compared with alprazolam and placebo. *Sleep, 28*(2), 187–193.

Hines, R., Keaney, D., Moskowitz, M. H., et al. (2002). Use of lidocaine patch 5% for chronic low back pain: A report of four cases. *Pain Medicine (Malden, Mass.), 3*(4), 361–365.

Ho, K. Y., Gan, T. J., & Habib, A. S. (2006). Gabapentin and postoperative pain—A systematic review of randomized controlled trials. *Pain, 126*(1–3), 91–101.

Ho, K. Y., Huh, B. K., White, W. D., et al. (2008). Topical amitriptyline versus lidocaine in the treatment of neuropathic pain. *The Clinical Journal of Pain, 24*(1), 51–55.

Hocking, G., & Cousins, M. J. (2003). Ketamine in chronic pain management: An evidence-based review. *Anesthesia and Analgesia, 97*(6), 1730–1739.

Hocking, G., Visser, E. J., Schug, S. A., et al. (2007). Ketamine: Does life begin at 40? *IASP Pain Clinical Updates, 15*(3), 1–6.

Hofmann-Kiefer, K., Eiser, T., Chappell, D., et al. (2008). Does patient-controlled continuous interscalene block improve early functional rehabilitation after open shoulder surgery? *Anesthesia and Analgesia, 106*(3), 991–996.

Hong, D., Conell-Price, J., Cheng, S., et al. (2008). Trandersmal nicotine patch for postoperative pain management: A pilot dose-ranging study. *Anesthesia and Analgesia, 107*(3), 1005–1010.

Horlocker, T. T., Wedel, D. J., Benzon, H., et al. (2003). Regional anesthesia in the anticoagulated patient: Defining the risks (the second ASRA consensus conference on neuraxial anesthesia and anticoagulation). *Regional Anesthesia and Pain Medicine, 28*(3), 172–197.

Hosking, R. D., & Zajicek, J. P. (2008). Therapeutic potential of cannabis in pain medicine. *British Journal of Anaesthesia, 101*(1), 59–68.

Howland, R. H. (2008). Understanding the clinical profile of a drug on the basis of its pharmacology: Mirtazapine as an example. *Journal of Psychosocial Nursing and Mental Health Services, 46*(12), 19–23.

Hsu, Y. W., Cortinez, L. I., Robertson, K. M., et al. (2004). Dexmedetomidine pharmacodynamics: Part I. *Anesthesiology, 101*(5), 1066–1076.

Huang, Y. M., Wang, C. M., Wang, C. T., et al. (2008). Perioperative celebrex administration for pain management after total knee arthroplasty—A randomized, controlled study. *BMC Musculoskeletal Disorders, 9*, 77.

Huang, Y. S., Lin, L. C., Huh, B. K., et al. (2007). Epidural clonidine for postoperative pain after total knee arthroplasty: A dose-response study. *Anesthesia and Analgesia, 104*(5), 1230–1235.

Hudetz, J. A., Patterson, K. M., Iqbal, Z., et al. (2009). Ketamine attenuates delirium after cardiac surgery with cardiopulmonary bypass. *Journal of Cardiothoracic and Vascular Anesthesia, 23*(5), 651–657.

Hugel, H., Ellershaw, J. E., & Dickman, A. (2003). Clonazepam as an adjuvant analgesic in patients with cancer-related neuropathic pain. *Journal of Pain and Symptom Management, 26*(6), 1073–1074.

Hunter, D. J., & Lo, G. H. (2008). The management of osteoarthritis: An overview and call to appropriate conservative treatment. *Rheumatic Diseases Clinics of North America, 34*(3), 689–712.

Hurley, R. W., Chatterjea, D., Feng, M. R., et al. (2002). Gabapentin and pregabalin can interact synergistically with naproxen to produce antihyperalgesia. *Anesthesiology, 97*(5), 1263–1273.

Hurley, R. W., Cohen, S. P., Williams, K. A., et al. (2006). The analgesic effects of perioperative gabapentin on postoperative pain: A meta-analysis. *Regional Anesthesia and Pain Medicine, 31*(3), 237–247.

Hurley, R. W., Lesley, M. R., Adams, M. C., et al. (2008). Pregabalin as a treatment for painful diabetic peripheral neuropathy: A meta-analysis. *Regional Anesthesia and Pain Medicine, 33*(3), 389–394.

Huskey, A. (2006). Cannabinoids in cancer pain management. *Journal of Pain & Palliative Care Pharmacotherapy, 20*(3), 43–46.

Ichimata, M., Ikebe, H., Yoshitake, S., et al. (2001). Analgesic effects of flecainide on postherpetic neuralgia. *International Journal of Clinical Pharmacology Research, 21*(1), 15–19.

Ichimata, M., Kitano, T., Ikebe, H., et al. (2001). Flecainide reverses neuropathic pain and suppresses ectopic nerve discharge in rats. *Neuroreport, 12*(9), 1869–1873.

Ikeda, K., Kobayashi, T., Kumanishi, T., et al. (2002). Molecular mechanisms of analgesia induced by opioids and ethanol: Is the GIRK channel one of the keys? *Neuroscience Research, 44*(2), 121–131.

Ilfeld, B. M., Ball, S. T., Gearen, P. F., et al. (2009). Health-related quality of life after hip arthroplasty with and without an extended-duration continuous posterior lumbarplexus nerve block: A prospective, 1-year follow-up of a randomized, triple-masked, placebo-controlled study. *Anesthesia and Analgesia, 109*(2), 586–591.

Ilfeld, B. M., & Enneking, F. K. (2002). A portable mechanical pump providing over four days of patient-controlled analgesia by perineural infusion at home. *Regional Anesthesia and Pain Medicine, 27*(1), 100–104.

Ilfeld, B. M., Gearen, P. F., Enneking, F. K., et al. (2006). Total knee arthroplasty as an overnight-stay procedure using continuous femoral nerve blocks at home: A prospective feasibility study. *Anesthesia and Analgesia, 102*(1), 87–90.

Ilfeld, B. M., Le, L. T., Ramjohn, J., et al. (2009). The effects of local anesthetic concentration and dose on continuous infraclavicular nerve blocks: A multicenter, randomized, observer-masked, controlled study. *Anesthesia and Analgesia, 108*(1), 345–350.

Ilfeld, B. M., Loland, V. J., Gerancher, J. C., et al. (2008). The effects of varying local anesthetic concentration and volume on continuous popliteal sciatic nerve blocks: A dual-center, randomized, controlled study. *Anesthesia and Analgesia, 107*(2), 701–707.

Ilfeld, B. M., Meyer, R. S., Le, L. T., et al. (2009). Health-related quality of life after tricompartment knee arthroplasty with or without an extended-duration continuous femoral nerve block: A prospective, 1-year follow-up of a randomized, triple-masked, placebo-controlled study. *Anesthesia and Analgesia, 108*(4), 1320–1325.

Ilfeld, B. M., Morey, T. E., & Enneking, F. K. (2002a). Continuous infraclavicular brachial plexus block for postoperative pain control at home. *Anesthesiology, 96*(6), 1297–1304.

Ilfeld, B. M., Morey, T. E., & Enneking, F. K. (2002b). Continuous popliteal sciatic nerve block for postoperative pain control at home. *Anesthesiology, 97*(4), 959–965.

Ilfeld, B. M., Morey, T. E., & Enneking, F. K. (2002c). The delivery rate accuracy of portable infusion pumps used for continuous regional analgesia. *Anesthesia and Analgesia, 95*(5), 1331–1336.

Ilfeld, B. M., Morey, T. E., & Enneking, F. K. (2003). Continuous infraclavicular perineural infusion with clonidine and ropivacaine compared with ropivacaine alone: A randomized, double-blinded, controlled study. *Anesthesia and Analgesia, 97*(3), 706–712.

Ilfeld, B. M., Morey, T. E., & Enneking, F. K. (2004). Infraclavicular perineural local anesthetic infusion. *Anesthesiology, 100*(2), 395–402.

Ilfeld, B. M., Morey, T. E., Wang, D., et al. (2002). Continuous popliteal sciatic nerve block for postoperative pain control at home. *Anesthesiology, 97*(4), 959–965.

Ilfeld, B. M., Morey, T. E., Wright, T. W., et al. (2003). Continuous interscalene brachial plexus block for postoperative pain control at home: A randomized, double-blinded, placebo-controlled study. *Anesthesia and Analgesia, 2003*(4), 1089–1095.

Ilfeld, B. M., Thannikary, L. J., Morey, T. E., et al. (2004). Popliteal sciatic perineural local anesthetic infusion. *Anesthesiology, 101*(4), 970–977.

Ilfeld, B. M., Wright, T. W., Enneking, F. K., et al. (2005). Total shoulder arthroplasty as an outpatient procedure using ambulatory perineural local anesthetic infusion: A pilot feasibility study. *Anesthesia and Analgesia, 101*(5), 1319–1322.

Ilkjaer, S., Bach, L. F., Nielsen, P. A., et al. (2000). Effect of preoperative oral dextromethorphan on immediate and late postoperative pain and hyperalgesia after total abdominal hysterectomy. *Pain, 86*(1), 19–24.

Infusion Nurses Society. (2006). *Infusion nursing standards of practice.* Norwood MA: Infusion Nurses Society.

Ingalls, N. K., Horton, Z. A., Bettendorf, M., et al. (2009). Randomized, double-blind, placebo-controlled trial using lidocaine patch 5% in traumatic rib fractures. *Journal of the American College of Surgeons, 210*(2), 205–209.

Institute for Safe Medication Practices (ISMP). (2006). Propofol sedation: Who should administer? *ISMP Medication Safety Alert! 4*(9), 1–2.

Ionescu, D., Badescu, C., & Acalovschi, I. (2007). Nicotine patch for the prevention of postoperative nausea and vomiting. *Clinical Drug Investigation, 27*(8), 559–564.

Irving, G., Jensen, M., Cramer, M., et al. (2009). Efficacy and tolerability of gastric-retentive gabapentin for the treatment of postherpetic neuralgia: Results of a double-blind, randomized, placebo-controlled clinical trial. *The Clinical Journal of Pain, 25*(3), 185–192.

Jackson, K., Ashby, M., Martin, P., et al. (2001). "Burst" ketamine for refractory cancer pain: An open-label audit of 39 patients. *Journal of Pain and Symptom Management, 22*(4), 834–842.

Jalowiecki, P., Rudner, R., Gonciarz, M., et al. (2005). Sole use of dexmedetomidine has limited utility for conscious sedation during outpatient colonoscopy. *Anesthesiology, 103*(2), 269–273.

Jeffs, S. A., Hall, J. E., & Morris, S. (2002). Comparison of morphine alone with morphine plus clonidine for postoperative patient-controlled analgesia. *British Journal of Anaesthesia, 89*(3), 424–427.

Jenkins, C. A., & Bruera, E. (2000). Difficulties in diagnosing neuropsychiatric complications of corticosteroids in advanced cancer patients: Two case reports. *Journal of Pain and Symptom Management, 19*(4), 309–317.

Jensen, P. G., & Larson, J. R. (2001). Management of painful diabetic neuropathy. *Drugs and Aging, 18*(10), 737–749.

Jensen, T. S. (2002). Anticonvulsants in neuropathic pain: Rationale and clinical evidence. *European Journal of Pain (London, England), 6*(Suppl. A), 61–68.

Jensen, T. S., & Baron, R. (2003). Translation of symptoms and signs into mechanisms in neuropathic pain. *Pain, 1021*(1–2), 1–8.

Jensen, T. S., & Finnerup, N. B. (2007). Management of neuropathic pain. *Curr Opin Support Palliat Care, 1*(2), 126–131.

Jimenez, N., Bradford, H., Seidel, K. D., et al. (2006). A comparison of a needle-free injection system for local anesthesia versus EMLA for intravenous catheter insertion in the pediatric patient. *Anesthesia and Analgesia, 102*(2), 411–414.

Jokela, R., Ahonen, J., Tallgren, M., et al. (2008). A randomized controlled trial of perioperative administration of pregabalin for pain after laparoscopic hysterectomy. *Pain, 134*(1–2), 106–112.

Jones, M. E. P., & Maze, M. (2001). Can we characterize the central nervous system actions of α2-adrenergic agonists? (Editorial I). *British Journal of Anaesthesia, 86*(1), 1–3.

Jose, V. M., Bhansali, A., Hota, D., et al. (2007). Randomized double-blind study comparing the efficacy and safety of lamotrigine and amitriptyline in painful diabetic neuropathy. *Diabetic Medicine, 24*(4), 377–383.

Joshi, W., Reuben, S. S., Kilaru, P. R., et al. (2000). Postoperative analgesia for outpatient arthroscopic knee surgery with intraarticular clonidine and/or morphine. *Anesthesia and Analgesia*, 90(5), 1102–1106.

Kaba, A., Laurent, S. R., Detroz, B. J., et al. (2007). Intravenous lidocaine infusion facilitates acute rehabilitation after laparoscopic colectomy. *Anesthesiology*, 106(1), 11–18.

Kajdasz, D. K., Iyengar, S., Desaiah, D., et al. (2007). Duloxetine for the management of diabetic peripheral neuropathic pain: Evidence-based findings from post hoc analysis of three multicenter, randomized, double-blind, placebo-controlled, parallel-group studies. *Clinical Therapeutics*, 29(Suppl.), 2536–2546.

Kakinohana, M., Higa, Y., Sasara, T., et al. (2004). Addition of ketamine to propofol-fentanyl anaesthesia can reduce postoperative pain and epidural analgesic consumption in upper abdominal surgery. *Acute Pain*, 5(2), 75–79.

Kamibayashi, T., & Maze, M. (2000). Clinical uses of α2-adrenergic agonists. *Anesthesiology*, 93(5), 1345–1349.

Kanai, A., Kumaki, C., Niki, Y., et al. (2009). Efficacy of a metered-dose 8% lidocaine pump spray for patients with post-herpetic neuralgia. *Pain Medicine (Malden, Mass.)*, 10(5), 902–909.

Kandler, D., & Lisander, B. (1993). Analgesic action of metoclopramide in prosthetic hip surgery. *Acta Anaesthesiologica Scandinavica*, 37(1), 49–53.

Kaniecki, R. (2008). Neuromodulators for migraine prevention. *Headache*, 48(4), 586–600.

Kannan, T. R., Saxena, A., Bhatnagar, S., et al. (2002). Oral ketamine as an adjuvant to oral morphine for neuropathic pain in cancer patients. *Journal of Pain and Symptom Management*, 23(1), 60–65.

Kapur, N., & Friedman, R. (2002). Oral ketamine: A promising treatment for restless leg syndrome. *Anesthesia and Analgesia*, 94(6), 1558–1559.

Karakaya, D., Baris, S., Ozkan, F., et al. (2004). Analgesic effectiveness of interpleural bupivacaine with fentanyl for post-thoracotomy pain. *Journal of Cardiothoracic and Vascular Anesthesia*, 18(4), 461–465.

Kararmaz, A., Kaya, S., Karaman, H., et al. (2003). Intraoperative intravenous ketamine in combination with epidural analgesia: Postoperative analgesia after renal surgery. *Anesthesia and Analgesia*, 97(4), 1092–1096.

Kardash, K. J., Beng, F. S., Tessler, M. J., et al. (2008). Single-dose dexamethasone reduces dynamic pain after total hip arthroplasty. *Anesthesia and Analgesia*, 106(4), 1253–1257.

Karp, J. F. (2004). Venlafaxine XR and chronic pelvic pain syndrome. *The Journal of Clinical Psychiatry*, 65(6), 880–881.

Karsdal, M. A., Henriksen, K., Arnold, M., et al. (2008). Calcitonin: A drug of the past or for the future? Physiologic inhibition of bone resorption while sustaining osteoclast numbers improves bone quality. *BioDrugs: Clinical Immunotherapeutics, Biopharmaceuticals and Gene Therapy*, 22(3), 137–144.

Kastrup, J., Bach, F. W., Petersen, P., et al. (1989). Lidocaine treatment of painful diabetic neuropathy and endogenous opioid peptides in plasma. *The Clinical Journal of Pain*, 5(3), 239–244.

Katz, J., Pennella-Vaughan, J., Hetzel, R. D., et al. (2005). A randomized, placebo-controlled trial of bupropion sustained release in chronic low back pain. *The Journal of Pain*, 6(10), 656–661.

Katz, N. P., Gammaitoni, A. R., Davis, M. W., et al. (2002). Lidocaine patch 5% reduces pain intensity and interference with quality of life in patients with postherpetic neuralgia: An effectiveness trial. *Pain Medicine (Malden, Mass.)*, 3(4), 324–332.

Katz, W. A., & Rothenberg, R. (2005). Section 4: Treating the patient in pain. *Journal of Clinical Rheumatology*, 11(Suppl. 2), S16–S27.

Kautio, A. L., Haanpaa, M., Saarto, T., et al. (2008). Amitriptyline in the treatment of chemotherapy-induced neuropathic symptoms. *Journal of Pain and Symptom Management*, 35(1), 31–39.

Kawamata, M., Sugino, S., Narimatsu, E., et al. (2006). Effects of systemic administration of lidocaine and QX-314 on hyperexcitability of spinal dorsal horn neurons after incision in the rat. *Pain*, 122(1–2), 68–80.

Kaweski, S. (2008). Topical anesthetic creams. *Plastic and Reconstructive Surgery*, 121(6), 2161–2165.

Kehlet, H. (2005). Preventive measures to minimize or avoid postoperative ileus. *Semin Colon Rectal Surg*, 16(4), 203–206.

Kehlet, H. (2006). Perioperative analgesia to prevent chronic postmastectomy pain. (Letter) *Anesthesia and Analgesia*, 103(2), 494–495.

Kehlet, H., Jensen, T. S., & Woolf, C. J. (2006). Persistent postsurgical pain: Risk factors and prevention. *Lancet*, 367(9522), 1618–1625.

Kehlet, H., & Wilmore, D. W. (2008). Evidence-based surgical care and the evolution of fast-track surgery. *Annals of Surgery*, 248(2), 189–198.

Kenney, P., Simpson, J., Koch, B., et al. (2006). A multi-center, randomized, double-blind, placebo-controlled trial to assess the efficacy and safety of lacosamide (200, 400, and 600 mg/day) in subjects with painful distal diabetic neuropathy. *The Journal of Pain*, 7(4), S45.

Kent, C. D., Kaufman, B. S., & Lowy, J. (2005). Dexmedetomidine facilitates the withdrawal of ventilatory support in palliative care. *Anesthesiology*, 103(2), 439–441.

Kerr, D., & Kohan, L. (2008). Local infiltration analgesia: A technique for control of acute postoperative pain following knee and hip surgery. *Acta Orthopaedica*, (7992), 174–183.

Keskinbora, K., & Aydinli, I. (2008). A double-blind randomized controlled trial of topiramate and amitriptyline either alone or in combination for the prevention of migraine. *Clinical Neurology and Neurosurgery*, 110(10), 979–984.

Keskinbora, K., Pekel, A. F., & Aydinli, I. (2007). Gabapentin and an opioid combination versus opioid alone for the management of neuropathic cancer pain: A randomized open trial. *Journal of Pain and Symptom Management*, 34(2), 183–189.

Khaliq, W., Alam, S., & Puri, N. K. (2007). Topical lidocaine for the treatment of postherpetic neuralgia. *Cochrane Database Systematic Reviews*, (2) CD004846.

Khojainova, N., Santiago-Palma, J., Kornick, C., et al. (2002). Olanzapine in the management of cancer pain. *Journal of Pain and Symptom Management*, 23(4), 346–350.

Khoromi, S., Cui, L., Nackers, L., et al. (2007). Morphine, nortriptyline and their combination vs. placebo in patients with chronic lumbar root pain. *Pain*, 130(1–2), 66–75.

Kiat Ang, C. K., Leung, D. Y. C., Lo, S., et al. (2006). Effect of local anesthesia and intravenous sedation on pain perception and vasovagal reactions during femoral arterial sheath after percutaneous coronary intervention. *International Journal of Cardiology*, 116(3), 321–326.

Kiefer, R. T., Rohr, P., Ploppa, A., et al. (2008). Efficacy of ketamine in anesthetic dosage for the treatment of refractory complex regional pain syndrome: An open-label phase II study. *Pain Medicine (Malden, Mass.)*, 9(8), 1173–1201.

Killgore, W. D., Rupp, T. L., Grugle, N. L., et al. (2008). Effects of dextroamphetamine, caffeine and modafinil on psychomotor vigilance test performance after 44 h of continuous wakefulness. *Journal of Sleep Research*, 17(3), 309–321.

Kim, S. I., Han, T. H., Kil, H. Y., et al. (2000). Prevention of postoperative nausea and vomiting by continuous infusion of subhypnotic propofol in female patients receiving intravenous patient-controlled analgesia. *British Journal of Anaesthesia*, 85(6), 898–900.

Kim, S. W., Shin, I. S., Kim, J. M., et al. (2008). Effectiveness of mirtazapine for nausea and insomnia in cancer patients with depression. *Psychiatry and Clinical Neurosciences*, 62(1), 75–83.

Kimos, P., Biggs, C., Mah, J., et al. (2007). Analgesic action of gabapentin on chronic pain in the masticatory muscles: A randomized controlled trial. *Pain*, 127(1–2), 151–160.

Kingery, W. S. (1997). A critical review of controlled clinical trials for peripheral neuropathic pain and complex regional pain syndrome. *Pain*, 72(2), 123–139.

Kiser, R. S., Cohen, H. M., Freedenfeld, R. N., et al. (2001). Olanzapine for the treatment of fibromyalgia symptoms. *Journal of Pain and Symptom Management*, 22(2), 704–708.

Kishore-Kumar, R., Max, M. B., Schafer, S. C., et al. (1990). Desipramine relieves postherpetic neuralgia. *Clinical Pharmacology and Therapeutics*, 47(3), 305–312.

Klepstad, P., Kaasa, S., Cherny, N., et al. (2005). Research Steering Committee of the EAPC: Pain and pain treatments in European palliative care units. A cross sectional survey from the European Association for Palliative Care Research Network. *Palliative Medicine*, 19(6), 477–484.

Klotz, U. (2006). Ziconotide–A novel neuron-specific calcium channel blocker for the intrathecal treatment of severe chronic pain—A short review. *International Journal of Clinical Pharmacology and Therapeutics*, 44(10), 478–483.

Knotkova, H., & Pappagallo, M. (2007). Adjuvant analgesics. *The Medical Clinics of North America*, 91(1), 113–124.

Knotkova, H., Pappagallo, M., & Szallasi, A. (2008). Capsaicin (TRPV1 agonist) therapy for pain relief: Farewell or revival? *The Clinical Journal of Pain*, 24(2), 142–154.

Koc, S., Memis, D., & Sut, N. (2007). The preoperative use of gabapentin, dexamethasone, and their combination in varicocele surgery: A randomized controlled trial. *Anesthesia and Analgesia*, 105(4), 1137–1142.

Kochar, D. K., Rawat, N., Agrawal, R. P., et al. (2004). Sodium valproate for painful diabetic neuropathy: A randomized double-blind placebo-controlled study. *QJM: Monthly Journal of the Association of Physicians*, 97(1), 33–38.

Kong, V. K., & Irwin, M. G. (2007). Gabapentin: A multimodal perioperative drug? *British Journal of Anaesthesia*, 99(6), 775–786.

Konstantatos, A., Silvers, A. J., & Myers, P. S. (2008). Analgesia best practice after cardiac surgery. *Anesthesiology Clinics*, 26(3), 591–602.

Koppert, W., Weigand, M., Neumann, F., et al. (2004). Perioperative intravenous lidocaine has preventive effects on postoperative pain and morphine consumption after major abdominal surgery. *Anesthesia and Analgesia*, 98(4), 1050–1055.

Korfitis, C., & Trafalis, D. T. (2008). Carbamazepine can be effective in alleviating tormenting pruritus in patients with hematologic malignancy. (Letter.) *Journal of Pain and Symptom Management*, 35(6), 571–572.

Kosson, D., Klinowiecka, A., Kosson, P., et al. (2008). Intrathecal antinociceptive interaction between the NMDA antagonist ketamine and the opioids, morphine and biphalin. *European Journal of Pain (London, England)*, 12(5), 611–616.

Kotarba, J. A. (1983). *Chronic pain: Its social dimensions* Beverly Hills: Sage Publications.

Kotlinska-Lemieszek, A., & Luczak, J. (2004). Subanesthetic ketamine: An essential adjuvant for intractable cancer pain. *Journal of Pain and Symptom Management*, 28(2), 100–102.

Krafft, R. M. (2008). Trigeminal neuralgia. *American Family Physician*, 77(9), 1291–1296.

Kranke, P., Eberhart, L. H., Roewer, N., et al. (2004). Single-dose parenteral pharmacological interventions for the prevention of postoperative shivering: A qualitative systematic review of randomized controlled trials. *Anesthesia and Analgesia*, 99(3), 718–727.

Kroenke, K., Krebs, E. E., & Bair, M. J. (2009). Pharmacology of chronic pain: A synthesis of recommendations from systematic reviews. *General Hospital Psychiatry*, 31(3), 206–219.

Kropeit, D., Scharfenecker, U., Schiltmeyer, B., et al. (2006). Lacosamide has low potential for drug-drug-interaction. *The Journal of Pain*, 7(4), S63.

Krymchantowski, A. V., Silva, M. T., Barbosa, J. S., et al. (2002). Amitriptyline versus amitriptyline combined with fluoxetine in the preventative treatment of transformed migraine: A double-blind study. *Headache*, 42(6), 510–514.

Kudoh, A., Takahira, Y., Katagai, H., et al. (2002). Small-dose ketamine improves the postoperative state of depressed patients. *Anesthesia and Analgesia*, 95(1), 114–118.

Kumar, A., Gupta, N. P., Hemal, A. K., et al. (2007). Comparison of three analgesic regimens for pain control during shockwave lithotripsy using Dornier Delta Compact lithotripter: A randomized clinical trial. *Journal of Endourology*, 21(6), 578–582.

Kumar, B., Kalita, J., Kumar, G., et al. (2009). Central poststroke pain: A review of pathophysiology and treatment. *Anesthesia and Analgesia*, 108(5), 1645–1657.

Kumar, R. (2008). Approved and investigational uses of modafinil: An evidence-based review. *Drugs*, 68(13), 1803–1839.

Kundu, S., & Achar, S. (2002). Principles of office anesthesia: Part II. Topical anesthesia. *American Family Physician*, 66(1), 99–102.

Kuo, C. P., Jao, S. W., Chen, K. M., et al. (2006). Comparison of the effects of thoracic epidural analgesia and i.v. infusion with lidocaine on cytokine response, postoperative pain and bowel function in patients undergoing colonic surgery. *British Journal of Anaesthesia*, 97(5), 640–646.

Kurella, M., Bennett, W. M., & Chertow, G. M. (2003). Analgesia in patients with ESRD: A review of available evidence. *American Journal of Kidney Diseases*, 42(2), 217–228.

Kvarnstrom, A., Karlsten, R., Quiding, H., et al. (2004). The analgesic effect of intravenous ketamine and lidocaine on pain after spinal cord injury. *Acta Anaesthesiologica Scandinavica*, 48(4), 498–506.

Labaille, T., Mazoit, J. X., Paqueron, X., et al. (2002). The clinical efficacy and pharmacokinetics of intraperitoneal ropivacaine for laparoscopic cholecystectomy. *Anesthesia and Analgesia*, 94(1), 100–105.

Lacy, C. F., Armstrong, L. L., & Goldman, M. P., et al. (Eds.), (2008). *Drug information handbook* (17th ed.). Hudson, OH: Lexi-Comp Inc.

Lainez, M. J. A., Pascual, J., Pascual, A. M., et al. (2003). Topiramate in the prophylactic treatment of cluster headache. *J Head Face Pain*, 43(7), 784–789.

Lalwani, K., Shoham, A., Koh, J. L., et al. (2005). Use of oxcarbazepine to treat a pediatric patient with resistant complex regional pain syndrome. *The Journal of Pain*, 6(10), 704–706.

Lamoure, J. (2007). *Does combining duloxetine and amitriptyline raise the risk for seizures? Medscape Pharmacists.* Available at http://www.medscape.com/viewarticle/554309 Accessed on April 24, 2007.

Larijani, G. E., Cypel, D., Gratz, I., et al. (2000). The efficacy and safety of EMLA cream for awake fiberoptic endotracheal intubation. *Anesthesia and Analgesia*, 91(4), 1024–1026.

Larijani, G. E., Goldberg, M. E., Hojat, M., et al. (2004). Modafinil improves recovery after general anesthesia. *Anesthesia and Analgesia*, 98(4), 976–981.

LaRoche, S. M. (2007). A new look at the second-generation antiepileptic drugs: A decade of experience. *The Neurologist*, 13(3), 133–139.

Lau, H., Patil, N. G., & Lee, F. (2003). Randomized clinical trial of postoperative subfascial infusion with bupivacaine following ambulatory open mesh repair of inguinal hernia. *Digestive Surgery*, 20(4), 285–289.

Lavelle, W., Lavelle, E. D., & Lavelle, L. (2007). Intra-articular injections. *The Medical Clinics of North America*, 91(2), 241–250.

Le, L. T., Loland, V. J., Mariano, E. R., et al. (2008). Effects of local anesthetic concentration and dose on continuous interscalene nerve blocks: A dual-center, randomized, observer-masked, controlled study. *Regional Anesthesia and Pain Medicine*, 33(6), 518–525.

LeBlanc, K. A., Bellanger, D., Rhynes, V. K., et al. (2005). Evaluation of continuous infusion of 0.5% bupivacaine by elastomeric pump for postoperative pain management after open inguinal hernia repair. *Journal of the American College of Surgeons*, 200(2), 198–202.

Lehman, K. (2005). Recent developments in patient-controlled analgesia. *Journal of Pain and Symptom Management*, 29(Suppl. 5), S72–S89.

Lema, M. J. (1996). Monitoring epidural local anesthetic action during the postoperative period. *Regional Anesthesia*, 21(Suppl. 6), 94–99.

Lena, P., Balarac, N., Lena, D., et al. (2008). Fast-track anesthesia with remifentanil and spinal analgesia for cardiac surgery: The effect on pain control and quality of recovery. *Journal of Cardiothoracic and Vascular Anesthesia*, 22(4), 536–542.

Leo, R. J. (2008). Safe analgesic use in patients with renal dysfunction. *Practical Pain Management*, 27, 12–22.

Leong, W. M., Lo, W. K., & Chiu, J. W. (2002). Analgesic efficacy of continuous delivery of bupivacaine by an elastomeric balloon infusor after abdominal hysterectomy: A prospective randomised controlled trial. *The Australian & New Zealand Journal of Obstetrics & Gynaecology*, 42(5), 515–518.

Lesser, H., Sharma, U., LaMoreaux, L., et al. (2004). Pregabalin relieves symptoms of painful diabetic neuropathy: A randomized controlled trial. *Neurology*, 63(11), 2104–2110.

Levendoglu, F., Ogun, C. O., Ozerbil, O., et al. (2004). Gabapentin is a first line drug for the treatment of neuropathic pain in spinal cord injury. *Spine*, 29(7), 743–751.

Lew, M. F. (2002). Review of the FDA-approved uses of botulinum toxins, including data suggesting efficacy in pain reduction. *The Clinical Journal of Pain*, 18(Suppl. 6), S142–S146.

Liberty, G., Gal, M., Halevy-Shalem, T., et al. (2007). Lidocaine-prilocaine (EMLA) cream as analgesia for hysterosalpingography: A prospective, randomized, controlled, double blinded study. *Human Reproduction (Oxford, England)*, 22(5), 1335–1339.

Liepe, K., Runge, R., & Kotzerke, J. (2005). Systemic radionuclide therapy in pain palliation. *The American Journal of Hospice & Palliative Care*, 22(6), 457–464.

Lin, P. L., Fan, S. Z., Huang, C. H., et al. (2008). Analgesic effect of lidocaine patch 5% in the treatment of acute herpes zoster: A double-blind and vehicle-controlled study. *Regional Anesthesia and Pain Medicine*, 33(4), 320–325.

Lin, T. F., Yeh, Y. C., Lin, F. S., et al. (2009). Effect of combining dexmedetomidine and morphine for intravenous patient-controlled analgesia. *British Journal of Anaesthesia*, 102(1), 117–122.

Lin, T. F., Yeh, Y. C., Yeh, Y. H., et al. (2005). Antiemetic and analgesic-sparing effects of diphenhydramine added to morphine intravenous patient-controlled analgesia. *British Journal of Anaesthesia*, 94(6), 835–839.

Lindstrom, P., & Lindblom, U. (1987). The analgesic effect of tocainide in trigeminal neuralgia. *Pain*, 28(1), 45–50.

List, T., Axelsson, S., & Leijon, G. (2003). Pharmacologic interventions in the treatment of temporomandibular disorders, atypical facial pain, and burning mouth syndrome: A qualitative systematic review. *Journal of Orofacial Pain*, 17(4), 301–310.

Liu, S. S., Richman, J. M., Thirlby, R. C., et al. (2006). Efficacy of continuous wound catheters delivering local anesthetic for postoperative analgesia: A quantitative and qualitative systematic review of randomized controlled trials. *Journal of the American College of Surgeons*, 203(6), 915–932.

Loblaw, D. A., Perry, J., Chambers, A., et al. (2005). Systematic review of the diagnosis and management of malignant extradural spinal cord compression: The Cancer Care Ontario Practice Guidelines Initiative's Neuro-Oncology Disease Site Group. *Journal of Clinical Oncology*, 23(9), 2028–2037.

Loblaw, D. A., Wu, J. S., Kirkbride, P., et al. (2007). Pain flare in patients with bone metastases after palliative radiotherapy— A nested randomized control trial. *Support Cancer Care*, 15(4), 451–455.

Lockhart, E. (2004). Topical combination of amitriptyline and ketamine for post herpetic neuralgia (abstract). *The Journal of Pain*, 5(Suppl. 1), 82.

Lockhart, E. (2006). Topical sterile lidocaine patch to reduce postoperative pain and decrease need for oral analgesics after inguinal heniorrhaphy (abstract). *The Journal of Pain*, 7(4), S59.

Loder, E., & Biondi, D. (2002). Use of botulinum toxins for chronic headaches: A focused review. *The Clinical Journal of Pain*, 18(Suppl. 6), S169–S176.

Loke, Y. K., Trivedi, A. N., & Singh, S. (2008). Meta-analysis: Gastrointestinal bleeding due to interaction between selective serotonin uptake inhibitors and non-steroidal anti-inflammatory drugs. *Alimentary Pharmacology & Therapeutics*, 27(1), 31–40.

Lussier, D., Huskey, A. G., & Portenoy, R. K. (2004). Adjuvant analgesics in cancer pain management. *The Oncologist*, 9(5), 571–591.

Lussier, D., & Portenoy, R. K. (2004). Adjuvant analgesics in pain management. In D. Doyle, G. Hanks, N. I. Cherny, & K. Calman (Eds.), *Oxford textbook of Palliative Medicine*. (3rd ed., pp. 349–378). New York: Oxford Press.

Lynch, M. E., & Clark, A. J. (2004). Comment on: Bell RF, Kalso K. Is intranasal ketamine an appropriate treatment for chronic non-cancer breakthrough pain? *Pain*, 110(3), 764.

Lynch, M. E, Clark, A. J., & Sawynok, J. (2003). A pilot study examining topical amitriptyline, ketamine, and a combination of both in the treatment of neuropathic pain. *The Clinical Journal of Pain*, 19(5), 323–328.

Lynch, M. E., Clark, A. J., Sawynok, J., et al. (2005). Topical 2% amitriptyline and 1% ketamine in neuropathic pain syndromes: A randomized, double-blind, placebo-controlled trial. *Anesthesiology*, 103(1), 140–146.

Lysakowski, C., Dumont, L., Czarnetzki, C., et al. (2007). Magnesium as an adjuvant to postoperative analgesia: A systematic review of randomized trials. *Anesthesia and Analgesia*, 104(6), 1532–1539.

Lysakowski, C., Dumont, L., Tramer, M. R., et al. (2003). A needle-free jet-injection system with lidocaine for peripheral intravenous cannula insertion: A randomized controlled trial with cost-effectiveness analysis. *Anesthesia and Analgesia*, 96(1), 215–219.

Lyseng-Williamson, K. A., & Siddiqui, M. A. (2008). Pregabalin: A review of its use in fibromyalgia. *Drugs*, 68(15), 2205–2223.

Macleod, A. D. (1998). Methylphenidate in terminal depression. *Journal of Pain and Symptom Management*, 16(3), 193–198.

MacPherson, R. D., Woods, D., & Penfold, J. (2008). Ketamine and midazolam delivered by patient-controlled analgesia in relieving pain associated with burns dressings. *The Clinical Journal of Pain*, 24(7), 568–571.

Magnano, D., Montalbano, R., Lamarra, M., et al. (2005). Ineffectiveness of local wound anesthesia to reduce postoperative pain after median sternotomy. *Journal of Cardiac Surgery*, 20(4), 314–318.

Maida, V., Ennis, M., Irani, S., et al. (2008). Adjunctive nabilone in cancer pain and symptom management: A prospective observational study using propensity scoring. *The Journal of Supportive Oncology*, 6(3), 119–124.

Maizels, M., & McCarberg, B. (2005). Antidepressants and antiepileptic drugs for chronic non-cancer pain. *American Family Physician*, 71(3), 483–490.

Malanga, G. A., Gwynn, M. W., Smith, R., et al. (2002). Tizanidine is effective in the treatment of myofasciale pain syndrome. *Pain Physician*, 5(4), 422–432.

Malanga, G. A., Reiter, R. D., & Garay, E. (2008). Update on tizanidine for muscle spasticity and emerging indications. *Expert Opinion on Pharmacotherapy*, 9(12), 2209–2215.

Manias, E., & Williams, A. (2008). Managing pain in chronic kidney disease: Patient participation in decision-making. *Journal of Advanced Nursing*, 61(2), 201–210.

Manning, B. H., Jianren, M., Frenk, H., et al. (1996). Continuous co-administration of dextromethorphan or MK-801 with morphine: Attenuation of morphine dependence and naloxone-reversible attenuation of morphine tolerance. *Pain*, 67(1), 79–88.

Mao, J., & Chen, L. L. (2000a). Gabapentin in pain management. *Anesthesia and Analgesia*, 91(3), 680–687.

Mao, J., & Chen, L. L. (2000b). Systemic lidocaine for neuropathic pain relief. *Pain*, 87(1), 7–17.

Mariano, E. R., Afra, R., Loland, V. J., et al. (2009). Continuous interscalene brachial plexus block via an ultrasound-guided posterior approach: A randomized, triple-masked, placebo-controlled study. *Anesthesia and Analgesia*, 108(5), 1688–1694.

Marmura, M. J., Passero, F. C., Jr., & Young, W. B. (2008). Mexiletine for refractory chronic daily headache: A report of nine cases. *Headache*, 48(10), 1506–1510.

Marret, E., Rolin, M., Beaussier, M., et al. (2008). Meta-analysis of intravenous lidocaine and postoperative recovery after abdominal surgery. *The British Journal of Surgery*, 95(11), 1331–1338.

Martin, B. R., & Wiley, J. L. (2004). Mechanism of action of cannabinoids: How it may lead to treatment of cachexia, emesis, and pain. *The Journal of Supportive Oncology*, 2(4), 305–316.

Martin, F., Cherif, K., Gentili, M. E., et al. (2008). Lack of impact of intravenous lidocaine on analgesia, functional recovery, and nociceptive pain threshold after total hip arthroplasty. *Anesthesiology*, 109(1), 118–123.

Martin-Sanchez, E., Furukawa, T. A., Taylor, J., et al. (2009). Systematic review and meta-analysis of cannabis treatment for chronic pain. *Pain Medicine (Malden, Mass.)*, 10(8), 1353–1368.

Martinez-Zapata, M. J., Roque, M., Alonso-Coello, P., et al. (2006). Calcitonin for metastatic bone pain. *Cochrane Database Systematic Reviews*, 3, CD003223.

Mason, L., Moore, R. A., Deery, S., et al. (2004). Systematic review of topical capsaicin for the treatment of chronic pain. *BMJ (Clinical Research Ed.)*, 328(7446), 991–994.

Mathew, N. T. (2001). Antiepileptic drugs in migraine prevention. *Headache*, 31(Suppl. 1), 18–25.

Mathiesen, O., Jacobsen, L. S., Holm, H. E., et al. (2008). Pregabalin and dexamethasone for postoperative pain control: A randomized controlled study in hip arthroplasty. *British Journal of Anaesthesia*, 101(4), 535–541.

Mathiesen, O., Moiniche, S., Dahl, J. B., et al. (2007). Gabapentin and postoperative pain: A qualitative and quantitative review, with focus on procedure. *BMC Anesthesiology*, 7, 6.

Mathiesen, O., Rasmussen, M. L., Dierking, G., et al. (2009). Pregabalin and dexamethasone in combination with paracetamol for postoperative pain control after abdominal hysterectomy: A randomized clinical trial. *Acta Anaesthesiologica Scandinavica*, 53(2), 227–235.

Max, M. B., Culnane, M., Schafer, S. C., et al. (1987). Amitriptyline relieves diabetic neuropathy pain in patients with normal or depressed mood. *Neurology*, 37(4), 589–596.

Max, M. B., Lynch, S. A., Muir, J., et al. (1992). Effects of desipramine, amitriptyline, and fluoxetine on pain in diabetic neuropathy. *The New England Journal of Medicine*, 326(19), 1250–1256.

Max, M. B., Schafer, S. C., Culnane, M., et al. (1988). Association of pain relief with drug side effects in postherpetic neuralgia: A single dose study of clonidine, codeine, ibuprofen and placebo. *Clinical Pharmacology and Therapeutics*, 43(4), 363–371.

Maxwell, C., Swift, R., Goode, M., et al. (2003). Advances in supportive care of patients with cancer and bone metastases: Nursing implications of zoledronic acid. *Clinical Journal of Oncology Nursing*, 7(4), 403–407.

May, A., Leone, M., Afra, J., et al. (2006). EFNS guidelines on the treatment of cluster headache and other trigeminal-autonomic cephalalgias. *European Journal of Neurology*, 13(10), 1066–1077.

Mays, T. A. (2006). Tricyclic antidepressants. In O. A. de Leon-Casasola (Ed.), *Cancer pain. Pharmacological, interventional and palliative care approaches* (pp. 305–316). Philadelphia: Saunders.

McCarberg, B. H. (2007). Cannabinoids: Their role in pain and palliation. *Journal of Pain & Palliative Care Pharmacotherapy*, 21(3), 19–28.

McCarthy, G. M., & McCarty, J. (1992). Effect of topical capsaicin in the therapy of painful osteoarthritis of the hands. *The Journal of Rheumatology*, 19(3), 604–607.

McCartney, C. J. L., Duggan, E., & Apatu, E. (2007). Should we add clonidine to local anesthetic peripheral nerve blockade? A qualitative systematic review of the literature. *Regional Anesthesia and Pain Medicine*, 32(4), 330–338.

McCartney, C. J. L., Sinha, A., & Katz, J. (2004). A qualitative systematic review of the role of N-methyl-D-aspartate receptor antagonists in preventive analgesia. *Anesthesia and Analgesia*, 98(5), 1385–1400.

McCleane, G. J. (1999). Intravenous infusion of phenytoin relieves neuropathic pain: A randomized, double-blinded, placebo-controlled, crossover study. *Anesthesia and Analgesia*, 89(4), 985–988.

McCleane, G. J. (2000). Topical application of doxepin hydrochloride, capsaicin and a combination of both produces analgesia in chronic human neuropathic pain: A randomized, double-blind, placebo-controlled study. *British Journal of Clinical Pharmacology*, 49(6), 574–579.

McCleane, G. J. (2002). Topical application of doxepin hydrochloride can reduce the symptoms of complex regional pain syndrome. *Injury*, 33(1), 88–89.

McCleane, G. J. (2007). Intravenous lidocaine: An outdated or underutilized treatment for pain? *Journal of Palliative Medicine*, 10(3), 798–805.

McCleane, G. J. (2008). Topical analgesic agents. *Clinics in Geriatric Medicine*, 24(2), 299–312.

McCleane, G. J. (2009a). Local anesthetics. In H. S. Smith (Ed.), *Current therapy in pain* (pp. 465–470). Philadelphia: Saunders.

McCleane, G. J. (2009b). Muscle relaxants. In H. S. Smith (Ed.), *Current therapy in pain* (pp. 470–475). Philadelphia: Saunders.

McKay, A., Gottschalk, A., Ploppa, A., et al. (2009). Systemic lidocaine decreased the perioperative opioid analgesic requirements but failed to reduce discharge time after ambulatory surgery. *Anesthesia and Analgesia*, 109(6), 1805–1808.

McQuaid, K. R., & Laine, L. (2008). A systematic review and meta-analysis of randomized, controlled trials of moderate sedation for routine endoscopic procedures. *Gastrointestinal Endoscopy*, 67(6), 910–923.

McQuay, H. J., Collins, S., Carroll, D., et al. (1999). Radiotherapy for the palliation of painful bone metastases. *Cochrane Database Systematic Reviews*, (2) CD001793.

McQuay, H. J., Poon, K. H., Derry, S., et al. (2008). Acute pain: Combination treatments and how we measure their efficacy. *British Journal of Anaesthesia*, 101(1), 69–76.

McQuay, H. J., Tramer, M., Nye, B. A., et al. (1996). A systematic review of antidepressants in neuropathic pain. *Pain*, 68(2–3), 217–227.

Mease, P. J., Clauw, D. J., Gendreau, R. M., et al. (2009). The efficacy and safety of milnacipran for treatment of fibromyalgia: A randomized, double-blind, placebo-controlled trial. *The Journal of Rheumatology*, 36(2), 398–409.

Mease, P. J., Russell, J., Kajdasz, D. K., et al. (2009). Long-term safety, tolerability, and efficacy of duloxetine in the treatment of fibromyalgia. *Seminars in Arthritis and Rheumatism*, Jan 17 [Epub ahead of print].

Medrik-Goldberg, T., Lifschitz, D., Pud, D., et al. (1999). Intravenous lidocaine, amantadine, and placebo in the treatment of sciatica: A double-blind, randomized, controlled study. *Regional Anesthesia and Pain Medicine*, 24(6), 534–540.

Mehrotra, B. (2009). Bisphosphonates—Role in cancer therapies. *Journal of Oral and Maxillofacial Surgery*, 67(5, Suppl. 1), 1–120.

Mehta, N. M., Malootian, A., & Gilligan, J. P. (2003). Calcitonin for osteoporosis and bone pain. *Current Pharmaceutical Design*, 9(32), 2659–2676.

Meier, G., & Buttner, J. (2007). *Peripheral regional anesthesia: An atlas of anatomy and techniques.* (2nd ed., English translation). New York: Thieme Medical Publishers.

Meier, T., Wasner, G., Faust, M., et al. (2003). Efficacy of lidocaine patch 5% in the treatment of focal peripheral neuropathic pain syndromes: A randomized, double-blind, placebo-controlled study. *Pain*, 106(1–2), 151–158.

Mellick, G. A. (1995). Hemifacial spasm: Successful treatment with felbamate. *Journal of Pain and Symptom Management*, 10(5), 392–395.

Mellick, G. A., & Mellick, L. B. (1995). Gabapentin in the management of reflex sympathetic dystrophy. *Journal of Pain and Symptom Management*, 10(4), 265–266.

Memis, D., Turan, A., Karamanlioglu, B., et al. (2004). Adding dexmedetomidine to lidocaine for intravenous regional anesthesia. *Anesthesia and Analgesia*, 98(3), 835–840.

Menigaux, C., Adam, F., Guignard, B., et al. (2005). Preoperative gabapentin decreases anxiety and improves early functional recovery from knee surgery. *Anesthesia and Analgesia*, 100(5), 1394–1399.

Menigaux, C., Fletcher, D., Dupont, X., et al. (2000). The benefits of intraoperative small-dose ketamine on postoperative pain after anterior cruciate ligament repair. *Anesthesia and Analgesia*, 90(1), 129–135.

Menza, M. A., Kaufman, K. R., & Castellanos, A. (2000). Modafinil augmentation of antidepressant treatment in depression. *The Journal of Clinical Psychiatry*, 61(5), 378–381.

Mercadante, S. (1996). Ketamine in cancer pain: An update. *Palliative Medicine*, 10(3), 225–230.

Mercadante, S., Arcuri, E., Tirelli, W., et al. (2000). Analgesic effect of intravenous ketamine in cancer patients on morphine therapy: A randomized, controlled, double-blind, crossover, double-dose study. *Journal of Pain and Symptom Management*, 20(4), 246–252.

Mercadante, S., Berchovich, M., Casuccio, A., et al. (2007). A prospective randomized study of corticosteroids as adjuvant drugs to opioids in advanced cancer patients. *The American Journal of Hospice & Palliative Care*, 24(1), 13–19.

Mercadante, S., Casuccio, A., Agnello, A., et al. (1999). Analgesic effects of nonsteroidal anti-inflammatory drugs in cancer pain due to somatic or visceral mechanisms. *Journal of Pain and Symptom Management*, 17(5), 351–356.

Mercadante, S., Casuccio, A., & Mangione, S. (2007). Medical treatment for inoperable malignant bowel obstruction: A qualitative systematic review. *Journal of Pain and Symptom Management, 33*(2), 217–223.

Mercadante, S., Ferrera, P., Villari, P., et al. (2004). Aggressive pharmacological treatment for reversing malignant bowel obstruction. *Journal of Pain and Symptom Management, 28*(4), 412–416.

Mercadante, S., Fulfaro, F., & Casuccio, A. (2001). The use of corticosteroids in home palliative care. *Supportive Care in Cancer, 9*(5), 386–389.

Mercadante, S., Villari, P., Ferrera, P., et al. (2009). Opioid switching and burst ketamine to improve the opioid response in patients with movement-related pain due to bone metastases. *The Clinical Journal of Pain, 25*(7), 648–649.

Meythaler, J. M., Clayton, W., Davis, L. K., et al. (2004). Orally delivered baclofen to control spastic hypertonia in acquired brain injury. *The Journal of Head Trauma Rehabililation, 19*(2), 101–108.

Meythaler, J. M., Guin-Renfroe, S., Brunner, R. C., et al. (2001). Intrathecal baclofen for spastic hypertonia from stroke. *Stroke, 32*(9), 2099–2109.

Meythaler, J. M., Guin-Renfroe, S., Johnson, A., et al. (2001). Prospective assessment of tizanidine for spasticity due to acquired brain injury. *Archives of Physical Medicine and Rehabilitation, 82*(9), 1155–1163.

Meythaler, J. M., Guin-Renfroe, S., Law, C., et al. (2001). Continuously infused intrathecal baclofen over 12 months for spastic hypertonia in adolescents and adults with cerebral palsy. *Archives of Physical Medicine and Rehabilitation, 82*(2), 155–161.

Miaskowski, C., Cleary, J., Burney, R., et al. (2005). *Guideline for the management of cancer pain in adults and children.* Glenview, IL: American Pain Society.

Michelet, P., Guervilly, C., Helaine, A., et al. (2007). Adding ketamine to morphine for patient-controlled analgesia after thoracic surgery: Influence on morphine consumption, respiratory function, and nocturnal desaturation. *British Journal of Anaesthesia, 99*(3), 396–403.

Milch, R. A. (2005). Neuropathic pain: Implications for the surgeon. *The Surgical Clinics of North America, 85*(2), 225–236.

Miller, A., & Price, G. (2009). Gabapentin toxicity in renal failure: The importance of dose adjustment. *Pain Medicine (Malden, Mass.), 10*(1), 190–192.

Miller, R. G. (2006). Osteoporosis in postmenopausal women. Therapy options across a wide range of risk for fracture. *Geriatrics, 61*(1), 24–30.

Minami, T., Bakoshi, S., Nakano, H., et al. (2001). The effects of capsaicin cream on prostaglandin-induced allodynia. *Anesthesia and Analgesia, 93*(2), 419–423.

Minton, O., Stone, P., Richardson, A., et al. (2008). Drug therapy for the management of cancer related fatigue. *Cochrane Database of Systematic Reviews,* (1) CD006704.

Mishra, S., Bhatnagar, S., Gupta, D., et al. (2009). Management of neuropathic cancer pain following WHO analgesic ladder: A prospective study. *Am J Hosp Palliat Med, 25*(6), 447–451.

Mistry, R. B., & Nahata, M. C. (2005). Ketamine for conscious sedation in pediatric emergency care. *Pharmacotherapy, 25*(8), 1104–1111.

Mitchell, A. C. (2001). An unusual case of chronic neuropathic pain responds to an optimum frequency of intravenous ketamine infusions. *Journal of Pain and Symptom Management, 21*(5), 443–446.

Mitchell, A. C., & Fallon, M. T. (2002). A single infusion of intravenous ketamine improves pain relief in patients with critical limb ischaemia: Results of a double blind randomised controlled trial. *Pain, 97*(3), 275–281.

Mitra, S. (2008). Opioid-induced hyperalgesia: Pathophysiology and clinical implications. *Journal Opioid Management, 4*(3), 123–130.

Moiniche, S., Mikkelsen, S., Wetterslev, J., et al. (1999). A systematic review of intra-articular local anesthesia for postoperative pain relief after arthroscopic knee surgery. *Regional Anesthesia and Pain Medicine, 24*(5), 430–437.

Monsivais, D., & McNeill, J. (2007). Multicultural influences on pain medication attitudes and beliefs in patients with nonmalignant chronic pain syndromes. *Pain Management Nursing, 8*(2), 64–71.

Moore, T. J., Walsh, C. S., & Cohen, M. R. (2004). Reported adverse event cases of methemoglobinemia associated with benzocaine products. *Archives of Internal Medicine, 164*(11), 1192–1196.

Morin, A. M., Kratz, C. D., Eberhart, L. H. J., et al. (2005). Postoperative analgesia and functional recovery after total-knee replacement: Comparison of a continuous posterior lumbar plexus (psoas compartment) block, a continuous femoral nerve block. And the combination of continuous femoral and sciatic nerve block. *Regional Anesthesia and Pain Medicine, 30*(5), 434–445.

Mortero, R. F., Clark, L. D., Tolan, M. M., et al. (2001). The effects of small-dose ketamine on propofol sedation: Respiration, postoperative mood, perception, cognition, and pain. *Anesthesia and Analgesia, 92*(6), 1465–1469.

Moss, J., & Glick, D. (2005). The autonomic nervous system. In R. D. Miller (Ed.), *Miller's anesthesia* (6th ed.)(pp. 617–677). Philadelphia: Elsevier.

Motsch, J., & Kamler, M. (1997). Alpha 2-adrenergic agonists. Use in chronic pain–a meta-analysis. *Schmerz (Berlin, Germany), 11*(5), 339–344.

Moulin, D. E., Clark, A. J., Gilron, I., et al. (2007). Pharmacological management of chronic neuropathic pain—Consensus statement and guidelines from the Canadian Pain Society. *Pain Research & Management, 12*(1), 13–21.

Movafegh, A., Soroush, A. R., Navi, A., et al. (2007). The effect of intravenous administration of dexamethasone on postoperative pain, nausea, and vomiting. *Anesthesia and Analgesia, 104*(4), 987–989.

Muehlbacher, M., Nickel, M. K., Kettler, C., et al. (2006). Topiramate in treatment of patients with chronic low back pain. A randomized, double-blind, placebo-controlled study. *The Clinical Journal of Pain, 22*(6), 526–531.

Muittari, P., & Kirvela, O. (1998). The safety and efficacy of intrabursal oxycodone and bupivacaine in analgesia after shoulder surgery. *Regional Anesthesia and Pain Medicine, 23*(5), 474–478.

Mulroy, M. F. (2002). Systemic toxicity and cardiotoxicity from local anesthetics: Incidence and preventive measures. *Regional Anesthesia and Pain Medicine, 27*(6), 556–561.

Multz, A. S. (2003). Prolonged dexmedetomidine infusion as an adjunct in treating sedation-induced withdrawal. *Anesthesia and Analgesia, 96*(4), 1054–1055.

Murcia Sanchez, E., Orts Castro, A., Perez Doblado, P., et al. (2006). Pre-emptive analgesia with pregabalin in laparascopic cholecystectomy. (Presentation) *European Journal of Pain (London, England)*, *10*(Suppl. 1), S198.

Murphy, D. B., McCartney, C. J. L., & Chan, V. W. S. (2000). Novel analgesic adjuncts for brachial plexus block: A systematic review. *Anesthesia and Analgesia*, *90*(5), 1122–1128.

Murphy, T. K., Siddall, P. J., & Griesing, T. (2007). Efficacy, by baseline severity of anxiety symptoms, of pregabalin for treating central neuropathic pain in patients with spinal cord injury. (Poster presentation.) *European Journal of Pain (London, England)*, *11*(Suppl. 1), S134–S135.

Nader, N. D., Li, C. M., Dosluoglu, H. H., et al. (2009). Adjuvant therapy with intrathecal clonidine improves postoperative pain in patients undergoing coronary artery bypass graft. *The Clinical Journal of Pain*, *25*(2), 101–106.

Nalamachu, S., Crockett, R. S., Gammaitoni, A. R., et al. (2006). A comparison of the lidocaine patch 5% vs naproxen 500 mg twice daily for the relief of pain associated with carpal tunnel syndrome: A 6-week, randomized, parallel-group study. *Medscape General Medicine*, *8*(3). Available at http://www.medscape.com/viewarticle/540341 Accessed August 16, 2006.

National Collaborating Centre for Chronic Conditions (NCC-CC). (2008). *Osteoarthritis: National clinical guideline for care and management in adults*. London: Royal College of Physicians. Available at http://www.nice.org.uk/nicemedia/pdf/CG059FullGuideline.pdf Accessed March 28, 2009.

Nesher, N., Ekstein, M. P., Paz, Y., et al. (2009). Morphine with adjuvant ketamine vs higher dose if morphine alone for immediate postthoractomy analgesia. *Chest*, *136*(1), 245–252.

NeurogesX, Inc. (2009). *Qutenza prescribing information*. Available at http://www.accessdata.fda.gov/drugsatfda_docs/label/2009/022395lbl.pdf Accessed February 1, 2010.

Newsome, S., Frawley, B. K., & Argoff, C. E. (2008). Intrathecal analgesia for refractory cancer pain. *Current Pain and Headache Reports*, *12*(4), 249–256.

Newton, H. B. (2007). Symptom management and supportive care of the patient with brain metastases. *Cancer Treatment and Research*, *136*, 53–73.

Ng, A., Swami, A., Smith, G., et al. (2002). The analgesic effects of intraperitoneal and incisional bupivacaine with epinephrine after total abdominal hysterectomy. *Anesthesia and Analgesia*, *95*(1), 158–162.

Ng, H. P., Nordstrom, U., Axelsson, K., et al. (2006). Efficacy of intra-articular bupivacaine, ropivacaine, or a combination of ropivacaine, morphine, and ketorolac on postoperative pain relief after ambulatory arthroscopic knee surgery: A randomized double-blind study. *Regional Anesthesia and Pain Medicine*, *31*(1), 26–33.

Nicholson, B. (2000). Gabapentin use in neuropathic pain syndromes. *Acta Neurologica Scandinavica*, *101*(6), 359–371.

Nielsen, J. B., & Sjogren, P. (2008). Clonidine in the treatment of cancer pain. *Ugeskrift for Laeger*, *170*(45), 3650–3653.

Nikolajsen, L., Finnerup, N. B., Kramp, S., et al. (2006). A randomized study of the effects of gabapentin on postamputation pain. *Anesthesiology*, *105*(5), 1008–1015.

Nilsson, S., Strang, P., Ginman, C., et al. (2005). Palliation of bone pain in prostate cancer using chemotherapy and strontium-89. A randomized phase II study. *Journal of Pain and Symptom Management*, *29*(4), 352–357.

Nishishinya, B., Urrutia, G., Walitt, B., et al. (2008). Amitriptyline in the treatment of fibromyalgia: A systematic review of its efficacy. *Rheumatology (Oxford)*, *47*(12), 1741–1746.

Novy, J., Stupp, R., & Rossetti, A. O. (2009). Pregabalin in patients with primary brain tumors and seizures: A preliminary observation. *Clinical Neurology and Neurosurgery*, *111*(2), 171–173.

Noyes, R., Brunk, S. F., Avery, D. H., et al. (1976). The analgesic properties of delta-9-tetrahydrocannabinal and codeine. *Clinical Pharmacology and Therapeutics*, *18*(1), 84–89.

Nurmikko, T. J., Serpell, M. G., Hoggart, B., et al. (2007). Sativex successfully treats neuropathic pain characterised by allodynia: A randomised, double-blind, placebo-controlled clinical trial. *Pain*, *133*(1–3), 210–220.

O'Brien, C. F. (2002). Treatment of spasticity with botulinum toxin. *The Clinical Journal of Pain*, *18*(Suppl. 6), S182–S190.

Obermann, M., Yoon, M. S., Sensen, K., et al. (2008). Efficacy of pregabalin in the treatment of trigeminal neuralgia. *Cephalagia*, *28*(2), 174–181.

O'Connor, A. B., Noyes, K., & Holloway, R. G. (2007). A cost-effectiveness comparison of desipramine, gabapentin, and pregabalin for treating postherpetic neuralgia. *Journal of the American Geriatrics Society*, *55*(8), 1176–1184.

Odom-Forren, J. (2006). The propofol debate continues. *Journal of Perianesthesia Nursing*, *21*(2), 77–78.

Odom-Forren, J. (2008). Perioperative patient safety and procedural sedation. *Periop Nurs Clin*, *3*(4), 355–366.

Odom-Forren, J., & Watson, D. (2005). *Practical guide to moderate sedation/analgesia*. St. Louis: Mosby.

Okabe, T., Takeda, S., Akada, S., et al. (2009). Postoperative intensive care unit drug fever caused by dexmedetomidine. *Anesthesia and Analgesia*, *108*(5), 1589–1591.

Olkkola, K. T., & Ahonen, J. (2008). Midazolam and other benzodiazepines. *Handbook of Experimental Pharmacology*, *182*(182), 335–360.

Olmos, M., Ballester, J. A., Vidarte, M. A., et al. (2000). The combined effect of age and premedication on the propofol requirements for induction by target-controlled infusion. *Anesthesia and Analgesia*, *90*(5), 1157–1161.

Olson, L. C., Hong, D., Conell-Price, J. S., et al. (2009). Transdermal nicotine patch is not effective for postoperative pain management in smokers: A pilot dose-ranging study. *Anesthesia and Analgesia*, *109*(6), 1987–1991.

Orhan, M. E., Yuksel, U., Bilgin, F., et al. (2007). Comparison of the local anesthetic effects of chlorpheniramine, midazolam, lidocaine, and normal saline after intradermal injection. *Medical Science Monitor*, *13*(4), PI7–PI11.

Otto, M., Bach, F. W., Jensen, T. S., et al. (2004). Valproic acid has no effect on pain in polyneuropathy: A randomized, controlled trial. *Neurology*, *62*(2), 285–288.

Owen, R. T. (2008). Milnacipran hydrochloride: Its efficacy, safety and tolerability profile in fibromyalgia syndrome. *Drugs Today*, *44*(9), 653–660.

Paech, M. J., Goy, R., Chua, S., et al. (2007). A randomized, placebo-controlled trial of preoperative oral pregabalin for postoperative pain relief after minor gynaecological surgery. *Anesthesia and Analgesia*, *105*(5), 1449–1453.

Paech, M. J., Pavy, T. J. G., Orlikowski, C. E. P., et al. (2004). Postcesarean analgesia with spinal morphine, clonidine, or their combination. *Anesthesia and Analgesia*, *98*(5), 1460–1466.

Paice, J. A., Ferrans, C. E., Lashley, F. R., et al. (2000). Topical capsaicin in the management of HIV-associated peripheral neuropathy. *Journal of Pain and Symptom Management*, *19*(1), 45–52.

Paisley, S., Beard, S., Hunn, A., et al. (2002). Clinical effectiveness of oral treatments for spasticity in multiple sclerosis: A systematic review. *Multiple Sclerosis (Houndmills, Basingstoke, England), 8*(4), 319–329.

Pandey, C. K., Bose, N., Garg, G., et al. (2002). Gabapentin for the treatment of pain in Guillain Barre syndrome: A double-blinded, placebo-controlled, crossover study. *Anesthesia and Analgesia, 95*(6), 1719–1723.

Pandey, C. K., Navkar, D. V., Giri, P. J., et al. (2005). Evaluation of the optimal preemptive dose of gabapentin for postoperative pain relief after lumbar diskectomy: A randomized, double-blind, placebo-controlled study. *J Neurosurg Anesthesiology, 17*(2), 65–68.

Pandey, C. K., Patra, P., Pant, K. C., et al. (2006). Gabapentin for the treatment of refractory dyesthetic pain after open cholecystectomy. *Anesthesia and Analgesia, 103*(1), 263.

Pandey, C. K., Priye, S., Ambesh, S. P., et al. (2004). Prophylactic gabapentin for prevention of postoperative nausea and vomiting in patients undergoing laparoscopic cholecystectomy: A randomized, double-blind, placebo-controlled study. *Journal of Postgraduate Medicine, 52*(2), 97–100.

Pandey, C. K., Priye, S., Singh, S., et al. (2004). Preemptive use of gabapentin significantly decreases postoperative pain and rescue analgesic requirements in laparoscopic cholecystectomy. *Canadian Journal of Anaesthesia, 51*(4), 358–363.

Pandey, C. K., Sahay, S., Gupta, D., et al. (2004). Preemptive gabapentin decreases postoperative pain after lumbar discoidectomy. *Canadian Journal of Anaesthesia, 51*(10), 986–989.

Pandey, C. K., Singhal, V., Kumar, M., et al. (2005). Gabapentin provides effective postoperative analgesia whether administered pre-emptively or post-incision. *Canadian Journal of Anaesthesia, 52*(8), 827–831.

Pandharipande, P. P., Ely, E. W., & Maze, M. (2006). Dexmedetomidine for sedation and perioperative management of critically ill patients. *Sem Anesthes Periop Med Pain, 25*(1), 43–50.

Pandharipande, P. P., Pun, B. T., Herr, D. L., et al. (2007). Effect of sedation with dexmedetomidine vs lorazepam on acute brain dysfunction in mechanically ventilated patients: The MENDS randomized controlled trial. *JAMA: The Journal of the American Medical Association, 298*(22), 2644–2653.

Panzer, O., Moitra, V., & Sladen, R. N. (2009). Pharmacology of sedative-analgesic agents: Dexmedetomidine, remifentanil, ketamine, volatile anesthetics and the role of peripheral mu antagonists. *Critical Care Clinics, 25*(3), 451–469.

Park, J. Y., Lee, G. W., Kim, Y., et al. (2002). The efficacy of continuous intrabursal infusion with morphine and bupivacaine for postoperative analgesia after subacromial arthroscopy. *Regional Anesthesia and Pain Medicine, 27*(2), 145–149.

Pasero, C. (2003a). Lidocaine patch 5%. *The American Journal of Nursing, 103*(9), 75–77.

Pasero, C. (2003b). Multimodal analgesia in the PACU. *Journal of Perianesthesia Nursing, 18*(4), 265–268.

Pasero, C. (2004a). Pathophysiology of neuropathic pain. *Pain Management Nursing, 5*(4), 3–8.

Pasero, C. (2004b). Perineural local anesthetic infusion. *The American Journal of Nursing, 104*(7), 89–93.

Pasero, C., Eksterowicz, N., Primeau, M., et al. (2007). American Society for Pain Management Nursing position statement: Registered nurse management and monitoring of analgesia by catheter techniques. *Pain Management Nursing, 8*(2), 48–54. Available at http://www.aspmn.org/Organization/documents/RegisteredNurseManagementandMonitoringof AnalgesiaByCatheterTechniquesPMNversion.pdf Accessed 3/12/09.

Pasero, C., & McCaffery, M. (1999). Procedural pain management. In M. McCaffery, & C. Pasero (Eds.), *Pain: Clinical manual* (2nd ed., pp. 362–398). St. Louis: Mosby.

Pasero, C., & McCaffery, M. (2005). Ketamine: Low doses may provide relief for some painful conditions. *The American Journal of Nursing, 105*(4), 60–64.

Pasero, C., & Wong, D. L. (1997). Using local anesthetics to control procedural pain. *The American Journal of Nursing, 97*(1), 17.

Patkar, A. A., Masand, P. S., Krulewicz, S., et al. (2007). A randomized, controlled, trial of controlled release paroxetine in fibromyalgia. *The American Journal of Medicine, 120*(5), 448–454.

Pawlik, M. T., Hansen, E., Waldhauser, D., et al. (2005). Clonidine premedication in patients with sleep apnea syndrome: A randomized, double-blind, placebo-controlled study. *Anesthesia and Analgesia, 101*(5), 1374–1380.

Peck, M., & Down, J. (2009). Use of sedatives in the critically ill. *Anaesthesia Intensive Care Medicine, 11*(1), 12–15.

Pelissier, T., Laurido, C., Kramer, V., et al. (2003). Antinociceptive interactions of ketamine with morphine or methadone in mononeuropathic rats. *European Journal of Pharmacology, 477*(1), 23–28.

Peng, P. W. H., Wijeysundera, D. N., & Li, C. C. F. (2007). Use of gabapentin for perioperative pain control—A meta-analysis. *Pain Research & Management, 12*(2), 85–91.

Perahia, D. G., Pritchett, Y. L., & Raskin, D. D. (2006). Efficacy of duloxetine in painful symptoms: An analgesic or antidepressant effect? *International Clinical Psychopharmacology, 21*(6), 311–317.

Perez, R. S. G. M., Kwakkel, G., Zuurmond, W. W. A., et al. (2001). Treatment of reflex sympathetic dystrophy (CRPS Type 1): A research synthesis of 21 randomized clinical trials. *Journal of Pain and Symptom Management, 21*(6), 511–526.

Perkins, K. A., Grobe, J. E., Stiller, R., et al. (1994). Effects of nicotine on thermal pain detection in humans. *Experimental and Clinical Psychopharmacology, 2*(1), 95–106.

Pernia, A., Mico, J. A., Calderon, E., et al. (2000). Venlafaxine for the treatment of neuropathic pain. *Journal of Pain and Symptom Management, 19*(6), 408–410.

Perrot, S., Javier, R. M., Marty, M., et al. (2008). Antidepressant use in painful rheumatic conditions. *Rheumatic Diseases Clinics of North America, 34*(2), 433–453.

Persec, J., Persec, Z., Bukovic, D., et al. (2007). Effects of clonidine preemptive analgesia on acute postoperative pain in abdominal surgery. *Collegium Antropologicum, 31*(4), 1071–1075.

Persson, J., Axelsson, G., Hallin, R. G., et al. (1995). Beneficial effects of ketamine in a chronic pain state with allodynia, possibly due to central sensitization. *Pain, 60*(2), 217–222.

Petty, S. J., Paton, L. M., O'Brien, T. J., et al. (2005). Effect of antiepileptic medication on bone mineral measures. *Neurology, 65*(9), 1358–1365.

Phillips, W. J., Gadiraju, S., Dickey, S., et al. (2007). Dexmedetomidine relieves pain associated with acute sickle cell crisis. (Letter.) *Journal of Pain and Symptom Management*, 34(4), 346–349.

Pinsker, W. (1998). Treatment of headache with bupropion. *Headache*, 38(1), 58.

Polomano, R. C., Rathmell, J. P., Krenzischek, D. A., et al. (2008). Emerging trends and new approaches to acute pain management. *Journal of Perianesthesia Nursing*, 23(Suppl. 1), S43–S53.

Pongrojpaw, D., Somprasit, C., & Chanthasenanont, A. (2008). The efficacy of lidocaine-prilocaine cream to reduce pain in genetic amniocentesis (abstract). *Acute Pain*, 10(1), 46.

Portenoy, R. K. (2000). Current pharmacotherapy of chronic pain. *Journal of Pain and Symptom Management*, 19(Suppl 1), S16–S20.

Portenoy, R. K., Murphy, T. K., Young, J., et al. (2006). Onset and duration of analgesia in combined analyses of clinical trials of pregabalin for painful DPN and PHN. *European Journal of Pain (London, England)*, 10(Suppl. 1), S119.

Portenoy, R. K., & Rowe, G. (2003). Adjuvant analgesic drugs. In E. Bruera & R. Portenoy (Eds.), *Cancer pain* (pp. 188–198). New York City: Cambridge University Press.

Porter, A. T., McEwan, A. J., Powe, J. E., et al. (1993). Results of a randomized phase-III trial to evaluate the efficacy of strontium-89 adjuvant to local field external beam irradiation in the management of endocrine resistant metastatic prostate cancer. *International Journal of Radiation Oncology Biology Physics*, 25(5), 805–813.

Porzio, G., Aielli, F., Verna, L., et al. (2006). Efficacy of pregabalin in the management of cetuximab-related itch. *Journal of Pain and Symptom Management*, 32(5), 397–398.

Poyhia, R., & Vainio, A. (2006). Topically administered ketamine reduces capsaicin-evoked mechanical hyperalgesia. *The Clinical Journal of Pain*, 22(1), 32–36.

Pritchett, Y. L., McCarberg, B. H., Watkin, J. G., et al. (2007). Duloxetine for the management of diabetic peripheral neuropathic pain: Response profile. *Pain Medicine (Malden, Mass.)*, 8(5), 397–409.

Prommer, E. E. (2006). Modafinil: Is it ready for prime time? *Journal of Opioid Management*, 2(3), 130–136.

Prommer, E. E. (2009). Topical analgesic combinations for bortezomib neuropathy. *Journal of Pain and Symptom Management*, 37(3), e3–e4.

Pulido, P. A., Colwell, C. W., Hoenecke, H. R., et al. (2002). The efficacy of continuous bupivacaine infiltration for pain management following orthopaedic knee surgery: Anterior cruciate ligament reconstruction and total knee arthroplasty. *Orthopaedic Nursing*, 21(1), 31–36.

Puntillo, K. A., White, C., Morris, A., et al. (2001). Patients' perceptions and responses to procedural pain: Results from Thunder Project II. *American Journal of Critical Care*, 10(4), 238–251.

Putzke, J. D., Richards, J. S., Kezar, L., et al. (2002). Long-term use of gabapentin for treatment of pain after traumatic spinal cord injury. *The Clinical Journal of Pain*, 18(2), 116–121.

Qin, H., Cai, J., & Yang, F. S. (2008). Could calcitonin be a useful therapeutic agent for trigeminal neuralgia? *Medical Hypotheses*, 71(1), 114–116.

Quan, D., Wellish, M., & Gilden, D. H. (2003). Topical ketamine treatment of postherpetic neuralgia. *Neurology*, 60(8), 1391–1392.

Quatraro, A., Minei, A., De Rosa, N., et al. (1992). Calcitonin in painful diabetic neuropathy. *Lancet*, 339(8795), 746–747.

Quilici, S., Chancellor, J., Lothgren, M., et al. (2009). Meta-analysis of duloxetine vs. pregabalin and gabapentin in the treatment of diabetic peripheral neuropathic pain. *BMC Neurology*, 9, 6.

Quisel, A., Gill, J. M., & Witherell, P. (2005). Complex regional pain syndrome: Which treatments show promise? *The Journal of Family Practice*, 54(7), 599–603.

Raber, M., Scattoni, M., Roscigno, F., et al. (2008). Topical prilocaine—lidocaine cream combined with peripheral nerve block improves pain control in prostatic biopsy: Results from a prospective randomized trial. (abstract) *Acute Pain*, 10(2), 97–98.

Radhakrishnan, M., Bithal, P. K., & Chaturvedi, A. (2005). Effect of preemptive gabapentin on postoperative pain relief and morphine consumption following lumbar laminectomy and discectomy: A randomized, double-blinded, placebo-controlled study. *Journal of Neurosurgical Anesthesiology*, 17(3), 125–128.

Railan, D., & Alster, T. S. (2007). Use of topical lidocaine for cosmetic dermatologic procedures. *Journal of Drugs in Dermatology*, 6(11), 1104–1108.

Ramsay, M. A. (2006). Bariatric surgery: The role of dexmedetomidine. *Sem Anesth Periop Med Pain*, 25(2), 51–56.

Rani, P. U., Naidu, M. U. R., Prasad, V. B. N., et al. (1996). An evaluation of antidepressants in rheumatic pain conditions. *Anesthesia and Analgesia*, 83(2), 371–375.

Rao, R. D., Michalak, J. C., Sloan, J. A., et al. (2007). North Central Cancer Treatment Group: Efficacy of gabapentin in the management of chemotherapy-induced peripheral neuropathy: A phase 3 randomized, double-blind, placebo-controlled, crossover trial (N00C3). *Cancer*, 110(9), 2110–2118.

Raskin, J., Pritchett, Y. L., Wang, F., et al. (2005). A double-blind, randomized multicenter trial comparing duloxetine with placebo in the management of diabetic peripheral neuropathic pain. *Pain Medicine (Malden, Mass.)*, 6(5), 346–356.

Raskin, J., Wiltse, C. G., Siegal, A., et al. (2007). Efficacy of duloxetine on cognition, depression, and pain in elderly patients with major depressive disorder: An 8-week, double-blind, placebo-controlled trial. *American Journal of Psychiatry*, 164(6), 900–909.

Rasmussen, M. L., Mathiesen, O., Dierking, G., et al. (2009). Multimodal analgesia with gabapentin, ketamine and dexamethasone in combination with paracetamol and ketorolac after hip arthroplasty: A preliminary study. *European Journal of Anaesthesiology*, (Epub ahead of print).

Rauck, R. L., Shaibani, A., Biton, et al. (2007). Lacosamide in painful diabetic peripheral neuropathy. *The Clinical Journal of Pain*, 23(2), 150–158.

Rawal, N. (2007). Postoperative pain relief using regional anaesthesia. *Curr Anaesth Crit Care*, 18(3), 140–148.

Rawal, N., Allvin, R., Axelsson, K., et al. (2002). Patient-controlled regional analgesia (PCRA) at home. *Anesthesiology*, 96(6), 1290–1296.

Rawal, N., Axelsson, K., Hylander, J., et al. (1998). Postoperative patient-controlled local anesthetic infusion at home. *Anesthesia and Analgesia*, 86(1), 86–89.

Ray, W. A., Griffin, M. R., Schaffner, W., et al. (1987). Psychotropic drug use and the risk of hip fracture. *The New England Journal of Medicine*, 316(7), 363–369.

Ray, W. A., Meredith, S., Thapa, B. P., et al. (2004). Cyclic antidepressants and the risk of sudden cardiac death. *Clinical Pharmacology and Therapeutics*, 75(3), 234–241.

Reddy, S., & Patt, R. B. (1994). The benzodiazepines as adjuvant analgesics. *Journal of Pain and Symptom Management,* 9(8), 510–514.

Reeves, A. I., So, E. L., Sharbrough, F. W., et al. (1996). Movement disorders associated with the use of gabapentin. *Epilepsia,* 37(10), 988–990.

Reeves, R. R., Beddingfield, J. J., & Mack, J. E. (2004). Carisoprodol withdrawal syndrome. *Pharmacotherapy,* 24(12), 1804–1806.

Reissig, J. E., & Rybarczyk, A. M. (2005). Pharmacologic treatment of opioid-induced sedation in chronic pain. *The Annals of Pharmacotherapy,* 39(4), 727–731.

Remerand, F., Le Tendre, C., Baud, A., et al. (2009). The early and delayed analgesic effects of ketamine after total hip arthroplasty: A prospective, randomized, controlled, double-blind study. *Anesthesia and Analgesia,* 109(6), 1963–1971.

Reves, J., Glass, P. S. A., Lubarsky, D. A., et al. (2005). Intravenous nonopioid anesthetics. In R. Miller (Ed.), *Miller's anesthesia.* (6th ed., pp. 317–378). Philadelphia: Churchill Livingstone.

Ribeiro, J. A., Sebastiao, A. M., & de Mendonca, A. (2002). Adenosine receptors in the nervous system: Pathophysiological implications. *Progress in Neurobiology,* 68(6), 377–392.

Rice, A. S. C., Maton, S., & Postherpetic Neuralgia Study Group (2001). Gabapentin in postherpetic neuralgia: A randomized, double-blind, placebo controlled study. *Pain,* 94(2), 215–224.

Richardson, C. F., Williams, D. W., & Kingham, J. G. (2002). Gabapentin induced cholestasis. *BMJ (Clinical Research Ed.),* 325(7365), 635.

Richman, J. M., Liu, S. S., Courpas, G., et al. (2006). Does continuous peripheral nerve block provide superior pain control to opioids? A meta-analysis. *Anesthesia and Analgesia,* 102(1), 248–257.

Richter, R. W., Portenoy, R., Sharma, U., et al. (2005). Relief of painful diabetic peripheral neuropathy with pregabalin: A randomized, placebo-controlled trial. *The Journal of Pain,* 6(4), 253–260.

Riker, R. R., Shehabi, Y., Bokesch, P. M., et al. (2009). Dexmedetomidine vs midazolam for sedation of critically ill patients. *JAMA,* 301(5), 489–499.

Rimback, G., Cassuto, G., & Tolleson, P. O. (1990). Treatment of postoperative paralytic ileus by intravenous lidocaine infusion. *Anesthesia and Analgesia,* 70(4), 414–419.

Rintala, D. H., Holmes, S. A., Courtade, D., et al. (2007). Comparison of the effectiveness of amitriptyline and gabapentin on chronic neuropathic pain in persons with spinal cord injury. *Archives of Physical Medicine and Rehabilitation,* 88(12), 1547–1560.

Ripamonti, C., & Dickerson, E. D. (2001). Strategies for the treatment of cancer pain in the new millennium. *Drugs,* 61(7), 955–977.

Ripamonti, C. I., Easson, A. M., & Gerdes, H. (2008). Management of malignant bowel obstruction. *European Journal of Cancer,* 44(8), 1105–1115.

Ripamonti, C., & Mercadante, S. (2004). How to use octreotide for malignant bowel obstruction. *The Journal of Supportive Oncology,* 2(4), 357–364.

Ripamonti, C., Mercadante, S., Groff, L., et al. (2000). Role of octreotide, scopolamine butylbromide, and hydration in symptom control of patients with inoperable bowel obstruction and nasogastric tubes: A prospective randomized trial. *Journal of Pain and Symptom Management,* 19(1), 23–34.

Robbins, W. (2000). Clinical applications of capsaicinoids. *The Clinical Journal of Pain,* 16(Suppl. 2), S86–S89.

Robinson, J. N., Sandom, J., & Chapman, P. T. (2004). Efficacy of pamidronate in complex regional pain syndrome type I. *Pain Medicine (Malden, Mass.),* 5(3), 276–280.

Robinson, R. G., Preston, D. F., Baxter, K. G., et al. (1993). Clinical experience with strontium-89 in prostatic and breast cancer patients. *Seminars in Oncology,* 20(3 Suppl. 2), 44–48.

Robinson, R. G., Preston, D. F., Schiefelbein, M., et al. (1995). Strontium-89 therapy for the palliation of pain due to osseous metastases. *JAMA: The Journal of the American Medical Association,* 274(5), 420–424.

Rog, D. J., Nurmikko, T. J., Friede, T., et al. (2005). Randomized, controlled trial of cannabis-based medicine in central pain in multiple sclerosis. *Neurology,* 65(6), 812–819.

Roldan-Marin, R., & de-al Barreda Becerril, F. (2009). Petechial and purpuric eruption induced by lidocaine/prilocaine cream: A rare side effect. *Journal of Drugs in Dermatology,* 8(3), 287–288.

Rolles, M. (2005). Early use of dexamethasone in malignant spinal-cord compression: A missed opportunity? *Clinical Oncology,* 17(2), 129–130.

Roque, M., Martinez-Zapata, M. J., Alonso-Coello, P., et al. (2003). Radioisotopes for metastatic bone pain. *Cochrane Database Systematic Reviews,* (4), CD003347.

Rorarius, M. G. F., Mennander, S., Suominen, P., et al. (2004). Gabapentin for the prevention of postoperative pain after vaginal hysterectomy. *Pain,* 110(1–2), 175–181.

Rosen, T. D. (2001). Olanzapine as an abortive agent for cluster headache. *Headache,* 41(8), 813–816.

Rosen, B., Bjorkman, A., & Lundborg, G. (2008). Improved hand function in a dental hygienist with neuropathy induced by vibration and compression: The effect of cutaneous anaesthetic treatment of the forearm. *Scandinavian Journal of Plastic and Reconstructive Surgery and Hand Surgery,* 42(1), 51–53.

Rosen, B., Bjorkman, A., Weibull, A., et al. (2009). Improved sensibility of the foot after temporary cutaneous anesthesia of the lower leg. *Neuroreport,* 20(1), 37–41.

Rosen, J., Pollock, B. G., Altieri, L., et al. (1993). Treatment of nortriptyline's side effects in elderly patients: A double-blind study of bethanechol. *The American Journal of Psychiatry,* 150(8), 1249–1251.

Rosenbaum, J. F., & Zajecka, J. (1997). Clinical management of antidepressant discontinuation. *The Journal of Clinical Psychiatry,* 58(Suppl. 7), 37–40.

Rosenberg, J. M., Harrell, C., Ristic, H., et al. (1997). The effect of gabapentin on neuropathic pain. *The Clinical Journal of Pain,* 13(3), 251–255.

Rosenblatt, W. H., Cioffi, A. M., Sinatra, R., et al. (1991). Metoclopramide: An analgesic adjunct to patient-controlled analgesics. *Anesthesia and Analgesia,* 73(5), 553–555.

Rosenstock, J., Tuchman, M., LaMoreaux, L., et al. (2004). Pregabalin for the treatment of painful diabetic peripheral neuropathy: A double-blind, placebo-controlled trial. *Pain,* 110(3), 628–638.

Rosner, H., Rubin, L., & Kestenbaum, A. (1996). Gabapentin adjunctive therapy in neuropathic pain states. *The Clinical Journal of Pain,* 12(1), 56–58.

Ross, J. R., Saunders, Y., Edmonds, P. M., et al. (2003). Systematic review of role of biphosphonates on skeletal morbidity in metastatic cancer. *BMJ (Clinical Research Ed.), 327*(7413), 469–474.

Rothenhausler, H. B., Ehrentraut, S., von Degenfeld, G., et al. (2000). Treatment of depression with methylphenidate in patients difficult to wean from mechanical ventilation in the intensive care. *The Journal of Clinical Psychiatry, 61*(10), 750–755.

Rowbotham, M. C., Davies, P. S., Verkempinck, C., et al. (1996). Lidocaine patch: Double-blind controlled study of a new treatment method for post-herpetic neuralgia. *Pain, 65*(1), 39–44.

Rowbotham, M. C., Duan, W. R., Thomas, J., et al. (2009). A randomized, double-blind, placebo-controlled trial evaluating the efficacy and safety of ABT-594 in patients with diabetic peripheral neuropathic pain. *Pain, 146*(3), 245–252.

Rowbotham, M. C., Harden, N., Stacey, B., et al. (1998). Gabapentin for the treatment of postherpetic neuralgia. *JAMA: The Journal of the American Medical Association, 280*(21), 1837–1842.

Rowbotham, M. C., Reisner, L. A., Davies, P. S., et al. (2005). Treatment response in antidepressant-naïve postherpetic neuralgia patients: Double-blind, randomized trial. *The Journal of Pain, 6*(11), 741–746.

Rowbotham, M. C., Stacey, B. R., Phillips, K., et al. (2007). A double-blind, randomized, placebo-controlled trial to evaluate time-to-onset of clinically meaningful pain relief in postherpetic neuralgia (PHN) patients treated with pregabalin. (Poster) *European Journal of Pain, 11*(Suppl. 1), S114.

Rozans, M., Dreisbach, A., Lertora, J. J. L., et al. (2002). Palliative uses of methylphenidate in patients with cancer: A review. *Journal of Clinical Oncology, 20*(1), 335–339.

Rozen, T. D. (2001). Antiepileptic drugs in the management of cluster headache and trigeminal neuralgia. *Headache, 41*(Suppl. 1), 25–33.

Rudich, Z., Peng, P., Dunn, E., et al. (2004). Stability of clonidine in clonidine-hydromorphone mixture from implanted intrathecal infusion pumps in chronic pain patients. *Journal of Pain and Symptom Management, 28*(6), 599–602.

Rudkin, L., Taylor, M. J., & Hawton, K. K. E. (2004). Strategies for managing sexual dysfunction induced by antidepressant medication. *Cochrane Database Systematic Reviews, (4)*, CD003382.

Ruegg, T. A., Curran, C. R., & Lamb, T. (2009). Use of buffered lidocaine in bone marrow biopsies: A randomized, controlled trial. *Oncology Nursing Forum, 36*(1), 52–60.

Ruoff, G. E. (2002). Challenges of managing chronic pain in the elderly. *Seminars in Arthritis and Rheumatism, 32*(3), 43–50.

Russell, I. J., Mease, P. J., Smith, T. R., et al. (2008). Efficacy and safety of duloxetine for treatment of fibromyalgia in patients with or without major depressive order: Results from a 6-month, randomized, double-blind, placebo-controlled, fixed-dose trial. *Pain, 136*(3), 432–444.

Rusy, L. M., Troshynski, T. J., & Weisman, S. J. (2001). Gabapentin in phantom limb pain management in children and young adults: Report of seven cases. *Journal of Pain and Symptom Management, 21*(1), 78–82.

Saarto, T., & Wiffen, P. J. (2007). Antidepressants for neuropathic pain. *Cochrane Database Systematic Reviews, (4)*, CD005454.

Sabatowski, R., Galvez, R., Cherry, D. A., et al. (2004). Pregabalin 1008-105 Study Group: Pregabalin reduces pain and improves sleep and mood disturbances in patients with post-herpetic neuralgia: Results of a randomised, placebo-controlled clinical trial. *Pain, 109*(1–2), 26–35.

Saber, A. A., Elgamal, M. H., Rao, A. J., et al. (2008). Early experience with lidocaine patch for postoperative pain control after laparoscopic ventral repair. *Int J Surg, 7*(1), 36–38.

Sakai, T., Tomiyasu, S., Ono, T., et al. (2004). Multiple sclerosis with severe pain and allodynia alleviated by oral ketamine. *The Clinical Journal of Pain, 20*(5), 375–376.

Saldana, M. T., Navarro, A., Perez, C., et al. (2010). A cost-consequences analysis of the effect of pregabalin in the treatment of painful radiculopathy under medical practice conditions in primary care settings. *Pain Practice, 10*(1), 31–41.

Salerno, A., & Hermann, R. (2006). Efficacy and safety of steroid use for postoperative pain relief. *The Journal of Bone Joint Surgery, 88-A*(6), 1361–1372.

Salinas, F. V., Liu, S. S., & Mulroy, M. F. (2006). The effect of single-injection femoral nerve block versus continuous femoral nerve block after total knee arthroplasty on hospital length of stay and long-term functional recovery within an established clinical pathway. *Anesthesia and Analgesia, 102*(4), 1234–1239.

Samson, D., Minville, V., Chassery, C., et al. (2007). Eutectic mixture of local anesthetic (EMLA) decreases pain during humeral block placement in nonsedated patients. *Anesthesia and Analgesia, 105*(2), 512–515.

Sanchez, B., Waxman, K., Tatevossian, R., et al. (2004). Local anesthetic infusion pumps improve postoperative pain after inguinal hernia repair: A randomized trial. *The American Surgeon, 70*(11), 1002–1006.

Sanders, R. D., & Maze, M. (2007). Alpha2-adrenoceptor agonists. *Current Opinion in Investigational Drugs (London, England: 2000), 8*(1), 25–33.

Sang Booher, S., Gilron, I., et al. (2002). Dextromethorphan and memantine in painful diabetic neuropathy and postherpetic neuralgia. *Anesthesiology, 96*(5), 1053–1061.

Santangelo, A., Testai, M., Barbagallo, P., et al. (2006). The use of bisphosphonates in palliative treatment of bone metastases in a terminally ill, oncological elderly population. *Archives of Gerontology and Geriatrics, 43*(2), 187–192.

Santiago-Palma, J., Fischberg, D., Kornick, C., et al. (2001). Diphenhydramine as an analgesic adjuvant in refractory cancer pain. *Journal of Pain and Symptom Management, 22*(2), 699–703.

Saper, J. R., Mathew, N. T., Loder, E. W., et al. (2007). A double-blind, randomized, placebo-controlled comparison of botulinum toxin type A injection sites and doses in prevention of episodic migraine. *Pain Medicine (Malden, Mass.), 8*(6), 478–485.

Sarhill, N., Walsh, D., Nelson, K. A., et al. (2001). Methyphenidate for fatigue in advanced cancer: A prospective open-label pilot study. *The American Journal of Hospice & Palliative Care, 18*(3), 187–192.

Sato, K., Higuchi, H., & Hishikawa, Y. (2008). Management of phantom limb pain and sensation with milnacipran. *The Journal of Neuropsychiatry and Clinical Neurosciences, 20*(3), 368.

Saulino, M., Burton, A. W., Danyo, D. A., et al. (2009). Intrathecal ziconotide and baclofen provide pain relief in seven patients with neuropathic pain and spasticity: Case reports. *Eur J Phys Rehabil Med*, 45(1), 61–67.

Sawyer, J., Febbraro, S., Masud, S., et al. (2009). Heated lidocaine/tetracaine patch (Synera, Rapydan) compared with lidocaine/prilocaine cream (EMLA) for topical anaesthesia before vascular access. *British Journal of Anaesthesia*, 102(2), 210–215.

Sawynok, J. (2003). Topically and peripherally acting analgesics. *Pharmacological Reviews*, 55(1), 1–20.

Sawynok, J., & Liu, X. J. (2003). Adenosine in the spinal cord and periphery: Release and regulation of pain. *Progress in Neurobiology*, 69(5), 313–340.

Schaub, E., Kern, C., & Landau, R. (2004). Pain on injection: A double-blind comparison of propofol with lidocaine pretreatment versus protocol formulated with long- and medium-chain triglycerides. *Anesthesia and Analgesia*, 99(6), 1699–1702.

Schiltmeyer, B., Kropeit, D., & Cawello, W., et al. (2006). No interaction between lacosamide and metformin. *The Journal of Pain*, 7(4), S63.

Schley, M., Topfner, S., & Wiech, K., et al. (2007). Continuous brachial plexus blockade in combination with the NMDA receptor antagonist memantine prevents phantom limb pain in traumatic upper limb amputees. *European Journal of Pain (London, England)*, 11(3), 299–308.

Schnider, T. W., Minto, C. F., & Shafer, S. L., et al. (1999). The influence of age on propofol pharmacodynamics. *Anesthesiology*, 90(6), 1502–1506.

Schug, S. A., Saunders, D., & Kurowski, I., et al. (2006). Neuraxial drug administration: A review of treatment options for anaesthesia and analgesia. *CNS Drugs*, 20(11), 917–933.

Schulte-Mattler, W. J., Krack, P., BoNTTH Study Group (2004). Treatment of chronic tension-type headache with botulinum toxin A: A randomized, double-blind, placebo-controlled multicenter study. *Pain*, 109(1–2), 110–114.

Schurr, M. J., Gordon, D. B., Pellino, T. A., et al. (2004). Continuous local anesthetic infusion for pain management after outpatient inguinal herniorrhaphy. *Surgery*, 136(4), 761–769.

Schwartzman, R. J., Alexander, G. M., Grothusen, J. R., et al. (2009). Outpatient intravenous ketamine for the treatment of complex regional pain syndrome: A double-blind placebo controlled study. *Pain*, 147(1–3), 107–115.

Schwartzman, R. J., Patel, M., Grothusen, J. R., et al. (2009). Efficacy of 5-day continuous lidocaine infusion for the treatment of refractory complex regional pain syndrome. *Pain Medicine (Malden, Mass.)*, 10(2), 401–412.

Schwarzkopf, K. R. G., Hoff, H., Hartmann, M., et al. (2001). A comparison between meperidine, clonidine and urapidil in the treatment of postanesthetic shivering. *Anesthesia and Analgesia*, 92(1), 257–260.

Scott, M. A., Letrent, K. J., Hager, K. L., et al. (1999). Use of transdermal amitriptyline gel in a patient with chronic pain and depression. *Pharmacotherapy*, 19(2), 236–239.

See, S., & Ginzburg, R. (2008). Skeletal muscle relaxants. *Pharmacotherapy*, 28(2), 207–213.

Segerdahl, M., Ekblom, A., Sandelin, K., et al. (1995). Perioperative adenosine infusion reduces the requirements for isoflurane and postoperative analgesics. *Anesthesia and Analgesia*, 80(6), 1145–1149.

Seib, R. K., & Paul, J. E. (2006). Preoperative gabapentin for postoperative analgesia: A meta-analysis. *Canadian Journal of Anaesthesia*, 53(5), 461–469.

Semenchuk, M. R., & Davis, B. (2000). Efficacy of sustained-release bupropion in neuropathic pain: An open-label study. *The Clinical Journal of Pain*, 16(1), 6–11.

Semenchuk, M. R., & Sherman, S. (2000). Effectiveness of tizanidine in neuropathic pain: An open-label study. *The Journal of Pain*, 11(4), 285–292.

Semenchuk, M. R., Sherman, S., & Davis, B. (2001). Double-blind, randomized trial of bupropion SR for the treatment of neuropathic pain. *Neurology*, 57(9), 1583–1588.

Sen, H., Sizlan, A., Yanarates, O., et al. (2009). A comparison of gabapentin and ketamine in acute and chronic pain after hysterectomy. *Anesthesia and Analgesia*, 109(5), 1645–1650.

Sen, S., Aydin, O. N., & Aydin, K. (2006). Beneficial effect of low-dose ketamine addition to epidural administration of morphine-bupivacaine mixture for cancer pain in two cases. *Pain Medicine (Malden, Mass.)*, 7(2), 166–169.

Serpell, M. G., & Neuropathic Pain Study Group. (2002). Gabapentin in neuropathic pain syndromes: A randomized, double-blind, placebo-controlled trial. *Pain*, 99(3), 557–566.

Sethna, N. F., Verghese, S. T., Hannallah, R. S., et al. (2005). A randomized controlled trial to evaluate S-Caine Patch for reducing pain associated with vascular access in children. *Anesthesiology*, 102(2), 403–408.

Setler, P. E. (2002). Therapeutic use of botulinum toxins: Background and history. *The Clinical Journal of Pain*, 18(Suppl. 6), S119–S124.

Shachor-Meyouhas, Y., Galbraith, R., & Shavit, I. (2008). Application of topical analgesia in triage: A potential for harm. *The Journal of Emergency Medicine*, 35(1), 39–41.

Shahani, R., Streutker, C., Dickson, B., et al. (2007). Ketamine-associated ulcerative cystitis: A new clinical entity. *Urology*, 69(5), 810–812.

Shaibani, A., Biton, V., Rauck, R., et al. (2009). Long-term oral lacosamide in painful diabetic neuropathy: A two-year open-label extension trial. *European Journal of Pain (London, England)*, 13(5), 458–463.

Shaibani, A., Fares, S., Selam, J. L., et al. (2009). Lacosamide in painful diabetic neuropathy: An 18-week double-blind placebo-controlled trial. *The Journal of Pain*, 10(8), 818–828.

Shaiova, L. (2005). The management of opioid-related sedation. *Current Pain and Headache Reports*, 9(4), 239–242.

Shakespeare, D., Boggild, M., & Young, C. A. (2003). Anti-spasticity agents for multiple sclerosis. *Cochrane Database Systematic Reviews*, (4), CD001332.

Shapiro, D., & Jarvik, M. E. (1998). Pain inhibition, nicotine, and gender. *Experimental and Clinical Psychopharmacology*, 6(1), 96–106.

Shapiro, R. E. (2008). Caffeine and headaches. *Current Pain and Headache Reports*, 12(4), 311–315.

Sharma, S., Rajagopal, M. R., Palat, G., et al. (2009). A phase II pilot study to evaluate use of intravenous lidocaine for opioid-refractory pain in cancer patients. *Journal of Pain and Symptom Management*, 37(1), 85–93.

Sheen, M. J., & Ho, S. T. (2008). Mirtazapine relieves postdural puncture headache. (Letter) *Anesthesia and Analgesia*, 107(1), 346.

Shemirani, N., Tang, D., & Friedland, D. R. (2010). Acute auditory and vestibular symptoms associated with heat and transdermal lidocaine. *The Clinical Journal of Pain*, 26(1), 58–59.

Sheth, R. (2005). Antiepileptic drugs enhance age-related osteoporosis. (Commentary.) *Neurology, 65*(9), 1343.

Shiau, J. M., Hung, K. C., Chen, H. H., et al. (2007). Combination of topical EMLA with local injection of lidocaine: Superior pain relief after Ferguson hemorrhoidectomy. *The Clinical Journal of Pain, 23*(7), 586–590.

Shiau, J. M., Su, H. P., Chen, H. S., et al. (2008). Use of a topical anesthetic cream (EMLA) to reduce pain after hemorrhoidectomy. *Regional Anesthesia and Pain Medicine, 33*(1), 30–35.

Shih, A., & Jackson, K. C. (2007). Role of corticosteroids in palliative care. *Journal of Pain & Palliative Care Pharmacotherapy, 21*(4), 69–76.

Siddall, P. J. (2005). Pain following spinal cord injury. In S. B. McMahon & M. Koltzenberg (Eds.), *Wall and Melzack's textbook of pain* (5th ed., pp. 1043–1055). Philadelphia: Elsevier.

Siddall, P. J., Cousins, M. J., Otte, A., et al. (2006). Pregabalin in central neuropathic pain associated with spinal cord injury: A placebo-controlled trial. *Neurology, 68*(24), 1792–1800.

Siddiqui, Z. I., Cepeda, S., Denman, W., et al. (2007). Continuous lumbar plexus block provides improved analgesia with fewer side effects compared with systemic opioids after hip arthroplasty: A randomized controlled trial. *Regional Anesthesia and Pain Medicine, 32*(5), 393–398.

Sidiropoulou, T., Buonomo, O., Fabbi, E., et al. (2008). A prospective comparison of continuous wound infiltration with ropivacaine versus single-injection paravertebral block after modified radical mastectomy. *Anesthesia and Analgesia, 106*(3), 997–1001.

Sigtermans, M. J., van Hilten, J. J., Bauer, M. C. R., et al. (2009). Ketamine produces effective and long-term pain relief in patients with complex regional pain syndrome type 1. *Pain, 145*(3), 304–311.

Silberstein, S. D. (2005). Topiramate in migraine prevention. *Headache, 45*(Suppl. 1), S57–S65.

Silberstein, S. D., & Collins, S. D. (1999). Safety of divalproex sodium in migraine prophylaxis: An open-label, long-term study. *Headache, 39*(9), 633–643.

Silberstein, S. D., Diener, H. C., Lipton, R. B., et al. (2008). Epidemiology, risk factors, and treatment of chronic migraine: A focus on topiramate. *J Head Face Pain, 48*(7), 1087–1095.

Silberstein, S. D., Lipton, R. B., Dodick, D. W., et al. (2007). Efficacy and safety of topiramate for the treatment of chronic migraine: A randomized, double-blind, placebo-controlled trial. *Headache, 47*(2), 170–180.

Silberstein, S. D., Neto, W., Schmitt, J., et al. (2004). Topiramate in migraine prevention: Results of a large, controlled trial. *Archives of Neurology, 61*(4), 490–495.

Silberstein, S. D., Saper, J., & Berenson, F., et al. (2008). Oxcarbazepine in migraine headache. *Neurology, 70*(7), 548–555.

Silver, M., Blum, D., Grainger, J., et al. (2007). Double-blind, placebo-controlled trial of lamotrigine in combination with other medications for neuropathic pain. *Journal of Pain and Symptom Management, 34*(4), 446–454.

Simmonds, M. K., Rashiq, S., Sobolev, I. A., et al. (2009). The effect of single-dose propofol injection on pain and quality of life in chronic daily headache: A randomized, double-blind, controlled trial. *Anesthesia and Analgesia, 109*(6), 1972–1980.

Simon, L. S., Lipman, A. G., Caudill-Slosberg, M., et al. (2002). *Guideline for the management of pain in osteoarthritis, rheumatoid arthritis, and juvenile chronic arthritis.* Glenview, IL: American Pain Society.

Simpson, D. M., Estanislao, L., Brown, S. J., et al. (2008). An open-label pilot study of high-concentration capsaicin patch in painful HIV neuropathy. *Journal of Pain and Symptom Management, 35*(3), 299–306.

Simpson, D. M., Olney, R., McArthur, J. C., et al. (2000). A placebo-controlled trial of lamotrigine for painful HIV-associated neuropathy. *Nerolology, 54*(11), 2115–2119.

Sindrup, S. H., Gram, L. F., Brosen, K., et al. (1990). The selective serotonin reuptake inhibitor paroxetine is effective in the treatment of diabetic neuropathy symptoms. *Pain, 42*(2), 135–144.

Sindrup, S. H., & Jensen, T. S. (2002). Pharmacotherapy of trigeminal neuralgia. *The Clinical Journal of Pain, 18*(1), 22–27.

Singelyn, F. J., Deyaert, M., Joris, D., et al. (1998). Effects of intravenous patient-controlled analgesia with morphine, continuous epidural analgesia, and continuous three-in-one block on postoperative pain and knee rehabilitation after unilateral total knee arthroplasty. *Anesthesia and Analgesia, 97*(1), 88–92.

Singelyn, F. J., Ferrant, T., Malisse, M. F., et al. (2005). Effects of intravenous patient-controlled analgesia with morphine, continuous epidural analgesia, and continuous femoral nerve sheath block on rehabilitation after unilateral total hip arthroplasty. *Regional Anesthesia and Pain Medicine, 30*(5), 452–457.

Singelyn, F. J., & Gouverneur, J. M. A. (2000). Extended "three-in-one" block after total knee arthroplasty: Continuous versus patient-controlled techniques. *Anesthesia and Analgesia, 91*(1), 176–180.

Singelyn, F. J., Seguy, S., & Gouverneur, J. M. A. (1999). Interscalene brachial plexus analgesia after open shoulder surgery: Continuous versus patient-controlled infusion. *Anesthesia and Analgesia, 89*(5), 1216–1220.

Singelyn, F. J., Vanderelst, P. E., & Gouverneur, J. M. A. (2001). Extended femoral nerve sheath block after total hip arthroplasty: Continuous versus patient-controlled techniques. *Anesthesia and Analgesia, 92*(2), 455–459.

Singh, K., Samartzis, D., Strom, J., et al. (2005). A prospective, randomized, double-blind study evaluating the efficacy of postoperative continuous local anesthetic infusion at the iliac crest bone graft site after spinal arthrodesis. *Spine, 30*(22), 2477–2483.

Siobal, M. S., Kallet, R. H., Kivett, V. A., et al. (2006). Use of dexmedetomidine to facilitate extubation in surgical intensive-care-unit patients who failed previous weaning attempts following prolonged mechanical ventilation: A pilot study. *Respiratory Care, 51*(5), 492–496.

Skinner, D. J., Epstein, J., & Pappagallo, M. (2009). Tramadol. In H. S. Smith (Ed.), *Current therapy in pain* (pp. 508–512). Philadelphia: Saunders.

Skryabina, E. A., & Dunn, T. S. (2006). Disposable infusion pumps. *American Journal of Health-System Pharmacy, 63*(13), 1260–1268.

Slatkin, N. E., Rhiner, M., & Bolton, T. M. (2001). Donepezil in the treatment of opioid-induced sedation: Report of six cases. *Journal of Pain and Symptom Management, 21*(5), 425–438.

Slonimski, M., Abram, S. E., & Zuniga, R. E. (2004). Intrathecal baclofen in pain management. *Regional Anesthesia and Pain Medicine, 29*(3), 269–276.

Smith, H. S., Audette, J., & Royal, M. A. (2002). Botulinum toxin in pain management of soft tissue syndromes. *The Clinical Journal of Pain, 18*(Suppl. 6), S147–S154.

Smith, H. S., Dubin, A., & Parikh, A. (2009). Post amputation pain disorders. In H. S. Smith (Ed.), *Current therapy in pain* (pp. 268–279). Philadelphia: Saunders.

Soares, L. G., & Chan, V. W. (2007). The rationale for a multimodal approach in the management of breakthrough cancer pain: A review. *The American Journal of Hospice & Palliative Care, 24*(5), 430–439.

Soderpalm, B. (2002). Anticonvulsants: Aspects of their mechanisms of action. *European Journal of Pain (London, England), 6*(Suppl. A), 3–9.

Solaro, C., Uccelli, M. M., Brichetto, G., et al. (2001). Topiramate relieves idiopathic and symptomatic trigeminal neuralgia. *Journal of Pain and Symptom Management, 21*(5), 367–368.

Sollazzi, L., Modesti, C., Vitale, F., et al. (2009). Preinductive use of clonidine and ketamine improves recovery and reduces postoperative pain after bariatric surgery. *Surgery for Obesity and Related Diseases, 5*(1), 67–71.

Sollevi, A., Belfrage, M., Lundeberg, T., et al. (1995). Systemic adenosine infusion: A new treatment modality to alleviate neuropathic pain. *Pain, 61*(1), 155–158.

Sommer, M., Bachmann, C. G., Liebetanz, K. M., et al. (2007). Pregabalin in restless legs syndrome with and without neuropathic pain. *Acta Neurologica Scandinavica, 115*(5), 347–350.

Spanos, S., Booth, R., Koenig, H., et al. (2008). Jet injection of 1% buffered lidocaine versus topical Ela-Max for anesthesia before peripheral intravenous catheterization in children. *Pediatric Emergency Care, 24*(8), 511–515.

Spielmans, G. I. (2008). Duloxetine does not relieve painful physical symptoms in depression: A meta-analysis. *Psychotherapy and Psychosomatics, 77*(1), 12–16.

Staats, P. S., Yearwood, T., Charapata, et al. (2004). Intrathecal ziconotide in the treatment of refractory pain in patients with cancer or AIDS. *JAMA: The Journal of the American Medical Association, 291*(1), 63–70.

Stacey, B. R., Barrett, J. A., Whalen, E., et al. (2008). Pregabalin for postherpetic neuralgia: Placebo-controlled trial of fixed and flexible dosing regiments on allodynia and time to onset of pain relief. *The Journal of Pain, 9*(11), 1006–1017.

Stacey, B. R., Dworkin, R. H., Murphy, K., et al. (2008). Pregabalin in the treatment of refractory neuropathic pain: Results of a 15-month open-label trial. *Pain Medicine (Malden, Mass.), 9*(8), 1202–1208.

Stahl, M., Meyer, C., Haas, E., et al. (2008). Leg ulcer progression caused by topical anesthesia with EMLA cream. *Journal der Deutschen Dermatologischen Gesellschaft* (English version), 6(7), 566–568.

Stahl, S. M., Grady, M. M., Moret, C., et al. (2005). SNRIs: Their pharmacology, clinical efficacy, and tolerability in comparison with other classes of antidepressants. *CNS Spectrum, 10*(9), 732–747.

Stanik-Hutt, J. A., Soeken, K. L., Belcher, A. E., et al. (2001). Pain experiences of traumatically injured patients in a critical care setting. *American Journal of Critical Care, 10*(4), 252–259.

Stanos, S. P. (2007). Topical agents for the management of musculoskeletal pain. *Journal of Pain and Symptom Management, 33*(3), 342–355.

Stein, A., Yassouridis, A., Szopko, C., et al. (1999). Intraarticular morphine versus dexamethasone in chronic arthritis. *Pain, 83*(3), 525–532.

Stevens, M. F., Werdehausen, R., Golla, E., et al. (2007). Does interscalene catheter placement with stimulating catheters improve postoperative pain or functional outcome after shoulder surgery? A prospective randomized and double-blinded trial. *Anesth Analg, 104*(2), 442–447.

Stojadinovic, A., Auton, A., Peoples, G. E., et al. (2006). Responding to challenges in modern combat casualty care: Innovative use of advanced regional anesthesia. *Pain Medicine (Malden, Mass.), 7*(4), 330–338.

Storey, P., Hill, H. H., St. Cuis, R., et al. (1990). Subcutaneous infusions for control of cancer symptoms. *Journal of Pain and Symptom Management, 5*(1), 33–41.

Straube, S. R., Moore, A., Derry, S., et al. (2009). Vitamin D and chronic pain. *Pain, 141*(1–2), 10–13.

Strichartz, G. R., & Berde, C. B. (2005). Local anesthetics. In R. D. Miller (Ed.), *Miller's anesthesia* (6th ed., pp. 573–603). Philadelphia: Elsevier.

Strumper, D., & Durieux, M. E. (2004). Antidepressants as long-acting local anesthetics. *Regional Anesthesia and Pain Medicine, 29*(3), 277–285.

Subramaniam, B., Subramaniam, K., Pawar, D. K., et al. (2001). Preoperative epidural ketamine in combination with morphine does not have a clinically relevant intra- and postoperative opioid-sparing effect. *Anesthesia and Analgesia, 93*(5), 1321–1326.

Subramaniam, K., Subramaniam, B., & Steinbrook, R. A. (2004). Ketamine as adjuvant analgesic to opioid: A quantitative and qualitative systematic review. *Anesthesia and Analgesia, 99*(2), 482–489.

Sullivan, E. E. (2006). The propofol controversy. *Journal of Perianesthesia Nursing, 21*(2), 128–130.

Sullivan, M. D., Bentley, S., Fan, M. Y., et al. (2009). A single-blind, placebo run-in study of duloxetine for activity-limiting osteoarthritis pain. *The Journal of Pain, 10*(2), 208–213.

Sumpton, J. E., & Moulin, D. E. (2001). Treatment of neuropathic pain with venlafaxine. *The Annals of pharmacotherapy, 35*(5), 557–559.

Suzuki, M., Haraguti, S., Sugimoto, K., et al. (2006). Low-dose intravenous ketamine potentiates epidural analgesia after thoracotomy. *Anesthesiology, 105*(1), 111–119.

Svendsen, K. B., Jensen, T. S., & Bach, F. W. (2004). Does the cannabinoid dronabinol reduce central pain in multiple sclerosis? Randomised double blind placebo controlled crossover trial. *British Medical Journal, 329*(7460), 253.

Svenson, J. E., & Abernathy, M. K. (2007). Ketamine for prehospital use: New look at an old drug. *The American Journal of Emergency Medicine, 25*(8), 977–980.

Sveticic, G., Gentilini, A., Eichenberger, U., et al. (2003). Combinations of morphine with ketamine for patient-controlled analgesia. *Anesthesiology, 98*(5), 1195–1205.

Swenson, J. D., Bay, N., Loose, E., et al. (2006). Outpatient management of continuous peripheral nerve catheters placed using ultrasound guidance: An experience in 620 patients. *Anesthesia and Analgesia, 103*(6), 1436–1443.

Taboada, M., Rodriguez, J., Bermudez, M., et al. (2009). Comparison of continuous infusion versus automated bolus for postoperative patient-controlled analgesia with popliteal sciatic nerve catheters. *Anesthesiology, 110*(1), 150–154.

Takrouri, M. S., Seraj, M. A., & Channa, A. B. (2002). Dexmedetomidine in intensive care unit: A study of hemodynamic changes. *Middle East Journal of Anesthesiology*, 16(6), 587–595.

Tang, R., Evans, H., Chaput, A., et al. (2009). Multimodal analgesia for hip arthroplasty. *The Orthopedic Clinics of North America*, 40(3), 377–387.

Tardy, D., Baldessarini, R. J., & Tazari, F. I. (2002). Effects of newer antipsychotics on extrapyramidal function. *CNS Drugs*, 16(1), 23–45.

Taricco, M., Adone, R., Pagliacci, C., et al. (2000). Pharmacological interventions for spasticity following spinal cord injury. *Cochrane Database of Systematic Reviews (Online)*, (2), CD001131.

Tarride, J. E., Gordon, A., Vera-Llonch, M., et al. (2006). Cost-effectiveness of pregabalin for the management of neuropathic pain associated with diabetic peripheral neuropathy and postherpetic neuralgia: A Canadian perspective. *Clinical Therapeutics*, 28(11), 1922–1934.

Tarumi, Y., Watanabe, S., Bruera, E., et al. (2000). High-dose ketamine in the management of cancer-related neuropathic pain. *Journal of Pain and Symptom Management*, 19(6), 405–407.

Tay, B. A., Ngan Kee, W. D., & Chung, D. C. (2001). Gabapentin for the treatment and prophylaxis of cluster headache. *Regional Anesthesia and Pain Medicine*, 26(4), 373–375.

Taylor, C. P. (2009). Mechanisms of analgesia by gabapentin and pregabalin—Calcium channel α2-δ ligands. *Pain*, 142(1–2), 13–16.

Taylor, M. J. (2006). Strategies for managing antidepressant-induced sexual dysfunction: A review. *Current Psychiatry Reports*, 8(6), 431–436.

Tei, Y., Morita, T., Shishido, H., et al. (2005). Lidocaine intoxication at very small doses in terminally ill cancer patients. *Journal of Pain and Symptom Management*, 30(1), 6–7.

Tetik, O., Islamoglu, F., Ayan, E., et al. (2004). Intermittent infusion of 0.25% bupivacaine through an intrapleural catheter for post-thoracotomy pain relief. *The Annals of Thoracic Surgery*, 77(1), 284–288.

Thomas, A. A., Nguyen, C. T., Dhar, N. B., et al. (2008). Topical anesthesia with EMLA does not decrease pain during vasectomy. *The Journal of Urology*, 180(1), 271–273.

Thorpe, S. J., Balakrishnan, V. R., & Cook, L. B. (1999). The safety of patient-controlled sedation. *Anaesthesia*, 52(12), 1144–1150.

Tiippana, E. M., Hamunen, K., Kontinen, V. K., et al. (2007). Do surgical patients benefit from perioperative gabapentin/pregabalin? A systematic review of efficacy and safety. *Anesthesia and Analgesia*, 104(6), 1545–1556.

Tiong, H. Y., Liew, L. C., Samuel, M., et al. (2007). A meta-analysis of local anesthesia for tranrectal ultrasound-guided biopsy of the prostate. *Prostate Cancer and Prostatic Diseases*, 10(2), 127–136.

To, T. P., Lim, T. C., Hill, S. T., et al. (2002). Gabapentin for neuropathic pain following spinal cord injury. *Spinal Cord*, 40(6), 282–285.

Todorov, A. A., Kolchev, C. B., & Todorov, A. B. (2005). Tiagabine and gabapentin in the management of chronic pain. *The Clinical Journal of Pain*, 21(4), 358–361.

Tofferi, J. K., Jackson, J. L., & O'Malley, P. G. (2004). Treatment of fibromyalgia with cyclobenzaprine: A meta-analysis. *Arthritis and Rheumatism*, 51(1), 9–13.

Tolle, T., Freynhagen, R., Versavel, M., et al. (2008). Pregabalin for relief of neuropathic pain associated with diabetic neuropathy: A randomized, double-blind study. *European Journal of Pain (London, England)*, 12(2), 203–213.

Tomkins, G. E., Jackson, J. L., O'Malley, P. G., et al. (2001). Treatment of chronic headache with antidepressants: A meta-analysis. *The American Journal of Medicine*, 111(1), 54–63.

Tramer, M. R., & Glynn, C. J. (2007). An evaluation of a single dose of magnesium to supplement analgesia after ambulatory surgery: Randomized controlled trial. *Anesthesia and Analgesia*, 104(6), 1374–1379.

Tremont-Lukats, I. W., Challapalli, V., McNicol, E. D., et al. (2005). Systemic administration of local anesthetics to relieve neuropathic pain: A systematic review and meta-analysis. *Anesthesia and Analgesia*, 101(6), 1738–1749.

Tremont-Lukats, I. W., Hutson, P. R., & Backonja, M. (2006). A randomized, double-masked, placebo-controlled pilot trial of extended IV lidocaine infusion for relief of ongoing neuropathic pain. *The Clinical Journal of Pain*, 22(3), 266–271.

Tripp, P., & Kuettel, M. (2006). In O. A. de Leon-Casasola (Ed.), *Cancer pain. Pharmacological, interventional and palliative care approaches* (pp. 465–480). Philadelphia: Saunders.

Tsavaris, N., Kopterides, P., Kosmas, C., et al. (2008). Gabapentin monotherapy for the treatment of chemotherapy-induced neuropathic pain: A pilot study. *Pain Medicine (Malden, Mass.)*, 9(8), 1209–1216.

Tumber, P. S., & Fitzgibbon, D. R. (1998). The control of severe cancer pain by continuous intrathecal infusion and patient controlled intrathecal analgesia with morphine, bupivacaine and clonidine. *Pain*, 78(3), 217–220.

Turan, A., Karamanlioglu, B., Memis, D., et al. (2004). Analgesic effects of gabapentin after spinal surgery. *Anesthesiology*, 100(4), 935–938.

Turan, A., Kaya, G., Karamanlioglu, B., et al. (2006). Effect of oral gabapentin on postoperative epidural analgesia. *British Journal of Anaesthesia*, 96(2), 242–246.

Turan, A., Memis, D., Karamanlioglu, B., et al. (2004). The analgesic effects of gabapentin in monitored anesthesia care for ear-nose-throat surgery. *Anesthesia and Analgesia*, 99(2), 375–378.

Turan, A., White, P. F., Karamanlioglu, B., et al. (2006). Gabapentin: An alternative to the cyclooxygenase-2 inhibitors for perioperative pain management. *Anesthesia and Analgesia*, 102(1), 175–181.

Turan, A., White, P. F., Karamanlioglu, B., et al. (2007). Premedication with gabapentin: The effect on tourniquet pain and quality of intravenous regional anesthesia. *Anesthesia and Analgesia*, 104(1), 97–101.

Turan, A., White, P. F., Koyuncu, O., et al. (2008). Transdermal nicotine patch failed to improve postoperative pain management. *Anesthesia and Analgesia*, 107(3), 1011–1017.

Ture, H., Sayin, M., Karlikaya, G., et al. (2009). The analgesic effect of gabapentin as a prophylactic anticonvulsant drug on postcraniotomy pain: A prospective randomized study. *Anesthesia and Analgesia*, 109(5), 1625–1631.

Turner, M. K., Hooten, M., Schmidt, J. E., et al. (2008). Prevalence and clinical correlates of vitamin D inadequacy among patients with chronic pain. *Pain Medicine (Malden, Mass.)*, 9(8), 979–984.

Twycross, R., Wilcock, A., Charlesworth, S., et al. (2003). Palliativedrugs.com therapeutic highlights: Gabapentin. *Indian J Palliat Care*, 9(2), 71–74.

Uceyler, N., Hauser, W., & Sommer, C. (2008). A systematic review on the effectiveness of treatment with antidepressants in fibromyalgia syndrome. *Arthritis and Rheumatism, 59*(9), 1279–1298.

Umino, M., Kohase, H., Ideguchi, S., et al. (2002). Long-term pain control in trigeminal neuralgia with local anesthetics using an indwelling catheter in the mandibular nerve. *The Clinical Journal of Pain, 18*(3), 196–199.

United States Food and Drug Administration (FDA). (2004). *CDER warning letter on topiramate.* Available at: http://www.fda.gov/cder/warn/2004/12547.pdf Accessed March 10, 2009.

United States Food and Drug Administration (FDA). (2005a). *Safety data on Cymbalta. Hepatic effects.* Available at: www.fda.gov/medwatch/SAFETY/2005/Cymbalta_Dear-HCP05OCT2005.FINALSIGNED.pdf Accessed February 21, 2009.

United States Food and Drug Administration (FDA). (2005b). *Gabitril (tiagabine) Dear Doctor letter.* Available at: http://www.fda.gov/medwatch/SAFETY/2005/gabitril_DHCP.htm Accessed March 10, 2009.

United States Food and Drug Administration (FDA). (2005c). *Dockets management. Removal from labeling for propofol.* Available at: http://www.fda.gov/ohrms/dockets/dockets/05p0267/05p0267.htm Accessed March 22, 2009.

United States Food and Drug Administration (FDA). (2007a). *Duloxetine prescribing information.* Available at: http://www.fda.gov/cder/foi/label/2007/021427s009s011s013lbl.pdf Accessed February 21, 2009.

United States Food and Drug Administration (FDA). (2007b). *Trileptal Medwatch.* Available at: http://www.fda.gov/medwatch/safety/2007/Aug_PI/Trileptal_PI.pdf Accessed March 13, 2009.

United States Food and Drug Administration (FDA). (2008). *Information on bisphosphonates.* Available at: http://www.fda.gov/cder/drug/infopage/bisphosphonates/ Accessed April 3, 2009.

Unlugenc, H., Gunduz, M., Guler, T., et al. (2005). The effect of pre-anaesthetic administration of intravenous dexmedetomidine on postoperative painin patients receiving patient-controlled morphine. *European Journal of Anaesthesiology, 22*(5), 386–391.

Ushida, T., Tani, T., Kanbara, T., et al. (2002). Analgesic effects of ketamine ointment in patients with complex regional pain syndrome type I. *Regional Anesthesia and Pain Medicine, 27*(5), 524–528.

Valdovinos, N. C., Reddin, C., Bernard, C., et al. (2009). The use of topical anesthesia during intravenous catheter insertion in adults: A comparison of pain scores using LMX-4 versus placebo. *Journal of Emergency Nursing, 35*(4), 299–304.

Valenzuela, R. C., & Rosen, D. A. (1999). Topical lidocaine-prilocaine cream (EMLA) for thoracostomy tube removal. *Anesthesia and Analgesia, 88*(5), 1107–1108.

Valero Marco, A. V., Martinez Castillo, C., & Macia Solera, L. (2008). Local anesthesia in arterial puncture: Nurses' knowledge and attitude. *Archivos de Bronconeumologia* (English Edition), *44*(7), 360–363.

Vallerand, A. H., Fouladbakhsh, J., & Templin, T. (2005). Patients' choices for the self-treatment of pain. *Applied Nursing Research, 18*(2), 90–96.

Van Amelsvoort, T., Bakshi, R., Devaux, C. B., et al. (1994). Hyponatremia associated with carbamazepine and oxcarbazepine therapy: A review. *Epilepsia, 35*(1), 181–188.

Van Elstraete, A. C., Tirault, M., Lebrun, T., et al. (2008). The median effective dose of preemptive gabapentin on postoperative morphine consumption after posterior lumbar spinal fusion. *Anesthesia and Analgesia, 106*(1), 305–408.

van Hilten, B. J., van de Beek, W. J., Hoff, J. I., et al. (2000). Intrathecal baclofen for treatment of dystonia in patients with reflex sympathetic dystrophy. *The New England Journal of Medicine, 343*(9), 625–630.

van Ophoven, A., Pokupic, S., Heinecke, A., et al. (2004). A prospective, randomized, placebo-controlled, double-blind study of amitriptyline for the treatment of interstitial cystitis. *The Journal of Urology, 172*(2), 533–536.

Vanotti, A., Osio, M., Mailland, E., et al. (2007). Overview on pathophysiology and newer approaches to treatment of peripheral neuropathies. *CNS Drugs, 21*(Suppl. 1), 3–12.

van Rijn, M. A., Munts, A. G., Marinus, J., et al. (2009). Intrathecal baclofen for dystonia of complex regional pain syndrome. *Pain, 143*(1–2), 41–47.

Van Schaeybroeck, P., Nuttin, B., Lagae, L., et al. (2000). Intrathecal baclofen for intractable cerebral spasticity: A prospective placebo-controlled, double-blind study. *Neurosurgery, 46*(3), 603–612.

Van Seventer, R., Feister, H. A., Young, J. P., Jr., et al. (2006). Efficacy and tolerability of twice-daily pregabalin for treating pain and related sleep interference in postherpetic neuralgia: A 13-week, randomized trial. *Current Medical Research and Opinion, 22*(2), 375–384.

van Tulder, M. W., Touray, T., Furlan, A. D., et al. (2003). Muscle relaxants for non-specific low-back pain. *Cochrane Database of Systematic Reviews (Online)*, (2), CD004252.

Vargo, J. J., Cohen, L. B., Rex, D. K., et al. (2009). Position statement: Nonanesthesiologist administration of propofol for GI endoscopy. *Gastroenterology, 137*(6), 2161–2167.

Venn, R. M., & Grounds, R. M. (2001). Comparison between dexmedetomidine and propofol for sedation in the intensive care unit: Patient and clinician perceptions. *British Journal of Anaesthesia, 87*(5), 684–690.

Ventafridda, V., Bonezzi, C., Caraceni, A., et al. (1987). Antidepressants for cancer pain and other painful syndromes with deafferentation component: Comparison of amitriptyline and trazadone. *Italian Journal of Neurological Sciences, 8*(6), 579–587.

Verdu, B., Decosterd, I., Buclin, T., et al. (2008). Antidepressants for the treatment of chronic pain. *Drugs, 68*(18), 2611–2632.

Vestergaard, K., Andersen, G., Gottrup, H., et al. (2001). Lamotrigine for central poststroke pain: A randomized controlled trial. *Neurology, 56*(2), 184–190.

Veves, A., Backonja, M., & Malik, R. A. (2008). Painful diabetic neuropathy: Epidemiology, natural history, early diagnosis, and treatment options. *Pain Medicine (Malden, Mass.), 9*(6), 660–674.

Vinik, A. I., Tuchman, M., Safirstein, B., et al. (2007). Lamotrigine for treatment of pain associated with diabetic neuropathy: Results of two randomized, double-blind, placebo-controlled studies. *Pain, 128*(1–2), 169–179.

Vintar, N., Rawal, N., & Veselko, M. (2005). Intraarticular patient-controlled regional anesthesia after arthroscopically assisted anterior cruciate ligament reconstruction: Ropivacaine/morphine/ketorolac versus ropivacaine/morphine. *Anesthesia and Analgesia, 101*(2), 573–578.

Virani, A., Mailis, A., Shapiro, L. E., et al. (1997). Drug interactions in human neuropathic pain pharmacology. *Pain, 73*(1), 3–13.

Visalyaputra, S., Lertakyamanee, J., Pethpaisit, N., et al. (1999). Intraperitoneal lidocaine decreases intraoperative pain during postpartum tubal ligation. *Anesthesia and Analgesia, 88*(5), 1077–1080.

Viscomi, C. M., & Rathmell, J. P. (1998). Pain management issues in the pregnant patient. In M. A. Ashburn & L. J. Rice (Eds.), *The management of pain* (pp. 363–381). New York: Churchill Livingstone.

Visser, E., & Schug, S. A. (2006). The role of ketamine in pain management. *Biomedicine & Pharmacotherapy, 60*(7), 341–348.

Vitale, V., Battelli, D., Gasperoni, E., et al. (2008). Intrathecal therapy with ziconotide: Clinical experience and considerations on its use. *Minerva Anestesiologica, 74*(12), 727–733.

Vitton, O., Gendreau, M., Gendreau, J., et al. (2004). A double-blind placebo-controlled trial of milnacipran in the treatment of fibromyalgia. *Hum Pyschopharmacol, 19*(Suppl. 1), S27–S35.

von Gunten, C. F., Eappen, S., Cleary, J. F., et al. (2007). Flecainide for the treatment of chronic neuropathic pain: A Phase II trial. *Palliative Medicine, 21*(8), 667–672.

Vossinakis, I. C., Stavroulaki, P., Paleochorlidis, I., et al. (2004). Reducing the pain associated with local anaesthetic infiltration for open carpal tunnel decompression. *The Journal of Hand Surgery, 29*(4), 399–401.

Vranken, J. H., Dijkgraaf, M. G. W., Kruis, M. R., et al. (2008). Pregabalin in patients with central neuropathic pain: A randomized, double-blind, placebo-controlled trial of a flexible-dose regimen. *Pain, 136*(1–2), 150–157.

Vranken, J. H., van der Vegt, M. H., Zuurmond, W. W. A., et al. (2001). Continuous brachial plexus block at the cervical level using a posterior approach in the management of neuropathic cancer pain. *Regional Anesthesia and Pain Medicine, 26*(6), 572–575.

Vranken, J. H., van Kan, H. J. M., & van der Vegt, M. H. (2006). Stability and compatibility of a meperidine—Clonidine mixture in portable pump reservoirs for the management of cancer pain syndromes. (Letter) *Journal of Pain and Symptom Management, 32*(4), 297–299.

Vurdelja, R. B., Budincevic, H., & Prvan, M. P. (2008). Central poststroke pain. *Lijecnicki Vjesnik, 130*(7–8), 191–195.

Wadhwa, A., Clarke, D., Goodchild, C. S., et al. (2001). Large-dose oral dextromethorphan as an adjunct to patient-controlled analgesia with morphine after surgery. *Anesthesia and Analgesia, 92*(2), 448–454.

Walia, K. S., Khan, E. A., Ko, D. H., et al. (2004). Side effects of antiepileptics—A review. *Pain Practice, 4*(3), 194–203.

Wallace, M. S., Barger, D., & Schulteis, G. (2002). The effect of chronic oral despiramine on capsaicin-induced allodynia and hyperalgesia: A double-blinded, placebo-controlled crossover study. *Anesthesia and Analgesia, 95*(4), 973–978.

Wallace, M. S., Galer, B. S., & Gammaitoni, A. R. (2006). Topical and oral anesthetics. In O. A. de Leon-Casasola (Ed.), *Cancer pain. Pharmacological, interventional and palliative care approaches* (pp. 327–335). Philadelphia: Saunders.

Wallace, M. S., Kosek, P. S., Staats, P., et al. (2008). Phase II, open-label, multicenter study of combined intrathecal morphine and ziconotide: Addition of ziconotide in patients receiving intrathecal morphine for severe chronic pain. *Pain Medicine (Malden, Mass.), 9*(3), 271–281.

Wallace, M. S., Magnuson, S., & Ridgeway, B. (2000). Efficacy of oral mexiletine for neuropathic pain with allodynia: A double-blind, placebo-controlled, crossover study. *Regional Anesthesia and Pain Medicine, 25*(5), 459–567.

Wang, L. K., Chen, H. P., Chang, P. J., et al. (2001). Axillary brachial plexus block with patient controlled analgesia for complex regional pain syndrome type I: A case report. *Regional Anesthesia and Pain Medicine, 26*(1), 68–71.

Wang, X., Xie, H., & Wang, G. (2006). Improved postoperative analgesia with coadministration of preoperative epidural ketamine and midazolam. *Journal of Clinical Anesthesia, 18*(8), 563–569.

Ware, M. A., Fitzcharles, M. A., Joseph, L., et al. (2010). The effects of nabilone on sleep in fibromyalgia : Results of a randomized controlled trial. *Anesthesia and Analgesia, 110*(2), 604–610.

Wasiak, J., & Cleland, H. (2007). Lidocaine for pain relief in burn injured patients. *Cochrane Database of Systematic Reviews (Online),* (3), CD005622.

Weaver, C. S., Hauter, W. E., Brizendine, E. J., et al. (2007). Emergency department procedural sedation with propofol: Is it safe? *Journal of Emergency Medicine, 33*(4), 355–361.

Webb, A. R., Skinner, B. S., Leong, S., et al. (2007). The addition of a small-dose ketamine infusion to tramadol for postoperative analgesia: A double-blinded, placebo-controlled, randomized trial after abdominal surgery. *Anesthesia and Analgesia, 104*(4), 912–917.

Weber, C., & Zulian, G. B. (2009). Malignant irreversible intestinal obstruction: The powerful association of octreotide to corticosteroids, antiemetics, and analgesics. *The American Journal of Hospice & Palliative Care, 26*(2), 84–88.

Webster, L. R., Fisher, R., Charapata, S., et al. (2009). Long-term intrathecal ziconotide for chronic pain: An open-label study. *Journal of Pain and Symptom Management, 37*(3), 363–372.

Webster, L. R., & Walker, M. J. (2006). Safety and efficacy of prolonged outpatient ketamine infusions for neuropathic pain. *American Journal of Therapeutics, 13*(4), 300–305.

Wedel, D. J., & Horlocker, T. T. (2005). Nerve blocks. In R. D. Miller (Ed.), *Miller's anesthesia.* (6th ed., pp. 1685–1717). Philadelphia: Elsevier.

Weinbroum, A. A., Bender, B., Nirkin, A., et al. (2004). Dextromethorphan-associated epidural patient-controlled analgesia provides better pain- and analgesics-sparing effects than dextromethorphan-associated intravenous patient-controlled analgesia after bone-malignancy resection: A randomized, placebo-controlled, double-blinded study. *Anesthesia and Analgesia, 98*(3), 714–722.

Welch, B. J., Graybeal, D., Moe, O. W., et al. (2006). Biochemical and stone-risk profiles with topiramate treatment. *American Journal of Kidney Diseases, 48*(4), 555–563.

Werner, M. U., Lassen, B., & Kehlet, H. (2002). Analgesic effects of dexamethasone in burn injury. *Regional Anesthesia and Pain Medicine, 27*(3), 254–260.

Werner, M. U., Perkins, F. M., Holte, K., et al. (2001). Effects of gabapentin in acute inflammatory pain in humans. *Regional Anesthesia and Pain Medicine, 26*(4), 322–328.

Wernicke, J. F., Wang, F., Pritchett, Y. L., et al. (2007). An open-label 52-week clinical extension comparing duloxetine with routine care in patients with diabetic peripheral neuropathic pain. *Pain Medicine (Malden, Mass.), 8*(6), 503–513.

Westfall, T. C., & Westfall, D. P. (2006). Adrenergic agonists and antagonists. In L. L. Brunton, J. S. Lazo & K. L. Parker (Eds.), *Goodman & Gilman's the pharmacological basis of therapeutics*. (11th ed.)(pp. 237–295). New York: McGraw-Hill.

Wheatley, G. H., 3rd, Rosenbaum, D. H., Paul, M. C., et al. (2005). Improved pain management outcomes with continuous infusion of a local anesthetic after thoracotomy. *The Journal of Thoracic and Cardiovascular Surgery, 130*(2), 464–468.

Wheeler, A. H., Goolkasian, P., & Gretz, S. S. (2001). Botulinum toxin A for the treatment of chronic neck pain. *Pain, 94*(3), 255–260.

White, P. F. (2005). The changing role of non-opioid analgesic techniques in the management of postoperative pain. *Anesthesia and Analgesia, 101*(Suppl. 5), S5–S22.

White, P. F., Rawal, S., Latham, P., et al. (2003). Use of a continuous local anesthetic infusion for pain management after median sternotomy. *Anesthesiology, 99*(4), 918–923.

White, P. F., Tufanogullari, B., Taylor, J., et al. (2009). The effect of pregabalin on postoperative anxiety and sedation levels: A dose-ranging study. *Anesthesia and Analgesia, 108*(4), 1140–1145.

Wiech, K., Kiefer, R. T., Topfner, S., et al. (2004). A placebo-controlled randomized crossover trial of N-methyl-D-aspartate acid receptor antagonist, memantine, in patients with chronic phantom limb pain. *Anesthesia and Analgesia, 98*(2), 408–413.

Wiffen, P. J., Collins, S., McQuay, H. J., et al. (2005). Anticonvulsant drugs for acute and chronic pain. *Cochrane Database of Systematic Reviews (Online)*, (3) CD001133.

Wiffen, P. J., McQuay, H. J., & Moore, R. A. (2005). Carbamazepine for acute and chronic pain in adults. *Cochrane Database of Systematic Reviews (Online)*, (3), CD005451.

Wiffen, P. J., McQuay, H. J., Rees, J., et al. (2005). Gabapentin for acute and chronic pain. *Cochrane Database of Systematic Reviews (Online)*, (3) CD005452.

Wiffen, P. J., & Rees, J. (2007). Lamotrigine for acute and chronic pain. *Cochrane Database of Systematic Reviews (Online)*, (2), CD006044.

Wijeysundera, D. N., Naik, J. S., & Beattie, S. (2003). Alpha-2 adrenergic agonists to prevent perioperative cardiovascular complications: A meta-analysis. *The American Journal of Medicine, 114*(9), 742–752.

Wild, G., Shinde, S., & Newton, M. (1999). Mixing of propofol and lidocaine. *British Journal of Anaesthesia, 83*(1), 193.

Wilhelm, I. R., Griessinger, N., Koppert, W., et al. (2005). High doses of topically applied lidocaine in a cancer patient. (Letter) *Journal of Pain and Symptom Management, 30*(3), 203–204.

Williams, B. A., Dang, Q., Bost, J. E., et al. (2009). General health and knee function outcomes from 7 days to 12 weeks after spinal anesthesia and multimodal analgesia for anterior cruciate ligament reconstruction. *Anesthesia and Analgesia, 108*(4), 1296–1302.

Williams, B. A., Kentor, M. L., Vogt, M. T., et al. (2006). Reduction of verbal pain scores after anterior cruciate ligament reconstruction with two-day continuous femoral nerve block: A randomized clinical trial. *Anesthesiology, 104*(2), 315–327.

Wilson, A. (2009). Regional analgesia and orthopaedic surgery. *Orthopaedics and Trauma, 23*(6), 441–449.

Wilson, J. A., Nimmo, A. F., Fleetwood-Walker, S. M., et al. (2008). A randomised double blind trial of the effect of pre-emptive epidural ketamine on persistent pain after limb amputation. *Pain, 135*(1–2), 108–118.

Windle, P. E., Kwan, M. L., Warwick, H., et al. (2006). Comparison of bacteriostatic normal saline and lidocaine used as intradermal anesthesia for placement of intravenous lines. *Journal of Perianesthesia Nursing, 21*(4), 251–258.

Wong, D. L. (2003). Topical local anesthetics. *The American Journal of Nursing, 103*(6), 42–45.

Wong, D. L., & Pasero, C. (1997). Reducing the pain of lidocaine. *The American Journal of Nursing, 97*(1), 17–18.

Wong, R. K. S., & Wiffen, P. J. (2002). Bisphosphonates for the relief of pain secondary to bone metastases. *Cochrane Database of Systematic Reviews (Online)*, (2), CD002068.

Wood, P. B. (2006). A reconsideration of the relevance of systemic low-dose ketamine to the pathophysiology of fibromyalgia. *The Journal of Pain, 7*(9), 611–614.

Wood, R. M. (2000). Ketamine for pain in hospice patients. *Int J Pharmaceutical Compounding, 4*(4), 253–254.

Woodrow, K. M., & Eltherington, L. G. (1988). Feeling no pain. Alcohol as an analgesic. *Pain, 32*(2), 159–163.

Woods, A. M., & DiFazio, C. A. (1995). Pharmacology of local anesthetics and related drugs. In J. J. Bonica, & J. S. McDonald (Eds.), *Principles and practice of obstetric analgesia and anesthesia*. (2nd ed., pp. 297–323). Baltimore: Williams & Wilkins.

Wright, J. L., Durieux, M. E., & Groves, D. S. (2008). A brief review of innovative uses for local anesthetics. *Current Opinion in Anaesthesiology, 21*(5), 651–656.

Wright, R. M., Roumani, Y. F., Boudreau, R., et al. (2009). Effect of central nervous system medication use on decline in cognition in community-dwelling older adults: Findings from the health, aging and body composition study. *Journal of the American Geriatrics Society, 57*(2), 243–250.

Wu, C. L., Berenholtz, S. M., Pronovost, P. J., et al. (2002). Systematic review and analysis of postdischarge symptoms after outpatient surgery. *Anesthesiology, 96*(4), 994–1003.

Wu, C. L., & Liu, S. S. (2009). Intravenous lidocaine for ambulatory anesthesia: Good to go or not so fast? *Anesthesia and Analgesia, 109*(6), 1718–1719.

Wu, C. L., Tella, P., Staats, P. S., et al. (2002). Analgesic effects of intravenous lidocaine and morphine on postamputation pain: A randomized double-blind, active placebo-controlled, crossover trial. *Anesthesiology, 96*(4), 841–848.

Wu, C. T., Borel, C. O., Lee, M. S., et al. (2005). The interaction effect of perioperative cotreatment with dextromethorphan and intravenous lidocaine on pain relief and recovery of bowel function after laparascopic cholecystectomy. *Anesthesia and Analgesia, 100*(2), 448–453.

Wu, E. Q., Birnbaum, H. G., Mareva, M. N., et al. (2006). Cost-effectiveness of duloxetine versus routine treatment for U.S. patients with diabetic peripheral neuropathic pain. *The Journal of Pain, 7*(6), 399–407.

Wulf, H., Gleim, M., & Mignat, C. (1994). The stability of mixtures of morphine hydrochloride, bupivacaine hydrochloride, and clonidine hydrochloride in portable pump reservoirs for the management of chronic pain syndromes. *Journal of Pain and Symptom Management, 9*(5), 308–311.

Wunsch, H., & Kress, J. P. (2009). A new era for sedation in ICU patients. *JAMA: The Journal of the American Medical Association, 301*(5), 542–543.

Wymer, J. P., Simpson, J., Sen, D., et al. (2009). Efficacy and safety of lacosamide in diabetic neuropathic pain. *The Clinical Journal of Pain, 25*(5), 376–385.

Wysowski, D. K., & Pollock, M. L. (2006). Reports of death with use of propofol (Diprivan) for nonprocedural (long-term) sedation and literature review. *Anesthesiology, 105*(5), 1047–1051.

Xia, Y., Chen, E., Tibbits, D. L., et al. (2002). Comparison of effects of lidocaine hydrochloride, buffered lidocaine, diphenhydramine, and normal saline intradermal injection. *Journal of Clinical Anesthesia, 14*(5), 339–343.

Xie, H., Wang, X., Liu, G., et al. (2003). Analgesic effects and pharmacokinetics of a low dose of ketamine preoperatively administered epidurally or intravenously. *The Clinical Journal of Pain, 19*(5), 317–322.

Xuerong, Y., Yuguang, H., Xia, J., et al. (2008). Ketamine and lornoxicam for preventing a fentanyl-induced increase in postoperative morphine requirement. *Anesthesia and Analgesia, 107*(6), 2032–2037.

Yaksh, T. L. (2006). Central pharmacology of nociceptive transmission. In S. B. McMahon & M. Koltzenberg (Eds.), *Wall and Melzack's textbook of pain.* (5th ed., pp. 271–414). Philadelphia: Elsevier.

Yaksi, A., Ozgonenel, L., & Ozgonenel, B. (2007). The efficiency of gabapentin therapy in patients with lumbar spinal stenosis. *Spine, 32*(9), 939–942.

Yamashita, S., Sato, S., Kakiuchi, Y., et al. (2002). Lidocaine toxicity during frequent viscous lidocaine use for painful tongue ulcer. *Journal of Pain and Symptom Management, 24*(5), 543–545.

Yamauchi, M., Asano, M., Watanabe, M., et al. (2008). Continuous low-dose ketamine improves the analgesic effects of fentanyl patient-controlled analgesia after cervical spine surgery. *Anesthesia and Analgesia, 107*(3), 1041–1044.

Yang, R. H., Wang, W. T., Chen, J. Y., et al. (2009). Gabapentin selective reduces persistent sodium current in injured type-A dorsal root ganglion neurons. *Pain, 143*(1), 48–55.

Yap, K. Y., Chui, W. K., & Chan, A. (2008). Drug interactions between chemotherapeutic regimens and antiepileptics. *Clinical Therapeutics, 30*(8), 1385–1407.

Yardeni, I. Z., Beilin, B., Mayburd, E., et al. (2009). The effect of perioperative intravenous lidocaine on postoperative pain and immune function. *Anesthesia and Analgesia, 109*(5), 1465–1469.

Yeh, C. C., Jao, S. W., Huh, B. K., et al. (2005). Preincisional dextromethorphan combined with thoracic epidural anesthesia and analgesia improves postoperative pain and bowel function in patients undergoing colonic surgery. *Anesthesia and Analgesia, 200*(5), 1384–1389.

Yiannakopoulos, C. K. (2004). Carpal ligament decompression under local anesthesia: The effect of lidocaine warming and alkalinisation on infiltration pain. *The Journal of Hand Surgery, 29*(1), 32–34.

Yosselson-Superstine, S., Lipman, A. G., & Sanders, S. H. (1985). Adjunctive antianxiety agents in the management of chronic pain. *Israel Journal of Medical Sciences, 21*(2), 113–117.

Younis, I., & Bhutiani, R. P. (2004). Taking the "ouch" out—effect of buffering commercial xylocaine on infiltration and procedure pain—a prospective, randomised, double-blind, controlled trial. *Annals of the Royal College of Surgeons of England, 86*(3), 213–217.

Yucel, A., Ozyalcin, S., Talu, G., et al. (2005). The effect of venlafaxine on ongoing and experimentally induced pain in neuropathic pain patients: A double blind, placebo controlled study. *European Journal of Pain (London, England), 9*(4), 407–416.

Yuen, K. Y., Shelley, M., Sze, W. M., et al. (2006). Bisphosphonates for advanced prostate cancer. *Cochrane Database of Systematic Reviews (Online),* (4), CD006250.

Yuen, V. M., Irwin, M. G., Hui, T. W., et al. (2007). A double-blind, crossover assessment of the sedative and analgesic effects of intranasal dexmedetomidine. *Anesthesia and Analgesia, 105*(2), 374–380.

Zaccara, G., Gangemi, P. F., & Cincotta, M. (2008). Central nervous system adverse effects of new antiepileptic drugs: A meta-analysis of placebo-controlled studies. *Seizure, 17*(5), 405–421.

Zacny, J. P., Coalson, D. W., Young, C. J., et al. (1996). Propofol at conscious sedation doses produces mild analgesia to cold pressor-induced pain in healthy volunteers. *Journal of Clinical Anesthesia, 8*(7), 459–474.

Zakine, J., Samarcq, D., Lorne, E., et al. (2008). Postoperative ketamine administration decreases morphine consumption in major abdominal surgery: A prospective, randomized, double-blind, controlled study. *Anesthesia and Analgesia, 106*(6), 1856–1861.

Zakrzewska, J. M., Chaudhry, Z., Nurmikko, T. J., et al. (1997). Lamotrigine (lamictal) in refractory trigeminal neuralgia: Results from a double-blind placebo controlled crossover trial. *Pain, 73*(2), 223–230.

Zaric, D., Boysen, K., Christiansen, C., et al. (2006). A comparison of epidural analgesia with combined continuous femoral-sciatic nerve blocks after total knee replacement. *Anesthesia and Analgesia, 102*(4), 1240–1246.

Zausig, Y. A., Zink, W., Keil, M., et al. (2009). Lipid emulsion improves recovery from bupivacaine-induced cardiac arrest, but not from ropivacaine- or mepivacaine-induced cardiac arrest. *Anesthesia and Analgesia, 109*(4), 1323–1326.

Zed, P. J., Abu-Laban, R. B., Chan, W. W. Y., et al. (2007). Efficacy, safety and patient satisfaction of propofol for procedural sedation and analgesia in the emergency department: A prospective study. *Can J Emerg Med, 9*(6), 421–427.

Zeigler, D., Pritchett, Y. L., Wang, F., et al. (2007). Impact of disease characteristics on the efficacy of duloxetine in diabetic peripheral neuropathic pain. *Diabetes Care, 30*(3), 664–669.

Zhang, W. Y. (2001). A benefit-risk assessment of caffeine as an analgesic adjuvant. *Drug Safety, 24*(15), 1127–1142.

Zieleniewski, W. (1990). Calcitonin nasal spray for painful diabetic neuropathy. *Lancet, 336*(8712), 449.

Zilbert, A. (2002). Topical anesthesia for minor gynaecological procedures: A review. *Obstetrical & Gynecological Survey, 57*(3), 171–178.

Zin, C. S., Nissen, L. M., Smith, M. T., et al. (2008). An update on the pharmacological management of post-herpetic neuralgia and painful diabetic neuropathy. *CNS Drugs*, 22(5), 417–442.

Zisook, S., Rush, A. J., Haight, B. R., et al. (2006). Use of bupropion in combination with serotonin reuptake inhibitors. *Biological Psychiatry*, 59(3), 203–210.

Zissis, N. P., Harmoussi, S., Vlaikidis, N., et al. (2007). A randomized, double-blind, placebo-controlled study of venlafaxine XR in out-patients with tension-type headache. *Cephalagia*, 27(4), 315–324.

Zuniga, R. E., Perera, S., & Abram, S. E. (2002). Intrathecal baclofen: A useful agent in the treatment of well-established complex regional pain syndrome. *Regional Anesthesia and Pain Medicine*, 27(1), 90–93.

Zuniga, R. E., Schlicht, C. R., & Abram, S. E. (2000). Intrathecal baclofen is analgesic in patients with chronic pain. *Anesthesiology*, 92(3), 876–880.

Appendix A Pain Resources on the Internet

Allison T. Nisbet and Jan L. Frandsen

Introduction and History

The Internet was created in 1969 to provide government scientists with a tool to send and receive information between collaborating sites, although it gradually expanded from being a government entity only. What we now know as the World Wide Web was created by European physicists who needed to send information to each other. They developed the hypertext markup language (HTML), which can be used to send and receive documents, sound, and live pictures—provided one has the software to perform these tasks. As a result of the High-Performance Computing Act of 1991, Internet access was made available to the public through telecommunications companies, information services, and other public access systems.

The information that was initially available to the public on the Internet was relatively limited, but today the Internet has more than 182 million sites on the World Wide Web alone, and from 2006 to 2007, the size of the Internet doubled (Netcraft, 2008). Furthermore, mailing lists, gopher sites, and other areas are accessible to the general public. One may liken Internet access to a gigantic, continuously expanding library. In addition, features such as chat rooms, newsgroups, and mailing lists bring together people from across the world to share and discuss experiences, information, and knowledge. More and more, the use of the Internet has become embedded in our daily lives and includes banking, bill paying, shopping, electronic learning (e-learning), electronic mail (e-mail), and posting personal blogs (opinions, comments). The degree to which information technology is used is growing every day. The volume of information—including medical information—continues to grow. Consequently the Internet attracts both health care professionals and patients.

Information about the Internet

As the internet has become more popular, the amount of information found there has grown proportionally. Most well-stocked bookstores or computer stores carry a variety of books written for all levels of usage on the subject of the Internet. Numerous magazines about the Internet are also available, and most computer magazines have columns, sections, or features devoted to the Internet and related topics. Of course, information about the Internet is available on the Internet itself.

Access to the Internet

Several ways are available to access the Internet. An increasing number of organizations have internal e-mail with a so-called "gateway" for sending and receiving e-mail via the Internet. Most higher-education facilities have Internet access and World Wide Web access. Most public libraries provide computers for their patrons to access the World Wide Web. Finally, one can subscribe to commercial online services or direct Internet service providers (ISPs), which can be accessed from a personal computer.

For those who want to access the Internet from home, many of the commercial online services and ISPs currently offer a flat fee or free access for those who subscribe to their service. These services and their features are reviewed regularly in computer or home/office magazines.

Selected Features of the Internet

The features that are most useful for both patients and health care professionals are primarily, but not limited to, e-mail, mailing lists, newsgroups, and the World Wide Web.

Electronic Mail (E-Mail)

Electronic mail (e-mail) is an effective way to communicate and exchange information and serves as an alternative to the use of the telephone and fax. Because e-mail can be composed, sent, and read at any time for both sender and receiver, it is very convenient and cost-effective. Furthermore, e-mail can be saved in an electronic form, such as on a writable CD (CD-RW) or a jump (flash) drive, similar to the way hard copy documents are filed in a filing cabinet.

If necessary, one can also transmit an e-mail with one or more documents attached to the message. This can be highly advantageous when two or more people are collaborating on a project, such as writing a scientific paper. The attached document can be formatted in many ways. Word-processing documents, software, slide presentation files, and photos can be transmitted this way. However, one should ensure that the receiver has the correct software to open or translate the attached document.

Mailing Lists

A mailing list contains the names and e-mail addresses of a group of individuals with similar interests for the purpose of sharing information over the Internet. The concept of a mailing list can be described as follows:

- A subscriber posts a question, comment, or some other information.
- The posting is then distributed to all subscribers.
- Subscribers to the group respond to the posting.
- The responses are then sent to the subscribers.

The members can act as a group by responding to the posting as though it was a regular personal e-mail message. The lists of available topics are almost unlimited. The resource list at the end of this appendix includes a few selected mailing lists related to pain management and a Web site where the reader can search for mailing lists geared toward a specific topic.

When subscribing to a mailing list, one must often follow a subscription policy. The subscription process varies a little from one mailing list to another, but when a mailing list is mentioned, details on the subscription procedure are generally included. Nicoll and Oulette (1997) provided some general rules on how to subscribe to mailing lists that still apply today. Subscriptions to mailing lists are free of surcharges; however, some health care mailing lists require that the subscriber be a health care professional.

Mailing lists transmit information to their subscribers as individual messages or in digest form. The digest form is distributed as one e-mail document containing all the messages sent to the mailing list over a given time period, such as 24 hours. The digest form might be preferable to the individual messages because some mailing lists may send 100 or more messages per day, which can be inconvenient and more time-consuming to read. Most mailing lists also provide the subscriber with access to archived messages.

Newsgroups

Thousands of newsgroups exist on the Internet, and as the Internet has grown, so has the number of these groups. One can compare newsgroups with any public (electronic) bulletin board. Newsgroups are located on a part of the Internet known as the Usenet. Unlike mailing lists, one does not subscribe to a newsgroup. Instead access is made through software provided by an ISP or through the use of commercial software. Newsgroups provide a unique opportunity for individuals to meet and communicate with each other. However, most newsgroups are not moderated, so the quality of information found there may not be as high as that of mailing lists.

Usenet groups related to medical topics are very active and provide a network and means of support for individuals with a particular illness, such as cancer. On some commercial information services, one can access forums that function similarly to the newsgroups. However, participation is limited to members of that particular service only.

As a health care professional, one must be careful when responding to messages related to medical or nursing advice in newsgroups because it could be considered practicing nursing or medicine across state lines. Should someone decide to take legal action based on advice given via the Internet, some insurance carriers might not provide coverage in the event of malpractice. Although a disclaimer at the end of a message does not free one from liability, it could be helpful.

File Transfer Protocol

File transfer protocol (FTP) is a method of transferring electronic files to a personal computer from a remote computer. A wide variety of services are available through FTP, and one can obtain everything from the text of Supreme Court opinions to computer freeware and shareware.

Gopher

The gopher is an alternative type of web browser that enables the Internet user to browse for resources. The gopher is really an electronic version of the library card catalog. However, once the gopher service locates the needed information, it can retrieve the file on the host computer.

World Wide Web

Many people think that the World Wide Web (also known as the Web and abbreviated as "www") and the Internet are the same entity. However, the Web is only one part of the entire Internet. Information on this part of the Internet is written in hypertext markup language (HTML) and uses a hypertext transfer protocol (http), a special protocol that allows the user not only to read text, but also to view

pictures and movies and hear sound. This information can be transmitted using either regular or cellular telephone lines or fiberoptic lines. In addition, http and HTML enable the user to connect to other areas in the same document, other documents on the same computer, other Web sites, or other file transfer protocol (FTP) servers. For example, the user can access the Web site of the American Pain Society (*http://www.ampainsoc.org*) (Figure A-1) and link (move) directly to the International Association for the Study of Pain (IASP), the American Society for Pain Management Nursing (ASPMN), or other professional organization Web sites, and from those sites can branch out to other sites.

The type of software that enables the user to access sites on the Internet is called a Web browser. These browsers provide a graphical interface between the personal computer and the Internet so that the personal computer can "read" files on the Web.

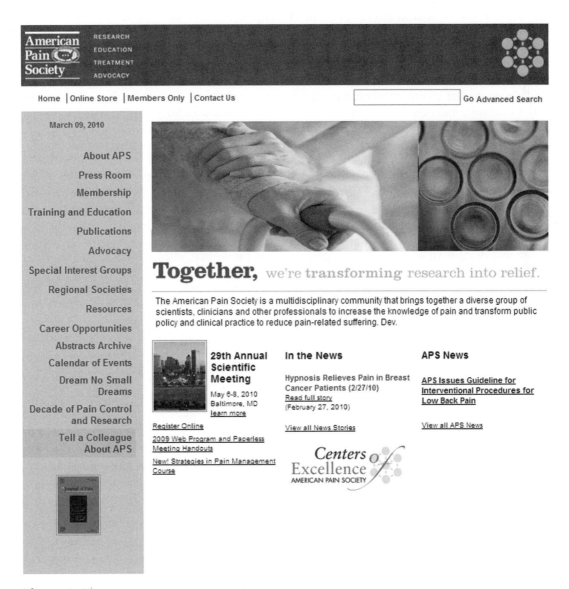

Figure A-1 | American Pain Society Web site home page.

The places where one can access information on the Web are called Web sites, which consist of one or more Web pages. The first page of a Web site, frequently referred to as the home page, often contains an index from which one can access other pages on the Web site via hyperlinks (see Figure A-1). Web addresses, also known as uniform resource locators (URLs), are used to simplify returning to a site. Because these addresses can be long and complicated, most Web browsers allow users to "bookmark" pages of interest.

Weblogs and Wikis

A weblog is defined as a "hierarchy of text, images, media objects and data, arranged chronologically, that can be viewed in an HTML browser" (Winer, 2003). It is often described simply as an online journal in which the content is presented unedited (non-peer reviewed) in the "voice" of one person. A wiki is best described as a weblog-like system that can be edited (such as Wikipedia). As such, a wiki generally consists of the edited (non–peer reviewed) voice of many persons. It is important for the user to understand the nature of weblogs and wikis to prevent misinterpretation of their information. For example, individuals seeking information regarding health care treatment may conduct online searches that yield results from both weblogs and wikis, and thus may contain personal opinion rather than evidence-based information. In addition, products are often advertised on weblogs and wikis and may detail "clinical outcomes" and personal testimonials that are not based in research. Health care professionals can reduce misunderstanding by educating patients and families about both the benefits and dangers of obtaining information from the World Wide Web.

Looking for Health Information on the Internet

The United States Department of Health and Human Services (U.S. DHHS, 2000) defines health literacy as "the degree to which individuals have the capacity to obtain, process, and understand basic health information and services needed to make appropriate health decisions." Given the vast amount of health information available online, looking for information on the Internet can be a daunting task, comparable to searching the card catalog at the library. However, because the Internet is an electronic database, one can search very large amounts of data in a very short time. For example, the keyword "pain" yields an impressive 239,000,000 sites. When the search is narrowed down to "acute pain," the number of sites decreases to 12,900,000.

Clearly the search should be narrowed to very specific terms, and more than one search may be necessary. Using the "help" function of the search engine to maximize its efficiency is strongly recommended. Some of the search engines' Web sites are listed in the selected list of Web sites at the end of this appendix.

Once the desired Web site has been located, one may wish to return to the site in the future without repeating the search. This can be done with the bookmark, or "favorite places," function on the Web browser. If more than one user is using the same browser, each person should have a different subset of bookmarks. A variety of Internet resources are listed at the end of this appendix.

Quality of Health Information on the Internet

In an early editorial in the *Journal of the American Medical Association,* Silberg, Lundberg, and Mussachio (1997) wrote, "Health care professionals and patients alike should view with equal parts delight and concern the exponential growth of the internet … The problem is not too little information but too much, vast chunks of it incomplete and not only in the medical arena." (p. 1244). The authors go so far as to call it "the world's largest vanity press," offering the warning "*Caveat lector et viewor*—let the reader and viewer beware."

If the Web is used as an information resource, the user must beware of its pitfalls. Much good information can be found on the Web, but the information should be scrutinized at least as carefully as one would do with other sources, such as journals and books. As mentioned, health care professionals need to let patients and families know that information from the Web may not be supported with sound scientific data, and some of the information may be false or deceptive. Additionally, it has been noted that health information found online is often incomplete and has poor readability, requiring at least a high school level of reading ability to understand content in both English and Spanish versions (Berland, Elliott, Morales, et al., 2001).

The Web presently remains a free-for-all, where anyone can post any information about any subject without the protection of the well-established standards applied to books and peer-reviewed journals. The industry continues to take a strong stand in developing ways to police this medium without legislation. Several initiatives involving government, industry, and professional organizations are being undertaken to improve the quality of medical information available on the Web. The National Library of Medicine and National Institutes of Health (2009), the United States Food and Drug Administration (U.S. FDA, 2005), and the American Association of Retired Persons (AARP, 2009) have all published online guides that may be used to evaluate health information Web sites. Assisting patients to become "Internet literate" as they seek out quality information available to them on the Internet is a crucial role of the health care professional. Some guidelines are listed in Box A-1. Additionally, health care professionals must be aware that a lack of access to Internet-sourced health information may represent an additional barrier to care for their patients and that issues of health literacy apply to this area of patient education as well (U.S. DHHS, 2009). Efforts to assist patients to identify available means to independently seek out quality health information encourage self-advocacy.

One resource to which health care professionals can confidently direct patients is "The Health On the Net Foundation (HON)" *(http://www.hon.ch/),* a nongovernmental organization whose mission is "to guide the growing community of healthcare consumers and providers on the World Wide Web to sound, reliable medical information and expertise" (HON, 2009). In this way, HON seeks to contribute to better and more accessible and cost-effective health care. Information on the organization's Web site is divided into content of interest to patients/individuals, medical professionals, and Web site publishers. Over 5000 links to quality health information, representing 72 countries, can be found at the HON site.

Mailing lists, Web sites, and e-mail addresses of interest to pain management clinicians and their patients are listed in Table A-1. The listing of a commercial Web site should not be considered an endorsement of the company or its products. The list was checked at the time of submission and found to be accurate, but addresses are subject to change by the provider of the service without prior notice.

Box A-1	Evaluating the Quality of Online Health Information

Questions to ask when evaluating health information found on the World Wide Web:*

- Who runs the site?
- Why have they created the site?
- What do they want from you? Do you have to pay to obtain information or products?
- Who is paying for the site?
- Does the site's information favor the sponsor?
- Is the information found on the site reviewed by experts?
- Where did the information come from?
- Does the site make unbelievable claims?
- Is the site up-to-date?
- Does the site ask for your personal information? If so, what will they do with it?

---

*Many of the answers to these questions can be found by using a Web site's sitemap, the "about us" page, or the main site page. An online tutorial, which gives examples of how to choose quality health information online, is available at the National Library of Medicine and National Institutes of Health's *Medline Plus* Web site.

As appears in Pasero, C., & McCaffery, M. (2011). *Pain assessment and pharmacologic management*, p. 823, St. Louis, Mosby. Data from National Library of Medicine (NLM) and National Institutes of Health (NIH). (2009). Evaluating Internet health information. Available at http://www.nlm.nih.gov/medlineplus/webeval/webeval.html. Accessed May 2, 2009. May be duplicated for use in clinical practice.

Table A-1	Selected List of Web Sites with Specific Application to the Pain Management Clinician

Sources for Pain-Related Information	Location
Agency for Health Care Policy and Research	*http://www.ahrq.gov*
Alliance of State Pain Initiatives	*http://www.aspi.wisc.edu*
Amedeo Medical Literature Service	*http://www.amedeo.com/*
Am J Nurs/Lippincott Nursing Center	*http://www.nursingcenter.com*
American Academy of Hospice and Palliative Care	*http://www.aahpm.org*
American Academy of Pain Management	*http://www.aapainmanage.org*
American Academy of Pain Medicine	*http://www.painmed.org*
American Academy of Neurology	*http://www.aan.com*
American Academy of Orofacial Pain	*http://www.aaop.org*
American Association of Neuroscience Nurses	*http://www.aann.org*
American Association for the Treatment of Opioid Dependence	*http://www.aatod.org*
American Cancer Society	*http://www.cancer.org*
American Chronic Pain Association	*http://www.theacpa.org*
American College of Apothecaries	*http://www.acainfo.org*
American College of Physician Homecare Guide for Advanced Cancer	*http://www.acponline.org/patients_families/end_of_life_issues/cancer/*
American Council for Headache Education	*http://www.achenet.org*

Continued

Table A-1 | Selected List of Web Sites with Specific Application to the Pain Management Clinician—cont'd

Sources for Pain-Related Information	Location
American Headache Society	http://www.americanheadachesociety.org
American Holistic Nurses Association	http://www.ahna.org
American Hospice Foundation	http://www.americanhospice.org
American Medical Association	http://www.ama-cmeonline.com
American Society of Interventional Pain Physicians	http://www.asipp.org
American Nurses Association	http://www.nursingworld.org
American Pain Foundation	http://www.painfoundation.org
American Pain Society	http://www.ampainsoc.org
American Pain Society & American Society for Pain Management Nursing List Serve Subscription	http://www.aspmn.org/Organization/listserv.htm
American Society of Anesthesiologists	http://www.asahq.org
American Society for Action on Pain	http://www.druglibrary.net/schaffer/asap/index.htm
American Society of Addiction Medicine	http://www.asipp.org
American Society of Pain Educators	http://www.paineducators.org
American Society for Pain Management Nursing	http://www.aspmn.org
American Society of PeriAnesthesia Nurses	http://www.aspan.org/
American Society of Regional Anesthesia & Pain Medicine	http://www.asra.com
Apparelyzed: Spinal Cord Injury Peer Support	http://www.apparelyzed.com/index.html
Arthritis Foundation	http://www.arthritis.org
Cancer Care	http://www.cancercare.org
Cancer-Pain.org	http://www.cancer-pain.org
Centers for Disease Control	http://www.cdc.gov
Center for Palliative Care Education	http://depts.washington.edu/pallcare/
Center to Advance Palliative Care	http://www.capc.org
Chronic Fatigue Immune Deficiency Syndrome Association of America	http://www.cfids.org/
Chronic Pain Association of Canada	http://www.chronicpaincanada.com
Chronic Pain Network™	http://www.chronicpainnetwork.com
City of Hope Pain and Palliative Care Resource Center	http://prc.coh.org/
CMEPain.com	http://www.cmepain.com
Complementary/Integrative Medicine (CIM) Education Resources	http://www.mdanderson.org/education-and-research/resources-for-professionals/clinical-tools-and-resources/cimer/
Emerging Solutions in Pain (ESP)	http://www.emergingsolutionsinpain.com
End of Life Nursing Education Consortium (ELNEC) Project through the American Association of Colleges of Nursing	http://www.aacn.nche.edu/ELNEC
Evidence-Based Medicine/Reference Sources	http://pain-topics.org/related_websites/#reference
Fibromyalgia Information Foundation	http://www.myalgia.com
Fibromyalgia Network	http://www.fmnetnews.com
Food and Drug Administration	http://www.FDA.gov
Gerontological Society of America	http://www.geron.org
Health On the Net Foundation	http://www.hon.ch/
Help for Headaches	http://www.headache-help.org
Hospice Foundation of America	http://www.hospicefoundation.org
Hospice & Palliative Nurses Association	http://www.hpna.org
International Association for the Study of Pain	http://www.iasp-pain.org
International Organizations (web links)	http://pain-topics.org/related_websites/#international
Last Acts (Robert Wood Johnson Foundation)	http://www.rwjf.org/pr/product.jsp?id=20938
The Mayday Pain Project	http://www.painandhealth.org
MD Anderson Cancer Center Pain Management Center	http://www.mdanderson.org/topics/paincontrol
MEDLINE	http://www.ncbi.nlm.nih.gov/pubmed/
Medscape	http://www.medscape.com
Memorial Sloan-Kettering Pain Control Program	http://www.mskcc.org/mskcc/html/474.cfm

Continued

| Table A-1 | Selected List of Web Sites with Specific Application to the Pain Management Clinician—cont'd |

Sources for Pain-Related Information	Location
Migraine Resource Network	*http://www.migraineresourcenetwork.com*
Morbidity and Mortality Weekly Report (MMWR)	*http://www.cdc.gov/mmwr/*
National Center for Complementary and Alternative Medicine	*http://www.nccam.nih.gov*
National Clearinghouse for Alcohol and Drug Information	*http://ncadi.samhsa.gov/*
National Council on Alcoholism and Drug Dependence	*http://www.ncadd.org*
National Foundation for the Treatment of Pain	*http://www.paincare.org*
National Fibromyalgia Association	*http://www.fmaware.org*
National Fibromyalgia Partnership	*http://www.fmpartnership.org*
National Fibromyalgia Research Association	*http://www.nfra.net*
National Headache Foundation	*http://www.headaches.org*
National Hospice Organization	*http://www.nho.org*
National Institute of Arthritis and Musculoskeletal and Skin Diseases	*http://www.niams.nih.gov/*
National Institutes of Health Pain Consortium	*http://painconsortium.nih.gov/*
National Institute for Nursing Research	*http://www.nih.gov/ninr*
National Library of Medicine	*http://www.nlm.nih.gov/*
National Organization for Rare Diseases (NORDO)	*http://www.rarediseases.org*
National Pain Education Council	*http://www.npecweb.org*
National Pain Foundation	*http://www.nationalpainfoundation.org*
National Palliative Care Research Center	*http://www.npcrc.org*
National Rehabilitation Information Center	*http://www.naric.com/*
National Shingles Foundation	*http://www.vzvfoundation.org*
National Vulvodynia Association	*http://www.nva.org*
The Neuropathy Association	*http://www.neuropathy.org*
Neurosciences on the Net	*http://www.neuroguide.com/*
Newsletter for Chronic Fatigue Syndrome	*http://www.cfs-news.org/cfs-news.htm*
North American Spine Society	*http://www.spine.org*
OncoLink	*http://cancer.med.upenn.edu/*
Oncology Nursing Society	*http://www.ons.org*
OncoPain Mailing List	A listserv for people coping with cancer pain. To subscribe, send an e-mail to *listserve@med.ucalgary.ca*; leave the subject line blank, and in the body of the message type: "subscribe oncopain ‹your first and last names›"
The Oxford Pain Internet Site	*http://www.medicine.ox.ac.uk/bandolier/booth/painpag/index2.html*
Pain and Policies Study Group	*http://www.painpolicy.wisc.edu*
Pain.com	*http://www.pain.com*
Pain Connection	*http://www.pain-connection.org*
PainEDU	*http://www.painedu.org*
Pain L Mailing List	A listserv for people coping with chronic pain. To subscribe, send an e-mail to *listserv@wvnvm.wvnet.edu*; leave the subject line blank, and in the body of the message type: "subscribe pain-l ‹your first and last names›"
PainKnowledge.org (National Initiative on Pain Control)	*http://www.painknowledge.org*
Pain and the Law	*http://www.painandthelaw.org*
Pain Management Online	*http://www.painmngt.com*
Pain Relief Network (PRN)	*http://www.painreliefnetwork.org*
Pain Treatment Topics	*http://pain-topics.org*
Power Over Pain Action Network	*http://www.painfoundation.org/poweroverpain/default.asp?file=network.htm*
Professional Journals, Magazines & Newsletters on Pain	*http://pain-topics.org/related_websites/#professional*

Continued

Table A-1	Selected List of Web Sites with Specific Application to the Pain Management Clinician—cont'd	
Sources for Pain-Related Information	**Location**
PROSPECT (**Pro**cedure **Spec**ific Postoperative Pain Managemen**t**)	*http://www.postoppain.org/*
PubMed (NLM Literature search engine)	*http://www.ncbi.nlm.nih.gov/PubMed*
Reflex Sympathetic Dystrophy Association of America	*http://www.rsds.org*
Sickle Cell Information Center	*http://www.scinfo.org/*
Sigma Theta Tau	*http://www.nursingsociety.org*
SpineUniverse	*http://www.spineuniverse.com*
Spondylitis Association of America	*http://www.spondylitis.org*
TMJ Association, Ltd.	*http://www.tmj.org*
Trigeminal Neuralgia Association	*http://www.endthepain.org*
Virtual Anaesthesia Textbook	*http://www.virtual-anaesthesia-textbook.com*
The Vulvar Pain Foundation	*http://www.vulvarpainfoundation.org*
WebMD Pain Management Health Center	*http://www.webmd.com/diseases_and_conditions/pain.htm*
World Wide Web search engine	*http://www.google.com*
World Wide Web search engine	*http://www.altavista.com*
World Wide Web search engine	*http://www.lycos.com*
World Wide Web search engine	*http://www.yahoo.com*

As appears in Pasero, C., & McCaffery, M. (2011). *Pain assessment and pharmacologic management*, pp. 823-826, St. Louis, Mosby. May be duplicated for use in clinical practice.

References

American Association of Retired Persons (AARP). (2009). *Checkups and prevention.* Available at http://www.aarp.org/health/staying_healthy/prevention/a2003-03-17-wwwhealth.html. Accessed April 29, 2009.

Berland, G. K., Elliott, M. N., Morales, L. M., et al. (2001). *Quality and readability in English and Spanish health information on the Internet: Accessibility.* Available at http://jama.ama-assn.org/cgi/reprint/285/20/2612. Accessed May 20, 2009.

Health On the Net Foundation (HON). (2009). *Mission and users.* Available at https://www.hon.ch/Global/HON_mission.html Accessed May 21, 2009.

National Library of Medicine (NLM) and the National Institutes of Health (NIH). (2009). *Evaluating Internet health information.* Available at http://www.nlm.nih.gov/medlineplus/webeval/webeval.html. Accessed May 2, 2009.

Netcraft. (2008). *October 2008 Web server survey.* Available at http://news.netcraft.com/archives/2008/10/29/october_2008_web_server_survey.html. Accessed May 21, 2009.

Nicoll, L. H., & Oulette, T. H. (1997). *Nurses' guide to the Internet.* Philadelphia: JB Lippincott.

Silberg, W. M., Lundberg, G. D., & Mussachio, R. A. (1997). Assessing, controlling and assuming the quality of medical information on the Internet: Caveat lector et viewor—Let the reader beware. *JAMA, 277*(15), 1244.

United States Department of Health and Human Services (DHHS). (2000). *Healthy People 2010: Understanding and Improving Health.* (2nd ed.). Washington, DC: U.S. Government Printing Office. Available at http://www.healthypeople.gov/Document/pdf/uih/2010uih.pdf. Accessed May 19, 2009.

United States Department of Health and Human Services (DHHS). Quick guide to health literacy. Available at http://www.health.gov/communication/literacy/quickguide/healthinfo.htm. Accessed May 5, 2009.

United States Food and Drug Administration (FDA). (2005). How to evaluate health information on the Internet. Available at http://www.fda.gov/Drugs/ResourcesForYou/Consumers/BuyingUsingMedicineSafely/BuyingMedicinesOvertheInternet/ucm202863.htm. Accessed June 3, 2010.

Winer, D. (2003). *Weblogs at Harvard Law, hosted by the Berkman Center for Internet & Society at Harvard Law School.* Available at http://blogs.law.harvard.edu/whatmakesaweblogaweblog.html. Accessed May 8, 2009.

Appendix B Clinical Aspects of the Use of Opioid Agreements for Chronic Noncancer Pain

Steven D. Passik and Kenneth L. Kirsh

UTILIZING written agreements that clearly state the roles of the prescribing clinician and the rules and expectations for the patient is helpful when structuring chronic noncancer pain treatment and is becoming more commonplace, despite a general lack of research attention (Brooke, 1998; Fishman, Kreis, 2002; Kowal, 1998). Agreements for patients in palliative care are also being discussed but are not widely used. Considerable controversy exists about the use of agreements with this population. This section focuses on noncancer pain, but many of the principles apply to patients with chronic cancer-related pain.

Numerous opioid agreements for chronic noncancer pain exist, but there is no universally accepted one (Passik, Kirsh, 2005). Many clinicians have found that it takes considerable time to development an agreement that meets the needs of their patient population and clinical setting. To offer guidance in the preparation of agreements, two sample forms are included in Figures B-1 and B-2. These are suggested by the American Academy of Pain Medicine (AAPM): "Consent for Chronic Opioid Therapy," (1999) (pp. 828-829) and "Long-Term Controlled Substances Therapy for Chronic Pain: Sample Agreement." (2001) (pp. 830-831). However, these probably will not meet the needs of all providers and patients in all clinical settings and may need to be modified and structured to fit individual practices and clinics.

Despite being poorly studied overall, recent research indicates that they can be useful and even be used successfully in primary care clinics (Hariharan, Lamb, Neuner, et al., 2007). A survey of internal medicine residents found that use of pain management agreements resulted in a greater level of confidence and a greater sense of reward as well as more positive attitudes toward treating patients with chronic noncancer pain (Fagan, Chen, Diaz, et al., 2008).

Clarifying Agreements versus Contracts

Before progressing further, it is imperative that common terminology be employed when discussing this topic. It is extremely common to have health professionals of all varieties and backgrounds interchangeably refer to these documents as either agreements or contracts. However, we must avoid this potential pitfall as nuances do matter greatly.

The terms *contract* and *agreement* both suggest an arrangement between two or more parties as to a specific course of action, such as something that is to be done or not done. An agreement can be anything from a mutual understanding to a binding obligation. Contracts are most often used in law and business for agreements that are legally enforceable. Thus contracts usually have legal and punitive connotations, suggesting a level of mistrust, whereas agreements imply that the parties have reached amicable arrangements that are freely accepted by all

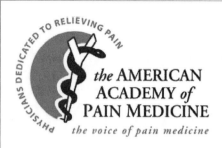

Consent for Chronic Opioid Therapy

A consent form from the **American Academy of Pain Medicine**

Dr. _____ is prescribing opioid medicine, sometimes called narcotic analgesics, to me for a diagnosis of _____.

This decision was made because my condition is serious or other treatments have not helped my pain.

I am aware that the use of such medicine has certain risks associated with it, including, but not limited to: sleepiness or drowsiness, constipation, nausea, itching, vomiting, dizziness, allergic reaction, slowing of breathing rate, slowing of reflexes or reaction time, physical dependence, tolerance to analgesia, addiction and possibility that the medicine will not provide complete pain relief.

I am aware about the possible risks and benefits of other types of treatments that do not involve the use of opioids. The other treatments discussed included:

_____

_____

_____

I will tell my doctor about all other medicines and treatments that I am receiving.

I will not be involved in any activity that may be dangerous to me or someone else if I feel drowsy or am not thinking clearly. I am aware that even if I do not notice it, my reflexes and reaction time might still be slowed. Such activities include, but are not limited to: using heavy equipment or a motor vehicle, working in unprotected heights or being responsible for another individual who is unable to care for himself or herself.

I am aware that certain other medicines such as nalbuphine (Nubain™), pentazocine (Talwin™), buprenorphine (Buprenex™), and butorphanol (Stadol™), may reverse the action of the medicine I am using for pain control. Taking any of these other medicines while I am taking my pain medicines can cause symptoms like a bad flu, called a withdrawal syndrome. I agree not to take any of these medicines and to tell any other doctors that I am taking an opioid as my pain medicine and cannot take any of the medicines listed above.

I am aware that addiction is defined as the use of a medicine even if it causes harm, having cravings for a drug, feeling the need to use a drug and a decreased quality of life. I am aware that the chance of becoming addicted to my pain medicine is very low. I am aware that the development of addiction has been reported rarely in medical journals and is much more common in a person who has a family or personal history of addiction. I agree to tell my doctor my complete and honest personal drug history and that of my family to the best of my knowledge.

Continued

Figure B-1 │ Consent for chronic opioid therapy.

I understand that physical dependence is a normal, expected result of using these medicines for a long time. I understand that physical dependence is not the same as addiction. I am aware physical dependence means that if my pain medicine use is markedly decreased, stopped or reversed by some of the agents mentioned above, I will experience a withdrawal syndrome. This means I may have any or all of the following: runny nose, yawning, large pupils, goose bumps, abdominal pain and cramping, diarrhea, irritability, aches throughout my body and a flu-like feeling. I am aware that opioid withdrawal is uncomfortable but not life threatening.

I am aware that tolerance to analgesia means that I may require more medicine to get the same amount of pain relief. I am aware that tolerance to analgesia does not seem to be a big problem for most patients with chronic pain, however, it has been seen and may occur to me. If it occurs, increasing doses may not always help and may cause unacceptable side effects. Tolerance or failure to respond well to opioids may cause my doctor to choose another form of treatment.

(Males only) I am aware that chronic opioid use has been associated with low testosterone levels in males. This may affect my mood, stamina, sexual desire and physical and sexual performance. I understand that my doctor may check my blood to see if my testosterone level is normal.

(Females Only) If I plan to become pregnant or believe that I have become pregnant while taking this pain medicine, I will immediately call my obstetric doctor and this office to inform them. I am aware that, should I carry a baby to delivery while taking these medicines, the baby will be physically dependent upon opioids. I am aware that the use of opioids is not generally associated with a risk of birth defects. However, birth defects can occur whether or not the mother is on medicines and there is always the possibility that my child will have a birth defect while I am taking an opioid.

I have read this form or have it read to me. I understand all of it. I have had a chance to have all of my questions regarding this treatment answered to my satisfaction. By signing this form voluntarily, I give my consent for the treatment of my pain with opioid pain medicines.

Patient signature _____ Date _____

Witness to above _____

Approved by the AAPM Executive Committee on January 14, 1999.

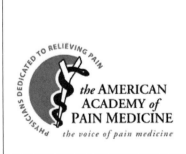

4700 W. Lake Avenue
Glenview, IL 60025-1485
847/375-4731
Fax 847/375-6477
E-mail info@painmed.org
Web site www.painmed.org

Figure B-1 | Cont'd.

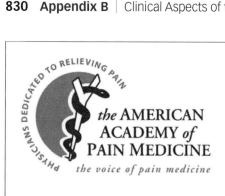

Long-Term Controlled Substances Therapy for Chronic Pain

SAMPLE AGREEMENT

*A consent form from the **American Academy of Pain Medicine***

The purpose of this agreement is to protect your access to controlled substances and to protect our ability to prescribe for you.

The long-term use of such substances as opioids (narcotic analgesics), benzodiazepine tranquilizers, and barbiturate sedatives is controversial because of uncertainty regarding the extent to which they provide long-term benefit. There is also the risk of an addictive disorder developing or of relapse occurring in a person with a prior addiction. The extent of this risk is not certain.

Because these drugs have potential for abuse or diversion, strict accountability is necessary when use is pro-longed. For this reason the following policies are agreed to by you, the patient, as consideration for, and a condition of, the willingness of the physician whose signature appears below to consider the initial and/or continued prescription of controlled substances to treat your chronic pain.

1. All controlled substances must come from the physician whose signature appears below or, during his or her absence, by the covering physician, unless specific authorization is obtained for an exception. (Multiple sources can lead to untoward drug interactions or poor coordination of treatment.)

2. All controlled substances must be obtained at the same pharmacy, where possible. Should the need arise to change pharmacies, our office must be informed. The pharmacy that you have selected is:

    _____ phone: _____.

3. You are expected to inform our office of any new medications or medical conditions, and of any adverse effects you experience from any of the medications that you take.

4. The prescribing physician has permission to discuss all diagnostic and treatment details with dispensing pharmacists or other professionals who provide your health care for purposes of maintaining accountability.

5. You may not share, sell, or otherwise permit others to have access to these medications.

6. These drugs should not be stopped abruptly, as an abstinence syndrome will likely develop.

7. Unannounced urine or serum toxicology screens may be requested, and your cooperation is required. Presence of unauthorized substances may prompt referral for assessment for addictive disorder.

Continued

Figure B-2 | Long-term controlled substances therapy for chronic pain: Sample agreement.

8. Prescriptions and bottles of these medications may be sought by other individuals with chemical dependency and should be closely safeguarded. It is expected that you will take the highest possible degree of care with your medication and prescriptions. They should not be left where others might see or otherwise have access to them.

9. Original containers of medications should be brought in to each office visit.

10. Since the drugs may be hazardous or lethal to a person who is not tolerant to their effects, especially a child, you must keep them out of reach of such people.

11. Medications may not be replaced if they are lost, get wet, are destroyed, left on an airplane, etc. If your medication has been stolen and you complete a police report regarding the theft, an exception may be made.

12. Early refills will generally not be given.

13. Prescriptions may be issued early if the physician or patient will be out of town when a refill is due. These prescriptions will contain instructions to the pharmacist that they not be filled prior to the appropriate date.

14. If the responsible legal authorities have questions concerning your treatment, as might occur, for example, if you were obtaining medications at several pharmacies, all confidentiality is waived and these authorities may be given full access to our records of controlled substances administration.

15. It is understood that failure to adhere to these policies may result in cessation of therapy with controlled substance prescribing by this physician or referral for further specialty assessment.

16. Renewals are contingent on keeping scheduled appointments. Please do not phone for prescriptions after hours or on weekends.

17. It should be understood that any medical treatment is initially a trial, and that continued prescription is contingent on evidence of benefit.

18. The risks and potential benefits of these therapies are explained elsewhere [and you acknowledge that you have received such explanation].

19. You affirm that you have full right and power to sign and be bound by this agreement, and that you have read, understand, and accept all of its terms.

_____   _____
Physician Signature   Patient Signature

_____   _____
Date   Patient Name (Printed)

Approved by the AAPM Executive Committee on April 2, 2001.

AAPM
4700 W. Lake Avenue
Glenview, IL 60025-1485
847/375-4731 Fax 847/375-6477
E-mail info@painmed.org
Web site http://www.painmed.org/

Figure B-2 | Cont'd.

parties and are open to change. Therefore the term *agreement* is used in this discussion, and use of the term *contract* is discouraged.

We must also remember that patients have certain rights, such as those stipulated by the Joint Commission on Accreditation of Healthcare Organizations (JCAHO, 1998). These include the right to considerate and respectful care, the right to effective pain management, and the right to make decisions about their medical care. A Bill of Rights for patients in pain states that a patient should be treated with respect at all times and not like a drug abuser (McCaffery, Pasero, 1999). An important consideration in evaluating written agreements is whether they violate these or other patients' rights. While some have postulated that the conditions found in many agreements are intimidating, convey mistrust, and are inflexible with regard to amount and frequency of opioid patients are allowed to take (Rose, 1996), we argue that utilizing agreements for all patients ultimately serves to protect them and actually empowers them as having responsibility as a partner in their own health care.

A related construct to the notion of an agreement is the term *consent*. When information is given to the patient verbally or in writing and is documented appropriately in the patient's record, it constitutes informed consent, and the signatures of the patient and clinician are not necessary (Bolen, 2006). However, some states have regulations or acts of law, such as the Intractable Pain Treatment Act, that require or recommend a signed consent form. (See Figure B-1 for an example.) Regardless of whether the consent is signed, the patient's medical record should reflect that informed consent was given. This also helps to cement the idea of the patient being an active participant in his or her health care.

The Philosophy Behind the Agreement: Education/Motivating versus Infantilizing

An opioid agreement (OA) can be nothing more than a piece of paper if it is signed, sealed, and placed in the patient's medical record and never discussed or examined again. Before their use became recognized as a more or less universal aspect of setting the stage for opioid pain management, OAs were often worse than a neglected piece of paper; rather they sometimes served as an infantilizing "invitation to get oneself discharged," drawn up and signed after a transgression by the patient angered the prescriber. At its best, an OA can be educational, informative, and even motivational if it helps the patient understand opioid therapy and how it differs from other drug therapies in which adherence to the rules of drug-taking are not nearly as emphasized (Table B-1). In addition, they can be helpful in reducing multiple prescribers and abuse, and clarifying goals of treatment (Fagan, Chen, Diaz,

et al., 2008; Manchikanti, Manchukonda, Damron, et al., 2006). At its worst, an OA is inflexible, tersely worded, and infantilizing. For example, the question "Why isn't it OK to raise my dose on my own?" is complex. The answer to such a question is grounded in the possibility of overdosing, the risk of addiction, the philosophy of acceptance and responsibility for living fully with chronic pain, the need for the patient to carry out drug trials in complex pain problems, the need to decentralize drug-taking as the only way to cope with pain, and many other complicated ideas, all of which are important aspects of the psycho-education of the chronic pain patient.

The agreement itself might not be able to cover all of the above-mentioned issues, but clearly it is a starting point, and an overly terse agreement lacking in flexibility and educational content is a missed opportunity for orienting the patient right from the initiation of treatment. We prefer an agreement with a preamble—one that points out the risks and benefits of opioid drugs and gives explanations for the "rules" that follow. This way, right from the start the parameters of opioid therapy are properly contextualized and can actually spawn a discussion of mutual goal setting. Otherwise, the possibilities mentioned above (expression of anger, estrangement, clinic vs. patient) are simply a poorly disguised exercise in protecting medical licensure and are readily obvious to the patient who may wonder why the prescribing clinician is questioning his or her good faith. See Table B-1 for more opioid agreement guidelines.

Universality and How the OA Is Given to the Patient

Clearly, if a clinic is to avoid bias and the accusation that they are consciously or unconsciously singling out only the problematic patients—or worse, patients of a certain age or ethnic group—the use of an OA should be clinicwide at the outset of opioid therapy. The agreement should be handed out and introduced as an exercise in mutual trust and goal setting by the clinic staff. Ideally, the OA would be introduced and discussed by the professional (not clerical) staff. Loading it into a stack of questionnaires, insurance forms, releases, and so on, to be filled out in the waiting area should be avoided. This is an opportunity to educate, not simply obtain another (unread, but signed) form for the chart.

Flexible Language

The language in the OA should be flexible. Otherwise, the staff is likely to be in violation of its agreement as often as the patient. There has been legal precedent for the successful suing of a pain prescriber for contributing to the addiction of his patient (Weiner, Wettstein, 1993) because he was

Table B-1 | General Guidelines to Consider When Using an Opioid Agreement (OA)

General Opioid Agreement Guidelines	
Do	**Avoid**
Clearly identify the provider who will be prescribing medications, along with office hours and contact information	Ignoring a listing of pertinent contact information
Have the OA explained by the physician	Having the clerical staff present the OA along with other clinic forms such as insurance paperwork
Use the OA as a talking tool to educate patients about pain and potential therapies as well as their responsibilities in the relationship	Making it another clinic sheet that is filed in the chart and largely forgotten
Use a preamble to set the stage for therapy	Using the OA as a preemptive means to infantilize the patient and as a threat that they will be "kicked out" of the practice
Use the OA early in the course of treatment, preferably on admission to the practice	Using the OA as a punitive measure for patients who have already misbehaved and setting limits for them when you are angry
Use OAs with all patients	Selecting only those patients who have proven to be noncompliant or just seem suspicious
Keep the language in the OA flexible	Using strong language that offers no flexibility for the clinician
Ensure that the reading level is appropriate, and consider developing a separate, low-literacy version if needed	Using overly technical language and medical jargon that is not normally used in daily conversation
Outline the goals of therapy and the responsibility of the prescriber	Making the OA a one-sided list of warnings and directions to be followed by the patient

As appears in Pasero, C., & McCaffery, M. (2011). *Pain assessment and pharmacologic management*, p. 833, St. Louis, Mosby. © 2011, Passik SD, Kirsh KL. May be duplicated for use in clinical practice.

in violation of his own agreement that stated that no early renewals of opioid prescriptions would be granted. Thus, "No early refills of opioid medications will be granted" should be replaced by: "Running out of your medication early is a complicated matter that can be confusing to your medical team. It could mean your pain is poorly controlled; it could mean you have been losing control over how you use your medications; or it could mean someone is borrowing or stealing your medications (among other possibilities)." Early refills are generally frowned upon since the response to a request for an early renewal is based on why the patient has run out early in the first place. This may be phrased as "Early renewals will be given at the discretion of your medical team." In addition, we must always remember that violations of the agreement might be due to a range of issues from misunderstanding, pseudoaddiction, chemical coping, or more illicit behaviors such as frank abuse or diversion (Pankratz, Hickam, Toth, 1989; Portenoy, 1994; Weissman, Haddox, 1989). As such, flexible language in the OA allows the clinician an opportunity to test these hypotheses and determine the true nature and cause of the infraction.

Another important point to consider when contemplating the language in an opioid agreement is the overall reading level required of the patient potentially signing the document. As a profound first step in exploring the literacy level required to comprehend opioid agreements, Roskos and colleagues (2007) examined 162 agreements for readability. Their findings should cause us to take notice, as the average reading level required nearly 14 years of education and were printed in a relatively small font size. In addition, technical medical language was often used along with other terms not considered part of typical daily conversation. To address this potential gap between providers and patients, Wallace and colleagues (2007) developed a low-literacy version of an opioid agreement. While only tested on a small sample of patients (n = 18), it nonetheless meets the needs of reducing readability to a seventh-grade reading level combined with larger font sizes and clear language.

Limit Setting

When to Do It?

One of the authors (SP) was fortunate to have been a psychology intern at the Payne Whitney Clinic of Cornell Medical Center and was, therefore, able to present cases to Dr. Otto Kernberg. Dr. Kernberg is one of the most famous and influential psychoanalytic thinkers on the treatment of personality disorders, and one who often employed limit setting in his work to curtail self-destructive and other acting out behaviors (Kernberg, 2004). One particular professor's rounds involved the inpatient management of the borderline personality disorder patient, and therapeutic interventions and limit setting were being discussed. In his intuitive way, he clearly picked up the staff's conscious and unconscious anger, and he sensed that their desire to ink a treatment "contract" was clearly a way for the staff to write out an invitation for discharge for the patient to sign. He warned to "never set limits when you are angry!" Dr. Kernberg's insights are important here, and not merely because OAs are an exercise in limit setting in some instances and that estimates exist that a very high percentage of chronic pain patients have personality disorders (Weisberg, Keefe, 1997; Weissberg, 1993). While universally employing OAs at the outset of opioid therapy in the clinic may diffuse some of this anger, the issue actually requires a further psychologic step back by the pain clinician. When did your OA originate in your clinic? Was it right after you were duped or burned? Is the legacy of one dishonest person going to make you infantilize or become estranged from your future patients? And is the language reflective of your desire to be an educator, caregiver, and motivator, or is it to be a heavy-handed enforcer?

Given that some of the patients treated with opioids may be known to have (or will come to be known to have) personality disorders, another principle of when to intervene may apply to OAs. Dr. Fred Pine, in a paper many years ago on psychologic work with the "ego weak" patient, recommended "striking while the iron is cold" (Mahler, Pine, Bergman, 1975). Following this principal, the timing of when to discuss and sign the opioid agreement might be best at the entry to clinic, even before opioids are contemplated for some patients. For some others, it might be best to sign the agreement sometime after an initial more liberal titration period so the patient feels cared for and somewhat better and avoids confusion about the rules.

Who Signs the OA?

Up to this point, we have been discussing a very traditional agreement that is signed by both the prescribing clinician and the patient. However, other models do exist and may prove to be even more valuable in the treatment context if they are at all feasible within the clinic and community setting. In the case of a patient referred to a specialty pain clinic by a primary care provider, it should be possible to have a tripartite or trilateral agreement wherein the patient, primary care provider, and pain specialist all sign an agreement (Fishman, Mahajan, Jung, et al., 2002). This can help lead to clarification of roles for

everyone involved as well as broaden avenues for cross-communication and collaboration. As recent research has shown (Wilkens, Belgrade, 2008), the satisfaction level of primary care providers with referrals to pain specialists has been relatively poor overall. While a trilateral agreement will not obviate all of this dissatisfaction, it does begin a dialogue and can help to address the issue.

Another novel possibility, potentially a quadrilateral agreement, would include pharmacists as part of the treatment team. Pharmacists are an often forgotten part of the health care equation, but ultimately control the flow of medication to communities. In addition, the role of pharmacists is changing in our society to include more medication oversight and guidance with patients (Tommasello, 2004). Since most agreements specify that a patient should choose one pharmacy and stick with it, it becomes possible to identify a potential pharmacist at the pharmacy where the patient chooses to fill his or her prescriptions. This again increases communication to all parties involved and helps the pharmacist to understand that legitimate prescriptions are being issued. It must be remembered that, in states with electronic reporting, pharmacists are typically required to enter all scheduled medications filled at their pharmacies and report this to state officials along with any potentially suspicious activity. Traditionally, this has caused a great deal of adversarial interactions between prescribers and pharmacists (Strickland, Huskey, Brushwood, 2007). With their inclusion in the agreement process, pharmacists can feel more comfortable filling scheduled prescriptions when an agreement and line of communication has been established.

Correlates to Urine Drug Screening

The decision to implement or not implement an OA shares some similarities clinically with the decision of whether or not to order a urine drug screen. Clinicians must control and monitor drug use in all patients, but there tends to be some selection bias with regard to the ordering and follow-up with urine drug screens. While urine toxicology screening has the potential to be a useful tool to the practicing clinician both for diagnosing potential abuse problems as well as monitoring patients with an established history of abuse, it should not be limited solely to those who are deemed problematic. Indeed, urine screens, like OAs, should be employed with all patients and explained as a tool to both protect the clinician as well as the patient. Simply put, a patient providing appropriate urine screens is able to show this as an objective measure of compliance to family, friends, and employers among others. For the main topic at hand, urine screens should be explained in the OA in just this fashion.

However, a chart review of the ordering and documentation of urine toxicology screens (UTSs) suggests that

UTSs are employed infrequently in tertiary care centers (Passik, Schreiber, Kirsh, et al., 2000). In addition, when urine tests are ordered, documentation tends to be inconsistent regarding the reasons for ordering as well as any follow-up recommendations based on the results. Indeed, the chart review found that nearly 40% of the charts surveyed listed no reason for obtaining the UTS, and the ordering provider could not be identified nearly 30% of the time. Staff education efforts can help to address this problem and may ultimately make urine toxicology screens a vital part of treating pain patients.

When ordering a UTS, it is important to remember that a clear understanding of these tests is critical. Although UTSs are an important tool, they should always be interpreted within the context of an individual patient and his or her circumstances. Unfortunately, prescribers using UTSs are often not proficient in interpretation of the results (Reisfield, Bertholf, Barkin, et al., 2007; Reisfield, Webb, Bertholf, et al., 2007). It is not uncommon for patients to be "discharged" or "fired" from a practice if their UTS is negative for the substances being prescribed. However, we must be aware of potential timing effects. For instance, if a patient is given hydromorphone and takes the last dose around 6 PM, has an office visit the next day at 10 AM, and provides a urine sample some time later, the UTS should come back negative. In this case, the patient had not taken any medication for 16 to 18 hours. Given that the half-life of hydromorphone is 2 to 3 hours, a total of 5 half-lives would be around 15 hours, and we should therefore expect a negative UTS. When questions arise, it is always best to contact the lab and ask for clarification on results.

Conclusion

In our review of the literature above, it might be correctly stated that there has never been an empirical study that has decisively shown that the use of an OA sets the stage for better outcomes in opioid therapy. But as you have read through this clinical section, it may be evident why this is so—has there to date been a study that has really captured the clinical nuances of language, attitude, timing, and context that can so subtly influence the pain clinician–pain patient relationship? Unfortunately, the development of such a study is unlikely. So, in the end, we hope to have made clinicians more thoughtful about their agreement and how they use it. Successful outcomes in pain management depend upon how well we motivate our patients to take responsibility for active participation in their recovery (Turk, Gatchel, 2002), and how they use their medications is one aspect of this. The OA can be a meaningless piece of paper, or it can be the codification of an ongoing dialogue that informs, motivates, and sets such a process in motion.

References

American Academy of Pain Medicine (AAPM). (1999). *Consent for Chronic Opioid Therapy*. (Review 2004). Available at www.painmed.org/pdf/opioid_consent_form.pdf. Accessed March, 12, 2009.

American Academy of Pain Medicine (AAPM). (2001). *Long-term controlled substances therapy for chronic pain: Sample agreement*. Available at http://www.painmed.org/pdf/controlled_substances_sample_agrmt.pdf. Accessed March, 18, 2009.

Bolen, J. (2006). Getting informed consent and agreement for treatment right: A legal perspective on key obligations for practitioners who use controlled substances to treat chronic pain. *Journal of Opioid Management*, 2(4), 193–200.

Brooke, C. (1998). Management of the hard to evaluate pain patient. *ASPMN Pathways*, 7(1), 14.

Fagan, M. J., Chen, J. T., Diaz, J. A., et al. (2008). Do internal medicine residents find pain medication agreements useful? *The Clinical Journal of Pain*, 24(1), 35–38.

Fishman, S. M., & Kreis, P. (2002). The opioid contract. *The Clinical Journal of Pain*, 18(Suppl 4), S70–S75.

Fishman, S. M., Mahajan, G., Jung, S. W., et al. (2002). The trilateral opioid contract. Bridging the pain clinic and the primary care physician through the opioid contract. *Journal of Pain and Symptom Management*, 24(3), 335–344.

Hariharan, J., Lamb, G. C., & Neuner, J. M. (2007). Long-term opioid contract use for chronic pain management in primary care practice. A five year experience. *Journal of General Internal Medicine*, 22(4), 485–490.

Joint Commission on Accreditation of Healthcare Organizations. (1998). *Hospital accreditation standards*. Oakbrook Terrace, IL: The Commission.

Kernberg, O. F. (2004). Perversion, perversity, and normality: Diagnostic and therapeutic considerations. In O. F. Kernberg (Ed.), *Aggressivity, narcissism, and self-destructiveness in the psychotherapeutic relationship: New developments in the psychopathology and psychotherapy of severe personality disorders*. New Haven, CT: Yale University Press.

Kowal, N. (1998). Evaluate patient outcomes. *ASPMN Pathways*, 7(1), 7.

Mahler, M., Pine, F., & Bergman, A. (1975). *The psychological birth of the human infant*. New York: Basic Books.

Manchikanti, L., Manchukonda, R., Damron, K. S., et al. (2006). Does adherence monitoring reduce controlled substance abuse in chronic pain patients? *Pain Physician*, 9(1), 57–60.

McCaffery, M., & Pasero, C. (1999). *Pain: Clinical manual*. St. Louis: Mosby.

Pankratz, L., Hickam, D., & Toth, S. (1989). The identification and management of drug-seeking behavior in a medical center. *Drug and Alcohol Dependence*, 24(2), 115–118.

Passik, S. D., & Kirsh, K. L. (2005). Managing pain in patients with aberrant drug-taking behaviors. *The Journal of Supportive Oncology*, 3(1), 83–86.

Passik, S. D., Schreiber, J., Kirsh, K. L., et al. (2000). A chart review of the ordering and documentation of urine toxicology screens in a cancer center: do they influence patient management? *Journal of Pain and Symptom Management*, 19(1), 40–44.

Portenoy, R. K. (1994). Opioid therapy for chronic nonmalignant pain: Current status. In H. L. Fields, & J. C. Liebeskind

(Eds.), *Progress in pain research and management*, vol. 1. Seattle: IASP Press.

Reisfield, G. M., Bertholf, R., Barkin, R. L., et al. (2007). Urine drug test interpretation: What do physicians know? *Journal of Opioid Management*, 3(2), 80–86.

Reisfield, G. M., Webb, F. J., Bertholf, R. L., et al. (2007). Family physicians' proficiency in urine drug test interpretation. *Journal of Opioid Management*, 3(6), 333–337.

Rose, H. L. (1996). Re: Formal treatment agreements for opioids in nonmalignant pain. *Journal of Pain and Symptom Management*, 12(4), 206–207.

Roskos, S. E., Keenum, A. J., Newman, L. M., et al. (2007). Literacy demands and formatting characteristics of opioid contracts in chronic nonmalignant pain management. *The Journal of Pain*, 8(10), 753–758.

Strickland, J. M., Huskey, A., & Brushwood, D. B. (2007). Pharmacist-physician collaboration in pain management practice. *Journal of Opioid Management*, 3(6), 295–301.

Tommasello, A. C. (2004). Substance abuse and pharmacy practice: What the community pharmacist needs to know about drug abuse and dependence. *Harm Reduct J*, 1(1), 3.

Turk, D. C., & Gatchel, R. J. (2002). *Psychological approaches to pain management: A practitioner's handbook*. New York: Guilford Press.

Wallace, L. S., Keenum, A. J., Roskos, S. E., et al. (2007). Development and validation of a low-literacy opioid contract. *The Journal of Pain*, 8(10), 759–766.

Weiner, B. A., & Wettstein, R. M. (1993). Professional liability. In B. A. Weiner, & R. M. Wettstein (Eds.), *Legal issues in mental health care*. New York: Springer.

Weisberg, J. N., & Keefe, F. J. (1997). Personality disorders in the chronic pain population: Basic concepts, empirical findings, and clinical implications. *Pain Forum*, 6(1), 1–9.

Weissberg, M. (1993). Multiple personality disorder and iatrogenesis: The cautionary tale of Anna O. *The International Journal of Clinical and Experimental Hypnosis*, 41(1), 15–34.

Weissman, D. E., & Haddox, J. D. (1989). Opioid pseudoaddiction—An iatrogenic syndrome. *Pain*, 36(3), 363–366.

Wilkens, J. R., & Belgrade, M. J. (2008). Do pain specialists meet the needs of the referring physician? A survey of primary care providers. *Journal of Opioid Management*, 4(1), 13–20.

Appendix C Use of Electronic Medical Records in Pain Management

Karen Kaiser

AN *electronic health record* is a broad term that includes portable electronic or web-based health records, electronic office-based care management systems, and *electronic medical record (EMR)* systems used by health care facilities such as acute, subacute, and long-term health care institutions. There are numerous synonyms for an electronic health record, with EMR being widely used. So, while some consider EMRs a subset of the electronic health record, others use the terms synonymously. The term *EMR* used in this Appendix applies to electronic systems implemented by institutions to store, share, and process patient information. While an EMR contains patient medical information found in a paper record, it also facilitates communication electronically and integrates clinical decision support. The latter is computer software consisting of a knowledge base that assists clinicians in making decisions about patient management. For example, clinical decision support systems include allergy checking, dose range checking, and drug interactions. See Box C-1 for terminology that will be used throughout this appendix and may be unfamiliar.

The implementation of an EMR system is expensive, resource intensive, and requires major changes in health care delivery processes, affecting routine daily activities of health care professionals. For this reason, EMRs have not been widely adopted. However, government, accrediting, and industry initiatives are providing the impetus for EMR implementation and moving the health care industry into the information age because of the numerous advantages over paper records (Pathways for medication safety, 2007; Leapfrog Group safety practices: Computerized physician order entry, 2009). EMR systems facilitate communication among health care professionals across care delivery sites, improve care coordination, increase patient safety, improve compliance with guidelines, and are useful in conducting research, auditing care process, assessing patient outcomes, and other activities (Cowell, 2007; Doran, Mylopoulos, Kushniruk, et al., 2007; Garg, Adhikari, McDonald, et al., 2005; Gruner, Ljutow, Schleinzer, et al., 2008; Hidle, 2007; Hunt, Haynes, Hanna, et al., 1998; Kaushal, Shojania, Bates, 2003; Nemeth, Wessell, Jenkins, et al., 2007; Wager, Lee, White, et al., 2000; Wolfstadt, Gurwitz, Field, et al., 2008).

Other than the use of pain diaries, little has been published about how the EMR can be used to safely and effectively assess and manage pain as well as meet accreditation requirements. Following is a discussion of how the EMR can help achieve these goals by using customized medication reconciliation; electronic dose range checking; medication order entry, preparation, and administration including range dose orders; pain documentation; and auditing pain processes.

Box C-1 | Terminology

Alert fatigue: The bypassing of computer warnings without consideration of their message to expedite computer order entry processes; usually caused by excessive numbers of alerts, many of which are not helpful.

Clinical decision support: Computer software consisting of a knowledge base that is used to assist clinicians in making choices about patient management, such as allergy checking, dose range checking, and drug interaction software.

Diluent: The amount of solution mixed with a medication to dilute it.

Drop-down box: A blank rectangle in the electronic record where the user can select one of a variety of prespecified responses by clicking on the three grayed out dots (...) in the right side of the box.

Dose range checking: The process by which the prescribed amount of a medication is checked against recommended upper and lower dose limits in a drug database.

eMAR: An electronic medication administration record, where drugs that have been prescribed are listed as an order sentence, with scheduled administration times if appropriate and a spot to electronically document administration.

Failure Effects Mode Analysis (FEMA): A process by which the consequences of actual or potential failures or errors that can be made in a process, design, or by an item are reviewed.

Free text field: A section where the prescriber can type any information he or she desires into that section up to the limit set by the computer program or programmer, as in a Comments section of a form.

Medication reconciliation: A process that occurs at times of transition between patient care settings in which medications that are currently being prescribed for a patient are checked against those that were taken in the previous care setting to minimize duplication, drug interactions, and omissions.

Order sentence: An electronic version of an order with all of its required components, such as a medication order that includes the drug, the dose, the route, the frequency (including time and as-needed [PRN] or scheduled dosing), and the reason for administration for PRN medications.

Order sets: Several related orders that can be retrieved as a group to facilitate ordering or discontinuing.

Prescriber medication order entry: The ordering of medications and associated dosing parameters by computer, including the electronic transfer of the order to the persons verifying, preparing, and administering the medication; also known as *physician order entry.*

Pump double-checks: The checking of the medication in the pump and pump settings independently by two different people to assess if the drug, diluent, concentration, dose, dosing parameters, and route are the same as ordered and on the pain management flow sheet.

Radio button: A small circle in front of or after listed items from which the user can choose one of the items in the list by clicking in the circle.

Reminder system: A visual or auditory signal that alerts the computer user that a task needs to be done or is overdue.

From Pasero, C., & McCaffery, M. (2011). *Pain assessment and pharmacologic management,* p. 838, St. Louis, Mosby. May be duplicated for use in clinical practice.

Designing Electronic Medical Record Systems for Pain Care

Numerous EMR systems are available for purchase or as free open source systems, including one that was developed for and is used extensively in the Veterans Administration Health Care System (VHA Office of Information VistA Computerized Patient Record System, 2009; Yellowlees, Marks, Hogarth et al., 2008). Available features vary, with some EMRs having more flexibility allowing for customization of the system based on the user's needs. Customization comes at an additional cost to the institution and may require hours of design work, testing, training, and evaluation prior to and after implementation. Fine-tuning may be necessary, and as system upgrades are available, design enhancements and new features may need implementation. However, anecdotal evidence suggests customization increases user compliance and satisfaction (Hidle, 2007; Whipple, Palchuk, Olsha-Yehiav et al., 2007).

Design and implementation teams consisting of professionals from multiple disciplines, such as nurses (e.g., advance practice, bedside, and pain nurses), information technology (IT) personnel, physicians, and pharmacists, are best suited to work through design decisions regarding pain management. IT personnel with a clinical background are invaluable members of the design team and should be requested as pain management is a high-volume and high-risk clinical phenomenon, regardless of the clinical setting. There are large percentages of patients in acute care settings, at home, in long-term care facilities, and in hospices who suffer from uncontrolled moderate to severe pain (see Chapter 1) (American Pain Foundation, 2008; Bercovitz, Decker, Jones, et al., 2008; Botti, Bucknall, Manias, 2004; Bradshaw, Empy, Davis, et al., 1087; Cohen, Easley, Ellis, et al., 2003; Dobratz, Burns, Oden, 1989; Green, 2008). Many require opioids, which have been identified by patient safety and accreditation organizations as high-risk, high-alert medications (Federico, 2007; The Joint Commission Sentinel Event #11 High-Alert Medications and Patient Safety, 2006). Even if opioids are not used, the numerous patient populations have differing needs and the varying responses to analgesics requires the ability to individualize pain assessment and management plans. Many pain therapies are complex. However, regardless of complexity, pain management is an interdisciplinary process. All of these increase the risk to the patient if there are errors. A well-designed EMR helps to address these issues.

It is important for the clinicians on the design team to understand paper-based system limitations, identify the safety measures developed to reduce error in paper-based systems, and translate these to IT professionals so that these aspects can be addressed in the various EMR components (e.g., pain assessment, order sets, and documentation). When developing safe, effective pain EMR components, design team members have to be able to think "out of the box," talk and walk through potential scenarios using the proposed design, and consider if a Failure Effects Mode Analysis (FEMA) should be undertaken to determine the optimum design.

Similar to paper-based systems, EMRs also have limitations that design team members and clinicians need to appreciate, such as the inability to calculate maximum doses of acetaminophen administered over a 24-hour period when single-entity acetaminophen and a combination opioid plus acetaminophen product are given concurrently. The team may need to "push the envelope" utilizing existing EMR system features to address the issue and maximize safety. Two examples are given. First, in the case of two orders for acetaminophen, cautions to the person administering these medications can be developed. Second, to prevent prescription of multiple sedating medications in patients cared for by the pain service, a rule can be developed to prevent non–pain service prescribers from ordering opioids and sedatives for pain service patients. Ease of use, patient safety, and integration of evidence-based or best-practice guidelines are guiding principles for design team members.

Even customizable systems come with prebuilt features that can be implemented out of the box (e.g., a post-pain response field for "as needed" [PRN] analgesics that triggers a reminder to the nurse to obtain the postanalgesic pain score). Prebuilt features may also be customizable to a degree (e.g., adding times based on drug and route of administration to the post–pain response field). Customization may be performed even after initial system implementation. So if the initial product does not meet the end user's needs, modifications should be discussed with IT specialists.

Although the institution's EMR IT design and implementation specialists will develop a wealth of knowledge, the EMR system vendor's staff and resources are more extensive and should be queried to answer difficult questions. Vendors also have user groups and Web sites where customized designs are shared. They can often provide contact information for individuals in comparable institutions who have grappled with similar design issues. E-mail list services such as is offered by the American Pain Society/American Society for Pain Management Nursing provide the ability to ask questions and receive screen shots of different designs as well as to dialogue with other users about how they addressed issues. These consultative mechanisms facilitate discussions about what individual institutions considered when making their design decisions, available options, and the pros and cons of these choices. List services and user groups also afford a mechanism to elicit support for submitting requests to the vendor about design changes. Vendors prioritize changes in their systems based on the number of design requests or concerns about system limitations from their users. So, if a system appears to lack desired features, has limitations, or is cumbersome, it is important to explore the avenues discussed above to create a user-friendly, safe, and efficient system.

Pain-Related Electronic Medical Record Components

Major EMR components integral to the assessment and management of pain are listed below. All are crucial to the provision of safe pain care.

- Medication reconciliation
- Dose range checking
- Medication order entry, preparation, and administration including range dose and interfaces with other electronic systems (medication dispensing cabinets)
- Documentation
- Quality monitoring and improvement activities

Each EMR component has unique design and implementation challenges, some of which may be exclusive to a specific EMR system. Select examples of generic issues associated with these EMR components and potential solutions with a major focus on patient safety are discussed in the following paragraphs.

Medication Reconciliation

The Joint Commission 2006 safety initiative called for reconciling medications when there is a change in a patient's care levels (The Joint Commission Addendum to Sentinel Event #35 Medication Reconciliation, 2006). The EMR can facilitate the process of medication reconciliation by reminding the clinician to perform the task and providing an accurate list of the patient's prescribed medications. Ideally, such a list would include essential elements of the prescription as well as information about the frequency of use for PRN and scheduled medications.

Well-designed EMR medication reconciliation can minimize the potential for withdrawal symptoms in individuals receiving long-term opioid therapy because between levels of care, the practitioner is provided with a list of active meds and their start dates and is required to make a decision about continuing or discontinuing each drug. For those knowledgeable in equi-analgesic conversions, medication reconciliation also provides information that can be used to determine dose conversions. This is an improvement over paper-based tracking of these changes that requires a review of several handwritten medication administration records, physician orders, or verbal reports. Obtaining this information prior to major status changes (e.g., preoperatively) is recommended.

Dose Range Checking

Dose range checking is one of the major error reduction features of EMR. It involves comparing the dose written by the prescriber against the dose in a drug database. Parameters such as minimum and maximum single dose limits and total daily dose can be compared. Database-recommended dose limits may be based upon parameters such as route of administration and patient-specific factors such as age, weight, and laboratory values (e.g., creatinine clearance). Doses exceeding database limits send an alert to the prescriber about the reason for the alert (e.g., dose exceeds the maximum recommended amount, or the intramuscular [IM] route is not recommended) and may suggest actions (e.g., use this dose only in opioid-tolerant individuals or consider another route of administration, respectively). Alerts that are overridden may also require the prescriber to provide a reason for overriding the alert (e.g., patient is opioid-tolerant).

Drug databases can include some inherent weaknesses that may or may not be corrected by customization. For example, they may contain routes of administration that are not used for pain management (e.g., hemodialysis catheters) or doses inconsistent with best-practice guidelines (e.g., a maximum single dose of 4 mg of intravenous [IV] hydromorphone, which exceeds guideline recommendations for opioid-naïve individuals) (American Pain Society, 2008). Some drug limitations may be set developing EMR rules outside of the dose range checking system, such as restricting the use of preservative-free morphine or other solutions to anesthesia prescribers or to the operating room (OR). Other major weaknesses in most, if not all, dose range–checking databases are the lack of automatic equianalgesic conversions during route or drug changes, inability to check for daily maximum cumulative doses when combination products (e.g., nonopioid + opioid formulations) are ordered, inability to customize limits based on patient status (e.g., higher dose limits allowed for opioid-tolerant individuals or for patients with ventilator-controlled respirations), and significant tolls on computer resources associated with multiple dose range–checking steps that can slow down

the system. When the proposed change has more negative implications than benefits, practitioners should be alerted of the EMR limitation, and a request for modification should be sent to the vendor.

Depending upon the database and the EMR system, analgesic information may be customizable. For example, route limitations may be possible, such as restricting preservative-free morphine to intrathecal or epidural administration only. Minimum and maximum single dose and total maximum daily dose limits can also be changed. Dose limits may be designed to vary based on age, weight, and patient-specific laboratory values, such as a specific creatinine clearance level when ketorolac is ordered (American Pain Society, 2003). In such instances, customization may require the IT staff to write multiple rules. For example, Rule 1 checks that the patient's age is within certain parameters, Rule 2 checks that the patient's weight is within the rule's specific parameters, and Rule 3 checks that a patient-specific laboratory value is within the designated range. To ensure safety, extensive testing and monitoring is recommended to determine what will happen if an individual rule and all possible combinations of rules are violated.

Attention to ensuring that customization is maintained during upgrades is imperative. Otherwise, as upgrades to the system or database occur, customized safety features may be lost. For example, if the IV hydromorphone single maximum dose limit is customized from 4 mg to 1 mg in an updated database, this customization can be overridden when upgrades are made. It is important to note that while dose range checking is a major safety feature, a phenomenon called "alert fatigue" whereby individuals are constantly bombarded with warnings (alerts) and begin to ignore them or breeze through them too quickly to comprehend and respond appropriately to them, is a real concern. Efforts to avoid unnecessary alerts are essential.

Medication Order Entry, Preparation, and Administration

With EMRs, prescribers can build simple orders from a list of options for each field associated with the order (i.e., medication, dose, route, and frequency). Or, the prescriber can select prebuilt order sentences (Figure C-1) that include drug, dose, route, and frequency; specific fields can be modified as needed. Order sets (Figure C-2) can also be developed that include prebuilt pain and adverse effect medication sentences, as well as assessment and monitoring parameters. This is particularly advantageous for complex order sets, such as for those written for specialized analgesic therapies (e.g., IV PCA, epidural analgesia, and nerve blocks) where a missing order may compromise patient care. In some systems, all currently active orders in a specific order set can be collected, so that the numerous associated orders can easily be reordered during medication reconciliation or discontinued when the specialized analgesic therapy is stopped.

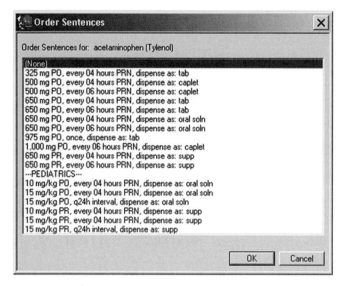

Figure C-1 | Order sentences.

© 2011, University of Maryland Medical Center.

A pitfall of the EMR is that prescriber-built orders may be indistinguishable from prebuilt orders to the eyes of anyone but the original prescriber. Since EMR orders are typed, they have the appearance of being written correctly. This is likely, at least in part, because there is no issue with legibility and missing dosing parameters. As an example, although modified-release opioids should be administered in scheduled around-the-clock doses, a prescriber-built order for PRN administration of an modified-release opioid may be perceived as being correct because it is typed and legible. Staff must be knowledgeable of this phenomenon.

As with dose range checking, prebuilt or institution-built order sentences may also be inconsistent with best-practice or evidence-based guidelines. Similarly, order sets built by non–pain service providers may be inconsistent with dose range–checking parameters and evidence-based information. To prevent this, prior to implementation of the system, order sentences should be assessed for consistency with evidence-based guidelines, whether they are individual order sentences or part of an order set. Consistency is important for safety and to prevent alert fatigue. As examples, order sentences and order sets should be assessed for issues such as follows.

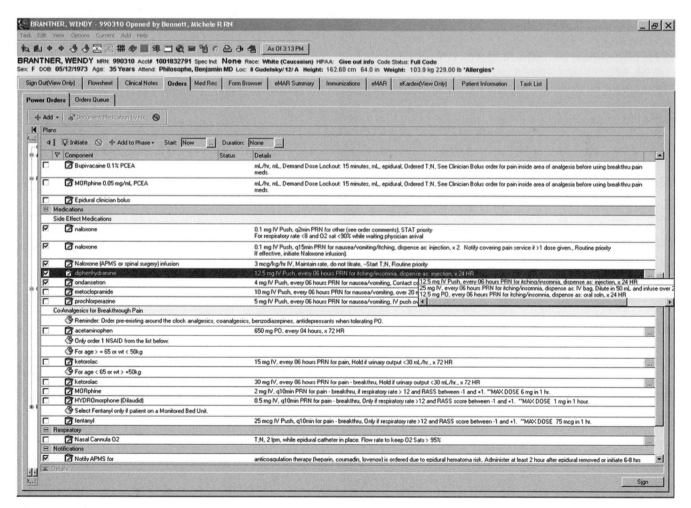

Figure C-2 | Epidural order set.

© 2011, University of Maryland Medical Center.

- Are long acting opioids scheduled for twice-daily (BID) dosing at unequal intervals or every 12 hours?
- Have the IM opioid administration sentences been deleted?
- Do the prebuilt IV opioid doses and frequencies use IM parameters, or is the dose and frequency divided in half as recommended (American Pain Society, 2008)?
- Are there low-dose naloxone sentences for opioid reversal?

The impact of evidence-based prebuilt analgesic order sets and sentences on patient outcomes (e.g., adverse effects and analgesic efficacy) is unknown, but if implemented, they should improve pain outcomes.

Customized Pain Management Orders and Alerts

A distinct advantage for pain services is the ability to develop customized alerts reminding other prescribers not to order analgesics and sedatives for patients cared for by the pain service, a step that can help prevent oversedation and life-threatening respiratory depression (Figure C-3). Choices have to be made about whether the alert should function merely as a reminder or be tied to a hard stop, preventing other prescribers from ordering medications. These alerts require the EMR system to recognize differences between

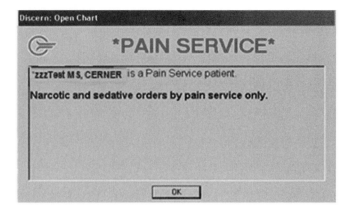

Figure C-3 | Pain service alert.

© 2011, University of Maryland Medical Center.

pain service prescribers and other prescribers, which requires collaboration between the pain service and the technology specialists to maintain an updated pain service prescriber list. Similarly, reminders for "No opioids or sedatives unless ordered by the Pain Service" can be constructed for nurses to see.

Order sentences can be customized as seen in Figure C-4. They can be constructed to require a reason for PRN

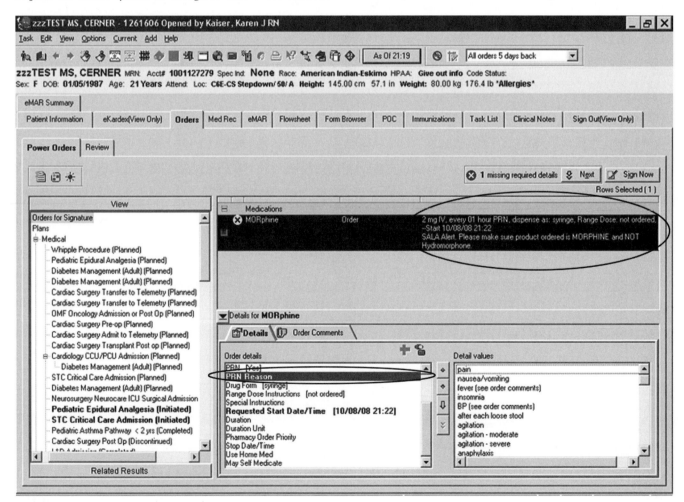

Figure C-4 | PRN reason and sound alike look alike (SALA) reminder.

© 2011, University of Maryland Medical Center.

medication administration (such as for pain, itching, or nausea), which can increase compliance with accreditation standards. Orders can be developed to include comments, specialized instructions, or reminders about sound-alike look-alike (SALA) drug alerts (e.g., morphine and hydromorphone, hydrocodone and hydromorphone, codeine and hydrocodone). Other related systems (e.g., medication dispensing cabinets) should be programmed to carry similar relevant messages (e.g., SALA alerts) for reinforcement.

Specialized instructions can also be customized for different health care providers. For example, pharmacists may see special admixture directions, and bedside nurses may see instructions such as "not to exceed acetaminophen limits" or "do not crush or chew" or parameters for administration of certain drugs (Figure C-5). However, lengthy orders may not display in their entirety, and parts may be obscured from the practitioner's view, requiring the user to take extra steps for the information to display. For example, the nurse may need to "hover" the computer's cursor over the order to see the complete order on the electronic medication administration record (eMAR).

Range dose orders, which individualize the medication dose to a patient's changing analgesic needs, may be constructed in accordance with policy and include guidance on how to consistently implement the order. For example, in Figure C-6, the prescriber is instructed to place the highest dose outside the parentheses, which facilitates EMR range dose checking of the highest amount of medication ordered; system limitations prevent dose range checking on information in the Comments section of an order. In Figure C-7, the prescriber is prompted to provide specific information about dosing.

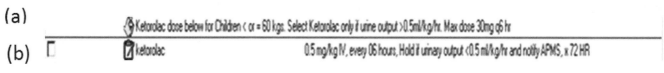

Figure C-5 | Notes to (a) prescribers and (b) nurses.

© 2011, University of Maryland Medical Center.

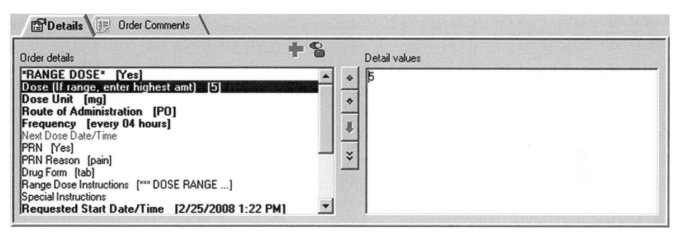

Figure C-6 | Range dose order prescriber highest dose prompt.

© 2011, University of Maryland Medical Center.

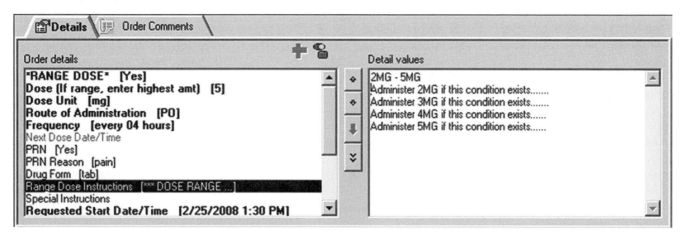

Figure C-7 | Range dose order prescriber range dose instruction prompt.

© 2011, University of Maryland Medical Center.

Safety Issues

There are differences between the paper record and the EMR that may impact safety. Some of these changes are significant to specific types of users, but differences may be subtle to other health care disciplines. In the paper record, the same medication order is seen by the prescriber, the pharmacist, and the nurse. In the EMR, there are different views for different disciplines based on the process being executed. Each of the three disciplines sees something different when performing their primary functions of ordering, preparing, and administering, respectively. Although the views are distinct for each purpose, design decisions made for one process may impact the view for another purpose and cause potential safety issues. For example, in some systems, in order for the pharmacist to have access to drug compounding information within the system, the diluent, rather than the drug, is the first item listed on the eMAR. Designs best suited for the pharmacist's drug verification and preparation may not result in the best display for the bedside nurse who administers the medication and vice versa. Regardless of the design decision made, one of the disciplines is put at risk for making an error. These "Catch-22" situations need to be reported to the vendor.

Views previously available on paper may not be readily available in the EMR, potentially resulting in patient harm or discomfort. For example, because there are no related pharmacy actions, the pharmacy may require that patient-controlled analgesia bolus orders be associated with the solution order instead of being placed as a separate order. In this case, the bolus order may be placed in the solution's Comments section, which is hidden from the nurse's view without hovering the computer's cursor over the order to see the comment's details. In response, the bolus dose may be delayed or not be given. In the case in which upper dose limits are programmed into the analgesic pump, such as in a computerized IV infusion with specialized features also known as a "Smart Pump," there are anecdotal reports where nurses have not seen the bolus order and mistakenly utilized the programmed upper dose bolus limit as the bolus dose. This could lead to overmedication of the patient.

When any design team member is concerned about a potentially significant adverse safety event (such as described in the previous paragraph) for which a resolution is not evident, additional expertise should be enlisted. The team should be led by a provider with an understanding of the problem, knowledge of the system, and without a stake in the outcome. Similarly, other system and process experts should be enlisted. The multidisciplinary team of stakeholders must evaluate actual and potential clinician responses to an existing order, as well as evaluate potential resolutions and the various clinician responses to the proposed changes. Once the group has made a decision that maximizes safety and patient comfort, plans for making the change, dissemination strategies, and a timely evaluation of the change (i.e., determination of whether the change resolved the issue and if unanticipated problems occurred as a result of the change) must be arranged.

Changes in Work Processes

Changes in the hospital staff's work processes are also required with the implementation of an EMR system (Kushniruk, Borycki, Kuwata, et al., 2006; Spence, Valenza, Taylor, 2007). These need to be well planned, communicated, and followed. To ensure safety while instituting these changes, best practices must be continued and not inadvertently abandoned. Some example of these work process changes and the potential impact follow.

Medications and the eMAR may be on separate portable utility carts. However, when preparing medications both carts need to be used concomitantly, which may be cumbersome. During administration of medications or double-checks of analgesic pump parameters, the order needs to be readily available, requiring access at the bedside to the computer or a current copy of the orders. Without the order and an identifiable medication at the bedside, it is difficult to assess the "5 Rights" (right patient, right drug, right dose, right time, and right route), which can increase the potential for error. Taking the required appropriate information to the bedside is a step that should not be abandoned, even if the patient is under isolation precautions. So, regardless of how cumbersome it is, computer access at the bedside with proper disinfection, as needed, or frequent downloads of current printed eMARs is necessary.

Some changes in processes are more subtle. For example, the nurse may receive an electronic notice that an opioid has been discontinued, but accepting this notice may take place on a screen that does not display the entire order, so the nurse may not readily recognize that an opioid the patient takes for chronic pain was discontinued prematurely without tapering the dose to prevent withdrawal. When the same discontinued medication is observed on the eMAR, the nurse may not be visually cued about the change, because discontinued medications drop to the bottom of the eMAR and are grayed out, making them more difficult to see than the text of current medications. In comparison, the visual cue of a crossed-out medication on a paper medication administration record that easily reminds all shifts about the medication change no longer exists. With an EMR, the nurse has to remember to actively look at all medication changes on the eMAR. Thus, it is important to make inspecting the eMAR during shift report a part of the normal routine with the advent of computerized prescriber order entry, which is the process of ordering, preparing, administering, and documenting medications using an electronic system instead of a paper system.

A major disadvantage of most EMR systems is the multistep process required for making changes or updating the system. For example, steps must be followed before the prescriber can order a nonformulary item. In some, if not all systems, first, the pharmacy or IT personnel must create a drug item that can be ordered by the prescriber. Next, the pharmacist must assure that the parameters (e.g., dose, route) of this item are correct. Then, the drug is made available by pharmacy or IT personnel for the prescriber to select (order). This process increases safety, but slows down the administration of care. In a fast-paced, quickly changing health care environment, a system that offers a quick response time and incorporates checks and balances to minimize harm from inadvertent errors is essential. When planning EMR implementation, expedited processes for adding a new formulary item at the point of care such as the one previously described must be developed. A decelerated, but similarly rigorous process can be developed for planned additions to the formulary.

Documentation

Pain documentation similar to those available in paper-based systems can be developed for EMR systems (Box C-2). A Pain Assessment/History form (Figure C-8), pain measurement tools (Figure C-9), and forms to document medication effectiveness such as a Pain Management Flow Sheet (Figure C-10) or graph depicting the pain score verses the pain management goal (Figure C-11) can be designed. Note that similar to paper-based tools, recreation of copyrighted information such as a pain measurement tool in the medical record requires the developer's permission and a notation of permission on the electronic form as seen in Figure C-9.

To enhance usability, forms should be short, without redundancy, and easy to complete, yet flexible. Radio buttons, check boxes, drop-down boxes, and Comments sections are helpful to achieve these goals. Radio buttons are small open circles in front of (or sometimes after) items in a horizontal and vertical list that can be selected. They function similar to a check box in that the user clicks in the circle or check box next to the desired response(s) from a list of several items that may be displayed in several columns. Radio buttons are useful when a single item is selected. Check boxes are useful when multiple selections are possible, such as selecting pain characteristics or the quality of pain (e.g., hot, burning, and electrical shock). Both generally take up more space on a form than a drop-down box. Neither the radio button nor the check box requires the user to do anything to see the items in the list. This is in contrast to the drop-down box. A drop-down box appears as an open space on the same line next to a category, and when the drop-down box is clicked on, several responses drop down in a list, from which the user selects one response. For example, several pain measurement tools may be listed, but only one is chosen and shown in the box. Comments boxes provide the most flexibility and allow the user to type in pertinent information but take up considerable space if the entire text is viewable. Saving space is important when designing forms; even simple, easy-to-complete forms can seem overwhelming and burdensome if they appear to be long.

Box C-2 | Resources

Electronic documentation: *http://healthit.ahrq.gov/ portal/server.pt?open=512&objID=650 parentn ame=CommunityPage&parentid=5&mode=2&i n_hi_userid=3882&cached=true*

Electronic documentation system: *http://www1.va.gov/ CPRSdemo/*

Strategies for reducing medication errors:
- Institute for Safe Medication Practices (Includes Failure Effects Mode Analysis): *http://www.ismp.org/ Tools/pathways.asp*
- Institute for Safe Medication Practices: *http://www.ismp.org*
- The Joint Commission: *http://www.jointcommission. org/SentinelEvents/*

From Pasero, C., & McCaffery, M. (2011). *Pain assessment and pharmacologic management,* p. 845, St. Louis, Mosby. May be duplicated for use in clinical practice.

Enhancements can be made to electronic forms that are not possible with paper-based forms. It is important to realize that the capability to make the enhancements depends on the system and the choices the institution makes during implementation of the system. Several examples of possible enhancements follow.

- Referrals are often necessary for people with pain and can be generated easily with the EMR by pressing a button (Figure C-12).
- EMR users can be required to provide information by making fields mandatory (e.g., provoking factors, quality of pain, region/radiation/relief, severity/ associated symptoms/medication side effects, and timing/onset/duration of pain).
- The nurse can be directed to select the appropriate pain measurement tool by choosing the category most appropriate for the patient (e.g., patient able to self-report, adult unable to self-report, neonate unable to self-report) on a Pain Assessment form as in Figure C-8.
- Behavioral pain measurement tools can be designed to calculate total sums, using the information from the individual data elements entered by the nurse (Figure C-13).
- Information from the electronic vital sign sheet and the eMAR can be automatically entered into the patient's pain management flow sheet.
- Documentation of analgesic pump parameter double-checks can be required.
- Reminders to obtain postanalgesic pain scores to evaluate medication effectiveness at specific time intervals based on drug formulation (e.g., injectable or transdermal) and route of administration (Figure C-14) can be programmed into the system.

PAIN ASSESSMENT / HISTORY

If initial pain complaint occurs after admission/initial visit, complete this form as a stand-alone form.

Date & Time 05/28/2009   0931   Deferred
- ○ Pt in excruciating pain, assess when pain is controlled
- ● Pt is not in excruciating pain
- ○ See TRU nursing assessment form

If patient unable to self-report, use History & Physical Exam, ROM, movement, and information from significant other to answer the following items.

*Location	*Side/Quadrant	*New Onset?	Comment
<MultiAlpha>	<MultiAlpha>	<Alpha>	

Pain Location

Where is the pain?

For the following items, assess patient's primary pain complaint. Consider other for secondary pain complaints.

Pain Characteristics

Describe the pain

- ☐ Aching
- ☐ Burning
- ☐ Crampy
- ☐ Crushing
- ☐ Dull
- ☐ Heaviness
- ☐ *Hot
- ☐ Gnawing
- ☐ Knife-like
- ☐ *Pain with touch
- ☐ *Piercing
- ☐ Pressure
- ☐ *Pricking
- ☐ Pulling
- ☐ Sharp
- ☐ *Shocklike
- ☐ *Shooting
- ☐ Stabbing
- ☐ Tenderness
- ☐ Throbbing
- ☐ *Tingling
- ☐ Unable to determine
- ☐ Other:

Consider an APMS consult (Order required) when selecting a pain characteristic with an asterisk.

Onset of Pain

When did it start?

- ○ Today
- ○ 1 day - 6 days
- ○ 1 week - 1 month
- ○ 1 month - 6 months
- ○ > 6 months
- ○ After injury
- ○ Post procedure-currently experiencing pain
- ○ Post procedure-currently not experiencing pain
- ○ Unknown
- ○ Other:

Provokes Pain

- ☐ None
- ☐ At rest
- ☐ Bending
- ☐ Contractions
- ☐ Coughing
- ☐ Lifting
- ☐ Lying down
- ☐ MD/RN physical exam/procedure
- ☐ Movement
- ☐ Sitting
- ☐ Staying in one position
- ☐ Unknown
- ☐ Other:

Pain Duration

How long does it last?

- ○ > 30 minutes to 1 hour
- ○ 1 min to 30 minutes
- ○ All day
- ○ During contractions
- ○ During procedure/exam
- ○ Fleeting < 1 min
- ○ Hours
- ○ Post procedure
- ○ Since injury
- ○ Unknown
- ○ Until pain med takes effect
- ○ Other:

Pain Frequency

How often within 24 hours?

- ○ Always
- ○ During contractions
- ○ During procedure
- ○ Most of the time
- ○ Post procedure
- ○ Rarely
- ○ Some of the time
- ○ Unknown
- ○ Other:

Pain Timing

What time of the day does it hurt?

- ☐ Morning
- ☐ Afternoon
- ☐ Night
- ☐ 24 Hours a day
- ☐ Anytime
- ☐ Intermittent
- ☐ During procedure/exam
- ☐ Before next scheduled pain med
- ☐ No pattern
- ☐ Unknown
- ☐ Other:

Relieves Pain

- ☐ Nothing
- ☐ Cold
- ☐ Distraction (TV, music, etc.)
- ☐ Heat
- ☐ Limit movement
- ☐ Medication
- ☐ Medication (See PACU/TRU/ED records)
- ☐ Re-position
- ☐ Rest
- ☐ Sitting
- ☐ Sucking (pediatric)
- ☐ TENS Unit
- ☐ Unknown
- ☐ Other:

Associated Symptoms

Any related pain problems?

- ☐ None
- ☐ Change in relationships
- ☐ Change in leisure activity/play
- ☐ Change in work habits
- ☐ Limitations with ADL
- ☐ Cognition changes
- ☐ Loss of appetite
- ☐ Loss of sleep
- ☐ Mood changes
- ☐ Nausea/vomiting
- ☐ No interference with ADL/sleep/play/Tx
- ☐ Unable to assess
- ☐ Other:

Pain Measurement Tools   1. Select the patient category below.

- ○ Patient can self report
- ○ Adult patient unable to self report
- ○ FLACC Non-neonates 0-18 can't self report
- ○ NICU post-op neonate (CRIES)
- ○ NICU neonate with procedural pain (PIPP)
- ○ Full term nursery neonate (NIPS)

2. Select the pain tool associated with the above category that was used.

If patient can self report
- ○ Faces Scale: 4-Adult   ○ Numerical/Verbal Rating Scale: 7-Adult   ○ Verbal Descriptor Scale: > 10 years

If patient cannot self report

Adult patient or unable to lighten sedation
- ○ Cognitively impaired and unable to self-report (adult : CNPI)   ○ Unable to lighten sedation/chemical paralysis-assume pain present

FLACC
- ○ FLACC (0 yrs.-7yrs.) unable to self report   ○ FLACC (0 yrs.-18 yrs.) for developmentally delayed children

NICU post-op neonate (CRIES)
- ○ CRIES: 32-60 weeks

NICU neonate with procedural pain (PIPP)
- ○ PIPP: <28 weeks to 44 weeks Post Conceptual Age

Full term nursery neonate (NIPS)
- ○ NIPS: 28-38 weeks

Please update patient/family education and plan of care forms

For example, pain issues exacerbated by:
1. Substance Abuse/History of substance abuse
2. Depression
3. In PEDS, also refer if parent requests more pain meds when child does not appear to be in pain
4. If patient exhibits withdrawn behavior or lack of cooperation with treatment.

By selecting this response, a notification will be sent to Social Work

- ○ Pain exacerbated by psychosocial/spiritual issues

Figure C-8 | Pain assessment history form.

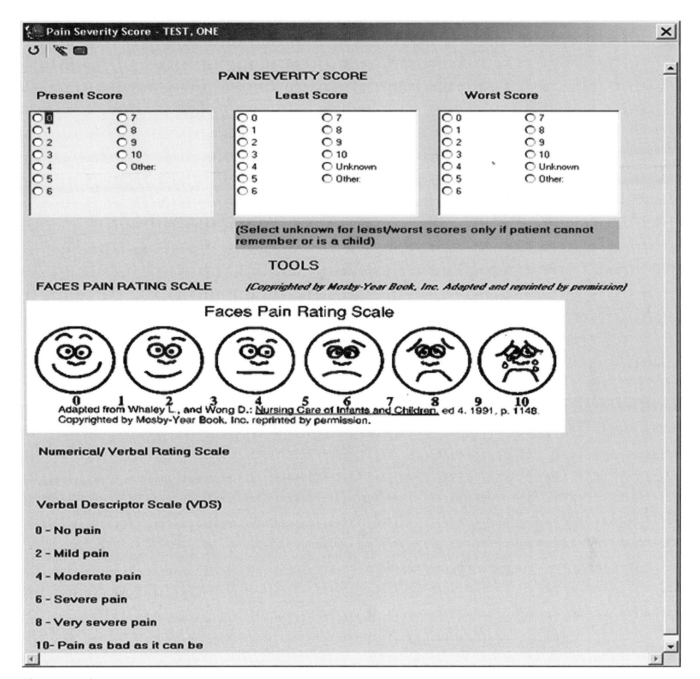

Figure C-9 | Pain measurement tools.

© 2011, University of Maryland Medical Center.

Besides enhancements to electronic pain documentation, there are some limitations. Like the enhancements, these are also system dependent. Some EMR systems only allow simple figures, such as a picture of a FACES pain measurement tool. An interactive body diagram upon which notations can be made indicating pain location, severity, and quality is preferred, but this enhancement may make electronic auditing difficult. Medication effectiveness documentation may have system limitations as well. For example, a reminder to obtain a postanalgesic pain score may be limited to PRN analgesics. This can cause confusion if there is no similar reminder for postanalgesic pain score assessment for scheduled medications.

There may be inflexibility when programming the time of the reminder (e.g., only one time allowed per route or drug; the time of the reminder must be less than 12 hours, which precludes programming an accurate peak effect for the fentanyl patch). There may also be limitations on the number of letters or words that can be displayed in drop-down box items and in a Comments section, respectively. When addressing the system limitations, the interdisciplinary team that develops pain documentation must carefully consider the effects of their choices on the clinician. In addition, the team must develop adequate ongoing clinician training and other strategies that address system limitations.

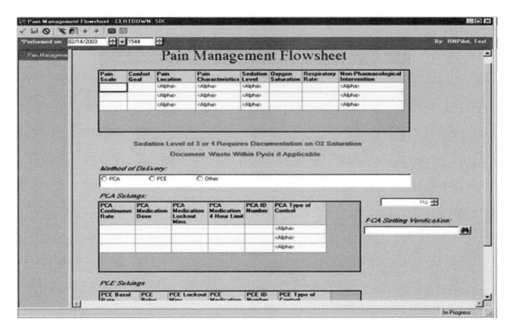

Figure C-10 | Pain management flow sheet.

© 2011, University of Maryland Medical Center.

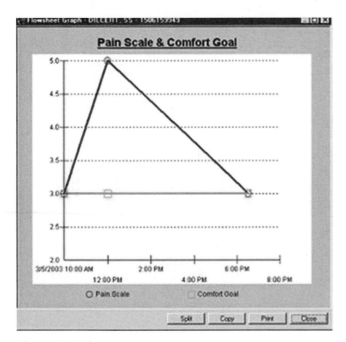

Figure C-11 | Pain management score verses pain management goal.

© 2011, University of Maryland Medical Center.

Pain Management Forms and Flow Sheets

Electronic pain management flow sheets that document preanalgesic and postanalgesic pain scores, pharmacologic and nonpharmacologic treatments, as well as the presence or absence of adverse effects using text or graphic display as shown in Figure C-10, had been designed but were not widely used at the time of this publication. Some parameters (e.g., respiratory rate, pain scores, sedation scores, medications, and doses) can be linked to other documentation forms in the EMR (e.g., vital sign record, eMAR) and may be pulled electronically into the pain management flow sheet or vice versa in some systems.

Paper-based pain management flow sheets and comprehensive pain assessment forms have been shown to increase the assessment of pain and effective management of pain (see Chapter 1) (McMillan, Williams, Chatfield, et al., 1988). Similar research is needed to demonstrate the effectiveness of electronic forms. One study in an outpatient clinic showed that compliance with documentation on an electronic pain assessment form by non-pain physicians was low because the form was burdensome

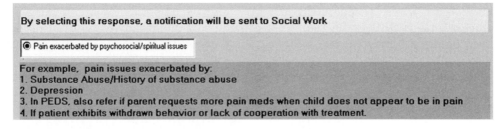

Figure C-12 | Psychosocial pain consult.

© 2011, University of Maryland Medical Center.

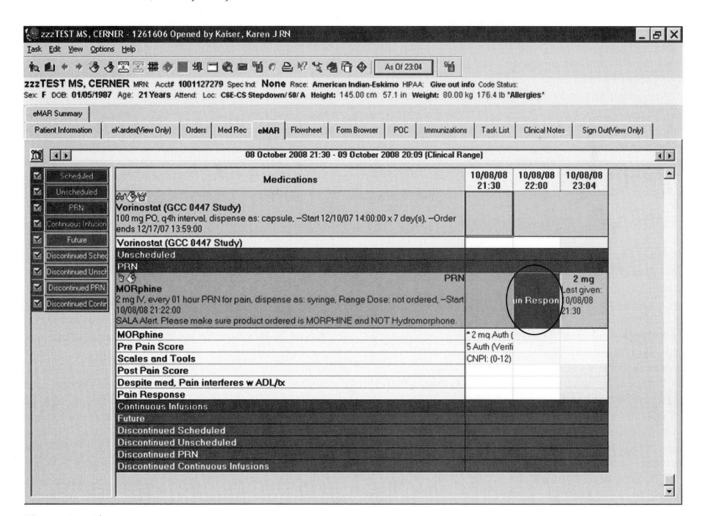

CHECKLIST OF NON-VERBAL PAIN INDICATORS

Date & Time 05/28/2009 0801   Assessment done by Kaiser, Karen J RN

	WITH MOVEMENT	AT REST	
Vocal complaints: Non-verbal		1	(Expression of pain, not in words, moans, groans, grunts, cries, gasps, sighs)
Facial grimaces/ winces		1	(Furrowed brow, narrowed eyes, tightened lips, jaw drop, clenched teeth, distorted expressions)
Bracing	1		(Clutching or holding onto side rails, bed, tray table, or affected areas during movement)
Restlessness		0	(Constant or intermittent shifting of position, rocking, intermittent or constant hand motions, inability to keep still)
Rubbing	1		(Massaging affected area)
Vocal complaints: Verbal		1	(Words expressing discomfort or pain-"ouch", "that hurts"; cursing during movement; or exclamations of protest-"stop", "that's enough")
Subtotal	2	3	

Patient's Total Score (Numerator) 5   The checklist of non-verbal pain indicators is a fraction. Note the numerator and the denominator

Tool's Total Score (Denominator) 12

Used with permission- Feldt, K.S. (1996)

Figure C-13 | Behavioral tool: self calculates.

© 2011, University of Maryland Medical Center.

Figure C-14 | Post pain response reminder: posted in blue at time of drug administration.

© 2011, University of Maryland Medical Center.

(Saigh, Triola, Link, 2006). In contrast, a pain clinic EMR utilized by a variety of disciplines received positive reviews (Gruner, Ljutow, Schleinzer, et al., 2008). Similar to electronic reminders used to document postanalgesic pain scores as described in the next section, reminders to perform assessments for specialty analgesic therapy, such as IV PCA or epidural analgesia, that are frequently documented on a pain management flow sheet are not well described in the literature. A static notation on an electronic care plan (eKardex) is described as part of the University of Maryland Center experience below, but it is not as likely to ensure compliance the way a timed reminder would function.

Great strides in compliance with accreditation standards are possible with electronic pain documentation, especially if responses are mandatory or the nurse receives reminders to perform certain tasks. However, to reduce user burden, mandatory documentation requirements should be used only when necessary. Forms should be short and eliminate redundancy. User feedback should be sought and applied to enhance utilization of the forms and improve user satisfaction. Reminder systems should also be integrated into the electronic medical record to assist with compliance with accreditation standards.

Quality Improvement and Research

When designing pain-related EMR forms (orders, medication reconciliation forms, and documentation forms) and processes (mandatory or discretionary; documentation requirements of analgesic pump double-checks), one must consider the reports needed to monitor compliance with pain-related regulatory and accreditation standards, as well as the data needed for quality improvement initiatives and prospective or retrospective research. Mandatory items on forms eliminate missing data, which is desirable when information is required to meet accreditation standards, but as mentioned, they should not be used excessively. Predetermined options, which are available with drop-down boxes, check boxes, and radio buttons, provide data that are more easily retrieved electronically and aggregated into a report compared with data written in comments fields. Comments section information, otherwise known as free-text data, is difficult to consolidate from multiple notes, as the health care provider can write anything desired. Free-text data is also subject to misspellings. Both make it difficult to aggregate the data and perform calculations for quality improvement and research.

With paper-based records, auditing is conducted by reviewing each chart by hand and calculating the percent of overall compliance (e.g., multiple records, multiple units) with accreditation standards. This can be extremely time-consuming, even when the results are entered into a database and overall compliance is calculated by machine predesigned report. Electronic auditing, where data is pulled from the EMR and collated electronically, is more efficient and frees up nursing time previously spent collecting data from the medical record and aggregating

(collating) the results. This is valuable time that can be used instead for developing process improvement actions.

To perform an electronic audit, an expert programmer, data analysis person, and report writer working in conjunction with a pain expert can develop the data extraction method, data calculations, and report format. Once each of these has been verified, repeat analyses using different time frames can be automated. This requires minimal nursing time expenditure compared with performing individual paper-based chart audits. All parties involved in the development of the audit need to be made aware of any changes to the electronic documentation forms, because the changes may affect future audit results.

Currently in the clinical setting, electronic auditing is limited primarily to use of data from fields where predetermined selections are available, such as radio buttons, check boxes, and drop-down boxes. Utilization of what is called "natural language" processing, which electronically searches rich narrative notes, determines the theme, and aggregates the data into a report, is time-consuming and requires sophisticated programming. Difficulties associated with natural language processing include searching and determining the meaning of free-text notes that contain misspellings or culturally specific nuances from notes written by multicultural health care providers. In addition, to audit a narrative record for pain information using natural language processing, the computer program must first identify that the nurse is writing about physical pain and not emotional pain. Once that task is complete, the program would have to examine what the nurse wrote, such as "the patient has 8/10 sharp, shooting, electrical shock pain in the left lower extremity." From this note, natural language processing would have to identify "8/10" as the pain score; "sharp, shooting, electrical shock" as pain characteristics, and "left lower extremity" as a location before it could determine if each of these elements of a pain assessment were included in the documentation. In contrast, if separate items and specific selections are provided for pain score, pain characteristics, and pain location, an electronic audit program would only need to be programmed to search each item and see if the nurse selected one response per item. In summary, the use of natural language processing in the clinical arena is likely to be a time-consuming and expensive proposition for some time. It is in its infancy, particularly with regard to monitoring of nurse-sensitive outcomes (Pakhomov, Jacobsen, Chute, et al., 2008).

Regardless of how the data is obtained (natural language processing or fixed responses) or its purpose (quality improvement or research), validation of the data is required to ensure that the data that is captured is indeed the data that was intended to be captured. Validation activities, such as verification through real-time or retrospective assessment of patient records and discussions with health care providers (e.g., nurses, nurse practitioners, physicians), can be used to identify potential clinical practice issues that need clarification or improving.

Well-designed forms with mandatory fields and standardized responses and reminders will facilitate the ability to obtain information retrospectively for quality improvement or research.

The University of Maryland Medical Center Experience

The author's place of employment, the University of Maryland Medical Center (UMMC), has had an EMR system since the mid-1990s. However, it was limited in scope (e.g., obstetrical area, simple physician orders, and simple nursing documentation). Housewide implementation was planned, but the company that produced the original EMR system was sold, and system upgrades and support were discontinued during the planning phase. A replacement system was purchased, and the functionality of the previous system was closely replicated at the time of implementation. With system expansion, considerable hospital resources were dedicated to converting critical patient information such as nursing intake assessment and laboratory and radiology results to electronic data; replacing an outdated pharmacy system and trauma documentation system; and developing prescriber order entry, especially medication order entry. These processes can facilitate access to information, reduce duplication of medical tests, and promote safety in the medication process (Cowell, 2007; Kaushal, Shojania, Bates, 2003; Wolfstadt, Gurwitz, Field, et al., 2008).

Award Incentive

Electronic or computerized prescriber order entry is the process by which orders are written by the prescriber in the electronic medical record and are electronically transmitted via computer to other associated computers, particularly computers in locations where the work associated with the order is performed. In the literature, this is also referred to as a *computerized physician order entry*. A computerized prescriber order entry includes orders for processes traditionally conveyed on paper and telephone, such as a patient's code status, dietary orders, laboratory, and x-rays. A specialized form of prescriber order entry is the computerized prescriber medication order entry, which is also known as the computerized physician medication order entry. In the computerized prescriber medication order entry, the prescriber's order is electronically transmitted: to the pharmacy system for pharmacy review, preparation, and dispensing; to a nurse's orders alert tab notifying the nurse of a new order; to the order's tab for viewing in the usual order format; and to the eMAR for the nurse to administer and document that the medication was administered.

Literature about the medication safety benefits of EMR systems played an important part in making prescriber medication order entry a high priority at the

UMMC. Attention to the Leapfrog group's yearly computerized medication order entry safety enhancements was a contributing factor in the system customization process at the UMMC. The Leapfrog Group, which consists of numerous Fortune 500 companies, recognizes and rewards systems that meet the group's yearly safety goals. Computerized prescriber order entry is integral to the organizational safety assessment that is required to be considered for the annual Leapfrog Award (Leapfrog Group safety practices: Computerized physician order entry, 2009). It is a contributing factor in the UMMC being a continued recipient of the award over consecutive years (Leapfrog Group safety practices: Computerized physician order entry, 2009).

Implementation

Introduction of EMR systems into the health care workplace is often completed in steps, particularly in the hospital setting. For example, dietary orders may precede laboratory orders, which may precede the computerized prescriber order entry. It may be months to years before the entire medical record is computerized. At the time of this publication, the University of Maryland was utilizing a combination of paper and electronic records. The nursing intake, patient care planning, and patient education are documented on computerized forms, but routine vital signs and daily nursing flow sheets (including pain management flow sheets and daily nursing documentation) are on paper.

Even when the system is completely implemented and there is no paper documentation, attention to the system is required. Similar to paper-based forms and associated processes, revisions are necessary. The UMMC's experience with implementation of a pain-related EMR as of the publication date is detailed in the following paragraphs.

Three things were imperative to the success of our pain electronic documentation. First, the University selected a multidisciplinary design team with knowledge about the functionality of the system. For example, the PhD-prepared nurse pain expert (the Appendix author) was one of numerous support persons from many disciplines trained for the implementation of the computerized physician order entry system. Second, the team sought and utilized input from stakeholders during the design process. For example, when developing nursing documentation forms, the Pain Task Force, a preexisting housewide nursing group charged with implementation and adherence to national pain standards, was and continues to be consulted or actively involved with IT professionals in the development and revision of forms. Third, all of the design team's work was conducted in a multidisciplinary fashion. For example, pain service nurse representatives, attending physicians, and a PhD-prepared pain expert worked with pharmacy and IT professionals to design and redesign prescriber order entry. The nursing representatives ensured that suggestions were evidence-based and applicable to all age groups and clinical settings as well as making sure data was in a format that could be easily extracted from the electronic record for auditing.

In conjunction with the IT Department, the Clinical Effectiveness Department at the UMMC, which consists of health analysts, the PhD-prepared pain expert, and other electronic documentation experts, initiated and validated electronic auditing for the following aspects of documentation and care to demonstrate compliance with accreditation requirements:

- Comprehensive pain assessment documentation
- Preanalgesic and postanalgesic pain score documentation
- Appropriate use of age-based pain assessment tools
- A static report, run several times daily, that searches current patients' EMRs for documentation in required documentation fields.

Successes

Great strides in compliance with accreditation standards have been made with electronic pain documentation at the UMMC. A major success was in the implementation of an electronic comprehensive pain assessment history form. In January 2002, approximately three months after implementation of a paper-based pain assessment history form, compliance with its completion was 28%. Over the course of a year and the use of various strategies, compliance increased to a steady state that ranged between 50% and 55%. In response to this low compliance rate, an electronic Pain Assessment/History Form was developed. The new form was designed to open up and display to the practitioner when a notation was made on the admission intake form stating the patient had pain on admission. Within two months after implementation of the compliance with the new Pain Assessment/History form, completion jumped to 85%, then dropped to 75% and plateaued. In an effort to improve compliance, additional enhancements were made over time based on suggestions from the Pain Task Force. Once all items on the form were

required for patients without excruciating pain on admission, compliance rates increased and plateaued at 90%. Audits by units showed that some patients admitted on the day of surgery or with excruciating pain on admission had incomplete forms (nurses have the option of delaying a comprehensive pain assessment in patients with uncontrolled pain upon admission). Capturing comprehensive pain assessments in these patients required changes in clinical processes as well as implementing a reminder system. To expedite patient flow, the postanesthesia care units agreed to complete forms for all surgical patients. In addition, the system was programmed to place a boxed red flag in front of the Pain Assessment/History Form name on the "index tab" that lists all chart elements when the form is incomplete (Figure C-15). When the form is complete, the boxed flag is blue (Figure C-16).

The UMMC has had similar success with preanalgesic pain score and postanalgesic pain score documentation. Preanalgesic pain score documentation has improved from 85% using paper documentation to 96% using electronic documentation. Postanalgesic pain score documentation has improved from approximately 79% using paper documentation to 87% with electronic documentation. The processes used to improve this documentation were analogous to those used to improve pain assessment history documentation. The Pain Task Force played an active role with these adaptations, required fields were used, reminder systems were implemented, nursing processes were changed, and the electronic form went through several adaptations. A synopsis of the changes is provided.

When computerized prescriber order entry was initiated at the UMMC, the vendor-developed preanalgesic and postanalgesic pain score forms were initiated. The preanalgesic form allows a preanalgesic pain score to be documented. The postanalgesic form provided a visual reminder to document a postanalgesic score. In this case, the visual cue is a blue flag posted on the eMAR for the time the nurse should obtain a postanalgesic pain score (at approximate peak effect of the administered analgesic) (see Figure C-14). The blue flag posts immediately after the nurse documents administration of the analgesic. The flag turns red, which

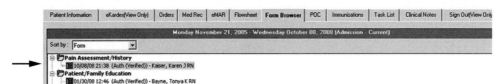

Figure C-15 | Incomplete pain assessment history form. Box turns red to indicate task is incomplete.

© 2011, University of Maryland Medical Center.

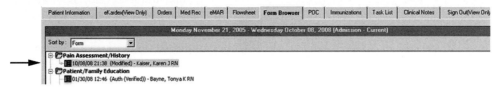

Figure C-16 | Complete pain assessment history form. Box turns blue to indicate task is complete.

© 2011, University of Maryland Medical Center.

indicates that the task is overdue if the nurse fails to document a postanalgesic pain score (Figure C-17). Due to system limitations at the time of implementation, this flag pertained only to PRN analgesics. Postanalgesic pain score documentation for PRN analgesics is consistently above 95%.

Pain Task Force members and staff notified the implementation team of the limitations of these forms. During the redesign process, the members of the Pain Task Force at the UMMC were instrumental in making several enhancements to the prebuilt tools for recording pain scores. The solution devised was more comprehensive and clinically useful than the original. This outcome was obtained by (a) face to face discussions with the information technology staff, (b) review of sequential animated drafts, and (c) evaluation of the final product.

For the preanalgesic form, the Pain Task Force requested the addition of an item that allows the selection and documentation of the pain measurement tool used to assess the presence of pain or pain severity. This encourages members of the health care team to consistently use the selected pain measurement tool for a particular patient, unless the patient's cognition level changes, necessitating a more appropriate tool. For example, if the patient could not self-report pain due to head trauma, a behavioral tool would be used until the patient was able to self-report pain, at which time a self-report tool such as a numerical rating scale or verbal descriptor scale would be used.

Pain Task Force members felt that to evaluate the analgesic's effectiveness, information on postanalgesic activities of daily living (ADL) was needed. So, for the postanalgesic form they requested a place to document pain interference with ADL and treatments (e.g., physical therapy, occupational therapy, respiratory treatment), which the nurse assesses when the postanalgesic pain score is obtained. The Pain Task Force also suggested reformatting the existing tool so that postanalgesic pain scores could be easily visualized for comparison with preanalgesic pain scores, when evaluating analgesic effectiveness (Figure C-18). Based on evaluation of the new forms, postanalgesic pain scores and documentation of pain interference have been made required fields for PRN analgesics. Besides encouraging assessment of the effectiveness of the analgesic and the overall pain treatment plan, the postanalgesic pain documentation form serves as a cue to remind the nurse to modify the care plan if pain interferes with ADLs or treatments.

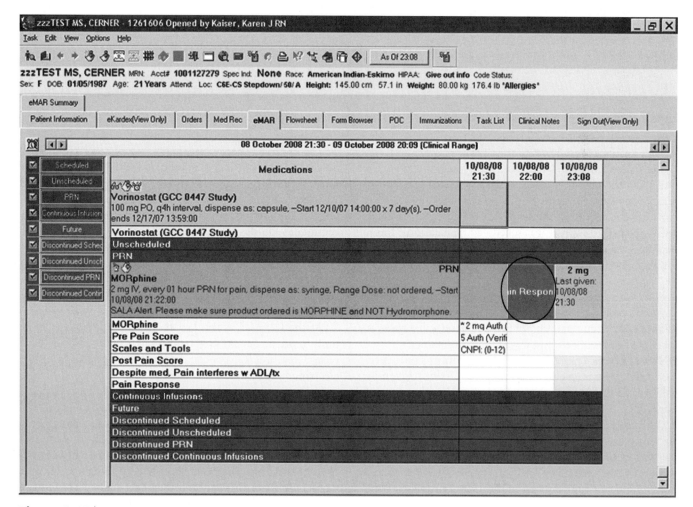

Figure C-17 | Post pain response overdue task reminder. Response box is red, indicating task is overdue.

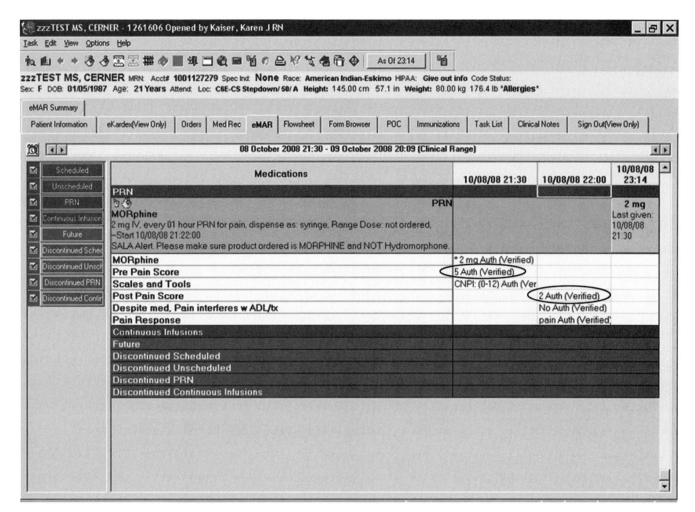

Figure C-18 | Post pain response documentation allows comparison of pre and post pain scores.

Because of system limitations, postanalgesic pain score documentation fields used to assess PRN analgesic effectiveness are not yet required for scheduled analgesics. As previously noted, there is also no visual reminder (i.e., blue or red flag) to reassess pain for scheduled medications. Based on Pain Task Force recommendations that it would provide a visual cue for documentation and system requirements, the customized PRN and scheduled analgesic electronic documentation forms are similar. The presence of the postanalgesic pain assessment fields did initially improve compliance with documentation of postanalgesic pain scores on scheduled medications, but it was not sustainable.

Postanalgesic pain score documentation for scheduled medications averages around 70%. Until a vendor solution to this limitation can be initiated with a version upgrade, a static report was developed and is run several times daily by the clinical units. The report searches current patients' EMRs for completion of required documentation fields. Nurses can use the report (particularly prior to or at change of shift or transfer) to ensure that their pain care and documentation are complete. Units that have integrated this into their daily clinical practice consistently score over 90% compliance with their posta-

nalgesic pain scores for scheduled medications on their monthly audits.

Static reminders such as the one described above are not as likely to ensure compliance the way a timed reminder would. Currently, we utilize a static notation on an electronic plan (eKardex) for assessment of pain for patients on specialized analgesic therapy. While we have seen an improvement in pain documentation of specialized analgesic therapy since our last audit, the audits are not directly comparative.

At the UMMC, several of the processes that were initially used in developing pain-related electronic medical record features have been successfully applied to other electronic processes at our facility, such as required fields, order sets, red reminder flags, and drug database customization. Similarly, electronic processes used in other situations have been applied to support pain-related best practices such as requiring documentation of fentanyl patch placement site(s) and subsequent patch removal. The UMMC has also used the EMR or data from it in a variety of ways to support other best pain management practices. We have used the data in process improvement activities, guiding refinements in the EMR system, and associated processes. For example, data in the EMR system have been used to assess and reduce IM opioid administration and inappropriate medication use (e.g., meperidine and propoxyphene) as well as discourage high doses of opioids in opioid-naïve patients via range-checking alerts. Many other pain-related safe practices and best practices are also easily assessed, implemented, supported, and evaluated using EMR technology.

Safeguards

There are many benefits to implementing an EMR system. Although EMR systems have been shown to decrease some errors, new types or causes of errors can surface as well (Campbell, Sittig, Ash, et al., 2006; Koppel, Metlay, Cohen, et al., 2005). However, many of these errors offer opportunities to make the EMR system and associated processes safer. Evaluation of how dose range checking alerts fire can provide an excellent opportunity to improve the system. For example, it may be discovered that only one of several alerts fire (e.g., weight but not age for ketorolac), or that the dose range is set too high for opioid-naïve patients (e.g., 0.8 to 4 mg), or that prescribers can order a drug to be administered via a route inconsistent with its purpose (e.g., duramorph intravenously rather than intraspinally). In these cases, revisions are necessary. However, numerous overrides of an alert may also be dangerous, as practitioners may not read the alert and instead automatically dismiss it (van der Sijs, Aarts, Vulto, et al., 2006). These situations require education or revision of the alert so that it serves its original purpose. Unsafe or inappropriate practices can be discouraged by limiting the routes of administration that the prescriber can order for a particular drug, provider, or clinical location (see Box C-2).

The EMR is sometimes seen as a comprehensive error reduction strategy, leading some to implicitly trust the information generated in the system, including orders. Health care practitioners may lapse into a false sense of security even though errors exist. Prebuilt order sentences that undergo dose range checking using noncustomized databases can look correct even though they are inconsistent with best-practice guidelines and may be unsafe. Also, it may be impossible to detect a custom-built order from an order that was prebuilt and carefully reviewed in a nonrushed, nonclinical environment.

Health care practitioners may not be trained for, understand the need for, or integrate new processes required by the EMR into clinical practice (Kushniruk, Borycki, Kuwata, et al., 2006; Spence, Valenza, Taylor, 2007; Tuttelmann, Luetjens, Nieschlag, 2006). For example, pharmacists and physicians may not realize that nursing staff do not receive dose range–checking alerts, and nurses may falsely think prescribers and pharmacists will respond appropriately to all dose range–checking alerts. There may also be changes in processes for some disciplines that are not readily apparent. For example, as previously described, the pharmacist, the nurse, and the physician see different screen views of the same medication order during the ordering, preparation, and administration process and thus have access to different information on their computer screens. Health care practitioners may operate under the assumption that the checks and balances that were in place with the paper-based system are still available with the EMR system, when, in fact, they no longer exist. It is imperative for staff to adjust to work flow process changes upon EMR implementation and to understand the work flow and processes of other disciplines to reduce error and improve patient safety (Salas, Wilson, Murphy, et al., 2008; Scott, Poole, Jayathissa, 2008).

Conclusion

As demonstrated above, the EMR has great potential to improve documentation and adherence to regulatory and accreditation standards and best-practice guidelines, as well as improve patient safety. Nurses are the practitioners with the greatest understanding of evidence-based pain guidelines and effective strategies to manage pain and minimize potential associated safety issues such as those discussed in this appendix. Most if not all pain specialists have developed safe processes for managing pain using paper-based medical record systems that can be applied to the EMR system. However, pain specialists usually see only a small percentage of their institution's patients. Based on the complexity of pain orders and the high-volume, high-risk (but low-potential) nature of errors associated with managing pain (some of which were demonstrated by examples provided in this appendix), it is recommended that pain practitioners take the initiative to become actively involved in and the primary owner of pain-related EMR development, implementation, and revisions. This includes creating a comprehensive medication reconciliation process, customized evidence-based dose range checking, safe and effective pain order sentences and order sets, appropriate alerts, electronic auditing procedures, and other processes that support best clinical practices. In addition, documentation processes that encourage thorough, adequate assessment and evaluation of pain relief interventions are essential. Pain practitioners should also ensure that there is consistency across institutional pain-related electronic technologies (e.g., Smart Pump technology, medication dispensing cabinets, and the EMR) to facilitate safety.

There is a general lack of research on pain-related EMRs. Until research can be conducted on this new technology, sharing information with colleagues about what strategies work best in the clinical setting and potential pitfalls associated with EMR is strongly encouraged. The overall goal is the development of streamlined safe, evidence-based, effective pain assessment and management from an interdisciplinary perspective using electronic technology.

References

American Pain Foundation. (2008). Overview of American pain surveys: 2005–2006. *Journal of Pain & Palliative Care Pharmacotherapy, 22*(1), 33–38.

American Pain Society. (2003). *Principles of analgesic use in the treatment of acute pain and cancer pain.* (5th ed.). Glenview, IL: American Pain Society.

American Pain Society. (2008). *Principles of analgesic use in the treatment of acute pain and cancer pain.* (6th ed.). Glenview, IL: American Pain Society.

Bercovitz, A., Decker, F. H., Jones, A., et al. (2008). End-of-life care in nursing homes: 2004 National Nursing Home Survey. *Natl Health Stat Report, 8*(9), 1–23.

Botti, M., Bucknall, T., Manias, E. (2004). The problem of postoperative pain: Issues for future research. *International Journal of Nursing Practice, 10*(6), 257–263.

Bradshaw, D. H., Empy, C., Davis, P., et al. (2008). Trends in funding for research on pain: A report on the National Institutes of Health grant awards over the years 2003 to 2007. *The Journal of Pain, 9*(12), 1077–1087.

Campbell, E. M., Sittig, D. F., Ash, J. S., et al. (2006). Types of unintended consequences related to computerized provider order entry. *Journal of the American Medical Informatics Association, 13*(5), 547–556.

Cohen, M. Z., Easley, M. K., Ellis, C., et al. (2003). Cancer pain management and the JCAHO's pain standards: An institutional challenge. *Journal of Pain and Symptom Management, 25*(6), 519–527.

Cowell, J. (2007). Improving patient safety by eliminating unsafe abbreviations from medication prescribing. *Alberta RN, 63*(8), 8–9.

Dobratz, M. C., Burns, K. M., & Oden, R. V. (1989). Pain in home hospice patients: An exploratory descriptive study. *The Hospice Journal, 5*(3–4), 117–133.

Doran, D. M., Mylopoulos, J., Kushniruk, A., et al. (2007). Evidence in the palm of your hand: Development of an outcomes-focused knowledge translation intervention. *Worldviews on Evidence-Based Nursing, 4*(2), 69–77.

Federico, F. (2007). Preventing harm from high-alert medications. *Joint Commission Journal on Quality and Patient Safety, 33*(9), 537–542.

Garg, A. X., Adhikari, N. K., McDonald, H., et al. (2005). Effects of computerized clinical decision support systems on practitioner performance and patient outcomes: A systematic review. *JAMA, 293*(10), 1223–1238.

Green, C. R. (2008). The healthcare bubble through the lens of pain research, practice, and policy: Advice for the new President and Congress. *The Journal of Pain, 9*(12), 1071–1073.

Gruner, A., Ljutow, A., Schleinzer, W., et al. (2008). Implementation of an electronic patient record. Experience in an interdisciplinary pain clinic. *Schmerz (Berlin, Germany), 22*(1), 24–33.

Hidle, U. (2007). Implementing technology to improve medication safety in healthcare facilities: A literature review. *The Journal of the New York State Nurses' Association, 38*(2), 4–9.

Hunt, D. L., Haynes, R. B., Hanna, S. E., et al. (1998). Effects of computer-based clinical decision support systems on physician performance and patient outcomes: A systematic review. *JAMA, 280*(15), 1339–1346.

Kaushal, R., Shojania, K. G., & Bates, D. W. (2003). Effects of computerized physician order entry and clinical decision support systems on medication safety: A systematic review. *Archives of Internal Medicine, 163*(12), 1409–1416.

Koppel, R., Metlay, J. P., Cohen, A., et al. (2005). Role of computerized physician order entry systems in facilitating medication errors. *JAMA, 293*(10), 1197–1203.

Kushniruk, A., Borycki, E., Kuwata, S., et al. (2006). Predicting changes in workflow resulting from healthcare information systems: Ensuring the safety of healthcare. *Healthcare Quarterly (Toronto, Ont.), 9*. Spec-8.

Leapfrog Group safety practices: Computerized physician order entry. Available at http://www.leapfroggroup.org/for_hospitals/leapfrog_safety_practices/cpoe. Accessed March 15, 2009. Last update 2009.

McMillan, S. C., Williams, F. A., Chatfield, R., et al. (1988). A validity and reliability study of two tools for assessing and managing cancer pain. *Oncology Nursing Forum, 15*(6), 735–741.

Nemeth, L. S., Wessell, A. M., Jenkins, R. G., et al. (2007). Strategies to accelerate translation of research into primary care within practices using electronic medical records. *Journal of Nursing Care Quality, 22*(4), 343–349.

Pakhomov, S. V., Jacobsen, S. J., Chute, C. G., et al. (2008). Agreement between patient-reported symptoms and their documentation in the medical record. *The American Journal of Managed Care, 14*(8), 530–539.

Pathways for medication safety. Available at http://www.ismp.org/Tools/pathways.asp. Accessed March 15, 2009. Last update 2007.

Saigh, O., Triola, M. M., & Link, R. N. (2006). Brief report: Failure of an electronic medical record tool to improve pain assessment documentation. *Journal of General Internal Medicine, 21*(2), 185–188.

Salas, E., Wilson, K. A., Murphy, C. E., et al. (2008). Communicating, coordinating, and cooperating when lives depend on it: tips for teamwork. *Joint Commission Journal on Quality and Patient Safety, 34*(6), 333–341.

Scott, I. A., Poole, P. J., & Jayathissa, S. (2008). Improving quality and safety of hospital care: A reappraisal and an agenda for clinically relevant reform. *Internal Medicine Journal, 38*(1), 44–55.

Spence, J., Valenza, J. A., & Taylor, D. (2007). Documentation of clinical workflow: A key step in a plan to facilitate implementation of an Electronic Patient Record. *AMIA Annual Symposium Proceedings, 11*, 1119.

The Joint Commission Addendum to Sentinel Event #35 Medication Reconciliation. (2006). Available at http://www.jointcommission.org/SentinelEvents/SentinelEventAlert/sea_35.htm. Accessed March 17, 2009.

The Joint Commission Sentinel Event #11 High-Alert Medications and Patient Safety. (2006). Available at http://www.jointcommission.org/SentinelEvents/SentinelEventAlert/sea_11.htm. Accessed March 18, 2009.

Tuttelmann, F., Luetjens, C. M., & Nieschlag, E. (2006). Optimising workflow in andrology: A new electronic patient record and database. *Asian Journal of Andrology, 8*(2), 235–241.

van der Sijs, H., Aarts, J., Vulto, A., et al. (2006). Overriding of drug safety alerts in computerized physician order entry. *Journal of AHIMA, 13*(2), 138–147.

VHA Office of Information VistA Computerized Patient Record System. Available at http://www1.va.gov/CPRSdemo/VHA-Office of Information. Accessed March 21, 2009. Last updated 2009.

Wager, K. A., Lee, F. W., White, A. W., et al. (2000). Impact of an electronic medical record system on community-based primary care practices. *The Journal of the American Board of Family Practice, 13*(5), 338–348.

Whipple, N. N., Palchuk, M. B., Olsha-Yehiav, M., et al. (2007). Supporting CMT and user customization in Clinical Documentation templates. *AMIA Annual Symposium Proceedings*, Oct 11, 1153.

Wolfstadt, J. I., Gurwitz, J. H., Field, T. S., et al. (2008). The effect of computerized physician order entry with clinical decision support on the rates of adverse drug events: A systematic review. *Journal of General Internal Medicine, 23*(4), 451–458.

Yellowlees, P. M., Marks, S. L., Hogarth, M., et al. (2008). Standards-based, open-source electronic health record systems: A desirable future for the U.S. health industry. *Telemedicine Journal and E-health, 14*(3), 284–288.

Appendix D Terminology

Chris Pasero and Margo McCaffery

The following terms were selected from the terminology found at the beginning of the chapters.

Acetaminophen Other generic names include *paracetamol* and *acetylparaaminophenol* (APAP). Also referred to as *aspirin-free*.

Addiction A chronic neurologic and biologic disease. As defined by pain specialists, it is characterized by behaviors that include one or more of the following: impaired control over drug use, compulsive use, continued use despite harm, and craving. Continued craving for an opioid and the need to use the opioid for effects other than pain relief. Physical dependence and tolerance are not the same as addiction.

Adjuvant analgesic A drug that has a primary indication other than pain (e.g., anticonvulsant, antidepressant, sodium channel blocker, and muscle relaxant) but is analgesic for some painful conditions. Sometimes referred to as *coanalgesic*.

Afferent Neuron that carries information to the central nervous system.

Agonist-antagonist A type of opioid (e.g., nalbuphine and butorphanol) that binds to the kappa opioid receptor site acting as an agonist (capable of producing analgesia) and simultaneously to the mu opioid receptor site acting as an antagonist (reversing mu agonist effects).

Allodynia Pain due to a stimulus that does not normally provoke pain such as touch. Typically experienced in the skin around areas affected by nerve injury, commonly seen with many neuropathic pain syndromes.

Analgesic ceiling A dose beyond which further increases in dose do not provide additional analgesia.

Antagonist Drug that competes with agonists for opioid receptor binding sites; can displace agonists, thereby inhibiting their action. Examples include naloxone, naltrexone, and nalmefene.

APAP: See "acetaminophen."

Bioavailability The extent to which a dose of a drug reaches its site of action.

Blood-brain barrier A barrier that exists between circulating blood and brain, preventing damaging substances from reaching brain tissue and cerebrospinal fluid.

Breakthrough dose (BTD) Also referred to as *supplemental dose* or *rescue dose*; the dose of analgesic taken to treat breakthrough pain.

Breakthrough pain (BTP) A transitory increase in pain that occurs on a background of otherwise controlled persistent pain.

Ceiling effect A dose above which further dose increments produce no change in effect.

Central disinhibition A central mechanism of neuropathic pain that occurs when control mechanisms along inhibitory (modulatory) pathways are lost or suppressed, leading to abnormal excitability of central neurons.

Central sensitization A key central mechanism of neuropathic pain; the abnormal hyperexcitability of central neurons in the spinal cord, which results from complex changes induced by the incoming afferent barrages of nociceptors.

Comfort-function goal The pain rating identified by the individual patient above which the patient experiences interference with function and quality of life, that is, activities that the patient needs or wishes to perform.

Controlled release See modified release.

Coxib NSAID that preferentially inhibits the cyclooxygenase (COX) isoenzyme COX 2. Examples are celecoxib and rofecoxib. The term is used interchangeably with *COX-2 selective NSAID*. The latter term will be used in this book.

Crescendo pain A period of rapid pain escalation often associated with increasing distress and functional impairment.

Cross excitation See ephaptic conduction.

Cross talk See ephaptic conduction.

Distribution half-life The time it takes a drug to move from the blood and plasma to other tissues. Distribution half-life differs from half-life (terminal) (see **half-life**).

DSM-IV *Diagnostic and Statistical Manual of Mental Disorders*. A guide for clinical practice that identifies mental disorders and lists diagnostic criteria. Revised edition exists, but the DSM-IV is the one most commonly used in the studies cited in this chapter.

Dysesthesia An unpleasant abnormal sensation (spontaneous or evoked) that is usually associated with neuropathic pain. It is usually described as "pins and needles" (e.g., a limb "falling asleep," burning, electric shock–like, tingling) and may be intermittent or continuous and experienced in an area of sensory loss. A dysesthesia should always be unpleasant, whereas a paresthesia should not be unpleasant. It may be difficult to differentiate dysesthesias from paresthesias.

Efferent Neuron that carries information away from the central nervous system.

Efficacy The extent to which a drug or another treatment "works" and can produce the effect in question—analgesia in this context. To determine whether this is the case, the treatment must be compared to another, typically a placebo, but sometimes an active comparator. Maximal efficacy refers to the maximum effect that can be produced by a drug, and comparative efficacy refers to the relative effects of two or more treatments compared at comparable treatment intensities.

Ephaptic conduction Also called cross-excitation or cross-talk; a peripheral mechanism that may sustain neuropathic pain through the creation of chemically-mediated connections between nerve fibers, causing the abnormal activation of nociceptive neurons, ultimately producing pain.

Extended release See modified release.

Faces Pain Scale-Revised (FPS-R) A series of 6 faces numbered 0, 2, 4, 6, 8, 10, beginning with a bland facial expression with subsequent faces increasing in expressions of distress. The patient is asked to point to the face that best reflects the intensity of his or her pain.

Half-life The time it takes for the plasma concentration (amount of drug in the body) to be reduced by 50%. After starting a drug or increasing its dose, four to five half-lives are required to approach a steady-state level in the blood, irrespective of the dose, dosing interval, or route of administration; after four to five half-lives, a drug that has been discontinued generally is considered to be mostly eliminated from the body.

Hand-off Communication The process by which nurses share pertinent information about their patients when care is transferred from one nurse to another.

Hydrophilic Readily absorbed in aqueous solution.

Hyperalgesia Increased pain response to noxious stimuli; decreased sensitivity to pain.

GABAergic Increased function of the gamma aminobutyric acid (GABA) (inhibitory) pathways; increased GABA function (GABAergic) may help to relieve neuropathic pain.

Immediate-release See short-acting.

Incomplete cross-tolerance Because similar drugs (like the mu agonists) have different intrinsic efficacies (how they produce effects after binding to a receptor) at the same receptors, and because each also interacts with a different group of receptor subtypes, a switch from one drug to another similar drug (e.g., from one mu agonist to another) is associated with a variable degree of tolerance to different effects; for example, in an animal model, tolerance to morphine's analgesic effect can be produced and be made very profound, but analgesia will reappear on switching to another mu agonist like hydromorphone.

Independent double-check process An individual, e.g., nurse or pharmacist, checks the analgesic, solution, concentration, dose, and/or programming of analgesic device against the written prescription without prompting from the person administering the analgesic or anyone else. This safety measure is implemented at specified (by institutional policy) intervals to ensure accuracy of drug delivery (e.g., prior to initiation of IV PCA).

Intellectual disability Type of developmental disability that involves cognitive impairment that is evident in childhood and continues throughout life. Sometimes referred to as *mental retardation*. An intellectual disability may or may not be accompanied by a physical disability.

Intractable In reference to pain that is unresponsive to all other recommended therapeutic options (e.g., first-line and second-line analgesics).

Intraspinal "Within the spine"; term referring to the spaces or potential spaces surrounding the spinal cord into which medications can be administered. Most often, the term is used when referring to the epidural and intrathecal routes of administration. Sometimes used interchangeably with the term *neuraxial*.

Lancinating Sudden stabbing or knifelike pain.

Lipophilic Readily absorbed in fatty tissues.

Malingering Intentionally produced symptom (e.g., pain) motivated by various factors, such as financial gain.

Medically ill patients Patients with existing debilitating pathologic condition/illness that may be progressive or stable, as opposed to those who have only the symptom of pain and are otherwise healthy.

Metabolite The product of biochemical reactions during drug metabolism.

Modified release Oral opioid analgesics that are formulated to release over a prolonged period of time; often used interchangeably with the terms **extended release, sustained release,** and **controlled release.** The term **modified release** will be used in this book to describe these drugs.

Mu agonist Any opioid that binds to the mu opioid receptor subtype and produces effects. Includes morphine and other opioids that relieve pain by binding to the mu receptor sites in the nervous system. Used interchangeably with the terms **full agonist, pure agonist,** and **morphine-like drug.**

Narcotic See **Opioid**. Obsolete term for **opioid**, in part because the government and media use the term loosely to refer to a variety of substances of potential abuse. Legally, controlled-substances classified as narcotics include opioids, cocaine, and various other substances.

Neuralgia Pain in the distribution of a nerve (e.g., sciatica, trigeminal neuralgia). Often felt as an electrical shock–like pain.

Neuropathic (pathophysiologic) pain Pain sustained by injury or dysfunction of the peripheral or central nervous system. Distinctly different from physiologic (nociceptive) pain.

Neuroplasticity The ability of the peripheral and central nervous systems to change both structure and function as a result of noxious stimuli.

NMDA N-methyl-D-aspartate. In this book the term is used in conjunction with drugs that are NMDA receptor antagonists or blockers, such as ketamine or dextromethorphan.

Nociceptive (physiologic) pain Pain that is sustained by ongoing activation of the sensory system that subserves the perception of noxious stimuli; implies the existence of damage to somatic or visceral tissues sufficient to activate the nociceptive system.

Nociceptor A primary afferent nerve that has the ability to respond to a noxious stimulus or to a stimulus that would be noxious if prolonged.

Nonopioid Used instead of **nonnarcotic**. Refers to acetaminophen and nonsteroidal antiinflammatory drugs (NSAIDs).

Normal release See short acting.

Numerical Rating Scale (NRS) Several types exist. The most commonly used NRS and the one used in this book consists of numbers placed along a horizontal line and asks the patient to rate pain from 0 to 10, with zero equaling no pain and 10 equaling the worst possible pain. Recommended for use in clinical practice. Can be presented verbally, but visual is preferred. This scale may also be presented on a vertical line.

NSAID An acronym for nonsteroidal antiinflammatory drug. (Pronounced "in said.") Also referred to as "aspirin like" drugs.

Opioid This term is preferred to **narcotic**. Opioid refers to codeine, morphine, and other natural, semisynthetic, and synthetic drugs that relieve pain by binding to multiple types of opioid receptors.

Opioid dose-sparing effect The dose of opioid may be lowered when another analgesic, such as a nonopioid or **adjuvant**, is added.

Opioid-induced hyperalgesia (OIH) A phenomenon clearly demonstrated in experimental models, but of uncertain significance in humans, by which exposure to the opioid induces increased sensitivity, or a lowered threshold, to the neural activity subserving pain perception; it is the "flip side" of analgesic tolerance, which is defined by the loss of analgesic activity due to exposure to the drug.

Opioid-naïve An opioid-naïve person has not recently taken enough opioid on a regular enough basis to become tolerant to the effects of an opioid.

Opioid rotation Switching from one mu agonist opioid to another; often used to treat analgesic tolerance or unmanageable and intolerable adverse effects.

Opioid-tolerant An opioid-tolerant person has taken opioids long enough at doses high enough to develop tolerance to many of the effects of the opioid, including analgesia and sedation, but there is no timeframe for developing tolerance.

Paresthesia Abnormal sensation, whether spontaneous or evoked, manifested by sensations of numbness, prickling, tingling, and heightened sensitivity that is typically not unpleasant.

Paroxysmal Sudden periodic attack or recurrence.

Peripheral sensitization A key peripheral mechanism of neuropathic pain that occurs when there are changes in the number and location of ion channels, in particular sodium channels abnormally accumulate in injured nociceptors producing a lower nerve depolarization threshold, ectopic discharges, and an increase in the response to stimuli.

Physical dependence Potential for withdrawal symptoms if the opioid is abruptly stopped or an antagonist is administered; not the same as **addiction**.

Placebo Any medication or procedure, including surgery, that produces an effect in a patient because of its implicit or explicit intent and not because of its specific physical or chemical properties.

Potency The dose required to produce a specified effect; relative potency is the ratio of the doses of two or more analgesics required to produce the same analgesic effect.

Preemptive analgesia Preinjury pain treatments (e.g., preoperative epidural analgesia and preincision local anesthetic infiltration) to prevent the establishment of peripheral and central sensitization of pain.

Primary afferent neuron See **nociceptor**.

Prodrug An inactive precursor of a drug, converted into its active form in the body by normal metabolic processes.

Protective analgesia An aggressive, sustained multimodal analgesic intervention administered perioperatively (e.g., local anesthetic block, acetaminophen, NSAID, and anticonvulsant initiated preoperatively and continued throughout the intraoperative and postoperative periods) and directed toward prevention of pathologic pain (e.g., persistent neuropathic postsurgical pain syndromes).

Pseudoaddiction A mistaken diagnosis of addiction in which patients exhibit behaviors often seen in addictive disease, such as escalating demands for larger doses of opioids, but actually reflect undertreated pain; may co-exist with the disease of addiction and drive relapse behaviors.

Refractory Nonresponsive or resistant to therapeutic interventions such as first- or second-line analgesics.

Self-report The ability of an individual to give a report, in this case, of pain, especially intensity. This is considered the "gold standard" of pain assessment. Patients may do this by marking on a scale such as the NRS, pointing to a number on a scale or a face. Head nodding and eye blinking can also be used to signal presence of pain and sometimes is used to rate intensity.

Sequential trials One drug is tried and if the results are unfavorable, it is discontinued and another drug is tried; a trial-and-error approach in which one drug after another is tried until the desired effects occur.

Short acting Oral opioid analgesics with a relatively fast onset of action (e.g., 30 minutes) and short duration (3 to 4 hours) and often referred to as *normal release* and inaccurately as *immediate release*. The term **immediate release** is particularly problematic because none of the oral opioid analgesics have an immediate onset of action. The term **short acting** will be used in this book.

Supraspinal Involving the brainstem or cerebrum.

Sustained release See **modified release**.

Sympathetically-maintained pain Pain that is identified through a very positive response to sympathetic nerve blocks; likely to be part of the syndrome known as complex regional pain syndrome (CRPS). Underlying mechanism is unclear but thought to be related to ephaptic conduction.

Systemic drug treatment; systemic administration Administration of a drug by a given route that allows absorption into the systemic circulation. Routes include oral, parenteral (IV, IM, SC), rectal, vaginal, topical application, transdermal, intranasal, and transmucosal. By contrast, the spinal route of administration deposits the drug directly into the central nervous system, minimizing the amount of drug that reaches the systemic circulation.

Tabetic pain A pain that is sharp, lightning in nature; also called lancinating pain.

Terminal half-life Provides an estimate of how fast a drug leaves the body; the time it takes for the amount of drug in the body to be reduced by 50%. Terminal half-life differs from distribution half-life (see above).

Titration Adjusting the amount (e.g., adjusting the dose of opioid).

Tolerance A process characterized by decreasing effects of a drug at its previous dose, or the need for a higher dose of drug to maintain an effect; not the same as **addiction**.

Upregulation An increase in a cellular component (e.g., the number of receptors), making the cells more sensitive to a particular drug or other agent.

Verbal Descriptor Scale (VDS) Several types exist. This pain intensity rating scale is a list of adjectives describing different levels of pain intensity. An example that can be placed on a 0 to 10 metric is: no pain (0), mild pain (2), moderate pain (4), severe pain (6), very severe pain (8), and most intense pain imaginable (10).

Verbal Numerical Scale (VNS) The NRS, often 0 to 5 or 0 to 10, is presented verbally, but studies suggest that the patient should also be shown a visual of the scale.

Visual Analog Scale (VAS) A horizontal (sometimes vertical) 10-cm line with word anchors at the extremes, such as "no pain" on one end and "pain as bad as it could be" or "worst possible pain" on the other end. Patient is asked to make a mark on the line to indicate intensity of pain, and the length of the mark from "no pain" is measured and recorded in centimeters or millimeters. Impractical for use in daily clinical practice.

Wind-up The progressive increase in response of central neurons that may be induced by high-intensity activity in the peripheral nociceptors that synapse on these neurons.

Terminology Related to Research

Anecdotal evidence Evidence derived from clinical observations, clinical experience, or published case reports.

Case reports Published reports of one or more patient cases describing patient experiences, circumstances, or situations that infer specific outcomes that are not based on any scientific method of study.

Case-control study A retrospective observational study used most often to evaluate risk factors that may help explain the appearance or presentation of a disease or condition. Subjects with a known disease or condition are matched with similar individuals who do not possess it. Various potential risk factors (e.g., age or sex) or lifestyle factors are then statistically evaluated to determine their levels of association with the disease or condition.

Cohort study A retrospective or prospective study in which a group of subjects who have a specific condition or receive a particular treatment are evaluated over time for a defined period. Data may be compared with another group of subjects who do not have the same condition or receive the same treatment, or subgroups within the cohort may be compared.

Controlled studies/trials Research studies that exert some or total control over the various treatment effects by using a comparison group (placebo group or comparator treatment group) and may use a single- or double-blind design, or random assignment of subjects.

Double-blind study Neither the investigator nor the subject know the critical aspects of the study (e.g., in a placebo-controlled trial, neither the person administering the intervention nor the subject receiving the intervention know if the intervention is experimental or placebo); used to reduce investigator and subject bias.

Meta-analysis Data analysis in which the results of several studies that address related research are combined and analyzed to arrive at one overall measurement of treatment effect.

Number needed to treat (NNT) A parameter that is often used in reporting the results of epidemiologic studies, clinical trials, systematic reviews, and meta-analyses. It is an estimate of how many people would need to receive an intervention to prevent one undesirable outcome or how many people need to receive a treatment in order that one derives a well-defined benefit (e.g., a 50% reduction in pain). NNT is calculated by using a formula that involves a known risk reduction or benefit analysis. Investigators typically determine and define the outcome that is used to compute the NNT for their study.

Open-label Both the investigators and subjects know what treatment subjects are receiving. An investigator studies the response to an analgesic in a sample of patients and follows them through the treatment phase, observing and recording the effects. A disadvantage of this study design is potential bias for patient selection, observations, and conclusions.

Placebo-controlled trial A study that compares a treatment to a placebo, which is a treatment with no known therapeutic value. The placebo typically resembles the active intervention and is used as the control to determine the active intervention's efficacy.

Randomized controlled trial (RCT) A study in which subjects are randomly assigned (by chance alone) to receive the various interventions in a study. Randomization increases the likelihood that factors that could influence the effects produced by a treatment

are distributed evenly across treatment groups, thereby limiting the risk of bias.

Relative risk (RR) A measure of the risk of a certain event happening in one group compared with the risk of the same event happening in another group. For example, in cancer research, relative risk is used in prospective (forward-looking) studies, such as cohort studies and clinical trials. A relative risk of 1 means there is no difference between groups in terms of their risk of cancer, based on whether or not they were exposed to a certain substance or factor, or how they responded to two treatments being compared. A relative risk of greater than 1 or less than 1 means that being exposed to a certain substance or factor either increases (relative risk greater than 1) or decreases (relative risk less than 1) the risk of cancer, or that the treatments being compared do not have the same effects (e.g., a relative risk of 2 would mean that those exposed to a certain substance or factor have twice the risk of cancer compared with those who are not exposed to a certain substance or factor). Relative risk is also often called *relative ratio*.

Reliability Regarding pain measures, it means that the scale consistently measures what it is intended to measure, such as pain intensity or presence of pain, from one time to the next.

Single-blind study The investigators know what treatment conditions to which subjects are assigned, but subjects are "blinded" (not aware) of what they are receiving.

Validity Regarding pain measures, it means that the tool accurately measures what it is intended to measure, such as pain intensity or presence of pain. A fundamental aspect of validity for pain rating scales is that they demonstrate sensitivity to changes in the magnitude of pain.

Index

Page numbers followed by *b*, *t*, and *f* indicate boxes, tables, and figures/forms respectively.

Subcutaneous administration, 399–401, 401*f*, 402*b*
Subjectivity, 20–24
Suboxone. *See* Buprenorphine
Substance abuse, 33–34
Substance dependence, 33–34
Substance misuse, 33–34
Subutex. *See* Buprenorphine
Sufentanil, 355–356
    intraspinal administration of, 418*t*, 420*t*, 425
    local anesthetics and, 425
    patient-controlled epidural analgesia, 421*t*, 425
Sulfa allergy, 208
Sulindac
    dosing of, 211*t*
    gastrointestinal event risks, 195*t*
Supraspinal, 279
Surgery
    aspirin discontinuation before, 234–235
    nonsteroidal antiinflammatory drugs discontinuation before, 234–235
    persistent pain after, 307–308, 430
Surgical wound healing, 238
Surrogate/proxy tools, 126–127
Swedish translation, of Faces Pain Scale-Revised, 69*f*
Switching of opioids. *See* Opioid switching
Symmetrel. *See* Amantadine
Sympathetically-maintained pain, 649
Synera, 729
Systemic drug treatment, 178, 279, 625

T
TAC, 730
Tagalong translation, of Numerical Rating Scale, 60*f*
Talwin. *See* Pentazocine
Tamil translation, of Faces Pain Scale-Revised, 69*f*
Tamper-resistant oral opioid formulations, 378
Tapentadol, 361–362
Targeted peripheral analgesia, 684
Tegretol. *See* Carbamazepine
Terminal half-life, 288–289, 331–332
Terminally ill patients
    delirium in, 503
    dyspnea in, 536–537
    pain in
        description of, 148
        management of, 535–537
Tetrahydrocannabinol, 651
Thai translation, of Faces Pain Scale-Revised, 69*f*
Thrombolysis, 439*t*
Thromboxane A₂
    acetaminophen effects on, 189–190
    nonsteroidal antiinflammatory drugs effect, 197, 204
Thunder Project II, 144
Tiagabine, 660
Titration, 178, 279, 625
Tizanidine, 648–650, 748*t*
TLC, 730
Tocainide, 667
Tofranil. *See* Imipramine
Tolerance
    addiction vs., 292
    characteristics of, 291–292
    definition of, 33, 178, 279, 291–292, 524, 625
    to opioids, 291–293, 295–296, 296*t*
    to pain, 24–25
    physical dependence vs., 292
    to respiratory depression, 292

Tolmetin
    dosing of, 211*t*
    gastrointestinal event risks, 195*t*
Tongan translation, of Numerical Rating Scale, 60*f*
Topical analgesics
    adjuvant, 628*t*
    advantages of, 684
    adverse effects of, 692
    anticonvulsants, 685*t*, 691
    antidepressants, 685*t*, 691
    capsaicin, 685*t*, 689–691
    clonidine, 685*t*, 691–692
    definition of, 684
    EMLA, 688, 727–728
    indications for, 692
    ketamine, 685*t*, 692
    lidocaine patch 5%, 684–688, 686*b*
    misconceptions about, 687
    older adults treated with, 687
    summary of, 692
Topical benzocaine, 730–731
Topiramate (Topamax), 659, 662–663, 665–666, 748*t*
Toradol. *See* Ketorolac
Total time interval, 460–461, 461*b*
Toxic epidermal necrolysis, 207–208
Trait anxiety, 32
Tramadol, 360–361, 365, 389
Transdermal, defined, 684
Transdermal clonidine, 648
Transdermal fentanyl patch, 390–396, 553*f*
    absorption, 390–391, 391*f*, 395–396
    adverse effects of, 395–396
    application sites for, 390, 395
    breakthrough doses, 449
    breakthrough pain during treatment with, 392
    in cachectic patients, 396
    cancer pain treated with, 394
    delivery systems for, 391–392, 391*f*
    disposal of, 395
    drug reservoir, 391–392, 391*f*
    hand-off communication regarding, 395
    heat exposure effects on, 395
    indications for, 392–394
    long-term use of, 394–395
    matrix, 391–392, 391*f*
    morphine switch to, 393*b*
    opioid switching to, 391, 392
    in opioid-naïve patients, 394
    pulmonary conditions, 396
    safety of, 394–395
Translations
    of Faces Pain Rating Scale-Revised, 69*f*
    of Numerical Rating Scale, 60*f*
    of Wong-Baker FACES Pain Rating Scale, 66*f*
Trauma-induced pain, 307
Treatment plans, 40
Triamcinolone, 647*t*
Tricyclic antidepressants, 637–638, 642–643
    adverse effects of, 642, 643
    cardiotoxicity of, 642
    dose of, 644–645
    hepatotoxicity concerns, 643
    indications for, 643–644
    mechanism of action, 641–642
    during pregnancy, 633
    summary of, 641
Trigeminal neuralgia, 658, 672
Trileptal. *See* Oxcarbazepine
Trixaicin. *See* Capsaicin
Turkish translation, of Faces Pain Scale-Revised, 69*f*
Tylenol No. 3, 184

Tylenol With Codeine. *See* Codeine with acetaminophen
Tylox. *See* Oxycodone, acetaminophen with

U
UDP-glucuronosyltransferases, 288
Ulcerations, nonsteroidal antiinflammatory drug-induced, 190
Unconscious patients
    awareness periods in, 148
    pain assessments in, 147–148
Undertreatment of pain, 46
University of Maryland Medical Center
    electronic medical record system, 851–855, 852*f*, 853*f*, 854*f*
Upregulation, 279, 625
Urdu translation, of Numerical Rating Scale, 60*f*
Urinary retention, 427, 502
Urine toxicology screens, 834–835

V
Vaginal administration, of opioids, 369*t*, 389–390
Valdecoxib, 201
Validity
    of Brief Pain Inventory, 159
    of Faces Pain Scale-Revised, 68, 96*t*, 159
    of Numerical Rating Scale, 57
    types of, 130*t*
    of verbal descriptor scales, 96*t*
Valium. *See* Diazepam
Valproic acid, 660, 748*t*
Vegetative patients
    definition of, 148
    pain in, 148
Venlafaxine, 640–641, 642, 748*t*
    patient medication information form, 781*f*
Verbal descriptor scales
    cognitively impaired older patient's use of, 94
    reliability of, 96*t*
    validity of, 96*t*
    visual analogue scale vs., 55
Veterans Health Administration study, 15, 19
Vicodin. *See* Hydrocodone, acetaminophen and
Vicoprofen, 184
Victoria Bowel Performance Scale, 490*f*
Vietnamese translation
    of FACES Pain Rating Scale, 66*f*
    of Numerical Rating Scale, 60*f*
Vimpat. *See* Lacosamide
Vistaril. *See* Hydroxyzine
Visual analogue scale, 55
    clinical practice use of, 55
    definition of, 55
    description of, 16*t*
    disadvantages of, 55
    horizontal, 55*f*
    verbal descriptor scale vs., 55
Vital signs
    nurses' willingness to record patients' reports of pain affected by, 26
    as reliable pain indicators, 27
Vitamin D, 745
Vomiting. *See* Postoperative nausea and vomiting

W
Wallisian translation, of Faces Pain Scale-Revised, 69*f*
Warfarin
    acetaminophen and, 189
    description of, 439*t*
Web sites, 821*f*, 822, 823*t*
Weblogs, 822

Dosing Guidelines for Selected Adjuvant Analgesics Used for Persistent (Chronic) Pain

Drugs/Routes	Usual Starting Dose (mg/day)	Usual Effective Dose Range (mg/day)	Dosing Schedule	Comments
Anticonvulsants				
gabapentin (Neurontin) PO	100-300	300-3600	q8h	First-line for neuropathic pain. May increase dose q3-4 days by amount equal to starting dose.
pregabalin (Lyrica) PO	100-150	150-600	q12h	First-line for neuropathic pain. May increase dose q3-4 days by amount equal to starting dose.
carbamazepine (Tegretol) PO	200	600-1200	q6-8h	Effective for trigeminal neuralgia.
clonazepam (Klonopin) PO	0.5	0.5-3	q8h	May be helpful for pain and anxiety associated with disease process.
topiramate (Topamax) PO	50-100	100-400	q12h	Effective for migraine. May increase dose by 25 mg weekly.
Antidepressants (Secondary Amines)				
desipramine (Norpramin) PO	10-25	50-150	hs	Secondary amines are first-line for neuropathic pain. Due to adverse effects, amitriptyline should be used only if a secondary amine is unavailable. Evaluate and titrate upward q3-5 days.
nortriptyline (Aventyl, Pamelor) PO	10-25	50-150	hs	
Antidepressants (Serotonin Norepinephrine Reuptake Inhibitors [SNRIs])				
duloxetine (Cymbalta)	30	60	q12h	First-line for neuropathic pain. Increase to 60 mg after 1 wk.
milnacipran (Savella)	12.5-25	50-100	q12h	Initiate with once-daily dosing, then increase to twice-daily dosing; doses > 200 mg/day have not been studied.
Corticosteroids				
dexamethasone (Decadron) PO	Low-dose regimen: 2-16 mg	Same	q6-12h	Long-term treatment with low doses is usually well tolerated in those with advanced medical illness. Indicated for acute episode of severe pain unresponsive to opioids. Risk of serious toxicity increases with dose, duration of therapy, and co-administration of NSAID.
	High-dose regimen: 100 mg then 96 mg in 4 divided doses	Same	q6h	
Local Anesthetics				
mexilitine (Mexitil) PO	150-200	900-1200	q8h	Third-line for neuropathic pain. Plasma concentrations should be followed to reduce risk of toxicity.
lidocaine IV	1-5 mg/kg	—	infusion	Brief infusion over 20-30 minutes. Analgesia occurs within 15-30 minutes. May be appropriate for rapidly escalating neuropathic pain.
lidocaine subcutaneous, IV	2.5-5 mg/kg/h	—	—	Continuous infusion
Others				
baclofen (Lioresal) PO	5-15	30-200	q8h	Indicated for neuropathic pain.
calcitonin subcutaneous, IV	25 IU	100-200 IU	qd	Calcitonin is indicated for various neuropathic pains, bone pain, and possibly osteoarthritis.
calcitonin nasal spray (Miacalcin)	200 IU	200-400 IU	qd	
clonidine transdermal (Catapres-TTS)	0.1/24h strength patch	0.2-0.6	q week patch change	Clonidine doses may be increased by 0.1 mg/day q3-5 days.
clonidine (Catapres) PO	0.1	0.2-0.6	qd	

h, Hour; *hs*, bedtime; *IU*, international unit; *q*, every; *qd*, every day.
For more complete information and references, see: Pasero, C., Polomano, R., Portenoy, R. K., et al. (2011). Adjuvant analgesics. In C. Pasero, & M. McCaffery. *Pain assessment and pharmacologic management*, St. Louis, Mosby.

Dosing Guidelines for Acetaminophen and Selected NSAIDs

Generic (Brand) Name(s)	Recommended Starting Oral Dose (mg)*	Dosing Schedule	Maximum Oral Dose (mg/day) Recommended**	Comments
acetaminophen (Tylenol, many others)	650	q4-6h	4000	Reduce dose or avoid in presence of chronic alcohol abuse/dependence and in those with hepatic dysfunction; no effect on bleeding time, but may produce dose-dependent increase in INR when taken concomitantly with warfarin.
aspirin (Bayer, many others)	650	q4-6h	4000	May not be as well tolerated as other NSAIDs.
celecoxib (Celebrex)	100-200	q12-24h	400	COX-2 selective NSAID; lower risk of GI toxicity compared with most other NSAIDs; avoid in those with high CV risk; once-daily dosing may be safer from CV perspective than twice-daily dosing.
choline magnesium trisalicylate	500-1000	q12h	4000	No effect on bleeding time.
diclofenac (Cataflam [short acting], Voltaren [delayed release], Voltaren-XR [modified release])	25-75	q8-12h	150	High COX-2 selectivity; also available in gel (Voltaren) and patch (Flector)
ibuprofen (Motrin, Advil, many others)	400-800	q6h	3200	Also available in cream and liquid.
ibuprofen (Caldolor) IV	400-800	q6h	3200	For acute pain and fever; must be diluted and given via IV infusion over 30-minute period.
ketoprofen	25	q6-8h	300	Available rectally and as a topical gel; also available in modified-release formulation (initially 100 mg/24h; increase to 200 mg/24h).
ketorolac (Toradol)	10	q6h	40	Use limited to 5 days.
ketorolac (Toradol) IV	≤ 30	q6h	≤ 120	Daily and maximum doses should be decreased by 50% for older adults.
nabumetone (Relafen)	1000	q12-24h	2000	Minimal effect on bleeding time.
naproxen (Naprosyn, Aleve)***	250-500	q12h	1500	Peak antiinflammatory effect may not be seen for 2-4 weeks of use.
salsalate (Disalcid)***	500-1000	q8-12h	4000	Minimal effect on bleeding time.

CV, Cardiovascular; *GI*, gastrointestinal; *h*, hour; *INR*, International Normalized Ratio; *IV*, intravenous; *q*, every.
*Should be reduced by one-half to two-thirds in the elderly, those on multiple drugs, or those with renal insufficiency.
**Data are lacking, but the dose listed is thought to be the maximum needed by most patients for analgesia and the dose beyond which adverse effects are more likely. Some patients require or tolerate less or more.
***Avoid full doses in older adults due to long half-life and increased risk of GI toxicity.
For more complete information and references, see: Pasero, C., Portenoy, R. K., & McCaffery, M. (2011). Nonopioid analgesics. In C. Pasero & M. McCaffery. *Pain assessment and pharmacologic management*, St. Louis, Mosby.

Indications for nonopioid analgesics:
- *Mild pain.* Start with a nonopioid. Acetaminophen or an NSAID alone often provides adequate relief.
- *Moderate to severe pain.* Pain of any severity may be at least partially relieved by a nonopioid, but an NSAID alone usually does not relieve severe pain.
- *Pain that requires an opioid, particularly postoperative pain, cancer-related bone pain, osteoarthritis, and rheumatoid arthritis.* Add a nonopioid for the opioid dose-sparing effect.

Gastroprotective therapies for prevention of ulcers in patients taking NSAIDs:
- Misoprostol (Cytotec).
- Proton pump inhibitor (e.g., esomeprazole [Nexium], lansoprazole [Prevacid], and omeprazole [Prilosec]).
- Though less effective than misoprostol and proton pump inhibitors, H₂ blocker (e.g., famotidine [Pepsid] and rantidine [Zantac]) may be used.

Preventive strategies when bleeding is a concern:
- Use an NSAID that has minimal or no effect on bleeding time, such as celecoxib (Celebrex), choline magnesium trisalicylate, salsalate (Disalcid), or nabumetone (Relafen).
- Use acetaminophen instead of a NSAID (may increase INR when taken concomitantly with warfarin).
- Celecoxib and others with no effect on bleeding time may be given preoperatively. Aspirin is stopped 1 week preoperatively in most patients; other NSAIDs, 2 to 3 days before surgery.

INR, International Normalized Ratio.

Analgesic	Parenteral (IM, SC, IV) Route[1,2] (mg)	PO Route[1] (mg)	Comments
Mu Opioid Agonists			
morphine	10	30	Standard for comparison. Multiple routes of administration. Available in short-acting and modified-release formulations. Active metabolite M6G can accumulate with repeated dosing in renal failure.
codeine	130	200 NR	Limited usefulness; IM has unpredictable absorption and high adverse effect profile; PO inferior to ibuprofen; usually compounded with nonopioid (e.g., Tylenol #3).
fentanyl	100 mcg (100 mcg/h transdermally ≈ 4 mg/h of IV morphine; 1 mcg/h transdermally ≈ 2 mg/24h of PO morphine)	—	Fast-acting, short half-life; at steady state, slow elimination from tissues can lead to prolonged half-life (up to 12 h). Start opioid-naïve patients on no more than 25 mcg/h transdermally. Transdermal fentanyl NR for acute pain management. Also available by oral transmucosal and buccal routes for breakthrough pain.
hydromorphone (Dilaudid)	1.5	7.5	Useful alternative to morphine. Metabolite may accumulate with long-term use. Available in high-potency parenteral formulation (10 mg/mL) useful for SC infusion; 3 mg rectal ≈ 650 mg aspirin PO. With repeated dosing (e.g., PCA), it is more likely that 2-3 mg parenteral hydromorphone = 10 mg parenteral morphine.
meperidine	75	300 NR	No longer recommended as a first-line opioid for the management of any type of pain due to potential toxicity from accumulation of metabolite, normeperidine. Normeperidine has 15-20 h half-life and is not reversed by naloxone. NR in older adults or patients with impaired renal function; NR by continuous IV infusion.
methadone (Dolophine)			For equianalgesia information on methadone, see Pasero, C., Quinn, T. E., Portenoy, R. K., et al. (2011). Opioid analgesics (Chapter 13). In C. Pasero, & M. McCaffery. *Pain assessment and pharmacologic management*, St. Louis, Mosby.
oxycodone	—	20	Used for moderate pain when combined with a nonopioid (e.g., Percocet, Tylox). Available as single entity in short-acting and modified-release (OxyContin) PO formulations; can be used like PO morphine for severe pain.
oxymorphone (Numorphan, Opana)	1	10 (PO and rectal)	Used for moderate to severe pain. Available in short-acting (Opana) and modified-release (Opana ER) formulations; can be used like PO morphine for severe pain.
Agonist-Antagonist Opioids (not recommended for severe, escalating pain; if used in combination with mu agonist opioids, may reverse analgesia and precipitate withdrawal in opioid-dependent patients)			
buprenorphine (Buprenex)	0.4	—	Not readily reversed by naloxone; NR for laboring patients. Available in sublingual formulations (Suboxone, Subutex) for treatment of opioid addictive disease.
butorphanol (Stadol)	2	—	Also available in nasal spray.
nalbuphine (Nubain)	10	—	

FDA, Food and Drug Administration; *NR*, not recommended; *PO*, oral; ≈, roughly equal to.
[1]Duration of analgesia is dose dependent; the higher the dose, usually the longer the duration.
[2]IV boluses may be used to produce analgesia that lasts approximately as long as IM or SC doses. However, of all routes of administration, IV produces the highest peak concentration of the drug, and the peak concentration is associated with the highest level of toxicity, e.g., sedation.
For more complete information and references, see: Pasero, C., Quinn, T. E., Portenoy, R. K., et al. (2011). Opioid analgesics (Chapter 13). In C. Pasero, & M. McCaffery. *Pain assessment and pharmacologic management*, St. Louis, Mosby.

Equianalgesic Chart:
Approximate equivalent doses of PO nonopioids and opioids for mild to moderate pain

Analgesic	PO Dosage (mg)
Nonopioids	
acetaminophen	650
aspirin (ASA)	650
ibuprofen	200-400
naproxen	275
ketoprofen	25 is superior to 650 ASA
Opioids[†]	
codeine	32-60
hydrocodone[††]	5
meperidine (Demerol)	50
oxycodone[†††]	3-5
propoxyphene (Darvon)	65-100

[†]Often combined with acetaminophen; avoid exceeding maximum total daily dose of acetaminophen (4000 mg/day).
[††]Combined with acetaminophen (e.g., Vicodin, Lortab).
[†††]Combined with acetaminophen (e.g., Percocet, Tylox). Also available alone as single entity short-acting and modified-release (OxyContin) oral formulations.

A Guide to Using Equianalgesic Charts

- Equianalgesic means approximately the same pain relief.
- The equianalgesic chart is a guideline for selecting doses in opioid-naïve patients. Doses and intervals between doses are titrated according to individuals' responses.
- The equianalgesic chart is helpful when switching from one drug to another, or switching from one route of administration to another.
- Dosages in the equianalgesic chart suggest a ratio for comparing the analgesic effects of one drug with those of another.
- For older adults, initially reduce the recommended adult opioid dose for moderate to severe pain by 25% to 50%.
- The longer a patient has been receiving opioids, the more conservative the starting doses of a **new** opioid should be.

For more complete information and references, see: Pasero, C., Portenoy, R. K., & McCaffery, M. (2011). Nonopioid analgesics. In C. Pasero, & M. McCaffery. *Pain assessment and pharmacologic management*, St. Louis, Mosby.